A Guide to Mastery
in Clinical Nursing

Joyce J. Fitzpatrick, PhD, MBA, RN, FAAN, FNAP, is an Elizabeth Brooks Ford Professor of Nursing, Frances Payne Bolton School of Nursing, Case Western Reserve University (CWRU) in Cleveland, Ohio, where she was the dean from 1982 through 1997. She is also an adjunct professor, Department of Geriatrics, Ichan School of Medicine, Mount Sinai Hospital, New York, New York. She earned a bachelor of science in nursing (Georgetown University), an MS in psychiatric–mental health nursing (The Ohio State University), a PhD in nursing (New York University), and an MBA (CWRU). She was elected a fellow of the American Academy of Nursing (AAN; 1981) and a fellow in the National Academies of Practice (1996). She received the *American Journal of Nursing* Book of the Year award 20 times. Dr. Fitzpatrick received the American Nurses Foundation Distinguished Contribution to Nursing Science Award for sustained commitment and contributions to the development of the discipline (2002). She was a Fulbright Scholar at University College Cork, Cork, Ireland (2007–2008), and was inducted into the Sigma Theta Tau International Research Hall of Fame (2014). In 2016, she was named a Living Legend of the AAN. Dr. Fitzpatrick's work is widely disseminated in nursing and health care literature; she has authored or edited more than 300 publications, including more than 80 books. She even served as a coeditor of the *Annual Review of Nursing Research* series, volumes 1 to 26, and she currently edits the journals *Applied Nursing Research, Archives of Psychiatric Nursing,* and *Nursing Education Perspectives,* the official journal of the National League for Nursing.

Celeste M. Alfes, DNP, MSN, RN, CNE, CHSE-A, is associate professor and director of the Center for Nursing Education, Simulation, and Innovation at the Frances Payne Bolton School of Nursing, Case Western Reserve University (CWRU) in Cleveland, Ohio. She earned a bachelor of science in nursing (University of Akron), master of science in nursing (University of Akron), and doctor of nursing practice (CWRU). With a background in critical care nursing, she has 20 years of experience teaching baccalaureate nursing students and has been instrumental in developing high-fidelity simulation programs nationally and internationally. She was instrumental in developing the Dorothy Ebersbach Academic Center for Flight Nursing, which features the nation's first high-fidelity Sikorsky S76® helicopter simulator adapted for interdisciplinary education and crew resource management. She received the National League for Nursing's Simulation Leader in Nursing Education award (2012) and the Joyce Griffin-Sobel Research award (2014). Her research incorporates interprofessional simulations to strengthen clinical reasoning and performance outcomes. Dr. Alfes currently serves as a reviewer for the National Science Foundation, is a co-investigator on funded research projects with the Laerdal Foundation of Norway and the U.S. Air Force Research Laboratory, is on the editorial board of *Applied Nursing Research,* and is a reviewer for the journals *Nursing Education Perspectives* and *Clinical Simulation in Nursing.*

Ronald L. Hickman, Jr., PhD, RN, ACNP-BC, FNAP, FAAN, is an associate professor and a board-certified acute care nurse practitioner at Frances Payne Bolton School of Nursing, Case Western Reserve University (CWRU) in Cleveland, Ohio. He earned a bachelor of arts in biology, a master of science (acute care nurse practitioner), and a doctor of philosophy in nursing from CWRU. He has received regional and national distinctions for his commitment and sustained contributions to nursing science and practice. Dr. Hickman is a nationally recognized nurse scientist and advanced practice nurse. In 2015, he was elected a fellow of the American Academy of Nursing and National Academies of Practice. With nearly two decades of clinical experience, he has provided evidence-based nursing care to patients and their families across tertiary care settings. He has authored more than 50 publications and numerous book chapters with a clinical focus, and serves as a contributing editor for the *American Journal of Critical Care.* As an associate editor of the *Guide to Mastery in Clinical Nursing,* Dr. Hickman's clinical expertise in the management of patients requiring life-sustaining care in emergency departments and intensive care units is highlighted in the book's content regarding emergency and critical care, medical–surgical care, and nurse anesthesia care.

A Guide to Mastery in Clinical Nursing

The Comprehensive Reference

Joyce J. Fitzpatrick, PhD, MBA, RN, FAAN, FNAP

Celeste M. Alfes, DNP, MSN, RN, CNE, CHSE-A

Ronald L. Hickman, Jr., PhD, RN, ACNP-BC, FNAP, FAAN

EDITORS

SPRINGER PUBLISHING COMPANY

Springer Publishing Company, LLC
11 West 42nd Street
New York, NY 10036
www.springerpub.com

Acquisitions Editor: Joseph Morita
Composition: Newgen KnowledgeWorks

ISBN: 978-0-8261-3234-5
ebook ISBN: 978-0-8261-3244-4

17 18 19 20 / 5 4 3 2 1

The author and the publisher of this Work have made every effort to use sources believed to be reliable to provide information that is accurate and compatible with the standards generally accepted at the time of publication. Because medical science is continually advancing, our knowledge base continues to expand. Therefore, as new information becomes available, changes in procedures become necessary. We recommend that the reader always consult current research and specific institutional policies before performing any clinical procedure. The author and publisher shall not be liable for any special, consequential, or exemplary damages resulting, in whole or in part, from the readers' use of, or reliance on, the information contained in this book. The publisher has no responsibility for the persistence or accuracy of URLs for external or third-party Internet websites referred to in this publication and does not guarantee that any content on such websites is, or will remain, accurate or appropriate.

Library of Congress Cataloging-in-Publication Data
Names: Fitzpatrick, Joyce J., 1944- editor. | Alfes, Celeste M., editor. | Hickman, Ronald L., editor.
Title: A guide to mastery in clinical nursing : the comprehensive reference / Joyce J. Fitzpatrick, Celeste M. Alfes,
   Ronald L. Hickman, editors.
Description: New York, NY : Springer Publishing Company, LLC, [2018] | Includes bibliographical references and index.
Identifiers: LCCN 2017039905 | ISBN 9780826132345 (paper back)
Subjects: | MESH: Nursing Care | Nursing Process
Classification: LCC RT41 | NLM WY 100.1 | DDC 610.73—dc23
LC record available at https://lccn.loc.gov/2017039905

Contact us to receive discount rates on bulk purchases.
We can also customize our books to meet your needs.
For more information please contact: sales@springerpub.com

Printed in the United States of America by McNaughton & Gunn.

Contents

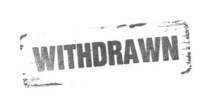

Contributors   *xiii*
Preface   *xxxi*
Acknowledgments   *xxxv*

I: EMERGENCY AND CRITICAL CARE NURSING

Section Editor: Theresa M. Campo

Abdominal Aortic Aneurysm   5
Vicki A. Keough

Abdominal Pain   8
Christopher J. Contino

Acid–Base Imbalances   10
Michael D. Gooch

Acute Abdomen   13
Susanna Rudy

Acute Coronary Syndrome   16
Andrea Efre

Acute Exacerbation of a Chronic Condition   19
Brenda L. Douglass

Acute Pancreatitis in Adults   21
Virginia Mangolds

Acute Respiratory Distress Syndrome   23
Kathleen C. Ashton

Acute Respiratory Failure   25
Breanna Hetland

Adrenal Insufficiency   28
Rachel K. Vanek

Back Pain   30
Sharon R. Rainer

Burns   33
Margaret Jean Carman

Burns: Classification and Severity   36
Melanie Gibbons Hallman and Lamon Norton

Chest Pain   39
Sharon R. Rainer

Child Abuse and Neglect   42
*Patricia M. Speck, Pamela Harris Bryant, Tedra S. Smith,
Sherita K. Etheridge, and Steadman McPeters*

Clostridium Difficile Infection   46
Anita Sundaresh

Continuous Veno-Venous Hemofiltration   48
Ian N. Saludares

Definitions of Emergency and Critical Care
Nursing   50
Nicole M. Hartman and Courtney Vose

Dental Emergencies   52
Melanie Gibbons Hallman and Lamon Norton

Disaster Response   55
Darlie Simerson

Disseminated Intravascular Coagulation   57
Joyce E. Higgins

Domestic Violence   59
*Patricia M. Speck, Diana K. Faugno, Rachell A. Ekroos,
Melanie Gibbons Hallman, Gwendolyn D. Childs,
Tedra S. Smith, and Stacey A. Mitchell*

Ear, Nose, and Throat Emergencies   63
Kathleen Bradbury-Golas

Elder Abuse and Neglect   66
*Patricia M. Speck, Richard Taylor, Stacey A. Mitchell,
Diana K. Faugno, and Rita A. Jablonski-Jaudon*

Encephalopathy   70
Deborah Vinesky

Endocrine Emergencies   72
Diane Fuller Switzer

Environmental Emergencies   75
Brittany Newberry

Extracorporeal Life Support   78
Grant Pignatiello, Katherine Hornack, and Julie E. Herzog

Fluid and Electrolyte Imbalances   81
Michael D. Gooch

Fluid Resuscitation   84
Laura Stark Bai

Heart Transplantation   86
S. Brian Widmar

Hepatic Failure   89
Leon Chen and Fidelindo Lim

Hepatitis   92
Ramona A. Sowers and Linda Carson

Hyperglycemia and Hypoglycemia   94
Laura Stark Bai

Hypertensive Crisis and Hypertension   96
Kathleen Bradbury-Golas

Hypothermia   99
Marian Nowak

Integumentary Emergencies   101
Susanna Rudy

Intra-Aortic Balloon Pump   104
Grant Pignatiello

Mental and Behavioral Health Emergencies   106
Lia V. Ludan

Neurotrauma   109
Anita Sundaresh

Obstetrical and Gynecological Emergency Care   112
Vicki Bacidore

Ophthalmic Emergencies   114
Shannon M. Litten

Orthopedic Emergencies in Adults   117
Cindy Kumar

Pediatric Emergencies   119
Rachel Tkaczyk

Psychiatric Disorders: Suicide, Homicide,
Psychosis   121
George Byron Peraza-Smith and Yolanda Bone

Respiratory Emergencies   124
Dustin Spencer

Return of Spontaneous Circulation With Hypothermia
Initiation   127
Laura Stark Bai

Seizures   129
Eric Roberts

Sepsis   131
Ronald L. Hickman, Jr.

Sexual Assault   133
Patricia M. Speck, Diana K. Faugno, Rachell A. Ekroos,
Melanie Gibbons Hallman, Sallie J. Shipman,
Martha B. Dodd, Qiana A. Johnson, and
Stacey A. Mitchell

Shock and Multiple Organ Dysfunction
Syndrome   139
Jennifer Wilbeck

Solid Organ Transplantation   141
Marcia Johansson

Spinal Cord Injury   143
Lamon Norton and Melanie Gibbons Hallman

Substance Use Disorders and Toxicological
Agents   146
Al Rundio

Thoracic Aortic Aneurysm   148
Megan M. Shifrin and Ronald L. Hickman, Jr.

Thrombocytopenia in Adults   150
Khoa (Joey) Dang

Thyroid Crisis   152
Cynthia Ann Leaver

Traumatic Brain Injury   155
Elizabeth Wirth-Tomaszewski

Traumatic Injury   158
Dustin Spencer

Urologic Emergencies   160
Kelley Toffoli

Ventilator-Associated Pneumonia   163
Nancy Jaskowak Cresse

Ventricular Assist Devices   165
S. Brian Widmar

The Violent Patient   168
Janet E. Reilly and Michael Wichowski

II: GERIATRIC NURSING

Section Editor: Evanne Juratovac

Age-Related Changes   174
Evanne Juratovac

Aging in Place   176
Evanne Juratovac

Caregivers   179
Evanne Juratovac

Delirium   181
Evanne Juratovac

Dementia   184
Lori Constantine

Elder Abuse, Neglect, and Exploitation   186
Sharon Ward-Miller

Falls   *188*
Uvannie Enriquez Castro

Frailty   *190*
Nirmala Lekhak and Evanne Juratovac

Infection   *192*
Irena L. Kenneley

Medication Reconciliation   *194*
Mary Jo Krivanek and Mary A. Dolansky

Nutrition   *197*
Marianna K. Sunderlin

Persistent Pain   *199*
Felvic Adriatico Javier

Pharmacokinetic Changes   *201*
Carli A. Carnish

Physical Activity   *204*
Michelle Borland

Polypharmacy   *206*
Maria A. Mendoza

Pressure Injury   *208*
Monica Cabrera, Lisa Torrieri, and Ekta Vohra

Sleep Disorders   *211*
Kerry Mastrangelo and Mary T. Quinn Griffin

Urinary Incontinence   *212*
Felvic Adriatico Javier

III: HEALTH SYSTEMS AND HEALTH PROMOTION

Section Editor: Deborah F. Lindell

HEALTH SYSTEMS

Advocacy   *216*
Ruth Ludwick and Margarete L. Zalon

Health Economics   *219*
Margarete L. Zalon and Ruth Ludwick

Health Policy   *222*
Ruth Ludwick and Angela Contant

Hospital Accreditation   *224*
Catherine S. Koppelman

Infection Prevention and Control   *226*
Irena L. Kenneley

Nursing Leadership   *229*
Catherine S. Koppelman

Nursing Management   *231*
Cynthia L. Danko

Nursing Process: Systems Approach   *234*
Shanina C. Knighton, Aniko Kukla, and Mary A. Dolansky

Patient Experience   *236*
Catherine S. Koppelman

Population Health   *238*
Deborah F. Lindell

Quality Improvement   *241*
Aniko Kukla, Mary A. Dolansky, and Shanina C. Knighton

Quality and Safety Education   *244*
Nadine M. Marchi

Social Determinants of Health   *246*
Rita M. Sfiligoj

Transitional Care Coordination   *248*
Nadine M. Marchi

HEALTH PROMOTION

Health Behavior   *250*
Deborah F. Lindell

Health Education   *253*
Rita M. Sfiligoj

Health Literacy   *255*
Joseph D. Perazzo

Self-Management   *257*
Marym M. Alaamri

Wellness   *259*
Elizabeth R. Click

IV: MEDICAL–SURGICAL NURSING

Section Editor: Jane F. Marek

Addison's Disease   *266*
Yolanda Flenoury

Amyotrophic Lateral Sclerosis   *268*
Mary Jo Elmo

Anemia in Adults   *270*
Kerry Mastrangelo and Mary T. Quinn Griffin

Atelectasis   *272*
Ashley L. Foreman

Atherosclerosis   *275*
Kari Gali

Benign Prostatic Hyperplasia   *277*
Kelly Ann Lynn

Bladder Cancer   *280*
Dianna Jo Copley

Bowel Obstruction   282
Kelly Ann Lynn and Jane F. Marek

Brain Tumors   285
Peter J. Cebull

Cardiomyopathy   287
Elsie A. Jolade

Chronic Kidney Disease   289
Mary de Haan

Chronic Obstructive Pulmonary Disease   292
Christina M. Canfield

Colorectal Cancer   294
Visnja Maria Masina and Crina V. Floruta

Coronary Artery Disease in Adults   296
Kate Cook and Mary T. Quinn Griffin

Cushing Syndrome   298
Yolanda Flenoury and Jane F. Marek

Deep Vein Thrombosis   300
Kelly K. McConnell

Diabetes Insipidus   303
Danielle M. Diemer

Diabetes Mellitus   304
Mary Beth Modic

Diverticular Disease   307
Rhoda Redulla

Endocarditis   310
Courtney G. Donahue and Celeste M. Alfes

Fractures   312
Joseph D. Perazzo

Gallbladder and Biliary Tract Disease   314
Andrea Marie Herr

Gastric Cancer   316
Una Hopkins and Jane F. Marek

Gastritis   319
Maria G. Smisek

Gastroesophageal Reflux Disease   321
Kelly Ann Lynn

Gout   323
Maria A. Mendoza

Guillain–Barré Syndrome   325
Kathleen Marsala-Cervasio

Heart Failure   327
Arlene Travis

Hemolytic Anemia   330
Rebecca M. Lutz and Charrita Ernewein

Heparin-Induced Thrombocytopenia   332
Bette K. Idemoto and Jane F. Marek

Hiatal Hernia   335
Maricar P. Gomez

Human Immunodeficiency Virus   337
Scott Emory Moore

Hypertension   339
Marian Soat

Hyperthyroidism   342
Colleen Kurzawa

Hypothyroidism   344
Karen L. Terry

Inflammatory Bowel Disease in Adults   347
Ronald Rock

Leukemia   349
Marisa A. Cortese

Liver Cancer   351
Shannon A. Rives

Lung Cancer   353
Helen Foley

Lymphoma   355
Marisa A. Cortese and Jane F. Marek

Multiple Sclerosis   357
Alaa Mahsoon

Myasthenia Gravis   360
Jennifer Gonzalez

Obesity   362
Kelly Ann Lynn

Osteoarthritis   365
Mary Variath

Osteomyelitis   367
Mary Variath and Jane F. Marek

Osteoporosis   369
Maria A. Mendoza

Paget's Disease   372
Jacqueline Robinson

Pancreatic Cancer   374
Jennifer E. Millman

Parkinson's Disease   376
Peter J. Cebull

Peptic Ulcer Disease   378
Lisa D. Ericson and Deborah R. Gillum

Pericarditis   381
Heidi Youngbauer

Peripheral Artery Disease   383
Gayle M. Petty

Pernicious Anemia   385
Edwidge Cuvilly

Polycythemia Vera   386
Sarine Beukian

Prostate Cancer   389
Erin H. Discenza

Rheumatoid Arthritis   391
Susan V. Brindisi

Sepsis   393
Sharon Stahl Wexler and Catherine O'Neill D'Amico

Sickle Cell Disease   396
Consuela A. Albright

Sleep Apnea   398
Deborah H. Cantero, Leslie J. Lockett, and
Rebecca M. Lutz

Spinal Stenosis and Disc Herniation   400
Steven R. Collier

Syndrome of Inappropriate Antidiuretic Hormone
Secretion   402
Carrie Foster

Systemic Lupus Erythematosus   405
Merlyn A. Dorsainvil

Thrombocytopenia   407
Maria A. Mendoza

Tuberculosis   409
Christina M. Canfield

Valvular Heart Disease   411
Rebecca Witten Grizzle

V: NEONATAL NURSING

Section Editor: Amy Bieda

ABO Incompatibility   416
Donna M. Schultz and Mary F. Terhaar

Acute Renal Failure   419
Christine Horvat Davey

Anemia of Prematurity   421
Barbara Greitzer Slone

Apnea of Prematurity   423
Amy Bieda

Bronchopulmonary Dysplasia   425
Amy Bieda

Decreased Pulmonary Blood Flow   428
Jennifer Johntony and Jodi Zalewski

Extremely Low-Birth-Weight Infant   431
Jenelle M. Zambrano

Gastroesophageal Reflux   433
Suzanne Rubin

Gastroschisis and Omphalocele   436
Beverly Capper

Hirschsprung's Disease   438
Anne M. Modic

Hydronephrosis   440
Charlene M. Deuber

Hyperbilirubinemia   442
Donna M. Schultz and Mary F. Terhaar

Hypertension   444
Mary F. Terhaar

Hypoglycemia   447
Tina Di Fiore

Hypoxic Ischemic Encephalopathy   449
Ke-Ni Niko Tien

Increased Pulmonary Blood Flow   452
Jennifer Johntony and Jodi Zalewski

Infant of a Diabetic Mother   454
Mary F. Terhaar

Intraventricular Hemorrhage   457
Helene M. Lannon

Late Preterm Infant   460
Donna A. Dowling

Meconium Aspiration Syndrome   462
Rae Jean Hemway

Necrotizing Enterocolitis   465
Charlene M. Deuber

Respiratory Distress Syndrome   467
Mary Ann Blatz

Retinopathy of Prematurity   469
Mary Ann Blatz

Sepsis   472
Karla Phipps

Substance Abuse/Opioid Withdrawal   475
Helene M. Lannon

Thermoregulation   477
Paula Forsythe

VI: NURSE ANESTHESIA

Section Editor: Sonya D. Moore

Adult Difficult Airway Management   482
Jennifer Nicholson and Ronald L. Hickman, Jr.

Anesthesia for Preeclampsia   484
Kerry L. Quisenberry

Anesthesia in Remote Locations   *487*
Angela Milosh

Anesthesia and Robotic Surgery   *489*
Angela Milosh

Anticoagulation and Anesthesia   *490*
Natalie Butchko and Aimee Dickman

Awake Craniotomy   *493*
*Rafiu Adeniji, Christopher Bibro, and
Natalie A. Slenkovich*

Cardiac Anesthesia   *495*
Christopher K. Ferguson

Enhanced Recovery After Anesthesia   *496*
Danielle T. Winch and Brian Garrett

Evoked Potentials   *498*
Melanie M. Stipp

Fluid and Transfusion Management in
Anesthesia Care   *501*
Andrew D. Lorenzoni and Justin R. Stegman

Liver Transplant and Anesthesia   *504*
*Kimberly M. Choudhary, Sonya D. Moore, and
Ronald L. Hickman, Jr.*

Malignant Hyperthermia   *506*
Colleen Thaxton Spencer and Elizabeth Demko

Morbid Obesity and Anesthesia   *508*
*Elizabeth Demko, Colleen Thaxton Spencer, and
Sonya D. Moore*

Neuromuscular Blockade Reversal:
Sugammadex   *511*
Britney A. Leonardi

One-Lung Ventilation   *512*
Monica M. Bitner, Brittany Hosler, and Jessica M. Tripi

Peripheral Nerve Blocks   *515*
Scott M. Urigel and Jeffrey E. Molter

Postoperative Nausea and Vomiting   *517*
Kimberly Kimble

Respiratory Depression and Patient-Controlled
Analgesia   *519*
Sonya D. Moore

Sickle Cell Disease and Anesthesia   *521*
*Mark A. Caldwell, Sonya D. Moore,
and Ronald L. Hickman, Jr.*

VII: OBSTETRICS AND WOMEN'S HEALTH

Section Editors: Maryann Clark and Mary Anne Gallagher

Breast Cancer and *BRCA*   *526*
Una Hopkins

Cervical Cancer   *528*
Godsfavour Guillet

Contraception   *532*
Latina M. Brooks

Endometriosis   *535*
Ingrid Apryl Spears

Episiotomy   *536*
Loraine O'Neill

Home Birth   *538*
Sabrina Nitkowski-Keever

Infertility   *541*
Tammy M. Lampley

Intimate Partner Violence   *544*
Marilyn E. Smith

In Vitro Fertilization   *546*
Donna Lynn Rose and Mary T. Quinn Griffin

Labor and Delivery   *548*
Carrie Gerber

Lactation   *550*
Jarold T. Johnston

Menopause   *554*
Maryann Clark

Motherhood   *556*
Stacen A. Keating and Miriam J. Chickering

Osteoporosis   *558*
Mary Variath

Ovarian Cancer   *561*
Kristine Cooper and Tasina Jones

Pelvic Pain   *563*
Loraine O'Neill

Perinatal Mood Disorders   *565*
Deepika Goyal

Polycystic Ovary Syndrome   *568*
Latina M. Brooks

Postpartum   *570*
Debra Bingham and Patricia Suplee

Postpartum Hemorrhage   *573*
Sabrina Nitkowski-Keever and Mary Anne Gallagher

Pregnancy   *576*
Miriam J. Chickering and Stacen A. Keating

Sexually Transmitted Infections   *578*
Maryann Clark

Skin Aesthetics   *581*
Erin Hennessey and Mary Anne Gallagher

VIII: PALLIATIVE CARE NURSING

Section Editor: Molly J. Jackson

Advance Directives in Palliative Care   586
*Marilyn Bookbinder, Joyce Palmieri, and
Molly J. Jackson*

Anorexia and Weight Loss   589
Janine Stage Galeski and Molly J. Jackson

Anxiety in Advanced Illness   592
Lori A. Fusco

Bowel Obstruction   594
Hilary Applequist

Communication   596
Anne M. Kolenic

Constipation   598
Angela M. Johnson

Delirium   600
Colleen Kurzawa

Diarrhea   603
Sheila Blank

Dysphagia   605
Marianna K. Sunderlin

Dyspnea   607
Katharine K. Cirino

Ethics   609
Laura Caramanica and Molly J. Jackson

Grief and Bereavement   611
Kathleen Leask Capitulo

Mucositis   614
Petique Oeflein

Persistent Pain   616
Brendon Bowers and Molly J. Jackson

Urinary Incontinence   617
Kathy J. Meyers and Molly J. Jackson

IX: PEDIATRIC NURSING

*Section Editors: Elizabeth Zimmermann
and Marguerite DiMarco*

Acute Renal Failure   622
Christine Horvat Davey

Appendicitis   624
Kerry D. Christy

Asthma   627
Laurine Gajkowski

Autism Spectrum Disorder   630
Sheila Blank and Celeste M. Alfes

Bronchiolitis Respiratory Syncytial Virus   632
Shannon Courtney Wong

Cancers of Childhood   634
Breanne M. Roche

Cerebral Palsy   636
Rachael Weigand

Cystic Fibrosis   639
Karen Vosper

Developmentally Appropriate Communication   641
Nanci M. Berman

Diabetes   643
Julia E. Blanchette

Failure to Thrive   646
Mary Alice Dombrowski

Inflammatory Bowel Disease   648
Sharon Perry

Obesity   650
Rosanna P. Watowicz

Oral Health   652
Marguerite DiMarco

Orthopedics   655
*Michelle Calabretta, Emily Canitia, and
Michelle A. Janas*

Seizure Disorder   657
Kathleen Maxwell

Sickle Cell Disease   660
Valerie Cachat

X: PERIOPERATIVE NURSING

Section Editor: Rebecca M. Patton

Ethics and Advocacy for Surgical Patients   666
Michelle McHugh Slater

Infection Control   668
Joan Rotnem and Rebecca M. Patton

Perioperative Patient Safety   671
Janet S. Duran

Surgical Interventions in Cancer Care   673
Carol Pehotsky, Mary Szostakowski, and Jacob Runion

Surgical Interventions in Parkinson's Disease   *675*
Karyn L. Boyar

Surgical Interventions Using Emerging
Technologies   *679*
*Carol Pehotsky, Mary Szostakowski, Jacob Runion,
Florin Sgondea, and Dena L. Salamon*

Traditional Surgical Interventions   *681*
Michelle McHugh Slater

XI: PSYCHIATRIC-MENTAL HEALTH NURSING

Section Editor: Jeffrey S. Jones

Anxiety Disorders   *686*
Susan Phillips

Bipolar Disorder   *688*
Julie A. Berg

Boundary Management   *690*
Jeffrey S. Jones

Dementia   *692*
Stephanie R. Martin

Depression   *694*
Jeffrey S. Jones

Eating Disorders   *696*
Kathryn E. Phillips

Impulse Control Disorders   *699*
Lisa L. Salser

Obsessive Compulsive Disorder   *702*
Susan Phillips

Posttraumatic Stress Disorder   *703*
Danette L. Core and Denise Chivington

Schizophrenia   *706*
Sharon L. Phillips

Substance Use Disorders   *708*
Chikodiri Gibson and Se Min Um

Suicide   *710*
Jeffrey S. Jones

Vulnerable Populations   *712*
Melanie S. Lint

Index   *715*

Contributors

Rafiu Adeniji, MSN, RN
Nurse Anesthesia Student
Frances Payne Bolton School of Nursing
Case Western Reserve University
Cleveland, Ohio

Marym M. Alaamri, MSN, RN
PhD Student
Frances Payne Bolton School of Nursing
Case Western Reserve University
Cleveland, Ohio

Consuela A. Albright, MSN, RN, FNP-BC, PPCNP-BC
Staff Nurse
Cleveland Clinic Children's Hospital for Rehabilitation
Cleveland, Ohio

Celeste M. Alfes, DNP, MSN, RN, CNE, CHSE-A
Associate Professor
Director, Center for Nursing Education, Simulation, and
    Innovation
Frances Payne Bolton School of Nursing
Case Western Reserve University
Cleveland, Ohio

Hilary Applequist, DNP, MSN, RN, APRN-NP, NP-C
Assistant Professor
DNP Program
Nebraska Methodist College
Omaha, Nebraska

Kathleen C. Ashton, PhD, RN, ACNS-BC
Clinical Professor of Nursing
College of Nursing and Health Professions
Drexel University
Philadelphia, Pennsylvania
Professor Emeritus
Rutgers, The State University of New Jersey
Camden, New Jersey

Laura Stark Bai, MS, RN, FNP-BC
Clinical Nurse Manager
Department of Emergency Medicine
Mount Sinai Hospital
New York, New York

Vicki Bacidore, DNP, RN, APRN, ACNP-BC, CEN, TNS
Assistant Professor of Nursing
Loyola University Chicago
Emergency Nurse Practitioner
Loyola University Medical Center
Maywood, Illinois

Julie A. Berg, MSN, RN, ANP-BC, PMHNP-BC
Certified Adult Psychiatric-Mental Health Nurse
    Practitioner
Certified Adult Nurse Practitioner
Department of Psychiatry
Louis Stokes Cleveland VA Medical Center
Cleveland, Ohio

Nanci M. Berman, MSN, RN
Assistant Professor
Lorain County Community College
Elyria, Ohio

Sarine Beukian, MSN, RN, AGACNP-BC
Cardiology Nurse Practitioner
Division of Cardiology
Department of Medicine
Bassett Medical Center, Affiliate of College of Physicians
    and Surgeons
Columbia University
New York, New York

Christopher Bibro, MSN, RN
Nurse Anesthesia Student
Frances Payne Bolton School of Nursing
Case Western Reserve University
Cleveland, Ohio

Amy Bieda, PhD, RN, APRN, PNP-BC, NNP-BC
Assistant Professor
Director, BSN Program
Lead Faculty, Neonatal Nurse Practitioner Program
Frances Payne Bolton School of Nursing
Case Western Reserve University
Cleveland, Ohio

Debra Bingham, DrPH, RN, FAAN
Executive Director
Institute for Perinatal Improvement
Washington, DC

Monica M. Bitner, MSN, RN
Nurse Anesthesia Student
Frances Payne Bolton School of Nursing
Case Western Reserve University
Cleveland, Ohio

Julia E. Blanchette, BSN, RN, CDE
PhD Student
Frances Payne Bolton School of Nursing
Case Western Reserve University
Cleveland, Ohio

Sheila Blank, MSN, RN
Licensed School Nurse
Clinical Instructor
Bitonte College of Health and Human Services
Department of Nursing
Youngstown State University
Youngstown, Ohio

Mary Ann Blatz, DNP, RN, RNC-NIC, IBCLC
Advanced Practice Nurse
NICU Nursing Research and Development
Neonatal Intensive Care Unit
Rainbow Babies and Children's Hospital
University Hospitals Cleveland Medical Center
Cleveland, Ohio

Yolanda Bone, DNP, RN, APRN, FNP-BC
W. Temple Webber Cancer Center
Christus St. Michael
Texarkana, Texas

Marilyn Bookbinder, PhD, RN, FPCN
Director of Quality and Performance Improvement
MJHS Institute for Innovation in Palliative Care
New York, New York

Michelle Borland, DNP, RN, CNE
Teaching Assistant Professor
Adult Health Department
West Virginia University
Morgantown, West Virginia

Brendon Bowers, BSN, RN
Nurse Clinician IIM
Radiation Oncology
Johns Hopkins Hospital
Baltimore, Maryland

Karyn L. Boyar, DNP, FNP-BC, RN
Assistant Clinical Professor
Rory Meyers College of Nursing
New York University
New York, New York

Kathleen Bradbury-Golas, DNP, RN, FNP-C, ACNS-BC
Associate Clinical Professor
Drexel University
Philadelphia, Pennsylvania
Family Nurse Practitioner
Virtua Medical Group
Hammonton Primary Care
Hammonton, New Jersey
Recovery Centers of America at Lighthouse
Mays Landing, New Jersey

Susan V. Brindisi, MS Ed, MA, MSN, RN, CHES, CRRN
Clinical Nurse Leader
Mount Sinai Health System
New York, New York

Latina M. Brooks, PhD, RN, CNP
Assistant Professor
Director, MSN Programs
Frances Payne Bolton School of Nursing
Case Western Reserve University
Cleveland, Ohio

Pamela Harris Bryant, DNP, RN, CRNP, AC-PC
Pediatric Nurse Practitioner
Assistant Professor
School of Nursing
University of Alabama at Birmingham
Birmingham, Alabama

Natalie Butchko, MSN, RN
Nurse Anesthesia Student
Frances Payne Bolton School of Nursing
Case Western Reserve University
Cleveland, Ohio

Monica Cabrera, MSN, RN, CNS, CWON
Nurse Clinician
Wound and Ostomy Nurse
New York–Presbyterian Hospital
Weill Cornell Medical Center
New York, New York

Valerie Cachat, MSN, RN, CPNP
Nurse Practitioner
Sickle Cell Anemia Center
Rainbow Babies and Children's Hospital
University Hospitals Cleveland Medical Center
Cleveland, Ohio

Michelle Calabretta, MSN, RN, CPNP-AC
Certified Pediatric Nurse Practitioner
Department of Pediatric Orthopaedics
University Hospitals Cleveland Medical Center
Cleveland, Ohio

Mark A. Caldwell, DNP, RN, CRNA, Col, USAFR (Ret.)
Assistant Director
Nurse Anesthesia Program
Frances Payne Bolton School of Nursing
Case Western Reserve University
Cleveland, Ohio

Theresa M. Campo, DNP, RN, FNP-C, ENP-C,
   FAANP, FAAN
Director Emergency Nurse Practitioner Track and Associate
   Clinical Professor
College of Nursing and Health Professions
Drexel University
Philadelphia, Pennsylvania
Emergency Nurse Practitioner
Atlanticare Regional Medical Center
Atlantic City, New Jersey

Christina M. Canfield, MSN, RN, APRN, ACNS-BC, CCRN-E
eHospital Program Manager
Cleveland Clinic
Cleveland, Ohio

Emily Canitia, MSN, RN, CPNP-AC/PC
Pediatric Nurse Practitioner
Pediatric Orthopedic Surgery
Rainbow Babies and Children's Hospital
University Hospitals Cleveland Medical Center
Cleveland, Ohio

Deborah H. Cantero, DNP, RN, ARNP, FNP-C
Assistant Professor
FNP Program Coordinator
School of Nursing and Health Sciences
Florida Southern College
Lakeland, Florida

Kathleen Leask Capitulo, PhD, RN, FAAN, FACCE,
   IIWCC, C-CNS
Chief Nurse Executive
James J. Peters VA Medical Center
Bronx, New York
Adjunct Professor
Icahn School of Medicine at Mount Sinai
New York, New York
Adjunct Associate Professor
Frances Payne Bolton School of Nursing
Case Western Reserve University
Cleveland, Ohio

Beverly Capper, MSN, RN, RNC-NIC
Assistant Director
BSN Program
Frances Payne Bolton School of Nursing
Case Western Reserve University
Cleveland, Ohio

Laura Caramanica, PhD, RN, CENP, ACHE, FAAN
Associate Professor in the Graduate Nursing Program
University of West Georgia
Marietta, Georgia

Margaret Jean Carman, DNP, RN, ACNP-BC,
   ENP-BC, FAEN
Emergency Nurse Practitioner
University of North Carolina Chapel Hill
Department of Emergency Medicine
Chapel Hill, North Carolina
Program Director
Adult-Gerontology Acute Care Nurse Practitioner Program
Georgetown University School of Nursing and Health Studies
Washington, DC

Carli A. Carnish, MSN, RN, CNP
Instructor
Clinical Placement Coordinator
Frances Payne Bolton School of Nursing
Case Western Reserve University
Cleveland, Ohio

Linda Carson, MSN, RN, APN
Retired Advanced Practice Nurse
Shore Medical Center
Somers Point, New Jersey

Uvannie Enriquez Castro, MPA, BSN, RN, NEA-BC
Patient Care Director
Hemodialysis & Apheresis Unit
New York–Presbyterian Hospital/Weill Cornell
New York, New York

Peter J. Cebull, MSN, RN, CNP
Nurse Practitioner
Frances Payne Bolton School of Nursing
Case Western Reserve University
Cleveland, Ohio

Leon Chen, DNP, RN, AGACNP-BC, CCRN, CEN
Clinical Assistant Professor of Nursing
Nurse Practitioner
Critical Care Medicine Service
Rory Meyers College of Nursing
New York University
Department of Anesthesiology and Critical Care Medicine
Memorial Sloan Kettering Cancer Center
New York, New York

Miriam J. Chickering, BSN, RN, IBCLC
Chief Executive Officer
Nurses International
Bethel, Minnesota

Gwendolyn D. Childs, PhD, RN
Associate Professor
School of Nursing
University of Alabama at Birmingham
Birmingham, Alabama

Denise Chivington, MSN, RN, PMHNP-BC, FNP-BC
Nurse Practitioner
Mental Health Specialty
Community Outpatient Clinics
Veterans Health Administration
Mental Health Specialty
Sandusky, Ohio

Kimberly M. Choudhary, MSN, RN, CPNP-AC/PC
Pediatric Surgery Nurse Practitioner
Rainbow Babies and Children's Hospital
University Hospitals Cleveland Medical Center
Cleveland, Ohio

Kerry D. Christy, CPNP AC/ PC, MSN, BSN, RN
Pediatric Surgery Nurse Practitioner
Rainbow Babies and Children's Hospital
University Hospitals Cleveland
    Medical Center
Cleveland, Ohio

Katharine K. Cirino, MSN, RN, ANP-BC, ACHPN
Nurse Practitioner
Hospice of the Western Reserve
Cleveland, Ohio

Maryann Clark, MSN, RNC-OB
Patient Safety Officer
Department of Obstetrics/Gynecology
Mount Sinai West
New York, New York

Elizabeth R. Click, ND, RN, CWP
Assistant Professor
Frances Payne Bolton School of Nursing
Medical Director
Case Western Reserve University
Cleveland, Ohio

Steven R. Collier, MS, RN, CNP
Nurse Practitioner
Department of Neurosurgery
Center for Spine Health
Cleveland Clinic
Cleveland, Ohio

Lori Constantine, DNP, RN, APRN, FNP-BC
Clinical Assistant Professor
West Virginia University School of Nursing
Morgantown, West Virginia

Angela Contant, MSN, RN, CEN, NEA-BC
Evidence-Based Practice Coordinator
Akron Children's Hospital
Kent, Ohio

Christopher J. Contino, DNP, RN, ENP-C, FNP-BC, CEN, CRN
Emergency Nurse Practitioner
Atlantic Emergency Associates
Atlantic City, New Jersey

Kate Cook, MSN, RN
DNP Student
Frances Payne Bolton School of Nursing
Case Western Reserve University
Cleveland, Ohio
Assistant Professor
Chamberlain University
Downers Grove, Illinois

Kristine Cooper, MSN, RN, AGPCNP-BC, OCN
Clinical Nurse III
Women's Oncology Unit M10
Memorial Sloan Kettering Cancer Center
New York, New York

Dianna Jo Copley, MSN, RN, APRN, ACCNS-AG, CCRN
Clinical Nurse Specialist
Cleveland Clinic
Cleveland, Ohio

Danette L. Core, MSN, RN, PMHCNS-BC, MLS, PCMH-C
Department of Veterans Affairs
Sandusky Outpatient Clinic
Sandusky, Ohio
Promedica BayPark Hospital
Oregon, Ohio

Marisa A. Cortese, PhD, RN, FNP-BC
Research Nurse Practitioner
White Plains Hospital—Center for Cancer Care
White Plains, New York

Nancy Jaskowak Cresse, DNP, MSN, RN, ANP-BC
Clinical Assistant Professor
Rutgers School of Nursing–Camden
Camden, New Jersey

Edwidge Cuvilly, MS, RN, ANP-BC, GNP, OCN
Nurse Practitioner
Bone Marrow Transplant
Weill Cornell Medicine
Division of Hematology & Medical Oncology
New York, New York

Catherine O'Neill D'Amico, PhD, RN, NEA-BC
Director
Programs and Operations
NICHE—Nurses Improving Care to Health System Elders
Rory Meyers College of Nursing
New York University
New York, New York

Khoa (Joey) Dang, MSN, RN, FNP-C
Assistant Professor/Assistant Director
College of Graduate Nursing
Western University of Health Sciences
Pomona, California

Cynthia L. Danko, DNP, MSN, RN
Instructor
Frances Payne Bolton School of Nursing
Case Western Reserve University
Cleveland, Ohio

Christine Horvat Davey, BSPS, BSN, RN
PhD Student
Frances Payne Bolton School of Nursing
Case Western Reserve University
Cleveland, Ohio

Mary de Haan, MSN, RN, ACNS- BC
Instructor
Frances Payne Bolton School of Nursing
Case Western Reserve University
Cleveland, Ohio

Elizabeth Demko, MSN, RN, CRNA
Co-Clinical Coordinator
University Hospitals Cleveland Medical Center
Cleveland, Ohio

Charlene M. Deuber, DNP, RN, NNP-BC, CPNP
Neonatal Nurse Practitioner
Newborn Care at Einstein Montgomery
    Medical Center
Children's Hospital of Philadelphia
East Norriton, Pennsylvania

Aimee Dickman, MSN, MN, BS, RN
Nurse Anesthesia Student
Frances Payne Bolton School of Nursing
Case Western Reserve University
Cleveland, Ohio

Danielle M. Diemer, MSN, RN, FNP-C
Nurse Practitioner
Department of Endocrinology
Cleveland Clinic
Cleveland, Ohio

Tina Di Fiore, MSN, RN
Clinical Nurse Specialist
Office of Advanced Practice Nursing
Cleveland Clinic Children's Hillcrest Hospital
Cleveland, Ohio

Marguerite DiMarco, PhD, RN, CPNP, FAAN
Associate Professor
Frances Payne Bolton School of Nursing
Case Western Reserve University
Cleveland, Ohio

Erin H. Discenza, MSN, RN
Instructor
Frances Payne Bolton School of Nursing
Case Western Reserve University
Cleveland, Ohio

Martha B. Dodd, DNP, RN, FNP-BC,
    SANE-A, SANE-P
Family Nurse Practitioner
Stephanie V. Blank Center for Safe and
    Healthy Children
Children's Healthcare of Atlanta
Atlanta, Georgia

Mary A. Dolansky, PhD, RN, FAAN
Associate Professor
Director of the QSEN Institute
Frances Payne Bolton School of Nursing
Case Western Reserve University
Cleveland, Ohio

Mary Alice Dombrowski, DNP, MSN, RN
Certified Family Nurse Practitioner
Department of Pediatric Gastroenterology, Hepatology, and
    Nutrition
Rainbow Babies and Children's Hospital
University Hospitals Cleveland Medical Center
Cleveland, Ohio

Courtney G. Donahue, MS, RN, FNP-BC, PCCN
Family Nurse Practitioner, Stroke NP
Department of Neurosciences
New York–Presbyterian Brooklyn Methodist Hospital
Brooklyn, New York

Merlyn A. Dorsainvil, DHSc, MS, MPH, RN
Assistant Professor
Department of Nursing
College of Technology of the City University of New York
Brooklyn, New York

Brenda L. Douglass, DNP, RN, APRN, FNP-C,
    CDE, CTTS
DNP Program Director
Assistant Clinical Professor
Department of Advanced Practice Nursing
Drexel University, College of Nursing &
    Health Professions
Philadelphia, Pennsylvania
Family Nurse Practitioner
Cape Regional Physician's Associates
Cape May, New Jersey

Donna A. Dowling, PhD, RN
Professor
Frances Payne Bolton School of Nursing
Case Western Reserve University
Cleveland, Ohio

Janet S. Duran, DNP, MSN, MHA, RN, LNC, ST
Director Perioperative Services
Cleveland Clinic
Fairview Hospital
Cleveland, Ohio

Andrea Efre, DNP, RN, ARNP, ANP, FNP-C
Owner
Healthcare Education Consultants
Tampa, Florida

Rachell A. Ekroos, PhD, RN, APRN-BC, AFN-BC,
    DF-IAFN, FAAN
Assistant Professor
School of Nursing
Affiliate Faculty
Center for Biobehavioral Interdisciplinary Science
University of Nevada, Las Vegas
Las Vegas, Nevada

Mary Jo Elmo, MSN, RN, CNP
Nurse Practitioner
Department of Surgery
University Hospitals Cleveland Medical Center
Cleveland, Ohio

Lisa D. Ericson, MSN, RN, FNP-BC
Assistant Professor
School of Nursing
Bethel College
Mishawaka, Indiana

Charrita Ernewein, DNP, RN, ARNP, FNP-C
Adjunct Professor
College of Nursing
South University
Valrico, Florida

Sherita K. Etheridge, MSN, RN, CPNP-PC
Nursing Instructor
Family, Community, and Health Systems
University of Alabama at Birmingham
Birmingham, Alabama

Diana K. Faugno, MSN, RN, CPN, SANE-A, SANE-P,
    FAAFS, DF-IAFN
Nurse Examiner
Barbara Sinatra Children's Center
Eisenhower Medical Center
Rancho Mirage, California

Christopher K. Ferguson, MSN, RN, CRNA
Nurse Anesthetist, Cardiothoracic Surgery
University Hospitals Cleveland Medical Center
Cleveland, Ohio

Joyce J. Fitzpatrick, PhD, MBA, RN, FAAN, FNAP
Elizabeth Brooks Ford Professor of Nursing
Frances Payne Bolton School of Nursing
Case Western Reserve University
Cleveland, Ohio

Yolanda Flenoury, MSN, RN, APRN-BC, CDE
Clinical Nurse Specialist
University Hospitals Cleveland Medical Center
Cleveland, Ohio

Crina V. Floruta, MSN, RN, ANP-BC, CWOCN
Nurse Practitioner—Colorectal Surgery
Cleveland Clinic
Cleveland, Ohio

Helen Foley, MSN, RN, AOCNS, ACHPN
Clinical Nurse Specialist Hematology/Oncology
Seidman Cancer Center
University Hospitals Cleveland Medical Center
Cleveland, Ohio

Ashley L. Foreman, DNP, RN, FNP-C
Family Nurse Practitioner
Chesapeake, Virginia

Paula Forsythe, MSN, RN
Clinical Nurse Specialist Neonatal Services
Neonatology Department
Rainbow Babies and Children's Hospital
University Hospitals Cleveland Medical Center
Cleveland, Ohio

Carrie Foster, MSN, RN, PNP
Surgical Hospitalist
Seattle Children's Hospital
Seattle, Washington

Lori A. Fusco, MSN, RN, CNE
Clinical Instructor
Department of Nursing
Youngstown State University
Youngstown, Ohio

Laurine Gajkowski, ND, RN, CPN
Instructor of Pediatric and Community Health Nursing
Frances Payne Bolton School of Nursing
Case Western Reserve University
Cleveland, Ohio
Staff Nurse
Rainbow Babies and Children's Hospital
University Hospitals Cleveland Medical Center
Cleveland, Ohio

Mary Anne Gallagher, MA, RN-BC
Director of Nursing
New York–Presbyterian Hospital
New York, New York
Adjunct Faculty
College of Nursing and Public Health
Adelphi University
Garden City, New York

Janine Stage Galeski, MSN, MA (Dipl. Kulturwirt), RN, FNP-BC
Instructor
Frances Payne Bolton School of Nursing
Case Western Reserve University
Cleveland, Ohio

Kari Gali, DNP, MSN, RN
CNP, Director of Quality and Population Health Design in Distance Health
Clinical Transformation
Cleveland Clinic
Cleveland, Ohio

Brian Garrett, DNP, RN, CRNA
Program Director
Grant Medical Center Nurse Anesthesia Program
Otterbein University
Westerville, Ohio

Carrie Gerber, MSN, RN
Clinical Coordinator for Labor and Delivery
Mount Sinai Hospital
New York, New York

Chikodiri Gibson, DNP, MBA, RN, ACNS, APN
Director of Nursing
Department of Psychiatry
Mount Sinai St. Luke's Hospital and
   Mount Sinai West Hospital
New York, New York

Deborah R. Gillum, PhD, RN, CNE
Dean of Nursing
Bethel College
Mishawaka, Indiana

Maricar P. Gomez, MSN, RN, FNP-BC, PCCN
Nurse Practitioner
Cleveland Clinic
Cleveland, Ohio
DNP Student
Frances Payne Bolton School of Nursing
Case Western Reserve University
Cleveland, Ohio

Jennifer Gonzalez, MSN, RN, APRN, AGCNS-BC
Clinical Nurse Specialist
University Hospitals Cleveland Medical Center
Cleveland, Ohio

Michael D. Gooch, DNP, RN, ACNP-BC, FNP-BC, ENP-BC, ENP-C, CFRN, CTRN, TCRN, CEN, NREMT-P
Assistant Professor of Nursing
Vanderbilt University School of Nursing
Flight Nurse
Vanderbilt University Medical Center's LifeFlight
Emergency Nurse Practitioner
TeamHealth Faculty
Middle Tennessee School of Anesthesia
Nashville, Tennessee

Deepika Goyal, PhD, MS, RN, FNP-C
Professor
Family Nurse Practitioner Program Director
The Valley Foundation School of Nursing
San Jose State University
San Jose, California

Mary T. Quinn Griffin, PhD, RN, FAAN, ANEF
Professor
Frances Payne Bolton School of Nursing
Case Western Reserve University
Cleveland, Ohio

Rebecca Witten Grizzle, PhD, MSN, RN, NP-C
Clinical Assistant Professor
College of Nursing
Sacred Heart University
Fairfield, Connecticut

Godsfavour Guillet, BSN, RN
Clinical Nurse Manager
Women's Health Unit
Women and Children's Services
Mount Sinai Hospital
New York, New York

Melanie Gibbons Hallman, DNP, RN, CRNP, CEN, FNP-BC
Instructor/Nurse Practitioner
School of Nursing
University of Alabama at Birmingham
Birmingham, Alabama

Nicole M. Hartman, DNP, MBA, RN, NEA-BC
Magnet Program Director
New York–Presbyterian/Columbia University Irving
   Medical Center
New York, New York

Rae Jean Hemway, MPA, BSN, RNC-NIC
Director of Pediatric Nursing
New York–Presbyterian Hospital
New York, New York

Erin Hennessey, DNP, RN, APRN
Nurse Practitioner, CEO
Owner of Blush Aesthetics, LLC
Perrysburg, Ohio

Andrea Marie Herr, MS, RN, ANP-BC
New York–Presbyterian Weill Cornell Medical Center
New York, New York

Julie E. Herzog, MSN, RN, ACNP-BC, CCRN, CSC
Acute Care Nurse Practitioner
Cardiothoracic Intensive Care Unit
University Hospitals Cleveland Medical Center
Cleveland, Ohio

Breanna Hetland, PhD, RN, CCRN-K
Assistant Professor
University of Nebraska Medical Center
College of Nursing
Omaha, Nebraska

Ronald L. Hickman, Jr., PhD, RN, ACNP-BC, FNAP, FAAN
Associate Professor and Assistant Dean for Research
Frances Payne Bolton School of Nursing
Case Western Reserve University
Cleveland, Ohio

Joyce E. Higgins, MSN, MBA, RN, CCRN
Staff Nurse
Florida Hospital Pepin Heart Institute
Tampa, Florida

Una Hopkins, DNP, RN, FNP-BC
Administrative Director
Center for Cancer Cure
White Plains Hospital
White Plains, New York

Katherine Hornack, MSN, RN, APRN, AGACNP-BC, CCRN
Nurse Practitioner II
University Hospitals Cleveland Medical Center
Cleveland, Ohio

Brittany Hosler, MSN, RN, CCRN
Nurse Anesthesia Student
Frances Payne Bolton School of Nursing
Case Western Reserve University
Cleveland, Ohio

Bette K. Idemoto, PhD, RN, ACNS-BC, CCRN
Clinical Nurse Specialist
University Hospitals Cleveland Medical Center
Cleveland, Ohio

Rita A. Jablonski-Jaudon, PhD, RN, CRNP, FAAN, FGSA
Nurse Practitioner
Memory Disorders Clinic
Professor
School of Nursing
University of Alabama Birmingham
Birmingham, Alabama

Molly J. Jackson, DNP, MSN, RN, AGNP-C, ACHPN
Assistant Professor
Director, Graduate Entry Program
Frances Payne Bolton School of Nursing
Case Western Reserve University
Cleveland, Ohio

Michelle A. Janas, MSN, RN, CPN
Advanced Clinical Nurse Coordinator
Pediatric Orthopedics
Rainbow Babies and Children's Hospital
University Hospitals Cleveland Medical Center
Cleveland, Ohio

Felvic Adriatico Javier, MBA, BSN, RN
DNP Student
Frances Payne Bolton School of Nursing
Case Western Reserve University
Cleveland, Ohio
Nurse Care Manager
Ambulatory Care Coordination/Care Management
New York–Presbyterian Weill Cornell Hospital
New York, New York

Marcia Johansson, DNP, RN, ARNP, ACNP-BC
Assistant Professor
Adult-Gerontology Acute Care Concentration Director
University of South Florida
Tampa, Florida

Angela M. Johnson, MSN, RN, NP-C
Nurse Practitioner
Optum Clinical Services
United Health Group
Cleveland, Ohio

Qiana A. Johnson, DNP, FNP-C
Family Nurse Practitioner
Children's Healthcare of Atlanta
Stephanie V. Blank Center for Safe and Healthy Children
Atlanta, Georgia

Jarold T. Johnston, Jr., MSN, RN, CNM, IBCLC
Assistant Professor of Nursing
Methodist University
Fayetteville, North Carolina

Jennifer Johntony, MSN, RN, CPNP-AC/PC
Pediatric Nurse Practitioner
The Congenital Heart Collaborative
Rainbow Babies and Children's Hospital
University Hospitals Cleveland Medical Center
Cleveland, Ohio

Elsie A. Jolade, DNP, EdM, RN, FNP-BC, ACNS, APRN, CCRN
Clinical Professor
Hunter College
School of Nursing
City University of New York
New York, New York

Jeffrey S. Jones, DNP, RN, PMHCNS-BC, CST, LNC
Psychiatric Clinical Nurse Specialist
Mansfield, Ohio

Tasina Jones, MSN, RN-BC, CNS, AOCNS
Clinical Nurse Specialist
Women's Oncology Unit
Memorial Sloan Kettering Cancer Center
New York, New York

Evanne Juratovac, PhD, RN, GCNS-BC
Assistant Professor
Frances Payne Bolton School of Nursing
Assistant Professor
School of Medicine
Faculty Associate
University Center on Aging and Health
Case Western Reserve University
Cleveland, Ohio

Stacen A. Keating, PhD, RN
Clinical Assistant Professor
Rory Meyers College of Nursing
New York University
New York, New York

Irena L. Kenneley, PhD, RN, CNE, CIC, FAPIC
Associate Professor/Faculty Development Director
Frances Payne Bolton School of Nursing
Case Western Reserve University
Cleveland, Ohio

Vicki A. Keough, PhD, RN, FAAN
Dean and Professor
Marcella Niehoff School of Nursing
Loyola University Chicago
Chicago, Illinois

Kimberly Kimble, MSN, RN, CRNA
Nurse Anesthesia Program
Frances Payne Bolton School of Nursing
Case Western Reserve University
Cleveland, Ohio

Shanina C. Knighton, PhD, RN
Post-Doctoral Fellow
Frances Payne Bolton School of Nursing
Case Western Reserve University
Cleveland, Ohio

Anne M. Kolenic, MSN, RN, AOCNS
Oncology Clinical Nurse Specialist
University Hospitals Seidman Cancer Center
Cleveland, Ohio

Catherine S. Koppelman, MSN, RN, NEA-BC
Consultant and Executive Coach
Nursing Leadership
Visiting Faculty
Frances Payne Bolton School of Nursing
Case Western Reserve University
Cleveland, Ohio

Mary Jo Krivanek, MPA, BSN, RN
Clinical Nurse Educator
Southwest General Health Center
Middleburg Heights, Ohio

Aniko Kukla, DNP, RN, CPNP-PC
Quality Manager
Quality Management Services
Salinas Valley Memorial Hospital
Salinas, California

Cindy D. Kumar, MSN, RN, AG-ACNP, FNP, ENP
Emergency Nurse Practitioner
TeamHealth
St. David's South Austin Medical Center Emergency
Department
Austin, Texas

Colleen Kurzawa, MSN, MFA, RN
PhD Student
Frances Payne Bolton School of Nursing
Case Western Reserve University
Cleveland, Ohio

Tammy M. Lampley, PhD, RN, CNE
Director
Nursing Education Program
Sacred Heart University
Fairfield, Connecticut

Helene M. Lannon, MSN, RN, APRN, NNP-BC
Neonatal Nurse Practitioner
Neonatal Intensive Care Unit
Pediatrix Medical Group of Nevada at
    Sunrise Children's Hospital
Las Vegas, Nevada

Cynthia Ann Leaver, PhD, RN, APRN, FNP-BC
Associate Dean of Faculty and Research
College of Nursing
United States University
San Diego, California

Nirmala Lekhak, PhD, RN
Assistant Professor
School of Nursing
University of Nevada Las Vegas
Las Vegas, Nevada

Britney A. Leonardi, MSN, RN, CRNA, CNE
Nurse Anesthesia Program
Frances Payne Bolton School of Nursing
Case Western Reserve University
Cleveland, Ohio

Fidelindo Lim, DNP, RN, CCRN
Clinical Assistant Professor of Nursing
Rory Meyers College of Nursing
New York University
New York, New York

Deborah F. Lindell, DNP, MSN, CNE, ANEF
Associate Professor
Frances Payne Bolton School of Nursing
Case Western Reserve University
Cleveland, Ohio

Melanie S. Lint, MSN, RN, APRN-CNS, PMHCNS-BC,
    CARN-AP
Adult Psychiatric Clinical Nurse Specialist
Columbus Springs East Hospital
Reynoldsburg, Ohio

Shannon M. Litten, DNP, RN, ARNP, ACNP-BC,
    FNP-BC, ENP-C
Lead Regional Director
American Academy of Emergency
    Nurse Practitioners
Adjunct Instructor in Nursing
Vanderbilt University School of Nursing
TEAMHealth
Emergency Nurse Practitioner
St. Mary's Medical Center
West Palm Beach, Florida

Leslie J. Lockett, MS, RNC, CNE, CMSRN
Director of RN-BSN Program
Instructor
College of Nursing
University of South Florida
Tampa, Florida

Andrew D. Lorenzoni, MSN, RN
Nurse Anesthesia Student
Frances Payne Bolton School of Nursing
Case Western Reserve University
Cleveland, Ohio

Lia V. Ludan, DNP, RN, FNP-BC
Family Nurse Practitioner
Department of Emergency
Cape Regional Medical Center
Cape May Courthouse, New Jersey
Penn Presbyterian Medical Center
Philadelphia, Pennsylvania

Ruth Ludwick, PhD, RN, CNS, FAAN
Professor Emeritus
Kent State University
Manager
Center for Clinical Research
University Hospitals Portage Medical Center
Kent, Ohio

Rebecca M. Lutz, DNP, RN, APRN, FNP-BC, PPCNP-BC
Assistant Professor
College of Nursing
University of South Florida
Tampa, Florida

Kelly Ann Lynn, MS, MA, RN
Manager
Center for Advanced Digestive Care
New York–Presbyterian Hospital
New York, New York

Alaa Mahsoon, MSN, RN
PhD Student
Frances Payne Bolton School of Nursing
Case Western Reserve University
Cleveland, Ohio

Virginia Mangolds, MSN, RN, FNP-C, ENP-C, BSED
Instructor
Emergency Medicine
Instructor
Graduate School of Nursing
Assistant Research Director
Department of Emergency Medicine
UMass Memorial Medical Center
Worcester, Massachusetts

Nadine M. Marchi, DNP, MSN, RN, CRRN, CNE
Instructor
Frances Payne Bolton School of Nursing
Case Western Reserve University
McGregor Faculty Scholar
QSEN Teaching Strategies Coordinator
Cleveland, Ohio

Jane F. Marek, DNP, MSN, RN
Assistant Professor
Frances Payne Bolton School of Nursing
Case Western Reserve University
Cleveland, Ohio

Kathleen Marsala-Cervasio, PhD, EdD, RN, ACNS-BC, CCRN
Associate Professor
Harriet Rothkopf Heilbrunn School of Nursing
Long Island University
Brooklyn Campus
Brookville, New York

Stephanie R. Martin, MSN, RN, APRN, CNS, ANCC
Clinical Nurse Specialist
Primary Care Mental Health Integration
U.S. Department of Veterans Affairs
Cleveland, Ohio

Visnja Maria Masina, MSN, RN, APRN, AGCNS-BC
Clinical Nurse Specialist
Cleveland Clinic
Cleveland, Ohio

Kerry Mastrangelo, DNP, RN, APRN, NP-C
Assistant Professor of Nursing
The Barbara H. Hagan School of Nursing
Molloy College
Rockville Center, New York

Kathleen Maxwell, MSN, RN, CNS, CNP
Family Nurse Practitioner
Pediatric Neurology
Rainbow Babies and Children's Hospital
University Hospitals Cleveland Medical Center
Cleveland, Ohio

Kelly K. McConnell, DNP, MSN, RN, AG-ACNP-BC
Assistant Professor
Frances Payne Bolton School of Nursing
Case Western Reserve University
Cleveland, Ohio

Steadman McPeters, DNP, RN, CRNP, CPNP-AC, RNFA
Assistant Professor
Director of Clinical Graduate Program Subspecialty
    Tracks and Dual Option & Acute Care Pediatric Nurse
    Practitioner Specialty Track Coordinator
Department of Family, Community, and Health Systems
School of Nursing
University of Alabama at Birmingham
Birmingham, Alabama

Maria A. Mendoza, EdD, RN, ANP, GNP-BC, CDE, CNE
Assistant Clinical Professor
Director
Nursing Education Master's and Advanced Certificate
    Programs
Rory Meyers College of Nursing
New York University
New York, New York

Kathy J. Meyers, MSN, RN, ACNS-BC
Project Manager
Frances Payne Bolton School of Nursing
Case Western Reserve University
Cleveland, Ohio

Jennifer E. Millman, BSN, RN
Clinical Practice Nurse
Advanced Endoscopy
Division of Gastroenterology
Weill Cornell Medical Center
New York, New York

Angela Milosh, DNP, RN, CRNA
Program Director
Cleveland Clinic School of Nurse Anesthesia
Frances Payne Bolton School of Nursing
Case Western Reserve University
Cleveland, Ohio

Stacey A. Mitchell, DNP, MBA, RN, SANE-A, SANE-P, FAAN
Clinical Associate Professor
Texas A&M University
College of Nursing
Bryan, Texas

Anne M. Modic, BSN, RN, BC-NNP
Neonatal Nurse Practitioner/Department of Neonatology
Rainbow Babies and Children's Hospital
University Hospitals Cleveland Medical Center
Cleveland, Ohio

Mary Beth Modic, DNP, RN, APRN-CNS, CDE
Diabetes Clinical Nurse Specialist
Department of Advanced Practice Nursing
Cleveland Clinic
Cleveland, Ohio

Jeffrey E. Molter, MSN, MBA, RN, CRNA
Director of Anesthesia
Findlay Surgery Center
Findlay, Ohio

Scott Emory Moore, PhD, RN, APRN,
  AGPCNP-BC
Postdoctoral Fellow
Frances Payne Bolton School of Nursing
Case Western Reserve University
Cleveland, Ohio

Sonya D. Moore, DNP, RN, CRNA
Assistant Professor
Nurse Anesthesia Program Director
Case Western Reserve University
Frances Payne Bolton School of Nursing
Cleveland, Ohio

Brittany Newberry, PhD, MSN, MPH, RN, APRN,
  FNP-BC, ENP-BC
Vice President of Education and
  Clinical Development
Nell Hodgson Woodruff School of Nursing
Emory University
Atlanta, Georgia

Jennifer Nicholson, MSN, RN, CRNA
Hillcrest Hospital–Cleveland Clinic
Instructor
Frances Payne Bolton School of Nursing
Nurse Anesthesia Program
Case Western Reserve University
Cleveland, Ohio

Sabrina Nitkowski-Keever, MSN, RN, RNC
Director Maternal Child Health
Maternal Child Health and Education
New York–Presbyterian Hudson Valley Hospital
Pleasant Valley, New York

Lamon Norton, DNP, RN, FNP, ACNP
Managing Partner
UEE Health Care Consulting Emergency
  Nurse Practitioner
Faculty
Samford University
Homewood, Alabama

Marian Nowak, DNP, MPH, RN, CSN, PN, FAAN
Assistant Professor
Rowan University Nursing Program
RN-BSN Program Coordinator
United Nations Nurse Delegate
CICIAMS Pan American President
Glassboro, New Jersey

Petique Oeflein, MSN, RN, FNP-C, ACHPN
Nurse Practitioner
Hospice and Palliative Care
Hospice of the Western Reserve
Cleveland, Ohio

Loraine O'Neill, MPH, RN
System Chief Patient Safety Officer
Department of Obstetrics and Gynecology
Mount Sinai Health System
Mount Sinai Medical Center
New York, New York

Joyce Palmieri, MS, RN, CHPN
Vice-President of Clinical Services
MJHS Hospice and Palliative Care
New York, New York

Rebecca M. Patton, DNP, MSN, RN, CNOR, FAAN
Lucy Jo Atkinson Scholar in Perioperative Nursing
Frances Payne Bolton School of Nursing; and
Case Western Reserve University
Past President, American Nurses Association
Cleveland, Ohio

Carol Pehotsky, DNP, RN, ACNS-BC, CPAN, NEA-BC
Associate Chief Nursing Officer
Surgical Services
Cleveland Clinic
Cleveland, Ohio

George Byron Peraza-Smith, DNP, RN, GNP-BC,
  AGPCNP-C, CNE
Associate Dean of Academic Affairs
United States University
San Diego, California

Joseph D. Perazzo, PhD, RN
Assistant Professor
College of Nursing
University of Cincinnati
Cincinnati, Ohio

Sharon Perry, MSN, RN, CPNP, CPN
Nurse Practitioner
Pediatric Gastroenterology, Hepatology, and Nutrition
Rainbow Babies and Children's Hospital
University Hospitals Cleveland Medical Center
Cleveland, Ohio

Gayle M. Petty, DNP, MSN, RN
Assistant Professor
Frances Payne Bolton School of Nursing
Case Western Reserve University
Cleveland, Ohio

Kathryn E. Phillips, PhD, MS, MA, RN, NP-BC
Assistant Professor
Fairfield University
Fairfield, Connecticut

Sharon L. Phillips, PhD, RN, PMHCNS-BC
Clinical Nurse Specialist
Louis Stokes Cleveland VA Medical Center
Warren Outpatient Clinic
Warren, Ohio

Susan Phillips, DNP, MPH, RN, APRN
Louis Stokes Cleveland VA Medical Center
Cleveland, Ohio

Karla Phipps, MSN, RN, APRN, NNP-BC
Neonatal Nurse Practitioner
Rainbow Babies and Children's Hospital
University Hospitals Cleveland Medical Center
Cleveland, Ohio

Grant Pignatiello, BSN, RN
PhD Candidate
Frances Payne Bolton School of Nursing
Case Western Reserve University
Cleveland, Ohio

Kerry L. Quisenberry, MSN, RN, CRNA
Clinical Coordinator
Nurse Anesthesia Program
Frances Payne School of Nursing
Case Western Reserve University
Cleveland, Ohio

Sharon R. Rainer, PhD, RN, APRN, FNP-BC
Assistant Professor
Thomas Jefferson University College of Nursing
Nurse Practitioner
Department of Emergency Medicine
Thomas Jefferson University
Philadelphia, Pennsylvania

Rhoda Redulla, DNP, RN-BC
Magnet® Program Director
Office of Nursing Excellence
New York–Presbyterian Hospital Weill Cornell
    Medical Center
New York, New York

Janet E. Reilly, DNP, RN, APRN-BC
Nurse Practitioner
Bellin Health Systems
Associate Professor
University of Wisconsin—Green Bay
Green Bay, Wisconsin

Shannon A. Rives, MSN, RN, ACNS-BC, CCRN, CMSRN
Clinical Nurse Specialist
Cleveland Clinic
Cleveland, Ohio

Eric Roberts, DNP, RN, FNP-BC, ENP-BC
Assistant Professor
Marcella Niehoff School of Nursing
Loyola University Chicago
Chicago, Illinois

Jacqueline Robinson, MSN, MBA, RN, ACNS-BC, CCRN
Simulation Manager
Frances Payne Bolton School of Nursing
Case Western Reserve University
Cleveland, Ohio

Breanne M. Roche, MSN, RN, CPNP, CPHON
Pediatric Nurse Practitioner
Rainbow Babies and Children's Hospital
University Hospitals Cleveland Medical Center
Cleveland, Ohio

Ronald Rock, MSN, RN, APRN, CNS
Nurse Manager/Clinical Nurse Specialist
Wound Ostomy Continence Nursing Department
Cleveland Clinic
Cleveland, Ohio

Donna Lynn Rose, DNP, RN
Senior Lecturer
School of Nursing
Old Dominion University
Norfolk, Virginia

Joan Rotnem, MSHA, BSN, RN, CNOR
Senior Perioperative Nurse Consultant
STERIS Corporation
Employee Health Nurse
Henderson Hospital
Henderson, Nevada

Suzanne Rubin, DNP, MPH, RN, CRNP-P
Nursery Pediatric Nurse Practitioner
Johns Hopkins Hospital
Baltimore, Maryland

Susanna Rudy, DNP, MFS, RN, AG-ACNP-BC, FNP-BC,
    ENP, CCRN
Faculty Instructor
Vanderbilt University School of Nursing
Vanderbilt University Medical Center
Emergency Department APRN
Nashville, Tennessee

Al Rundio, PhD, DNP, RN, APRN, CARN-AP, NEA-BC,
    FNAP, FIAAN, FAAN
Associate Dean for Nursing
Chief Academic Nursing Officer
Clinical Professor of Nursing
Drexel University
College of Nursing & Health Professions
Philadelphia, Pennsylvania

Jacob Runion, MBA, BSN, RN, CNOR
Director of Nursing
Cleveland Clinic
Cleveland, Ohio

Dena L. Salamon, BSN, RN
Nurse Manager
Cleveland Clinic
Cleveland, Ohio

Lisa L. Salser, MSN, RN, PMHCNS-BC
Department of Veterans Affairs
Louis Stokes Cleveland VA Medical Center
Cleveland, Ohio

Ian N. Saludares, MPA, BSN, RN,
    CCRN-K, NEA-BC
ICU/CCU—Nurse Manager
New York Presbyterian—Lawrence Hospital
Bronxville, New York

Donna M. Schultz, DNP, RN, APRN, NNP-BC
Neonatal Nurse Practitioner
Mednax Medical Group
Baylor University Medical Center & The Tots Clinic
Dallas, Texas

Rita M. Sfiligoj, DNP, MSN, MPA, RN
Instructor
Frances Payne Bolton School of Nursing
Case Western Reserve University
Cleveland, Ohio

Florin Sgondea, BSN, RN
Robotic Coordinator
Cleveland Clinic
Cleveland, Ohio

Megan M. Shifrin, DNP, RN, ACNP-BC
Assistant Professor
School of Nursing
Vanderbilt University
Director of the AGACNP Intensivist Focus
Nashville, Tennessee

Sallie J. Shipman, EdD, MSN, RN, CNL
Assistant Professor
School of Nursing
Family, Community, and Health Systems
University of Alabama at Birmingham
Birmingham, Alabama

Darlie Simerson, DNP, RN, APN, FNP-BC, CEN
Assistant Professor
Marcella Niehoff School of Nursing
Loyola University Chicago
Maywood, Illinois
Family Nurse Practitioner
Northwestern Convenient Care Centers
Northwestern Medicine Central DuPage Hospital
Winfield, Illinois

Michelle McHugh Slater, DNP, MSN, RN, CNOR
Associate Professor of Nursing
Ursuline College
Veterans Affairs Quality Scholar
Louis Stokes Cleveland VA Medical Center
Cleveland, Ohio

Natalie A. Slenkovich, MSN, RN, CCRN
Nurse Anesthesia Student
Frances Payne Bolton School of Nursing
Case Western Reserve University
Cleveland, Ohio

Barbara Greitzer Slone, MS, MPH, RN, CPNP
Chief Nurse Practitioner
Neonatal Intensive Care Unit
Department of Pediatrics
New York University Winthrop Hospital
Mineola, New York

Maria G. Smisek, MSN, RN-BC
Doctoral Student
Frances Payne Bolton School of Nursing
Case Western Reserve University
Cleveland, Ohio

Marilyn E. Smith, PhD, RN, PMHNP-BC, APRN
Clinical Professor
School of Nursing
West Virginia University
Morgantown, West Virginia

Tedra S. Smith, DNP, RN, CRNP, CPNP-PC, CNE
Assistant Professor
School of Nursing
University of Alabama at Birmingham
Birmingham, Alabama

Marian Soat, MSN, RN, APRN, CCNS, CCRN
Clinical Nurse Specialist
Department of Advance Practice Nursing
Cleveland Clinic
Cleveland, Ohio

Ramona A. Sowers, DNP, RN, FNP-BC, ANP-BC
Family Nurse Practitioner
Neurodiagnostic, Sleep Apnea Clinic
Durham, North Carolina
Adjunct Faculty
Nursing @Simmons Online Programs
School of Nursing and Health Sciences
Simmons College
Boston, Massachusetts

Ingrid Apryl Spears, MSN, BS, RN
Bronx, New York

Patricia M. Speck, DNSc, APN, APRN, FNP-BC, DF-IAFN, FAAFS, FAAN
Professor and Coordinator
Advanced Forensic Nursing Department of Family, Community, & Health Systems
School of Nursing
University of Alabama at Birmingham
Birmingham, Alabama

Colleen Thaxton Spencer, MSN, RN, CRNA
Co-Clinical Coordinator
University Hospitals of Cleveland Medical Center
Cleveland, Ohio

Dustin Spencer, DNP, RN, NRP, NP-C, PMHS, ENP-BC, CNL
Assistant Professor of Nursing
Davenport University
Grand Rapids, Michigan
Lead Advanced Practice Clinician
American Physician Partners
Lancaster, South Carolina

Justin R. Stegman, MSN, BS, RN
Nurse Anesthesia Student
Frances Payne Bolton School of Nursing
Case Western Reserve University
Cleveland, Ohio

Melanie M. Stipp, MSN, RN, CCRN
Nurse Anesthesia Student
Frances Payne Bolton School of Nursing
Case Western Reserve University
Critical Care Registered Nurse
Cleveland Clinic
Cleveland, Ohio

Anita Sundaresh, MS, BSN, RN
Adult Nurse Practitioner
New York Presbyterian Hospital
New York, New York
Adjunct Faculty Member
Adelphi University for Graduate Nursing
Garden City, New York

Marianna K. Sunderlin, MSN, RN, ACNS-BC
Nurse Educator
American Psychiatric Nurses Association
Adjunct Faculty, Wright State University
Beavercreek, Ohio

Patricia Suplee, PhD, RN, RNC-OB
Associate Professor
Rutgers School of Nursing-Camden
Camden, New Jersey

Diane Fuller Switzer, DNP, ARNP, RN, FNP-BC, ENP-B,C ENP-C, CCRN, CEN, FAEN
Assistant Clinical Professor
Seattle University College of Nursing
Seattle, Washington

Mary Szostakowski, MSN, RN, CNOR
Nurse Manager
Department of Urology and Gynecology
Cleveland Clinic
Cleveland, Ohio

Richard Taylor, DNP, RN, CRNP, APN-BC
Associate Scientist
University of Alabama at Birmingham
Center of Palliative and Supportive Care
Assistant Professor
School of Nursing
Department of Acute, Chronic, and Continuing Care
University of Alabama at Birmingham
Birmingham, Alabama

Mary F. Terhaar, DNSC, RN, ANEF, FAAN
Associate Dean for Academic Affairs
Arline H. and Curtis F. Garvin Professor
Frances Payne Bolton School of Nursing
Case Western Reserve University
Cleveland, Ohio

Karen L. Terry, DNP, MSN, RN, NP-C, GNP-BC
Nurse Practitioner
Mercy Health Physicians Lorain Geriatrics
Amherst, Ohio

Ke-Ni Niko Tien, MSN, RN, APRN, NNP-BC
Nurse Practitioner
Neonatal Intensive Care Unit
Cleveland Clinic
Cleveland, Ohio

Rachel Tkaczyk, MSN, RN, CPNP-AC/PC-BC
Pediatric Nurse Practitioner
Assistant Clinical Professor
Drexel University
Philadelphia, Pennsylvania

Kelley Toffoli, DNP, RN, FNP-BC
Drexel University
Philadelphia, Pennsylvania

Lisa Torrieri, MSN, RN, FNP, CWON
Nurse Clinician
Wound and Ostomy Nurse
New York–Presbyterian Hospital
Weill Cornell Medical Center
New York, New York

Arlene Travis, MSN, RN, ANP-BC
Nurse Clinician
Mount Sinai Hospital
New York, New York
Adjunct Assistant Professor
Pace University Lienhard School of Nursing
New York, New York

Jessica M. Tripi, MSN, RN
Nurse Anesthesia Student
Frances Payne Bolton School of Nursing
Case Western Reserve University
Cleaveland, Ohio

Se Min Um, BSN, RN-BC
Nurse Manager
Addiction Institute at Mount Sinai West
New York, New York

Scott M. Urigel, MSN, RN, CRNA
Western Reserve Anesthesia Education
Western Reserve Anesthesia Associates
Painesville, Ohio
Case Western Reserve University
Cleveland, Ohio
Middle Tennessee School of Anesthesia
Madison, Tennessee
Developer, Block Buddy mobile application

Rachel K. Vanek, MSN, RN, CNP
Acute Care Nurse Practitioner
Pulmonary Critical Care Medicine
Medical Intensive Care Unit
University Hospitals Cleveland Medical Center
Cleveland, Ohio

Mary Variath, MSN, RN
Instructor
Frances Payne Bolton School of Nursing
Case Western Reserve University
Cleveland, Ohio

Deborah Vinesky, MSN, RN
Assistant Professor
Cuyahoga Community College
Cleveland, Ohio
DNP Student
Frances Payne Bolton School of Nursing
Case Western Reserve University
Cleveland, Ohio

Ekta Vohra, BSN, RN, CWON
Nurse Clinician
Wound and Ostomy Nurse
New York–Presbyterian Hospital
Weill Cornell Medical Center
New York, New York

Courtney Vose, DNP, MBA, RN, APRN, NEA-BC
Vice President and Chief Nursing Officer
New York–Presbyterian/Columbia University Irving
    Medical Center/Allen/Ambulatory
    Care Network; and
Clinical Instructor
Columbia University School of Nursing
New York, New York

Karen Vosper, BSN, RN, CPN
Advanced Clinical Nurse
Cystic Fibrosis Center
Cleveland, Ohio

Sharon Ward-Miller, MA, RN, PMHCNS-BC
Patient Care Director
Personality Disorders Unit
New York–Presbyterian Hospital–Westchester Division
White Plains, New York

Rosanna P. Watowicz, PhD, RD, LD
Assistant Professor
Department of Nutrition
School of Medicine
Case Western Reserve University
Cleveland, Ohio

Rachael Weigand, MSN, RN, CPN P-PC
Nurse Practitioner
Heart Center
Akron Children's Hospital
Brecksville, Ohio

Sharon Stahl Wexler, PhD, RN, FNGNA
Associate Professor
Pace University
Lienhard School of Nursing
New York, New York

Michael Wichowski, BSN, RN
Hospital Supervisor
St. Nicholas Hospital
Sheboygan, Wisconsin

S. Brian Widmar, PhD, RN, ACNP-BC, CCRN, FAANP
Director
Adult-Gerontology Acute Care Nurse
    Practitioner Program
Vanderbilt University School of Nursing
Nashville, Tennessee

Jennifer Wilbeck, DNP, RN, ACNP, FNP, ENP, FAANP
Associate Professor
Vanderbilt University School of Nursing
Nashville, Tennessee

Danielle T. Winch, DNP, RN, CRNA
Adjunct Faculty
Grant Medical Center
Otterbein University
Dublin, Ohio

Elizabeth Wirth-Tomaszewski, DNP, RN, CRNP, CCRN, ACNP-BC, ACNPC
Assistant Clinical Professor and Track Director
Adult Gerontology Acute Care Nurse
    Practitioner Program
College of Nursing and Health Professions
Drexel University
Philadelphia, Pennsylvania

Shannon Courtney Wong, MSN, RN, CPNP
Instructor
Frances Payne Bolton School of Nursing
Case Western Reserve University
Cleveland, Ohio

Heidi Youngbauer, MSN, RN
Adjunct Professor
Department of Nursing
Sacred Heart University
Onalaska, Wisconsin

Jodi Zalewski, MSN, RN, CPNP-AC
Pediatric Nurse Practitioner
The Congenital Heart Collaborative
University Hospitals Cleveland Medical Center
Cleveland, Ohio

Margarete L. Zalon, PhD, RN, ACNS-BC, FAAN
Professor of Nursing
Director, Online MS in Health Informatics Program
University of Scranton
Scranton, Philadelphia

Jenelle M. Zambrano, DNP, RN, CNS, CCNS, CCRN
Director, Professional Practice and Development
Fountain Valley Regional Hospital and
    Medical Center
Fountain Valley, California

Elizabeth Zimmermann, DNP, MSN, RN, CHSE
Instructor of Pediatric and Community
    Health Nursing
Frances Payne Bolton School of Nursing
Case Western Reserve University
Cleveland, Ohio

There are many transitions that generalist nurses make during their careers as professional nurses. The first transition is graduation from a prelicensure nursing education program that prepares them to sit for the National Council Licensure Examination—Registered Nurse, the NCLEX-RN® examination. Once the graduates of a prelicensure nursing program have passed the NCLEX, they apply for state licensure and provide nursing under the Nurse Practice Act, legislation that governs the professional nursing practice in each state. According to the National Council of State Boards of Nursing (NCSBN), "licensure is the process by which boards of nursing grant permission to an individual to engage in nursing practice after determining that the applicant has attained the competency necessary to perform a unique scope of practice. Licensure is necessary when the regulated activities are complex and require specialized knowledge and skill, and independent decision making. The licensure process determines if the applicant has the necessary skills to safely perform a specified scope of practice by predetermining the criteria needed and evaluating licensure applicants to determine if they meet the criteria" (NCSBN, 2017a, para. 1, p. 1).

Although there are some variations in practice requirements across states in the United States and its territories, there is a great deal of consistency in the expectation that the individuals licensed as registered nurses (RNs) are generalists who, without additional education or licensing, can practice across a wide range of specialties in nursing. Thus, a RN who has practiced in a medical–surgical unit can transition to a pediatric unit and practice without additional required credentialing. Some areas of professional practice, although still considered in the scope of practice of the generalist RN, have stipulations that are imposed by the institutions or educational programs to ensure the quality of care delivered by RNs in specialized areas of clinical care. To practice in a critical care emergency department, for example, it might be expected that the RN has already worked for a specific period in a general medical–surgical unit.

Although there are no explicit rules across states and institutions, there is some conventional wisdom that often leads new RN generalists to provide nursing care to medical–surgical patients. However, there continues to be divided opinion among nurse educators and clinical nurse leaders regarding the necessity of this grounding of novice RN generalists in medical–surgical units. Some advocates would encourage new RNs to follow their passions. Thus, if they wanted to work in a critical care unit, they could undoubtedly find an opportunity to provide care to the critically ill in a hospital. This is especially true in underserved communities, such as rural areas and public hospitals located in inner cities.

Transition to professional nursing practice is one of the major areas of concern for both nurse educators and clinical nurse leaders, who are employing new registered nurse graduates. New registered nurses are entering health care environments that are facing complex challenges. In the current health care climate, health care organizations are under pressure to operate lean and with efficiency as a result of the recent changes in policy and regulatory oversight. As new RNs, the complex needs of patients with multimorbidity, a state of having two or more chronic conditions, are challenging and require thoughtful care planning. In addition to the high demands of complex patients and families, new graduate RNs also experience the complexities of navigating generational diversity in the workforce, performance anxiety, peer bullying, and lack of sufficient mentoring, which affect their ability to deliver safe and effective nursing care (Hofler & Thomas, 2016). Altogether, the new graduate nurse is vulnerable to compassion fatigue and burnout, which may result in increased attrition. Furthermore, there is documentation indicating that the rate of turnover of new RNs is high if they are not adequately prepared for the challenges they face in the clinical environment (Hofler & Thomas, 2016; Missen, McKenna, & Beauchamp, 2014).

There are excellent resources to assist the new RN in making the transition to professional practice. For

TABLE P.1	NCSBN Transition to Practice Courses and Competencies
COURSE	**COMPETENCIES**
Course 1: Communication and Teamwork	Develop a situational awareness that helps your team operate more effectively and prevents harm to patients.
Course 2: Patient- and Family-Centered Care	Promote your patients' recovery by incorporating their culture and values while engaging their support network.
Course 3: Evidence-Based Practice	Make a real contribution to your team as you access, share, and implement the latest research.
Course 4: Quality Improvement	Participate in processes that continuously improve the outcomes of care.
Course 5: Informatics	Effectively use technology to create usable information that supports the practice of nursing.
Course for Preceptors: Helping Nurses Transition to Practice	Foster the growth of new graduate nurses by embracing the role of a teacher, coach, and protector.

example, NCSBN Transition to Practice program is a 6-month program consisting of five courses for new RNs (NCSBN, 2017b). The courses and competencies for the NCSBN program are included in Table P.1.

Another general preparation program for new RNs transitioning to practice is the Quality and Safety Education for Nurses (QSEN) program. QSEN addresses the challenge of preparing future nurses with the knowledge, skills, and attitudes (KSAs) necessary to continuously improve the quality and safety of the health care systems in which they work. Core QSEN competencies, KSAs, teaching strategies, and faculty development resources have been developed to assist in this transition (QSEN, 2017). The QSEN competency areas include patient-centered care, teamwork and collaboration, evidence-based practice, quality improvement, safety, and informatics.

Although transition to practice is an important area, many other transitions can occur for RNs as they decide to move from one clinical practice area to another. Rather than focus on the general clinical components included in the transition-to-practice programs, we thought it was equally important to assist the generalist RN in transitioning from one clinical area to another. Therefore, this book is also for those who want to know the primary clinical problems that RNs may encounter in each of the selected clinical areas.

To begin, we invited key leaders in clinical content areas to serve as content editors. These content editors identified the expert clinicians in their field to author entries for that specialty. The clinical content areas included are emergency and critical care nursing, geriatric nursing, health systems and health promotion, medical–surgical nursing, neonatal nursing, nurse anesthesia, obstetrics and women's health, palliative care nursing, pediatric nursing, perioperative nursing, and psychiatric mental health nursing. The book includes a comprehensive compendium of clinical nursing content areas. There is no previous work of this nature published as a reference book. Our objective is to provide detailed information on the most important topics in clinical nursing practice for both new RNs and those transitioning to a new clinical area. Each clinical content area includes the key clinical nursing problems encountered in generalist nursing practice, followed by an overview of each clinical problem, pertinent clinical background, clinical aspects for the nurse (assessment, nursing management and clinical implications, and outcomes), and a summary. Key references are provided for each entry, including both classic references and current citations from clinical and research literature.

All of the clinical areas included in this book focus on the generalist RN, except for nurse anesthesia practice. There are four types of advanced practice nurses (APNs), and the certified registered nurse anesthetist is one of these. The other three APN groups are certified nurse-midwives, nurse practitioners, and clinical nurse specialists. Although we did not include any specific attention to clinical problems for the other groups of APNs, there is content relevant for the novice APN. For example, the newly prepared and certified nurse midwife might never have encountered a childbearing woman with cervical cancer. Thus, the entry on cervical cancer in the women's health section would be especially instructive to a certified nurse-midwife in transition to this new practice area.

We believe that this compilation will also be useful to clinical nursing faculty teaching beginning students. Although there are a number of comprehensive textbooks available in each clinical content area, this reference provides information that is both concise and practical for students as they enter each clinical area. The entries can also be used to evaluate the basic knowledge that the students need to have about the clinical nursing problems identified.

In summary, this book has particular relevance to several groups of nurses. Nurse faculty will find it useful as a synopsis for clinical problems encountered in a specific clinical area. For clinicians transitioning to new clinical areas it will be a ready resource for key clinical problems that they may encounter in the new area. Moreover, newly licensed RNs will find that this guide to clinical mastery will chart their way in addressing the important clinical problems that their patients experience.

Joyce J. Fitzpatrick
Celeste M. Alfes
Ronald L. Hickman, Jr.

Hofler, L., & Thomas, K. (2016). Transition of new graduate nurses to the workforce: Challenges and solutions in the changing health care environment. *North Carolina Medical Journal*, 77(2), 133–136. doi:10.18043/ncm .77.2.133

Missen, K., McKenna, L., & Beauchamp, A. (2014). Satisfaction of newly graduated nurses enrolled in transition-to-practice programmes in their first year of employment: A systematic review. *Journal of Advanced Nursing*, 70(11), 2419–2433. doi:10.1111/jan.12464

National Council of State Boards of Nursing. (2017a). About nursing licensure. Retrieved from https://www .ncsbn.org/licensure.htm

National Council of State Boards of Nursing. (2017b). Courses in the transition to practice program. Retrieved from https://learningext.com/new-nurses

Quality and Safety in Nursing Education. (2017). QSEN Institute. Retrieved from http://qsen.org/about-qsen

Acknowledgments

The editors would like to acknowledge the following individuals:

The section editors for their work in identifying authors and editing the submissions in their respective sections of the book; the authors of all of the entries for their clinical expertise and their contributions; Mary Anne Gallagher, doctoral student at Case Western Reserve University (CWRU), for her work in identifying several authors who contributed entries for many of the sections, and her editing of the final entries for the Obstetrics and Women's Health section; CWRU BSN students Hanna Potter and Jennie He for assisting with reference checking for the editorial team, and CWRU BSN student Claire Miller for credential checking for all contributors.

The Springer Publishing staff, in particular Joseph Morita, Joanne Jay, Lindsay Claire, and Rachel Landes, for their attention to detail in the editing and production of the book.

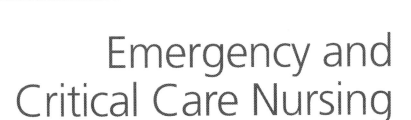

Emergency and Critical Care Nursing

Nursing care in the emergency care and critical care settings is quite complex and challenging due to heightened acuity of patients in need of evidence-based care. Emergency nurses provide high-quality care to patients with injuries and illness across all age groups regardless of ethnicity, culture, socioeconomic status, or religious beliefs. Nurses need to have the ability to identify life-threatening or potentially life-threatening problems while working in an area of "controlled chaos." The emergency care setting offers numerous opportunities to practice in emergency departments, urgent care, correction facilities, prehospital and interhospital transports (i.e., ambulance, rotor and fixed wing aircraft), and trauma centers.

Critical care nurses also provide high-quality complex care to patients with life-threatening problems. They use their skills and knowledge to rapidly identify subtle changes and intervene in patients with multifaceted and complicated conditions. The intensive care setting may focus on specific types of problems such as cardiac care, trauma, organ transplantation, medical, surgical, or burns. Nurses in all emergency and critical settings are continually challenged to maintain their knowledge and skills to deliver care to their patients and families.

Core to nursing care is caring for the patient and included in that care is integrating families into care. When families are vested in the care of their loved ones it has numerous benefits to both the patient and the family members. This partnership approach is growing rapidly across the United States in both the emergency and critical care setting. Studies have shown that family presence during resuscitation helps family members to see that "everything has been done" to save the patient's life whether successful or not. Family presence during all aspects of care also affords the family member a sense of hope and investment in assisting the patient to regain a healthy state. The patient and family experience in the emergency and critical care setting can have lasting effects on both.

When patients are in the critical care setting it can have a negative effect on the patient as well as the family members, even with a positive outcome. The lasting cognitive, physical, and mental effects can be overwhelming and difficult to deal with. There is a syndrome known as postintensive care syndrome (PICS) and nurses caring for these patients need to be astute and proactive to help patients and family members to cope and get the counseling they may need. The cause of PICS is unknown but may be mitigated with communication and information given throughout the course of treatment.

Whether caring for patients in the emergency or critical care settings, nurses are paramount to the interdisciplinary team caring for patients in actual or potential life-threatening situations. They are the professionals providing the majority of interaction with patients and family members. Continuity of care from the emergency setting to the critical care setting is imperative for providing high-quality care to patients.

Emergency care and critical care nursing are fast-paced settings requiring foundational knowledge to implement evidence-based practice to prevent life-limiting consequences for patients. This unit includes contemporary clinical topics that are representative of what nurses will encounter in emergency departments or intensive care units. Common conditions are discussed regarding burns, pain, injuries and trauma, systemic disorders, violence, mental health, metabolic disorders as well as trends in life-sustaining care for the acutely ill patients and their families.

- Abdominal Aortic Aneurysm *Vicki A. Keough*
- Abdominal Pain *Christopher J. Contino*
- Acid–Base Imbalances *Michael D. Gooch*
- Acute Abdomen *Susanna Rudy*
- Acute Coronary Syndrome *Andrea Efre*
- Acute Exacerbation of a Chronic Condition *Brenda L. Douglass*
- Acute Pancreatitis in Adults *Virginia Mangolds*
- Acute Respiratory Distress Syndrome *Kathleen C. Ashton*
- Acute Respiratory Failure *Breanna Hetland*
- Adrenal Insufficiency *Rachel K. Vanek*
- Back Pain *Sharon R. Rainer*
- Burns *Margaret Jean Carman*
- Burns: Classification and Severity *Melanie Gibbons Hallman and Lamon Norton*
- Chest Pain *Sharon R. Rainer*
- Child Abuse and Neglect *Patricia M. Speck, Pamela Harris Bryant, Tedra S. Smith, Sherita K. Etheridge, and Steadman McPeters*
- *Clostridium Difficile* Infection *Anita Sundaresh*
- Continuous Veno-Venous Hemofiltration *Ian N. Saludares*
- Definitions of Emergency and Critical Care Nursing *Nicole M. Hartman and Courtney Vose*
- Dental Emergencies *Melanie Gibbons Hallman and Lamon Norton*
- Disaster Response *Darlie Simerson*
- Disseminated Intravascular Coagulation *Joyce E. Higgins*
- Domestic Violence *Patricia M. Speck, Diana K. Faugno, Rachell A. Ekroos, Melanie Gibbons Hallman, Gwendolyn D. Childs, Tedra S. Smith, and Stacey A. Mitchell*
- Ear, Nose, and Throat Emergencies *Kathleen Bradbury-Golas*
- Elder Abuse and Neglect *Patricia M. Speck, Richard Taylor, Stacey A. Mitchell, Diana K. Faugno, and Rita A. Jablonski-Jaudon*
- Encephalopathy *Deborah Vinesky*
- Endocrine Emergencies *Diane Fuller Switzer*
- Environmental Emergencies *Brittany Newberry*
- Extracorporeal Life Support *Grant Pignatiello, Katherine Hornack, and Julie E. Herzog*
- Fluid and Electrolyte Imbalances *Michael D. Gooch*
- Fluid Resuscitation *Laura Stark Bai*

- Heart Transplantation *S. Brian Widmar*
- Hepatic Failure *Leon Chen and Fidelindo Lim*
- Hepatitis *Ramona A. Sowers and Linda Carson*
- Hyperglycemia and Hypoglycemia *Laura Stark Bai*
- Hypertensive Crisis and Hypertension *Kathleen Bradbury-Golas*
- Hypothermia *Marian Nowak*
- Integumentary Emergencies *Susanna Rudy*
- Intra-Aortic Balloon Pump *Grant Pignatiello*
- Mental and Behavioral Health Emergencies *Lia V. Ludan*
- Neurotrauma *Anita Sundaresh*
- Obstetrical and Gynecological Emergency Care *Vicki Bacidore*
- Ophthalmic Emergencies *Shannon M. Litten*
- Orthopedic Emergencies in Adults *Cindy Kumar*
- Pediatric Emergencies *Rachel Tkaczyk*
- Psychiatric Disorders: Suicide, Homicide, and Psychosis *George Byron Peraza-Smith and Yolanda Bone*
- Respiratory Emergencies *Dustin Spencer*
- Return of Spontaneous Circulation With Hypothermia Initiation *Laura Stark Bai*
- Seizures *Eric Roberts*
- Sepsis *Ronald L. Hickman, Jr.*
- Sexual Assault *Patricia M. Speck, Diana K. Faugno, Rachell A. Ekroos, Melanie Gibbons Hallman, Sallie J. Shipman, Martha B. Dodd, Qiana A. Johnson, and Stacey A. Mitchell*
- Shock and Multiple Organ Dysfunction Syndrome *Jennifer Wilbeck*
- Solid Organ Transplantation *Marcia Johansson*
- Spinal Cord Injury *Lamon Norton and Melanie Gibbons Hallman*
- Substance Use Disorders and Toxicological Agents *Al Rundio*
- Thoracic Aortic Aneurysm *Megan M. Shifrin and Ronald L. Hickman, Jr.*
- Thrombocytopenia in Adults *Khoa (Joey) Dang*
- Thyroid Crisis *Cynthia Ann Leaver*
- Traumatic Brain Injury *Elizabeth Wirth-Tomaszewski*
- Traumatic Injury *Dustin Spencer*
- Urologic Emergencies *Kelley Toffoli*
- Ventilator-Associated Pneumonia *Nancy Jaskowak Cresse*
- Ventricular Assist Devices *S. Brian Widmar*
- The Violent Patient *Janet E. Reilly and Michael Wichowski*

■ ABDOMINAL AORTIC ANEURYSM

Vicki A. Keough

Overview

Aortic aneurysms can become a serious and lethal health crisis. Prior to 2010, aortic aneurysms were the primary cause of death of 15,000 Americans, and were a comorbid condition associated with approximately 17,000 deaths nationwide (Centers for Disease Control and Prevention [CDC], 2016; Go et al., 2014; Hoyert, 2012). Aortic aneurysms disproportionately affect males. Although about one third of aortic aneurysms occur among females, a majority of aortic aneurysms occur among males aged 65 years and older (Kent et al., 2010; Ramanath, Oh, Sundt, & Eagle, 2009). The U.S. Preventive Services Task Force (2005) estimated that aneurysms that occur in the abdominal aorta, abdominal aortic aneurysms (AAAs), annually affect 3.9% to 7.2% of men and 1% to 1.3% of women older than 50 years (LeFevre, 2014). Each year, approximately 55,000 Americans undergo an abdominal aneurysm repair and approximately 1.7 million Americans are screened for abdominal aneurysms (Cowan et al., 2006; LeFevre, 2014). Therefore, nursing care of patients with an AAA is focused on the assessment of disease and symptom progression and implementation of evidence-based care to prevent premature disability or death.

Background

The aorta is the largest artery and blood vessel in the human body, and it extends from the top of the right ventricle to the bifurcation of the iliac arteries in the lower pelvis. The abdominal aorta begins at the diaphragm and extends to the iliac arteries. An aneurysm occurs wherever there is an outpouching and weakness in an arterial vessel. The weakened area of the arterial vessel wall is persistently exposed to shearing forces from blood constantly pumped from the left ventricle through the vascular system. The normal diameters of the abdominal aorta are 1.7 cm in males and 1.5 cm in females (Aggarwal, Qamar, Sharma, & Sharma, 2011; Howell & Rabener, 2016).

When the pressure in the artery exceeds the ability of the weak vessel wall to maintain its integrity, a tear in the vessel wall can occur, causing an outpouching and disruption of the arterial vessel's wall integrity. In the emergent case, the vessel can rupture resulting in sudden, massive blood loss. In a less extreme case, the vessel wall can become weak and bulge, increasing in diameter. Risk of abdominal aortic rupture occurs when the diameter is greater than 3 cm. The Joint Council for the American Association for Vascular Surgery and Society for Vascular Surgery has published an estimation of the risk for rupture of an AAA ranging from 0% risk of rupture when the AAA diameter is less than 4 cm to 30% to 50% risk of rupture when the diameter is greater than or equal to 8 cm (Brewster et al., 2003). The rate at which the AAA expands is also a consideration. If a small AAA expands 0.5 cm or more over 6 months, there is a high rate of rupture. When discovered early enough, very often the vessel can be repaired (Aggarwal et al., 2011; Hirsch et al., 2006; Howell & Rabener, 2016).

Prevention is the best treatment for success. The U.S. Preventive Services Task Force (2005) recommends screening for AAA for males between the ages of 65 and 75 years with a history of smoking and for women of the same age with a history of smoking and hypertension. Having a family history of AAA, as well as a history of either coronary artery disease or atherosclerosis, is indicative of early screening for an AAA. In addition, a family history of repair of AAA in a first-degree relative dramatically increases the risk of AAA. Early detection, surveillance, and appropriate treatment can significantly attenuate the morbidity and mortality associated with AAA.

In cases of hypertension, atherosclerosis, and a positive family or smoking history, there are several less common contributing factors that predispose adults to an AAA. In adults, infants, and children, AAA has been associated with "seatbelt syndrome," whereby the seatbelt can cause injury to the abdominal aorta during a high-speed crash. Other possible causes of AAA include cystic medial necrosis, trauma, and syphilis. Finally, a *Chlamydia pneumoniae* infection has been implicated as a causative factor in weakening of the abdominal aortic wall (Guirguis-Blake & Wolff, 2005; Keisler & Carter, 2015; Kokje, Hamming, & Lindeman, 2016; Kurosawa, Matsumura, & Yamanouchi, 2013; LeFevre, 2014; Motte, 2015; Salo, Soisalon-Soininen, Bondestam, & Matilla, 1999).

Clinical Aspects

ASSESSMENT

As the mainstay of therapy is focused on screening and rapid intervention, early detection is essential. AAAs can occasionally be found on a physical examination; however, this occurs in only about 50% of confirmed cases. It is more difficult to palpate AAAs if the patient is obese. When a palpable AAA mass is found, it is most likely in the epigastric and left hypochondriac area of the abdomen (Howell & Rabner, 2016). Auscultation is another physical assessment technique that is helpful in the diagnosis of AAA. The presence of a bruit over the abdominal aorta should alert the clinician to do further tests for AAA (Aggarwal et al., 2011). Palpating distal pulses, such as popliteal and pedal, gives the nurse an indication of distal perfusion. In addition, the nurse should examine the skin for signs of adequate perfusion such as warmth, pink color, and good capillary refill. Ominous signs that the skin is not being perfused adequately are cool, pale skin, diaphoresis, and mottling (Aggarwal et al., 2011; Hirsch et al., 2006).

The majority of AAAs are found serendipitously. Often, adults with an AAA present without signs or symptoms until the vessel wall has ruptured and their circumstances are life-threatening. AAAs are often detected during abdominal imaging studies, such as CT, ultrasound, or MRI, as part of a workup for an unrelated complaint. The most common symptom of an AAA is pain and tenderness around the abdomen, flank, or back. Some patients also report epigastric discomfort and altered bowel elimination. Pain on palpation is predictive of a serious risk for rupture. If AAA is suspected, the clinician should be careful not to palpate too vigorously in order to prevent a rupture. A ruptured AAA represents a medical emergency. Once the AAA ruptures, patients often report severe, sharp abdominal or back pain, and a pulsatile abdominal mass may appear. AAA rupture is associated with severe hypotension resulting from hypovolemic shock and consequently results in manifestations such as mottled skin, decreased level of consciousness, diaphoresis, and oliguria. The abdomen may become distended with ecchymosis or a palpable hematoma. For patients who present with clinical findings consistent with a ruptured AAA, half of these patients will survive (Aggarwal et al., 2011; Creager & Loscalzo, 2008; Harris, Faggioli, Fiedler, Curl, & Ricotta, 1991; Keisler & Carter, 2015).

NURSING INTERVENTIONS, MANAGEMENT, AND IMPLICATIONS

Interventions for AAA are focused on serial observation, medical management, and surgical repair or endovascular stenting. Observation can be tricky.

The American College of Cardiology/American Heart Association (ACC/AHA) guidelines recommend monitoring aneurysms that are 3 to 4 cm in diameter every 2 to 3 years and those with a diameter of 4.0 to 5.4 cm should be monitored every 6 to 12 months (Hirsch et al., 2006).

Medical management is focused on smoking cessation; management of hypertension, atherosclerosis and coronary artery diseases; treatment of infection; and surveillance. As infection has been implicated as a possible cause of AAA, the administration of pathogen-specific antibiotics has demonstrated some success in treating aneurysms (Kurosawa et al., 2013). Pharmacologic interventions that have been used in the treatment of AAAs that are not within standards for surgical or endovascular repair include managing hypertension, atherosclerosis, and antibiotics (Baxter, Terrin, & Dalman, 2008; Hirsch et al., 2006; Kurosawa et al., 2013).

Surgical or endovascular repair is recommended for patients with an AAA measuring 5.5 cm or greater that is asymptomatic, patients who are symptomatic, and for those patients with an aneurysm that increased in size at a rate greater than 0.5 cm over 6 months (Hirsch et al., 2006). Poor long-term survival for surgical AAA repair has been associated with end-stage renal disease, chronic lung disease, and cardiovascular disease (Khashram, Williman, Hider, Jones, & Roake, 2016). In general, patients do well after an AAA repair.

A ruptured AAA presents a life-threatening emergency. Once the nurse has completed a thorough assessment and AAA is suspected, the provider must be alerted to the emergency. As it is often an emergent life-threatening situation, keeping the patient calm and informing the family of the emergent nature of the repair is of high priority. Nursing interventions include providing adequate oxygenation, cardiovascular support in the form of fluid (blood and/or blood products), vasopressors, and emergent transport to repair the ruptured artery. Managing of extreme anxiety and pain is crucial at this time. Keeping the family informed and providing family-centered care are critical as the patient is facing a life-threatening emergency.

However, if the AAA has been identified as stable, then educating the patient and family about the risk factors, signs, and symptoms of an expanding or ruptured AAA is important. The patients and their families must be given clear and specific follow-up instructions that include follow-up appointments and instructions for ameliorating the risk factors for AAA such as smoking cessation, healthy eating, and close adherence to medication. The patient and family should be informed of the seriousness of the disease. Patients and their families should also understand that they can lead a normal and healthy life as long as they reduce or eliminate risk factors and follow-up as instructed.

OUTCOMES

The goals of nursing care with a patient with an AAA are focused on positive patient outcomes and prevention of complications. Early identification and intervention of an AAA are foundational to emergency nursing. Performing a rapid but thorough health history, including past medical history and risk factors, and physical examination will assist the nurse in not only identification of an AAA but also other life-threatening disorders. Nurses must closely monitor these patients for abrupt changes in mental status, vital signs, and symptoms in order to prevent complications.

Summary

Emergency and critical care nurses play a vital role in the early detection of AAAs as they can often be discovered during the initial nursing assessment. If the AAA is discovered before rupture, quick diagnosis and immediate intervention can be a lifesaving measure. Once the AAA has progressed to the point of rupture, a life-threatening emergency exists. Even in the best of circumstances, once a rupture has occurred, survival is only about 50%. It is important for the emergency or critical care nurse to have knowledge of the pathophysiology, signs, symptoms, and quick interventions for AAA so that they can intervene appropriately. In addition, knowledge of the best practice recommendations for AAA screening, prevention, and treatment is essential for emergency nurses.

Aggarwal, S., Qamar, A., Sharma, V., & Sharma, A. (2011). Abdominal aortic aneurysm: A comprehensive review. *Experimental Clinical Cardiology*, 16(1), 11–15.

Baxter, B. T., Terrin, M. C., & Dalman, R. L. (2008). Medical management of small abdominal aortic aneurysms. *Circulation*, 117, 1883–1889.

Brewster, D. C., Cronenwett, J. L., Hallett, J. W., Johnston, K. W., Kupski, W.C., & Matsumura, J. S. (2003). Guidelines for the treatment of abdominal aortic aneurysms. Report of a subcommittee of the Joint Council of the American Association for Vascular Surgery and Society for Vascular Surgery. *Journal of Vascular Surgery*, 37, 1106–1117.

Centers for Disease Control and Prevention. (2016). Deaths, percent of total deaths, and death rates for the 15 leading causes of death in 5-year age groups, by race, and sex: United States, 2013. Retrieved from https://www.cdc.gov/nchs/data/dvs/lcwk1_2013.pdf

Cowan, J. A., Dimick, J. B., Henke, P. K., Rectenwald, J., Stanley, J. C., & Upchurch, G. R., Jr. (2006). Epidemiology of aortic aneurysm repair in the United States from 1993–2003. *Annals of the New York Academy of Sciences*, 1082, 1–10.

Creager, M. A., & Loscalzo, J. (2008). Diseases of the aorta. In A. S. Fauci, E. Braumwald, D. L. Kasper, S. L. Hauser, D. L. Longo, J. L. Jameson, & J. Loscalzo (Eds.), *Harrison's principles of internal medicine* (17th ed., pp. 736–738). Columbus, OH: McGraw-Hill.

Go, A. S., Mozaffarian, D., Roger V. L., Benjamin E. J., Berry J. D., Blaha, M. J., . . . Turner, M. B. (2014). Heart disease and stroke statistics—2013 update: A report from the American Heart Association. *Circulation*, 127, e6–e245.

Guirguis-Blake, J., & Wolff, T. A. (2005). Screening for abdominal aortic aneurism. *American Family Physician*, 71, 2154–2155.

Harris, L. M., Faggioli, G. L., Fiedler, R., Curl, G. R., & Ricotta, J. J. (1991). Ruptured abdominal aortic aneurysms: Factors affecting mortality rates. *Journal of Vascular Surgery*, 14, 812–818.

Hirsch, A. T., Haskal, Z. J., Hertzer, N. R., Bakal, C. W., Creager, M. A., Halpern, J. L., . . . Riegel, B. (2006). ACC/AHA 2005 Practice Guidelines for the management of patients with peripheral arterial disease (lower extremity, renal, mesenteric, and abdominal aortic): A collaborative report from the American Association for Vascular Surgery/Society for Vascular Surgery, Society for Cardiovascular Angiography and Interventions, Society for Vascular Medicine and Biology, Society of Interventional Radiology, and the ACC/AHA Task Force on Practice Guidelines (Writing Committee to Develop Guidelines for the Management of Patients With Peripheral Arterial Disease): Endorsed by the American Association of Cardiovascular and Pulmonary Rehabilitation; National Heart, Lung, and Blood Institute; Society for Vascular Nursing; Trans-Atlantic Inter-Society Consensus; and Vascular Disease Foundation. *Circulation*, 113, e463–e654.

Howell, C. M., & Rabener, M. J. (2016). Abdominal aortic aneurysm: A ticking time bomb. *Journal of the American Association of Physician Assistants*, 26, 3.

Hoyert, D. L. (2012). National vital statistics reports. NCHS. *National Vital Statistics Reports*, 61, 1–52.

Keisler, B., & Carter, C. (2015). Abdominal aortic aneurysm. *American Family Physician*, 91(8), 538–543.

Kent, K. C., Zwolak, R. M., Egorova, N. N., Riles, T. S., Manganaro, A., Moskowitz, A. J., & Greco, G. (2010). Analysis of risk factors for abdominal aortic aneurysm in a cohort of more than 3 million individuals. *Journal of Vascular Surgery*, 52, 539–548.

Khashram, M., Williman, J. A., Hider, P. N., Jones, G. T., & Roake, J. A. (2016). Systematic review and meta-analysis of factors influencing survival following abdominal aortic aneurysm repair. *European Journal of Vascular and Endovascular Surgery*, 51, 203–215.

Kokje, V. B., Hamming, J. F., & Lindeman, J. H. (2016). Pharmaceutical management of small abdominal aortic aneurysms: A systematic review of the clinical evidence. *European Journal of Vascular and Endovascular Surgery*, *51*(1), 64–75. doi:10.1016/j.ejvs.2015.09.006

Kurosawa, K., Matsurmura, J. S., & Yamanouchi, D. (2013). Current status of medical treatment for abdominal aortic aneurysm. *Circulation*, *77*, 2860–2866.

LeFevre, M. I. (2014). Screening for abdominal aortic aneurysm: U.S. Preventive Services Task Force recommendation statement. *Annals of Internal Medicine*, *161*, 281–290.

Motte, S. (2015). What is the evidence to support screening for abdominal aortic aneurysm and what is the role of the primary care physician? *Radiology Clinics of North America*, *53*(6), 1209–1224. doi:10.1016/j.rcl.2015.06.007

Ramanath, V. S., Oh, J. K., Sundt, T. M., & Eagle, K. A. (2009). Acute aortic syndromes and thoracic aortic aneurysm. *Mayo Clinic Proceedings*, *84*(5), 465–481.

Salo, J. A., Soisalon-Soininen, S., Bondestam, S., & Matilla, P. S. (1999). Familial occurrence of abdominal aortic aneurysm. *Annals of Internal Medicine*, *130*, 637–642.

U.S. Preventive Services Task Force. (2005). Screening for abdominal aortic aneurysm: Recommendation statement. *Annals of Internal Medicine*, *142*, 198–202.

■ ABDOMINAL PAIN

Christopher J. Contino

Overview

Abdominal pain is a complicated complaint in the emergency care setting. The chief complaint of abdominal pain comprises approximately 5% to 10% of emergency department visits annually (Kendall & Moreira, 2016). The most recent data from the Centers for Disease Control and Prevention (CDC) indicates that 8.1% of patients who seek care in an emergency department have a chief complaint of stomach or abdominal pain, which translates into more than 11 million visits related to the complaints of abdominal pain (CDC, 2011). Although many cases of abdominal pain are not life-threatening and are self-limited, there are a multitude of cases that may require emergent intervention from emergency room nurses.

Background

Abdominal pain comprises a significant portion of emergency department visits annually (Kendall & Moreira, 2016). Although abdominal pain affects all patient populations, there are key demographics that may have a more significant course, and include the *elderly*, defined as those older than 65 years, and immunocompromised patients, such as individuals living with HIV. Individuals from these at-risk populations have disproportionately higher rates of mortality and morbidity compared to younger adults with a functioning immune system. In the emergency department, nurses are usually the first point of contact for the patients, and it is important that they are able to recognize life-threatening emergencies and care for the patients appropriately (Cole, Lynch, & Cugnoni, 2006).

The abdomen can be broadly divided into four quadrants: right upper, left upper, right lower, and left lower. In addition, the epigastric area, just under the xiphoid process, is a key area for assessment. Understanding the location of pain may help in determining the cause of the origin of the pain. Right upper quadrant pain may be due to cholecystitis, hepatitis, or ulcers. Left upper quadrant pain may involve the spleen or stomach. Right lower quadrant pain may be appendicitis or diverticulitis, and left lower quadrant pain may be from colitis or diverticulitis. Depending on the gender of the patient, lower abdominal pain can stem from genitourinary processes such as ectopic pregnancy and pelvic inflammatory disease in the female, or testicular disease in the male patient. Diffuse abdominal pain can occur from a multitude of causes (Penner, Mary, & Majumdar, 2016).

The differential diagnoses of abdominal pain can vary widely and include causes arising from the abdominal or extra-abdominal etiologies (O'Brien, 2015). The complete discussion of all causes of abdominal pain is vast and exceeds the scope of this entry; therefore, this discussion will focus on the most common causes of life-threatening abdominal pain. These include bowel obstruction, abdominal aortic aneurism, bowel perforation, ectopic pregnancy, placental abruption, splenic rupture, mesenteric ischemia, and myocardial infarction.

Pediatric patients with abdominal pain pose a challenge with diagnosis and may vary widely with age. In the infant through toddler years, patients may not be able to adequately describe their pain. Many of the differential diagnoses remain salient; however, in the very young infant, consider pyloric stenosis, intussusception, Hirschsprung's disease, and Meckel's diverticulitis. Pediatric patients may become dehydrated faster than adults, so fluid balance is key. Also, pediatric patients can cardiovascular compensate longer than adults; however, when the decompensation occurs, it happens rapidly.

Assess a pediatric patient frequently and thoroughly, and keep a high index of suspicion for serious disease.

Clinical Aspects

ASSESSMENT

The key to managing patients with a chief complaint of abdominal pain is performing a thorough history and physical examination that can narrow the list of suspicious etiologies. As with all patient encounters, an initial assessment should focus on airway, breathing, and circulation (ABC), and generate a rapid sense of whether the patient is critically ill or unstable before proceeding to further assessment. Any abnormalities during the initial evaluation should be addressed immediately, and only after this should further assessment be performed. Findings that may indicate that a patient is critical include tachycardia, hypertension, fever, extreme tenderness, abdominal rigidity, or pain elicited by minor touch. In these cases, it is important to ensure that the provider is aware and is at the bedside to evaluate the patient concurrently.

Once it has been established that the patient is otherwise stable, a thorough history and physical examination may commence. All patients should receive a thorough SAMPLE history, which includes signs and symptoms, allergies, medications, past illnesses, last oral intake, and events leading up to the present illness. The patient's pain should be characterized utilizing the OPQRST mnemonic, which evaluates onset, provocative and palliative factors, quality, radiation, site or location, associated signs and symptoms, and time. In case of abdominal pain, the location of pain may help to narrow the differential diagnosis, although it should not be relied on as many etiologies of abdominal pain can vary from patient to patient. The character and nature of the pain can also help to narrow the diagnosis. There are three main types of pain described as visceral, somatic, and referred. Visceral pain is typically described as dull and hard to localize, and it usually originates from solid organs and the walls of hollow organs. Somatic pain is usually described as sharp and can be localized, and is usually caused by inflammation, ischemia, or peritoneal irritation. Referred pain is pain that is felt at a location distant from its originating source. This is a key concept to remember as several potentially life-threatening disease processes may be felt as abdominal pain but do not originate in the abdominal area; a key example of this would be myocardial ischemia presenting as epigastric pain.

NURSING INTERVENTIONS, MANAGEMENT, AND IMPLICATIONS

Initial nursing interventions should ensure that the ABC status is adequate and secure. All undifferentiated abdominal pain patients should have nothing by mouth (NPO) in case surgery may be necessary. Patients should have intravenous (IV) access secured, preferably with a large-bore IV catheter in the antecubital region. This is important should fluid resuscitation be necessary and many diagnostic imaging modalities require this for IV contrast administration. The nurse should prepare to obtain diagnostic samples of blood and urine. Local protocol should dictate when and how to obtain the samples. Laboratory evaluation should be tailored to the individual patient to avoid unnecessary testing; however, in some clinical settings, there are established nursing protocols that should dictate the nurse's plan of care. It is important to note that in the case of abdominal pain, all females of childbearing age should receive a rapid test for pregnancy, as a potentially life-threatening diagnosis of ectopic pregnancy may be the cause of pain or pregnancy may prohibit certain diagnostic medical imaging tests from being performed. An emergency department adage is to always consider a female of childbearing age with abdominal pain to have an ectopic pregnancy until proven otherwise.

OUTCOMES

When discussing any clinical disease process, it is important to discuss outcomes. With regard to abdominal pain, the main outcome in the emergency department setting is rapid exclusion of life-threatening causes of pain that require emergent intervention. This includes timely diagnosis; early consultation with specialists, including surgery; and collaboration with ancillary departments. Pain control is also a significant outcome measure (Kendall & Moreira, 2016). Once an appropriate physical exam has been conducted, pain control should be a priority. Pain should be assessed and reassessed frequently by utilizing a standard pain scale. The ultimate outcome is to reduce mortality and morbidity.

Summary

Abdominal pain is a common complaint in the emergency department, with a wide variety of potential causes. Although a large portion of patients with abdominal pain do not have a specific cause of their pain, there are a few disease processes that are immediately life-threatening. It is crucial that emergency department nurses are able to recognize the spectrum of possible causes of pain, recognize unstable or ill patients, and institute appropriate interventions. The key to most abdominal pain complaints is a thorough history and physical examination, with assistance from appropriate labs and imaging as necessary. Be aware of special populations such as the elderly, immunocompromised, and women of childbearing age.

Centers for Disease Control and Prevention. (2011). National Hospital Ambulatory Medical Care Survey: 2010 emergency department summary tables (pp. 1–39). Retrieved from https://www.cdc.gov/nchs/data/ahcd/nhamcs_emergency/2011_ed_web_tables.pdf

Cole, E., Lynch, A., & Cugnoni, H. (2006). Assessment of the patient with acute abdominal pain. *Nursing Standard*, 20(39), 67–75.

Kendall, J. L., & Moreira, M. E. (2016). Evaluation of the adult with abdominal pain in the emergency department. In R. Hockberger & J. Grayzel (Eds.), *UptoDate* (pp. 1–51). Retrieved from https://www.uptodate.com/contents/evaluation-of-the-adult-with-abdominal-pain-in-the-emergency-department

O'Brien, M. C. (2015). Gastrointestinal emergencies. In J. Tintinalli, J. S. Stapczynski, O. J. Ma, D. Cline, R. K. Cydulka, & G. Meckler (Eds.), *Tintinalli's emergency medicine: A comprehensive study guide* (8th ed.). New York, NY: McGraw-Hill.

Penner, R., Mary, F., & Majumdar, S. (2016). Evaluation of the adult with abdominal pain. In A. Auerbach, M. Aronson, & H. N. Sokol (Eds.), *UptoDate* (pp. 1–31). Retrieved from https://www.uptodate.com/contents/evaluation-of-the-adult-with-abdominal-pain

■ ACID–BASE IMBALANCES

Michael D. Gooch

Overview

Acid–base balance is key for all physiological processes and functions. An imbalance occurs when the pH falls outside the normal range and leads to organ dysfunction, for example, coagulopathy, electrolyte disturbances, and organ failure. The potential of hydrogen (pH) is a measure of the concentration of hydrogen ions (H^+) in the body and is based on a 0-to-14 scale. There is an inverse relationship between the pH and H^+ concentration: The lower the number, the higher the H^+ concentration of the body fluid. An acid–base imbalance, acidosis, results from an accumulation of acids or a loss of base and is often defined as a pH less than 7.35. Whereas, alkalosis is often specified as a pH greater than 7.45 and occurs due to an excess amount of base/alkali or deficiency of the body's acids. A prolonged pH of less than 6.8 or greater than 7.8 is not compatible with life (Berend, de Vries, & Gans, 2014; Hall, 2016; Kamel & Halperin, 2017).

Acid–base imbalances may occur in patients of any age and result from numerous processes, including pulmonary and renal disease, toxicological and endocrine emergencies, and shock (Berend et al., 2014; Gooch, 2015). Identification and management of these imbalances are important to reduce complications and improve patient outcomes. Nurses should be able to recognize the diagnostics needed to properly identify an imbalance, the associated clinical manifestations, and initial management of these derangements.

Background

For equilibrium to be maintained, there must be a balance between the intake or production and the excretion of both acids and bases. Acid is used to describe any compound capable of donating an H^+. A base is a substance capable of accepting an H^+ (Hall, 2016; Kamel & Halperin, 2017). Without acid–base balance, the pH will not be maintained at a level that supports homeostasis. Acids can be classified as carbonic or respiratory and noncarbonic or metabolic acids. Metabolic acids include ketones and lactate, which often results from the oxidation or metabolism of carbohydrates, proteins, and fats. Foods containing phosphates and sulfates also contribute to the metabolic acid load. Carbonic acid (H_2CO_3) is a weak acid that plays a major role in this balance. Bicarbonate (HCO_3^-) is the body's primary base. Bicarbonate is formed during the metabolism of some fruits and vegetables, and by the kidneys (Gooch, 2015; Hall, 2016; Kamel & Halperin, 2017).

There are three processes that regulate acid–base balance. First is the chemical buffer system. This process can quickly alter the pH by reversibly changing the concentration and state of H^+. In the setting of acidosis, H^+ is combined with a buffer. As the concentration decreases or, in the case of alkalosis, it is released from the buffer. Bicarbonate is the most abundant extracellular buffer. This reaction is summarized by the formula: $H_2CO_3 \leftrightarrow H^+ + HCO_3^-$. Phosphate and proteins, including hemoglobin, are key intracellular buffers (Cho, 2017; Gooch, 2015; Hall, 2016; Kamel & Halperin, 2017).

In addition to the chemical buffering system, there is physiological buffering or compensation. Carbon dioxide (CO_2) is a by-product of the body's metabolic processes. There is a direct relationship between the H^+ concentration and the CO_2 level, and an inverse relationship between the CO_2 level and the pH. The medulla and chemoreceptors regulate the respiratory rate in response to changes in the H^+ concentration. As CO_2 levels increase, the respiratory rate increases to blow off more CO_2, lowering the level and increasing the pH. As the respiratory rate slows, the CO_2 concentration increases and the pH decreases. This buffer can quickly adjust the CO_2 level to compensate for an imbalance over minutes to hours, though it is not as potent as chemical buffering (Gooch, 2015; Hall, 2016; Kamel & Halperin, 2017).

Lastly, the kidneys regulate the excretion of noncarbonic acids and H^+, as well as the reabsorption of almost 100% of the excreted HCO_3^-. The kidneys produce HCO_3^- during the excretion of ammonium, if needed, to maintain a normal pH. Unlike the lungs, the renal or metabolic pathway is much slower and may take hours to days to complete the process. The lungs expel 150 times more acid each day than the kidneys (Rice, Ismail, & Pillow, 2014). If there is an increase in the H^+ concentration, the kidneys can increase the excretion of acids and increase the reabsorption and production of HCO_3^- to help stabilize the pH. Just the opposite can occur if there is an accumulation of HCO_3^-. This entire balance process is demonstrated by the formula: $CO_2 + H_2O \leftrightarrow H_2CO_3 \leftrightarrow H^+ + HCO_3^-$. Carbonic anhydrase, an enzyme found primarily in red blood cells, the lungs, and renal tubules, increases the rate of these reactions. In the case of lung or renal disease, these physiological buffer systems are altered (Gooch, 2015; Hall, 2016; Kamel & Halperin, 2017).

Clinical Aspects

Imbalances are categorized as metabolic or respiratory in nature. Evaluation of the patient's blood gas is needed to properly identify the imbalance. An arterial blood gas is not always needed and in most patients a venous gas is acceptable. Primary respiratory imbalances affect the pH because of an altered CO_2 level (normal range: 35–45 mmHg), in which primary metabolic imbalances are due to an altered HCO3- level (normal range: 22–26 mEq/L). A patient may present with one of four acid–base imbalances, referred to as a *simple imbalance*, or a combination of metabolic and respiratory imbalances, referred to as a *mixed imbalance*. A primary imbalance is most often accompanied by secondary compensation of the physiological buffer systems; however, this compensation may not be enough to return the pH to a normal range (Berend et al., 2014; Cho, 2017; Hall, 2016; Kamel & Halperin, 2017).

Respiratory acidosis often develops due to impaired gas exchange or hypoventilation from pulmonary disease or injury, or altered central nervous system control, for example, an opioid or sedation agent. If there is impaired exhalation of CO_2, there will be an increase in the H^+ concentration and a drop in the pH leading to acidosis. Respiratory alkalosis develops from hyperventilation. As the CO_2 level decreases due to the increased respiratory rate, the pH increases due to a drop in the H^+ concentration. Hyperventilation can be related to hypoxia, the stress response, or could be iatrogenic, for example, incorrect mechanical ventilation (Al-Jaghbeer & Kellum, 2014; Cho, 2017; Gooch, 2015; Hall, 2016; Kamel & Halperin, 2017).

Respiratory imbalances are best managed by managing the airway. As with any patient, the history and physical exam are essential to identifying the cause, managing the patient, and preventing complications. In the setting of a respiratory acidosis, measures may be needed to improve ventilations, gas exchange, and expiration of CO_2. This may include beta agonists, assisting ventilations, or administration of a reversal agent, for example, naloxone (Narcan), to improve the respiratory rate and effort. For the patients with hyperventilation, which has led to a respiratory alkalosis, the respiratory rate should be slowed. The nurse should consider reasons why the patient is hyperventilating and address the cause, not just the rate, for example, hypoxia, anxiety, and pain. Hyperventilation may be compensatory for an impending metabolic acidosis, for example, Kussmaul's respirations (Cho, 2017; Gooch, 2015; Kamel & Halperin, 2017). Once the cause of the respiratory imbalance is identified, the disarrangement can usually be quickly reversed.

A metabolic acidosis results from the buildup of acids or the loss of base, leading to an increase in the H^+ concentration that shifts the pH downward. This may result from renal impairment, that is, renal failure, in which the kidneys are unable to excrete acids or reabsorb and produce adequate amounts of bicarbonate. Metabolic acidosis is often defined based on the anion gap, which represents the difference between the measured serum cations and anions. It may be calculated using this formula: sodium – (chloride + bicarbonate). A normal gap is considered by some to be 8 ± 4 mEq/L; this as well as the formula varies from lab to lab. A nongap acidosis results from bicarbonate loss due to gastrointestinal, renal, or iatrogenic causes. Bicarbonate is lost as a result of excessive vomiting or diarrhea. Hyperchloremia, which leads to increased renal excretion of bicarbonate, may result from excessive administration of intravenous (IV) normal saline solution (iatrogenic) or renal tubular acidosis (Al-Jaghbeer & Kellum, 2014; Berend et al., 2014; Cho, 2017; Gooch, 2015; Hall, 2016; Kamel & Halperin, 2017; Rice et al, 2014).

An anion gap metabolic acidosis results from the increased production or accumulation of noncarbonic acids, which cannot be buffered by the respiratory system. A gap indicates there are anions present that are not evaluated during routine laboratory analysis. A mnemonic sometimes used to recall common causes of a gap acidosis is CAT MUDPILES: carbon monoxide, cyanide, alcoholic ketoacidosis, toluene, methanol, metformin, uremia, diabetic ketoacidosis, propylene glycol, ingestion of iron or isoniazid, lactic acidosis, ethylene glycol, and salicylates (Al-Jaghbeer & Kellum, 2014; Cho, 2017; Gooch, 2015; Rice et al., 2014). As these anions accumulate, they shift the pH downward, impair the body's buffering systems, and disrupt cellular activities.

The initial management of a patient with a metabolic acidosis should focus on restoring perfusion with IV fluids and identifying the cause. Improving cellular and especially renal perfusion will improve energy production and elimination of acids. The specific treatment will depend on the cause of the acidosis. The administration of IV sodium bicarbonate is rarely indicated and should only be used in the setting of severe acidosis, that is, a pH less than 7.0 with organ dysfunction (Al-Jaghbeer & Kellum, 2014; Berend et al., 2014; Cho, 2017, 2014; Gooch, 2015; Kamel & Halperin, 2017; Rice et al., 2014).

The last imbalance is metabolic alkalosis, which develops as the result of excessive acid loss or accumulation of base, shifting the pH upward. The causes of this imbalance are separated based on the urine chloride level: low—referred to as saline or chloride responsive or elevated—referred to as saline or chloride unresponsive. Saline-responsive conditions are often due to an increase in bicarbonate due to a loss of hydrochloric acid, chloride, and potassium caused by excessive vomiting, diarrhea, or suctioning, or from diuresis. Saline-unresponsive alkalosis is less common and is often related to the excess production or intake of mineralocorticoids (Al-Jaghbeer & Kellum, 2014; Berend et al., 2014; Cho, 2017; Gooch, 2015; Hall, 2016; Kamel & Halperin, 2017; Soifer & Kim, 2014).

The management of a metabolic alkalosis also varies with the cause. If the patient has a chloride-responsive condition, the administration of IV normal saline may be indicated to restore renal perfusion and replace chloride. In the setting of a chloride-unresponsive alkalosis, acetazolamide (Diamox), a carbonic anhydrase inhibitor, is sometimes administered to increase urinary bicarbonate excretion (Al-Jaghbeer & Kellum, 2014; Berend et al., 2014; Cho, 2017; Gooch, 2015; Kamel & Halperin, 2017; Soifer & Kim, 2014).

Summary

Acid–base balance is essential to maintaining normal cellular function. Given the narrow range of a normal pH, a small change may lead to organ dysfunction. A patient may have a simple or a mixed imbalance. Analysis of the pH, CO_2, and HCO_3^- from the blood gas and assessment findings help identify the problem and guide treatment to correct the imbalance. Most respiratory imbalances are corrected by managing the airway and improving gas exchange. Metabolic problems are corrected based on the cause, but often involve restoring vascular volume and restoring perfusion. Acid–base imbalances are associated with various diseases and may be encountered in any patient. Prompt recognition and management are essential to limiting complications and improving patient outcomes.

Al-Jaghbeer, M., & Kellum, J. A. (2015). Acid–base disturbances in intensive care patients: Etiology, pathophysiology and treatment. *Nephrology, Dialysis, Transplantation, 30*(7), 1104–1111. doi:10.1093/ndt/gfu289

Berend, K., de Vries, A. P. J., & Gans, R. O. B. (2014). Physiological approach to assessment of acid-base disturbances. *New England Journal of Medicine, 371*(15), 1434–1445. doi:10.1056/NEJMra1003327

Cho, K. C. (2017). Electrolyte and acid–base disorders. In M. A. Papadakis, S. J., McPhee, & M. W. Rabow (Eds.), *Current medical diagnosis and treatment 2017* (56th ed., pp. 884–912). New York, NY: McGraw-Hill.

Gooch, M. D. (2015). Identifying acid-base and electrolyte imbalances. *Nurse Practitioner, 40*(8), 37–42. doi:10.1097/01.NPR.0000469255.98119.82

Hall, J. E. (2016). *Guyton and hall textbook of medical physiology* (13th ed.). Philadelphia, PA: Elsevier.

Kamel, K. S., & Halperin, M. L. (2017). *Fluid, electrolytes, and acid-base physiology: A problem-based approach* (5th ed.). Philadelphia, PA: Elsevier.

Rice, M., Ismail, B., & Pillow, M. T. (2014). Approach to metabolic acidosis in the emergency department. *Emergency*

Medicine Clinics of North America, 32(2), 403–420. doi:10.1016/j.emc.2014.01.002

Soifer, J. T., & Kim, H. T. (2014). Approach to metabolic alkalosis. *Emergency Medicine Clinics of North America*, 32(2), 453–463. doi:10.1016/j.emc.2014.01.005

■ ACUTE ABDOMEN

Susanna Rudy

Overview

An acute abdomen can be defined as a sudden or spontaneous onset of severe nontraumatic abdominal pain lasting longer than 6 hours and typically less than 24 hours, which can be associated with potentially life-threatening intra-abdominal pathology in a relatively healthy person. The acute abdomen can be caused by the progression of nontraumatic disorders that are benign or self-limited to conditions that require emergent surgical intervention. A thorough history and focused physical exam will be the cornerstone of diagnoses and treatment of a presenting acute abdominal complaint.

Background

Acute abdominal pain (AAP) has been generally defined as nontraumatic abdominal pain of limited duration. It is the most common diagnosis for emergency department (ED) visits, accounting for approximately 7.7% of 130 million ED visits in 2013. It is also the number one listed diagnosis for ED visits in women aged 15 to 65 years and the third leading diagnosis in men and women older than 65 years who present to the ED (Centers for Disease Control and Prevention, 2013; Cervellin et al., 2016; Jiang, Weiss, & Barrett, 2017; Macaluso & McNamara, 2012).

The incidence of adults presenting with AAP symptoms to the ED has steadily increased across the past two decades and is expected to maintain an upward trajectory with the influx of the newly insured into the health care system (Skinner, Blanchard, & Elixhauser, 2014). Nonsurgical cases of abdominal pain account for nearly 30% of inpatient hospital admissions (Cervellin et al., 2012). The primary symptom in an acute abdomen is most often how the pain is expressed or presents. Although many cases are benign, a rapid onset of severe pain can indicate a serious medical

problem. The differential diagnoses of abdominal pain can be a challenge and therefore, the type and location of the pain are indicators of the direction to take when narrowing down a diagnosis (Papadakis & McPhee, 2017). Not all pain is the same; the different types are rooted within our embryologic development and are expressed differently, dependent on the organ or structure innervated. Pain can be caused by infection, inflammation, obstruction, muscle contraction, or decreased blood flow to the organs.

The type and location of pain is a helpful diagnostic tool. Visceral pain originates from innervations of nociceptors within the abdominal organs that respond to stretch and contraction, distention or ischemia such as gas, bloating, and microvascular occlusion. This pain is often difficult to pinpoint, characterized as dull, aching, colicky, gnawing, vague, and creating a nauseating sensation. Visceral pain in the upper epigastric area of the abdomen may reflect disorders of the stomach, duodenum, pancreas, and liver (Macaluso & McNamara, 2012). Umbilical pain may indicate disorders of the small intestine, upper colon, or appendix. Lower abdominal suprapubic visceral pain may be related to the lower colon or issues with the aorta, bladder, or kidneys. Somatic pain is described as sharp, stabbing, and localized and is triggered by noxious stimulation of the nerves lining the peritoneal cavity. Blood or chemical irritants from a perforated bowel or ruptured ectopic pregnancy can lead to peritonitis, a painful acute abdomen and a life-threatening condition if treatment is delayed. Referred pain is a perception of pain distant from the source. Some abdominal pain can be referred, or felt in another area due to irritation to the same nerve distribution. Examples of referred pain are kidney stones that are felt in the groin, and free air or blood causing irritation to the diaphragm that may be felt in the shoulder. A perforated stomach, bowel, or ruptured appendix, ectopic pregnancy, and abdominal aortic aneurysm (AAA) are life-threatening surgical emergencies requiring urgent diagnosis and management. Intestinal obstruction and pancreatitis can also present as an acute abdomen requiring prompt diagnosis and medical management to prevent deterioration in status.

The time of onset of pain and severity can determine progression. A severe and sudden onset of pain could indicate an intra-abdominal catastrophe such as a dissecting or ruptured AAA, perforated ulcer, or torsion. Gradual, insidious onset of pain can be seen with inflammatory disease and infections as well as mechanical obstructions such as volvulus and mesenteric ischemia from occlusions. Referred pain, and patterns of pain, may be diagnostic but any persistent pain should raise concern for a potentially life-threatening process. Noting exertional or alleviating factors can also help lead to a diagnosis. Abdominal pain relieved or exacerbated by eating fatty or spicy foods could indicate gallbladder or peptic ulcer disease. Pain exacerbated by jarring, jumping up and down, ambulation, or with coughing can be indicative of peritoneal irritation from free fluid in the abdomen (Macaluso & McNamara, 2012).

Abdominal pain accompanied by the time of onset of associated symptoms, such as nausea, vomiting, diarrhea, or urinary retention, can also indicate a primary intra-abdominal pathology and help narrow the differential list. In an acute abdomen, pain will typically precede vomiting but not in all cases. Vomiting should be evaluated for the presence of blood or bile. Vomiting is rarely seen in large-bowel obstructions but is almost always present in small-bowel obstructions, which can progress to feculent emesis as the obstruction progresses (Macaluso & McNamara, 2012). Diarrhea is common with abdominal complaints but is serious in conditions that can cause an acute abdomen such as mesenteric ischemia, appendicitis, and colon and bowel obstructions. Absence of bowel sounds (BS), inability to pass flatus, and blood in stool can indicate serious underlying conditions that can lead to an acute abdomen.

Clinical Aspects

ASSESSMENT

A structured approach must be used with any patient with abdominal pain. A thorough history and physical examination are a priority and will guide the overall management and determine the necessary lab and diagnostic tests to rule out any life-threating causes for presentation.

Previous medical, surgical, and social history should be queried from the nonsedated patients. A previous history of abdominal surgery in patients presenting with acute abdomen raises concerns of obstruction from adhesions. Underlying medical conditions, such as metabolic derangements, toxic ingestions, autoimmune diseases, diabetic ketoacidosis, and illicit drug use, can affect the heart as well as the integrity of the gastrointestinal (GI) tract and obstruction of the mesenteric arterial circulation, which may result in GI bleeding, decreased motility, and bowel ischemia (Macaluso & McNamara, 2012). An atypical presentation of abdominal pain is of greater concern in patients who abuse narcotics, have a history of gastric

bypass, and those who are immunocompromised due to medication or underlying immune system pathology (Makrauer & Greenberger, 2016).

Comprehensive nursing care involves an overall assessment of the patient with AAP. A toxic-appearing patient may present with altered mental status, be anxious, diaphoretic, in severe pain, have a distended and rigid abdomen with severe pain indicating the possibility of a surgical abdomen, and signs of shock. This presentation warrants immediate stabilization, surgical consultation, and further diagnostic and lab workup (Jacobs & Silen, 2016).

Evaluation begins with a history of presenting illness and an assessment of pain in terms of location, quality or character, onset, intensity, presence of radiation, duration, progression, exacerbating and alleviating factors, as well as determining the presence of associated symptoms, reviewing the medical and surgical history, and conducting a thorough focused physical examination. Physical assessment involves evaluating the patients overall general appearance, vital signs, and assessment of the abdomen through inspection, auscultation, percussion, and palpation (Macaluso & McNamara, 2012; Makrauer & Greenberger, 2016).

A focused visual inspection of the exposed abdomen is done to evaluate for the presence of masses, pulsations, symmetry, scarring from previous injury or surgery, ecchymosis, distention, or ascites. Auscultation of an acute abdomen may reveal high, low-pitched, or absent BS. Often of low utility and reliability, absent BS can be a late sign indicating ileus, bowel obstruction, or an ominous finding in abdominal catastrophe (Macaluso & McNamara, 2012). Percussion of the abdomen can illicit pain in peritonitis as well as differentiate tympany between small- and large-bowel obstructions. Palpation of the abdomen should be conducted with the patient supine and the knees in a flexed position to help relax the abdominal muscles. Palpation will help identify the location of pain; determine the presence of a rigid abdomen, guarding, and rebound tenderness, all of which are indications of an acute abdomen. In addition, nurses should be familiar with the specialty abdominal examination techniques used by providers to identify the etiology of abdominal pain, which include but are not limited to Carnett's sign, cough test, closed eyes sign, Murphy's sign, psoas sign, obturator sign, and Roving's sign (Jacobs & Silen, 2016; Macaluso & McNamara, 2012; Papadakis & McPhee, 2017).

Appropriate lab techniques and diagnostics are dictated by the physical exam and presenting symptoms; however, many are of limited value in evaluating a patient with AAP due to the high rate of false-negative results. The baseline lab tests to consider are urinalysis, urine pregnancy test in women of childbearing age, a complete metabolic panel (CMP), complete blood count (CBC) with differential, liver function tests (LFTs), lipase, prothrombin time (PT)/partial thromboplastin time (PTT), and international normalized ratio (INR), lactate, blood cultures if sepsis is suspected, arterial blood gas (ABG), and a type and screen if the patient has an acute abdomen and surgery is anticipated (Jacobs & Silen, 2016; Makrauer & Greenberger, 2016; Papadakis & McPhee, 2017).

Initial diagnostic imaging exams are dictated by the location of pain. Plain abdominal films are of limited value in the acute abdomen. Abdominal ultrasonography (US) can be used as a focused assessment with sonography for trauma (FAST) and has the advantages of rapid point-of-care testing, is less expensive than a contrast scan, and has no risk of exposure to radiation or contrast dye that can adversely affect the kidneys (Jacobs & Silen, 2016; Makrauer & Greenberger, 2016; O'Brien, 2016). A CT scan with contrast is recommended over US in certain cases of AAP. Reliance on this advanced medical imaging is commonplace in part due to a high degree of sensitivity (89%) and a specificity of approximately 77%, increasing the chances of identifying the underlying condition when compared with ultrasound (Brownson & Mandell, 2014; Cartwright & Knudson, 2015; Gans, Pols, & Boermeester, 2015).

NURSING INTERVENTIONS, MANAGEMENT, AND IMPLICATIONS

Nursing care of patients with an acute abdomen centers on reliance on prompt identification of an acute intra-abdominal emergency and identification of signs and symptoms of early sepsis. Competence in IV insertion and nursing-related procedural skills will facilitate treatment for stabilizing hemodynamics, facilitating labs, diagnostics, and antibiotic administration, as well as placement of a nasogastric tube for gastric decompression and management of nausea with an antiemetic. Attention to guidelines for GI and deep vein thrombosis (DVT) prophylaxis in preparation for emergent surgical intervention or admission is standard of care.

The management of abdominal pain management is a priority and an achievable goal for optimizing patient care. Addressing pain management is one of the most important contributing factors to removing barriers to care. Research indicates that pain medication should not be withheld from patients experiencing AAP as pain relief can help remove the physical and emotional barriers associated with pain that can limit obtaining an accurate history and physical exam (Thomas, 2013). Family-centered care should be encouraged for overall compassionate support of the patient and family.

OUTCOMES

Early recognition of the acute abdomen with surgical consultation is helpful for both patient and surgeon in establishing a definitive diagnosis for prompt treatment and management for improving patient outcomes and decreasing mortality. Evidence-based identification of an acute abdomen with intra-abdominal sepsis has a 50% mortality rate; if sepsis progresses and results in multiple organ failure (three organs), the mortality rate approaches 100% (Arumugam et al., 2015). Ongoing assessment and serial repeat examination of the patient can trend toward improvement with current management or identify failed therapy. When a diagnosis remains in question, the patient should be continually observed in a monitored ED setting or admitted under observation. Patients who are found to be stable enough to discharge should be given strict instructions to return immediately for any worsening of symptoms, persistent pain beyond 8 hours, the development of a fever, or new-onset vomiting that could indicate the progression of an early appendicitis or bowel obstruction (Brownson & Mandell, 2014; Macaluso & McNamara, 2012).

Summary

AAP is the most common presenting symptom in the ED. An acute abdomen is associated with severe and sudden onset of abdominal pain with associated symptoms with an onset of less than 24 hours, likely requiring surgical intervention. Rapid assessment and diagnosis are priority. Despite advances in medical technology and diagnostics, a delay in the diagnosis and treatment of an acute abdomen can adversely affect outcomes, leading to misdiagnosis, increased morbidity and mortality, and subsequent medicolegal litigation (Macaluso & McNamara, 2012).

Arumugam, S., Al-Hassani, A., El-Menyar, A., Abdelrahman, H., Parchani, A., Peralta, R., . . . Al-Thani, H. (2015). Frequency, causes and pattern of abdominal trauma: A 4-year descriptive analysis. *Journal of Emergencies, Trauma, and Shock, 8*(4), 193–198. doi:10.4103/0974-2700.166590

Brownson E. G., & Mandell, K. (2014) The acute abdomen. In G. M. Doherty (Ed.), *Current diagnosis*

& *treatment: Surgery* (14th ed., Chapter 21). New York, NY: McGraw-Hill. Retrieved from http://accessmedicine .mhmedical.com/content.aspx?bookid=1202&section id=71519979

Cartwright, S., & Knudson, M. (2015, April 1). Diagnostic imaging of acute abdominal pain in adults. *American Family Physician, 91*(7), 452–459. Retrieved from http:// www.aafp.org/afp/2015/0401/p452.html

Centers for Disease Control and Prevention. (2013). Emergency department visits. Retrieved from https:// www.cdc.gov/nchs/data/ahcd/nhamcs_emergency/2013_ ed_web_tables.pdf

Cervellin, G., Mora, R., Ticinesi, A., Meschi, T., Comelli, I., Catena, F., & Lippi, G. (2016). Epidemiology and outcomes of acute abdominal pain in a large urban emergency department: Retrospective analysis of 5,340 cases. *Annals of Translational Medicine, 4*(19), 362. doi:10.21037/atm.2016.09.10

Gans, S. L., Pols, M. A., & Boermeester, M. A. (2015). Guideline for the diagnostic pathway in patients with acute abdominal pain [Review Article]. *Digestive Surgery, 32*(1), 23–31. doi:10.1159/000871583

Jacobs, D. O., & Silen, W. (2016). Abdominal pain. In D. L. Kasper, A. S. Fauci, S. L. Hauser, D. Longo, J. Jameson, & J. Loscalzo (Eds.), *Harrison's manual of medicine* (19th ed., pp. 154–157). New York: NY: McGraw-Hill.

Jiang, H. J., Weiss, A. J., & Barrett, M. L. (2017). Characteristics of emergency department visits for superutilizers by payer, 2014. [Statistical Brief #221]. Retrieved from https://www.hcup-us.ahrq.gov/reports/statbriefs/ sb221-Super-Utilizer-ED-Visits-Payer-2014.pdf

Macaluso, C. R., & McNamara, R. M. (2012). Evaluation and management of acute abdominal pain in the emergency department. *International Journal of General Medicine, 5*, 789–797. doi:10.2147/IJGM.S25936

Makrauer, F. L., & Greenberger, N. J. (2016). Acute abdominal pain: Basic principles & current challenges. In N. J. Greenberger, R. S. Blumberg, & R. Burakoff (Eds.), *Current diagnosis & treatment: Gastroenterology, hepatology, & endoscopy* (3rd ed., Chapter 1). New York, NY: McGraw-Hill. Retrieved from http://accessmedicine .mhmedical.com/content.aspx?bookid=1621&Section id=105181134

O'Brien, M. C. (2016). Acute abdominal pain. In J. E. Tintinalli (Ed.), *Tintinalli's emergency medicine: A comprehensive study guide* (8th ed.). New York, NY: McGraw-Hill. Retrieved from http://accessmedicine.mhmedical.com .proxy.library.vanderbilt.edu/book.aspx?bookid=1658

Papadakis, M. A., & McPhee, S. J. (2017). *Current medical diagnosis and treatment*. New York, NY: McGraw-Hill.

Skinner, H. G, Blanchard, J, & Elixhauser, A. (2014). Trends in emergency department visits, 2006–2011 [Statistical Brief #179]. Retrieved from https://www.hcup-us.ahrq .gov/reports/statbriefs/sb179-Emergency-Department -Trends.pdf

Thomas, S. H. (2013). Management of pain in the emergency department [Review Article]. *International Scholarly Research Notices [ISRN] Emergency Medicine, 2013*. doi:10.1155/2013/583132

■ ACUTE CORONARY SYNDROME

Andrea Efre

Overview

Acute coronary syndrome (ACS) is an umbrella term used to describe a range of coronary artery emergencies, including myocardial infarction (MI) and unstable angina (UA). It is caused by a sudden reduction or blockage of blood flow to the cardiac muscle, frequently caused by atherosclerosis, and most prevalent in older adults. The blockage limits blood flow to the myocardium (heart muscle) that usually causes chest pain. The treatment goal is to improve blood flow (revascularization) as quickly as possible and may be achieved with pharmacology or interventional cardiac catheterization depending on the available facilities. Rapid identification of diagnostic criteria and initiation of emergency treatment by the nurse is essential to save the coronary muscle, prevent further cardiac damage, and improve outcomes.

Background

ACS refers to a spectrum of conditions that are divided into three categories:

1. ST-elevation MI (STEMI), also known as *acute myocardial infarction (AMI)*

2. Non-ST elevation MI (NSTEMI)

3. UA

The latter two categories of NSTEMI and UA were combined into a new title of non-ST elevation ACS (NSTE) in the American Heart Association and American College of Cardiologists 2014 practice guidelines to emphasizes the continuum between UA and NSTEMI (Amsterdam et al., 2014). Therefore, you may see the terms and treatment plans used interchangeably. Almost three quarters of all ACS patients present as NSTE-ACS (greater than 625,000 patients annually) in the United States (Amsterdam et al., 2014). As a common presentation of coronary heart disease, NSTE-ACS is the leading cause of global cardiovascular morbidity and mortality (Rodriguez & Mahaffey, 2016).

Risk factors associated with ACS are the same as those involved in coronary heart disease and include age, gender, family history, smoking, hypertension, dyslipidemia, physical inactivity, obesity, diabetes mellitus, and recreational drugs such as cocaine. An estimated 15.5 million Americans older than 20 years of age have CHD, and from that number 550,000 have MIs annually, and 200,000 have recurrent attacks (Mozaffarinini et al., 2016). The older adult is most at risk from ACS. In the United States, the average age at the first MI is 65 years for men and 72 years for women (Mozaffarinini et al., 2016).

The cause of ACS is typically related to the formation of a thrombus that occludes the coronary vessel and prevents blood flow to the myocardium. The STEMI suggests that the coronary artery is fully occluded and is the most life-threatening and time-sensitive presentation of ACS. In NSTEMI or UA, the thrombus may partially or intermittently occlude the coronary artery, which is why the symptoms may be less severe or difficult to determine. The limited coronary blood flow is most often characterized by sternal or central chest pain.

Diagnosis of ACS is determined by the 12-lead EKG findings and serum cardiac enzymes. A 12-lead EKG should be performed and interpreted in 10 minutes of symptom onset or arrival to the emergency facility (Amsterdam et al., 2014). The EKG determine whether there is an acute injury to the myocardium identified by ST-elevation, T wave changes, or a new onset of left bundle branch block. The STEMI has elevations of ST segment in grouped leads on the 12-lead EKG, which identify the location of the affected myocardium and the coronary artery most likely involved. No ST elevations are noted in NSTEMI or UA, but it should be noted that ST depression or T wave inversions may be present in either.

Cardiac biomarkers are released into the blood when myocardial tissue damage (necrosis) occurs, and are found in both STEMI and NSTEMI. The biomarkers of troponin, myoglobin, and creatine kinase may remain elevated in the circulation following the infarction, but troponin has a longer period of detection (up to 10 days) and is thought to be the more sensitive and specific of the other biomarkers (Roffi et al., 2015). No increase in serum biomarkers is found in UA.

Immediate identification and differentiation of STEMI or NSTE-ACS are needed to define the treatment plan. Rapid intervention is necessary to restore coronary blood flow with percutaneous coronary intervention (PCI) in a cardiac catheterization laboratory. Delays in treatment enhance the progression of the coronary blockage, which leads to the loss of myocardial muscle and a potential cardiac arrest or death.

Clinical Aspects

ASSESSMENT

Acute, central (substernal) chest pain is the typical primary symptom of ACS. The pain may radiate to the left arm, shoulders, back, neck, jaw, or abdomen. It is important to ask open-ended questions and ask the patient to describe the chest pain and any other symptoms. Establish the location, onset, duration, and characteristics of the pain. Both STEMI and NSTE-ACS are most commonly present as a pressure-type chest pain that typically occurs at rest or with minimal exertion, and lasting for more than 10 minutes, whereas angina is typically relieved in 5 minutes of stopping the offending activity or with short-acting nitroglycerin (Amsterdam et al., 2014).

Determine whether there are associated symptoms such as shortness of breath, diaphoresis, lightheadedness, nausea, vomiting, or apprehension. Also, ask the patient whether anything aggravates or relieves the symptoms, what they were doing at the time of symptom onset, and whether they have attempted any treatments before telling you about the pain. When a patient arrives in the emergency room it is common that he or she has attempted treatments at home (e.g., taking other people's prescriptions, or using illicit drugs to self-medicate), they may not openly offer this information initially without probing questions being asked.

Women, older adults, patients with diabetes, or patients with a history of heart failure may present with more subtle symptoms often without severe chest pain, which makes the diagnosis much more challenging and may lead to delay in treatment. Symptoms include shortness of breath, fatigue, lethargy, indigestion, anxiety, or sleep disturbances. If chest pain is present, it may be atypical and be reported as numbness, burning, or stabbing pain.

The physical examination should remain relatively unchanged from before the onset of the symptom. It is advisable to reassess the heart and lungs to identify deterioration, for example, rales on lung examination and development of S3 heart sound (found in fluid overload) suggest pulmonary edema or heart failure. Finding new murmurs or S4 heart sound (related to a noncompliant ventricle) could be caused by cardiac ischemia and should be further evaluated.

A change in vital signs may be noted in ACS, such as tachycardia, hypotension, hypertension, tachypnea, and possibly decreased oxygen saturation. Continuous cardiac monitoring for dysrhythmias and ST or T wave changes identify lethal rhythms or evolution of the ischemia. EKG changes are related to the location of myocardial impairment and lack of blood flow. If the right coronary artery is occluded, then ST changes may be noted in the inferior leads (II, III, and AVF), plus atrial dysrhythmias may be seen because of the lack of blood supply to the right atria, the sinoatrial node, or atrioventricular node. These rhythms may include new-onset atrial fibrillation, tachycardia, bradycardia, or a heart block. If the circumflex artery is involved the ST changes are usually noted in the lateral leads (I, AVL, V5, and V6). If the left coronary artery is affected by occlusion, anterior changes are seen in the 12-lead EKG throughout the chest leads (V1–V4), plus the left ventricle may be affected causing ventricular arrhythmias, including the life-threatening ventricular tachycardia or ventricular fibrillation.

NURSING INTERVENTIONS, MANAGEMENT, AND IMPLICATIONS

The goal for the management of STEMI is PCI, which should be performed within 90 minutes of arrival to the emergency facility (or from the symptom onset if inpatient). If PCI is not available, arrangements should be made to transfer the patient to a facility that can perform PCI in 120 minutes. If the transfer takes longer than 2 hours, then a fibrinolytic agent (such as tenecteplase, reteplase, or alteplase) should be administered and arrangements made to transfer for PCI in 3 to 24 hours (O'Gara et al., 2013). Primary PCI is also considered reasonable in patients with STEMI if there is clinical or EKG evidence of ongoing ischemia between 12 and 24 hours after symptom onset (O'Gara et al., 2013).

Dual antiplatelet therapy with aspirin and platelet inhibitors (known as *P2Y12 inhibitors*) is used in the initial treatment of STEMI and remains the cornerstone for the treatment of NSTE-ACS (Rodriguez & Mahaffey, 2016). An aspirin loading dose of 325 mg is given, followed by 81 mg daily, and loading doses of clopidogrel 300 mg to 600 mg followed by daily doses of 75 mg. If desired, prasugrel or ticagrelor may be used instead of clopidogrel.

Adjunct pharmacological treatments for ischemia to decrease myocardial oxygen demand and increase myocardial oxygen supply are considered. These include nitrates (sublingual or intravenous), antiplatelet therapy, morphine, and beta-blockers. Beta-blockers should be avoided if cocaine use is suspected, or in patients with vasospastic angina (Roffi et al., 2015).

Following a successful PCI, the expected outcome of the ACS patient is to be discharged home with education on lifestyle modifications, medication compliance, and committing to cardiac rehabilitation and continued care. Underlying disorders, such as hypertension, diabetes mellitus, or dyslipidemia, need to be controlled. Beta-blockers, ACE inhibitors, angiotensin receptor blockers (ARB), and statins are often prescribed. Lifestyle modifications to reduce overall cardiovascular risk include smoking cessation, regular physical activity, weight reduction in patients with high body mass index, and dietary changes to include reduced intake of salt and saturated fat, and increase in fruit, vegetables, wholegrain cereals, and fish (Amsterdam et al., 2014; O'Gara et al., 2013).

OUTCOMES

A rapid assessment by the nurse ensures early intervention and improved outcomes. Delays in assessment, diagnosis, or intervention can be prevented with the use of standing orders and algorithms to initiate care. Cardiogenic shock may occur in up to 3% of NSTE-ACS patients, for whom immediate PCI is most often used for revascularization (Roffi et al., 2015). Primary PCI is also indicated for cardiogenic shock or acute severe heart failure in STEMI patients, irrespective of time delay from onset (O'Gara et al., 2013). Revascularization with PCI is not always possible, such as in multiple vessel diseases, or difficult positioning of the coronary occlusion. For those who are not candidates for PCI or fibrinolytic therapy, emergency coronary artery bypass graft (CABG) in 6 hours of symptom onset may be considered in STEMI (O'Gara et al., 2013).

Summary

In summary, the priority of the nurse is to rapidly gather accurate information, including symptoms, vital signs, physical assessment, and a 12-lead EKG. Initial treatments should be started during the assessment period, including continuous cardiac monitoring, supplemental oxygen, dual antiplatelet therapy, and consideration of nitroglycerine administration if available and the patient is normotensive. Early intervention improves outcomes and therefore contacting the provider and transmitting a copy of the 12-lead EKG if the provider is not physically available speeds up the diagnostic process. Every effort should be made to reach the revascularization goal to undergo PCI within 90 minutes of symptom onset.

Amsterdam, E. A., Wenger, N. K., Brindis, R. G., Casey, D. E., Ganiats, T. G., Holmes, D. R., . . . Zieman, S. J.; American College of Cardiology; American Heart Association Task Force on Practice Guidelines; Society for Cardiovascular Angiography and Interventions; Society of Thoracic Surgeons; American Association for Clinical Chemistry. (2014). 2014 AHA/ACC guideline for the management of patients with non-ST-elevation acute coronary syndromes: A report of the American College of Cardiology/American Heart Association Task Force on Practice Guidelines. *Journal of the American College of Cardiology, 64*(24), e139–e228.

Jacobs, A. K., Kushner, F. G., Ettinger, S. M., Guyton, R. A., Anderson, J. L., Ohman, E. M., . . . Somerfield, M. R. (2013). ACCF/AHA clinical practice guideline methodology summit report: A report of the American College of Cardiology Foundation/American Heart Association Task Force on Practice Guidelines. *Journal of the American College of Cardiology, 61*(2), 213–265.

Mozaffarian, D., Benjamin, E. J., Arnett, D. K., Blaha, M. J., Cushman, M., Das, S. R., . . . Turner, M. B.; American Heart Association Statistics Committee and Stroke Statistics Subcommittee. (2016). Heart disease and stroke statistic—2016 update: A report from the American Heart Association. *Circulation, 133*(4), e38–e360. doi:10.1161/cir.0000000000000350

O'Gara, P. T., Kushner, F. G., Ascheim, D. D., Casey, D. E., Chung, M. K., DeLemos, J. A., . . . Yancy, C. W.; American College of Cardiology Foundation/American Heart Association Task Force on Practice Guidelines. (2013). 2013 ACCF/AHA guidelines for the management of ST-elevation myocardial infarction: A report of the American college of cardiology foundation/American Heart Association Task Force on Practice Guidelines. *Circulation, 127*(4), e362–e425. doi:10.1161/CIR.0b013e3182742cf6

Rodriguez, F., & Mahaffey, K. W. (2016). Management of patients with NSTE-ACS: A comparison of the recent AHA/ACC and ESC guidelines. *Journal of the American College of Cardiology, 68*(3), 313–321.

Roffi, M., Patrono, C., Collet, J. P., Mueller, C., Valgimigli, M., Andreotti, F., . . . Windecker, S. (2015). 2015 ESC guidelines for the management of acute coronary syndromes in patients presenting without persistent ST-segment elevation. *Revista Espanola de Cardiologia, 68*(12), 1125.

■ ACUTE EXACERBATION OF A CHRONIC CONDITION

Brenda L. Douglass

Overview

Across the United States, chronic health conditions have escalated over the past decade. In 2016, about one in four Americans had more than one chronic health condition and for individuals aged 65 years and older, prevalence rises to three in four Americans (Centers for Disease Control and Prevention [CDC], 2016, November 14). According to the National Health Council (2016), a chronic condition is defined as a disease lasting 3 months or more. Chronic health conditions have a profound impact on quality of life, often leading to premature disability. Chronic conditions cause heightened rates of mortality and considerable economic burdens to the patient, family, and society (CDC, 2016a). An acute exacerbation of a chronic condition occurs when there is an increase in severity of the chronic condition over baseline symptoms and physiologic decline.

Chronic conditions and acute exacerbations are often preventable, thus presenting an opportunity for nursing professionals to intervene to restore an individual's health status and provide education on the prevention of future exacerbations. One of the most common chronic conditions with episodes of acute exacerbations in the setting of emergency or critical care is chronic obstructive pulmonary disease (COPD). The recognition and management of patients with an acute exacerbation of COPD is the principal focus of this discussion.

Background

The clinical trajectory of adults with COPD is often marked with acute exacerbations requiring hospitalization. An acute exacerbation of COPD is an event characterized by worsening respiratory symptoms beyond the normal daily variations and lending to a change in the medication regimen (World Health Organization [WHO], 2017). Acute exacerbations of COPD are critical events that denote physiologic instability and worsening in the obstructive ventilation, which contributes to an increase in an individual's risk of death (Global Initiative for Chronic Obstructive Lung Disease [GOLD], 2017; Wedzicha, 2015). Risk factors for COPD exacerbation include advanced age, duration of COPD, productive cough, chronic mucous hypersecretion, history of exacerbations and antibiotic use, COPD-related hospitalization in the prior year, and one or more comorbid conditions (Stoller, 2017). Comorbidities, such as cardiovascular disease, diabetes mellitus, and hypertension, are common in patients with COPD, further raising the risk of the need for hospitalization and mortality (GOLD, 2017; Stoller, 2017).

Acute exacerbations of COPD are typically classified by the range of the severity of dyspnea, from mild (e.g., increased dyspnea or cough), moderate (e.g., chest tightness, wheezing), to severe worsening in dyspnea (e.g., hypoxemia, acute respiratory failure; GOLD, 2017; Stoller, 2017). In 70% of cases, COPD exacerbations are associated with acute respiratory infections (Stoller, 2017). COPD exacerbations are disabling, necessitate urgent medical care and hospitalizations, as well as heighten an individual's risk of death (CDC, 2016b; GOLD, 2017). In addition to devastating personal costs, there is a significant societal burden associated with COPD exacerbations with direct costs estimated at $32 billion and indirect costs at $20.4 billion (CDC, 2016b).

According to the Global Initiative for Chronic Obstructive Lung Disease (GOLD) guidelines (2017), goals of therapy in the management of COPD exacerbations are directed at minimizing the negative impact of the current exacerbation and to prevent recurrent episodes. The severity of the exacerbation and underlying disease determines whether the patient can be managed in an inpatient or outpatient setting (GOLD, 2017). About 80% of patients experiencing COPD exacerbations can be managed in the outpatient setting with pharmacologic therapies (GOLD, 2017). Classification of the level of severity for the COPD exacerbation is crucial to optimal intervention. COPD exacerbations are classified into three categories: (a) mild (administration of short-acting beta agonist [SABA]), (b) moderate (administration of a SABA, antibiotic, and/or oral corticosteroid), and (c) severe (pharmacologic management and/or positive ventilation; GOLD, 2017). Acute respiratory failure associated with severe COPD exacerbations mandates aggressive intervention, such as those often delivered in the emergency and critical care settings.

Clinical Aspects

ASSESSMENT

To guide nursing care, a comprehensive assessment of signs and symptoms is recommended to determine the level of airflow limitation and presence of comorbid health issues during an acute exacerbation of COPD. Emphasis on assessing the severity of symptoms as changes from the individual's baseline symptom profile is recommended. Specifically, nurses should assess for worsening dyspnea, wheeze, increased cough, sputum characteristics, work of breathing, mental status, and indications of an upper respiratory infection. This information should be used to classify the severity of the COPD exacerbation (e.g., mild, moderate, or severe), as well as the frequency of and time since last acute exacerbation: a thorough review of preexisting comorbid conditions

(e.g., pneumonia, cardiovascular disease, obstructive sleep apnea, respiratory failure requiring mechanical ventilation) and assessment for symptoms of comorbid conditions (e.g. chest pain/ pressure, peripheral edema), environmental factors (e.g., smoking history, exposure to smoke and other pollutants), and current medication regimen with attention to medications for the management of COPD, including medication dosages, devices, adherence, and responsiveness to these therapies. On physical examination, attention to vital signs (e.g., blood pressure, heart rate, respiratory rate, level of consciousness) may help to inform a nurse's ability to specify the severity of the COPD exacerbation. To further specify the severity of an acute exacerbation, pulse oximetry, arterial blood gas analysis, and a chest radiograph are useful objective and diagnostic measures that guide nursing care for individuals with a COPD exacerbation.

NURSING INTERVENTIONS, MANAGEMENT, AND IMPLICATIONS

Nursing interventions provide opportunities to set goals in the clinical management of chronic conditions manifested by an acute exacerbation. An emphasis is placed on prevention, early recognition, and engaging the patient through patient-centered care (CDC, 2016a; GOLD, 2017). Providing education to patients on self-management goals to include in early recognition of worsening symptoms and when to seek medical care is integral to prevent or minimize impairment. Key points to effective nursing management include assessment of severity and providing the level of intervention necessary according to evidence-based guidelines for the most optimal treatment strategy (GOLD, 2017).

OUTCOMES

Acute exacerbations of chronic conditions, such as COPD, are often intertwined with comorbid conditions, precipitated by triggers, and present complexities in care of the patient with chronic conditions (GOLD, 2017). The delivery of nursing care from a holistic perspective, blending in physical, emotional, and spiritual care with integration of evidence-based practices, presents an opportunity to improve the health outcomes of individuals experiencing an acute exacerbation of COPD.

Summary

An acute exacerbation of COPD is a leading cause of death in the United States (CDC, 2016a). COPD exacerbations have negative impact on an individual's health and quality of life—leading to premature disability and shortened life spans (CDC, 2016a; GOLD, 2017). The cost of chronic conditions and acute exacerbations of chronic disease pose an economic burden to the nation. Acute exacerbation of COPD provides an illustration of a chronic health condition in which prevention and early intervention are key to improving health outcomes.

Centers for Disease Control and Prevention. (2016a). Chronic disease prevention and health promotion. Retrieved from https://www.cdc.gov/chronicdisease

Centers for Disease Control and Prevention. (2016b). Chronic obstructive pulmonary disease (COPD). Retrieved from https://www.cdc.gov/copd/index.html

Global Initiative for Chronic Obstructive Lung Disease. (2017). Global strategy for the diagnosis, management and prevention of COPD, GOLD 2017 report. Retrieved from http://goldcopd.org

Han, M. K., Dransfield, M., & Martinez, F. (2016). Chronic obstructive pulmonary disease: Definition, clinical manifestations, diagnosis, and staging. In J. Stoller & H. Hollingsworth (Eds.), *UpToDate*. Retrieved from http://www.uptodate.com/contents/chronic-obstructive-pulmonary-disease-definition-clinical-manifestations-diagnosis-and-staging

National Health Council. (2016). About chronic health conditions. Retrieved from http://www.nationalhealthcouncil.org/newsroom/about-chronic-conditions

Stoller, J. (2017). Management of exacerbations of chronic obstructive pulmonary disease. In P. Barnes & H. Holingsworth (Eds.), *UpToDate*. Retrieved from http://www.uptodate.com/contents/management-of-exacerbations-of-chronic-obstructive-pulmonary-disease

Wedzicha, J. (2015). Mechanisms of chronic obstructive pulmonary disease exacerbations. *Annals of the American Thoracic Society*, *12*(2), 157–159. doi:10.1513/AnnulsATS.201507-427AW

World Health Organization. (2017). Chronic respiratory diseases. Retrieved from http://www.who.int/respiratory/copd/en

■ ACUTE PANCREATITIS IN ADULTS

Virginia Mangolds

Overview

Acute pancreatitis (AP) is an inflammatory process of the pancreas involving the activation of intrapancreatic enzymes that further exacerbate pancreatic tissue injury and altered organ function. The diagnosis of AP is made using elevations in pancreatic enzymes, clinical symptoms, and a variety of diagnostic imaging. Nursing care for adults with AP is focused on hemodynamic monitoring, prevention of pancreatic stimulation, electrolyte monitoring, pain control, identifying and treating local complications in the pancreas, identifying and treating multisystem failure, emotional support, patient education and discharge preparation with outpatient support if necessary (Burns, 2014; Krenzer, 2016).

Background

AP is the most common gastrointestinal diagnosis for acute hospitalizations in the United States. In fact, more than 270,000 annual admissions were attributed to AP in 2012 and the estimated cost of these hospitalizations totaled $2.6 billion (Peery et al., 2012). Despite the need for inpatient care, the mortality rate of patients with AP is 2% to 10%, which is related to shock, anoxia, hypotension, or fluid or electrolyte imbalance. This high mortality rate may be attributed to the 10% to 30% of patients exhibiting severe AP associated with pancreatic and peripancreatic necrosis (Talukdar, Clemens, & Vege, 2012).

The diagnosis of AP is made by fulfilling two of the three following criteria: (a) abdominal pain; (b) elevated serum lipase or amylase (more than three times the upper limit of normal); and (c) characteristic findings of AP on imaging, usually contrast-enhanced CT (Banks et al., 2013). Gallstones and chronic alcohol abuse account for 90% of AP. Drug-induced causes have been linked to metronidazole, tetracycline, azathioprine, and estrogens. Other less common etiologies are vascular, genetic, infectious, autoimmune, traumatic, and idiopathic, and may include hyperlipidemia, hypercalcemia, and pancreatic neoplasms (Burns, 2014). Laboratory evaluation and treatment consist of obtaining and analyzing multiple laboratory values, including amylase, lipase, complete blood cell count with differential, electrolytes, blood urea nitrogen (BUN), creatinine, glucose, coagulation studies, lactate, calcium, magnesium, albumin, and liver enzymes (Van Leeuwen & Bladh, 2015).

Common diagnostic imaging consists of ultrasound, CT and CT angiography (CTA; Catanzano, 2009) and/or MRI (Tenner, Baillie, DeWitt, Vege, & American College of Gastroenterology, 2013). Imaging recommendations indicate that ultrasound should be the initial diagnostic study (Catanzano, 2009; Krenzer, 2016; Sarr, 2013), which is particularly sensitive to AP as a result of cholelithiasis. CT imaging is recommended for later in the course of the disease, for patients whose symptoms do not improve or worsen (Catanzano, 2009; Sarr, 2013). Early in the course of the disease, CT findings may be minimal or absent. CT is used with contrast to confirm an unclear diagnosis and to evaluate the extent of damage to the pancreas and surrounding area. It can be used to separate the pancreatic parenchyma from the surrounding duodenum and to evaluate for pancreatic necrosis. It is also useful for identifying and evaluating a suspected or known pancreatic mass. CTA may be performed in cases of known pancreatic neoplasm; complicated pancreatitis, such as pancreatic necrosis, abscess, or hemorrhage; or evaluation of pseudocyst formation (Catanzano, 2009).

The classification of severity has been broken down to mild, moderately severe, and severe (Sarr, 2013). Mild AP is associated with nonorgan failure and lack of local or systemic complication. Moderately severe AP is associated with organ failure that resolves in 48 hours (transient) and local or systemic complications without persistent organ failure. Severe AP is associated with persistent single or multiple organ failure for more than 48 hours (Banks et al., 2013; Krenzer, 2016).

Clinical Aspects

According to Ackley, Ladwig, and Makic (2017), based on the North American Nursing Diagnosis Association International (NANDA International), patients being cared for in the inpatient setting may benefit from the following nursing diagnosis and treatment, based on the assess, diagnose, plan, implement care, evaluate the outcomes (ADPIE) plan and from making necessary improvements in (a) ineffective breathing pattern, (b) deficient fluid volume, (c) acute pain, (d) diarrhea, (e) nausea, and (f) ineffective denial.

ASSESSMENT

Ineffective breathing pattern occurs when inspiration and/or expiration does not provide adequate ventilation. Monitor respiratory rate, depth, and ease of respiration; note the amount of anxiety associated with dyspnea; attempt to determine whether the client's dyspnea is physiological or psychological; note the rapidity of the development of dyspnea, which may be an indicator of the severity of the condition. Treatment of dyspnea includes positioning the patient in an upright or semi-Fowler's position, and administering oxygen as ordered.

Deficient fluid volume occurs when there is decreased intravascular, interstitial, and/or intracellular fluid. Monitor for thirst, restlessness, headaches, and difficulty concentrating. Notify the provider of any indication of deficient fluid volume, and assist in adjusting the fluid replacement as indicated.

NURSING INTERVENTIONS, MANAGEMENT, AND IMPLICATIONS

To identify acute pain, perform a comprehensive assessment of pain, which includes location, characteristics, onset/duration, frequency, quality, intensity, and severity of pain. Work with the medical provider to ensure adequate pain control.

Diarrhea is the passage of loose, unformed stools. Document frequency and amount of stool. Follow dietary orders as written by the patient's providers and notify them if the diarrhea continues, despite of their diet.

Nausea is a subjective, phenomenon of an unpleasant feeling in the back of the throat and stomach, which does not result in vomiting. Implement appropriate dietary measures, such as NPO (nothing by mouth) status as appropriate, small frequent meals, and low-fat meals.

Ineffective denial is the conscious or unconscious attempt to disavow knowledge or meaning of an event to reduce anxiety and/or fear, leading to the detriment of health. Assess the patient's and family's understanding of the illness, treatments, and expected outcomes. Aid the patient in making choices regarding treatment and actively invite him or her into the decision-making process.

OUTCOMES

Outcomes to aim for, using nursing diagnoses, are related to breathing patterns, urine output, pain control, diarrhea control, nausea and vomiting control, and active participation in outpatient treatment programs if the AP is related to substance abuse (Ackley et al., 2017). Specifically, the suggested outcomes include that (a) the patient demonstrates a breathing pattern that supports blood gas results within his or her normal parameters; (b) maintains urine output of 0.5 mL/kg/hour; (c) maintains normal blood pressure, heart rate, and body temperature; (d) maintains elastic skin turgor and moist mucous membranes and orientation to person, place, and time; (e) expresses satisfaction with pain control; (f) has solid, formed stool with defecation; (g) has the ability to tolerate normal oral intake without vomiting; (h) seeks out appropriate health care attention when needed; and (i) actively engages in a treatment program related to identified "substance abuse" if applicable (Ackley et al., 2017).

Summary

AP is the most common gastrointestinal cause for acute hospitalization with more than 270,000 annual admissions and an estimated cost of $2.6 billion. The classification of severity has been broken down to mild, moderately severe, and severe. The diagnosis includes clinical, laboratory, and diagnostic findings. Nursing outcome goals can be used to evaluate the patient's progression toward reaching a normal functioning and a good health status.

Ackley, B. J., Ladwig, G. B., & Makic, M. F. (2017). *Nursing diagnosis handbook—An evidence-based guide to planning care* (11th ed.). St. Louis, MO: Elsevier.

Banks, P. A., Bollen, T. L., Dervenis, C., Gooszen, H. G., Johnson, C. D., Sarr, M. G., . . . Acute Pancreatitis Classification Working Group. (2013). Classification of acute pancreatitis—2012: Revision of the Atlanta classification and definitions by international consensus. *Gut*, 62(1), 102–111. doi:10.1136/gutjnl-2012-302779

Burns, S. M. (2014). *AACN essentials of critical care nursing* (3rd ed.). New York NY: McGraw-Hill.

Catanzano, T. M. (2009). *How to think like a radiologist—Ordering imaging studies*. New York, NY: Cambridge University Press.

Krenzer, M. E. (2016). Understanding acute pancreatitis. *Nursing*, 46(8), 34–40. doi:10.1097/01.NURSE.0000484959.78110.98

Peery, A. F., Dellon, E. S., Lund, J., Crockett, S. D., McGowan, C. E., Bulsiewicz, W. J., . . . Shaheen, N. J. (2012). Burden of gastrointestinal disease in the United States: 2012 update. *Gastroenterology*, 143(5), 1179–1187; e1171–e1173. doi:10.1053/j.gastro.2012.08.002

Sarr, M. G. (2013). 2012 revision of the Atlanta classification of acute pancreatitis. *Polish Archives of Internal Medicine*, 123(3), 118–124.

Talukdar, R., Clemens, M., & Vege, S. S. (2012). Moderately severe acute pancreatitis: prospective validation of this new subgroup of acute pancreatitis. *Pancreas*, 41(2), 306–309. doi:10.1097/MPA.0b013e318229794e

Tenner, S., Baillie, J., DeWitt, J., Vege, S. S.; American College of, G. (2013). American College of Gastroenterology guideline: Management of acute pancreatitis. *American Journal of Gastroenterology*, 108(9), 1400–1415; 1416. doi:10.1038/ajg.2013.218

Van Leeuwen, A. M., & Bladh, M. L. (2015). *Davis's comprehensive handbook of laboratory and diagnostic tests with nursing implications* (6th ed.). Philadelphia, PA: F. A. Davis.

■ ACUTE RESPIRATORY DISTRESS SYNDROME

Kathleen C. Ashton

Overview

In the spectrum of illnesses associated with the respiratory system, acute respiratory distress syndrome (ARDS) is one of the most life-threatening and potentially fatal acute respiratory conditions. Formerly known as adult respiratory distress syndrome, ARDS results from either direct or indirect trauma to the lungs and affects both children and adults who are hospitalized with other conditions. It can also occur following an acute medical problem or procedure. The nursing care for patients with ARDS is primarily supportive and includes monitoring positive pressure ventilation, avoiding fluid overload, as well as a careful assessment and evaluation of the patient's treatment response. Based on the current literature, the mortality rate for ARDS is approximately 30%, and survivors of ARDS suffer high rates of morbidity (Mehta & Povoa, 2017; Sweeney & McAuley, 2016).

Background

Several conditions are implicated in the development of ARDS, including sepsis, smoke inhalation, near-drowning, severe pneumonia, major trauma, and any conditions resulting in a profound systemic inflammatory response. Sepsis is a leading cause of ARDS that tends to stimulate a systemic inflammatory response (Vidyasagar, 2016). In general, there are a variety of pathophysiologic conditions that activate the innate immune response, which in turn activates a physiologic reaction to that and, as a result, releases proinflammatory substances into the bloodstream to combat the infection or aid the recovery from a traumatic injury. An otherwise protective process, a systemic inflammatory response can have broad effects on the blood vessels, in particular the pulmonary vessels, which experience increased permeability. As the changes in the permeability of pulmonary vessels lead to the diffusion of fluid into alveoli, it reduces the affected alveoli's ability to promote blood oxygenation effectively. As more alveoli are affected, hypoxemia can be captured on chest imaging as bilateral pulmonary infiltrates that are not fully associated with heart failure (Mehta & Povoa, 2017).

First described by Ashbaugh, Bigelow, Petty, and Levine (1967), ARDS is classified as noncardiogenic pulmonary edema that leads to decreased lung compliance and hypoxia (Vidyasagar, 2016). The American–European Consensus Conference (AECC) defined the syndrome in 1994, and the Berlin Definition was established in 2011 by a panel convened by the European Society of Intensive Care Medicine, the American Thoracic Society, and the Society of Critical Care Medicine (Raneri et al., 2012). The Berlin Definition was validated in more than 4,000 patients' data (Sweeney & McAuley, 2016) and delineates the three stages of ARDS, mild, moderate, and severe, based on the degree of hypoxemia with the associated mortality for each stage. The corresponding mortality rates are 27% for mild, 32% for moderate, and 47% for the severe stage (Fanelli et al., 2013).

Risk factors for the development of ARDS include numerous illnesses and injuries, both pulmonary and systemic with pneumonia being the most common risk factor (Sweeney & McAuley, 2016). Pneumonia and aspiration have the highest associated mortality in ARDS. There are currently about 200,000 cases of ARDS reported annually in the United States.

Over the past 50 years, there have been numerous studies addressing the pathogenesis and clinical aspects of the syndrome, including underlying mechanisms, biomarkers, genetic predisposition, risk factors, epidemiology, and treatment. Genetics is now recognized to play a role in the predisposition to the development of ARDS (Fanelli et al., 2013). Despite the plethora of research studies, there are currently very few effective therapies for ARDS, other than the use of protective lung strategies (Fanelli et al., 2013).

Clinical Aspects

ASSESSMENT

Critical care nurses are the frontline nurses regarding the surveillance of the progression of ARDS. The assessment of patients for changes in the respiratory status is an ongoing responsibility of the nurses to alert physicians and others to changes in the patient's ability to effectively deliver oxygenated blood to the tissues. Breath sounds must be assessed at frequent intervals to ascertain any changes that could signal an increase in fluid and the effects of inflammation. Oxygen saturation, as

measured by pulse oximetry, is a crucial measurement to assist in recognition of changes. Invasive lines to measure pressure changes and fluid status are a mainstay of critically ill patients in intensive care units. Individuals may begin to show signs of respiratory compromise even before they land in an intensive care unit, so it is imperative that nurses assess patients to look for signs showing that they could be developing ARDS.

NURSING INTERVENTIONS, MANAGEMENT, AND IMPLICATIONS

The treatment for ARDS is supportive and centered on mechanical ventilation. In the setting of lung injury associated with ARDS, this modality can treat both the condition and contribute to lung injury, too. However, the positive pressure mechanical ventilation is the cornerstone of management; it can also incite lung injury and contribute to both the morbidity and mortality seen in ARDS (Fanelli et al., 2013). Thus, a judicious management of positive pressure ventilation is recommended among patients with ARDS.

Results of recent studies point to the use of lower tidal volumes and maintenance of plateau pressures in a specified range to reduce mortality and provide a survival benefit (Fanelli et al., 2013, p. 327). Tidal volumes of 6 mL/kg are now recommended as opposed to 10 mL/kg used previously (Vidyasagar, 2016). Lower tidal volumes help prevent ventilator-induced lung injury (VILI) caused by volutrauma (Vidyasagar, 2016). One recent and very significant change in ventilator strategy is the acceptance of lesser arterial oxygen tension (PaO_2) in the range of 85% to 90% for patient survival and hemodynamic stability (Vidyasagar, 2016). Lower tidal volumes and acceptance of lesser oxygen tension reduce lung overdistension and help prevent additional injury.

Another problem of management is the cyclic opening and closing of small airways and alveolar units, known as *atelectatic trauma*. Clinical trials have measured the effects of using higher levels of positive-end expiratory pressure (PEEP). The results are inconclusive, but there is limited evidence that higher (between 5 and 9 cm H_2O) levels of PEEP may reduce mortality (Fanelli et al., 2013).

Many other unconventional therapies are also used to manage ARDS, with varying success. Prone positioning exploits gravity and repositioning of the heart in the thorax to promote lung reexpansion and improve ventilation, thus improving oxygenation. Its impact on mortality remains controversial (Fanelli et al., 2013). The recent PROSEVA (Proning Severe ARDS Patients) trial demonstrated a significant benefit in mortality with the use of ventilation in the prone position (Scholten, Beitler, Prisk, & Malhotra, 2017).

High-frequency oscillatory ventilation (HFOV) is a technique that delivers extremely small tidal volumes using a relatively high mean airway pressure at high respiratory frequencies to avoid tidal overstretch (Fanelli et al., 2013). In two large multicenter clinical trials, HFOV failed to demonstrate improvement in survival, and its use is currently quite controversial (Fanelli et al., 2013).

In the case of severe hypoxemia and respiratory failure, extracorporeal membrane oxygenation (ECMO) is used as a rescue therapy. The objective is to overcome severe hypoxemia and respiratory acidosis while maintaining the lungs in a state of complete rest (Fanelli et al., 2013). However, ECMO is a scarce and expensive resource available only in major specialty centers. Regarding pharmacologic interventions, neuromuscular blockade and sedatives are often administered to decrease the patient's work of breathing, thereby improving respiratory mechanics and lowering oxygen consumption (Sweeney & McAuley, 2016).

As ARDS is a form of pulmonary edema, fluid therapy is an essential component of management. Fluids are provided for resuscitation and organ rescue during the early stages of the illness, followed by fluid unloading (deresuscitation)—either spontaneous or induced—after hemodynamic stability has been achieved (Sweeney & McAuley, 2016). The nursing role in intake and output measurement is paramount is this aspect of management.

OUTCOMES

Individuals who survive ARDS have significant morbidity and look on the clinicians to provide interventions to reduce the sequelae. Survivors experience exercise limitation, physical and psychological sequelae, decreased physical quality of life, and increased costs and use of health care services that may persist for 5 years or more (Mehta & Povoa, 2017). Interventions are aimed at identifying modifiable risk factors and addressing specific needs such as rehabilitation, nutrition, and support for caregivers.

Summary

ARDS is an acute process that can occur rapidly. Nursing vigilance can contribute to early identification and excellence in management to reduce morbidity and mortality. Prevention includes vaccination and other methods to reduce predisposing factors.

Ashbaugh, D. G., Bigelow, D. B., Petty, T. L., & Levine, B. E. (1967). Acute respiratory distress in adults. *Lancet, 12*(2), 319–323.

Fanelli, V., Vlachou, A., Ghannadian, S., Simonetti, U., Slutsky, A. S., & Zhang, H. (2013). Acute respiratory distress syndrome: New definition, current and future therapeutic options. *Journal of Thoracic Disease, 5*(3), 326–334.

Mehta, S., & Povoa, P. (2017). Long-term physical morbidity in ARDS survivors. *Intensive Care Medicine, 43*(1), 101–103.

Raneri, V. M., Rubenfeld, G. D., Thompson, B. T., Ferguson, N. D., Caldwell, E., Fan, E., . . . Slutsky, A. S.; ARDS Definition Task Force. (2012). ARDS definition task force: Acute respiratory syndrome: The Berlin definition. *Journal of the American Medical Association, 307*, 2526–2533.

Scholten, E. L., Beitler, J. R., Prisk, G. K., & Malhotra, A. (2017). Treatment of ARDS with prone positioning. *Chest, 151*(1), 215–224.

Sweeney, R. M., & McAuley, D. F. (2016). Acute respiratory distress syndrome. *Lancet, 388*(10058), 2416–2430.

Vidyasagar, S. (2016). Emerging concepts in acute respiratory distress syndrome: Implications for clinicians. *Journal of Clinical Science and Research, 5*, 202–204. doi:10.15380/22775706.JCSR.16.09.001

■ ACUTE RESPIRATORY FAILURE

Breanna Hetland

Overview

Acute respiratory failure (ARF) is characterized by a sudden onset of respiratory distress. It occurs when the lungs fail to maintain adequate exchange of oxygen and carbon dioxide to meet the body's metabolic needs. ARF is classified as either hypoxemic (insufficient oxygen) or hypercapnic (excessive carbon dioxide). It may result from inadequate air movement, insufficient gas diffusions in the alveoli, and/or poor pulmonary blood flow. Conditions, such as pneumonia, chronic obstructive pulmonary disease (COPD), acute respiratory distress syndrome (ARDS), and congestive heart failure (CHF), commonly lead to ARF (Fourneir, 2014; Peter, 2016; Rehder, Turi, & Cheifetz, 2014).

In the United States, the number of hospitalizations for ARF has increased to approximately 2 million each year. Although a reduction in inpatient mortality has been noted, ARF still carries an annual cost of more than $50 billion (Stefan et al., 2013). Due to the two different types of ARF, knowledge of the physiologic cause of ARF is crucial to selecting appropriate treatments. Targeted management of ARF is dependent on the extent and duration of symptoms, but nursing management should focus on providing symptom support until the underlying cause of ARF can be identified and treated (Fourneir, 2014; Peter, 2016; Rehder et al., 2014).

Background

Respiration, the act of inhaling and exhaling air to transport oxygen to the lung alveoli, includes (a) ventilation, (b) oxygenation, (c) perfusion, (d) ventilation/perfusion relationship. Ventilation, the movement of air in and out of the lungs through inspiration and expiration, is affected by airway compliance and airway resistance. Oxygenation involves the exchange of carbon dioxide and oxygen at the alveoli. Perfusion is the movement of blood through the pulmonary capillaries. The ventilation/perfusion relationship encompasses the balance between the amount of air reaching the alveoli (ventilation) and the amount of blood reaching the alveoli (perfusion). These processes involve the conducting airways (nose, pharynx, larynx, trachea, bronchi, bronchioles, and terminal bronchioles), alveoli (tiny sacs within the lungs where gas exchange occurs), pulmonary circulation (portion of the cardiovascular system that oxygenates the blood), and respiratory pump (thorax, respiratory musculature, and nervous system). They are regulated by neurological, chemical, and mechanical control systems within the body, and dysfunction in any of these control systems can lead to ARF (Fourneir, 2014; Peter, 2016; Rehder et al., 2014).

ARF is classified as hypoxemic, a lack of circulating oxygen in the blood characterized by an arterial oxygen concentration of PaO_2 less than 60 mmHg, or hypercapnic, an excess of circulating carbon dioxide in the blood, characterized by an atrial carbon dioxide concentration of $PaCO_2$ greater than 40mmHg. Hypoxemic ARF occurs in conditions that cause lung atelectasis and those that lead to fluid in the lungs such as pulmonary edema, pneumonia, alveolar hemorrhage, ARDS. Hypercapnic ARF happens when there is hypoperfusion of the respiratory muscles during shock states as well as when processes in the central nervous system (CNS), peripheral nerves, muscles, neuromuscular junction, or alveoli

malfunction. These conditions include: CNS depression (drug overdose, stroke), spinal cord infections or transection, peripheral nerve weakness (Guillain–Barré Syndrome), chest wall deformities, muscle weakness (myasthenia gravis, hypokalemia, hypophosphatemia), and alveolar hypoventilation (COPD, cystic fibrosis, airway obstruction, pulmonary fibrosis) (Fourneir, 2014; Peter, 2016; Rehder et al., 2014).

ARF is the most frequent reason for admission of hospitalized patients to the intensive care unit with 2.5% of cases requiring ventilatory support. ARF requires an average hospital length of stay of 7.1 days and results in more than 350,000 in-hospital deaths each year. The most common etiologies noted in hospitalized patients with ARF include: pneumonia, CHF, COPD, ARDS, asthma, drug ingestion, trauma, and sepsis. Mortality rates were highest in patients 85 years of age and older (Stefan et al., 2013). Patients with severe ARF requiring mechanical ventilation report a multitude of distressing symptoms, including anxiety, pain, delirium, and lack of sleep (Puntillo et al., 2010). In addition, after hospital discharge, patients report symptoms of posttraumatic stress disorder (PTSD) and rate their quality of life significantly lower than comparative controls (Bienvenu et al., 2013).

Clinical Aspects

ASSESSMENT

Clinical signs of acute respiratory distress are often nonspecific, but early detection through comprehensive nursing assessment can help prevent progression to ARF. Tachypnea and shortness of breath are often the first signs of respiratory distress. Clinical indications of worsening condition include nasal flaring, use of accessory muscles, paradoxical abdominal movements, prolonged expiratory phase, expiratory grunting, cyanosis, decrease in pulse oximetry despite increasing the administration of supplemental oxygen, anxiety, diminished lung sounds, inability to speak in full sentences, tripod positioning to further expand the chest, feelings of impending doom, and altered mental status. In addition to clinical presentation, pulse oximetry, arterial blood gasses, and capnography are important physiologic measurements to consider (Fourneir, 2014; Peter, 2016; Rehder et al., 2014).

The goals of treatment for ARF depend on its pathophysiologic cause, but should aim to treat the underlying cause of the respiratory failure, improve oxygen delivery to the tissues, decrease oxygen demand in the tissues, reduce the production of carbon dioxide, promote the elimination of carbon dioxide, and limit damaging therapies. Treatment of the underlying cause may include antibiotics (infection), steroids and bronchodilators (acute asthma, COPD), medications to reverse CNS or peripheral nerve problems that caused the respiratory failure (i.e., Narcan for a drug overdose). Oxygen delivery to the tissues can be enhanced by applying supplemental oxygen through low-flow devices, high-flow devices, or noninvasive or invasive mechanical ventilation. Ventilator support may be required for patients with severe or hypoxic respiratory failure with progressing respiratory fatigue. Extracorporeal life support may also be necessary to treat ARF when conventional ventilatory strategies are not sufficient. In addition to supplemental oxygen delivery, it is important to maintain hemoglobin and optimize cardiac output as well as reduce fever and control sepsis in order to decrease oxygen demand of the tissues (Fourneir, 2014; Peter, 2016; Rehder et al., 2014).

Carbon dioxide production can be reduced, controlling excess motor activity (anticonvulsants for seizures). The elimination of carbon dioxide can be promoted by increasing respiratory drive (reduce sedatives; give CNS stimulants) and improving lung mechanics. Upright positioning, analgesics for chest pain, bronchodilators and bronchial hygiene for airway resistance, and interventions to reduce abdominal distention can all improve lung mechanics. In addition, respiratory muscle performance can be enhanced by ensuring adequate oxygenation and tissue perfusion, correcting electrolyte abnormalities, and administering medications to improve diaphragmatic contractility. Special care should be given to limit therapies that may potentially damage lung tissue such as using high oxygen concentrations for protracted periods and failing to implement lung-protective ventilator strategies (Fourneir, 2014; Peter, 2016; Rehder et al., 2014).

NURSING INTERVENTIONS, MANAGEMENT, AND IMPLICATIONS

When caring for a patient with ARF, it is imperative to perform continuous assessments and provide appropriate symptom support measures to promote relaxation and facilitate oxygenation. Supplemental oxygen should be applied immediately and the airway must be evaluated for patency. The airway should be clear of secretions or mechanical obstructions and the head of bed upright. If a patient continues to decompensate,

an oral or nasal airway may be placed and mechanical ventilation applied. The need for mechanical ventilation should be assessed with attention to the clinical scenario, rate of clinical deterioration, and the patient's response to previously attempted therapies (Fourneir, 2014; Peter, 2016; Rehder et al., 2014).

OUTCOMES

Nurses must be aware of physiologic symptoms of inadequate tissue oxygenation, such as angina and mental status changes, as well as conditions that may impair oxygen delivery. It is important to turn the patient regularly to maintain the ventilation/perfusion relationship. Efforts to minimize and remove secretions in addition to liberal use of an incentive spirometer will maximize tissue oxygenation and help prevent atelectasis. Malnutrition can impair respiratory muscle function and reduce ventilator drive. Patients with ARF can easily become malnourished due to increased metabolic demands and inadequate nutrition intake, therefore nutritional expertise should be sought. Lastly, nurses should offer the patient and family pertinent education related to medications, the purpose of nursing measures, signs of clinical decompensation, patient risk factors, and appropriate follow-up (Fourneir, 2014; Peter, 2016; Rehder et al., 2014).

Summary

Treating ARF requires knowledge of the specific mechanisms that cause respiratory failure and a systematic approach to supportive symptom management. As the number of ARF cases continues to rise, nurses must be acutely aware of the signs, symptoms, and appropriate nursing interventions for ARF in order to reduce the morbidity and mortality related to ARF (Fourneir, 2014; Peter, 2016; Rehder et al., 2014).

Bienvenu, O. J., Gellar, J., Althouse, B. M., Colantuoni, E., Sricharoenchai, T., Mendez-Tellez, P. A., . . . Needham, D. M. (2013). Post-traumatic stress disorder symptoms after acute lung injury: A 2-year prospective longitudinal study. *Psychological Medicine, 43*(12), 2657–2671. doi:10.1017/S0033291713000214

Fourneir, M. (2014). Caring for patients in respiratory failure. *American Nurse Today, 9*(11), 18–23.

Peter, J. V. (2016). Acute respiratory failure. *Clinical Pathways in Emergency Medicine,* 167–178. Retrieved from https://link.springer.com/chapter/10.1007/978-81-322-2710-6_13/fulltext.html

Puntillo, K. A., Arai, S., Cohen, N. H., Gropper, M. A., Neuhaus, J., Paul, S. M., & Miaskowski, C. (2010). Symptoms experienced by intensive care unit patients at high risk of dying. *Critical Care Medicine, 38*(11), 2155–2160. doi:10.1097/CCM.0b013e3181f267ee

Rehder, K. J., Turi, J. L., & Cheifetz, I. M. (2014). Acute respiratory failure. *Pediatric Critical Care Medicine,* 401–411. Retrieved from https://link.springer.com/chapter/10.1007/978-1-4471-6362-6_31

Stefan, M. S., Shieh, M. S., Pekow, P. S., Rothberg, M. B., Steingrub, J. S., Lagu, T., & Lindenauer, P. K. (2013). Epidemiology and outcomes of acute respiratory failure in the United States, 2001 to 2009: A national survey. *Journal of Hospital Medicine, 8*(2), 76–82. doi:10.1002/jhm.2004

■ ADRENAL INSUFFICIENCY

Rachel K. Vanek

Overview

Adrenal insufficiency (AI) can be an acute or chronic illness affecting patients in the acute care, office, long-term care, or home care settings. It can either be a primary disorder due to destruction of the adrenal cortex or a secondary disorder due to disruption of hypothalamic–pituitary functions. Its signs and symptoms are a consequence of the failure of the hypothalamic–pituitary–adrenal axis (HPA) to secrete adequate amounts of essential hormones and of the adrenal gland to respond properly. It is a rare disease, often undiagnosed, thought to occur in one person in 100,000; it occurs equally in men and women in the United States. It is often an overlooked disorder that has myriad symptoms that mimic other acute and chronic illnesses (National Organization for Rare Disorders, 2017).

Background

The Endocrine Society's clinical practice guidelines define primary adrenal insufficiency as "the inability of the adrenal cortex to produce sufficient amounts of glucocorticoids and/or mineralocorticoids. It is a severe and potentially life-threatening condition due to the central role of these hormones in energy, salt, and fluid homeostasis" (Bornstein et al., 2016, p. 367).

This hypothalamic–pituitary–adrenal axis is essential for the regulation of homeostasis and an individual's stress response. Any alteration affecting a component of the HPA axis can lead to insufficient adrenal hormone secretion. Under physiologic conditions, the HPA axis is regulated by negative feedback control mechanisms. When there is insufficient circulating cortisol, the hypothalamus secretes corticotropin-releasing hormone, which stimulates the release of adrenocorticotropic hormone (ACTH) from the anterior pituitary. ACTH affects the cortex of the adrenal gland to stimulate the secretion of cortisol until there is an adequate concentration of circulating cortisol to maintain homeostasis (Charmandari, Nicolaides, & Chrousos, 2014.)

In primary AI, the adrenal cortex is either destroyed or does not function properly. This can be caused by infiltrative disease destroying the adrenal cortex. Bleeding into the adrenal gland, systemic fungal or bacterial infection, HIV infection, tuberculosis, autoimmune disease, metastatic disease, and amyloidosis can result in adrenal destruction. Secondary AI occurs when damage to the hypothalamus or pituitary gland occurs. Surgery to remove the pituitary, radiation to the pituitary, tumors of the hypothalamus, metastatic disease involving the pituitary or hypothalamus, chronic systemic steroid use, and pituitary necrosis are some examples of pathological states that can lead to the development of secondary deficiency of adrenal hormones. These disorders can be seen in pediatric and adult populations (Oelkers, 1996).

AI can have vague and insidious symptoms and signs. They often overlap with symptoms of other disorders and can be difficult to characterize as caused by AI alone. In general, AI symptoms impact quality of life by rendering the patient at baseline tired, weak, dizzy from orthostasis, anorexic, and depressed. The patient can have skin changes, constipation, diarrhea, loss of libido, arthralgia, myalgia, and electrolyte disturbances. Acutely, the patient can have fever, abdominal pain, mental status changes, encephalopathy, delirium, and shock. Refractory hypotension can lead to multisystem organ dysfunction and failure (Bornstein et al., 2016).

Clinical Aspects

ASSESSMENT

History of the patient or family may reflect fatigue, loss of energy, perhaps recent infection, or pregnancy. Heat or cold intolerance can also be a common complaint. Recent changes in appetite, bowel habits, or abdominal pain are common. Dizziness is often a trigger prompting patients to seek medical care. Physical exam may reveal patients with evidence of recent weight loss. Their skin may be very dry or have changes in pigmentation, such as hyperpigmentation in areas of skin exposed to the sun or constant friction (think "waistband, socks"). Blood pressure and heart rate should be checked with the patient sitting and standing to evaluate orthostasis. Mucous membranes may be dry and appear dusky in color. Patients may have loss of axillary or pubic hair (Bornstein et al., 2016).

Laboratory findings may reveal hyponatremia, hypoglycemia, and hyperkalemia. Chloride may also be elevated. Elevated blood urea nitrogen and creatinine due to dehydration may also be noticed. Hemoglobin usually is normal but in up to 15% of the patients with AI normocytic anemia may occur. An early-morning cortisol level may be collected and, if it is less than 10, AI should be considered (Oelkers, 1996).

An ACTH stimulation test may also be done. In this test, the patient's baseline cortisol is measured. The patient is then given a dose of intravenous ACTH and cortisol is checked at 30 and 60 minutes. If the levels increase above 20 mcg/mL, then adrenal function is normal. Plasma ACTH, renin, or aldosterone levels may be measured as well in patients who are not in extremis. Laboratory studies to rule out autoimmune disease may also be ordered. Abdominal CT can be performed to evaluate for disruptions in adrenal anatomy. The test can identify enlarged, calcified, or acute hemorrhage in the adrenal glands (Oelkers, 1996).

NURSING INTERVENTIONS, MANAGEMENT, AND IMPLICATIONS

Risk for falls and risk for injury may be related to volume depletion. Oftentimes, changing position slowly and allowing time for equilibration lessens this risk while the disorder is being evaluated. Once treatment has commenced, orthostatic changes should improve.

Ongoing monitoring of orthostatic blood pressure and pulse helps assess response. Assessing adequate oral hydration and administering any ordered intravenous fluids while monitoring for signs of fluid overload are within the nursing realm. Proper administration of glucocorticoid and mineralocorticoid is key to treatment. The patient must be taught signs of symptoms of treatment failure, how and when to take medications, and what symptoms to report to the health care provider (National Organization for rare disorders, 2017).

Weight loss and poor appetite are key signs of nutritional imbalance and should begin to improve with treatment. Weighing patients, assessing for weight loss, and appetite changes are part of the ongoing nursing assessment. The patient may have a knowledge deficiency of AI as a new diagnosis or even as a previously existing problem (The Complete List of NANDA Nursing Diagnosis for 2012–2014, with 16 New Diagnoses, 2014. The nurse should assess the patient's knowledge and provide education for a positive outcome. Key education requirements for patients are proper medication management, when to call the provider, side effects, and warning signs of infection. Patients must be taught to keep an up-to-date medication list for all providers who participate in their care. Informing other providers of the diagnosis of AI will allow proper treatment during surgery or other interventions that can precipitate an adrenal crisis. Patients and their caregivers need to recognize signs of adrenal crisis and know what to do to intervene (Charmandari et al., 2014).

OUTCOMES

Nurses should be astute to the subtle signs of renal insufficiency (RI) on laboratory analysis to help identify the patient with RI and help to prevent progression to kidney injury and chronic failure. These signs may not be apparent but the nurse can use measures that encourage RI from occurring or progressing through hydration, avoidance of renal damaging medication administration, and diet. These measures can promote positive outcomes.

Summary

AI is a rare disorder that can lead to life-threatening symptoms related to the actions of the HPA axis, the most severe being refractory hypotension leading to organ damage. Nursing actions and management are key to establishing proper diagnosis and supporting recovery. Proper administration and timing of diagnostic tests are essential. Restoration of volume and correction of electrolyte disturbances facilitate resumption of life activities and improved satisfaction with the improved quality of life. Teaching the patients and their caregivers about the diagnosis, treatment aims, medications actions, and warning signs of failing treatment are all essential to positive outcomes.

Bornstein S. R., Allolio B., Arlt W., Barthel A., Don-Wauchope A., Hammer G. D., . . . Tory D. J. (2016). Diagnosis and treatment of primary adrenal insufficiency: An Endocrine Society clinical practice guideline. *Journal of Clinical Endocrinology and Metabolism*, 101(2), 364–389.

Charmandari E., Nicolaides N. C., & Chrousos G. P. (2014). Adrenal insufficiency. *Lancet, 383*(9935), 2152–2167.

The Complete list of NANDA nursing diagnoses for 2012–2014, with 16 new diagnoses. (2014). Retrieved from http://www.kc-courses.com/fundamentals/week2 process/nanda2012.pdf

National Organization for Rare Disorders. (2015). Addison's disease. Retrieved from https://rarediseases.org/rare -diseases/addisons-disease

Oelkers, W. (1996). Adrenal insufficiency. *New England Journal of Medicine, 335*(16), 1206–1212.

■ BACK PAIN

Sharon R. Rainer

Overview

Back pain is one of the most common conditions for which patients seek medical treatment from a health care professional. Most people older than 18 years experience at least one episode of acute low-back pain (ALBP) during a lifetime. According to data from the National Electronic Injury Surveillance System, the incidence of back pain is 139 per 100,000 person-years in the United States. According to the Centers for Disease Control and Prevention's (CDC) National Center for Health Statistics (NCHS), 28.4% of adults older than 18 years had experienced lower back pain in the previous 3 months (Ma, Chan, & Carruthers, 2014). In addition, approximately 6 million people annually are evaluated in emergency departments (EDs) for back pain (Perina, 2017).

Back pain is costly to treat and manage. Along with high incidence and prevalence, back pain is the third most costly medical condition followed by cancer and heart disease (Perina, 2017). The cost of treatment increases considerably with chronicity. The economic impact of chronic low-back pain (CLBP) includes decreased function and mobility that results in lost productivity, high treatment costs, and disability payments. Chronic back pain (CBP) is the most common cause of disability in Americans younger than 45 years (Allen & Hulbert, 2009). Each year, 3% to 4% of the U.S. population is temporarily disabled, and 1% of the working-age population is totally and permanently disabled due to back pain (Ma et al., 2014). Low-back pain (LBP) is the second most frequent reason to visit an outpatient office, the fifth most common cause for hospitalization, and the third most frequent reason for a surgical procedure (Wheeler & Berman, 2016). Estimates of the cost of back pain treatment and management have reached $100 to $200 billion annually (Allen & Hulbert, 2009, p. 1067; Ma et al., 2014, p. 4).

Background

ALBP is defined as pain with duration of less than 6 weeks in the posterior area between the costal angles and gluteal folds (Kinkade, 2007). Typically, in adults, the first episode of LBP will occur between the ages of 20 and 40 and resolve within 6 to 12 weeks (Kinkade, 2007). Episodes of LBP may be nonspecific in nature or may be the result of an underlying illness or injury. Most acute episodes of musculoskeletal LBP are self-limited and resolve quickly requiring minimal interventions. Typically, strains and sprains of the back are described as nonspecific. However, pain associated with the condition can be moderate to severe and in some cases debilitating, causing the patient limited activity and mobility and lost time from work. Moreover, within 1 to 2 years, recurrent back pain occurs in approximately 25% to 62% of patients (Casazza, 2012).

Pain that persists longer than 3 months is defined as CLBP (Allen & Hulbert, 2009, p. 1067). As with ALBP, CLBP can be related to an underlying chronic condition. Sometimes, the underlying chronic condition may be serious in nature and therefore patients warrant a careful clinical evaluation. In many cases, CLBP impacts a patient's quality of life. It is common for psychosocial issues to play a role in treatment of patients with CLBP. Patients with chronic, persistent pain that is not well controlled may experience clinical, psychological, and social problems associated with chronic pain. The consequences of unrelieved pain include limitations in daily activities, lost work productivity, reduced quality of life, and stigma (Dowell, Haegerich, & Chou, 2016). Patients with CLBP may also experience a reduced sense of control, disturbed mood, negative self-efficacy, anxiety, and other mental health disorders (Last & Hulbert, 2009), including opioid use disorder (Dowell et al., 2016). Opioids are commonly prescribed to patients with CLBP in spite of a lack of evidence to support the efficacy of these medications. In fact, opioids are commonly prescribed for adults with both acute and chronic pain. An estimated 20% of patients seen by a primary care provider with noncancer pain will obtain an opioid prescription (Dowell et al., 2016).

Clinical Aspects

ASSESSMENT

A careful and accurate focused health history and physical examination are essential for all patients experiencing back pain. A thorough evaluation of a patient's symptoms by a clinician is essential to identify potentially serious underlying causes of back pain. Generally, back pain can be placed into four broad categories. They are nonspecific LBP, including sprains/strains; pain associated with radiculopathy or spinal stenosis (spine related); referred pain from a nonspinal source such as aortic aneurysm, gynecologic, or renal conditions; and pain associated with another cause such as cancer, arthritis, or infection (Last & Hulbert, 2009).

Although back pain associated with a serious underlying pathology is rare, health care providers (HCPs) are obligated to assess patients for "red flags," which are symptoms that raise clinical suspicion of a serious underlying etiology (Casazza, 2012). Red flags will prompt a clinician to investigate further, initiate aggressive treatment, and/or make a referral to the ED or spine specialist. Examples of chief complaints involving LBP that raise clinical suspicion about serious red flags include significant trauma such as motor vehicle crash, falls in the elderly, falls from significant heights in younger patients, and heavy lifting in patients with osteoporosis (Casazza, 2012).

Likewise, patients with back pain need to be assessed for the presence or absence of sciatica indicating a mechanical spinal condition, which in some cases may be serious, and indicates a need for a specialist referral. Sciatica or sciatic neuralgia is defined as pain in the distribution of the sciatic nerve often associated with a lumbar herniated disc (Stafford, Peng, & Hill, 2007). It is important to differentiate between leg pain and sciatica that involves pain traveling below the knee. Neurological symptoms, including progressive motor or sensory deficits in the extremities, raise serious concerns and may indicate the need for urgent surgical intervention. Patients need to be assessed quickly for signs of cauda equina syndrome (CES). CES is a rare but serious condition that results from pressure and swelling of the nerves at the end of the spinal cord. CES is a medical emergency requiring urgent surgical intervention to relieve pressure of the spinal nerves (Spector, Madigan, Rhyne, Darden, & Kim, 2008). Without emergency intervention, patients with CES may experience adverse results, including paralysis, impaired bladder and/or bowel control, difficulty walking, and/or other neurological and physical problems. Although CES is an uncommon condition, it is important that patients are screened quickly for signs of the disorder. Signs and symptoms include bowel and bladder dysfunction or urinary retention, loss of anal sphincter tone, saddle anesthesia, progressive leg weakness, bilateral sciatica, or numbness in the legs. Decreased rectal tone may be a relatively late finding. Early signs and symptoms of a developing postoperative CES are often attributed to common postoperative findings. Therefore, HCPs in the perioperative setting are urged to have a high level of suspicion of potential CES in postoperative spine patients with back and/or leg pain refractory to analgesia, especially with urinary retention (Spector et al., 2008).

Additional assessment of the patient with back pain includes a thorough history of any cancer that may have metastasized to bone and risk factors for suspected spinal infections. Spinal infections are of high clinical suspicion in patients injecting intravenous (IV) drugs such as heroin and crack cocaine. A complete health history must also specifically include questions about bone health (osteoporosis, arthritis, prior fractures, or injuries), fever, weight loss, and any prior imaging to help determine whether any underlying cause can be identified (Wheeler & Berman, 2016).

The goal of a focused history and physical examination is to help clinicians stratify patients into back pain categories—nonspecific, spine related, referred from nonspine source, or other causes as described previously. Clinicians are obligated to identify and treat the cause of back pain. One important test to help identify a possible herniated disc is the straight leg raise (SLR). The SLR is a screening test used by clinicians to detect a herniated lumbar disk and it has high sensitivity and moderate specificity (Perina, 2017). The test is performed with the patient sitting or lying; however, the supine position is preferred. The knee is kept extended while the clinician raises one leg at a time to assess for pain in the posterior leg radiating below the knee caused by irritation or inflammation of the sciatic nerve. The SLR test is positive only when the maneuver elicits pain that radiates to below the knee. It is not considered a positive test, indicating a possible herniated disc, if the pain remains localized in the back or there is pain in the hamstrings when the leg is raised. In addition to the SLR, the patient should have strength and reflexes in the lower extremities assessed as part of a thorough physical examination. The basic examination of a patient with back pain includes observation of movement and palpation of the spine for tenderness, range of motion of the back and extremities; SLR; and neurological examination, including deep tendon reflexes, muscle strength, and sensation in the lower extremities.

NURSING INTERVENTIONS, MANAGEMENT, AND IMPLICATIONS

Providing nursing care to patients with back pain can be challenging across all settings. The aim of treatment for LBP is to provide adequate pain care and improve function, reduce time away from work or activities, and develop coping strategies in the event of chronic, persistent pain or surgical intervention (Casazza, 2012). Most often, clinicians will not order imaging, such as radiographs, for patients presenting with back pain in the absence of trauma and red-flag symptoms. If the clinician suspects a serious underlying condition, he or she will order an MRI, which is the study of choice. CT is an alternative diagnostic test when MRI is contraindicated or unavailable. Radiography may be helpful to screen for serious conditions but usually has little diagnostic value. If spinal infection is suspected, the clinician may order laboratory tests. These tests would likely include a complete blood count with differential, erythrocyte sedimentation rate (ESR), and C-reactive protein (CRP) level. In the case of nonspecific LBP, clinicians will not typically order any laboratory testing or imaging; however, in some cases of LBP that are not clearly musculoskeletal, a urinalysis may be useful. Other laboratory studies are rarely needed unless the clinician strongly suspects a disorder other than back pain (Kinkade, 2007).

Treatment of back pain depends on the suspected underlying cause. Generally, patients with back pain are treated conservatively and surgical referral is a last resort. Treatment for CBP encompasses conservative management with both pharmacological and nonpharmacological pain care. Remaining active with exercise and physical therapy may be beneficial for patients with CLBP (Perina, 2017). Recommended first-line treatment for nonspecific back pain includes nonsteroidal anti-inflammatory drugs (NSAIDs) and acetaminophen. There is conflicting evidence about NSAIDs being more effective than acetaminophen in the treatment of ALBP. Used by patients in recommended dosages, acetaminophen can be a helpful adjunct that avoids the renal and gastrointestinal toxicities of NSAIDs (Perina, 2017). This is a particularly important consideration for the treatment of back pain in older adults who are at higher risk for adverse drug reactions. For patients experiencing sciatica, opioids may be required to control pain when first-line medications fail. Tramadol (Ultram) is an analgesic that has weak opioid and serotonin–norepinephrine-reuptake inhibitor (SNRI) activity. Studies show some short-term improvements in pain and function with Tramadol but there is a lack of evidence to support long-term use in chronic pain sufferers. Opioids should be considered a second- or third-line analgesic for a short period of time. It is important to note that studies have shown no

significant advantage of opioid use in symptom relief or return to work when compared with NSAIDs or acetaminophen (Kinkade, 2007).

Muscle relaxants are another class of drugs that may be prescribed in the treatment of back pain. Patients may be prescribed cyclobenzaprine (Flexeril) in the first 1 to 2 weeks of treatment. There is some evidence that suggest skeletal muscle relaxants lead to better relief of symptoms when used with NSAIDs. However, studies do not show benefit of long-term use of muscle relaxants to treat CBP. The use of benzodiazepines and carisoprodol (Soma) carries risk of dependency. Clinicians will often refer people with CLBP to pain management and/or a spine specialist.

Nurses are an important and integral part of the interprofessional team involved in the care of patients with LBP. Often, nurses have a significant impact on a patient's ability to self-manage their pain. Education around self-management is important to help prevent back pain relapses and in managing pain that lasts longer than 3 months. Patient education that has shown to have some benefit in preventing CLBP includes exercise and activity, promoting weight loss where indicated, increasing overall physical conditioning, recognizing and avoiding aggravating factors, the natural history of the disease, and expected time frame for improvement in pain and function (Kinkade, 2007; Perina, 2017).

OUTCOMES

Back pain relapses are common and the socioeconomic burden of CBP is sizable. Therefore, efforts to prevent relapse and reduce the incidence of chronic pain are of great importance in addressing quality of care and improved outcomes for patients with back pain. Strategies aimed at preventing injuries that cause initial back pain episodes and preventing CBP improve outcomes. The U.S. Preventive Services Task Force (USPSTF) and the COST B13 Working Group on European Guidelines for Prevention in LBP have synthesized the evidence for treatment and management of back pain. Of note, back belts that patients may commonly wear, especially in occupations with heavy lifting, have not been proven to prevent back injuries. An interprofessional approach to treating and managing back pain will improve outcomes. Patients have access to an enormous amount of information on the Internet about back pain treatments. HCPs must be ready to discuss evidence-based approaches to prevention, treatment, and management. In addition to physical therapy, massage and yoga therapy may be treatments patients inquire about and want to try. There is insufficient evidence to recommend for or against massage therapy for ALBP (Casazza, 2012). Yet, for chronic pain, it may be helpful. Moreover, one form of yoga has been shown to have benefit. A therapeutic form of yoga, Viniyoga, may provide relief to CBP. Research has shown that a 6-week course of yoga decreased medication use and provided more pain relief than exercise and self-care strategies for nonspecific back pain (Last & Hulbert, 2009). Clinicians who are aware of these and other therapies will help patients make informed decisions and engage them in shared decision making about their care.

Summary

The evaluation and treatment of back pain occurs along a continuum in most cases from the initial treatment aimed at alleviating the pain associated with an acute episode to improving pain and function with adequate pain care for patients experiencing CBP. It is important for HCPs in all settings to thoroughly assess patient's back pain even if the pain is chronic. There are a variety of causes of back pain and some may be serious requiring immediate intervention. It is also important to document and openly discuss patient expectations about pain care, self-care, alternative therapies, and return to their previous level of activity. Discussing and documenting goals and expectations at each encounter helps to provide continuity of care. HCPs must be vigilant in helping patients understand prevention strategies for back pain and how to recognize red flags that require urgent intervention.

Allen, A. R., & Hulbert, K. (2009). CLBP: Evaluation and management. *American Family Physician*, 79(12), 1067–1074.

Casazza, B. A. (2012). Diagnosis and treatment of ALBP. *American Academy of Family Physicians*, 85(4), 343–350.

Dowell, D., Haegerich, T. M., & Chou, R. (2016). CDC guideline for prescribing opioids for chronic pain—United States. *Journal of the American Medical Association*, 315(15), 1624. doi:10.1001/jama.2016.1464

Kincade, S. (2007). Evaluation and treatment of acute low back pain. *American Family Physician*, 75(8), 1181–1188.

Last, A. R., & Hulbert, K. (2009). CLBP: Evaluation and management. *American Family Physician*, 79(12), 1067–1074.

Ma, V. Y., Chan, L., & Carruthers, K. J. (2014). Incidence, prevalence, costs, and impact on disability of common conditions requiring rehabilitation in the United States: Stroke, spinal cord injury, traumatic brain injury, multiple sclerosis, osteoarthritis, rheumatoid arthritis, limb loss, and back pain. *Archives of Physical Medicine and Rehabilitation*, 95(5), 986–995. doi:10.1016/j.apmr.2013.10.032

Perina, D. G. (2017). Mechanical back pain. *Medscape*. Retrieved from http://emedicine.medscapre.com/article/822462-guidelines

Spector, L. R., Madigan, L., Rhyne, A., Darden, B., & Kim, D. (2008). Cauda equina syndrome. *Journal of the American Academy of Orthopaedic Surgeons*, 16(8), 471–479.

Stafford, M. A., Peng, P., & Hill, D. A. (2007). Sciatica: A review of history, epidemiology, pathogenesis, and the role of epidural steroid injection in management. *British Journal of Anaesthesia*, 99(4), 461–473. doi:10.1093/bja/aem238

Wheeler, A. H., & Berman, S. A. (2016). LBP and sciatica: Overview, pathophysiology, characteristics of pain-sensitive structures. *Medscape*. Retrieved from http://emedicine.medscape.com/article/1144130-overview

■ BURNS

Margaret Jean Carman

Overview

Burns is a traumatic tissue injury resulting from the application of thermal, electrical, chemical, or radiation sources to the body. The epithelial layers serve to promote temperature and fluid regulation, protect the body from infection, and provide ongoing sensory input from the environment. Significant injury results in a massive inflammatory response, with capillary leakage and fluid and electrolyte losses from the vascular space. Untreated hypovolemic shock and inhalation injuries often lead to an early death, whereas delayed deaths from burns occur chiefly because of infection. Nursing care of the individual with burn injuries extends across a trajectory from resuscitation to recovery and rehabilitation to promote a functional and emotionally secure future.

Background

Burn injuries lead to more than 3,000 deaths across the United States and 265,000 globally each year (American Burn Association [ABA], 2016; World Health Organization [WHO], 2016). The majority of fatalities result from residential fires, making primary prevention an important aspect of the nursing role. Sixty percent of the individuals requiring hospital admission are transferred to one of the 128 burn centers in the United States. Early identification of patients who meet the criteria for transfer is essential. Criteria include greater than 10% total body surface area (TBSA) burns in patients younger than 10 or older than 50 years of age, or more than 20% TBSA in people between 10 years and 50 years; full-thickness burns on more than 5% of the TBSA at any age; significant electrical burns, including lightning injuries; significant chemical burns; inhalation injuries, and burns occurring in an individual with significant comorbidities that may complicate treatment or recovery (ABA, 2016).

The vast majority of burn injuries involve thermal injury (77%), followed by chemical or contact (11%) and electrical (3%) etiologies (ABA, 2016). The acute phase of injury includes rapid assessment and initial resuscitation to prevent burn shock, although the ongoing care is focused on prevention and treatment of infection and promoting restoration of normal physiological function.

Burn injuries are a global problem. The risk of injury is greatest in underdeveloped countries, in populations of lower socioeconomic standing. Adult women and children aged 1 year to 9 years are most susceptible to injury, which can often be linked to environmental or behavioral factors. Open-fire cooking or lack of industrial standards in some countries increases the exposure to potential toxins or thermal hazards, increasing the risk of injury. Adequate supervision of children and injury prevention are key to decreasing the incidence of burns, particularly in middle and lower income countries (WHO, 2016). Behavioral factors, such as substance abuse, alcoholism, and tobacco abuse, are major contributors to the incidence of burns and may play a role in the mechanism of injury (WHO, 2016).

Clinical Aspects

Initial burn care includes actions to stop the burning process. For thermal injuries, cool water or moisten gauze saline should be used. Ice or cold water are avoided to prevent hypothermia or further damage to the injured tissue. Constricting items or those that may continue to convey heat should be immediately removed.

For patients with chemical or radiation injuries, consider consultation with a poison control center before decontamination. Chemicals remaining on the skin may compromise the safety of the providers and should be brushed off, as the use of water may activate the offending agent. Secure any information available on the substance and communicate this, to ensure that appropriate decontamination of chemical or radiation exposures can be executed.

ASSESSMENT

Rapid assessment, stabilization, and transfer to a designated burn center (if appropriate) are the initial priorities. The patient should be immediately assessed for associated trauma or inhalation injuries, which can cause rapid decompensation and loss of airway patency. Blast injuries or burns occurring in a confined space are at risk for inhalation injury; carbonaceous sputum or particles in the oropharynx, involvement of the face or neck, singed facial hair (including eyebrows and nasal hair), altered mentation, increased work of breathing, or hoarseness indicate airway compromise and the possible need for proactive intubation (American College of Surgeons Committee on Trauma).

Exposure to vaporized agents in the burning environment may result in carbon monoxide (CO) poisoning; clinical signs include a headache, nausea, and confusion. The classic finding of cherry-red skin discoloration is uncommon and not a reliable clinical indicator of CO poisoning; pulse oximetry is also unreliable, given that CO displaces oxygen from binding with the hemoglobin molecule, affecting saturation readings (Bozeman, Myers, & Barish, 1997). Other inhaled agents, such as cyanide, are commonly found in household items and should be considered for potential poisonous exposure.

Determination of the wound depth and TBSA burned are used to calculate fluid resuscitation and patient management. Superficial (first degree) burns affect two to three layers of the epidermis and are not included in the determination of TBSA. Superficial burns are painful and have pink or red coloration with no blistering. Partial-thickness (second degree) burns extend through the epidermis and into the dermal layer, affecting local vascular and nerve structures. These wounds may be further described as deep-partial-thickness burns and may result in the need for skin grafting. Partial-thickness burns result in the formation of blisters or bullae because of the leakage of plasma, swelling, and red discoloration, with severe pain. The remaining blood supply allows for blanching of the skin surface to pressure. Deep-partial-thickness injuries may progress to full thickness, particularly if the wound becomes infected. Secondary injury from tissue ischemia and the inflammatory response results in this further tissue loss.

Full-thickness injuries extend through the dermal layer, causing coagulation of blood vessels and destruction of deep structures, including hair follicles, sweat glands, and nerves. This increases the risk for thermal deregulation, infection, and massive fluid and electrolyte losses, leading to hypovolemic shock. Full-thickness injuries have a leathery, white, or waxy appearance because of the loss of vascularity, termed *eschar*. The wounds do not blanch to pressure, and while cutaneous sensation is lost, severe pain may be experienced because of inflammation in the adjacent, viable tissue. Circumferential injuries should be noted, as these may require fasciotomy to preserve circulation.

TBSA may be assessed using several well-validated tools, including the rule of nines or rule of palms. Although these tools provide an easy and rapid means for estimation, the Lund and Browder method provides increased accuracy and accounts for developmental age (Shariati & Mirhaghi, 2014). It is important to recognize that no tool provides an exact measurement. Digital, computer-based technologies will likely become the future standard of care to better determine the extent of the injury (Zuo, Medina, & Tredget, 2017).

NURSING INTERVENTIONS, MANAGEMENT, AND IMPLICATIONS

Fluid losses because of a burn injury can lead to massive dehydration, shock, and electrolyte abnormalities. Patients with more than 20% TBSA require fluid resuscitation over the first 24 hours post-injury (American College of Surgeons Committee on Trauma, 2008). The Parkland or modified Brooke formulas are most commonly used to calculate volume requirements, based on TBSA and patient weight. Crystalloid replacement is the initial standard for fluid resuscitation, with lactated Ringer's solution most commonly given to prevent metabolic acidosis. Albumin may be included in the resuscitation of certain patient populations and is often used to maintain colloidal pressures in the vascular space (ABA, 2011; Serio-Melvin et al., 2017; Wang et al., 2014).

Traditional methods for the estimation of fluid requirements can lead to overresuscitation or "fluid creep," resulting in increased morbidity and mortality from burn injuries. Complications include compartment syndromes, respiratory failure, and ocular hypertension (Pruitt, 2000; Saffle, 2016). Protocols for adjustment of fluid resuscitation are beneficial for prevention as compared to standard formulas (Cancio, Salinas, & Kramer, 2016). Urine output is an important measure of successful fluid replacement and is used to guide ongoing fluid administration. The standard goal for urine output is 0.5 to 1.0 mL/kg/hr, whereas evidence supports a more liberal target of 0.25 to 0.5 mL/kg/hr (Cancio et al., 2016).

The extent of electrical injuries may not be evident on assessment. Cardiac monitoring should be instituted, and the patient observed for cardiac dysrhythmias. Entrance and exit wounds may be visible as electrical current typically flows to the ground; the patient may display delayed appearance of tissue necrosis along this path. Rhabdomyolysis is common in burns, and more so with electrical injury (Coban, 2014).

Analgesia is critical to the nursing care of the burn patient. Intramuscular medications should be avoided initially to avoid sequestration in the peripheral tissues, because of impaired circulation and the risk for delayed mobilization, leading to potential overdose. Opioid medications are appropriate to treat acute pain, and nonsteroidal anti-inflammatory drugs are used for pain as well as limiting the severity of the inflammatory reaction.

Normal stress responses may lead to paralytic ileus or curling ulcer; gastrointestinal prophylaxis should be instituted for the critically ill, although adequate nutrition via enteral or parenteral routes should be considered early on to promote healing.

Infection is the most common cause of delayed death following a burn injury. Tetanus immunization status should be assessed early on (ABA, 2011). Wound management, including excision of eschar, skin grafting, or the use of biologic skin substitutes provides some degree of prevention (ABA, 2016; Israel, Greenhalgh, & Gibson, 2017). Antimicrobial dressings include silver or antibiotic-based preparations. Systemic antimicrobials are often required for bacterial or fungal infections. As recovery can be a long process in severe burns, the risk of developing antibiotic resistance is substantial.

Preservation or restoration of mobility and function through splinting and regular repositioning begin from the time of admission. Collaboration with physical and occupational therapy is the key. Compression devices, such as ACE wraps and customized garments to promote venous return and limit keloid formation can impact cosmetic appearance, lymphatic drainage, and range of motion.

Nursing care should include an ongoing assessment for signs of depression, posttraumatic stress disorder (PTSD), and other effects of altered body image. Patients experience a wide range of emotions ranging from depression to resilience (Kool, Geenen, Egberts, Wanders, & Van Loey, 2017). Attendance to the emotional aspects of burn injury and recovery can affect the patient's trajectory and quality of life for many years.

Summary

Burn injuries represent trauma to the largest and one of the most multifunctional organs of the body. Loss of skin integrity affects nearly every system in the body, rapidly leading to shock and death unless treated appropriately. Nursing care of the burn victim requires timely and effective intervention to maintain and restore thermal regulation, offer resistance from infection, attain fluid and electrolyte balance, and to address the physiological and emotional complications of injury. Although injury management is the most obvious role for nursing, primary prevention and community education should remain a priority for the professional nurse.

American Burn Association. (2011). Advanced burn life support (ABLS) provider course manual. Retrieved from https://evidencebasedpractice.osumc.edu/Documents/Guidelines/ABLSProviderManual_20101018.pdf

American College of Surgeons Committee on Trauma. (2008). *Advanced trauma life support for doctors: ATLS student course manual* (8th ed.). Chicago, IL: American College of Surgeons.

Bozeman, W. P., Myers, R. A., & Barish, R. A. (1997). Confirmation of the pulse oximetry gap in carbon monoxide poisoning. *Annals of Emergency Medicine, 30*(5), 608–611.

Cancio, L. C., Salinas, J., & Kramer, G. C. (2016). Protocolized resuscitation of burn patients. *Critical Care Clinics, 32*(4), 599–610.

Coban, Y. K. (2014). Rhabdomyolysis, compartment syndrome and thermal injury. *World Journal of Critical Care Medicine, 3*(1), 1–7.

Israel, J. S., Greenhalgh, D. G., & Gibson, A. L. (2017). Variations in burn excision and grafting: A survey of the American Burn Association. *Journal of Burn Care & Research, 38*(1), e125–e132.

Kool, M. B., Geenen, R., Egberts, M. R., Wanders, H., & Van Loey, N. E. (2017). Patients' perspectives on quality of life after burn. *Burns*, S0305–4179(16), 30497-1. doi:10.1016/j.burns.2016.11.016

Pruitt, B. A. (2000). Protection from excessive resuscitation: "Pushing the pendulum back." *Journal of Trauma, 49*(3), 567–568.

Saffle, J. (2016). Fluid creep and over-resuscitation. *Critical Care Clinics, 32*(4), 587–598. doi:10.1016/j.cc.c.2016.06.007

Serio-Melvin, M. L., Salinas, J., Chung, K. K., Collins, C., Graybill, J. C., Harrington, D. T., . . . Cancio, L. C. (2017). Burn shock and resuscitation: Proceedings of a symposium conducted at the meeting of the American Burn Association, Chicago, IL, 21 April 2015. *Journal of Burn Care & Research, 38*(1), e423–e431.

Shariati, S. M., & Mirhaghi, A. (2014). A comparison of burn size estimation methods' accuracy applied by medical students. *Future of Medical Education Journal, 8*(4), 36–40.

Wang, C. H., Hsieh, W. H., Chou, H. C., Huang, Y. S., Shen, J. H., Yeo, Y. H., . . . Lee, C. C. (2014). Liberal versus restricted fluid resuscitation strategies in trauma patients: A systematic review and meta-analysis of randomized controlled trials and observational studies. *Critical Care Medicine, 42*(4), 954–961.

World Health Organization. (2016). Burns. Retrieved from http://www.who.int/mediacentre/factsheets/fs365/en

Zuo, K. J., Medina, A., & Tredget, E. E. (2017). Important developments in burn care. *Plastic and Reconstructive Surgery, 139*(1), 120e–138e.

■ BURNS: CLASSIFICATION AND SEVERITY

Melanie Gibbons Hallman
Lamon Norton

Overview

Burns result from thermal, electrical, chemical, mechanical, or radioactive injury to tissues. The extent of burn depth varies from superficial, involving the epidermis, to deeper structures, including muscle, bone, and organs, particularly the lungs (Stavrou et al., 2014). The cardiovascular and nervous systems are significantly impacted by electrical and lightning insults, potentially resulting in immediate cardiac or respiratory arrest (Moore, 2015b). Each year, more than 265,000 deaths occur worldwide related to burns, producing life-altering changes for victims and their families (Zuo, Medina, & Tredget, 2017). Serious burns result in a cascade of physiological responses that can influence morbidity and mortality for affected patients (Jewo & Fadeyibi, 2015).

Background

Annually, more than 500,000 people in the United States are evaluated in emergency departments for burns. Forty thousand people are hospitalized and an estimated 3,400 victims die (Rowan et al., 2015). Burn risk is highest in children. Younger children are more likely to sustain scald burns, whereas children older than 6 years of age are more likely to experience burns from flames. The length of time that tissues are exposed to a burn source, the intensity of the source, and skin thickness determine the degree of burn (Rau, Spears, & Petruska, 2014).

The most common etiologies of burns are thermal (flame, steam, scalds), electrical (alternating current [AC] and direct current [DC], lightning), and chemical (alkaline and acid). Burns impart injury by damaging skin surfaces, by impairing airways and lungs via inhalation burns, and by ingesting chemicals or objects capable of causing mucosal burns. Multiple organs, tissues, and body systems are susceptible to burns as primary or secondary injuries. Complications of burn shock, infection, respiratory compromise, and multisystem organ failure may result in death (Stavrou et al., 2014). Prevention or rapid correction of these complications is essential to achieving desirable outcomes for burn victims.

Thermal burns may directly affect only the epidermis and dermis, or may involve deeper structures of fat, muscle, and bone. The extent of injury caused by electrical burns is determined by the type of electrical current, either low voltage (less than 1,000 volts) or high voltage (more than 1,000 volts). Severity is also determined by the length of time the victim is in contact with an electrical current. Lower voltage and less time exposed to the electrical source usually causes less severe injury (Moore, 2015b). Chemical burns require early identification and rapid decontamination and treatment. The concentration and acidity or alkalinity of a chemical, combined with the length of time the skin or mucosa is exposed to the agent, determine the significance of a chemical burn (Moore, 2015a).

Burn depth is categorized as first (superficial), second (partial thickness), and third degree (full thickness), with a deepest fourth degree category being possible (Zuo et al., 2017). First-degree burns commonly are superficial and involve the epidermis only, requiring little or no treatment. Second-degree burns include both superficial and deep partial-thickness burns. Superficial partial-thickness burns include injuries to the epidermis and the outermost dermis. Redness, swelling, and discomfort or pain accompany. Deep partial-thickness burns damage both the epidermal and dermal layers, causing necrosis and intercellular edema, resulting in blister formation. Second-degree burns are typically more painful than first-degree burns, with loss of skin integrity and subsequent fluid depletion. Full-thickness burns damage the epidermis, dermis, and subcutaneous tissue. Tissue necrosis evolves, producing eschar (leathery, sloughing, dead tissue) and leaving no protective barrier for remaining structures. Eschar increases the risk for bacterial infection in burns. Edema, inflammation, and vasodilation accompany this type of burn, and little or no sensation remains (Rau et al., 2014). Complications, including shock, infection, respiratory compromise, and multisystem organ failure, are common in burn injuries and evolve during the acute phase of injury (Stavrou et al., 2014).

Clinical Aspects

Determining the percentage of total body surface area (TBSA) and depth of burns is the first step in burn resuscitation (Stavrou et al., 2014). Selection of appropriate resuscitation fluid and the correct amount to infuse over the first 24 hours following burn injury directly affect burn wound healing and chances for survival (Cancio, 2014). There are multiple tools available to calculate the approximate area of burns in the prehospital and acute-phase settings. The rule of nines, modified Lund and Browder chart, and Parkland formula are among the most common measurement systems used for this purpose. More advanced methods for determining burn extent, such as laser Doppler imaging, may be initiated 2 to 5 days following preliminary burn resuscitation in order to avoid over-resuscitation with fluids, which poses an additional danger to patient outcomes (Martin, Lundy, & Rickard, 2014). The starting point for fluid resuscitation is typically between 2 and 4 mL/kg/TBSA/24 hr (Lundy et al., 2016).

Evaluation and definitive management of airway, breathing, circulation, and fluid resuscitation are the most crucial elements of care for burn patients with life-threatening injuries. Early intubation is imperative for patients sustaining airway burns. A detailed history of injury, including time; mechanism; voltage, if electrical source of injury; details of decontamination for chemical sources; a chemical safety data sheet if available; associated trauma; syncope; smoke exposure; abuse potential; and prehospital treatment should be obtained. Wet linens should be rapidly replaced with sterile dry linens. All jewelry and clothing should be removed, and careful evaluation of nonburn injuries should be done. Placement of urinary catheter and nasogastric tube should be accomplished during the reassessment phase of care (Cancio, 2014).

Multiple factors must be considered following the acute phase of burn resuscitation. Hypothermia is an early complication of burns. The greater the surface area burned, the more vulnerable the patient is to development of hypothermia. It is important that the patient be kept warm and dry in order to conserve energy expended from the postburn hypermetabolic state. Persistent hypermetabolism and muscle wasting in extensive burns requires early nutritional reinforcement, but balancing calories and the composition of nutrients must be individualized to avoid overconsumption and increased risk for hyperglycemia (Rowan et al., 2015). Pruritus (itching) is an unfortunate and very common result of burns. It occurs in almost every pediatric burn patient and in as much as 87% of affected adults. Itching may not respond favorably to anti-inflammatory drugs and other analgesics (Stavrou et al., 2014). Optimal management of pruritus should be addressed after patient stabilization during hospitalization and in discharge planning.

Contractures manifest related to loss of skin elasticity and pose great risk of loss of physical function. Mobilization of joints should begin as soon as possible during hospitalization. Essentially, every body system and organ can be affected following a significant burn injury. Duodenal ulcers, anemia, hypermetabolic syndrome, insulin resistance, and liver dysfunction may develop in response to injury. In addition, other common sequelae, including central nervous system inflammation, cardiac dysfunction, and respiratory compromise, may develop. Compartment syndrome from circumferential burns may develop acutely, necessitating escharotomy or fasciotomy in any area of the body. Kidneys may be damaged by lactic acidosis and urine myoglobin production (Rau et al., 2014). Elevation in urine myoglobin levels is commonly associated with rhabdomyolysis, an associated complication of significant burn injuries (Moore, 2015b). Monitoring urine output is important to guiding titration of fluid resuscitation. It is important that IV fluids for burn resuscitation be initiated early, and that fluid intake and output be accurately measured, recorded, and reported. The urine output goal for adults is 30 to 50 mL/hr, and for children, weighing 30 kg or less, 1 mL/kg/hr (Lundy et al., 2016).

Deep vein thrombosis (DVT) prevention strategies should begin immediately in burn patients, since these injuries result in a hypercoagulable state (Zuo et al., 2017). Nurses should anticipate initiation of anticoagulant prophylaxis therapy. Burn severity impacts the degree of pain that patients experience. Long-term pain and sensory dysfunction accompany more extensive burns. Acutely burned patients may experience pain in the form of many abnormal sensations, including burning, dullness, itching, and dysesthesia (Rau et al., 2014). Frequent pain assessment and response to specific medications are important to determine the most effective pain treatment options for individual patients.

Prevention of infection in burn patients is crucial to survival. Burn sepsis typically presents within the first week postinjury. The most common causes of burn sepsis include pneumonia, central vascular access devices, and burn-injured skin. It is essential that health care workers maintain sterile technique and adhere to strict infection control practices while caring for burn patients. Antibiotic selection is carefully determined by specimen cultures to avoid pathogen resistance (Zuo et al., 2017). Significant burn wounds often require wound debridement and advanced wound care. Skin grafting is necessary for almost all full-thickness burns. Aesthetic changes related to deeper burns can have lasting effects on mental, emotional, and social well-being. Anxiety and depression are common especially within the first year after injury. Symptoms of posttraumatic stress disorder may emerge during the recovery process (Stavrou et al., 2014). Psychosocial support is essential in provision of holistic patient care and to improve long-term outcomes.

Rapid communication with a regional burn center is advised by American Burn Association guidelines for patients with burn extent greater than 10% of total body surface area. Patients with inhalation injuries; burns associated with trauma; burns of the hands, feet, perineum, genitalia, or over major joints regardless of surface area burned; any third-degree burn; electrical, chemical, or lightning injuries; pediatric patients; and special needs patients, including those with social, emotional, or rehabilitation needs, require consultation with a burn center (Cancio, 2014).

Summary

Burn injuries pose significant challenges related to acute and long-term care. Nurses should remain current and knowledgeable regarding burn pathophysiology, assessment and treatment significant to this patient population. Awareness of the most current evidence-based care available to burn patients assists nurses in providing them relative and efficient care.

Cancio, L. C. (2014). Initial assessment and fluid resuscitation of burn patients. *Surgical Clinics of North America*, *94*(4), 741–754.

Jewo, P. I., & Fadeyibi, I. O. (2015). Progress in burns research: A review of advances in burn pathophysiology. *Annals of Burns and Fire Disasters*, *28*(2), 105.

Lundy, J. B., Chung, K. K., Pamplin, J. C., Ainsworth, C. R., Jeng, J. C., & Friedman, B. C. (2016). Update on severe burn management for the intensivist. *Journal of Intensive Care Medicine*, *31*(8), 499–510.

Martin, N. A. J., Lundy, J. B., & Rickard, R. F. (2014). Lack of precision of burn surface area calculation by UK armed forces medical personnel. *Burns*, *40*, 246–250.

Moore, K. (2015a). Hot topics: Chemical burns in the emergency department. *Journal of Emergency Nursing*, *41*(4), 364–365.

Moore, K. (2015b). Hot topics: Electrical injuries in the emergency department. *Journal of Emergency Nursing*, *41*(5), 455–456.

Rau, K. K., Spears, R. C., & Petruska, J. C. (2014). The prickly, stressful business of burn pain. *Experimental Neurology*, *261*, 752–756.

Rowan, M. P., Cancio, L. C., Elster, E. A., Burmeister, D. M., Rose, L. F., Natesan, S., . . . Chung, K. K. (2015). Burn wound healing and treatment: Review and advancements. *Critical Care*, *19*(1), 243–255.

Stavrou, D., Weissman, O., Tessone, A., Zilinsky, I., Holloway, S., Boyd, J., & Haik, J. (2014). Health related quality of life in burn patients—a review of the literature. *Burns*, *40*(5), 788–796.

Zuo, K. J., Medina, A., & Tredget, E. E. (2017). Important developments in burn care. *Plastic and Reconstructive Surgery*, *139*(1), 120e–138e.

■ CHEST PAIN

Sharon R. Rainer

Overview

Chest pain is a common chief complaint that adult patients may present with across all clinical practice settings. In the absence of trauma, chest pain is a symptom of an underlying problem or condition that can range from life-threatening to benign. Nontraumatic chest pain is among the most common reasons patients seek medical attention, including calls to 9-1-1 to active emergency medical services (EMS) for suspected heart attacks. The evaluation of patients presenting with chest pain in all practice settings, including the emergency department, is challenging as there are several possible causes for the chest pain, some of which may prove fatal (Gupta & Munoz, 2016). In some cases, chest pain may be chronic; typically chest pain is an acute presenting symptom that necessitates rapid and careful assessment by the nurses and the health care team.

Background

Cardiovascular disease, including ischemic heart disease, is the leading cause of death for both men and women in the United States and worldwide (Kochanek, Murphy, Xu, & Arias, 2014). More than half of the deaths that occur as a result of heart disease are in men. *Heart disease* is a term used to describe several conditions, many of which are related to plaque buildup in the walls of the coronary arteries. Every year, approximately 2 million Americans have a heart attack or stroke and, as a result of these conditions, more than 600,000 die from cardiovascular disease (Kochanek et al., 2014). Due to the fact that chest pain is a common symptom of heart disease, acute chest pain must always be considered cardiovascular in nature until proven otherwise.

Chest pain generally falls into two broad categories: cardiac and noncardiac chest pain. Myocardial ischemia, injury, or infarct is the category in which an interruption in blood flow to the heart to some degree causes cardiac chest pain. It is synonymous with the condition angina pectoris and is a concern for all patients presenting with chest pain until there is a reasonable degree of clinical certainty established by a clinician that the chest pain is originating from a noncardiac source. Other cardiopulmonary causes of chest pain may include diseases of the aorta, pneumonia, pulmonary embolism, pleurisy, and pneumothorax and these conditions may be life-threatening and cause serious harm to patients if left undiagnosed and if a delay in treatment ensues. Underlying noncardiopulmonary conditions that may present with chest pain include gastrointestinal diseases; musculoskeletal problems; and psychological problems, including anxiety/panic attacks, depression, and cocaine use (Kontos, Diercks, & Kirk, 2010).

Acute coronary syndrome (ACS) is a constellation of clinical signs and symptoms encompassing myocardial ischemia, injury, and infarct. ACS includes unstable angina, non–ST-segment elevation myocardial infarctions (non-STEMI), and ST-segment elevation myocardial infarction (STEMI). Chest pain may be the presenting symptom of ACS. Angina is chest pain or discomfort caused when your heart muscle does not get enough oxygen-rich blood. ACS occurs when the patient has underlying coronary artery disease (CAD). CAD is defined as the formation of an atherosclerotic plaque in one or more of the coronary arteries that restricts flow of blood and oxygen delivery to the cardiac tissue.

ACS can result in reversible or irreversible cardiac injury or necrosis. Due to the high-risk nature of ACS, the American Heart Association (AHA) and the American College of Cardiology (ACC) recently updated practice guidelines and performance measure to help clinicians adhere to a standard of care for patients who present with symptoms of ACS (Amsterdam et al., 2014).

In addition, noncardiac chest pain may have similar presenting features as cardiac chest pain and also has multiple causes requiring careful evaluation. During the initial evaluation, the clinician may determine that ACS is less likely than other noncardiac causes of chest pain but should be considered. The mnemonic CHEST PAIN is often used to recall some of the common causes of noncardiac chest pain (Newberry, Barnett, & Ballard, 2005): C (costochondritis, cocaine abuse), H (herpes zoster, hyperventilation), E (esophagitis/esophageal spasm), S (aortic valve stenosis), T (trauma), P (pulmonary embolism, pneumonia, pneumothorax, pericarditis, pancreatitis), A (angina/aortic dissection/aortic aneurysm), I (infarction/intervertebral disk disease), N (neuropsychiatric disorders [i.e., anxiety, depression]).

Clinical Aspects

ASSESSMENT

A nurse's diagnostic accuracy requires careful attention to history, especially attributes of pain, to determine cardiac causes of pain. The use of the PQRST mnemonic helps shed light on symptoms that may indicate cardiac chest pain—provokes/palliates/precipitating factors; quality; region/radiation; severity/associated symptoms; time/temporal relations (Newberry et al., 2005). However, neither quality nor intensity of chest pain is ever a sufficient attribute to rule in or rule out an underlying cardiac cause. Typically, clinicians rely on a comprehensive history and physical examination of the patient with chest pain in order to develop a list of differential diagnoses that may include cardiac and noncardiac reasons for the symptom (McConaghy & Oza, 2013). In addition, clinicians will often apply a validated clinical decision rule to predict heart disease as a cause of chest pain.

Risk factors are important considerations when obtaining a patient's history. Several evidence-based tools exist to help clinicians identify and predict CAD as the cause of chest pain (McConaghy & Oza, 2013). The risk factors typically used to identify those with CAD are as follows: age/gender (55 years and older in men or 65 years or older in women); known CAD, occlusive vascular disease, or cerebrovascular disease; pain that is worse with exercise; pain not reproducible by palpation; and patient assumption that pain is of cardiac origin. A recent study identified that only 1% of those patients with none or one of these clinical features had CAD, whereas 63% of the patients with four or five of the features had CAD. The study further suggests that patients with chest pain and four or five of these components require urgent workups for chest pain and suspected ACS (McConaghy & Oza, 2013).

A nurse may be the first member of the health care team to identify and document risk factors associated with heart disease to help inform the history and physical exam done by clinicians. These risk factors are broadly categorized as medical conditions, behaviors, family history, and other factors (Kochanek, et al., 2014). Medical conditions include hypertension, hypercholesterolemia, and diabetes. Behaviors refer to those risk factors considered to be modifiable. These risk factors include diet, exercise, obesity, and tobacco and alcohol use. Family history, age, gender, and ethnicity are nonmodifiable, genetic characteristics that may predispose a patient to heart disease.

Therefore, it is important to determine those patients at risk for CAD who may be experiencing signs and symptoms of ACS. Chest pain may be the main symptom; however, it may not be present at all or may be vague in nature. Nurses should assess for other symptoms of ACS, including the following (O'Donnell, Mckee, O'Brien, Mooney, & Moser, 2012):

■ Substernal pain that occurs with exertion and alleviates with rest

■ Chest pain lasting for 20 minutes or longer

■ Dull, heavy pressure in or on the chest

■ Sensation of a heavy object on the chest

■ Chest pain radiating to the back, neck, jaw, left arm, or shoulder, right arm, or back

■ Chest pain affected by inspiration

■ Chest pain not reproducible with chest palpation

■ Accompanying diaphoresis

■ Pain initiated by stress, exercise, large meals, sex, or any activity that increases the body's demand upon the heart for blood

■ Fatigue

■ Extreme fatigue or edema after exercise

■ Shortness of breath

■ Levine's sign: Chest discomfort described as a clenched fist over the sternum (the patient will clench his or her fist and rest it on or over his or her sternum)

■ Angor animi: Fear of impending doom or death

■ Pain high in the abdomen or chest, nausea and extreme fatigue after exercise, back pain, and edema can occur in anyone but are more common in women

■ Nausea, lightheadedness, or dizziness

The 12-lead EKG is the test of choice in the initial evaluation of patients with chest pain (Hollander, Than, & Mueller, 2016; Overbaugh, 2009). ST-segment changes (elevation or depression), new-onset left bundle branch block, presence of Q waves, and new-onset T wave inversions increase the likelihood of ACS or acute MI. Nurses are not responsible for interpreting the EKG; however, rapid identification of ischemia, injury, and infarct is important so that treating clinicians or EMS can be rapidly alerted. The AHA/ACC recommends that patients presenting with acute chest pain symptom have a 12-lead EKG performed and interpreted by a health care provider within 10 minutes of the patient's arrival to the emergency department (Amsterdam et al., 2014).

NURSING INTERVENTIONS, MANAGEMENT, AND IMPLICATIONS

Providing nursing care to patients with chest pain can be challenging across all practice settings due to the broad range of underlying possible diseases that may exist. A nurse who obtains vital signs, including temperature, heart rate, blood pressure, respiration rate, oxygen saturation, and pain intensity, as close to the onset of chest pain as possible is making a significant contribution to the identification of a life-threatening emergency. A systematic approach is essential to determine whether the patient is stable or unstable. Tachycardia and hypotension are indicative of important hemodynamic changes that may be associated with an acute MI, cardiogenic shock, pulmonary embolism, pericarditis with tamponade, or tension pneumothorax. Acute aortic emergencies, such as aortic dissection, may present with severe hypertension but may be associated with hypotension when there is coronary arterial compromise or dissection into the pericardium. Tachycardia and hypoxia may indicate a pulmonary cause of the chest pain. The presence of low-grade fever is usually nonspecific but may be found in patients with acute MI and thromboembolism in addition to infection. Therefore, an accurate set of vital signs completed and documented in a timely manner is an important nursing intervention contributing to the workup of patients with chest pain (Overbaugh, 2009).

When a patient is diagnosed with angina, the nurse will carry out interventions to decrease damage to the heart muscle. Initial drug therapies that may be ordered include aspirin, oxygen, nitroglycerin, and morphine. Nurses often use the mnemonic MONA to recall these initial treatments, although MONA does not specify the correct order of administration. Patients with suspected ACS are often ordered 325 mg of aspirin by mouth as soon as possible after symptoms begin, unless contraindicated (Newberry et al., 2005; Overbaugh, 2009).

Signs and symptoms of ACS are not sufficient to make a clinical diagnosis, so clinicians rely on diagnostic testing. Identifying life-threatening ischemia, infarct, and injury is important in the initial evaluation of chest pain. Nurses are instrumental in facilitating the workup of chest pain patients. This may involve identifying risk factors and changes in symptoms. In addition, as the EKG and history and physical examination are often insufficient alone in diagnosing acute MI and ACS, clinicians in the acute setting will order blood tests to measure the concentration of cardiac troponin, a biomarker for cardiac injury and ischemia (Hollander et al., 2016).

Patient education focused on prevention of cardiovascular disease in all age groups is an important nursing intervention. By educating both the young and old on identifying and lowering modifiable risk factors related to cardiovascular disease, nurses promote health and prevent complications of heart disease. Interventions to help patients adhere to a cardiac-prudent diet, exercise, avoiding tobacco, managing stress, and controling diseases like hypertension and diabetes are part of a thorough intervention geared toward patients with chest pain and suspected CAD.

OUTCOMES

Chest pain represents a high-volume, high-risk clinical problem across all practice settings. Some 20 million patients in North America and Europe present to emergency departments annually with symptoms suggestive of ACS (Hollander et al., 2016). Rapid and careful early identification of those most at risk of dying from an acute MI or ACS is the goal of quality health care delivery. In order to save lives, nurses must be vigilant in identifying patients with chest pain and possible ACS as well as facilitate the workup of noncardiac reasons for chest pain. In some outpatient or community clinical settings, the nurse may need to activate the EMS for patients experiencing chest pain so that a thorough investigation into the cause can be conducted by an emergency clinician. In other clinical settings, such as in patient units or the emergency department, rapid prioritization of the patient with chest pain to ensure that vital signs and an EKG are safely and quickly obtained is imperative to facilitating the thorough assessment and treatment of the patient.

Summary

Chest pain is a common presenting symptom of patients who may be experiencing a host of underlying medical conditions. Although most patients presenting with chest pain are not having an acute MI, determining the cause of their chest pain warrants a careful medical and nursing evaluation. Given that the causes of chest pain can range from musculoskeletal disorders to life-threatening MI, and deadly aortic dissection or pulmonary embolism, nurses on the front lines must have a high level of suspicion about potentially life-threatening causes. Nurses are likely to be the first health care professional to encounter patients with chest pain. Therefore, the nurse must exercise vigilance and diligence in facilitating rapid clinical evaluation of all patients with chest pain in order to save lives and expedite the identification of the underlying cause.

Amsterdam, E. A., Wenger, N. K., Brindis, R. G., Casey, D. E., Ganiats, T. G., Holmes, D. R., . . . Zieman, S. J. (2014). 2014 AHA/ACC guideline for the management of patients with non-ST-elevation acute coronary syndromes: A report of the American College of Cardiology/American Heart Association Task Force on Practice Guidelines. *Circulation*, *130*(25), e344–e426. doi:10.1161/cir.0000000000000134

Gupta, R., & Munoz, R. (2016). Evaluation and management of chest pain in the elderly. *Emergency Medicine Clinics of North America*, *34*(3), 523–542. doi:10.1016/j.emc.2016.04.006

Hollander, J. E., Than, M., & Mueller, C. (2016). State-of-the-art evaluation of emergency department patients presenting with potential acute coronary syndromes. *Circulation*, *134*(7), 547–564. doi:10.1161/circulationaha.116.021886

Kochanek K. D., Murphy S. L., Xu J., & Arias, E. (2014). *Mortality in the United States, 2013. NCHS data brief, no. 178*. Hyattsville, MD: National Center for Health Statistics, Centers for Disease Control and Prevention, U.S. Department of Health and Human Services.

Kontos, M. C., Diercks, D. B., & Kirk, J. D. (2010). Emergency department and office-based evaluation of patients with chest pain. *Mayo Clinic Proceedings*, *85*(3), 284–299. doi:10.4065/mcp.2009.0560

McConaghy, J. R., & Oza, R. S. (2013). Outpatient diagnosis of acute chest pain in adults. *American Family Physician*, *87*(3), 177–182.

Newberry, L., Barnett, G. K., & Ballard, N. (2005). A new mnemonic for chest pain assessment. *Journal of Emergency Nursing*, *31*(1), 84–85. doi:10.1016/j.jen.2004.10.005

O'Donnell, S., McKee, G., O'Brien, F., Mooney, M., & Moser, D. K. (2012). Gendered symptom presentation in acute coronary syndrome: A cross sectional analysis. *International Journal of Nursing Studies*, *49*(11), 1325–1332. doi:10.1016/j.ijnurstu.2012.06.002

Overbaugh, K. J. (2009). Acute coronary syndrome. *American Journal of Nursing*, *109*(5), 42–52. doi:10.1097/01.naj.0000351508.39509.e2

■ CHILD ABUSE AND NEGLECT

Patricia M. Speck
Pamela Harris Bryant
Tedra S. Smith
Sherita K. Etheridge
Steadman McPeters

Overview

For a majority of states (46 out of 50), child abuse and neglect are serious public health problems. Among states contributing to a report published in 2014, there were 6.6 million children involved in 3.6 million reports of child abuse and neglect nationwide; authorities validated 2.2 million or 61%, with an incidence rate of 29 per 1,000 children (U.S. Department of Health and Human Services [HHS], 2016, p. ix). Professionals who have contact with children as part of their job are mandatory reporters responsible for over 45% of the reported cases (p. ix). Of the children evaluated, the majority had one report (83%), and some had two or more reports (16%; p. x). The children with validated experiences were neglected (75%) and physically abused (17%), but if the child experienced both, only one category counted toward maltreatment (p. x). Other types of maltreatment comprise the remaining percentage of validated reports. The mortality rate was 2.13 deaths per 100,000, or 1,546 fatalities (p. x). Boys had a higher fatality rate than girls (2.48 vs. 1.82 per 100,000), and Caucasians died more frequently (43%), followed by different minority populations of children (African American—30.3%; Hispanic—15.1%; p. x). The financial impact of abuse and neglect of children in 2008 was $124 billion (Fong, Brown, Florence, & Mercy, 2012). Perpetrators of child abuse and neglect were mostly women (54.1%), White (48.8%), mistreating two or more children (HHS, 2016, p. x).

Background

The Child Abuse Prevention and Treatment Act (CAPTA), with reauthorization, defined behaviors as acts of child abuse and neglect as:

Any recent act or failure to act on the part of a parent or caretaker which results in death, serious physical or emotional harm, sexual abuse or exploitation; or an act or failure to act, which presents an imminent risk of serious harm. (p. viii)

Maltreatment includes psychological maltreatment (emotional abuse), neglect (including endangerment), and physical and sexual abuse (HHS, 2016). The Justice for Victims of Trafficking Act of 2015 (JVTA) requires states to report the number of identified sex-trafficked children younger than 18 years, allowing states to provide services and report identified victims up to age 24 years (Civic Impulse, 2017). Of the adults rescued at 18 years of age, overwhelmingly, their introduction to the industry began between the ages of 12 and 14 years. These legislative mandates at the national and state levels are helpful to the registered nurses responsible for evaluating injury in pediatric populations and reporting suspicions of abuse or neglect.

The children most at risk for child abuse and neglect are in chaotic or traumatized families, many experiencing social and personal environments not conducive to development or emotional health. Disparities and social determinants as risk factors diminish attainment of health outcomes. Social determinants include the environment and attitudes, exposure to crime and

violence, disease and access to health care, and personal and support systems (Office of Disease Prevention and Health Promotion, 2017). Chronic stress in environments, whether from the individual's disease, the family, the community, or the system, increases hormonal dysregulation predisposing the child to increased risk of violence and disease (McEwen, 1998).

Building on the stress and adaptation theories of the 1990s, emerging science focuses on epigenetic transference of cellular environments that predisposes offspring to poor health outcomes (Whitman & Kondis, 2016). In fact, physically and sexually victimized children display at least one mental health disorder by age 18 (Silverman, Reinherz, & Giaconia, 1996), which passes on to their children, and is predictive of future victim experiences.

A tool to measure adverse childhood experiences (ACEs) validated that there is a connection between ACEs and health outcomes, including early death (Felitti et al., 1998). The research continues. Diseases, once thought to be a result of genetics, may be a result of physical changes following significant ACEs; in fact, the impact of ACEs affects all human body systems where earlier stress results in risk behaviors, chronic disease, and early death (Anda et al., 2009; Brown et al., 2009).

Pregnant women and their developing fetus(s), newborns, infants, and children exposed to violence experience elevated stress hormones and begin a quest to escape or calm the "fear" response. The neuroendocrine system creates the brainstem irritation response (fear) to a threat and the hormonal sequelae of several hormonal pathways, including the hypothalamic–pituitary–adrenal (HPA) axis (Malenka, Nestler, & Hyman, 2009). The resulting "fight-or-flight" response causes an elevation in stress hormones, cascading and triggering other hormones in the stressed environment of the body. The hormones in the stress response originate from the primitive emotional midbrain, stimulated by the brain stem in response to fear, resulting in a constellation of symptoms, called general adaptation syndrome (GAS; Selye, 1974). *The victim responds normally to abnormal stresses.* However, the stress hormones change end-organ function. Today, research documents change in response to chronic stress, for example, digestion, immune system, mood, anxiety, energy storage (fat), and other deleterious alterations, specifically in a child's brain architecture, affecting learning, behavior, and long-term health (Child Welfare Information Gateway, 2015). The child is handicapped socially and developmentally by the exposure, usually without sensitive identification and intervention to mitigate the normal response to serious stresses in the family. The health outcomes include behavioral aberrations, hypertension, obesity, autoimmune diseases, poor school performance, adoption of risk behaviors (with subsequent disease or injury), and others. Understanding the underlying physiology of stress and trauma in childhood prepares registered nurses to address obvious symptoms that lead to future poor health choices and outcomes.

Clinical Aspects

It is important that practicing registered nurses recognize that child abuse or neglect is caused by a parent (HHS, 2016). Each state defines child abuse differently, but all states follow federal legislation, so the practicing registered nurse must be familiar with state legislation related to reporting child maltreatment. If there is a suspicion of child abuse, the registered nurse (caring for a pediatric patient) is a mandatory reporter in every state and all U.S. territories (HHS, 2016; Parrish, 2016).

Nurses must receive *education* about abuse and neglect to successfully screen and document developmental milestones at all ages and developmental stages. The first requirement is to understand elements of abuse and neglect, which include emotional abuse, such as belittling the child to outright screaming obscenities; physical abuse, such as pinching, pushing, slapping, and shoving the child at any developmental age or chronologic age; and outcomes from the abuses, which include depression, self-injurious behavior, suicide, or homicide (HHS, 2016).

Screening for stresses and developmental milestones identifies at-risk children and gives the registered nurse an opportunity to provide anticipatory guidance and intervention (Larkin, Shields, & Anda, 2012), which may include reporting the event(s) to the state's child services agency. Registered nurses caring for pediatric populations need a strong institutional policy and procedure for the management of abused and neglected pediatric patients, as well as the skills to identify, mitigate, and prevent early relational stresses between the child and his or her primary parent or caretaker. The ACEs questions, when considered a vital sign and asked at every visit, provide the opportunity to intervene on multiple levels. The answers to the questions help the nurse monitor to prevent child abuse and neglect. The assessment domains for pediatric registered nurse providers include the areas of "language,

literacy, and math," but also "interpersonal interaction and opportunities for self-expression" (Snow & Van Hemel, 2008, p. 22). Guidelines and validated tools for assessment at each developmental stage prepare the registered nurse provider to assist nonoffending parents with a comprehensive plan for intervention to mitigate the impact of abuse and neglect. Functional approaches for nurses require special training in the assessment of all children, including challenges and deficits in abilities. Parents from a variety of cultures, including minority and immigrant families, also positively respond to the anticipatory guidance provided by the registered nurses.

Using the totality of nursing education, the registered nurse as an expert in growth and development of children, incorporates Maslow's hierarchy of needs to include trusting one's environment at all developmental stages. When the closest caregiver (usually a parent) is unable or unwilling to provide the nurture, recognition is the first step to planning the necessary interventions to protect the safety of the child. Recommending prevention and parenting programs for at-risk families is a good first step, including home visitation or more frequent visits or phone calls to check on mother and child well-being. This is particularly important for the teen mother, who may be surviving a chaotic upbringing, experiencing the predictable high-risk behaviors of adolescence, and teen pregnancy.

All child assessments should be head to toe and include all mucous membrane areas (ears, eyes, nose, and throat and anogenital). The expectation with each visit is that the child evaluation includes behavior and skin injuries, asking about the manner and cause of the injury detected, and, if serious or inconsistent, reasons for delay in identification and treatment. The registered nurse assessment for child abuse or neglect is descriptive only, documenting objective information and monitoring activity between mother or caregiver and infant or child. If registered nurses are the first to suspect abuse or neglect, they are mandated reporters, regardless of other professionals' opinions. Not all injury or neglect is intentional, so the institutions designated to complete the comprehensive evaluation of the child, family, and social situation, while trying for all, are mandated to exercise legal authority over the child's safety. Throughout the process, the registered nurse's role is therapeutic and helpful, explaining the process of reporting and providing clarity to the process of the investigation. Nurses work with the institutional team to provide nursing care, assessment, and documentation, important for the safety and planning of the pediatric patient. In event of child removal from the home, the registered nurse's role is to comfort the nonoffending parent, provide community resources, and explain (to their ability) processes through anticipatory guidance.

Summary

Children depend on safe and secure environments created by their parent or caregiver to provide the love and support needed at all developmental stages and ages. Child abuse and neglect represent an inability of the responsible adult to nurture the child. During pregnancy, the stress of the mother transfers to the fetus and can result in spontaneous abortion; after delivery, lack of maternal nurture arrests the infant's development and changes the brain architecture, so the child is unable to navigate a learning environment. Stress creates anxiety in older children, which leads to the overproduction of stress hormones, crippling the capacity of the children to move through Maslow's basic hierarchical steps toward adulthood and independence.

Domestic violence, poverty, trafficking of human families, war, drug use (covered in other entries), neglect, and abuse by parent or caregivers create additional stress responses in the infant and child that doom the child to adopt risky behaviors beginning as young as 6 or 8 years of age. Registered nurses are in the position to recognize the child subjected to violence and the subsequent stress this causes. The developmental milestones provide clues for the pediatric registered nurses to begin the inquiry into ACEs, scales measuring depression and anxiety, and other validated methods for assessing mother and child. Recognition of the health signs of hypertension, obesity, risk behavior, mental health diagnoses, neglect, and other signs of fear in an infant or child provide the opportunity for all registered nurses to intervene, report, and participate in interprofessional team collaboration to create safe and secure environments for all children.

Anda, R. F., Dong, M., Brown, D. W., Felitti, V. J., Giles, W. H., Perry, G. S., . . . Dube, S. R. (2009). The relationship of adverse childhood experiences to a history of premature death of family members. *BMC Public Health, 9*, 106. doi:10.1186/1471-2458-9-106

Brown, D. W., Anda, R. A., Tiemeier, H., Felitti, V. J., Edwards, V. J., Croft, J. B., & Giles, W. H. (2009). Adverse childhood experiences and the risk of premature mortality. *American Journal of Preventive Medicine 37*(5), 389–396. doi:10.1016/j.amepre.2009.06.021

Child Welfare Information Gateway. (2015). *Understanding the effects of maltreatment on brain development.* Washington, DC: U.S. Department of Health and Human Services, Children's Bureau.

Civic Impulse. (2017). H.R. 181—114th Congress: Justice for Victims of Trafficking Act of 2015. Retrieved from https://www.govtrack.us/congress/bills/114/hr181

Felitti, V. J., Anda, R. F., Nordenberg, D., Williamson, D. F., Spitz, A. M., Edwards, V., . . . Marks, J. S. (1998). Relationship of childhood abuse and household dysfunction to many of the leading causes of death in adults: The adverse childhood experiences (ACE) study. *American Journal of Preventive Medicine, 14*, 245–258. doi:10.1016/S0749-3797(98)00017-8

Fang, X., Brown, D. S., Florence, C., & Mercy, J. A. (2012). The economic burden of child maltreatment in the United States and implications for prevention. *Child Abuse & Neglect, 36*(2), 156–165. doi:10.1016/j.chiabu.2011.10.006

Larkin, H., Shields, J. J., & Anda, R. F. (2012). The health and social consequences of adverse childhood experiences (ACE) across the lifespan: An introduction to prevention and intervention in the community. *Journal of Prevention and Intervention in the Community, 40*(4), 263–270. doi:10.1080/10852352.2012.707439

Malenka, R. C., Nestler, E. J., & Hyman, S. E. (2009). Neural and neuroendocrine control of the internal milieu. In A. Sydor & R. Y. Brown (Eds.), *Molecular neuropharmacology: A foundation for clinical neuroscience* (pp. 246, 248–259). New York, NY: McGraw-Hill Medical.

McEwen, B. S. (1998). Stress, adaptation, and disease: Alostasis and allostatic load. *Annals of the New York Academy of Sciences, 840*, 33–44. doi:10.1111/j.1749-6632.1998.tb09546.x

Office of Disease Prevention and Health Promotion. (2017). Determinants of health. In *Healthy People 2020.* Retrieved from https://www.healthypeople.gov/2020/about/foundation-health-measures/Determinants-of-Health#social

Parrish, R. (2016). Legal system intervention in cases of child maltreatment. In A. P. Giardino, L. Shaw, P. M. Speck, & E. R. Giardino (Eds.), *Recognition of child abuse for the mandated reporter* (pp. 321–356). St. Louis, MO: STM Learning.

Selye, H. (1974). *Stress without distress.* Philadelphia, PA: Lippincott.

Silverman, A. B., Reinherz, H. Z., & Giaconia, R. M. (1996). The long-term sequelae of child and adolescent abuse: A longitudinal community study. *Child Abuse & Neglect, 20*(8), 709–723.

Snow, C. E., & Van Hemel, S. B. (2008). *Early childhood assessment: Why, what, and how.* Washington, DC: National Research Council of the National Academies.

U.S. Department of Health & Human Services, Administration for Children and Families, Administration on Children, Youth and Families, Children's Bureau. (2016).

Child maltreatment, 2014. Retrieved from http://www .acf.hhs.gov/programs/cb/research-data-technology/ statistics-research/child-maltreatment

Whitman, B. V., & Kondis, J. (2016). Understanding the short-term and long-term effects of child abuse. In A. P. Giardino, L. Shaw, P. M. Speck, & E. R. Giardino (Eds.), *Recognition of child abuse for the mandated reporter* (pp. 165–178). St. Louis, MO: STM Learning.

■ *CLOSTRIDIUM DIFFICILE* INFECTION

Anita Sundaresh

Overview

Clostridium difficile, commonly referred to as *C. difficile* or *C. diff*, is an infectious pathogen that can result in life-threatening inflammation of the colon. The presence of symptoms, such as diarrhea and colonoscopic findings consistent with pseudomembranous colitis, or a positive stool specimen stool for *C. difficile* toxins or toxigenic C, establish a diagnosis of a *C. difficile* infection (Cohen et al., 2010). Early pharmacologic treatment and meticulous hand hygiene are essential components of nursing care for the patient with a *C. difficile* infection (CDI; Fernanda et al., 2015).

Background

C. difficile is a gram-positive anaerobic bacterium. It is transmitted from patients through the hands of health care personnel or in the environment by the ingestion of spores (Lessa, Gould, & Mc Donald, 2012). "Disruption of normal gut flora, typically by exposure to antimicrobials, allows *C. difficile* to proliferate, causing a broad spectrum of clinical manifestations that can range from asymptomatic carriage to diarrhea of varying severity to fulminant colitis and even death" (Lessa et al., 2012, p. 65). Fluid secretion, inflammation, and mucosal damage develop leading to diarrhea if the strain is toxigenic, namely, toxin A and B, resulting in a condition called *pseudomembranous colitis* (Barbut & Petit, 2001). The average incubation period for *C. difficile* is 1 to 20 days, and this pathogen is resistant to most disinfectants, heat, and some alcohol-based antiseptic agents. Therefore, the most effective strategy for *C. difficile* prevention is judicious and frequent handwashing with soap and water (Agha, 2010).

The mode of transmission of *C. difficile* is the fecal–oral route. Contributing factors to the development of CDI are broad-spectrum antibiotics, such as penicillin, penicillin associated with a beta-lactamase inhibitor, cephalosporin, and clindamycin, which alter the composition of the intestinal flora or gut microbiome (Barbut & Petit, 2001). Some other risk factors are medications and performance of nonsurgical gastrointestinal procedures such as a nasogastric tube, stool softeners, and antiulcer medications (Barbut & Petit, 2001).

Populations of individuals who are most at risk are patients in acute- or long-term care settings (Barbut & Petit, 2001). Patients with a CDI may present with unexplained leukocytosis and complain of abdominal pain. Owing to the toxigenic effects of the *C. difficile*, an innate immune response ensues, resulting in leukocytosis. As the severity of the infection worsens, patients may develop abdominal pain or distention related to a colonic ileus or toxic dilatation (Barbut & Petit, 2001). Complications of severe *C. difficile* colitis include dehydration, bowel perforation, hypotension, renal failure, systemic inflammatory response syndrome, sepsis, and death (Cohen et al., 2010). The risk of CDI is greater in the elderly population and disproportionately affects elderly females more frequently than their male counterparts (Agha, 2010).

A colectomy can be considered in patients who are severely ill. If surgical management is deemed necessary, then a subtotal colectomy preserving the rectum can be performed. The serum lactate levels have been shown to predict the perioperative mortality, in which higher serum lactate levels are associated with a high probability of death (Cohen et al., 2010). Having a subtotal colectomy can impact a patient's quality of life because CDI can be debilitating (Cohen et al., 2010). "*C. difficile* accounts for 20%–30% of cases of antibiotic-associated diarrhea and is the most commonly recognized cause of infectious diarrhea in health care settings" (Cohen et al., 2010, p. 435). The management of CDI cost $55.2 million and involved 55,380 inpatient hospital stays in Massachusetts from the years 1999 to 2003 (Cohen et al., 2010).

Clinical Aspects

ASSESSMENT

Assessing the patient with suspected or documented *C. difficile* begins with a health history and physical examination. The history should include number of bowel movements, color, odor, onset of changes, and any hospitalizations and recent medications, especially antibiotics. Stools should be collected for analysis and the number, color, consistency, and odor should also be documented.

NURSING INTERVENTIONS, MANAGEMENT, AND IMPLICATIONS

It is important for nurses to understand the diagnosis and treatment of CDI as it is the leading cause of hospital-associated illness affecting the health care system (Surawicz et al., 2013). Patients who are experiencing high-volume diarrhea with a recent history of antibiotic exposure should be presumed to have CDI. Stool specimens should be collected to verify the presence of the pathogen. Stringent contact precautions and hand hygiene should be implemented to prevent the transmission of the pathogen.

Hand hygiene is a critical aspect of the clinical care of a patient with a CDI that can mitigate transmission of the pathogen to others. It is important for nurses to perform hand hygiene to prevent *C. difficile* spores from reaching patients. Donning gowns and gloves before entering the patients' rooms can also be an effective barrier method. The use of disposable thermometers for patients who have CDI can reduce the spread of CDI (Rupnik, Wilcox, & Gerding, 2009).

Restrictive use of antibiotics should be the number one priority for preventing CDI. It is also important to wear vinyl gloves or to cohort patients with CDI to control outbreaks. "Control measures include strict antibiotic policy, a high degree of suspicion of *C. difficile*, prompt diagnosis, isolation, and treatment of infected patients, and implantation of enteric precautions" (Barbut & Petit, 2001, p. 409). It is important to maintain contact precautions until diarrhea has resolved (Cohen et al., 2010).

Nurses are encouraged to provide evidence-based supportive care for patients who are infected with *C. difficile*. Treatment should include intravenous fluid resuscitation, electrolyte replacement, and pharmacological venous thromboembolism prophylaxis. It is strongly recommended to discontinue use of any antimicrobial agent. Patients who have mild to moderate disease should be treated with metronidazole 500 mg orally three times a day for 10 days. Failure to respond to metronidazole in 5 to 7 days should prompt providers to switch treatment to vancomycin. Patients who are severely affected by CDI should be treated with vancomycin 125 mg four times a day for 10 days. Nurses should know the dosage recommendations to anticipate the medication needs of patients affected with CDI (Surawicz et al., 2013).

It is necessary to control and prevent the transmission of *C. difficile* in the hospital. The incidence of CDI can be decreased if hospitals institute a hospital-based infection control program. It is not recommended to routinely screen for CDIs to reduce the risk of the infection. Contact precautions should be initiated once a patient is confirmed to have a CDI. All health care workers and visitors should incorporate hand hygiene and use of gloves and gowns on entering the room of infected patients. It is also beneficial for nurses to use single-use disposable equipment to prevent the transmission of the disease. Disinfecting environmental surfaces with an Environmental Protective Agency (EPA)-recommended disinfectant can help to stop the spread of infection. Isolating the patients to a private room or combining patients with people who have *C. difficile* is recommended (Surawicz et al., 2013).

OUTCOMES

An early diagnosis of a CDI can significantly enhance a patient's mortality risk, and an effective use of contact precautions, as well as hand hygiene, can mitigate the likelihood of transmission of the pathogen to others. The adherence to evidence-based practice and clinical guidelines have also shown to minimize the transmission of *C. difficile*. Health care workers must comply with hand hygiene to prevent the transmission of the disease. It is necessary to maintain contact precautions until diarrhea is resolved. Given the variance in clinical manifestations of CDIs, nurses must be aware that the most judicious strategy to prevent a CDI is the appropriate administration of an antimicrobial therapy, and for patients with a CDI hand hygiene, contact precautions, and administration of the pathogen-specific antibiotic aid in reducing the patient's mortality risk (Cohen et al., 2010).

Summary

The delivery of nursing care must focus on reducing infections among the elderly and screening patients who are affected by CDI. Tools must be developed to identify virulence factors for CDIs, especially in the toxin-variant strains (Rupnik et al., 2009). Studies must also be conducted in populations that were previously considered at low risk, such as children and pregnant women. Separate studies must be conducted among patients who have mild and severe CDI. Further studies need to be done on the use of probiotics as a preventative measure for CDI. "Lack of standardization of preparations, including quality control to minimize variations in bacterial counts during storage, and the possibility of inducing bacteremia or fungaemia remain drawbacks of probiotic use" (Rupnik et al., 2009, p. 534).

Agha, M. (2012). Epidemiology and pathogenesis of *C. difficile* and MRSA in the light of current NHS control policies: A policy review. *Annals of Medicine and Surgery*, *1*, 39–43.

Barbut, F., & Petit, J. C. (2001). Epidemiology of *Clostridium difficile*-associated infections. *Clinical Microbiology and Infection*, *7*(8), 405–410.

Cohen, S. H., Gerding, D. N., Johnson, S., Kelly, C. P., Loo, V. G., McDonald, L. C., . . . Wilcox, M. H.; Society for Healthcare Epidemiology of America; Infectious Diseases Society of America. (2010). Clinical practice guidelines for *Clostridium difficile* infection in adults: 2010 update by the Society for Healthcare Epidemiology of America (SHEA) and the Infectious Diseases Society of America (IDSA). *Infection Control and Hospital Epidemiology*, *31*(5), 431–455.

Fernanda, C. L., Yi, M., Wendy, M. B., Zintars, G., Ghinwa, K. D., John, R. D., . . . Clifford, L. M. (2015). Burden of Clostridium difficile infection in the United States. *New England Journal of Medicine*, *372*, 825–834.

Lessa, F. C., Gould, C. V., & McDonald, L. C. (2012). Current status of *Clostridium difficile* infection epidemiology. *Clinical Infectious Diseases*, *55*(Suppl. 2), S65–S70.

Rupnik, M., Wilcox, M. H., & Gerding, D. N. (2009). *Clostridium difficile* infection: New developments in epidemiology and pathogenesis. *Nature Reviews Microbiology*, *7*(7), 526–536.

Surawicz, C. M., Brandt, L. J., Binion, D. G., Ananthakrishnan, A. N., Curry, S. R., Gilligan, P. H., . . . Zuckerbraun, B. S. (2013). Guidelines for diagnosis, treatment, and prevention of *Clostridium difficile* infections. *American Journal of Gastroenterology*, *108*(4), 478–498; quiz 499.

■ CONTINUOUS VENO-VENOUS HEMOFILTRATION

Ian N. Saludares

Overview

Renal-replacement therapies (RRTs) represent a cornerstone in the management of severe acute kidney injury. This area of intensive care and nephrology has undergone significant improvement and evolution in recent years. Continuous RRTs have been a major focus of new technological and treatment strategies. RRT is being used increasingly in the intensive care unit (ICU), not only for renal indications but also for other organ-supportive strategies. Continuous veno-venous hemofiltration (CVVH) is one of the methods used in RRT. RRTs are an extracorporeal blood-purification therapy intended to compensate for impaired renal function over relatively short periods of time (Ronco et al., 2015).

This short-term treatment is used in ICU patients with acute or chronic renal failure. Usually, hemodialysis is typically done for patients with kidney failure. However, if the patient has low blood pressure or other contraindications for hemodialysis, CVVH may be a necessary alternative. Access to the circulation for CVVH is a large-bore dual-lumen central venous catheter designated for hemodialysis. CVVH is used in the critical care setting for patients with volume-overload, hemodynamically unstable conditions with azotemia or uremia (Astle, 2017).

Background

Acute kidney injury is associated with substantial morbidity and mortality (Bagshaw, George, & Bellomo, 2007) It is a common finding among patients in the ICU and is an independent predictor of mortality. Acute kidney injury that is severe enough to result in the use of renal-replacement therapy affects approximately 5% of the patients admitted to the ICU and is associated with a mortality rate of 60% (Uchino, 2005).

The optimal approach to RRT, as well as the optimal intensity and timing of such therapy in critically ill patients remains unclear. In one single-center, randomized, controlled study in which continuous RRT was the sole treatment approach, survival improved when the intensity of therapy was increased from an assigned effluent rate of 20 mL/kg of body weight per hour to either 35 or 45 mL/kg/hr (Bellomo, 2009).

CVVH was designed as an RRT for patients with acute renal failure. It is often chosen over intermittent hemodialysis when blood pressure instability is a problem, and CVVH is more efficient than peritoneal dialysis. CVVH is a technique characterized by a veno-venous circuit and a pump to perfuse the hemofilter. CVVH is suited to individualization of ultrafiltration and solute clearance in patients with acute renal failure and volume overload, specifically when there is impaired cardiovascular function or where arterial access is problematic.

RRTs are indicated in the following circumstances: patients with high-risk for hemodynamic instability who do not tolerate the rapid fluid shifts that occur with hemodialysis, in those who require large amounts of hourly intravenous (IV) fluids or parenteral nutrition, and in those who need more than the usual 3- to 4-hour hemodialysis treatment to correct the metabolic imbalances of acute renal failure. CVVH is used when patients primarily need excess fluid removed, whereas continuous veno-venous hemodialysis (CVVHD) is used when patients also need waste products removed because of uremia (Snyder, 2013).

In general, it appears that the decision to use RRT is affected by strongly held physician beliefs as well as a number of patient and organizational characteristics. Patient characteristics may include age, gender, race, illness acuity, and comorbidities. Organizational characteristics vary depending on the country, type of institution, type of ICU, type of physician or insurance provider, and the perceived cost of therapy. However, the strength of association of these characteristics with the decision to use RRT is not fully understood. Furthermore, large epidemiological studies are needed to establish the factors that are most important in determining practice patterns, and whether there are important access-to-care issues with this therapy (Ostermann et al., 2016).

Clinical Aspects

Basic knowledge is required to understand the principles of diffusion, ultrafiltration, osmosis, oncotic and hydrostatic pressures, and how they pertain to fluid and solute management during RRT (Astle, 2017). CVVH uses a hemofilter dialyzer that acts as an artificial kidney. This is a semipermeable membrane that creates two separate compartments: the blood compartment and the dialysis solution compartment.

ASSESSMENT

Patient assessment should include baseline vital signs, including hemodynamic parameters, weight, a review of current medications, laboratory values; assessments of neurological, vascular and nutritional status should also be conducted. The appraisal of the vascular access catheter insertion site for signs and symptoms of infection should also be included in the patient assessment. The insertion site can provide a portal entry for organisms, which may result in septicemia if unrecognized and treated. The patency of the vascular access catheter should also be assessed for adequate blood flow on aspiration and flushing, which is necessary during treatment to facilitate optimal fluid and solute removal. It is also important to note that the placement of the vascular access may compromise circulation to the distal parts of the access limb, which is why assessment of adequate circulation should also be completed.

NURSING INTERVENTIONS, MANAGEMENT, AND IMPLICATIONS

Continuous venovenous RRT is achieved with a pump system. The blood pump provides the pressure that drives the extracorporeal system. The most common sites used for vascular access catheters are the internal jugular, subclavian, and femoral veins. During continuous RRT, a dialysate, which is composed of water, a buffer usually lactate or bicarbonate, and various electrolytes, is used. Heparin citrate is often used during continuous RRT to prevent clotting of the extracorporeal circuit during treatment.

Some of the key parameters that should be documented during CVVH include (a) date and time of treatment initiation, mode of therapy, filter change; (b) condition of the vascular access regarding patency and quality of blood flow; (c) date and time of vascular access catheter insertion and dressing change; and (d) condition of insertion site and any signs or symptoms of infection. It is also very important to document vital signs and hemodynamic parameters before, during, and after the procedure. Status of pulse distal to vascular access site should also be noted. Most important, documentation of patient's response to treatment, hourly fluid balance calculation, daily weight, laboratory values before and after the treatment should be recorded.

OUTCOMES

CVVH is a temporary treatment for patients with acute renal failure who are unable to tolerate hemodialysis and are unstable. This is an extracorporeal blood purification therapy intended to substitute for impaired renal function over an extended period and is applied, or aimed at being applied, 24 hours per day. Although continuous RRT (CRRT) is a resource-intensive and expensive technology, it remains the default modality of support most frequently used for severely ill patients at high risk for death (Wald, 2014). CVVH uses the principles of ultrafiltration, hydrostatic pressure, and convection to remove both fluid and solutes from the patient. Owing to the large loss of fluid that occurs in this mode, the patient requires a replacement fluid to be programmed in the filter. The filter ensures that the amount programmed as the fluid replacement rate is the amount of fluid that is lost during hemofiltration, to ensure that the patient keeps an even balance.

Summary

The demand for CRRT is growing. The North American region is outpacing the global demand for CRRT. global demand for CRRT. The reason being the presence of a large number of major players in this area and the rising prevalence of kidney failure because of rising diabetes, cancer, and other chronic diseases ("Global Continuous Renal Replacement Therapy Market Insights," 2017).

Astle, S. M. (2017). Continuous renal replacement therapies. In D. L. Wiegand (Ed.), *AACN procedure manual for high acuity, progressive and critical care* (7th ed., pp. 1054–1055). St. Louis, MO: Elsevier.

Bagshaw, S. M., George, C., & Bellomo, R.; ANZICS Database Management Committee. (2007). Changes in the incidence and outcome for early acute kidney injury in a cohort of Australian intensive care units. *Critical Care, 11*(3), R68.

Bellomo, R. (2009). Intensity of continuous renal-replacement therapy. *New England Journal of Medicine, 361,* 1627–1638.

Global Continuous Renal Replacement Therapy Market Insights, Opportunity, Analysis, Market Shares and Forecast 2017–2023. (2017). Retrieved from http://www.researchandmarkets.com/reports/3774875/global-continuous-renal-replacement-therapy#relb0

Ostermann, M., Joannidis, M., Pani, A., Floris, M., De Rosa, S., Kellum, J. A., & Ronco, C.; 17th Acute Disease Quality Initiative (ADQI) Consensus Group. (2016). Patient selection and timing of continuous renal replacement therapy. *Blood Purification, 42*(3), 224–237.

Ronco, C., Ricci, Z., De Backer, D., Kellum, J. A., Taccone, F. S., Joannidis, M., . . . Vincent, J. L. (2015). Renal replacement therapy in acute kidney injury: Controversy and consensus. *Critical Care, 19,* 146.

Snyder, A. C. (2013). Patient management: Renal system. In D. K. Patricia Gonce Morton (Ed.), *Critical care nursing: A holistic approach* (p. 646). Philadelphia, PA: Wolter Kluwer Health–Lippincott Williams & Wilkins.

Uchino, S, K. J. (2005). Acute renal failure in critically ill patients: A mulitnational, mulicenter study. *Journal of the American Medical Association, 294*(7), 813–818.

Wald, R. S. S. (2014). The association between renal replacement therapy modality and long-term outcomes among critically ill adults with acute kidney injury. *Critical Care Medicine, 42*(4), 868–877.

■ DEFINITIONS OF EMERGENCY AND CRITICAL CARE NURSING

Nicole M. Hartman
Courtney Vose

Overview

Caring for critically ill patients, either emergently or over a period, requires advanced clinical knowledge, broader technical skills, and the ability to work calmly to manage crisis in an often-turbulent environment. In the emergency room, *crisis* refers to the immediate danger the patient experiences from either illness or injury. In the critical care setting, crisis refers to the complex care required to sustain life. In both situations, the registered nurses caring for these patients must possess the skills required to safely move the patient beyond the crisis. Knowledge of how the specialties of emergency room and critical nursing developed will enhance the skills of these crisis care clinicians.

Background

Emergency nursing is a specialty in which nurses are trained to care for patients in the critical time frame related to their illness or injury. A skill set these nurses must possess is the ability to quickly discern the criticality of the situation, as they are often the first clinicians to evaluate the patient. Emergency nurses must be comfortable functioning autonomously because they are at the front line and regularly start treatment. They are the ones who most frequently mobilize the care team emergently, urgently, or nonurgently. Physicians and providers rely on their judgment to determine the speed at which they need to respond in treatment arenas that are often overcrowded. The ability to appropriately triage patients is arguably the most crucial skill needed by all emergency nurses. In addition, these nurses provide vital support to the family and friends of their patients to help them work through the stress of loss, grief, or uncertainty. The importance of this skill set cannot be overemphasized.

Emergency nurses are best described as generalists, not specialists. They often provide emergent care for every age patient, from birth to death. They also must know about every specialty in order to assess, triage, and stabilize patients before they are transferred to specialty care areas like an intensive care unit. It is because of these diverse patient care experiences that emergency nursing attracts nurses from all specialties. It is no longer a perquisite to have critical care or pre-hospital experience.

Emergency nursing is a modern concept. Until the early 20th century, care was provided when the patient was injured or became ill and emergency departments (EDs) did not exist (Solheim, 2016). During World War II, the Korean War, and the Vietnam War, emergent care provided to soldiers demonstrated that rapid and acute care makes a difference in patient outcomes (Solheim, 2016). The success of these urgent-care venues led to growth of hospitals and emergency treatment spaces throughout the 20th century. These urgent-care spaces evolved from "rooms" to departments as the need for access to emergency and primary health care grew.

The postwar patient population was changing due to the development of EDs and the advent of medications, such as penicillin. Patients who used to die from critical illness were now able to survive, but required intensive care while in the hospital (Fairman & Lynaugh, 1998). Critical care nursing can trace its roots back to Florence Nightingale (1860), as she advocated for seriously ill patients to be grouped together in a quiet section of the hospital ward. This concept was more widely adopted by hospitals in the 1950s during extensive reorganization of hospital wards to allow for more efficient care of patient populations.

Changes in the 1960s and 1970s with health care technology increased the complexity of care patients received in the hospital. The number of hospitals with designated critical care areas was increasing and becoming the new standard of care. Nurses were now caring for patients recovering from open heart surgery, severe trauma, and various disease processes that used to end the patient's life. It became apparent that these complex patients required more focused one-on-one nursing care in addition to the medical technology support they were receiving (Fairman & Lynaugh, 1998).

The complexity of these critically ill patients' cases required more time, technology, and skill from their nurses and doctors. The idea of one nurse per patient was born of necessity. It simply took that much time for nurses to provide care and monitor these complex patients. The environment needed to be spacious enough for the equipment required to sustain life and for patients to be seen and treated (Fairman &

Lynaugh, 1998). But grouping these patients together also presented new issues for nurses. The emotional toll that caring for the critically ill patients takes on the caregiver was a new concept. Nurses were often overwhelmed with the emotions they experienced more than the complexity of care they were providing (Fairman & Lynaugh, 1998).

The modern-day critical care unit owes much of its design and operation to the struggles of the 1950s and 1960s. Advancements were made of necessity and have become the evidence used to push the specialty of critical care nursing forward. The formation of the American Association of Critical-Care Nurses (AACN) in the 1960s has given this group of nurses a single voice to help shape the delivery of critical care.

Today, the AACN Synergy Model for Patient Care drives critical care nurses to deliver complex care that is focused on patients and families. This model focuses on the synergy that occurs when patient and family needs guide the formation of competencies for nursing care (Hardin & Kaplow, 2017). The characteristics of critically ill patients and families lead to skill development that will allow for optimal patient outcomes. It is this synergy between the nurses and the patients and their families that promotes healing in a safe environment (Hardin & Kaplow, 2017).

Clinical Aspects

The Emergency Nurses Association (ENA) is the only professional nursing association dedicated to defining the future of emergency nursing and emergency care through advocacy, expertise, innovation, and leadership (ENA, 2016). Emergency nursing was formally recognized as a specialty by the American Nurses Association (ANA) in partnership with the ENA in 2011. They wrote that

emergency nursing was the care of individuals across their life span, which is episodic, typically short-term, and occurs in all settings.

Emergency nurses function in EDs, urgent care centers, and on advanced life support ambulances and helicopters most frequently. They also work in roles inclusive of entrepreneurs, forensic nurses, jobs with the federal government, cruise ship nurses, humanitarian nurses, disaster nurses, camp nurses, and on-set nurses (Solheim, 2016).

Advanced degrees and certifications are available for emergency nurses. They may advance their education and become clinical nurse specialists (CNSs) or nurse practitioners (NPs). Per the ENA (2016), these advanced practice nurses (APNs) are uniquely prepared to develop and apply theory, conduct research, educate health care providers and consumers, and develop standards of practice that contribute to optimum outcomes. The American Academy of Emergency Nurse Practitioners (AAENP) is an organization that represents emergency nurse practitioners (ENPs). The APNs practicing in the emergency setting care for patients autonomously and collaboratively providing assessment, diagnosis, interventions, evaluations, and interpretation of diagnostic studies.

There are currently two board certifications in emergency nursing: (a) certified emergency nurse (CEN) and (b) certified pediatric emergency nurse (CPEN). There are other certifications in subspecialties like certified flight registered nurse (CFRN) and certified transport registered nurse (CTRN). ENPs also have two routes to board certification. The American Nurses Credentialing Center offers board certification through professional portfolio, and the American Academy of Nurse Practitioners Certification Board offers board certification through examination.

Critical care nursing has transformed over history, not only in competencies for nurses, but also in the types of subspecialties that have developed. The AACN offers board certification as critical care registered nurse (CCRN) adult, pediatric, and neonatal. There are also certifications specific to various subspecialties, such as cardiac and progressive care. The role of the nurse has changed in the critical care setting, but direct care nurse is still the most common role. This includes providing care for patients in various subspecialties, such as cardiac, neurological, surgical, pediatric, and neonatal intensive care units (Urden, 2016).

The CNS has emerged as a predominate APN in the critical care setting. The CNS serves as an educator providing clinical teaching, research development, leadership, and consultative skills to nurses in the numerous intensive care settings. The CNS is often designated by specialty, such as neurology CNS. In addition, a CNS can serve as a case manager for specific critical care populations, such as stroke patients (Urden, 2016).

Another common role for APNs in the critical care setting is the NP. These nurses receive specialized training to manage the care of designated patients, including diagnosis and treatment. They may have prescriptive authority based on the state's nurse practice laws. The NPs are often a consistent presence for many patients and families, as they interact with the patient throughout all aspects of care (Urden, 2016). These roles demonstrate the need for highly skilled, specialized nurses caring for critically ill patients.

Summary

EDs and critical care units require nurses with special education, enhanced skills, and behavioral characteristics that allow them to work calmly under stress to care for complex patient populations. The significant improvements made in health care technology are allowing sicker patients to be treated and to live longer. Nurses caring for critically ill patients accept the challenges these patients present and develop a critical care specialty. In addition, the role of the APN allows nurses to provide care in different ways, such as a CNS or NP. These advancements in nursing for emergent and critically ill patients are truly life-changing.

American Nurses Association & Emergency Nurses Association. (2011). American Nurses Association recognizes emergency nursing as specialty practice. Retrieved from http://www.nursingworld.org/FunctionalMenuCategories/MediaResources/PressReleases/2011-PR/ANA-Recognizes-Emergency-Nursing-Specialty-Practice.pdf

Emergency Nurses Association. (2016). Retrieved from https://www.ena.org/Pages/default.aspx

Fairman, J., & Lynaugh, J. (1998). *Critical care nursing: A history.* Philadelphia: University of Pennsylvania Press.

Hardin, S. R., & Kaplow, R. (2017). *Synergy for clinical excellence: The AACN synergy model for patient care* (2nd ed.). Burlington, MA: Jones & Bartlett.

Nightingale, F. (1860). *Notes on nursing: What it is, and what it is not.* Philadelphia, PA: Wilder Publications.

Solheim, J. (2016). *Emergency nursing: The profession, the pathway, the practice.* Indianapolis, IN: Sigma Theta Tau International.

Urden, L. D. (2016). Caring for the critically ill patient. In L. D. Urden, K. M. Stacy, & M. E. Lough (Eds.), *Priorities in critical care nursing* (7th ed., pp. 1–9). St. Louis, MO: Elsevier Mosby.

■ DENTAL EMERGENCIES

Melanie Gibbons Hallman
Lamon Norton

Overview

Common dental injuries include chipped or fractured teeth, luxation, and tooth avulsion affecting primary and permanent teeth. Approximately 33% of adults and 25% of school-age children experience dental trauma (DiAngelis et al., 2012). A systematic approach to evaluation of dental injury, correct diagnosis, and determination of urgency of care are important to tooth survival (Keels et al., 2014). Mouth cellulitis, including dental abscesses are a common reason for patients to seek emergency care (Allareddy, Rampa, Lee, Allareddy, & Nalliah, 2014). Nurses play an important role in triage and history acquisition, assessment, provision of care, and education for patients experiencing dental trauma and infections.

Background

Dental conditions typically seen in emergency departments include trauma related to accidents, athletics, and violence. Treatment is determined by degree of severity, type of injury, and dental location (American Association of Endodontists, 2017). Most oral injuries arise before age 10 and occur less frequently after age 30. Dental injuries are seen in young males more than females, possibly related to higher risk-taking behavior. The anterior teeth are at highest risk of injury. Dental trauma can be costly not only financially but also in time lost at work and school and in health care manpower and expenses (Andersson, 2013).

Preschool children are prone to falls, often resulting in oral injuries. In school-age children, sports and direct contusions are the common causes of dental injury. Child abuse may be a factor in dental injuries sustained by children (Hicks, Green, & Van Wicklin, 2016). Motor vehicle accidents and assaults are common causes of dental injuries in adolescents and young adults. Studies reveal that alcohol contributes to injuries experienced in these age groups, most often occurring during leisure time and on weekends (Andersson, 2013).

Injury to permanent dentition requires professional attention. Dental avulsion occurs when a tooth is displaced from the socket, usually due to trauma. This condition affects dental ligament cells, nerves, and blood supply, as well as the bone and gingiva (Hicks et al., 2016). Survival of an avulsed tooth is time-dependent. Dental concussion is caused by contusion and results in tooth tenderness. Increased mobility and bleeding at the tooth/gum interface are not associated with this injury. Dental fractures may affect the crown, root, or dental alveoli (sockets). Individual tooth or group tooth mobility raises

suspicion for fracture. Luxation may present with abnormal tooth mobility or as a tooth locked into a displaced position. The tooth may be partially avulsed, or impacted into the alveolus with bleeding usually present. Injuries to primary dentition typically require minimal or no treatment (Keels et al., 2014), whereas permanent teeth often require treatment. Failure to appropriately address dental injuries and abscesses can result in physical, psychological, and financial detriment to patients, which may be lifelong (DiAngelis et al., 2012). A periodontal abscess consists of localized pockets of infection that form around a tooth causing erythema and pain, often accompanied by palpable swelling. The tooth itself may be healthy. Patients with dental abscesses are commonly afebrile and if the abscess is left untreated, a local infection may progress to cellulitis and possibly a systemic infection (Hodgdon, 2013; Veerasathpurush, Rampa, Lee, Allaerddy, & Malliah, 2014).

Clinical Aspects

ASSESSMENT

A concise medical and dental history, including tetanus status, current medications, and medication allergies, should be acquired. The mechanism of injury is important to determining potential associated head injury or physical abuse. It is crucial to inquire whether the patient experienced loss of consciousness, headache, dizziness, nausea, or vomiting. These symptoms may indicate a concussion or other brain insult. If head injury is suspected, the patient's cervical spine should be assessed and protected until evaluated and cleared by a provider. If tooth or mouth contamination is suspected, the need for tetanus booster and antibiotic prophylaxis should be considered (Keels et al., 2014). Rapid assessment and treatment are crucial to tooth survival in avulsion injuries affecting permanent teeth.

NURSING INTERVENTIONS, MANAGEMENT, AND IMPLICATIONS

Care should focus on keeping patients calm and comfortable and determining whether the affected tooth is primary or permanent. Do not touch the root of the tooth; only handle by the crown (the white end of the tooth) wearing gloves and using gauze. Determine how long the tooth has been out of socket. If the tooth remains dry greater than 1 hour before being replanted or placed in a physiologic transport medium such as milk, saliva, saline, tissue culture medium, or Hank's balanced storage solution (HBSS), the tooth is considered likely nonviable. Never rub the tooth to get it clean. Immediately notify a provider if an avulsed tooth is still potentially viable in order to expedite its care and remain within the 1-hour window. Place the avulsed tooth in available physiologic medium if this has not already been initiated, even if it is more than 1 hour out of socket. If an avulsed tooth was replanted before arrival at the emergency department, the patient may gently bite down on a gauze pad to maintain stability if he or she is alert and mature enough to follow instructions. The patient should remain upright. Replantation does not guarantee long-term tooth survival (Andersson et al., 2012). Tooth avulsion injuries are common in children. Completely avulsed primary teeth should not be replanted. The nurse should inquire whether the tooth was found. If not found, radiographs should be ordered to ensure that the tooth was not inhaled, swallowed, or impacted (Keels et al., 2014).

Dental concussions of primary and permanent teeth do not require immediate treatment. The patient or caregiver should be informed to observe for darkening of an injured tooth over a period of days to months following injury. This would indicate possible pulpal necrosis and require immediate dental evaluation. Dental crown fractures require early referral to a dentist, especially if the pulp is exposed. Many fractures require dental splinting, which must be managed by a dental professional. The less mature the permanent tooth, the worse the prognosis (Keels et al., 2014).

Luxation injuries are categorized by the direction in which the tooth is displaced. Mild luxation may not require treatment, but notable displacement may require gentle repositioning by a medical or dental provider. The tooth is usually tender to touch or to tapping and presents with varying degrees of increased mobility. Increased tooth sensitivity is common. Bleeding at the tooth/gum interface is often seen (DiAngelis et al., 2012).

Injuries to primary dentition in children are common. The roots of primary teeth are closely approximated to evolving permanent teeth. An impaction injury to a primary tooth can pose a risk of injury to the adjacent evolving permanent tooth. Patients sustaining primary tooth impaction should be urgently referred to a dental provider for evaluation. Some luxation injuries to primary teeth often heal spontaneously (Malmgren et al., 2012).

Dental injuries and abscesses commonly result in patient anxiety and pain. Frequently assess the patient's airway patency and maintain bleeding control. Calm the patient and make him or her as comfortable as possible. Reassure him or her and keep him or her informed of activities and the ongoing plan of care. Assessment of pain status is a key component of care for the patient experiencing a dental injury or infection. Nonaspirin analgesics may provide substantial relief of dental pain (Hicks et al., 2016). Request pain medication when indicated, ensuring no allergy exists. Notify the medical provider if the patient's pain intervention is not effective. Ice pack application may be painful related to dental nerve injury. A heat pack may serve to be more soothing for pain. Anticipate antibiotic administration in cases of dental fracture, tooth avulsion, and dental abscess. Absent or decreased pain, reduction of swelling and bleeding, and decreased anxiety are desirable outcomes following dental trauma.

Summary

Patients sustaining dental injuries and abscesses often seek care in emergency departments. Nurses play a vital role in assessment, care, and treatment for these patients. Providing discharge instructions that are understandable and individualized to patient and caregiver literacy level is crucial to achieving desirable outcomes for these patients. Providing resource options for timely dental follow-up care is necessary.

Allareddy, V., Rampa, S., Lee, M. K., Allareddy, V., & Nalliah, R. P. (2014). Hospital-based emergency department visits involving dental conditions: Profile and predictors of poor outcomes and resource utilization. *Journal of the American Dental Association*, 145(4), 331–337.

American Association of Endodontists. (2016). Traumatic dental injuries. Retrieved from http://www.aae.org/patients/treatments-and-procedures/traumatic-dental-injuries.aspx

Andersson, L. (2013). Epidemiology of traumatic dental injuries. *Journal of endodontics*, 39(3), S2–S5.

Andersson, L., Andreasen, J. O., Day, P., Heithersay, G., Trope, M., DiAngelis, A. J., & Hicks, M. L. (2012). International Association of Dental Traumatology guidelines for the management of traumatic dental injuries: 2. Avulsion of permanent teeth. *Dental Traumatology*, 28(2), 88–96.

DiAngelis, A. J., Andreasen, J. O., Ebeleseder, K. A., Kenny, D. J., Trope, M., Sigurdsson, A., . . . Lenzi, A. R. (2012). International Association of Dental Traumatology guidelines for the management of traumatic dental injuries: 1. Fractures and luxations of permanent teeth. *Dental Traumatology, 28*(1), 2–12.

Hicks, R. W., Green, R., & Van Wicklin, S. A. (2016). Dental avulsions: Review and recommendations. *Nurse Practitioner, 41*(6), 58–62.

Hodgdon, A. (2013). Dental and related infections. *Emergency Medicine Clinics of North America, 31*(2), 465–480.

Keels, M. A., Segura, A., Boulter, S., Clark, M., Gereige, R., Krol, D., & Slayton, R. (2014). Management of dental trauma in a primary care setting. *Pediatrics, 133*(2), e466–e476.

Malmgren, B., Andreasen, J. O., Flores, M. T., Robertson, A., DiAngelis, A. J., Andersson, L., . . . Malmgren, O. (2012). International Association of Dental Traumatology guidelines for the management of traumatic dental injuries: 3. Injuries in the primary dentition. *Dental Traumatology, 28*(3), 174–182.

Veerasathpurush, A., Rampa, S., Lee, M. K., Allaerddy, V., & Malliah, R. (2014). Hospital-based emergency department visits involving dental conditions. *Journal of the American Dental Association, 145*(5), 331–337.

■ DISASTER RESPONSE

Darlie Simerson

Overview

Disaster response in the emergency department (ED) begins with disaster preparedness in partnership with the community. The Department of Homeland Security (DHS) developed the National Response Framework to facilitate national preparedness for any events deemed to pose the greatest risk to our nation. Four phases identified were mitigation, preparedness, response, and recovery (DHS, 2016). These phases start at the community level and extend into the ED, the entry point of care to the hospital. Emphasis is placed on preparation for the hazards that each community is most at risk of experiencing. The ED and community resources, including first responders and public health departments, rely heavily on each other to function efficiently and effectively. Our nation has been through several recent natural disasters and terrorist events in which lessons have been learned on best practices to use in handling disasters. Issues specific to the ED include disaster triage, personnel safety, symptom surveillance, patient surge capacity, throughput, and clinical management preparedness for all potential hazards (Emergency Nurses Association [ENA], 2013).

Background

Disasters are catastrophic events that may cause injury or loss of life. There are both man-made and natural disasters that include environmental, chemical, biological, and nuclear incidences. When humans are adversely affected, the ED is customarily the desired point of care. Often disasters cause a disruption of services within the ED, which necessitates careful allocation of resources with essential functions taking priority. An emergency operations plan (EOP) is mandated by The Joint Commission (TJC) for all hospitals and is activated to accommodate a surge in patient numbers in the ED. Disaster training drills are the recommended modality for members of the community and ED to interact and take part in disaster simulations. This allows for all members of the team to become familiar with their role in the EOP. These drills also provide an opportunity for identification of training needs and for assessment of the level of preparedness (TJC, 2014).

It is important that ED nurses are prepared to anticipate many of the possible disaster scenarios. Prior training in the management of all hazards is necessary to prevent the ED from becoming overwhelmed in a sudden event. Nurses in the ED play a pivotal role in symptom surveillance, triage, and patient surge management during a disaster response. They are often the first member of the ED team to encounter the patient and the first to discover a hazard exposure. Nurses must take on a leadership role in implementing the EOP. It is important that they are prepared for this role by being familiar with the plan and how to access specific hazard information. Personnel safety is paramount to prevent more casualties from being added to the already heavy burden caused by the disaster. Use of personal protective equipment (PPE) and making PPE available to others when necessary is the first priority. The need for patient isolation and decontamination must be quickly recognized and initiated.

Clinical Aspects

Specific hazards of concern in the ED include injuries secondary to natural disasters and chemical contamination as well as illness secondary to biological exposures. The first priority is to protect others, including the nurse, from injury or contamination. PPE should be readily available and training should be provided to the nurses before the incident. Isolation and contamination needs should be identified in triage if at all possible to prevent further spread throughout the ED. Resources, such as safety data sheets, must be easily accessible at the point of initial contact so that nurses can quickly acquire treatment guidelines for chemical and other known exposures. Some other important resources are the Centers for Disease Control and Prevention (CDC) and the local public health department.

ASSESSMENT

Disaster triage for mass casualties determines resource requirements such as ED staffing numbers and bed availability. This is an assignment for nurses experienced in triage procedures. The EOP includes guidelines that are implemented to aid in identification of the patient level of severity and the appropriate location for treatment. This is particularly true of trauma-related disasters in which isolation and decontamination are not necessary. It is of paramount importance that prior preparation, through EOP drills, has occurred so that ED staff are able to handle a surge in patient numbers in a sudden disaster. Additional ED nurse responsibilities include surge discharge of noncritical patients and increased throughput of stabilized patients to other hospital treatment areas in order to increase ED bed availability.

Anticipatory training is recommended for ED nurses in preparation for those hazards most likely to be seen in the ED. It is impossible to know everything about all hazards but the ED nurses should know where to quickly access information. Types of disasters with the potential to result in a large influx of ED patients include bioterrorism, chemical emergencies, radiation emergencies, natural disasters or severe weather, and infectious outbreaks. In addition, particular attention is directed to vulnerable populations such as children, elderly, chronically ill, and mentally ill (ENA, 2013).

Although not all inclusive, anthrax, botulism, plague, and smallpox are considered to be the most likely encountered bioterrorism agents. The CDC provides specific information regarding management of infection or exposure. It is important that ED nurses recognize an unusual increase in patients with the same symptoms, especially fever, respiratory, or gastrointestinal complaints. An unusual pattern or uncharacteristic timing to the symptoms should be noted (CDC, 2016).

Chemical emergencies can result from a vast number of sources. When these are hazmat events, there is customarily communication from first responders indicating the type of exposure. The CDC and regional poison control centers are excellent resources for management information. Decontamination may be dry or wet depending on the chemical and is sometimes carried out at the scene of the exposure. Identification of the type of chemical is key to the treatment needed.

Radiation emergencies have the potential to quickly overwhelm the ED. Use of PPE is essential for nurses and other ED staff. Decontamination is necessary to lessen the risk of acute skin injury, to lower the risk of internal contamination, and to reduce the risk of contamination to health care providers. Removal of all clothing can reduce contamination on the patient up to 90% (U.S. Department of Health and Human Services, 2016). Further decontamination occurs by washing the patient. Contaminated water collected afterward must be properly disposed of as in dedicated ED decontamination showers.

Natural disasters or severe weather may include hurricanes, tornados, and flooding. These may result in mass casualties from trauma. Events such as these have the potential to cause a sudden surge in patients arriving in the ED with a large variety of injuries. Again, ED nurses must rely on previous training and the EOP to manage resource availability. The sequela of these events may be a rapid failure in health care areas that are less prepared for disasters such as nursing homes, clinics, and dialysis centers. The ED may be the only available resource for care following a catastrophic event.

Last of all are the infectious outbreaks. Surveillance is an important aspect of ED nursing as mentioned in the bioterrorism section. ED nurses are in a unique position to recognize reoccurring symptoms presenting to the ED. In recent years, an Ebola outbreak in West Africa has raised our awareness of the potential for an epidemic and the need to screen patients for possible exposure. Recent travel information has become a familiar part of initial information obtained on all patients entering the ED. Use of PPE for personnel protection and proper use of isolation techniques are the mainstays of infection management.

Summary

Disaster response in the ED can be determined by a vast number of potential agents. Although impossible to have in-depth knowledge regarding each, it is important for ED nurses to recognize the need to protect personnel and act quickly to address immediate patient needs to lessen sequelae. It is the responsibility of ED nurses to participate in preparedness exercises and continuing education in anticipation of taking a leadership role in the event of a disaster.

Centers for Disease Control and Prevention. (2016). Emergency preparedness and response. Retrieved from https://emergency.cdc.gov/hazards-specific.asp

Department of Homeland Security. (2016). *National response framework* (3rd ed.). Retrieved from https://www.fema.gov/media-library/assets/documents/117791

Emergency Nurses Association. (2013). Position statement: Disaster and emergency preparedness for all hazards. Retrieved from https://www.ena.org/SiteCollection Documents/Position%20Statements/AllHazards.pdf

The Joint Commission. (2014). Emergency management resources: New and revised requirements. Retrieved from https://www.jointcommission.org/emergency_ management.aspx

United States Department of Health and Human Services. (2016). Radiation emergency medical management. Retrieved from https://www.remm.nlm.gov/ext_contami nation.htm

■ DISSEMINATED INTRAVASCULAR COAGULATION

Joyce E. Higgins

Overview

Disseminated intravascular coagulation (DIC) is a secondary syndrome resulting in the activation of clotting and thrombolytic systems that impair tissue perfusion and result in devastating end-organ damage (Wada, Matsumoto, & Yamashita, 2014). The extent of organ destruction related to the imbalances in the coagulation and fibrin activity that result in DIC and the primary etiologic mechanism, such as an infection (Asakura, 2014). Although there are many causes, sepsis in combination with DIC has a higher mortality rate and can be very difficult to manage in the critically ill adult (Ishikura et al., 2014).

Background

According to the Scientific Standards Committee (SSC) formed in the International Society on Thrombosis and Hemostasis (ISTH; 2001), DIC is defined as an acquired syndrome, characterized by the intravascular activation of coagulation and the loss of localization coming from different causes. It can originate from and cause damage to the microvasculature that, if sufficiently severe, can produce organ dysfunction (Taylor, Toh, Hoots, Wada, & Levi, 2001).

Organ dysfunction is a latent characteristic of systemic inflammatory response syndrome (SIRS) and sepsis. The inflammatory response causes circulatory instability throughout the body. When SIRS is not a locally managed inflammation in the body, it is referred to as *sepsis*. Sepsis is identified as a failure of two or more body systems that can lead to organ failure. Sepsis in the adult can increase in severity when combined with the coagulopathy disorders of DIC (Davis, Miller-Dorey, & Jenne, 2016; Ishikura et al., 2014; Okamoto, Tamura, & Sawatsubashi, 2016). Early detection and management of DIC with sepsis can help decrease client mortality.

Several studies use the British Committee for Standards in Haematology (BCSH), Japanese Society of Thrombosis and Hemostasis (JSTH), Italian Society for Thrombosis and Hemostasis (SISET), and the ISTH/SSC as collaborative guideline recommendations for diagnosis and treatment plans in DIC (Wada et al., 2013). As DIC is not a primary condition, a combination of tests and treatments are needed to achieve a successful outcome. The use of a scoring system and treatment of the underlying disease process is highly recommended across all guidelines to assist in the treatment and a decrease in mortality (Wada et al., 2013, 2014). The severity of the clients' ailments can be scored using the Sequential Organ Failure Assessment (SOFA), Acute Physiological and Chronic Health Evaluation (APACHE II), or Japanese Association for Acute Medicine as in a study by Ishikura et al. (2014), which identified sepsis-induced DIC in classifications of mild, moderate, and severe. Each classification had more complications and brought on higher mortality.

There are different types of DIC, such as bleeding, massive bleeding, fibrin growth related to tumors, and organ failure. Each type presents with different characteristics, bleeding is a slow or constant leaking from coagulation; massive uncontrolled bleeding as occurs in surgery, ruptured placenta, or aortic aneurysms; hyperfibrinolysis from tumor growth as seen in leukemia; and hypercoagulation or hyperfibrinolysis as found in organ failure with sepsis (Wada et al., 2014). Sepsis is the decompensation of two or more organ systems that can be difficult to overcome, especially with the presentation of DIC.

Sepsis is diagnosed based on the cellular inflammatory response in the body increasing the tissue factor (TF) and preventing fibrinolysis because of an accumulation of plasminogen activator inhibitor type-1 (PAI-1). This causes a growth of fibrin in capillaries and small vessels called *microemboli* or *clots* that destroy cell structures. The destruction of cells leads to organ failure, and multiple organ failures can lead to death (Ishikura et al., 2014; Wada et al., 2014).

The clients in intensive care units (ICUs) are more susceptible to the development of DIC because of SIRS. The underlying disease process of some of these diagnoses are an infection, burn surgeries, hepatitis, acute pancreatitis, and rhabdomyolysis (Asakura, 2014). The inflammatory response releases neutrophils, histones, cathepsin G, and neutrophil extracellular traps (NETs) that bind together to defeat the infection. This adds to the activation of the coagulation cascade causing a buildup of cells in the vasculature (Davis et al., 2016). According to Okamoto et al. (2016), DIC in sepsis is defined by escalation of the inflammation and its collection of released responses along with the coagulation pathways. The coagulation complication in combination with thrombocytopenia increases the risk of intracranial hemorrhage by 88%, further increasing mortality (Levi & Hunt, 2015).

Clinical Aspects

The treatment of DIC is divided as mentioned previously by the SSC of the ISTH. The SSC recommendations are for a collaboration of tests and treatment of the underlying cause. As DIC is a secondary syndrome, the nurse needs to be alert for changes that can arise both gradually and suddenly.

ASSESSMENT

Constant monitoring of vital signs and assessment requires ICU admission. Overt signs of bleeding can be hematuria, hemoptysis, bleeding from old puncture sites, and change in the level of consciousness (LOC). Signs of alteration in coagulation causing an embolic development can include but are not limited to purpura, petechiae, cyanosis, gangrene, chest pain, acute myocardial infarction, respiratory distress, abdominal pain and/or distention, constipation, and change of LOC. Frequent clinical and laboratory measurements are required for a proper evaluation of DIC (Levi & Hunt, 2015).

Laboratory markers of low platelets, increased prothrombin time (PT), increased activated partial thromboplastin time (a PTT), prolonged fibrinogen, and fibrin degradation products (D-dimer) vary in the reliability to diagnose DIC (Levi, 2014). Each test is reflective of other disease processes and not specific to DIC. Other laboratory studies, such as thromboelastography (TEG), can be used to assess coagulation factor function, as well as platelet function, clot strength, and fibrinolysis. The use of TEG can help the health care team determine the pharmacologic interventions that might be most beneficial to patients with DIC (Levi & Hunt, 2015).

NURSING INTERVENTIONS, MANAGEMENT, AND IMPLICATIONS

Treatment using heparin is useful for both the inflammatory response of platelets, histones, and the NETs, as well as, altering the thrombin of the clotting factors (Davis et al., 2016). The anticoagulated agent heparin has a short acting half-life making it easier to adjust in high-risk clients who are more likely to bleed. Several ongoing studies have shown to have beneficial responses using both low-dose heparin and molecular weight-based dosing for treatment of sepsis and DIC-related sepsis (Davis et al., 2016; Okamoto et al., 2016).

Additional treatments include transfusion of clotting factors, such as platelet concentration (PC), fresh frozen plasma (FFP), and fibrinogen as cryoprecipitate. Not all the guidelines recommend blood product infusion, although doing so helps with patients who have active bleeding and also replenishes the diminishing factors in the clotting cascade (Davis et al., 2016). Red blood cell (RBC) transfusion is used with massive blood loss related to trauma, surgery, and in DIC if necessary (Davis et al., 2016).

Antithrombin (AT) is a glycoprotein made in the liver inhibiting thrombin activity and clotting cascade factors (Davis et al., 2016). The AT is significantly depleted in DIC. Japan reflects several studies of DIC using AT treatment. Okamoto et al.'s (2016) randomized multicenter control trial with treatment using moderate AT dosing ranges showed a decrease in DIC scores and faster recovery. Not all guidelines recommend the use of AT administration for the treatment of DIC, although in Japan, Tagami, Matsui, Horiguchi, Fushimi, and Yasunaga (2014) showed a decrease in the 28-day mortality with AT dosage in severe pneumonia and DIC.

Current and future studies are ongoing to validate treatment and diagnostics for DIC. The guideline recommendations of ISTH/SSC, SISET, BCSH, and JSTH and scoring systems can assist with building strategies for future comparison in trials to benefit clients.

OUTCOMES

Prevention of DIC is the priority nursing outcome. It is imperative to institute early and rapid interventions to correct the underlying offender and prevent further damage. DIC can be devastating and is truly life-threatening. Evaluating the patient for early signs is key in preventing this disorder.

Summary

DIC is a diversely complicated secondary disease. The diagnosis and treatment can be a long process. All experts do not agree on the treatment modalities. However, they do concur that it is more beneficial to the high-risk clients of the ICU to diagnose and treat early-onset symptoms and underlying causes of DIC. No single laboratory measurement identifies DIC. It takes a combination of assessment, skill, and diagnostic testing to identify and treat DIC. Nursing personnel can continue to stay abreast of the clinical changes in the client that may trigger DIC. They can collaborate to treat the inflammatory response system and replace the products of the coagulation pathway as needed to decrease severity and mortality of the client.

Asakura, H. (2014). Classifying types of disseminated intravascular coagulation: Clinical and animal models. *Journal of Intensive Care, 2*(1), 20.

Davis, R. P., Miller-Dorey, S., & Jenne, C. N. (2016). Platelets and coagulation in infection. *Clinical & Translational Immunology, 5*(7), e89.

Ishikura, H., Nishida, T., Murai, A., Nakamura, Y., Irie, Y., Tanaka, J., & Umemura, T. (2014). New diagnostic strategy for sepsis-induced disseminated intravascular coagulation: A prospective single-center observational study. *Critical Care, 18*(1), R19.

Levi, M. (2014). Diagnosis and treatment of disseminated intravascular coagulation. *International Journal of Laboratory Hematology, 36*(3), 228–236.

Levi, M., & Hunt, B. J. (2015). A critical appraisal of point-of-care coagulation testing in critically ill patients. *Journal of Thrombosis and Haemostasis, 13*(11), 1960–1967.

Okamoto, K., Tamura, T., & Sawatsibashi, Y. (2016). Sepsis and disseminated intravascular coagulation. *Journal of Intensive Care, 4,* 4–23. doi:10.1186/s40560-016-0149-0

Tagami, T., Matsui, H., Horiguchi, H., Fushimi, K., & Yasunaga, H. (2014). Antithrombin and mortality in severe pneumonia patients with sepsis-associated disseminated intravascular coagulation: An observational nationwide study. *Journal of Thrombosis and Haemostasis, 12*(9), 1470–1479.

Taylor, F. B., Toh, C. H., Hoots, W. K., Wada, H., & Levi, M.; Scientific Subcommittee on Disseminated Intravascular Coagulation of the International Society on Thrombosis and Haemostasis. (2001). Towards definition, clinical and laboratory criteria, and a scoring system for disseminated intravascular coagulation. *Thrombosis and Haemostasis, 86*(5), 1327–1330.

Wada, H., Matsumoto, T., & Yamashita, Y. (2014). Diagnosis and treatment of disseminated intravascular coagulation (DIC) according to four DIC guidelines. *Journal of Intensive Care, 2*(1), 15.

Wada, H., Thachil, J., Di Nisio, M., Mathew, P., Kurosawa, S., Gando, S., . . . Toh, C. H. (2013). Guidance for diagnosis and treatment of disseminated intravascular coagulation from harmonization of the recommendations from three guidelines. *Journal of Thrombosis and Haemostasis, 11,* 761–767. doi:10.1111/jth.12155

■ DOMESTIC VIOLENCE

Patricia M. Speck
Diana K. Faugno
Rachell A. Ekroos
Melanie Gibbons Hallman
Gwendolyn D. Childs
Tedra S. Smith
Stacey A. Mitchell

Overview

Domestic violence (DV), also known as *family* or *intimate partner violence*, is obvious in the Code of Hammurabi (1780 BCE), ancient laws designed to guide male heads of household in the infliction of punishment to control members of their family and property (King, 2008). Legal thinking evolved, and in the 1700s, a legal decision curtailed carte blanche violence against wives, apprentices, and children by defining the "Rule of Thumb," which was a common law limiting penalties to a whip or stick size—no bigger than the man's thumb! In 1871, first to deny Great Britain's custom of wife beating, the State of Alabama prosecuted a husband for assault and battery, codifying the wife's citizen rights and protections under the U.S. Constitution (Supreme Court of Alabama, 1871, p. 3). Although greater society believes that DV is a "family matter," legislation passed since the 1970s squarely identifies DV behavior as assault, warranting criminal justice intervention (Erez, 2002). Important to nurses referring victims, DV legislation guarantees victims access to community support programs funded by the

Family Violence Prevention and Services Act (Family Violence Prevention and Services Programs, 2016).

Background

There is a demonstrated association between DV and immediate and long-term health, social, and economic consequences (DuMonthier & Dusenbery, 2016) taking the form of "physical assault, psychological abuse, social abuse, financial abuse, or sexual assault" (Kaur & Garg, 2008, p.74). The economic impact in the United States is between $4 billion and $9 billion, with $6.3 billion in direct medical and mental health care costs (Breiding et al., 2014; Hughes & Brush, 2015). For RNs charged with the evaluation and referral of patients at risk for DV, the evidence is mixed, and further study is needed about the cost-benefit of identification and the effectiveness of referral (O'Doherty et al., 2015). No one factor contributes to DV, but there are linkages for male and female offenders with a history of DV, depression, social isolation, antisocial behavior, and substance abuse (Capaldi, Knoble, Shortt, & Kim, 2012), in which single lifestyle and separation from partner create vulnerability, and marriage is protective of women. Nursing practice is fundamental in the prevention of DV, where there is clear understanding of the contributing factors and coordinating resources necessary for change in communities.

Estimating the incidence of DV is difficult as victims do not report and when they do, recording of the event reflects community language, not consistent with national data terms (Fernandes-Alcantara, 2014). Victims also may fear the law enforcement response, particularly in small communities where everyone is known, there is shame, or they experience fear of increasing abuse after disclosure. Research demonstrates that DV is very common, both men and women experience victimization (sexual, physical, and psychological), but women are victimized more often than men, and minority women more than nonminority women (Breiding et al., 2014).

DV creates chaos in traumatized families whereby offenders isolate and economically deprive the partner of employment, financial decisions, and control of funds (DuMonthier & Dusenbery, 2016). The children of victims of DV are most at risk for child abuse and neglect, many experiencing personal environments of social isolation, not conducive to normal development or emotional health (Bair-Merritt, Blackstone, & Feudtner, 2006). Disparities and social determinants create complex risk factors in DV environments that diminish attainment of health. Those environments and attitudes include exposure to crime and violence, disease, and lack of access to health care and personal and support systems (Braveman & Gottlieb, 2014; Chung et al., 2016), with isolation and lack of social support (Capaldi et al., 2012).

Building on the stress and adaptation theories of the 1990s, chronic stress in DV environments increases hormonal dysregulation predisposing the family members to increased risk of violence and disease, and early death (Felitti et al., 1998; McEwen, 1998). Pregnant women and their developing fetus(s), newborns, infants, and children exposed to DV experience elevated stress hormones and begin a quest to escape or calm the "fear" response (a comprehensive explanation of the biophysiology appears in the Child Abuse and Neglect entry). For the adolescent and adult subjected to DV, similar biological responses increase risk of aberrant and risk-taking behaviors (Hyman, Malenka, & Nestler, 2006; McEwen & Seeman, 1999). Understanding the underlying biophysiology of stress and trauma responses of the adolescent or adult DV victims prepares the RN to address obvious anxiety, mood, and depression symptoms that lead to poor health choices and outcomes (Felitti et al., 1998; McEwen, 1998).

Clinical Aspects

The incidence and prevalence of DV ensures that nurses will care for patients in a DV situation, because half the women they serve experience psychological aggression by an intimate partner, and a third experience physical aggression (Breiding et al., 2014). However, there are many challenges to obtaining a history of DV from patients. The social beliefs are barriers, particularly when communities believe it is a "family" matter. Other barriers to asking about or disclosing DV information is that it is a sensitive topic, reflecting personal shame and self-blame in victims, and where providers lack training about how to ask and what to do (Campbell, Sharps, Sachs, & Yam, 2003; Connor, Nouer, Speck, Mackey, & Tipton, 2013; O'Doherty et al., 2015). There is an economic and emotional dependency in patients, and for some, insecurity reflects their inability to support their families (Gutmanis, Beynon, Tutty, Wathen, & MacMillan, 2007). Nurses need to recognize DV's mental and physical health outcomes, which are directly related to the biology of trauma and include depression, anxiety, posttraumatic stress disorder, psychosis, inability to trust others, self-harm, and a host of psychosomatic conditions (Stewart & Vigod, 2017), as well as heart disease, obesity, hypertension, obstructive lung diseases, and stroke (Felitti et al., 1998; McEwen, 1998).

Nurses receiving concept-based education about forensic nursing might experience a simulation using DV as an exemplar. There are eight concepts in a routine nursing inquiry, which include "preparedness, self-confidence, professional supports, abuse inquiry, practitioner consequences of asking, comfort following disclosure, practitioner lack of control, and practice pressures" (Gutmanis et al., 2007, p. 4). When interviewed, DV victims acknowledged wanting health care professionals who were "nonjudgmental, nondirective, and individually tailored, with an appreciation of the complexity of partner violence" and health care providers who were able to listen, express concern, empathy, and support (Feder, Hutson, Ramsay, & Taket, 2006, p. 34). Women's perceptions of health care provider interactions depended on the woman's readiness to address the issue and trust of a health care provider (Feder et al., 2006). With didactic and simulation preparation, variability in health care practices diminishes and the identification, plans for intervention with trauma-informed and patient-centered care improves, all necessary support DV victims and their families throughout disclosure (Gutmanis et al., 2007).

ASSESSMENT

A number of screening tools exist and include Abuse Assessment Screen/Abuse Assessment Screen-Disability (AAS/AASD); Humiliation, Afraid, Rape, and Kick (HARK); Hurt, Insulted, Threatened, or Screamed Questionnaire (HITS); Partner Abuse Interview; Partner Violence Screen; Suicide Assessment Five-step Evaluation (SAFE-T); STaT; Women Abuse Screening Tool (WAST); WAST Short Form; and Women's Experience with Battering Scale. However, of these, only three are validated to assess all three areas of abuse—physical, sexual, and psychological—and they are AAS, HARK, and WAST (Arkins, Begley, & Higgins, 2016). These tools are useful for nurses in many settings, including emergency departments, surgical areas, perinatal care, and mental health. It is suspected that other practice areas are amenable to screening, but need validated tools in their populations that are reliable and "screen for all three types of abuse" (Arkins et al., 2016, p. 233). The tools noted are not generalizable, therefore testing in

unique communities and cultures is recommended. Lethality assessments are sensitive and provide a tool to first responders estimating the risk of near lethal and deadly violence (Campbell et al., 2003; Campbell, Webster, & Glass, 2009). The lethality scales do not predict who will die from DV; therefore, consider their use in health care practices carefully.

NURSING INTERVENTIONS, MANAGEMENT, AND IMPLICATIONS

The RN is in a position to speak frankly and comfortably with the patient about all health risks, including DV. When suspected, the nurse should therapeutically explore the possibility of the patient's vulnerability to DV, past experiences, and current situation. If the patient does disclose, the nurse should advise the patient about options to reporting. If he or she does not disclose, anticipatory guidance about community resources is warranted. For both the discloser and nondiscloser, the nurse should strongly advise the escape/elopement from the abuser to be secret and deliberate. Unfortunately, when victims threaten to leave the abuser or announce they will leave the abuser or they leave, the abuser is at greatest risk to commit murder of the partner, their children, other family members, and animals.

The RN and the institutional team provide trauma-informed and patient-centered care, assessment, and documentation, important for the safety and postencounter planning of the patient and family. If the RN is the first to suspect DV, he or she should consider counseling the patient to connect with DV community resources while the patient is with him or her. The nurse alerts hospital social workers and community collaborators, who have experience with DV and institutional relationships through memorandum. The RN assessment for DV or other forensic nursing presentations is descriptive only, documenting objective information and addressing anxiety and fear through the creation of a safe environment. Throughout the process, the RN role is therapeutic and helpful, explaining each step in the process and providing clarity to the legal investigation.

OUTCOMES

The patient should be cautioned to work with the community resources to plan and prepare, leaving the relationship only when the first opportunity presents, without fanfare, fights, or threats, which raise the lethality index. Of note, if the offender is aware of the plans to leave, all providers at the institution and in the community are at risk; there is also an increased risk of partner and family harm. Institutions need safety policies and procedure plans, where active shooter training applies to DV offenders, especially when the victim prepares to elope from the relationship. Of course, when the victim requires urgent or emergent care, procedures that deidentify the name and location are prudent.

Summary

Safety is a human desire, and families depend on health care providers to supply information about their health and welfare. In DV, chaos ensues with physical, sexual, and psychological stresses unknown to those outside the relationship. During the relationship-building phases that trap victims, the time between events and apologies keep some people with their partners. Others are trapped in slave-like conditions, never experiencing pleasant times, instead experiencing toxic trauma bonding with a boyfriend trafficker. The continuum of violence creates stress and health outcomes contributing to economic deprivation and insecurity, fear for DV victims themselves and their families, and eventually for their survival. The nurse is positioned to begin a conversation about violence and its impact on health, as well as options that patients may accept from a comprehensive community response, with reassurance and anticipatory guidance for the victims perceived and real dangers. For nurses, it is wise to recognize the importance of existing danger for the care provider and coworkers who facilitate elopement, where vicarious trauma and structural change require attention to ensure trauma-informed and patient-centered care. Finally, recognize that adults have liberties to return to the abuser (see the Child Abuse and Neglect entry if you suspect children are at risk); it is to be hoped that there will be another opportunity to influence the victim's decision to escape.

Arkins, B., Begley, C., & Higgins, A. (2016). Measures for screening for intimate partner violence: A systematic review. *Journal of Psychiatric and Mental Health Nursing*, 23(3–4), 217–235. doi:10.1111/jpm.12289

Bair-Merritt, M. H., Blackstone, M., & Feudtner, C. (2006). Physical health outcomes of childhood exposure to intimate partner violence: A systematic review. *Pediatrics*, 117(2), 278–290. doi:10.1542/peds.2005-1473

Braveman, P., & Gottlieb, L. (2014). The social determinants of health: It's time to consider the causes of the causes. *Public Health Reports*, 129(Suppl. 2), 19–31.

Breiding, M. J., Smith, S. G., Basile, K. C., Walters, M. L., Chen, J., & Merrick, M. T. (2014). Prevalence and characteristics of sexual violence, stalking, and intimate partner violence victimization—National Intimate Partner and Sexual Violence Survey, United States, 2011. Retrieved from https://www.cdc.gov/mmwr/pdf/ss/ss6308.pdf

Campbell, J. C., Sharps, P. W., Sachs, C., & Yam, M. L. (2003). Medical lethality assessment and safety planning in domestic violence cases. *Clinics in Family Practice*, 5(1), 101–112.

Campbell, J. C., Webster, D. W., & Glass, N. (2009). The danger assessment: Validation of a lethality risk assessment instrument for intimate partner femicide. *Journal of Interpersonal Violence*, 24(4), 653–674. doi:10.1177/0886260508317180

Capaldi, D. M., Knoble, N. B., Shortt, J. W., & Kim, H. K. (2012). A systematic review of risk factors for intimate partner violence. *Partner Abuse*, 3(2), 231–280. doi:10.1891/1946-6560.3.2.231

Chung, E. K., Siegel, B. S., Garg, A., Conroy, K., Gross, R. S., Long, D. A., . . . Fierman, A. H. (2016). Screening for social determinants of health among children and families living in poverty: A guide for clinicians. *Current Problems in Pediatric and Adolescent Health Care*, 46(5), 135–153. doi:10.1016/j.cppeds.2016.02.004

Connor, P. D., Nouer, S. S., Speck, P. M., Mackey, S. N., & Tipton, N. G. (2013). Nursing students and intimate partner violence education: Improving and integrating knowledge into health care curricula. *Journal of Professional Nursing*, 29(4), 233–239. doi:10.1016/j.profnurs.2012.05.011

DuMonthier, A., & Dusenbery, M. (2016). Intersections of domestic violence and economic security. Retrieved from https://iwpr.org/wp-content/uploads/2017/01/B362-Domestic-Violence-and-Economic-Security-1.pdf

Erez, E. (2002). Domestic violence and the criminal justice system: An overview. *Online Journal of Issues in Nursing*, 7(1), 4.

Family Violence Prevention and Services Programs. (2016). Final rule. *Federal Register*, 81(212), 76446–76480.

Feder, G. S., Hutson, M., Ramsay, J., & Taket, A. R. (2006). Women exposed to intimate partner violence: Expectations and experiences when they encounter health care professionals: A meta-analysis of qualitative studies. *Archives of Internal Medicine*, 166(1), 22–37. doi:10.1001/archinte.166.1.22

Felitti, V. J., Anda, R. F., Nordenberg, D., Williamson, D. F., Spitz, A. M., Edwards, V., . . . Marks, J. S. (1998). Relationship of childhood abuse and household dysfunction to many of the leading causes of death in adults. The Adverse Childhood Experiences (ACE) Study. *American Journal of Preventive Medicine*, 14(4), 245–258.

Fernandes-Alcantara, A. L. (2014). Family Violence Prevention and Services Act (FVPSA): Background and funding. Retrieved from https://fas.org/sgp/crs/misc/R42838.pdf

Gutmanis, I., Beynon, C., Tutty, L., Wathen, C. N., & MacMillan, H. L. (2007). Factors influencing identification of and response to intimate partner violence: A survey of physicians and nurses. *BMC Public Health*, 7, 12. doi:10.1186/1471-2458-7-12

Hughes, M. M., & Brush, L. D. (2015). The price of protection. *American Sociological Review*, 80(1), 140–165. doi:10.1177/0003122414561117

Hyman, S. E., Malenka, R. C., & Nestler, E. J. (2006). Neural mechanisms of addiction: The role of reward-related learning and memory. *Annual Review of Neuroscience*, 29, 565–598. doi:10.1146/annurev.neuro.29.051605.113009

Kaur, R., & Garg, S. (2008). Addressing domestic violence against women: An unfinished agenda. *Indian Journal of Community Medicine*, 33(2), 73–76. doi:10.4103/0970-0218.40871

King, L. W. (2008). The Code of Hammurabi. Retrieved from http://avalon.law.yale.edu/ancient/hamframe.asp

McEwen, B. S. (1998). Stress, adaptation, and disease: Allostasis and allostatic load. *Annals of the New York Academy of Sciences*, 840, 33–44. doi:10.1111/j.1749-6632.1998.5b09546.x

McEwen, B. S., & Seeman, T. (1999). Protective and damaging effects of mediators of stress. Elaborating and testing the concepts of allostasis and allostatic load. *Annals of the New York Academy of Sciences*, 896, 30–47.

O'Doherty, L., Hegarty, K., Ramsay, J., Davidson, L. L., Feder, G., & Taft, A. (2015). Screening women for intimate partner violence in healthcare settings. *Cochrane Database of Systematic Reviews*, 2015(7), CD007007. doi:10.1002/14651858.CD007007.pub3

Stewart, D. E., & Vigod, S. N. (2017). Mental health aspects of intimate partner violence. *Psychiatric Clinics of North America*, 40(2), 321–334. doi:10.1016/j.psc.2017.01.009

Supreme Court of Alabama. (1871). Fulgham v. The State Ala. 1871. Retrieved from http://faculty.law.miami.edu/zfenton/documents/Fulghamv.State.pdf

■ EAR, NOSE, AND THROAT EMERGENCIES

Kathleen Bradbury-Golas

Overview

Ear, nose, and throat (ENT) disorders are common daily occurrences seen in the emergency department. Most of these disorders are primary care conditions, ranging from foreign objects, trauma, to infection and are usually non–life-threatening. Emergency care for ENT disorders, regardless of age, is focused on an accurate assessment of the complaint, associated symptoms, and priority management of airway and breathing patterns.

ENT disorders can occur separately or in combination with one or more other organ systems. For example, the common cold may include nasal congestion and sinus pressure, sore throat, and ear popping or pain, whereas bacterial pharyngitis may include only a sore throat and fever. All are capable of leading to more dangerous complications (i.e., pneumonia) when not treated accordingly.

Background

Ear, nose, and throat problems are one of the most common causes for which a person seeks medical care. These problems are more common in children than adults, due to their wider and more horizontal Eustachian tubes and an underdeveloped immunity (Surapaneni & Sisodia, 2016). Otitis media (middle/inner ear infection) remains one of the most common infections in children, affecting up to 75% of children at least once between the ages of 5 and 11 years (Liese et al., 2015). The occurrence of otitis media decreases markedly after age 6, with other head, face, and sinus conditions causing secondary otalgia in adults (Dains, Baumann, & Scheibel, 2016).

ENT disease can be caused by a variety of microorganisms with rhinoviruses as the leading cause of the common cold in all age groups. Acute pharyngitis, sinusitis, and otitis media are mainly associated with respiratory viruses and common bacteria. The most common bacterial agent for pharyngitis is *Group A beta-hemolytic Streptococcus* (GABS), accounting for 20% to 40% of cases in children, but only 10% of cases in adults (Cohen, Bertille, Cohen, & Chalumeau, 2016). Unfortunately, overuse of antibiotics for viral infections has led to antibiotic resistance, especially with *Streptococcus pneumoniae*, thereby complicating treatment. According to the Centers for Disease Control and Prevention (CDC; 2015), antibiotic adverse drug events are responsible for one out of five emergency department visits and over half of antibiotics prescribed for acute respiratory infections are inappropriate. In 2009, the United States spent $10.7 billion on combined inpatient and outpatient antibiotic use (CDC, 2015).

In addition to common upper respiratory infections, foreign object removal is often a common reason for visiting the emergency department. The nostrils and ears are prime locations for a foreign object to be found, with luck, before infection has taken place. A ruptured tympanic membrane (eardrum) can occur from either excessive fluid behind the ear due to infection or trauma from foreign objects (i.e., cotton swabs). The ear is the organ of hearing as well as equilibrium, therefore loss of hearing or vertigo and dizziness are also signs of possible issues within this system. Due to the vastness of symptomology within the many different disorders, a thorough nursing assessment is the starting point for differentiation of the cause of clinical manifestations.

Clinical Aspects

ASSESSMENT

Completing an accurate history and assessment is a critical component of nursing care and begins the process of clinical reasoning and triage. Utilizing the acronym OLDCART will assist the nurse in determining the onset and duration of the illness; major system affected; characteristics, including associated symptoms; activities that might make it worse; factors that have helped relieve the symptoms; and when during the day the symptoms are worse or better (Bickley, 2017). OLDCART stands for onset, location, duration, characteristics, alleviating factors, relieving factors, and timing. Specific medical history for comorbid conditions that increase complication risk and social history, such as immunization status, tobacco and alcohol use, and exposure to childcare/preschool, will be necessary to obtain. Many studies in developing countries have reported that socioeconomic status, especially poor living conditions, poor nutrition, and overcrowding increase the incidence of acute respiratory infections in the pediatric population, which in turn increases mortality risk (Chen, Williams, & Kirk, 2014; Ide & Uchenwa-Onyenegecha, 2015). In addition to determining complication risk, history will also help determine treatment modalities and additional teaching/health promotion needs.

The ears are complex sensory organs of hearing and balance. When assessing "ear pain" or otalgia, note that the pain can be primary (coming from the ear itself) or secondary (from other regions). Causes of primary otalgia include infections, inflammation, or foreign body, whereas causes of secondary otalgia include jaw, dental, and periodontal problems, along with infections of the nasopharyngeal areas. Otitis media (infection of the middle/inner ear) and otitis

externa (infection of the ear canal or "swimmer's ear") are two examples of primary otalgia. Otitis media usually presents with a sharp pain, fever, feeling of fullness, and possible hearing loss. Children will often be irritable and pull on the affected ear. Otitis externa presents with pain upon movement of the tragus or jawline, purulent discharge from the ear canal, and possible hearing loss.

When assessing hearing loss or dizziness and vertigo, the nurse should note how the onset has occurred—sudden or gradual. Dizziness or vertigo is second only to back pain of adults seeking medical help (Rhoads & Petersen, 2014). Disorders, such as cerumen impaction, foreign body, labyrinthitis (inflammation of the inner ear), ruptured tympanic membrane, and Ménière's disease, should be considered.

The nose and sinuses are responsible for filtering/warming the air, primary site for inspiration and expiration, and the sense of smell and speech sounds. Nasal congestion, discharge, and sinus pressure or pain are the most common complaints offered. However, appetite and taste are also often disrupted with nasal disorders. It is essential for the nurse to assess for nasal discharge (rhinorrhea) including thickness, color, duration, and another other associated symptoms. Nasal discharge and sinus pressure are often primary symptoms of the common cold. Sinusitis is a sinus inflammation, with many possible causes, including infection, chemical irritants, cocaine use, and dental abscesses. Sinus pain, purulent nasal drainage, and fever are the most common symptoms. Allergic rhinitis (nasal membrane inflammation) is an allergic response to an environmental allergen (i.e., dust, pollen) and exhibits watery nasal drainage, congestion, sneezing, and sore throat. Foreign bodies in the nose occur most often in the pediatric population and aspiration of the object is a major concern. Other pediatric considerations should include careful assessment of the respiratory status as children may present with difficulty breathing and stridor. Epistaxis (nose bleed or hemorrhage) can occur from many different reasons, including but not limited to nose picking, nasal trauma (such as nasal fracture), hypertension and anticoagulant and inhalant use. Herbal therapies contribute to epistaxis as items such as ginkgo biloba increase the risk of bleeding through antiplatelet activity.

The mouth and oropharynx aid in speech, provide taste sensation, act as a passageway for air, and pass food into the esophagus. The most common complaint within the oropharyngeal area is a sore throat or pharyngitis. Again, assessing for other associated symptoms will assist in differentiating possible causes. Sore throats caused by bacterial infections usually occur suddenly; viral infections are more gradual in onset. The most common bacterial cause of pharyngitis is *group A beta-hemolytic Streptococcus* infection. Along with a sore throat, the patient will present with fever, hoarseness, enlarged lymph nodes, halitosis, and malaise. A "rapid strep" or throat culture may be indicated for these patients. If an abscess forms around the tonsil area (peritonsillar abscess), it must be treated immediately to prevent airway obstruction.

NURSING, INTERVENTIONS, MANAGEMENT, AND IMPLICATIONS

During triage, it is essential for the nurse to complete a full history and begin the clinical reasoning process to differentiate the possible causes of the illness/complaint. At this time, the nurse will be instrumental in determining the acuity level of each patient, ensuring that patients are treated accordingly. In the case of foreign object removal, the nurse should prepare for removal through suction, irrigation, alligator forceps, or ear curette. If the health care provider is unable to remove the object, an ENT specialist may need to be consulted. Cerumen impaction removal requires irrigation with warm water and peroxide. Epistaxis will require direct pressure to the bridge of nose, ice application, and possible nasal packing and cauterization. For all procedures, the emergency department nurse should be knowledgeable of the procedure and protocol.

Most ENT infections are treated using a variety of prescribed and over-the-counter medications. Therapeutic interventions include decongestants, antipyretics, pain medication, and antibiotic therapy, when indicated. Decongestants are contraindicated for all patients with hypertension and heart disease due to their vasoconstriction effect.

Antibiotic therapy can be either systemic or topical (Emergency Nurses Association, 2013). Penicillin is the standard systemic antibiotic prescribed, with macrolides (i.e., erythromycin) being prescribed if the patient has a penicillin allergy. Accurate dosing, especially with the pediatric patient, is necessary; therefore, the nurse needs to double check the amount/dose to ensure patient safety. For topical antibiotic administration, as with ear infections and the use of otic antibiotics, the nurse should make sure the drops are warm before administration. In instances when the ear canal is extremely edematous, an ear wick may be used to facilitate delivery of topical medications into the medial canal. For inflammatory reactions, as with seasonal allergies, antihistamines may be prescribed. These medications can also be administered either systemically or topically.

Patient and family education is essential for maximizing outcomes. Instructing the patient and family on completing the full antibiotic course; side effects of any of the medications; proper medication techniques; gargling with warm salt water; keeping ear (s) dry through use of plug(s); using steam, warm compresses, or humidifiers to loosen secretions; good handwashing; and increasing fluid intake should all be addressed upon discharge (Emergency Nurses Association, 2013).

OUTCOMES

The overall goal of therapy for most ENT disorders is resolution of symptoms within 7 to 14 days. Should symptoms continue past that time period, the patient may need a referral to ENT specialist. Chronic sinusitis occurs when the sinus ostia is remodeled leading to changes in the clearance mechanisms of the nares. Though rare now in the United States, *Streptococcal* pharyngitis may develop into a more serious complication, such as acute glomerulonephritis or rheumatic fever. Acute otitis media or blockage of the Eustachian tube can lead to a persistently draining perforation of the tympanic membrane (chronic otitis media). Once treatment has been initiated in the emergency department, the patient should be referred to his or her primary care provider for follow-up evaluation.

Summary

ENT disorders are common everyday occurrences. Most can be effectively treated with early intervention. In rare circumstances, when not detected or treated early, diseases, such as cancer or systemic infections, can cause death. Good history taking and differentiation of symptoms, subsequent nursing care, prescribed pharmacotherapy, and discharge education are essential elements of patient care management and health promotion.

Bickley, L. S. (2017). *Bates' guide to physical examination and history taking* (12th ed.). Philadelphia, PA: Lippincott.

Centers for Disease Control and Prevention. (2015). Fast facts about antibiotic resistance. Retrieved from http://www.cdc.gov/getsmart/community/about/fast-facts.html

Chen, Y., Williams, E., & Kirk, M. (2014). Risk factors for acute respiratory infection in the Australian community.

PLOS ONE, 9(7), e101440. doi:10.1371/journal .pone.0101440

Cohen, J., Bertille, N. Cohen, R., & Chalumeau, M. (2016). Rapid antigen detection test for group A streptococcus in children with pharyngitis. *Cochrane Database of Systematic Reviews*, 2016, CD010502. doi:10.1002/ 14651858.CD010502.pub2

Dains, J., Baumann, L., & Scheibel, P. (2016). *Advanced health assessment and clinical diagnosis in primary care* (5th ed.). St. Louis, MO: Elsevier.

Emergency Nurses Association. (2013). *Sheehy's manual of emergency care* (7th ed.). St. Louis, MO: Mosby

Ide, L., & Uchenwa-Onyenegecha, T. (2015). Burden of acute respiratory tract infections as seen in University of Port Harcourt Teaching Hospital Nigeria. *Journal of US–China Medical Science*, 12, 158–162. doi:10.17265/ 1548-6648/2015.04.003

Liese, J. G., Giaquinto C., Carmona A., Larcombe J. H., Garcia-Sicilia, J., . . . Rosenlund, M. R. (2015). Incidence and clinical presentation of acute otitis media in children aged <6 years in European medical practices. *Epidemiologic Infection*, 142(8), 1778–1788.

Rhoads, J., & Petersen, S. (2014). *Advanced health assessment and diagnostic reasoning* (2nd ed.). Burlington, MA: Jones & Bartlett.

Surapaneni, H., & Sisodia, S. (2016). Incidence of ear, nose and throat disorders in children: A study in a teaching hospital in Telangana. *International Journal of Otorhinolaryngology and Head and Neck Surgery*, 2(1), 26–29.

■ ELDER ABUSE AND NEGLECT

Patricia M. Speck
Richard Taylor
Stacey A. Mitchell
Diana K. Faugno
Rita A. Jablonski-Jaudon

Overview

In 1900, those 65 years and older were one in 25 (3.1 million) persons in the United States and by 2060, one in four (98.2 million) persons in the United States will be older than 65 years (National Criminal Justice Reference Service, 2017; U.S. Census Bureau, 2017), and the oldest old, who are aged 85 and older, will be 25% of all elders 65 years and older and 5% of the total U.S. population in 2013 (U.S. Census Bureau, 2011, 2017). In the elderly population, women outnumber men, with approximately 10% of elders 65 to 74 years, residing in institutions; by age 85 to 100, 50% reside in nursing homes (U.S. Census Bureau, 2011). Emotional

elder abuse by care staff (40%; Pillemer & Moore, 1989) and physical abuse (40%) by nonresidents are prevalent (Bloemen, Rosen, Clark, Nash, & Mielenz, 2015). With the gradual increase in elder parent placement in institutions, increasing numbers of dependent elders foretell that most practicing nurses in 2030 will care for older persons. An unknown portion of their patients will be targeted for or will experience neglect, abuse, and/or exploitation (Alzheimer's Association, 2017; National Clearinghouse of Abuse in Later Life, 2013).

Background

The lack of a universal definition of elder abuse has diminished the accuracy in reporting the incidence and prevalence of this public health problem (J. Hall, Karch, & Crosby, 2016). Many definitions are descriptions of behaviors by offenders, matching legal definitions of the crimes. The Centers for Disease Control and Prevention's Violence Division defines *elder abuse* as:

- *Physical Abuse:* The intentional use of physical force that results in acute or chronic illness, bodily injury, physical pain, functional impairment, distress, or death.

- *Sexual Abuse or Abusive Sexual Contact:* Forced or unwanted sexual interaction (touching and nontouching acts) of any kind with an older adult [including incapacitated older adult].

- *Emotional or Psychological Abuse:* Verbal or nonverbal behavior that results in the infliction of anguish, mental pain, fear, or distress.

- *Neglect:* Failure by a caregiver or other responsible person to protect an elder from harm, or the failure to meet needs for essential medical care, nutrition, hydration, hygiene, clothing, basic activities of daily living or shelter, which results in a serious risk of compromised health and safety.

- *Financial Abuse or Exploitation:* The illegal, unauthorized, or improper use of an older individual's resources by a caregiver or other person in a trusting relationship, for the benefit of someone other than the older individual.(Centers for Disease Control and Prevention, 2016, paras 2, 3, 4, 5, 6)

The incidence and prevalence of elder neglect, abuse, and exploitation is unknown (National Institute of Justice, 2015). The reporting incidence and prevalence is divided into community-residing older persons and older persons in residential care facilities where

11% reported an experience of emotional, physical, sexual abuse, or neglect in the past year. In residential care facilities, caretakers primarily abuse older persons with critical remarks and humiliation; however, recent research highlighted resident-to-resident abuse and the need for training of care providers to mitigate or diminish future events (J. Hall et al., 2016; National Institute of Justice, 2015). Physical and mental health change in an older person creates vulnerability to neglect, abuses, and exploitation (National Institute of Justice, 2015). Abuse may include intentional isolation or abandonment, food insecurity, financial exploitation, emotional and psychological abuses, as well as physical and sexual assaults (National Council on Aging, n.d.). In persons with dementia, the elder person may resist care because dementia's neurodegeneration heightens perception of threats (Jablonski, Therrien, & Kolanowski, 2011; Jablonski, Therrien, Mahoney, et al., 2011). Care-resistant behavior increases exponentially as the dementia worsens (Jablonski, Therrien, & Kolanowski, 2011; Jablonski, Therrien, Mahoney, et al., 2011). In holistic palliative care (PC), elders, declining due to end-of-life factors, are at significantly higher risk of victimization by caregiver perpetrators of abuse (Jayawardena & Liao, 2006). For the dependent older person recently enrolled in PC, instead of improved quality of life and a "good death" (which is the intention of PC), abusive relationships in a private home are now serendipitously observed by RNs (Fisher, 2003), who are mandated reporters.

Calculating incidence and prevalence in a population of diverse elderly is complex. A sample of community-dwelling older persons nationally ($N = 5777$) found 11.4% ($n = 589$) experienced mistreatment in the past year, including "neglect and emotional, physical, and sexual abuse" (Acierno et al., 2010, p. 293), providing an opportunity for nursing to raise awareness and develop prevention interventions, particularly in high-risk racial and ethnic minorities (Beach, Schulz, Castle, & Rosen, 2010; DeLiema, Gassoumis, Homeier, & Wilber, 2012). *The Crimes Against the Elderly*, 2003–2013 (Morgan & Mason, 2014), reports a nonfatal violent crime rate of 3.6 per 1,000 and property crime rate of 72.3 per 1,000 for this 10-year period, providing opportunity for anticipatory guidance from RNs with safety concerns for community-dwelling elders.

Older persons have U.S. constitutional guarantees, including a right to self-determination (J. Hall, 2016, p. 37), including the right to self-neglect. This right to self-determination is more complex when dementia is present; for instance, family and formal caregivers may misinterpret the perception of threat as an exercise in autonomy (J. A. Adams, Bailey, Anderson, & Docherty, 2011). RNs behaviors may also contribute to failure to administer necessary treatments or medications because the person with dementia "refused," when in fact, the nurses' approaches triggered the care-refusal behavior (Jablonski, Kolanowski, Winstead, Jones-Townsend, & Azuero, 2016).

Disparities and social determinants as risk factors diminish attainment of health. Social determinants include the environment and attitudes, exposure to crime and violence, disease and access to health care, financial and food security, and personal and caregiver support systems (Leff, Kao, & Ritchie, 2015; National Criminal Justice Reference Service, 2017). Chronic stress in environments increases allostatic load risk, in which situational elevations in the allostatic load following abuse are also responsible for an increase in mortality following trauma in the elderly (Lachs, Williams, O'Brien, Pillemer, & Charlson, 1998) and contribute to the estimated additional $5.3 billion health expenditures, not to mention the prosecution, law enforcement, corrections, and other ongoing expenses in pursuit of justice (A. Hall et al., 2016).

Epigenetics is gaining favor as the explanation for intergenerational poor health outcomes, in which brain trauma from emotional or physical abuse or violence by intimates and family may predict future generation's diseases and focal dementias in older persons (Klengel, Pape, Binder, & Mehta, 2014).

Adverse childhood experience (ACE) scores are recommended as a routine vital sign, and provide insight about life experiences and health states (Felitti et al., 1998; Lachs et al., 1998), where ACEs correlate with all human body system diseases. ACEs explain the impact of a history of abuses in a population of persons in PC who report increased distress and anxiety (Probst, Wells-DiGregorio, & Marks, 2013) and experience somatic and mental health disorders, chronic disease, and early death (Probst et al., 2013). For example, elderly Holocaust survivors reexperience memories as dementia progresses (La Ganga, 2007) and Hurricane Katrina spiked elder death rates for several years (V. Adams, Kaufman, Van Hattum, & Moody, 2011).

The victims of elder neglect, abuse, or exploitation initially respond in a normal fashion to psychological stressors or traumatic events. However, the neuroendocrine system creates a sudden brainstem irritation response (fear) activating the hypothalamic–pituitary–adrenal axis, and when high hormonal levels cooccur with comorbid disease states in older persons, internal crisis of disease and stress leads to death (Christakis & Allison, 2006; Elwert & Christakis, 2008; Selye, 1974). Understanding the underlying physiology of stress and trauma prepares the RNs to recognize maladaptive and negative symptoms in chronically victimized elderly (Selye, 1956, 1974) and intercede with evidence-based interventions (Schneiderman, Ironson, & Siegel, 2005).

Clinical Aspects

ASSESSMENT

Screening the older person identifies at-risk elders and provides RNs an opportunity for anticipatory guidance and intervention (The Hartford Institute for Geriatric Nursing, 2017). The RNs caring for elder populations need a strong institutional policy and procedure reflecting the domains in geriatric care, which include skills in screening, identification, and management of abused and neglected older patients, and an interprofessional comprehensive plan to establish a safe environment for the older person to mitigate the impact of abuse and neglect (National Research Council, 2008, p. 22).

A nursing assessment includes the physical examination and emotional aspects of an older person's behavior with his or her caregiver, capacity to understand what happened, and a head-to-toe physical examination, which includes all skin and mucous membrane areas. The RNs consider other causes of injury, including bleeding diseases, medication side effects, falls, or previous assaults (including rape and domestic violence). The RNs document the assessment for elder neglect, abuse, or exploitation using descriptive terms only, such as color, size, and location. If the RNs are the first to suspect abuse or neglect, they are mandated reporters, regardless of others' opinions (Falk, Baigis, & Kopac, 2012; A. Hall et al., 2016). The RNs who objectively and comprehensively document the history and physical findings will fare well as "fact" witnesses in any criminal trial. Not all neglect or injury is intentional, so anticipating and educating family caregivers can prevent future neglect or injury. Throughout the assessment process, the RN role is therapeutic and supportive, mitigating mental health exacerbations (anger, depression, anxiety; Brown, 2012; Y. H. Chen, Lin, Chuang, & Chen, 2017).

NURSING INTERVENTIONS, MANAGEMENT, AND IMPLICATIONS

Nursing management after identification of elder abuse or neglect includes understanding that older persons have a lifetime of experiences with effective methods for integrating new information (Y. Chen & Blanchard-Fields, 1997). The RNs explain the process of reporting and provide clarity to the organizational processes such as mandating reporting. The RNs work with the institutional team to provide nursing care, assessment, and documentation, which are important for the safety and planning for the elder patient. When the closest caregiver (usually a child) is unable or unwilling to provide nurture and safety, recommending prevention or respite programs for at-risk families is a good first step, including more frequent home visitations or phone calls to check on the older persons and their caretaker's well-being (Bomba, 2006; Shugarman, Fries, Wolf, & Morris, 2003; Stark, 2012). The RNs understand that chaotic upbringing and/or abuses create hostility, which may result in self-injury, depression, or suicide or death (Johnson, 2016; Schulz & Sherwood, 2008). In the event the elder is deemed unable to return to his or her home, the RN's role is to comfort the older person, allow the older person to vent his or her feelings, and provide community resources to the family.

Elder abuse is defined differently by state laws, but all states follow federal legislation of the Elder Justice Act (2010), so the practicing RNs must be familiar with their state laws related to reporting elder neglect, abuse, or exploitation. If there is a suspicion of elder abuse, the RNs are obligated by law in most states to report to adult protective services and local law enforcement, which will address the criminal aspects of the case (Burgess, 2006).

Summary

Elder persons depend on safe and secure environments to live out their years. Elder neglect, abuse, and exploitation represent intentional crimes against them, primarily by family members, acquaintances, and other caretakers. Rarely do strangers gain access to older persons. Domestic violence, poverty, trafficking of human persons, war, drug use (covered in other entries), as well as neglect, abuse, and exploitation by family or caregivers create additional stress. Stress response following neglect, abuse, and exploitation creates a burden on the elder's existing disease states through overproduction of stress hormones. The stress hormones cripple the elder's capacity to overcome the trauma reaction, and sometimes the elders die before they can process the trauma.

RNs are in the position to recognize the elder subjected to violence and identify the subsequent stress reactions by using the nursing process. The RNs practicing with older persons should have serial vital signs in the elder's health record, including historical ACEs, scales measuring depression and anxiety, cognitive assessments, and other validated methods for assessing the older persons and their caretaker. The RNs ask the questions related to life events, important to the older person desiring nostalgia. Recognition of stress responses, including uncontrolled hypertension, diabetes, mental health exacerbation while on medication, neglect, and other signs of fear in the older person provide the opportunity for all RNs to intervene, report, and participate in interprofessional team collaboration to create safe, supportive, and secure environments for all older persons and their caretakers (Dong et al., 2011).

Acierno, R., Hernandez, M. A., Amstadter, A. B., Resnick, H. S., Steve, K., Muzzy, W., & Kilpatrick, D. G. (2010). Prevalence and correlates of emotional, physical, sexual, and financial abuse and potential neglect in the United States: The National Elder Mistreatment Study. *American Journal of Public Health*, 100(2), 292–297. doi:10.2105/AJPH.2009.163089

Adams, J. A., Bailey, D. E., Anderson, R. A., & Docherty, S. L. (2011). Nursing roles and strategies in end-of-life decision making in acute care: A systematic review of the literature. *Nursing Research and Practice*. doi:10.1155/2011/527834

Adams, V., Kaufman, S. R., Van Hattum, T., & Moody, S. (2011). Aging disaster: Mortality, vulnerability, and long-term recovery among Katrina survivors. *Medical Anthropology*, 30(3), 247–270. doi:10.1080/01459740.2011.560777

Alzheimer's Association. (2017). 2017—Alzheimer's disease, facts, and figures. *Alzheimers Dementia*, 13, 325–373.

Beach, S. R., Schulz, R., Castle, N. G., & Rosen, J. (2010). Financial exploitation and psychological mistreatment among older adults: Differences between African Americans and non-African Americans in a population-based survey. *The Gerontologist*, 50(6), 744–757. doi:10.1093/geront/gnq053

Bloemen, E. M., Rosen, T., Clark, S., Nash, D., & Mielenz, T. J. (2015). Trends in reporting of abuse and neglect to long term care ombudsmen: Data from the National Ombudsman Reporting System from 2006 to 2013. *Geriatric Nursing*, 36(4), 281–283. doi:10.1016/j.gerinurse.2015.03.002

Bomba, P. A. (2006). Use of a single page elder abuse assessment and management tool: A practical clinician's approach to identifying elder mistreatment. *Journal of Gerontological Social Work*, 46(3–4), 103–122. doi:10.1300/J083v46n03_06

Brown, L. (2012). *Assessing, intervening, and treating traumatized older adults*. Paper presented at the Biennial Trauma Conference: Addressing Trauma across the Lifespan: Integration of Family, Community, and Organizational Approaches, Florida.

Burgess, A. W. (2006). *Elderly victims of sexual abuse and their offenders* (p. 157). Boston College, Boston, MA: National Institutes of Justice Office of Justice Programs.

Centers for Disease Control and Prevention. (2016). Elder abuse: Definitions. Retrieved from https://www.cdc.gov/violenceprevention/elderabuse/definitions.html

Chen, Y., & Blanchard-Fields, F. (1997). Age differences in states of attributional processing. *Psychology and Aging*, 12(4), 694–703. doi:10.1037/0882-7974.12.4.694

Chen, Y.-H., Lin, L.-C., Chuang, L.-L., & Chen, M.-L. (2017). The relationship of physiopsychosocial factors and spiritual well-being in elderly residents: Implications for evidence-based practice. *Worldviews on Evidence-Based Nursing*. Advance online publication. doi:10.1111/wvn.12243

Christakis, N. A., & Allison, P. D. (2006). Mortality after the hospitalization of a spouse. *New England Journal of Medicine*, 354(7), 719–730. doi:10.1056/NEJMsa050196

DeLiema, M., Gassoumis, Z. D., Homeier, D. C., & Wilber, K. H. (2012). Determining prevalence and correlates of elder abuse using promotores: Low-income immigrant Latinos report high rates of abuse and neglect. *Journal of the American Geriatrics Society*, 60(7), 1333–1339. doi:10.1111/j.1532-5415.2012.04025.x

Dong, X. Q., Simon, M. A., Beck, T. T., Farran, C., McCann, J. J., Mendes de Leon, C. F., . . . Evans, D. A. (2011). Elder abuse and mortality: The role of psychological and social wellbeing. *Gerontology*, 57(6), 549–558.

Elwert, F., & Christakis, N. A. (2008). Variation in the effect of widowhood on mortality by the causes of death of both spouses. *American Journal of Public Health*, 98(11), 2092. doi:10.2105/AJPH.2007.114348

Falk, N. L., Baigis, J., & Kopac, C. (2012, August 14). Elder mistreatment and the Elder Justice Act. *Online Journal of Issues in Nursing*, 17(3), 7. doi:10.3912/OJIN.Vol17No03PPT01

Felitti, V. J., Anda, R. F., Nordenberg, D., Williamson, D. F., Spitz, A. M., Edwards, V., . . . Marks, J. S. (1998). Relationship of childhood abuse and household dysfunction to many of the leading causes of death in adults. The Adverse Childhood Experiences (ACE) Study. *American Journal of Preventive Medicine*, 14(4), 245–258.

Fisher, C. (2003). The invisible dimension: Abuse in palliative care families. *Journal of Palliative Medicine*, 6(2), 257–264.

Hall, A., McKenna, B., Dearie, V., Maguire, T., Charleston, R., & Furness, T. (2016). Educating emergency department nurses about trauma informed care for people presenting with mental health crisis: A pilot study. *BMC Nursing*, 15(1), 21. doi:10.1186/s12912-016-0141-y

Hall, J., Karch, D. L., & Crosby, A. (2016). Elder abuse surveillance: Uniform definitions and recommended core data elements. Retrieved from https://www.cdc.gov/violenceprevention/pdf/EA_Book_Revised_2016.pdf

The Hartford Institute for Geriatric Nursing (Producer). (2017, May 1). Elder mistreatment training manual and protocol. Retrieved from https://consultgeri.org/education-training/e-learning-resources/elder-mistreatment-training-manual-and-protocol

Jablonski, R. A., Kolanowski, A., Winstead, V., Jones-Townsend, C., & Azuero, A. (2016). Maturation of the MOUTh intervention: From reducing threat to relationship-centered care. *Journal of Gerontological Nursing*, 42(3), 15–23.

Jablonski, R. A., Therrien, B., & Kolanowski, A. (2011). No more fighting and biting during mouth care: Applying the theoretical constructs of threat perception to clinical practice. *Research and Theory for Nursing Practice*, 25(3), 163–175.

Jablonski, R. A., Therrien, B., Mahoney, E. K., Kolanowski, A., Gabello, M., & Brock, A. (2011). An intervention to reduce care-resistant behavior in persons with dementia during oral hygiene: A pilot study. *Special Care in Dentistry*, 31(3), 77–87.

Jayawardena, K. M., & Liao, S. (2006). Elder abuse at end of life. *Journal of Palliative Medicine*, 9(1), 127–136.

Johnson, L. (2016). Pushed to the edge: Caregivers who kill. Retrieved from https://www.agingcare.com/articles/caregivers-kill-parents-commit-suicide-150336.htm

Klengel, T., Pape, J., Binder, E. B., & Mehta, D. (2014). The role of DNA methylation in stress-related psychiatric disorders. *Neuropharmacology*, 80, 115–132. doi:10.1016/j.neuropharm.2014.01.013

Lachs, M. S., Williams, C. S., O'Brien, S., Pillemer, K. A., & Charlson, M. E. (1998). The mortality of elder mistreatment. *Journal of the American Medical Association*, 280(5), 428–432.

La Ganga, M. (2007). Fearing the Nazis again. *Los Angeles Times*, August 23. Retrieved from http://articles.latimes.com/2007/aug/23/local/me-rachel23

Leff, B., Kao, H., & Ritchie, C. (2015). How the principles of geriatric care can be used to improve care for medicare patients. *Journal of the American Society on Aging*, 39(7), 99–105.

Morgan, R., & Mason, B. (2014). Crimes against the elderly, 2003–2013: Special Report, U.S. Department of Justice, Bureau of Justice Statistics. November. Retrieved from https://www.bjs.gov/content/pub/pdf/cae0313.pdf

National Clearinghouse of Abuse in Later Life. (2013). An overview of elder abuse: A growing problem. Retrieved from http://www.ncdsv.org/images/NCALL_Overview-of-elder-abuse-a-growing-problem_2013.pdf

National Council on Aging. (n.d.). Elder abuse facts. Retrieved from https://www.ncoa.org/public-policy-action/elder-justice/elder-abuse-facts

National Criminal Justice Reference Service. (2017). Special feature: Elder abuse. Retrieved from https://www.ncjrs.gov/elderabuse

National Institute of Justice. (2015). Extent of elder abuse victimization. Retrieved from https://www.nij.gov/topics/crime/elder-abuse/Pages/extent.aspx

National Research Council. (2008). Early childhood assessment: Why, what, and how? In Committee on Developmental Outcomes and Assessments for Young Children, C. E. Snow, & S. B. Van Hemel (Eds.), *Board on children, youth and families, board on testing and assessment, division of behavioral and social sciences and education*. Washington, DC: National Academies Press.

Pillemer, K., & Moore, D. W. (1989). Abuse of patients in nursing homes: Findings from a survey of staff. *The Gerontologist*, 29(3), 314–320.

Probst, D. R., Wells-Di Gregorio, S., & Marks, D. R. (2013). Suffering compounded: The relationship between abuse history and distress in five palliative care domains. *Journal of Palliative Medicine*, 16(10), 1242–1248. Retrieved from https://doi.org/10.1089/jpm.2012.0619

Rhodes, J., Chan, C., Paxson, C., Rouse, C. E., Waters, M., & Fussell, E. (2010). The impact of hurricane Katrina on the mental and physical health of low-income parents in New Orleans. *American Journal of Orthopsychiatry*, 80(2), 237–247. doi:10.1111/j.1939-0025.2010.01027.x

Schneiderman, N., Ironson, G., & Siegel, S. D. (2005). Stress and health: Psychological, behavioral, and biological determinants. *Annual Review of Clinical Psychology*, 1, 607–628. doi:10.1146/annurev.clinpsy.1.102803.144141

Schulz, R., & Sherwood, P. R. (2008). Physical and mental health effects of family caregiving. *American Journal of Nursing*, 108(Suppl. 9), 23–27. doi:10.1097/01.NAJ.0000336406.45248.4c

Selye, H. (1956). *The stress of life*. New York, NY: McGraw-Hill.

Selye, H. (1974). *Stress without distress*. Philadelphia, PA: Lippincott.

Shugarman, L. R., Fries, B. E., Wolf, R. S., & Morris, J. N. (2003). Identifying older people at risk of abuse during routine screening practices. *Journal of the American Geriatrics Society*, 51(1), 24–31.

Stark, S. (2012). Elder abuse: Screening, intervention, and prevention. *Nursing*, 42(10), 24–29; quiz 29–30. doi:10.1097/01.nurse.0000419426.05524.45

U.S. Census Bureau. (2011). Sixty-five plus in the United States. Retrieved from https://www.census.gov/population/socdemo/statbriefs/agebrief.html

U.S. Census Bureau. (2017). Older Americans month: May 2017. Retrieved from https://www.census.gov/content/dam/Census/newsroom/facts-for-features/2017/cb17-ff08.pdf

■ ENCEPHALOPATHY

Deborah Vinesky

Overview

Encephalopathy is a general term that means brain disease, damage, or malfunction; the defining characteristic is an altered mental state. Encephalopathy most often occurs as a secondary complication of a primary neurological problem. Neurological problems can result from infections, trauma and physical injuries, genetics, environmental influences, and nutrition-related causes. Early treatment of most causes can decrease, eliminate, or stop the symptoms related to encephalopathy (Davis, 2015). The development of effective therapies that prevent and treat encephalopathy requires an understanding of its pathologic and physiologic processes (Williams, 2013).

Background

The National Institute of Neurological Disorders and Stroke (NINDS, 2017) defines encephalopathy as:

Encephalopathy is a term for any diffuse disease of the brain that alters brain function or structure. Encephalopathy may be caused by infectious agent (bacteria, virus, or prion), metabolic or mitochondrial dysfunction, brain tumor or increased pressure in the skull, prolonged exposure to toxic elements (including solvents, drugs, radiation, paints, industrial chemicals, and certain metals), chronic progressive trauma, poor nutrition, or lack of oxygen, or blood flow to the brain. Care of the patient with encephalopathy presents unique challenges because generally it is manifested by an altered state accompanied by physical manifestations. (NINDS, 2017)

There are two distinct categories of encephalopathy: acute and chronic. The chronic encephalopathies are characterized by chronic mental status change that are slowly and insidiously progressive. In addition, they usually result from permanent and usually irreversible structural changes in the brain itself. In contrast, acute encephalopathy is characterized by a functional alteration of mental status due to systemic factors. It may be reversible when the abnormalities are corrected, and a full return to baseline mental status is expected. Acute encephalopathy can be further described as toxic, metabolic, or toxic-metabolic (Pinson, 2015).

Toxic encephalopathy can occur following exposure to acute or chronic neurotoxins. Neurotoxins include chemical compounds of chemotherapy, heavy metals, pesticides, and industrial and cleaning solvents. Exposure to toxins can lead to a variety of neurological symptoms, characterized by memory loss, visual disturbances, and an altered mental status. Metabolic encephalopathy, or toxic-metabolic encephalopathy, is a category of encephalopathy describing abnormalities related to water, electrolytes, vitamins, and other chemicals that have the potential to adversely affect brain function. Neurotoxins are chemical agents affecting the transmission of chemical signals between neurons, at any step in neural transmission.

"Delirium" and "acute encephalopathy" are virtually two different terms that essentially represent the same condition. Delirium describes the mental manifestation, whereas encephalopathy is the underlying pathophysiologic process. Manifestations of delirium include reduced awareness of the environment, cognitive impairment, emotional disturbances, and changes in behavior. Changes in behavior include hallucinations, restlessness, agitation or combative behavior, lethargy, and disturbed sleep patterns. The *Diagnostic and Statistical Manual of Mental Disorders*, Fifth Edition (DSM-5; American Psychiatric Association, 2013), does not use encephalopathy in its definition and classification of delirium (Pinson, 2015). Historically, delirium has been considered a manifestation of generalized cerebral metabolic insufficiency and may result in a combination of abnormal blood flow, abnormal energy metabolism, abnormal neurotransmission, and abnormal cellular maintenance processes (Williams, 2013).

Clinical Aspects

ASSESSMENT

Care of the patient will vary depending on the etiology of the encephalopathy. Altered mental status is the hallmark of encephalopathy; the initial approach should be systematic and should focus on stabilization. In many patients, particularly the elderly, there exists some preexisting degree of chronic and ongoing cognitive impairment, dementia, or psychiatric illness. Various infections, including bacteria, viruses, prions, and parasites, can cause temporary or permanent brain damage leading to encephalopathy. Restricted oxygen supply to the brain, alcohol abuse, metabolic disease, tumors, prolonged inhalation of toxic chemicals, exposure to radiation, and drug abuse can lead to encephalopathy.

The most important part of the workup will be the history and physical examination, including vital signs. If the patient is alert and cooperative, and/or there are family members present, information should be obtained, including current medical illness, medications (recent and present), or possible ingestion of toxins. Data are obtained that will aid in ruling out causes that have the potential to harm the patient, and those that are correctable. Acute change in mental status is a symptom and must be monitored for and documented appropriately. Once the patient is stabilized, an assessment based on a systems approach should be conducted, utilizing previously gained information related to the patient's history (Parmley & Neeley, 2017).

NURSING INTERVENTIONS, MANAGEMENT, AND IMPLICATIONS

Hospitalized patients suffering from encephalopathy have complex nursing needs. These same patients are susceptible to poor quality of care that has the potential to affect their quality of life. Nursing is challenged with recognizing and addressing the unique needs of this special population. Misinterpretation of the needs of this vulnerable population may result in the patients receiving suboptimal care with further decline in cognitive functioning (Joosse, Palmer, & Lang, 2013).

OUTCOMES

The primary outcome of evidence-based strategies is to minimize the patient's risk and exposure to toxins that may contribute to manifestation of encephalopathy. Nursing care should focus on the assessment of patient's mental status and change in behaviors, which include aimless wandering, agitation, impaired balance and gait, and interrupted sleep and rest. Given the altered mental status, a central clinical symptom of encephalopathy, nursing care should be also focused on maintaining a safe environment of care for patients with this medical condition.

To aid the nurse in providing quality care, it is necessary to be able to synthesize and translate evidence-based practice into best practices to be used at the bedside. Early assessment and preventive measures are useful in maintaining function and preventing decline. Functional impairment and behavioral symptoms include inability to initiate meaningful activity, disorientation and anxiety, apathy, repetitive vocalization, resistiveness, combativeness, and dietary issues like food refusal; all interfere with nursing care (Joosse et al., 2013). Electronic support services provide clinical support for patient care services. These services promote evidence-based early recognition, risk assessment, identification of problems, and selection of appropriate nursing interventions and outcomes (Joosse et al., 2013).

Summary

Encephalopathy most often occurs secondary to a complication of a primary neurological problem.

Care of the patient with encephalopathy is dependent upon its etiology. Hospitalized patients suffering from acute and chronic encephalopathy have complex nursing needs requiring astute assessment skills, based on a systems approach once the patient is stabilized. Recognizing and addressing the unique needs of this population will promote optimal quality of care. With a focus on promoting independence and controlling risk factors, a decline in cognitive functioning will be prevented. Safety is of the utmost importance in this population, as is early assessment and instituting preventive measures.

American Psychiatric Association. (2013). *Diagnostic and statistical manual of mental disorders* (5th ed.). Arlington, VA: American Psychiatric Publishing.

Davis, C. P. (2015). Encephalopathy. Retrieved from http://www.medicinenet.com/encephalopathy/article.htm

Joosse, L. L., Palmer, D., & Lang, N. (2013). Caring for elderly patients with dementia: Nursing interventions. *Nursing Research and Reviews*, 3, 107–117.

National Institute of Neurological Disorders and Stroke. (2017). Encephalopathy information page. Retrieved from https://www.ninds.nih.gov/Disorders/All-Disorders/Encephalopathy-Information-Page

Parmley, C. L., & Neeley, R. (2017). Acute altered mental status, mental status changes, depressed mental status, lethargic, obtunded, altered level of consciousness. *Clinical Reviews, 27*(2).

Pinson, R. (2015). Encephalopathy. American College of Physicians Hospitalist. Retrieved from https://acphospitalist.org/archives/2015/01/coding.htm

Williams, S. (2013). Pathophysiology of encephalopathy and delirium. *Journal of Clinical Neurophysiology, 30*(5), 435–437.

■ ENDOCRINE EMERGENCIES

Diane Fuller Switzer

Overview

Endocrine emergencies are life-threatening conditions that require early and prompt identification, assessment, and aggressive pharmacologic and nursing interventions to prevent adverse consequences such as death. The endocrine system is very complex and although integrated, individual organ dysfunction has a unique presentation and requires specialized pharmacologic and nursing management to correct the imbalance as it impacts all the body systems.

Although the endocrine system consists of the hypothalamus, pituitary, thyroid, parathyroid, adrenals, pancreas, testes, and ovaries, this chapter focus on specific emergencies and nursing management related to the pancreas, thyroid, and adrenal glands. These emergencies include diabetic ketoacidosis (DKA), hyperosmolar hyperglycemia syndrome (HHS), hypoglycemia, thyrotoxicosis, and adrenal crisis.

Background

Diabetes mellitus is a complex, chronic condition identified by hyperglycemia resulting in macrovascular, microvascular, and neuropathic complications. Although the disease affects 29 million or 9.3% of the U.S. population, 8.1 million are unaware that they have the disease (Centers for Diseases Control and Prevention [CDC], 2012; Sease & Shealy, 2016). This disease is caused by a defect in insulin whereby the body does not make enough of it or is unable to use it, resulting in hyperglycemia. There are four classifications: type 1 an autoimmune disorder, type 2 insulin resistance or impaired insulin release, gestational, and secondary (genetic defects, drug induced, infections; Clutter, 2016; Sease & Shealy, 2016). The incidence of type 2 diabetes mellitus (T2DM), which accounts for 90% of diabetes mellitus, is expected to increase with an aging population, sedentary lifestyle, and rising obesity. In 2012, T2DM affected 11.2 million people aged 65 years or older, and 34.9% of the U.S. population were diagnosed with obesity (CDC, 2012; Sease & Shealy, 2016).

DKA is defined as a manifestation of severe insulin deficiency, often associated with stress and activation of counterregulatory hormones, resulting in hyperglycemia, dehydration, and electrolyte abnormalities resulting in a metabolic acidosis, which can lead to life-threatening metabolic derangements, myocardial depression, hypotension, coma, and death (Clutter, 2016; Sanuth, Bidlencik, & Volk, 2014; Sease & Shealy, 2016; Westerberg, 2013). Although DKA tends to affect younger populations with type 1 diabetes mellitus (T1DM), it may occur in individuals with T2DM who have ketosis-prone diabetes. In an individual with undiagnosed diabetes mellitus, DKA may be the presenting symptom. The most common causes of DKA are an infection, new-onset diabetes mellitus, and an interruption of insulin therapy, trauma, myocardial infarction (MI), and physiologic stressors (Clutter, 2016; Lenahan & Holloway, 2015; Sanuth et al., 2014;

Sease & Shealy, 2016; Westerberg, 2013). It is listed as a primary diagnosis in approximately 7 patients per 1,000 hospital discharges, associated with an average length of stay of 3.4 days, with an annual expenditure estimated at $2.4 billion, and the incidence continues to rise (American Diabetes Association [ADA], 2016; CDC, 2012; Gosmanov, Gosmanova, & Kitabchi, 2015).

HHS is a life-threatening condition similar to DKA with hyperglycemia and dehydration but without acidosis or ketonuria. This condition occurs more often in older adults with T2DM and is expected to increase in incidence (Gosmanov et al., 2015; Lenahan & Holloway, 2015). Often, patients are unaware they have T2DM as they have not been diagnosed with it. The common causes of HHS include disease states such as infection (pneumonia), silent MI, cerebral vascular accident (CVA), and medications such as steroids, or thiazide diuretics (Clutter, 2016; Gosmanov et al., 2015; Lenahan & Holloway, 2015).

DKA and HHS share similar symptoms such as malaise, fatigue, recent illness or infections, but DKA is differentiated from HHS in that the onset of symptoms occurs across several days with nausea, vomiting, diffuse abdominal pain, increase in thirst, and sweet smelly breath (acetone). As DKA worsens, Kussmaul respirations (deep breaths because of an anion gap metabolic acidosis with respiratory compensation) may develop and confusion and drowsiness may be present. Lab results demonstrate an elevated glucose level less than 600, and positive ketones in urine. HHS has a gradual onset over several days to weeks and may present with dehydration, stupor, coma, elevated glucose more than 600, but without ketones in the urine. DKA is more common, usually with (T1DM), in a younger population (aged 20–29 years) with mortality of 5% to 10%. HHS is less common, usually occurs with T2DM, but can be T1DM, more severe illness with an older population (aged 57–70 years) and a higher mortality of 10% to 20% (ADA, 2016; Clutter, 2016; Gosmanov et al., 2015; Lenahan & Holloway, 2015).

Hypoglycemia occurs when the blood glucose level is 60 to 70 mg/dL or lower, usually affects patients with T1DM, but can occur with or without diabetes as a result of too much insulin or hypoglycemic medications, a delay or decrease in food intake, increase in exercise, alcohol, chronic kidney disease, liver failure, or sepsis. Hypoglycemia is common. In 2014, there were a total of 14.2 million emergency department visits for hypoglycemia; 245,000 (CDC, 2017) in the hospital setting are associated with a higher mortality rate (ADA, 2016;

Clutter, 2016; Lenahan & Holloway, 2015; Westerberg, 2013). Hypoglycemia should be considered with any individual who has risk factors and who presents or develops symptoms of hypoglycemia such as a headache, confusion, shakiness, anxiety, sweating, tachycardia, irritability, drowsiness, or unresponsiveness.

Thyrotoxicosis is caused by excess thyroid hormone released from the thyroid gland, with clinical presentations of autonomic hyperactivity such as nervousness, tremor, palpitations, tachycardia, irritability, and increased perspiration. Graves' disease is the most common cause (60%–80%), with clinical features of exophthalmos, eyelid retraction, periorbital edema, proptosis, and diffuse thyroid enlargement. Thyrotoxicosis in the elderly usually occurs from toxic thyroid nodules or multinodular goiter. If left untreated, it can progress to an acute life-threatening condition called *thyroid storm* that is evidenced by a high fever, tachycardia, tachypnea, dehydration, delirium, and coma (Katz, 2016).

Adrenal crisis, or acute adrenal insufficiency, occurs when the body is unable to respond to excessive physiologic stress with an increase of endogenous cortisol (Dang, Chen, Pucino, & Calis, 2016). Adrenal crisis can occur in patients who have chronic adrenal insufficiency and do not receive sufficient glucocorticoid replacement in times of stress, in patients who have bilateral adrenal infarction, and in the critically ill, especially those in septic shock. Abrupt discontinuation or rapid tapering of glucocorticoid steroids can precipitate an adrenal crisis as well. These patients progress to circulatory collapse without immediate glucocorticoid replacement, and require volume resuscitation, correction of electrolyte abnormalities, and search for a precipitant such as an infection (Dang et al., 2016).

Clinical Aspects

ASSESSMENT

When caring for the patient with DKA, a detailed history from the individual or family member regarding the onset of symptoms, if onset is acute or gradual, type of symptoms (malaise, fatigue, anorexia, fever, chills, nausea, vomiting, abdominal pain, chest pain, increase in thirst [polydipsia], and/or urination [polyuria], weight loss, recent illnesses, stressors [surgery/infection/MI], medications [noncompliance], substance abuse, alcohol intake, comorbid conditions, living conditions, and history of previous or similar episodes)

is necessary to determine the type of endocrine emergency the individual may be experiencing.

Frequent assessment of cardiovascular status (blood pressure, heart rate, temperature, color, volume status or perfusion as assessed by skin turgor, color, extremity pulses, warmth, and capillary refill) is necessary to prevent hypotension and maintain organ and tissue perfusion. The initial respiratory assessment must be performed to observe for Kussmaul respirations, tachypnea, shortness of breath, and oxygen saturation. Auscultation of the lungs can identify adventitious or absent breath sounds, which may be an indication of pneumonia or fluid overload. A chest x-ray can confirm whether an infectious process or fluid overload is present in the cardiopulmonary system. A renal system assessment is necessary to monitor for urine output following fluid resuscitation and correction of electrolyte abnormalities (hyperglycemia, hypokalemia), and nonanion gap metabolic acidosis. The neurological system is assessed for mental status changes that may indicate cerebral edema. The integumentary system should be assessed for signs of dehydration, infection, perfusion, color, and warmth.

The treatment of DKA requires large amounts of fluid resuscitation, insulin infusion, potassium replacement, and closure of the anion gap metabolic acidosis. Close attention to the potassium shift with insulin administration, prevention of hypoglycemia, hypokalemia, and complications associated with these electrolyte abnormalities (altered mental status, cerebral edema, EKG changes) are dependent on frequent nursing assessments and nursing interventions to correct the abnormalities.

HHS is similar to DKA with hyperglycemia, dehydration, and electrolyte losses, but without acidosis or ketonuria. As with DKA, the treatment and nursing care are similar with intravenous fluid resuscitation, cardiac monitoring, frequent electrolyte and serum glucose checks with electrolyte replacement, and to prevent a rapid reduction in serum glucose reduction, which may precipitate cerebral edema.

Hypoglycemia can occur with or without diabetes. Any patient who presents with an altered mental status or unresponsiveness, or develops mental status changes during hospitalization, requires immediate evaluation and nursing intervention to correct the hypoglycemia. Frequent nursing assessments of patients at risk, and providing patient education regarding diet, exercise, and frequent blood sugar monitoring to increase awareness of hypoglycemia triggers and symptoms help prevent complications.

NURSING INTERVENTIONS, MANAGEMENT, AND IMPLICATIONS

Successful management of endocrine emergencies is dependent on early and frequent nursing assessments to search for precipitating events such as infection, medications, and stressors. As these presentations may mimic neurologic, psychiatric, or substance abuse disorders, it is important that the nurse perform an accurate assessment, including history, physical exam, and response to nursing interventions, to determine the underlying cause for the alteration in a mental and physical presentation. Priority nursing-related problems include confusing presentations, so the nurse must search for and treat the precipitating event. This involves correction of volume deficits with fluid resuscitation and monitoring fluid status with frequent vital signs, including blood pressure, heart rate, respiratory rate, temperature, and urine output. Electrolyte abnormalities need to be corrected to promote fluid and acid–base balance. Frequent assessment of mental status is the key to determine whether a worsening condition is developing or if the patient is not responding to the current therapy. The administration of pharmacologic interventions requires close attention to maintain hemodynamic stability ensuring oxygenation and perfusion of organs and tissues.

OUTCOMES

The expected outcomes of evidence-based nursing care for endocrine emergencies are to prevent complications that may lead to adverse outcomes with an increase in morbidity and mortality. Structured order sets for the management of these conditions employ "best practice" and high-quality, evidence-based, safe patient care, so that these individuals can be stabilized safely and quickly, have a short hospital stay, and receive patient education to prevent future hospitalizations.

Summary

Adults with endocrine emergencies present with metabolic derangements in fluid and acid–base balance with unstable hemodynamics and altered mental status, which can progress to coma and death. Complications can be prevented with frequent nursing assessments and initiation of aggressive evidence-based nursing interventions. Adherence to hospital protocol-based treatment algorithms may prevent adverse outcomes.

American Diabetes Association. (2016). Standards of medical care in diabetes—2016. *Diabetes Care, 38*(Suppl. 1), S4–S93. Retrieved from http://care.diabetesjournals.org/content/suppl/2015/12/21/39.Supplement_1.DC2/2016-Standards-of-Care.pdf

Centers for Diseases Control and Prevention. (2017). Diabetes, data, and trends. Retrieved from https://www.cdc.gov/diabetes/pdfs/data/statistics/national-diabetes-statistics-report.pdf

Clutter, W. E. (2016). Endocrine diseases. In P. Bhat, A. Dretler, M. Gdowski, R. Ramgopal, & D. Williams (Eds.), *The Washington manual of medical therapeutics* (35th ed., pp. 758–778). Philadephia, PA: Wolters Kluwer/Lippincott Williams & Wilkins.

Dang, D. K., Chen, J. T., Pucino, Jr. F., & Calis, K. A. (2016). Chapter 45: Adrenal gland disorders. In M. A. Chisholm-Burns, T. L. Schwinghammer, & B. G. Wells (Eds.), *Pharmacotherapy, principles, and practice* (4th ed., pp. 695–710). New York, NY: McGraw-Hill.

Gosmanov, A. R., Gosmanova, E. O., & Kitabchi, A. E. (2015). Hyperglycemic crises: Diabetic ketoacidosis (DKA), and hyperglycemic hyperosmolar state (HHS). In L. J. De Groot, G. Chrousos, K. Dungan, K. R. Feingold, A. Grossman, J. M. Hershman . . . A. Vinik (Eds.), *Endotext* [Internet]. South Dartmouth, MA: MDText.com. Retrieved from https://www.ncbi.nlm.nih.gov/books/NBK279052

Katz, M. D. (2016). Thyroid disorders. In M. A. Chisholm-Burns, T. L. Schwinghammer, & B. G. Wells (Eds.), *Pharmacotherapy, principles, and practice* (4th ed., pp. 679–694). New York, NY: McGraw-Hill.

Lenahan, C. M., & Holloway, B. (2015). Differentiating between DKA and HHS. *Journal of Emergency Nursing, 41*(3), 201–207. Retrieved from http://www.jenonline.org

Sanuth, B., Bidlencik, A., & Volk, A. (2014). Management of acute hyperglycemic emergencies: Focus on diabetic ketoacidosis. *AACN Advanced Critical Care, 25*(3), 197–202. Retrieved from http://aacn.org

Sease, J., & Shealy, K. (2016). Diabetes mellitus. In M. A. Chisholm-Burns, T. L. Schwinghammer, & B. G. Wells (Eds.), *Pharmacotherapy, principles, and practice* (4th ed., pp. 651–678). New York, NY: McGraw-Hill.

Westerberg, D. (2013). Diabetic ketoacidosis: Evaluation and treatment. *American Family Physician, 87*(5). Retrieved from http://www.aafp.org/afp

■ ENVIRONMENTAL EMERGENCIES

Brittany Newberry

Overview

Environmental emergencies are common reasons for patients to seek care in the emergency department (ED)

and the risk of becoming ill or injured during travel or recreation depends on many factors (Brunette, 2016). These injuries can happen at home, work, or recreational settings. Environmental injuries and emergencies are varied and require the clinician to have a high index of suspicion and focused history taking and assessment skills. Patients who experience environmental emergencies may have differing levels of prehospital care and may have additional complications such as exposure, heavily contaminated wounds, and/or prolonged extrication times (Lipman et al., 2014).

Environmental emergencies include, but are not limited to, envenomation and poisoning injuries, high altitude and decompression illnesses, and thermoregulation injuries. Prevention is an important aspect of reducing the morbidity and mortality associated with environmental emergencies. Environmental emergencies can also include day-to-day illnesses that can occur in the wilderness such as abdominal pain, stroke, and myocardial infarction.

Background

There are many types of environmental emergencies and the types of injuries/illnesses seen often depend on the area of practice. Some environmental injuries are more common in certain areas, such as envenomation, high altitude and decompression illnesses, and thermoregulation injuries, and clinical staff should be aware of emergencies that are common to their geographic area. Other emergencies, such as poisoning, occur in more widespread geographic areas.

Envenomation injuries can occur anywhere and are not uncommon events. Physical response to an envenomation may vary from a mild local reaction to severe systemic and/or anaphylactic reactions (Ittyachen, Abdulla, Anwarsha, & Kumar, 2015). Clinicians need to be familiar with venomous animals in their geographic area to rapidly recognize and treat these potential life-threatening injuries. Envenomation injuries can occur from spiders, scorpions, insects, snakes, marine animals, bees, or wasps. Each vector contains a unique toxin that requires rapid identification and potential specific treatment. A thorough history is important for these patients.

Poisoning injuries can be accidental or intentional. Oftentimes these injuries are the result of substance abuse by patients for recreational purposes (Vallersnes, Jacobsen, Ekeberg, & Brekke, 2016). However, children and adults can also be the victim of unintentional poisoning because of ingestion or exposure. Suicide attempts should generally be considered for these patients. A thorough history from the patient and any knowledgeable friends or family members are essential. The clinician should not hesitate to contact poison control to ensure that proper treatment is being initiated.

High altitude and decompression illnesses: More than 100 million people visit altitudes greater than 8,000 feet every year. Acute mountain sickness (AMS) can occur in unsuspecting healthy people and is usually a benign illness. However, at times, AMS may progress to life-threatening events such as high altitude cerebral edema (HACE) or high altitude pulmonary edema (HAPE; Netzer, Strohl, Faulhaber, Gatterer, & Burtscher, 2013). Clinicians working in potential exposure areas need to have astute assessment skills to recognize subtle changes or deterioration in condition for these patients.

Decompression illnesses consist of decompression sickness (DCS) and pulmonary overinflation syndrome (POIS). These illnesses occur when divers ascend too rapidly without giving time for carbon dioxide to properly off-gas from the blood. POIS has the additional complication of causing ruptured alveoli in the lungs, which then causes the extravasation of air bubbles into the tissues (Hall, 2014). Decompression illnesses are most commonly seen in coastal areas where diving is a popular recreational or occupational activity.

Thermoregulation injuries include the two extremes of hypothermia and hyperthermia. Each is a deviation from the body's ability to maintain homeostasis of temperature because of environmental or metabolic factors. Acute hypothermia can result from exposure or metabolic derangement and requires normalization. Severe hypothermia can lead to coagulopathy, cardiac arrest, and even death (Katrancha & Gonzalez, 2014).

Heat-related illnesses can be exercise induced or result from exposure to extreme temperatures or certain medications (Canel, Zisimopoulou, Besson, & Nendaz, 2016). Exertional heat illness (EHI) includes heat edema, heat cramps, heat syncope, and heat exhaustion and can lead to exertional heat stroke (EHS), which is a medical emergency (Pryor, Bennett, O'Connor, Young, & Asplund, 2015). EHS can lead to rhabdomyolysis, electrolyte imbalances, organ failure, and death if not treated.

Clinical Aspects

ASSESSMENT

Any envenomation injury or poisoning patient should have his or her vital signs monitored carefully and assessed for any signs of allergic reaction or anaphylaxis.

Poisoning patients from substance abuse should be assessed for any evidence of self-harm and receive appropriate monitoring and counseling if required. In addition, patients should be screened for substance abuse and potential withdrawal symptoms. High-altitude and decompression illnesses: Signs of AMS may include a headache, dizziness, vomiting, anorexia, fatigue, and/or insomnia, which usually occurs between 6 and 36 hours of high-altitude exposure.

NURSING INTERVENTIONS, MANAGEMENT, AND IMPLICATIONS

Envenomation injury or poisoning need rapid identification of the vector or substance, which is important to help guide treatment. Depending on the injury, treatment may consist of cold compresses, antihistamines, steroids, fluid resuscitation, antivenom, surgical intervention, and/or pain medications. A great number of insects, snakes, and other animals are venomous and can create complex and even fatal manifestations (Haddad, Amorim, Haddad, & Costa- Cardoza, 2015). Ensure that poison control has been contacted and that treatment recommendations are followed.

Rapid assessment and identification of potential substances are important to determine the best treatment. However, any life-threatening situations should be treated emergently. Patients should have the vital signs consistently monitored and airway, breathing, and circulation (ABCs) continuously assessed. These patients may be discharged home, transferred to another facility, observed, or admitted depending on the severity of their symptoms. Patient and/or parent education is an important facet of discharging poisoning patients, as prevention is paramount.

The treatment for AMS is descent. Signs, such as ataxia, hallucinations, confusion, vomiting, decreased activity, or severeunbearable headache, should cause the clinician to consider HACE. Ataxia is the hallmark sign of HACE. HAPE symptoms include dyspnea at rest, cough, weakness, and chest tightness. The patient may also have central cyanosis, frothy sputum, and crackles/wheezing in at least one lung field, tachypnea, and tachycardia. HAPE is most often misdiagnosed as pneumonia pointing to the importance of taking a thorough history (Netzer et al., 2013). Mild AMS can be treated with cessation of ascension and symptomatic treatment until the symptoms are resolved. HAPE and HACE should be treated with immediate descent and evacuation, oxygen therapy, and appropriate medications depending on the symptoms and severity.

Decompression illnesses (DCS and POIS) are best prevented with the regulated and monitored ascent to the water surface. Greater depth and longer dive times put divers at greater risk for decompression illness. Symptoms of DCS include joint pain (particularly in the shoulder) that is not worsened with the range of motion. POIS manifestations can include arterial gas embolism (AGE), pneumothorax, mediastinal emphysema, and/or subcutaneous emphysema. All of these symptoms result from overdistention and rupture of lung alveoli from expanding gases during ascent (Hall, 2014). Treatment primarily entails hyperbaric oxygen therapy but may require additional respiratory support for severe barotrauma.

Patients who experience acute nontherapeutic hypothermia should be rewarmed even in the absence of vital signs. Patients with a core body temperature of less than 32°C should have active rewarming via heated blankets, heating pads, radiant heat, warm baths, or forced warm air (Giesbrecht, 2000). During rewarming, monitor patients, as removal from the cold environment may result in peripheral vasodilation potentially leading to hypotension, inadequate coronary perfusion, and/or ventricular fibrillation (Brown, Brugger, Boyd, & Paal, 2012). Patients who experience frostbite should have the affected areas rapidly rewarmed in warm water with the temperatures ranging from 37°C to 39°C (Nygaard et al., 2017). During rewarming, be prepared to assess the patient for and treat pain.

People who have had EHI in the past are more prone to experience heat-related illnesses and complications at subsequent exposures (Pryor et al., 2015). The classic triad of EHS is core body temperature more than 105°F, central nervous system dysfunction, and hot skin (often with anhidrosis). Other signs may include tachycardia, hypotension, tachypnea, rales, nausea, vomiting, diarrhea, cutaneous vasodilation, renal failure because of rhabdomyolysis, and coagulopathy. Immediate treatment for EHS is removal from the heat stressor and ABCs, rapid cooling for body temperature more than 105°F, aggressive fluid administration for any blood pressure (BP) less than 90/60, rehydration with isotonic fluids, and correction of electrolyte imbalances. Laboratory studies should be monitored carefully until the patient returns to baseline. Patients who experience EHS need thorough education about their illness, when to return to the ED, and how to prevent heat-related illnesses in the future.

OUTCOMES

Patients who are exposed to environmental emergency require immediate and deliberate care. Nurses working in emergency settings should first assess the patient to begin to differentiate a probable source of the injury. Because patients exposed to an environmental emergency can rapidly decompensate, it is critical that patients, family members, and emergency medical technicians be queried to gain information about the patient's condition. Stabilization and definitive care is needed to attenuate the progression of the injury.

Summary

Environmental injuries are common reasons for patients to seek care in the ED setting. Clinicians must have a high index of suspicion and initiate a thorough history and assessment. In addition, the clinician should be familiar with common environmental injuries in their geographic area to facilitate the rapid recognition and treatment of these injuries. All injuries should begin with the rapid assessment and treatment of ABCs and the recognition and treatment of associated life- or limb-threatening conditions such as anaphylaxis, neurovascular compromise, and hemorrhage.

Brown, D. J., Brugger, H., Boyd, J., & Paal, P. (2012). Accidental hypothermia. *New England Journal of Medicine, 367*(20), 1930–1938.

Brunette, G. W. (2016). *CDC health information for international travel.* New York, NY: Oxford University Press.

Canel, L., Zisimopoulou, S., Besson, M., & Nendaz, M. (2016). Topiramate-induced severe heatstroke in an adult patient: A case report. *Journal of Medical Case Reports, 10,* 95.

Giesbrecht, G. G. (2000). Cold stress, near drowning and accidental hypothermia: A review. *Aviation, Space, and Environmental Medicine, 71*(7), 733–752.

Haddad, V., Amorim, P. C., Haddad, W. T., & Cardoso, J. L. (2015). Venomous and poisonous arthropods: Identification, clinical manifestations of envenomation, and treatments used in human injuries. *Revista da Sociedade Brasileira de Medicina Tropical, 48*(6), 650–657.

Hall, J. (2014). The risks of scuba diving: A focus on decompression illness. *Hawai'i Journal of Medicine & Public Health, 73*(11, Suppl. 2), 13–16.

Ittyachen, A. M., Abdulla, S., Anwarsha, R. F., & Kumar, B. S. (2015). Multi-organ dysfunction secondary to severe wasp envenomation. *International Journal of Emergency Medicine, 8,* 6.

Katrancha, E. D., & Gonzalez, L. S. (2014). Trauma-induced coagulopathy. *Critical Care Nurse, 34*(4), 54–63.

Lipman, G. S., Weichenthal, L., Stuart Harris, N., McIntosh, S. E., Cushing, T., Caudell, M. J., . . . Auerbach, P. S.

(2014). Core content for wilderness medicine fellowship training of emergency medicine graduates. *Academic Emergency Medicine, 21*(2), 204–207.

Netzer, N., Strohl, K., Faulhaber, M., Gatterer, H., & Burtscher, M. (2013). Hypoxia-related altitude illnesses. *Journal of Travel Medicine, 20*(4), 247–255.

Nygaard, R. M., Lacey, A. M., Lemere, A., Dole, M., Gayken, J. R., Lambert Wagner, A. L., & Fey, R. M. (2017). Time matters in severe frostbite: Assessment of limb/digit salvage on the individual patient level. *Journal of Burn Care & Research, 38*(1), 53–59.

Pryor, R. R., Bennett, B. L., O'Connor, F. G., Young, J. M., & Asplund, C. A. (2015). Medical evaluation for exposure extremes: Heat. *Wilderness & Environmental Medicine, 26*(4, Suppl), S69–S75.

Vallersnes, O. M., Jacobsen, D., Ekeberg, Ø., & Brekke, M. (2016). Outpatient treatment of acute poisoning by substances of abuse: A prospective observational cohort study. *Scandinavian Journal of Trauma, Resuscitation and Emergency Medicine, 24,* 76.

■ EXTRACORPOREAL LIFE SUPPORT

Grant Pignatiello
Katherine Hornack
Julie E. Herzog

Overview

Extracorporeal life support (ECLS) is a variation of cardiopulmonary bypass that provides support to the lungs and/or heart for patients in the intensive care unit (ICU) (Gaffney, Wildhirt, Griffin, Annich, & Radomski, 2010). According to the most recent data available from the Extracorporeal Life Support Organization (ELSO) registry, approximately 86,000 individuals have received ECLS, with 30% of these individuals being adults (ELSO, 2017). ECLS is a complex treatment modality for individuals experiencing severe critical illness; thus, the nursing care of this unique cohort entails rigorous monitoring of physiological parameters, thorough analysis of the clinical situation, and adapt management and advocacy of the family's psychosocial experience.

Background

ECLS, an expansion of the commonly known extracorporeal membrane oxygenation (ECMO), describes all extracorporeal, life support treatments (e.g., oxygenation, carbon dioxide removal, and hemodynamic support) that are used in the management of the critically ill patient suffering from severe pulmonary or cardiorespiratory failure. Broadly, there are two main categories of ECLS: venous–venous (VV) and venous–arterial (VA; Gaffney et al., 2010; Makdisi & Wang, 2015). VV ECLS is used as an advanced respiratory support modality that is indicated when the lungs' oxygenation capabilities are impaired as a result of physiologic insult (e.g., acute respiratory distress syndrome, pulmonary contusion, inhalation injury, lung transplantation, and status asthmaticus). VV ECLS consists of the implantation of a large catheter into a large vein (femoral or internal jugular) and the superior vena cava or right atrium; deoxygenated blood is then pulled from one of the catheters, cycled through an oxygenator, and returned to the patient through the right atrium.

Conversely, VA ECLS provides both respiratory and hemodynamic support. Indicated in situations in which the heart is unable to provide sufficient cardiac output despite inotropic and afterload-reducing support (e.g., cardiogenic shock, pulmonary embolism, cardiomyopathy, acute coronary syndrome, etc.), VA ECLS functions similarly to VV ECLS, except the oxygenated blood is returned to the arterial system through the femoral, axillary, carotid, or ascending aortic arteries—not relying on the left side of the heart to circulate independently.

ECLS is indicated for the critically ill patient who demonstrates profound respiratory and/or cardiac insufficiency that is refractory to other clinical treatments. Thus, ECLS is available to critically ill patients of all ages—from neonates to adults. However, a review of the available data suggests ECLS demonstrates the greatest effectiveness when implemented in neonatal and pediatric populations. According to the ECLS Organization (ELSO) registry, ECLS is used 3.5 and 2.5 times more often in neonatal populations than pediatric and adult populations, respectively (ELSO, 2017). In neonatal populations, VV and VA ECLS mortality is approximately 15% and 36%, respectively with 73% of VV and 40% of VA surviving to hospital discharge or transfer from the ICU. Mortality rates do not appear to differ in pediatric populations, as approximately 70% of pediatric patients survive ECLS treatment, regardless of ECLS type (i.e., VV or VA); however, pediatric patients who receive VV ECLS are more likely to survive to be discharged (57% vs. 50%; ELSO, 2017).

In adults, ECLS associated-mortality depends on the indication of ECLS initiation. Like the pediatric and neonatal population, survival rates are higher in adults who receive VV ECLS when compared to adults who receive

VA ECLS (66% vs. 56%; ELSO, 2017). However, the use of VA ECLS for severe cardiogenic shock or cardiac arrest demonstrates more discouraging outcomes, with survival rates ranging from 20% to 30% (Makdisi & Wang, 2015). Furthermore, the complications associated with ECLS therapy are numerous, with end-organ system damage and infection being a common risk (Zangrillo et al., 2013). Therefore, it is consensually noted that before ECLS is initiated, the full clinical perspective of the patient be taken into perspective, as ECLS is a costly and resource-intensive treatment modality often necessitating a prolonged ICU length of stay (Aubron et al., 2013; Gaffney et al., 2010; Munshi, Telesnicki, Walkey, & Fan, 2014). Furthermore, the complications associated with ECLS initiation and management potentiate the risk of chronic critical illness—which is associated with its unique array of management complexities and increased morbidity and mortality.

Clinical Aspects

ASSESSMENT

A team approach is essential in managing patients who require ECLS. Most ECLS care is provided in tertiary-level ICUs with specially trained health care personnel, including critical care physicians, perfusion clinicians, advanced practice clinicians, nurses, respiratory therapists, and surgeons (Williams, 2013). A large portion of the nursing care is evaluating for complications. Complications associated with a patient on ECLS are cannula dislodgement, bleeding, intracranial bleeding, sepsis, air emboli, renal injury, disseminated intravascular coagulation, vascular complications, and decubitus ulcers (Gay, Ankney, Cochran, & Highland, n.d.). Thus, goals of nursing care are multifaceted in nature and require thorough assessment skills.

The incidence of neurological injury is approximately 16% in neonatal patients and 10% among adult and pediatric populations. The injury is precipitated by the nature of the underlying pathology, which commonly includes hypoxia and hypoperfusion, as well as coagulopathies related to anticoagulation therapy. Types of neurological injury include seizure, hemorrhage, infarction, and brain death (Mehta & Ibsen, 2013). Frequent neurological assessments should be performed to evaluate for deviations from the patient's baseline. Patients on ECLS often require sedation and may need neuromuscular blockade. Therefore, the neurological assessment includes evaluation of pupillary reflexes, peripheral sensory/motor function, sedation monitoring, and peripheral nerve stimulation reactivity. Changes from the patient's baseline commonly indicate further diagnostic imaging such as EEG or CT.

Cardiovascular nursing assessment focus may vary among patients receiving VV or VA ECLS. As the ECLS serves as the perfusion source, assessing peripheral and central perfusion is necessary (Chung, Shiloh, & Carlese, 2014). Vital signs and hemodynamic parameters are continuously monitored; hemodynamic parameters include mean arterial pressure, cardiac output/index, central venous pressure, pulmonary artery pressure, systemic vascular resistance, and mixed venous oxygen saturation level (SvO_2). SvO_2 levels, which represent peripheral oxygen consumption, are used to adjust ECLS circuit flow rates and should remain more than 60% (Gay et al., n.d.). The nursing assessment includes cardiac rhythm monitoring and neurovascular extremity evaluation. Further nursing management includes monitoring the therapeutic impact of and for complications related to vasopressor and inotropic medications.

Most patients receiving ECLS require continuous mechanical ventilation. Thus, nursing assessments should include continuous pulse oximetry, endotracheal tube position, breath sounds, and the quantity and quality of pulmonary secretions. Ventilation goals focus on resting the lungs by limiting tidal volumes (less than 4 mL/kg predicted body weight [PBW]), plateau pressures (20–25 cmH_2O), and respiratory rate while maintaining elevated positive end-expiratory pressure (PEEP) levels (greater than or equal to 10 cm H_2O; Schmidt et al., 2014). Ventilator and ECLS flow settings are adjusted from the frequent monitoring of arterial and venous blood gases.

NURSING INTERVENTIONS, MANAGEMENT, AND IMPLICATIONS

Monitoring of the ECLS circuit is often a shared responsibility between the perfusion clinician and nurse. For example, monitoring of the inflow and outflow cannulas should be routinely assessed for bleeding and placement stability; bleeding or unstable cannula sites should be reported to the perfusion clinician and ICU team. The nurse should evaluate oxygenator function by monitoring blood gas values. The ECLS catheters should be evaluated for rhythmic shaking, known as *chattering*, which may indicate hypovolemia or improper cannula placement (Chung et al., 2014). The bedside nurse should be aware of the ECLS flow rates, oxygenator, and sweep settings for integration into the interpretation of laboratory values and assessment findings.

Regarding the genitourinary system, hourly urine output should be monitored—acute renal failure occurs in 70% to 85% of patients receiving ECLS, often necessitating dialysis. Moreover, the nurse should monitor for electrolyte abnormalities (Chen, Tsai, Fang, & Yang, 2014). The gastrointestinal system must be monitored for signs of ischemia or bleeding; stool should be assessed for color and consistency. Notably, patients receiving ECLS commonly receive gastric ulcer prophylaxis through proton pump antagonists or histamine antagonists (Zangrillo et al., 2013).

A patient receiving ECLS has vast hematologic and integumentary considerations. Anticoagulation is required during ECLS to prevent clot formation in the circuit related to blood–surface interactions; however, bleeding is the most common complication of ECLS (Bartlett, 2016). Serial hematologic laboratory testing, including activated clotting time, anti-factor Xa activity levels, activated partial thromboplastin time, complete blood counts, fibrinogen, and lactate dehydrogenase (Annich, 2015). Owing to anticoagulation and the invasive nature of the ECLS cannulas, monitoring for bleeding is imperative. Patients on ECLS receive many blood product transfusions to keep appropriate intravascular volume in addition to optimizing oxygen-carrying capacity (Sen et al., 2016). Patients receiving ECLS are at an increased risk of integumentary complications secondary to immobility—increasing the risk for pressure ulcer development. Ideally, the patient's body position should be changed every 2 hours with pressure points supported by a dry, wrinkle-free surface.

Summary

ECLS serves as an effective treatment modality for the patient suffering from severe pulmonary or cardiorespiratory failure. Care of the patient receiving ECLS is complex, requiring interdisciplinary cooperation and competent nursing care—with an emphasis on continuously analyzing the patient's clinical presentation and monitoring for complications. As the health care industry witnesses advances in vascular access, ECLS circuitry, anticoagulation therapy, and patient management, Bartlett (2016) envisions outcomes associated with ECLS therapy to improve, introducing health care to a population of ECLS patients he describes as "awake, extubated, spontaneously breathing (patients), without systemic anticoagulation, managed in step-down units, general care, or even at home" (p. 10). As ECLS therapy continues to evolve, nursing care remain as a primary determinant in ensuring positive patient outcomes.

Annich, G. (2015). Extracorporeal life support: The precarious balance of hemostasis. *Journal of Thrombosis and Haemostasis*. Retrieved from http://onlinelibrary.wiley.com/doi/10.1111/jth.12963/full

Aubron, C., Cheng, A. C., Pilcher, D., Leong, T., Magrin, G., Coper, D. J., . . . Pellegrino, V. (2013). Factors associated with outcomes of patients on extracorporeal membrane oxygenation support: A 5-year cohort study. *Critical Care, 17*(2), R73. doi:10.1186/cc12681

Bartlett, R. H. (2016). ECMO: The next ten years. *Egyptian Journal of Critical Care Medicine, 4*(1), 7–10. doi:10.1016/j.ejccm.2016.01.003

Chen, Y.-C., Tsai, F.-C., Fang, J.-T., & Yang, C.-W. (2014). Acute kidney injury in adults receiving extracorporeal membrane oxygenation. *Journal of the Formosan Medical Association, 113*(11), 778–785.

Chung, M., Shiloh, A. L., & Carlese, A. (2014). Monitoring of the adult patient on venoarterial extracorporeal membrane oxygenation. *Scientific World Journal, 2014,* 393258. doi:10.1155/2014/393258

Extracorporeal Life Support Organization. (2017). Retrieved from https://www.elso.org

Gaffney, A. M., Wildhirt, S. M., Griffin, M. J., Annich, G. M., & Radomski, M. W. (2010). Extracorporeal life support. *British Medical Journal, 341,* c5317. doi:10.1136/bmj.c5317

Gay, S. E., Ankney, N., Cochran, J. B., & Highland, K. B. (n.d.). Critical care challenges in the adult ECMO patient. *Dimensions of Critical Care Nursing, 24*(4), 15762–15764. Retrieved from http://www.ncbi.nlm.nih.gov/pubmed/16043975

Mehta, A., & Ibsen, L. M. (2013). Neurologic complications and neurodevelopmental outcome with extracorporeal life support. *World Journal of Critical Care Medicine, 2*(4), 40–47.

Schmidt, M., Pellegrino, V., Combes, A., Scheinkestel, C., Cooper, D. J., & Hodgson, C. (2014). Mechanical ventilation during extracorporeal membrane oxygenation. *Critical Care, 18*(1), 203.

Sen, A., Callisen, H. E., Alwardt, C. M., Larson, J. S., Lowell, A. A., Libricz, S. L., . . . Ramakrishna, H. (2016). Adult venovenous extracorporeal membrane oxygenation for severe respiratory failure: Current status and future perspectives. *Annals of Cardiac Anaesthesia, 19*(1), 97–111.

Williams, K. E. (2013). Extracorporeal membrane oxygenation for acute respiratory distress syndrome in adults. *AACN Advanced Critical Care, 24*(2), 149–158; quiz 159.

Zangrillo, A., Landoni, G., Biondi-Zoccai, G., Greco, M., Greco, T., Frati, G., . . . Pappalardo, F. (2013). A meta-analysis of complications and mortality of extracorporeal membrane oxygenation. *Critical Care and Resuscitation, 15*(3), 172–178. Retrieved from http://www.ncbi.nlm.nih.gov/pubmed/23944202

■ FLUID AND ELECTROLYTE IMBALANCES

Michael D. Gooch

Overview

Fluid and electrolyte balance is essential for homeostasis. Fluid balance ensures adequate cellular perfusion and function and is the key to maintaining electrolyte balance as well. Sodium (Na^+), potassium (K^+), calcium (Ca^{2+}), and magnesium (Mg^{2+}) play key roles in maintaining cell membrane stability, muscle contractions, cardiac and neuronal conduction, and bone health. This balance may be altered by numerous processes, including numerous medications, diseases, alterations in the pH, and nutrition. A thorough history, including medication review, physical examination, and analysis of laboratory data, is often needed to identify an imbalance, assess for complications, and formulate a plan of care. Nurses should be able to recognize the diagnostics needed to properly identify an imbalance, the associated clinical manifestations, and initial management of these derangements.

Background

Water makes up 50% to 60% of our total body weight, though this varies by age, gender, and muscle and fat composition (Hall, Matlock, Ward, Gray, & Clayden, 2016; Harring, Deal, & Kuo, 2014; Kamel & Halperin, 2017). Water is contained in various compartments and can be shifted around if needed by the body. The intracellular space accounts for two thirds of our total body water. The remainder is extracellular and includes intravascular (plasma) and interstitial spaces. Water balance is regulated by the hypothalamic–neurohypophyseal–renal axis; during acute illness this axis is often altered leading to imbalances in many hospitalized patients (Knepper, Kwon, & Nielsen, 2015). By releasing vasopressin or antidiuretic hormone (ADH), altering the thirst response, and altering renal water excretion, this axis works to maintain a serum osmolality of 280 to 295 mmol/kg, as with any lab the accepted values vary. Osmolality is a measure of the concentration of solutes in a solution (Hall et al., 2016; Harring et al., 2014; Kamel & Halperin,

2017). The higher the osmolality, the higher the concentration of solutes. Osmolality must be balanced between intracellular and extracellular compartments to maintain equilibrium and cell membrane integrity (Kamel & Halperin, 2017; Sterns, 2015). Sodium is the primary extracellular solute and directly influences osmolality, as well as how fluids shift among the body's compartments. Fluid movement is also influenced by plasma proteins, glucose, and other electrolytes.

Sodium is the most abundant extracellular cation, with an accepted normal range of 135 to 145 mEq/L. Hyponatremia is considered the most common electrolyte imbalance encountered in the hospitalized patient (Cho, Kim, Hong, Joo, & Kim, 2017). It is estimated that 15% of admitted adults have hyponatremia with an overall mortality rate of 3% to 29% (Harring et al., 2014). The degree of hyponatremia is often assessed based on the serum and urine Na+ concentrations and osmolality. Isotonic hyponatremia (osmolality 280–295 mmol/kg) is characterized by a normal serum osmolality and may result from elevated serum lipids or proteins. Hypertonic hyponatremia (osmolality greater than 295 mmol/kg) may be caused by hyperglycemia or osmotic diuretics (Cho et al., 2017; Craig, Baker, & Rodd, 2015; Harring et al., 2014; Kamel & Halperin, 2017).

The most common problem is hypotonic hyponatremia (osmolality less than 280 mmol/kg). Hypotonic patients can be further categorized as hypovolemic, euvolemic, and hypervolemic. Hypovolemia occurs when there is a loss of both water and Na+ from the body, for example, excessive gastrointestinal (GI) or genitourinary (GU) losses. The Na+ loss usually exceeds the water loss, and these patients often appear dehydrated. Euvolemia occurs when excess free water is gained, most often related to ADH release or function, and there is no excess of serum Na+. This may include hypothyroidism; cortisol insufficiency; syndrome of inappropriate antidiuretic hormone (SIADH); exogenous free water intake; and use of certain drugs, including thiazide diuretics and 3,4-methylenedioxymethamphetamine (MDMA, ecstasy). As the free water is gained, the serum Na+ is lowered, but there is usually no loss of Na+. However, the patient does not appear dehydrated or volume overloaded. Hypervolemia occurs when there is an increased retention of both body water and Na+, often because of renal disease, heart failure, or cirrhosis. Water is retained more than Na+, leading to a decrease in the serum Na+. These patients usually appear volume overloaded (Cho et al.,

2017; Craig et al., 2015; Harring et al., 2014; Kamel & Halperin, 2017; Sterns, 2015).

Hypernatremia is most often associated with a decrease in free water intake that leads to cellular dehydration and an increased osmolality. This can be seen in patients with a decreased thirst reflex and those without easy access to water, for example, those with limited mobility, extremes of age, and in comatose states. It is also associated with diabetes insipidus (DI); because of the lack of ADH, the kidneys cannot adequately regulate water balance. Excess water loss worsens hypernatremia, but unless the thirst reflex is altered or there is limited access to water, insufficient free water intake is the primary cause of hypernatremia (Cho et al., 2017; Craig et al., 2015; Harring et al., 2014; Kamel & Halperin, 2017).

Potassium is the most abundant intracellular cation with an accepted serum range of 3.5 to 5.0 mEq/L. Potassium plays a key role in maintaining the resting membrane potential of cardiac and muscle cells. Hypokalemia may be related to an increased loss from the GI or GU tract, cellular shifts from alkalosis and beta-2 stimulation, or inadequate dietary intake. Hypomagnesemia can also lead to hypokalemia. Hyperkalemia may result from medications that increase K+ levels, inadequate excretion as seen in renal failure, cellular shifts seen with acidosis and significant tissue trauma, or maybe a measurement error because of cell hemolysis from the lab draw, often referred to as *pseudohyperkalemia* (Combs & Buckley, 2015; Gooch, 2015; Hall et al., 2016; Kamel & Halperin, 2017; Medford-Davis & Rafique, 2014).

Calcium plays an essential role in neuromuscular function and bone health. A normal Ca^{2+} level is often considered to be 8.5 to 10.5 mg/dL or an ionized level of 4.6 to 5.3 mg/dL. About half of the serum Ca^{2+} is bound to proteins; the remainder is free or ionized. Almost all (99%) of the body's Ca^{2+} is stored in the bones. Hypocalcemia most often results from inadequate intake or GI absorption, a chronic kidney disease that results in vitamin D deficiency, hypoparathyroidism, or from massive blood transfusions. In the setting of hypoalbuminemia, hypocalcemia may be noted and is often considered a pseudohypocalcemia. Evaluating the ionized Ca^{2+} level can help determine whether a true imbalance exists. Hypercalcemia most often develops from hyperparathyroidism or in cases of higher levels; malignancy is a prime cause. It is estimated that 20% to 30% of cancer patients experience hypercalcemia (Chang, Radin, & McCurdy, 2014; Cho et al., 2017; Gooch, 2015; Hall et al., 2016; Love & Buckley, 2015).

Magnesium is the second most common intracellular cation and plays a similar role to Ca²⁺ in regard to the nervous system. When outside the normal range of 1.8 to 2.5 mg/dL, it may influence K⁺ and Ca²⁺ levels. Hypomagnesemia is more common and often results from altered dietary intake or absorption or increased urinary excretion. Hypermagnesemia is rare and often associated with renal failure, but could be related to medications that increase the magnesium levels (Cho et al., 2017; Chang et al., 2014; Love & Buckley, 2015).

Clinical Aspects

ASSESSMENT

It is common for acutely ill patients to have one or more imbalance. The nurse should be observant for risk factors and signs or symptoms of these imbalances. Imbalances in electrolytes can result in symptoms or clinical manifestations that are not exclusive to a particular electrolyte. Often, to link the clinical manifestations associated with an electrolyte imbalance, laboratory data need to identify the imbalance and inform the treatment plan. The patient may have altered mental status, weakness, headache, or seizures. Management is guided by the lab values, clinical findings, and rapidity with which the symptoms started. Hypovolemia should be corrected as the patient's condition allows. In the stable hyponatremic patient, free water restrictions may be all that is required to stabilize the patient. In the unstable seizing patient, a bolus of hypertonic (3%) saline may be required. In most patients, increasing the serum Na⁺ by 4 mEq/L is all that is needed to reduce cerebral edema and resolve the seizures. In patients with SIADH or hypervolemic hyponatremia, a vasopressin antagonist may be administered to block ADH receptors in the kidneys and limit the reabsorption of water (Cho et al., 2017; Craig et al., 2015; Gooch, 2015).

NURSING INTERVENTIONS, MANAGEMENT, AND IMPLICATIONS

Hypernatremia may be managed with isotonic intravenous (IV) fluids initially to restore perfusion. Loop diuretics may be used in volume overloaded patients to increase the excretion of water and Na⁺. In the setting of DI, desmopressin (DDAVP) may be given. An important caveat to the management of Na⁺ imbalances is that the level should not be rapidly changed. If the serum Na⁺ is increased too quickly, osmotic demyelination or central pontine myelinolytic may occur. If the serum Na⁺ is reduced too rapidly, cerebral edema often develops. A guideline to prevent complications is to correct the level by no more than 1 to 2 mEq/L/hr and no more than 10 mEq/day (Cho et al., 2017; Craig et al., 2015; Gooch, 2015; Sterns, 2015). The more chronic the condition, the slower the correction.

Any patient suspected of having a K⁺ imbalance should have his or her EKG quickly assessed. Patients may experience muscle cramps or weakness, which could progress to respiratory failure. Flattened or inverted T waves, the appearance of U waves, and ST depression are often seen with hypokalemia. Hypokalemic management is also based on severity and may require oral or IV K⁺ replacement. In the setting of hypomagnesemia, the Mg²⁺ imbalance will have to be corrected first (Cho et al., 2017; Combs & Buckley, 2015; Gooch, 2015; Medford-Davis & Rafique, 2014).

Of the electrolyte imbalances, hyperkalemia is the most lethal. If there is a concern for hyperkalemia, the EKG should quickly be assessed for the presence of peaked T waves, a prolonged PR interval, or a widened QRS. If these EKG changes are present, IV Ca²⁺ should be administered to stabilize the resting membrane potential of the cardiac cells and prevent life-threatening arrhythmias. Treatment should not be delayed while awaiting lab values. Hyperkalemia is managed in two ways. First, high-dose albuterol, insulin with glucose, or sodium bicarbonate may be given to shift the K⁺ back in the cells temporarily. Subsequently, the excessive K⁺ should be eliminated. This is most effectively accomplished through hemodialysis, but loop diuretics or cation exchange resins may also be used with caution (Cho et al., 2017; Combs & Buckley, 2015; Gooch, 2015; Medford-Davis & Rafique, 2014).

Hypocalcemia causes neuromuscular excitability, including muscle spasms, paresthesias, hyperactive deep tendon reflexes (DTRs), and eventually, seizures. The EKG should also be assessed for a prolonged QT interval and bradycardia. Symptomatic patients may be managed with oral or IV Ca²⁺ replacement. Patients with hypercalcemia may have lethargy, muscle weakness, hypoactive DTRs, and at higher levels a shortened QT and widened QRS may be noted on the EKG. Patients may develop atrioventricular blocks, which can progress to cardiac arrest in levels more than 15 mg/dL. Initially, IV fluids should be given to restore renal perfusion. Depending on the severity of the patient, hemodialysis may be used to remove the excess Ca²⁺. In less severe cases, the patient may be given a loop diuretic, a bisphosphonate, a glucocorticoid, or calcitonin (Chang et al., 2014; Cho et al., 2017; Gooch, 2015; Love & Buckley, 2015).

Lastly, patients with low serum Mg^{2+} levels present similarly to those with hypokalemia and hypocalcemia and have weakness and muscle cramps. This can progress to neuromuscular and cardiac irritability. Treatment is focused on replacement with oral or IV Mg^{2+} depending on the patient's condition. Hypermagnesemia is similar to hypercalcemia, and patients experience blunted neuromuscular effects, including lethargy, paralysis, decreased DTRs, and eventually hypotension, cardiac and respiratory compromise. Calcium may be administered to antagonize the Mg^{2+} and reverse neuromuscular weakness. If needed, dialysis is effective at removing the excess electrolyte in severe cases (Chang et al., 2014; Cho et al., 2017; Love & Buckley, 2015).

Summary

Fluid and electrolyte balance is critical to maintaining all the body functions. Sodium and water have an important relationship and imbalances are common in patients with acute problems. Patients with Na^+ imbalances often present with neurological changes and the imbalance cannot be aggressively corrected. Potassium is crucial for cardiac and muscle function and an imbalance can be life-threatening, and often requires rapid identification and correction to prevent complications. Calcium and Mg^{2+} both play an important role in neuromuscular function and can affect cardiac function as well. Nurses should evaluate for these imbalances in the acutely ill patient, recalling that the patient may have more than one. Labs are often helpful, but history and physical examination findings are also important to identify the imbalance and manage the derangement.

Chang, W.-T., Radin, B., & McCurdy, M. T. (2014). Calcium, magnesium, and phosphate abnormalities in the emergency department. *Emergency Medicine Clinics of North America, 32*(2), 349–366.

Cho, K.-C., Kim, J.-J., Hong, C.-K., Joo, J.-Y., & Kim, Y. B. (2017). Perimesencephalic nonaneurysmal subarachnoid hemorrhage after clipping of an unruptured aneurysm. *World Neurosurgery, 102*, 694.e15–694.e19.

Combs, D. J., & Lu, Z. (2015). Sphingomyelinase D inhibits store-operated Ca2+ entry in T lymphocytes by suppressing ORAI current. *Journal of General Physiology, 146*(2), 161–172.

Craig, S. A., Baker, S. R., & Rodd, H. D. (2015). How do children view other children who have visible enamel defects? *International Journal of Paediatric Dentistry, 25*(6), 399–408.

Gooch, M. D. (2015). Identifying acid-base and electrolyte imbalances. *Nurse Practitioner, 40*(8), 37–42.

Hall, J. E., Matlock, J. V., Ward, J. W., Gray, K. V., & Clayden, J. (2016). Medium-ring nitrogen heterocycles through migratory ring expansion of metalated ureas. *Angewandte Chemie, 55*(37), 11153–11157.

Harring, T. R., Deal, N. S., & Kuo, D. C. (2014). Disorders of sodium and water balance. *Emergency Medicine Clinics of North America, 32*(2), 379–401.

Kamel, K. S., & Halperin, M. L. (2017). *Fluid, electrolytes, and acid–base physiology: A problem-based approach* (5th ed.). Philadelphia, PA: Elsevier.

Knepper, M. A., Kwon, T. H., & Nielsen, S. (2015). Molecular physiology of water balance. *New England Journal of Medicine, 372*(14), 1349–1358.

Love, J. W., & Buckley, R. G. (2015). Disorders of calcium, phosphate, and magnesium metabolism. In A. B. Wolfson (Ed.), *Harwood-Nuss' clinical practice of emergency medicine* (6th ed., pp. 1052–1057). Philadelphia, PA: Wolters Kluwer.

Medford-Davis, L., & Rafique, Z. (2014). Derangements of potassium. *Emergency Medicine Clinics of North America, 32*(2), 329–347.

Sterns, R. H. (2015). Disorders of plasma sodium. *New England Journal of Medicine, 372*(13), 1269.

■ FLUID RESUSCITATION

Laura Stark Bai

Overview

Intravenous fluid resuscitation is one of the most common treatments in acute medical care (Myburgh, 2015). It is used as a therapy in adults and children for a range of medical problems, including dehydration, sepsis, diabetic ketoacidosis (DKA) and hyperglycemic hyperosmolar state (HHS) trauma, burns, acute pancreatitis, and more. There are two types of fluids that are used for fluid resuscitation. Crystalloids are isotonic solutions composed of ions that are capable of passing through semipermeable membranes, such as a capillary wall. The examples include normal saline, Ringer's lactate, or dextrose 5% in water. Colloid solutions, conversely, consist of insoluble molecules, which enhance therapeutic expansion of intravascular spaces. An example of a colloid solution is albumin or fresh frozen plasma. Isotonic saline (0.9%), referred to as *normal saline*, is a crystalloid solution and the most commonly used intravenous fluid in the world (Myburgh, 2015).

Background

Fluid resuscitation is an important element in the treatment plan in many medical ailments. Crystalloid and colloid solutions are infused into the intravascular space to correct metabolic and electrolyte abnormalities, as well as manage hypotension and hypoperfusion through fluid expansion in the vascular space (Katz & Choukalas, 2013). Although fluid resuscitation is safe and effective, there are complications that must also be considered to maintain patient safety.

Sepsis is one of the more serious conditions that require proper fluid resuscitation, affecting an estimated 300 cases per 100,000 population (Mayr, Yende, & Angus, 2014). To correct sepsis-induced hypoperfusion, current guidelines recommend administration of crystalloid fluids for hypotension and elevated lactate at a dose of 30 mL/kg for adults and 20 mL/kg for children (Waltzman, 2015). Initiation of fluids should occur immediately on the recognition of sepsis, and total fluid administration should be complete in 3 hours as part of the treatment bundle (Rosini & Srivastava, 2013). This is important, as early fluid resuscitation has been linked to decreased mortality in patients with severe sepsis and septic shock (Lee et al., 2014).

Fluid resuscitation is a mainstay in the treatment of DKA and HHS to lower blood sugar levels, correct electrolyte levels, and ensure hemodynamic stability. Patients in DKA may be in deficit of 3 to 5 mL of fluid and need fluid resuscitation with an initial 1 L bolus of normal saline, followed by continuous infusion for maintenance therapy. When blood sugar levels stabilize below 250 mg/dL, then dextrose 5% is added to the infusion. Fluid replacement is also essential in HHS, as the fluid deficit is up to 10 L or more. The recommendation for fluid therapy is an initial 500 mL bolus of normal saline followed by 1 to 2 L over 2 hours. The total amount of fluid administered in the first 12 hours should be half of the estimated fluid loss. It is important that the correct rate of infusion is monitored, as too rapid a correction of hyperosmolality from fluid resuscitation can lead to cerebral edema.

Fluid loss and dehydration are one of the most serious issues as a result of a burn injury because of fluid shifts from the intravascular spaces. Therefore, fluid resuscitation is essential in the effective treatment of this patient population to maintain tissue oxygenation, correct hypovolemia, and improve survival. There are multiple formulas available to calculate the amount of fluid given in the first 24 to 48 hours based on the percentage of surface area burned and patient weight. Children, elderly patients, and patients with inhalation injury may require additional fluid requirements (Mitchell et al., 2013). Each formula has its recommendation on the type of fluid administered (Haberal, Abali, & Karakayali, 2010). It is important to be aware of an institution's policy for the treatment of burn patients.

Fluid therapy is a central part of the treatment of acute pancreatitis because of hypovolemia from vasodilation, capillary leakage, edema, and vomiting that may lead to decreased tissue damage if untreated. Prompt and aggressive fluid resuscitation is recommended to decrease morbidity and mortality. Specifically, 250 to 500 mL/hr should be administered to patients with pancreatitis, except patients with comorbidities putting them at risk for fluid overload. However, in practice, an estimated 3.5 to 4.5 L of fluids are typically administered in the first 24 hours. Fluid status should be reassessed every 6 to 8 hours by checking urinary output, heart rate, blood urea nitrogen (BUN) hematocrit, and central venous pressure (CVP; Bortolotti, Saulnier, Colling, Redheuil, & Preau, 2014).

Fluid resuscitation is also important in reducing morbidity and mortality in trauma and hemorrhagic shock, especially in the first 24 hours. However, new guidelines point toward lower target blood pressures in trauma patients for guiding fluid resuscitation. Current guidelines indicate less use of crystalloids and earlier use of plasma and platelets and allowance of permissive hypotension before bleeding control (Carrick, Leondard, Slone, Mains, & Bar-Or, 2016).

Care must be taken with fluid resuscitation as to avoid complications. With aggressive fluid administration, patients may be at risk for fluid overload, which may exhibit as orthopnea, dyspnea on exertion, shortness of breath, and extremity swelling. Fluid overload is reversible with the use of diuretics or dialysis to remove excess fluid.

Clinical Aspects

ASSESSMENT

Nursing assessment for patients in need of fluid resuscitation focus on assessment for signs and symptoms of fluid volume deficit. Physical examination includes assessment of skin turgor, mucous membranes, mental status, neck veins, and urine output to assess for hydration and volume status. Nurses should pay close attention to vital signs, particularly blood pressure and heart rate, as hypotension and tachycardia may indicate hypovolemia. Lab values that should be considered as part of the assessment include BUN, creatinine, specific gravity, and hematocrit. Important information to obtain the patient's history includes a full medical history, particularly for renal, cardiac, or liver disease, because of the risk of fluid overload. In addition, history of present illness, weight, and current medication list should also be gathered.

NURSING INTERVENTIONS, MANAGEMENT, AND IMPLICATIONS

Nursing problems that should be considered are fluid volume deficit, the risk for ineffective tissue perfusion, and risk for impaired skin integrity.

Interventions include careful and timely administration of prescribed crystalloid or colloid fluids. Monitoring of urine output, blood pressure, heart rate, specific gravity, electrolytes and renal function tests, and body weight are also paramount to treatment.

OUTCOMES

Nursing interventions for patients requiring fluid resuscitation focus on achieving goals for increasing fluid intake, eliminating signs of dehydration, maintaining blood pressure and urine output, proper electrolyte balance, and normal kidney function.

Summary

Fluid resuscitation is an important aspect of treatment for multiple medical conditions. Protocols for the amount and type of fluid and the time over which they should be administered vary based on the goals of therapy and patient weight. It is important for nurses to be aware of plans for fluid resuscitation and the rationale behind the therapy. Nurses must also closely monitor the patient status, vital signs, and laboratory values to evaluate the effectiveness of therapy. Deviations from the expected plan of care should be escalated to the medical care teams.

Bortolotti, P., Saulnier, F., Colling, D., Redheuil, A., & Preau, S. (2014). New tools for optimizing fluid resuscitation in acute pancreatitis. *World Journal of Gastroenterology*, 20(43), 16113–16122.

Carrick, M. M., Leonard, J., Slone, D. S., Mains, C. W., & Bar-Or, D. (2016). Hypotensive resuscitation among trauma patients. *BioMed Research International, 2016*, 8901938.

Haberal, M., Sakallioglu Abali, A. E., & Karakayali, H. (2010). Fluid management in major burn injuries. *Indian Journal of Plastic Surgery, 43*(Suppl.), S29–S36.

Katz, J., & Choukalas, C. (2013). Goal directed fluid resuscitation: A review of hemodynamic, metabolic, and monitoring based goals. *Current Anesthesiology Reports, 3*(2), 98–104.

Lee, S. J., Ramar, K., Park, J. G., Gajic, O., Li, G., & Kashyap, R. (2014). Increased fluid administration in the first three hours of sepsis resuscitation is associated with reduced mortality: A retrospective cohort study. *Chest, 146*(4), 908–915.

Mayr, F. B., Yende, S., & Angus, D. C. (2014). Epidemiology of severe sepsis. *Virulence, 5*(1), 4–11.

Mitchell, K. B., Khalil, E., Brennan, A., Shao, H., Rabbitts, A., Leahy, N. E., . . . Gallagher, J. J. (2013). New management strategy for fluid resuscitation: Quantifying volume in the first 48 hours after burn injury. *Journal of Burn Care & Research, 34*(1), 196–202.

Myburgh, J. A. (2015). Fluid resuscitation in acute medicine: What is the current situation? *Journal of Internal Medicine, 277*(1), 58–68.

Rosini, J. M., & Srivastava, N.; Surviving Sepsis Campaign. (2013). The 2012 guidelines for severe sepsis and septic shock: An update for emergency nursing. *Journal of Emergency Nursing, 39*(6), 652–656.

Waltzman, M. L. (2015). Pediatric shock. *Journal of Emergency Nursing, 41*(2), 113–118.

■ HEART TRANSPLANTATION

S. Brian Widmar

Overview

Heart transplantation is a surgical procedure for the treatment of end-stage heart failure or structural heart disease (McCalmont & Velleca, 2017). A total of 66,737 heart transplants have been performed since 1988, with 3,191 performed in 2016 alone (Organ Procurement and Transplantation Network, 2017). Important nursing considerations for care in the heart transplant recipient include assessment of normal alterations in anatomy and physiology, the administration and management of antirejection or immunosuppressant medications, monitoring for signs and symptoms of organ rejection and infection, and reduction of risk for opportunistic and hospital-acquired infections (Costanzo et al., 2010; Welbaum, 2015).

Background

Heart failure is a chronic, progressive clinical syndrome that develops from a structural or functional cardiac abnormality that reduces ventricular filling or ejection (McCalmont & Velleca, 2017). There are an estimated 6.5 million Americans living with heart failure, and of those, around 960,000 new heart failure cases are diagnosed annually (Writing Group et al., 2016). The causes of heart failure are numerous, including cardiomyopathy (secondary to ischemic heart disease, valvular disease, or hypertension), infections, metabolic disorders, electrolyte deficiencies, nutritional disorders, systemic diseases (e.g., connective tissue disorders, amyloidosis), and exposure to toxic substances (e.g., alcohol or illicit drug use, radiation therapy, chemotherapy, or chemical exposures; McCalmont & Velleca, 2017).

Across the trajectory of the heart failure syndrome, advanced, "end-stage" heart failure, or stage D heart failure, is classified as being refractory to optimized medical therapy and requires specialized interventions to improve symptoms and reduce risk of mortality (Hunt et al., 2001). Options for therapy in stage D heart failure include heart transplantation; chronic mechanical circulatory support; chronic inotropes; experimental surgery or drugs; and end-of-life care, or hospice (Hunt et al., 2001). Heart transplantation is indicated when heart failure symptoms persist and there is evidence of end-organ dysfunction despite optimized medical therapy, or when refractory angina cannot be relieved through surgical revascularization or optimized medical therapy (McCalmont & Velleca, 2017). Other indications for heart transplantation include refractory life-threatening arrhythmias or congenital heart disease with progressive heart failure that cannot be corrected through surgical repair (McCalmont & Velleca, 2017). Since 1988, around 2,000 to 3,000 heart transplants have been performed each year (Organ Procurement and Transplantation Network, 2017).

Research studies have shown an improvement in patient quality of life after transplantation (Grady, Jalowiec, & White-Williams, 1996). In addition to improvement in quality of life, heart transplantation has demonstrated an increase in life expectancy, and has shown to be cost-effective, adding an average of 8.5 years of life with less than $800,000 per quality-adjusted life year (QALY) relative to medical therapy (Writing Group et al., 2016). From 2008 to 2010, the 1-year survival rate for heart transplant recipients was 89.6%, and the 5-year survival rate was 77% (Colvin et al., 2017).

Major causes of posttransplant morbidity include renal dysfunction, hypertension, diabetes, osteoporosis, hyperlipidemia, and gout (Kittleson & Kobashigawa, 2014). Major causes of postoperative mortality in the heart transplant recipient include rejection, infection, cardiac allograft vasculopathy, and malignancy (Kittleson & Kobashigawa, 2014). The incidence of acute rejection in the first year after transplantation was 23% among recipients who underwent transplant between 2013 and 2014 (Colvin et al., 2017). The most common cause of death in the first postoperative year was infection, followed by cardiovascular/cerebrovascular disease (Colvin et al., 2017). Malignancy was less frequently seen as a cause of death and was reported as the cause in 1.7% of deaths after 5 postoperative years (Colvin et al., 2017).

Clinical Aspects

Postoperatively, the heart transplant recipient has specific assessment findings related to the transplant surgery and will have a greater risk for rejection due to the postoperative immune response, and an increased risk for infection, due to the introduction of immunosuppression therapy. Immunosuppression drug therapy may increase postoperative morbidity due to drug-related side effects. Specific assessment findings and implications for care are discussed here.

Heart rate and blood pressure must be closely monitored. When excised from the donor, the transplanted heart is "denervated," meaning the sympathetic and parasympathetic nerve fibers are severed. This anatomical variant affects the resting and responsive heart rate. The normal resting heart rate in the heart transplant patient is generally higher than the normal range, usually 90 to 110 beats per minute (McCalmont & Velleca, 2017). Heart rates outside of this range should be reported. It is important to note that medications that act on the vagus nerve (atropine, digoxin) will be ineffective and should not be used (Moore-Gibbs & Bither, 2015).

The transplanted heart does not respond quickly to stress that requires an abrupt increase in heart rate to maintain adequate cardiac output (e.g., orthostatic hypotension, hypovolemia, etc.). Patients may become orthostatic if quickly transitioning from bed to chair and should be allowed to dangle before attempting transfer. Lastly, due to denervation, many heart transplant patients with myocardial ischemia or myocardial infarction will not feel the chest pain associated with angina, so clinical manifestations of ischemia or infarction, such as ST segment depression or elevation on electrocardiogram, patient complaints of shortness of breath, fatigue, and so on, should be closely monitored (McCalmont & Velleca, 2017).

Often, a heart transplant recipient may not exhibit signs and symptoms of rejection, and because of this, routine surveillance for rejection is standard practice in hospitals (McCalmont & Velleca, 2017). An endomyocardial biopsy (EMB) is the key diagnostic test used in grading the severity of rejection, and treatment is usually directed based upon results (Moore-Gibbs & Bither, 2015). However, in some heart transplant patients, signs and symptoms of rejection may be similar to the signs and symptoms of heart failure, especially if cardiac output is decreased. Pulse quality, the presence of edema, decreased urine output, and other signs and symptoms of heart failure (e.g., shortness of breath, hypotension, weight gain, activity intolerance, lethargy, and general malaise) should be closely monitored in the heart transplant recipient and should be reported. Hypertension is fairly common in heart transplant patients, most often due to immunosuppressant therapies (Moore-Gibbs & Bither, 2015).

Standard immunosuppressant therapy in the heart transplant recipient includes a three-drug approach, usually initiated at the time of transplantation. These drugs include a calcineurin inhibitor (tacrolimus or cyclosporine), an antimetabolite (mycophenolate mofetil), and corticosteroids (McCalmont & Velleca, 2017). Corticosteroids are often weaned to a low daily dose, or are weaned gradually to eventually be discontinued. Nurses should be familiar with their hospital's specific corticosteroid-tapering protocol, as these may vary across transplant programs (Moore-Gibbs & Bither, 2015).

Many patients will have renal dysfunction secondary to heart failure at the time of transplantation, and this can be exacerbated by hypovolemia and hypotension intraoperatively, as well as from nephrotoxic effects of immunosuppression therapy and antibiotic regimens postoperatively (McCalmont & Velleca, 2017). Oliguria or anuria should be promptly reported, as should electrolyte abnormalities, elevated blood urea nitrogen (BUN), and creatinine levels. Judicious use of volume administration or vasoactive medication therapy to maintain a mean arterial pressure between 60 and 80 mmHg may be necessary. Placement of a Foley catheter may be required to closely monitor urine output (McCalmont & Velleca, 2017).

Due to immunosuppressant therapy, heart transplant patients are at an increased risk for community-acquired infections, opportunistic infections, and nosocomial infections (McCalmont & Velleca, 2017). Corticosteroid therapy may reduce the patient's ability to produce pyrogens, and, as a result, the patient's body temperature may be lower than normal. Small increases in body temperature should be noted and reported. A temperature greater than 100.4°F may be used as a threshold for drawing blood cultures (McCalmont & Velleca, 2017).

Strict handwashing and proper technique is probably the most effective intervention for reducing hospital-acquired infections (McCalmont & Velleca, 2017). Wound care, dressing and device site care per hospital protocol, and the timely removal of any invasive lines or indwelling catheters as early as possible are vitally important to reducing risk of nosocomial infection (Moore-Gibbs & Bither, 2015). Perioperative antibiotics should be administered to reduce the incidence of surgical site infections. Additional antibiotic regimens will be used as prophylaxis against opportunistic infections such as cytomegalovirus, *Pneumocystis jiroveci*, or oral candidiasis (McCalmont & Velleca, 2017).

Summary

Heart transplantation is a surgical intervention indicated in patients with advanced, end-stage heart failure, which has been shown to increase life expectancy and improve heart failure symptoms and quality of life. However, due to physiologic alterations secondary to the operative procedure, and its required postoperative medication therapies, heart transplant recipients are at an increased risk for hemodynamic alterations, organ rejection, and increased potential for opportunistic and nosocomial infections. Nurses must be aware of the implications of these changes upon hemodynamic function and the suppressed immune response, and should closely monitor for signs and symptoms associated with organ rejection and infection, to ensure patient safety and adequately anticipate and provide appropriate interventions and care.

Colvin, M., Smith, J. M., Skeans, M. A., Edwards, L. B., Uccellini, K., Snyder, J. J., . . . Kasiske, B. L. (2017). OPTN/SRTR 2015 annual data report: Heart. *American Journal of Transplantation*, 17(S1), 286–356.

Costanzo, M. R., Dipchand, A., Starling, R., Anderson, A., Chan, M., Desai, S., . . . Lung Transplantation, G. (2010). The International Society of Heart and Lung Transplantation Guidelines for the care of heart transplant recipients. *Journal of Heart and Lung Transplantation*, *29*(8), 914–956. doi:10.1016/j.healun.2010.05.034

Grady, K. L., Jalowiec, A., & White-Williams, C. (1996). Improvement in quality of life in patients with heart failure who undergo transplantation. *Journal of Heart and Lung Transplantation*, *15*(8), 749–757.

Hunt, S. A., Baker, D. W., Chin, M. H., Cinquegrani, M. P., Feldman, A. M., & Francis, G. S. (2001). ACC/AHA guidelines for the evaluation and management of chronic heart failure in the adult: Executive summary. A report of the American College of Cardiology/American Heart Association Task Force on Practice Guidelines (Committee to revise the 1995 Guidelines for the Evaluation and Management of Heart Failure): Developed in collaboration with the International Society for Heart and Lung Transplantation; endorsed by the Heart Failure Society of America. *Circulation*, *104*(24), 2996–3007.

Kittleson, M. M., & Kobashigawa, J. A. (2014). Long-term care of the heart transplant recipient. *Current Opinion in Organ Transplantation*, *19*(5), 515–524. doi:10.1097/ MOT.0000000000000117

McCalmont, V., & Velleca, A. (2017). Heart transplantation. In S. Cupples, S. Lerret, V. McCalmont, & L. Ohler (Eds.), *Core curriculum for transplant nurses* (pp. 307– 412). Philadelphia, PA: Mosby.

Moore-Gibbs, A., & Bither, C. (2015). Cardiac transplantation: Considerations for the intensive care unit nurse. *Critical Care Nursing Clinics of North America*, *27*(4), 565–575. doi:10.1016/j.cnc.2015.07.005

Organ Procurement and Transplantation Network. (2017). National data, from U.S. Department of Health and Human Services. Retrieved from https://optn.transplant.hrsa.gov

Welbaum, C. (2015). Caring for patients with solid organ transplants. *American Nurse Today*, *10*(9). Retrieved from https://www.americannursetoday.com/ caring-patients-solid-organ-transplants

Writing Group, M., Mozaffarian, D., Benjamin, E. J., Go, A. S., Arnett, D. K., Blaha, M. J., . . . Stroke Statistics. (2016). Executive summary: Heart disease and stroke statistics—2016 update: A report from the American Heart Association. *Circulation*, *133*(4), 447–454. doi:10.1161/ CIR.0000000000000366

■ HEPATIC FAILURE

Leon Chen
Fidelindo Lim

Overview

The liver is an organ that is indispensable in maintaining the body's homeostasis. Therefore, hepatic failure (HF) is a critical condition that impacts multiple organ systems and is directly correlated with heightened estimates of mortality. Acute hepatic failure (AHF) is often described as "a severe liver injury, potentially reversible in nature with the onset of hepatic encephalopathy within eight weeks of the first symptoms in the absence of pre-existing liver disease" (Bernal & Wendon, 2013, p. 2525). Although the immediate effects of AHF can lead to neurological, respiratory, cardiovascular, renal, endocrinological, and coagulation dysfunctions, chronic liver disease is characterized by progressive hepatic injury that changes normal anatomy and physiology, and leads to complication that presents unique challenges (Singh, Gupta, Alkhouri, Carey, & Hanouneh, 2016).

Background

HF can be categorized as either acute or chronic. AHF is characterized by a rapid liver dysfunction and is notable for acute jaundice, encephalopathy, and coagulopathy in a patient with no previous diagnosis of liver disease. AHF can then be subdivided into categories based on the interval of symptom onset. Categories include hyperacute (symptoms onset less than 7 days), acute (8–28 days) and subacute (28 days to 28 weeks; Kim & Kim-Shluger, 2016). Drug-induced hepatitis from acetaminophen toxicity is the most common cause of AHF in the United States, followed by viral infections such as hepatitis A, B, C, and E virus. HF can also be caused by ischemic injuries in the setting of circulatory failure (Bernal & Wendon, 2013). With the failure of liver function, systemic complications ensue.

Hepatic encephalopathy (HE) is characterized by altered mental status in the setting of fulminant HF. The pathogenesis of this condition is poorly understood, but is likely multifactorial and leads to cerebral edema (Bernal & Wendon, 2013). The factors that contribute to cerebral edema include the breakdown of the blood–brain barrier, the release of neurotoxins, and osmotic alterations. Previously it was thought that the altered mental status was purely because of the build-up of serum ammonia under decreased hepatic clearance. However, the process is now believed to be more complex, although a serum ammonia level of over 200 mmol/L is highly predictive of cerebral edema (Kim & Kim-Shluger, 2016). Cerebral edema in AHF, if untreated, ultimately causes intracranial hypertension. The mortality of HF-associated intracranial hypertension is high and is the leading cause of death worldwide among liver failure patients (Romero-Gómez, Montagnese, & Jalan, 2013).

Respiratory failure because of altered mental status or metabolic derangement can occur in the setting of fulminant HF. In addition, because of the dysfunction in the immune system seen in HF, patients are at a higher risk for infection and up to one third of the patients develop acute respiratory disease syndrome and requires invasive respiratory support (Bernal & Wendon, 2013; Kim & Kim-Shluger, 2016).

Circulatory failure occurs because of the dysfunctional liver, clearance of vasoactive metabolites is decreased as a result there is vasoplegia and profound vasodilation. The result is a decrease in systemic vascular resistance and an alteration of cardiac output. The deceased vascular resistance increases cardiac output, and places increased demand on the heart. In some cases, this leads to high-output cardiac failure (Bernal & Wendon, 2013; Kim & Kim-Shluger, 2016). Often patients who have AHF are baseline hypovolemic because of poor oral intake and nausea/vomiting. In these cases, a decreased vascular resistance exacerbates an already low cardiac output state and leads to further cardiac circulatory compromise (Lee, 2012).

Renal failure can occur in up to 50% of patients with AHF. The cause of renal failure can be the toxic insult that caused the original HF or the alteration in volume status and circulatory failure. With the decrease in cardiac output, renal perfusion pressure decreases and the organ suffers from ischemic damage (Bernal & Wendon, 2013; Kim & Kim-Shluger, 2016). Maintaining euvolemia is crucial to sustaining renal function although renal-replacement therapy is often required to support the patient's kidney functions.

Profound hypoglycemia can be seen in AHF patients because of an impaired gluconeogenesis and glycogenolysis, both of which are essential in maintaining euglycemia through breaking down glycogen storage or formulating serum glucose (Lee, 2012).

The liver produces a cascade of coagulation factors, including factors II, VII, IX, and X along with factors C and S. With the disruption of the liver function, the production of coagulation factors is decreased and often these patients are prone to bleeding (Bernal & Wendon, 2013; Kim & Kim-Shluger, 2016).

Chronic hepatic failure (CHF) is the progressive fibrosis of liver tissue through chronic injury. Excessive alcohol consumption is implicated in the majority of the cases. However, autoimmune disease, such as Wilson's disease, can also lead to chronic liver disease. The anatomy of the liver is altered with scarring and stricture of the vasculature. This disruption leads to conditions such as portal hypertension (PH), esophageal varices, and spontaneous bacterial peritonitis (SBP; Bernal & Wendon, 2013; Kim & Kim-Shluger, 2016).

The progressive structural changes that cause PH include fibrosis, nodule formation, and vascular thrombosis inside the liver. All of these result in an increased vascular resistance in the portal venous system and pressure overload in vessels that drain into the system. PH is the main cause of complications such as esophageal varices and SBP (Mehta et al., 2014).

Fifty percent of patients with the chronic liver disease or cirrhosis develop esophageal varices. This distended esophageal vein is a resultant of increased portal venous pressure, and the severity of the varices is correlated with the severity of the underlying liver disease. Major esophageal variceal bleeding occurs in approximately 6% to 76%, and depending on the literature and mortality rates, approaches 20% (Kim & Kim-Shluger, 2016).

One of the most common complications of cirrhosis is ascites. This condition develops in 58% of patients within 10 years of diagnosis of cirrhosis, and these patients have a 1-year mortality of 15% and a 5-year mortality rate of 44% (Kim & Kim-Shluger, 2016). Ascites is the buildup of fluid because of an inadequate venous return at the portal system. This protein-rich fluid often becomes infected and causes SBP. SBP is diagnosed in 12% of all hospitalized patients with ascites and carries a mortality rate of 33% (Kim & Kim-Shluger, 2016). If left unrecognized and untreated, it is an extremely deadly complication of cirrhosis or chronic liver disease.

Clinical Aspects

The prevention, care, and cure of HF are complex and challenging. As in the management of any condition, better outcomes are achieved with collaborative, evidence-based, and patient-centered care. The American Association for the Study of Liver Diseases (AASLD) issued a data-supported position paper to inform the management of AHF and HE (Lee, Larson, & Stravitz, 2011; Vilstrup et al., 2014).

ASSESSMENT

Altered mental status, coagulopathy, and rapid clinical decline are the primary considerations in HF. The nurse should assess the patient for confusion, jaundice, petechiae, spider angiomas, melena, hematemesis, ascites, and peripheral edema. The key recommendations from the AASLD position paper include (Lee et al., 2011):

- Obtain details concerning all prescription and nonprescription drugs, herbs, and dietary supplements taken over the past year.

- To exclude Wilson disease, obtain ceruloplasmin, serum and urinary copper levels, slit lamp examination for Kayser–Fleischer rings, hepatic copper levels when liver biopsy is feasible, and total bilirubin/alkaline phosphatase ratio.

- Liver biopsy is recommended when autoimmune hepatitis is suspected.

- In patients who have a previous cancer history or massive hepatomegaly, consider underlying malignancy and obtain imaging and liver biopsy to confirm the diagnosis.

- Liver biopsy may be appropriate to attempt to identify a specific etiology if the etiological remains elusive after extensive initial evaluation.

- Periodic surveillance cultures are recommended to detect bacterial and fungal pathogens as early as possible.

- Monitor and trend serum ammonia, metabolic profile, complete blood count, and coagulation profile (activated partial thromboplastin time [aPTT], partial thromboplastin time [PTT], and international normalized ratio [INR]).

HF inevitably affects every body system. The nurse needs to assess the patient's renal, respiratory, integumentary, and cardiac status while monitoring him or her.

NURSING INTERVENTIONS, MANAGEMENT, AND IMPLICATIONS

Taking into account the patient's overall scenario, relevant nursing diagnoses in HF include risk for injury related to delirium, substance intoxication, and delirium tremens; fatigue related to malnutrition; imbalanced nutrition: insufficient nutrients related to a loss of appetite, nausea, and vomiting; risk for deficient fluid volume; ineffective protection related to impaired blood coagulation and bleeding.

Nursing interventions in AHF are geared toward preventing and responding to life-threatening complications such as esophageal varices, bleeding, HE, hepatorenal syndrome, malnutrition, and SBP (Gluud, Vilstrup, & Morgan, 2016). Highlights from the 2014 AASLD guidelines in the management of HF (Lee et al., 2011) and HE include (Vilstrup et al., 2014):

- For patients with known or suspected acetaminophen overdose in 4 hours of presentation, give activated charcoal just before starting N-acetylcysteine dosing.

- Lactulose is the first choice for treatment and prevention of episodic overt HE.

- Neomycin and metronidazole are choices for the treatment of HE.

- Seizure activity should be treated with phenytoin and benzodiazepines with short half-lives. Prophylactic phenytoin is not recommended.

- In the absence of intracranial pressure (ICP) monitoring, frequent (hourly) neurological evaluation is recommended to identify early evidence of intracranial hypertension.

- Mannitol bolus (0.5–1.0 g/kg body weight) is recommended as first-line therapy for increase in ICP. The prophylactic administration of mannitol is not recommended.

- Replacement therapy for thrombocytopenia and/or prolonged prothrombin time is recommended only in the setting of hemorrhage or previous invasive procedures.

Current research does not justify the routine use of parenteral nutrition, enteral nutrition, or oral nutritional supplements in patients with liver disease (Koretz, Avenell, & Lipmann, 2012). The comprehensive nursing care of the patient draws on current guidelines related to hemodynamic monitoring, fluid management, blood transfusion, and infection control.

OUTCOMES

Expected positive outcomes include excretion of excess fluid (reduced ascites and edema), the absence of respiratory distress, prompt resolution of bleeding episodes and HE, hepatic function test will return to normal or baseline, and the client will adhere to lifestyle modifications to improve and maintain hepatic health. The highest quality of life should be restored if possible.

Summary

Although AHF is a rare condition, expert nursing is essential in preventing life-threatening complications such as coagulopathy and HE. The precise etiology of HF should be addressed to guide collaborative management, particularly for patients with HE. The nurse should be vigilant in protecting the patient's liver from further damage from medications and other comorbidities. As patients may deteriorate rapidly, arranging care in a center with expertise in managing patients with HF will secure the best possible outcomes for these patients.

Bernal, W., & Wendon, J. (2013). Acute liver failure. *New England Journal of Medicine, 369*(26), 2525–2534.

Kim, B., & Kim-Schluger, L. (2016). Liver failure: Acute and chronic. In J. M. Oropello, S. M. Pastores, & V. Kvetan (Eds.), *Lange critical care* (1st ed., pp. 469–480). New York, NY: McGraw-Hill.

Koretz, R. L., Avenell, A., & Lipman, T. O. (2012, May). Nutritional support for liver disease. *Cochrane Database of Systematic Reviews.* doi:10.1002/14651858.CD008344 .pub2

Lee, W. M. (2012). Acute liver failure. *Seminars in Respiratory and Critical Care Medicine, 33*(1), 36–45.

Lee, W. M., Larson, A. M., & Stravitz, R. T. (2011). AASLD position paper: The management of acute liver failure: Update 2011. Retrieved from https://www.aasld.org/ sites/default/files/guideline_documents/alfenhanced.pdf

Mehta, G., Gustot, T., Mookerjee, R. P., Garcia-Pagan, J. C., Fallon, M. B., Shah, V. H., . . . Jalan, R. (2014). Inflammation and portal hypertension—The undiscovered country. *Journal of Hepatology, 61*(1), 155–163.

Romero-Gómez, M., Montagnese, S., & Jalan, R. (2015). Hepatic encephalopathy in patients with acute decompensation of cirrhosis and acute-on-chronic liver failure. *Journal of Hepatology, 62*(2), 437–447.

Singh, T., Gupta, N., Alkhouri, N., Carey, W. D., & Hanouneh, I. (2016). In reply: Acute liver failure. *Cleveland Clinic Journal of Medicine, 83*(8), 557.

Vilstrup, H., Amodio, P., Bajaj, J., Ferenci, P., Mullen, K. D., Weissenborn, K., & Wong, P. (2014). Hepatic encephalopathy in chronic liver disease: 2014 Practice Guideline by the American Association for the Study of Liver Diseases and the European Association for the Study of the Liver. *Hepatology, 60*(2), 715–735.

■ HEPATITIS

Ramona A. Sowers
Linda Carson

Overview

Hepatitis is a term used for a variety of viral, bacterial, and noninfectious causes of inflammation of the liver. It is believed to have been first described by Hippocrates. Some persons have no symptoms, whereas others may develop fever, headache, malaise, anorexia, nausea, vomiting, diarrhea, abdominal pain, clay-colored stools, pruritus, dark-colored urine, and jaundice of the skin, sclera, and mucous membranes. Known causes of hepatitis include heavy alcohol and/or drug use; toxins such as carbon tetrachloride; medications, prescribed or over-the-counter such as acetaminophen; herbal and dietary supplements; and medical conditions, including genetic disorders, poor hygiene, environmental conditions, and viruses. According to the World Health Organization (WHO), hepatitis is a major public health problem globally, with more than 1,000,000 deaths annually from viral hepatitis. The Centers for Disease Control and Prevention (CDC) also notes that the most common forms of hepatitis in the United States are viral.

Background

There are several types of hepatitis that are related to viral infections. The first of these types of hepatitis is hepatitis A (HAV), which is highly contagious. The usual transmission is oral–fecal, either person to person or by consumption of contaminated food or water. Microscopic amounts have been found on objects that infected persons have come in contact with. HAV infection has an incubation period that averages 28 days and is generally a self-limited illness that does not progress to a chronic condition. A decrease in the number of outbreaks can be accredited to extensive education regarding handwashing and food preparation as well as the global use of HAV immunization. Lifelong immunity occurs following an infection or after receiving the HAV vaccine. (CDC, 2017).

Hepatitis B (HBV) was previously known as *serum hepatitis*. Transmission occurs when blood, serum, or other bodily fluids from an infected person enter the body of someone who is uninfected. This may be through sexual contact, sharing needles and syringes, mother to baby during birth, or poor infection control in health facilities. Symptoms may occur any time between 2 weeks and 6 months postexposure. The illness may be acute or short term but can become chronic with 15% to 25% of infected patients developing cirrhosis, liver cancer, and liver failure. Treatment is supportive. HBV vaccine is effective in preventing the disease (CDC, 2017).

Hepatitis C (HCV) is a serious blood-borne illness previously called *non-A, non-B hepatitis*. Infection occurs through exposure to infected blood and blood products, solid organ transplantation before 1992, shared needles or other equipment used to inject drugs, and unprotected sex with multiple sexual partners who are infected. Mayo Clinic experts estimate that one third of the global population is infected, most undetected for decades as they are not clinically ill. In the United States, approximately 2% of the population is infected (Krebbeks & Cunningham, 2013). The federal government has recommended screening for HCV in persons born between 1945 and 1965. HCV is the most common cause of liver transplantation (Glund & Glund, 2009). Diagnosis is often made during routine medical testing. HCV can now be "successfully cured" with the recent treatment options of antiviral medications such as Harvoni (ledipasvir/sofosbuvir). To date, there is no vaccine available to provide immunity against HCV (CDC, 2017).

Hepatitis D, "delta hepatitis," is uncommon in the United States. It is caused by the hepatitis D virus (HDV) and only occurs in individuals also infected with the hepatitis B virus. HDV is an incomplete virus that needs HBV to replicate. It can be acute, short term, or long-term chronic. It is transmitted percutaneously or through mucosal contact with infected blood. The incubation period is 65 to 104 days. Treatment is supportive and currently there is no vaccine to provide immunity (CDC, 2017).

Hepatitis E virus (HEV) infection is self-limiting and does not result in chronic illness. It is rare in the United States but common in many parts of the world such as Asia and Africa. Transmission is through ingestion of fecal matter, even microscopic amounts, usually associated with a contaminated water supply in countries with poor sanitation. Incubation period is 16 to 65 days. There is no vaccine. As with HAV, good hygiene and handwashing as well as avoiding any contact with the HEV virus is the best method of prevention (CDC, 2017).

Clinical Aspects

Viral hepatitis has two components: the active phase, which is seen in all five forms of the virus, and the chronic phase of the disease, seen only in hepatitis B, C, and D. The five viruses known to cause the various forms of viral hepatitis cause many of the same symptoms in the infected patient during the acute phase. Symptoms are dependent on the cause and severity of liver involvement. The most commonly reported signs and symptoms include complaints of anorexia, low-grade fever, significant abdominal pain, generalized fatigue and malaise, nausea and vomiting, jaundice (having a yellow hue to the mucous membranes and skin), dark-colored urine and clay-colored stools, and unexplained arthralgia or joint pain.

Many patients in the chronic phases of hepatitis B and C remain asymptomatic. It can take decades following exposure for the patient to become symptomatic.

ASSESSMENT

A focused health history will determine the patient's risk factors for hepatitis: age (more than 75% of patients with HCV were born between 1945 and 1965); medications, prescribed (sulfonamides, phenothiazides) and over-the-counter (acetaminophen); travel; alcohol use; exposure to toxins; sexual history; any known exposure (health care worker with needlestick); long-term dialysis; blood transfusion or solid organ transplant before 1992; use of clotting factor concentrates before 1987; use of injected illegal drugs; and HIV. Diagnostic studies, including complete blood count (CBC), urinalysis, and liver function studies (LFTs), will provide insight into the liver status. An acute viral hepatitis panel is used to help detect and/or diagnose acute liver infection and inflammation that is due to one of the three most common hepatitis viruses: HAV, HBV, or HCV (CDC, 2017).

- Hepatitis A antibody, immunoglobulin M (IgM)—These antibodies typically develop 2 to 3 weeks after first being infected and persist for about 2 to 6 months. Hepatitis A IgM antibodies develop early in the course of infection, so a positive hepatitis A IgM test is usually considered diagnostic for acute hepatitis A in a person with signs and symptoms.

- Hepatitis B core antibody, IgM—This is an antibody produced against the hepatitis B core antigen. It is the first antibody produced in response to a hepatitis B infection and, when detected, may indicate an acute infection. It may also be present in people with chronic hepatitis B when flares of disease activity occur.

- Hepatitis B surface antigen (HBsAg)—This is a protein present on the surface of the hepatitis B virus. It is the earliest indicator of an acute infection but may also be present in the blood of those chronically infected.

- Hepatitis C antibody—This test detects antibodies produced in response to an HCV infection. It cannot distinguish between an active or previous infection. If positive, it is typically followed up with other tests to determine whether the infection is a current one.

Additional studies may include the following:

- HAV antibody, total and HBV core antibody, total—These tests detect both IgM and immunoglobulin G (IgG) antibodies and may be used as part of the panel to determine whether someone has had a previous infection.

- HBV surface antibody—The test for this antibody may sometimes be included in a panel to help determine whether an infection has resolved or a person has developed the antibody after receiving the hepatitis B vaccine and achieved immunity for protection against HBV (National Library of Medicine, 2014).

NURSING INTERVENTIONS, MANAGEMENT, AND IMPLICATIONS

The goals of the nursing intervention and management during the acute phase are to decrease demand on the liver, minimize complications, and prevent transmission of the infecting virus by providing education about the disease process, treatment, and prognosis. Appropriate hand hygiene and personal protective equipment is used to prevent the transmission of all hepatitis viruses. Monitoring of the patient should include vital signs, pain assessment, cardiac status via EKG and telemetry, and urinary output. Auscultation of the heart and lungs will help provide an accurate assessment of the patient's current cardiopulmonary status.

During the chronic phase of viral hepatitis, nursing interventions will be no different than those for any other patient requiring medical care: vital signs, height, weight, and pain assessment are required.

OUTCOMES

The patient's vital signs will return to baseline, urinary output will be greater or equal to 30 mL/hr, indicating normalizing renal function, and all peripheral pulses will be palpable, indicating return of adequate circulatory perfusion. SaO$_2$ saturation on room air will return to greater than 90% or there will be reduction in the required supplemental oxygen required by the patient. The patient's mental status will return to baseline, indicating that cerebral perfusion has occurred. The patient and his or her family members will be able to answers questions regarding the prevention and transmission of viral hepatitis, during both the acute phase and the chronic phase.

Summary

Hepatitis can be caused by viral, bacterial, and noninfectious conditions that precipitate inflammation of the liver. Symptom severity is dependent on the amount of liver involvement. Today's challenge is to identify at-risk patients for vaccination, testing, and treatment utilizing current medical guidelines (Krebbeks & Cunningham, 2013). Vaccination is effective in preventing HAV and HBV. Advances in antiviral therapy can halt and even reverse the progression of liver disease and decrease mortality in patients infected with HBV and HCV (Zhou et al., 2016).

Centers for Disease Control and Prevention. (2017, May 16). Viral hepatitis. Retrieved from https://www.cdc.gov/hepatitis

Krebbeks, V., & Cunningham, V. (2013). A DNP nurse-managed hepatitis C clinic, improving quality of life for those in a rural area. *Online Journal of Rural Nursing, 13*(1). Retrieved from http://rnojournal.binghamton.edu/index.php/RNO/article/view/104

National Library of Medicine. (2014, November 20). Hepatitis viral panel. Retrieved from http://www.nlm.nih.gov/medlineplus

Zhou, K., Fitzpatrick, T., Walsh, N., Kim, J. Y., Chou, R., Lackey, M., . . . Tucker J. D. (2016). Interventions to optimize the care continuum for chronic viral hepatitis: A systematic review and meta-analysis. *Lancet, 16*(12), 1409–1422.

■ HYPERGLYCEMIA AND HYPOGLYCEMIA

Laura Stark Bai

Overview

Hyperglycemia and hypoglycemia are two terms that refer to abnormalities in blood sugar levels. Hyperglycemia occurs when blood sugar is higher than the normal range for a patient and hypoglycemia is when blood sugar is lower than the normal range. Both conditions are not diseases in themselves but are associated with a greater disease process that requires prompt medical attention. They are each associated with different symptoms and occur for different reasons. Most often, hyperglycemia and hypoglycemia are complications of diabetes mellitus, which affects approximately 9.3% of Americans.

Background

Hyperglycemia is a deviation of one's blood sugar level above the normal range. For healthy individuals, normal blood sugar is approximately 70 to 99 mg/dL when fasting. Postprandial blood sugar, which is taken 2 hours after a meal consumption, should be less than 140 mg/dL. Blood sugar that is tested and results in a number higher than this is indicative of hyperglycemia. Both adults and children can develop hyperglycemia. It is difficult to assess the incidence of hyperglycemia because of its wide range of causes. However, glucose levels can vary from 40% to 90% based on the testing threshold used to define hyperglycemia (Viana, Moraes, Fabbrin, Santos, & Gerchman, 2014). Hyperglycemia has multiple causes, including stress, medications (i.e., steroids), excess consumption of carbohydrates, inactivity, illness, infection, and surgery. Most often, it is caused by two serious, and potentially fatal, complications of diabetes mellitus (DM).

Diabetic ketoacidosis (DKA) is an acute condition that is associated with blood sugar levels of about 250 to 600 mg/dL, severe metabolic acidosis, hyperosmolality, and ketonemia. It most commonly affects patients with type 1 DM but is often seen in patients with type 2 DM. Mortality rates range from about 1% to 5%, based on the patient's age and comorbidities (Nyenwe & Kitabchi, 2016). Hyperglycemic hyperosmolar state (HHS) is similar to DKA with its presence of hyperglycemia and hyperosmolality. However, HHS is associated with blood glucose levels more than 600 mg/dL, severe dehydration without ketosis, and is most often seen in elderly patients with type 2 DM (Pasquel & Umpierrz, 2014). Although the incidence of HHS is not known, it accounts for fewer than 1% of hospitalizations for patients who have DM. The mortality rate is estimated to be 10% to 20% (Pasquel & Umpierrz, 2014).

Both DKA and HHS are most often precipitated by lack of/or inadequate levels of insulin in the blood or infectious processes. They can both also be attributed to other bodily stressors, such as myocardial infarction, stroke, or pancreatitis. Symptoms include polyuria, polydipsia, polyphagia, nausea, vomiting, weakness, abdominal pain, dehydration, confusion, and lethargy and/or coma. Treatment focuses on correction of hyperglycemia and electrolyte imbalances, as well as rehydration. In extreme circumstances, patients may require a critical level of care if intubation or hourly blood sugar checks are indicated. DKA is considered resolved when blood sugar is below 200 mg/dL plus two of the following three criteria: anion gap less than 12 mEq/L, serum bicarbonate more than 15 mEq/L, or venous pH more than 7.3 (Van Ness-Otunnu & Hack, 2013). HHS is resolved when serum osmolality returns to normal range and vital signs and mentation return to baseline (Van Ness-Otunnu & Hack, 2013).

Hypoglycemia occurs when an individual's blood sugar drops below the normal range to 69 mg/dL or less. Symptoms include diaphoresis, hunger, weakness, lightheadedness, shaking, anxiety, seizures, nausea, and vomiting. In some cases, patients may even experience stroke-like symptoms, such as blurry vision, confusion, or slurred speech. The most common causes of hypoglycemia are DM, particularly when patients decrease their food consumption, increase activity levels, or overdose on insulin administration. Other causes include overproduction of insulin after a meal, excess alcohol consumptions, anorexia, pregnancy, dumping syndrome, and medical conditions that affect the heart, liver, or kidneys. Treatment for hypoglycemia is based on the precipitating cause of the decrease in blood sugar levels. Typically, a 15-g dose of a carbohydrate, such as orange juice, increases blood sugar levels. Commercially prepared glucose products are also available and can be used for hypoglycemia. However, if a person is not alert enough to orally consume glucose, dextrose can be administered parenterally.

The key to prevention of hyperglycemia and hypoglycemia is proper health maintenance. Patients who are at risk for these conditions should be careful to maintain consistency in their diets and exercise routines. Avoiding carbohydrates and sugars in excessive quantities will help to avoid hyperglycemia. Frequent monitoring of blood sugar levels with adherence to a proper medication regimen as prescribed by a physician is also crucial.

Clinical Aspects

ASSESSMENT

When assessing patients with suspected hyperglycemia or hypoglycemia, assessment and maintenance of airway, breathing, and circulation are of vital importance, as coma and death are symptoms of both. Subsequently, a finger stick for blood sugar level is crucial to identify hyperglycemia or hypoglycemia quickly. Furthermore, serum electrolytes, serum osmolality, urinalysis, complete blood count, pH, arterial blood gas, and an electrocardiogram are needed to help identify the cause of the syndrome and guide nursing interventions and treatment. In addition, if the patient is conscious or if a third party is available, a thorough history of present illness, past medical history, surgical history, and a list of medications should be obtained to gather precipitating information that can inform a cause. Further assessment should evaluate the adequacy of circulation, activity level, elimination, knowledge deficits, pain, fluid and nutrition status, and respiratory status.

NURSING INTERVENTIONS, MANAGEMENT, AND IMPLICATIONS

When it comes to hypoglycemia and hypoglycemia, nurses play a very important role. Some patients may have a knowledge deficit that requires education by a nurse on how to properly manage blood sugar. Patients are also at risk for multiple issues secondary to hyperglycemia and hypoglycemia, such as infection, skin integrity, the risk for falls, the risk for altered sensory perception, fluid volume deficit, fluid and electrolyte imbalance, ineffective therapeutic regimen, and altered or imbalanced nutrition.

Although medical treatment is different, the nursing interventions for hyperglycemia and hypoglycemia are largely focused on health maintenance and self-monitoring. Nursing interventions include monitoring of blood sugar levels, diet management, and education, monitoring for signs and symptoms of hyperglycemia or hypoglycemia and electrolyte imbalance, and administration of blood glucose lowering or elevating agents as indicated.

Treatment for hyperglycemia focuses lowering blood sugar, correcting electrolyte imbalances, and rehydration. In critical cases, patients may require endotracheal intubation and strict nursing management to monitor glucose and electrolyte levels. Treatment for hypoglycemia is usually a 15-g dose of a carbohydrate, such as orange juice, to increase blood sugar levels. However, if a person is not alert enough to orally consume glucose, it can be administered intramuscularly or intravenously. Long-term management of both hyperglycemia and hypoglycemia involves proper medication administration, diet, and activity management, which should be discussed with a primary care physician and possibly a registered dietician. Hemoglobin A1c (HbA1c) should be monitored as well to track blood sugar trends over a 2- to 3-month period to determine compliance with/or effectiveness of treatment for people at risk for hyperglycemia.

OUTCOMES

With rapid recognition and treatment initiation, morbidity and mortality associated with hyperglycemia and hypoglycemia can be reduced. A thorough history and physical in conjunction with the appropriate assessment and laboratory testing must be completed to rule out all possible precipitating causes of hyperglycemia and hypoglycemia (Van Ness-Otunnu & Hack, 2013). By following the recommended guidelines for the management of each syndrome, a positive prognosis can be expected.

Summary

Hyperglycemia and hypoglycemia are two syndromes associated with deviation from normal blood sugar levels. Although multiple factors can cause each, they are both most often caused by the complications of DM.

Either condition can ultimately be fatal, however, with proper nursing and medical management, resolution is very achievable. Prevention is key through close management of medications, diet, and activity level.

Nyenwe, E. A., & Kitabchi, A. E. (2016). The evolution of diabetic ketoacidosis: An update of its etiology, pathogenesis, and management. *Metabolism: Clinical and Experimental, 65*(4), 507–521.

Pasquel, F. J., & Umpierrez, G. E. (2014). Hyperosmolar hyperglycemic state: A historic review of the clinical presentation, diagnosis, and treatment. *Diabetes Care, 37*(11), 3124–3131.

Van Ness-Otunnu, R., & Hack, J. B. (2013). Hyperglycemic crisis. *Journal of Emergency Medicine, 45*(5), 797–805.

Viana, M. V., Moraes, R. B., Fabbrin, A. R., Santos, M. F., & Gerchman, F. (2014). Assessment and treatment of hyperglycemia in critically ill patients. *Revista Brasileira de terapia Intensiva, 26*(1), 71–76.

■ HYPERTENSIVE CRISIS AND HYPERTENSION

Kathleen Bradbury-Golas

Overview

A hypertensive crisis is a sudden and severe rise in blood pressure (BP). There are two types of hypertensive crises—both require immediate medical attention (American Heart Association, 2016). Hypertensive urgency occurs when the BP reading is equal to or greater than 180/110 mmHg, and remains there for two or more readings within a 10-minute span without indication of end-organ damage. The hypertensive patient may be asymptomatic or exhibit symptoms of headache, shortness of breath, or epistaxis. A hypertensive emergency (previously referred to as *malignant hypertension*) occurs with a persistent systolic BP (SBP) reading of 180 mmHg or a diastolic BP (DBP) reading of 120 mmHg. Symptoms include altered level of consciousness, confusion, stupor, chest pain, and possible stroke symptoms. In general, hypertension, defined as a BP reading higher than 140/90 mmHg on two or more occasions, can be attributed to many causes such as pain, anxiety, tobacco smoking, obesity, illicit drug use, excessive alcohol or salt use, and age.

If the BP is not maintained at a normal reading (less than 140/90), whether it is slightly elevated over a long period or severely elevated for a short period of time, the sequelae can result in myocardial infarction, heart failure, cardiomyopathy, aortic dissection, intracranial infarction/hemorrhage, retinal hemorrhage/infarct, and renal damage/failure (Stafford, Will, & Brooks-Gumbert, 2012). Emergency nursing care for adults with hypertensive crises is focused on early recognition, prompt evaluation, and emergency pharmacotherapy initiation for BP reduction in order to avoid permanent end-organ damage.

Background

In 2009, the American Heart Association (2016) estimated that 77.9 million Americans older than 20 years had some degree of hypertension. According to the Centers for Disease Control and Prevention (CDC), hypertension affects approximately 32% of the American population, averaging one in every three American adults (CDC, 2015). Having hypertension costs the United States more than $48 billion yearly and increases the risk of heart disease and stroke, the leading causes of death in the United States (CDC, 2015). Hypertension is more prevalent in adults older than 55 years (gender equal at this age), African Americans, those individuals who are overweight or obese due to lack of physical activity and high sodium intake, and those who have the genetic predisposition for the disease (National Institutes of Health, 2015). Because only 50% of patients known to have hypertension maintain adequate control of their BP, the resulting end-organ damage can occur markedly with time.

Most patients who suffer from hypertensive crises are known hypertensive patients, with poor or inadequate control (Marik, 2015). However, hypertensive crises can also occur from preeclampsia/eclampsia, pheochromocytoma (adrenal tumor), primary aldosteronism, hyperthyroidism, Cushing syndrome (excess glucocorticoid), or central nervous system disorders (head trauma or brain tumors).

Hypertension and prehypertension in children and adolescents have been increasing due to the strong association of high BP and increased weight and obesity within this population. The National Institutes of Health guidelines (2005) continue to define hypertension in children and adolescents as SBP and/or DBP, that is, on repeated measurement, at or above the 95th percentile. BP between the 90th and 95th percentile in childhood has been designated "high normal." However, secondary hypertension (disorders such as pheochromocytoma, Turner syndrome, coarctation of the aorta, or diabetes) is more common in children than in adults (National Institutes of Health, 2005; Rodriquez-Cruz & Pantnana, 2015). Therefore, all pediatric/adolescent

patients with elevated BPs should be assessed for an underlying disorder causing the hypertension.

Clinical Aspects

ASSESSMENT

Completing an accurate history and assessment is a critical component of nursing care. Obtaining a full history of other comorbid conditions, such as hyperlipidemia, diabetes mellitus, coronary artery disease, renal disease, and sleep apnea is crucial when assessing a patient with a hypertensive crisis. In addition, current medications and obtaining recall of previous BP readings will assist in determining medication compliance.

All patients should be questioned regarding their use of over-the-counter medications and other drugs, including cocaine, methamphetamines, phencyclidine, and alcohol. In addition, patients who take monoamine oxidase inhibitors (MAOIs) are at increased risk for serious medication interactions, as combined use of MAOIs and other antidepressants can lead to a hypertensive reaction (Stafford et al., 2012). Prolonged use of nonsteroidal anti-inflammatories, decongestants, oral contraceptives, and various herbal products (i.e., bitter orange and ephedra) can also lead to a hypertensive crisis.

The physical assessment should focus on changes in the following body systems: cardiac (BP in both arms, heart rate, abnormal heart sounds [S3, S4, gallop], and volume status), vascular (carotid, aortic or renal bruits, edema), respiratory (adventitious breath sounds [crackles], oxygen saturation), and neurological (focal changes as commonly seen in cerebral vascular accidents, seizures; Batchelor, Gillman, Goodin, & Schwytzer, 2015). The nurse will need to be knowledgeable of various diagnostic indicators to assist in determining the degree of organ damage that has occurred. These include 12-lead electrocardiogram (myocardial infarction, ischemic changes, ventricular hypertrophy); urinalysis for blood, protein, glucose, and microalbumin; renal function tests (blood urea nitrogen and creatinine); and radiographs (chest x-ray for left ventricular/cardiac enlargement; Emergency Nurses Association, 2013). CT scans and echocardiography may also be indicated depending on presenting symptomatology.

NURSING INTERVENTIONS, MANAGEMENT, AND IMPLICATIONS

Distinguishing between the two hypertensive crises is essential to ensuring that proper treatment is initiated.

During triage, it is essential for the nurse to differentiate hypertensive emergency from urgency to allow for quick initiation of treatment. Patients presenting with a hypertensive emergency should immediately receive a rapid-acting, titratable intravenous antihypertensive agent within a critical/emergency care area for BP reduction (Marik, 2015). During this time, the BP should be monitored continuously, which may require the insertion and use of an arterial line. Urine output is also monitored hourly to ensure adequate renal perfusion. The patient is assessed as per protocol and by physiologic response to determine response to therapy and extent of end-organ damage (Emergency Nurses Association, 2013).

Patients with hypertensive urgency, without other serious symptoms, should have their BP reduced slowly with an oral antihypertensive agent within a 24- to 48-hour period. Rapid-onset oral antihypertensive agents, such as clonidine, labetalol, or captopril, are often used for gradual, short-term reduction of BP while being observed in either an observational unit or emergency department, though treatment rarely requires hospitalization. Once stabilized, the patient will be changed to a long-term antihypertensive agent, stabilized, and then monitored in the outpatient primary care setting.

OUTCOMES

The initial goal of therapy for a hypertensive emergency is to reduce the mean arterial pressure by 25% over the first 24 to 48 hours. In contrast, there is no evidence to suggest a benefit from rapidly reducing the BP in patients with hypertensive urgency. Actually, too rapid a reduction in this state could yield organ damage from hypoperfusion.

Classifications of medications often used for rapid reduction of BP include nitrates (i.e., nitroprusside and nitroglycerin), beta-adrenergic blockers (i.e., labetolol and atenolol), calcium channel blockers (i.e., nicardipine, dilitazem, verapamil), and angiotensin-converting enzyme inhibitors (i.e., enalapril; Bisognano, 2015). Hydrazine is the preferred agent for pregnant patients. The nurse should have a thorough knowledge of the action, administration techniques, side effects, and adverse reaction for all medications that he or she administers. Associated end-organ effects may require specific treatment for specific disorders.

Long-term prognosis and outcomes depend upon patient compliance with medications and the extent of secondary end-organ damage. Once the patient's BP is reduced to a therapeutic level, the nurse should provide education on lifestyle modifications, medication adherence, and health care compliance.

Summary

Hypertension remains the "silent" killer of vascular disease here in the United States. In the essential form, hypertension has no symptoms, yet it continues to damage multiple organ sites throughout the body when not treated. Hypertensive crisis results for many different reasons, which include but are not limited to poor BP control, noncompliance with antihypertensive medications, and secondary physiologic disorders. Early recognition, differentiation in triage, and subsequent nursing care and pharmacotherapy are essential elements in reducing the short- and long-term complications that can occur in hypertensive crisis.

American Heart Association (2016). Hypertensive crisis: When you should call 9-1-1 for high blood pressure. Retrieved from https://www.heart.org/HEARTORG/Conditions/HighBloodPressure/AboutHighBloodPressure/Hypertensive-Crisis_UCM_301782_Article.jsp#.WDMfh03fN1s

Batchelor, N., Gillman, P., Goodin, J., & Schwytzer, D. (2015). *Medical surgical nursing* (4th ed.). Silver Spring, MD: American Nurses Association.

Bisognano, J. (2015). Malignant hypertension. *Medscape.* Retrieved from http://emedicine.medscape.com/article/241640-overview#a5

Centers for Disease Control and Prevention. (2015). High blood pressure facts. Retrieved from http://www.cdc.gov/bloodpressure/facts.htm

Emergency Nurses Association. (2013). *Sheehy's manual of emergency care* (7th ed.). St. Louis, MO: Mosby

Marik, P. (2015). *Hypertensive crises, Part III. Evidence-based critical care* (pp. 429–443). Cham, Switzerland: Springer International Publishing. doi:10.1007/978-3-319-11020-2_28

National Institutes of Health. (2005). Diagnosis, evaluation, and treatment of high blood pressure in children and adolescents. Retrieved from https://www.nhlbi.nih.gov/files/docs/resources/heart/hbp_ped.pdf

National Institutes of Health. (2015). Exploring high blood pressure. Retrieved from http://www.nhlbi.nih.gov/health/health-topics/topics/hbp/atrisk

Rodriquez-Cruz, E., & Pantnana, S. (2015). Pediatric hypertension. Retrieved from http://emedicine.medscape.com/article/889877-overview

Stafford, E., Will, K., & Brooks-Gumbert, A. (2012). Management of hypertensive urgency and emergency. *Clinician Reviews, 22*(10), 20. Retrieved from http://www.mdedge.com/clinicianreviews/article/79156/nephrology/management-hypertensive-urgency-and-emergency

■ HYPOTHERMIA

Marian Nowak

Overview

Hypothermia is defined as a core body temperature of 95°F (35°C). Hypothermia occurs when the heat loss to the environment cannot be compensated by the heat produced by the body (*Free Medical Dictionary*, 2016). It is a potentially life-threatening condition. Exposure to extreme cold is a leading cause of preventable weather-related mortality. Variables that increase the risk for hypothermia-related death include advanced age, mental illness, male gender, and drug intoxication.

Nursing care for adults with hypothermia is focused on the early recognition of the deleterious effects of the exposure to low temperatures and the gradual rewarming to mitigate the body's defense of peripheral vasoconstriction. Accurate nursing assessment and response can optimize the effectiveness of an individual's ability to recover from this potential life-threatening condition (Lewis, Dirksen, Heitkemper, & Bucher, 2014).

Background

Extreme cold weather resulting in hypothermia is associated with excess morbidity and mortality. Moreover, it may result in death because it can exacerbate preexisting chronic conditions (including cardiovascular and respiratory diseases). A total of 13,419 deaths occurred from hypothermia during the period of 2003 to 2014; an unadjusted annual rate ranged from 0.3 to 0.5 per 100,000 persons. Data concerning hypothermia-related deaths for the United States overall were obtained from the Centers for Disease Control and Prevention's (CDC's) multiple cause-of-death files and "hypothermia" defined as any death with an underlying or contributing cause of death from exposure to excessive natural cold. Males accounted for 9,050 (67%) decedents (CDC, 2015). Mortality rates were highest among persons of advanced age. Several studies suggest that alcohol usage or drug poisoning contributes to a 10% increase in the cause of death in hypothermic patients. During 2006 to 2010, 10,649 deaths of U.S. residents were attributed to weather-related causes. This includes exposure to excessive natural heat, heat stroke, and sun stroke, which contributed to 3,332 (31%) of these deaths, and exposure to extreme environmental temperatures, a significant reduction in a person's core body temperature, or both was cited for 6,660 (63%) of deaths (Berko, Deborah, Saha, & Ingram, 2014).

Among deaths attributed to natural cold during 2006 to 2010, the death rate for infants was 1 death per million, which was higher than the rate for children aged 5 to 14 years but lower than the rate for persons aged 25 and over. Cold-related death rates were lowest for children aged 5 to 14 years of age (0.2 deaths per million) and increased progressively with age, as was the case for heat-related mortality, with rates increasing from 1.3 to 7.8 deaths per million among persons aged 15 to 74. The cold-related death rates for persons aged 75 and over are substantially higher than the rates for younger persons: 15.5 deaths per million among persons aged 75 to 84 and 39.6 deaths per million among persons aged 85 and older (Berko et al., 2014).

Persons with conditions that impair thermoregulatory function and those taking various medications are more susceptible to the effects of cold. Subpopulations at risk for cold-related mortality include older adults, infants, males, Black persons, and persons with preexisting chronic medical conditions. Alcoholics, persons using recreational drugs, homeless persons, and those with inadequate winter clothing or home heating are at increased risk of cold-related mortality. Other persons at risk include those who live in places with rapid temperature changes, large shifts in nighttime temperatures, or are at high elevations (Berko et al., 2014). Most body heat is lost in the form of radiant heat. *Radiant heat* refers to the heat given off by the body in the form of waves through the air (Lewis et al., 2014).

The greatest loss is from the head, lungs, and thorax. Severe environmental conditions, such as freezing temperatures, prolonged exposure to cold weather, cold winds, inadequate clothing, and exhaustion, predispose clients to hypothermia. Wet clothing increases evaporation heat loss up to five times and emersion in cold water increases evaporation up to 25 times (Iowa Great Lakes Water Safety Council, 2016).

Peripheral vasoconstriction is the body's first defense mechanism to attempt to compensate for heat loss. As cold temperature persists, shivering occurs in an attempt to produce heat. To prevent body cooling and hypothermia of seriously ill or injured casualties during transportation, casualty coverings must provide adequate thermal insulation against cold, wind, and moisture. Studies indicate that variables that affect the development of hypothermia include the time of exposure as determined by temperature and wind speed (Jussila, Rissanen, Parkkola, & Anttonen, 2014).

Clinical Aspects

ASSESSMENT

Assessment findings vary with the severity of the condition. Hypothermia may mimic cerebral or metabolic disturbances. Presenting symptoms may include ataxia, confusion, and withdrawal (Lewis et al., 2014)

Patients With Mild Hypothermia

Assessment findings also vary with the severity of the condition. Patients with mild hypothermia (93.2°F–96.8°F) often display shivering, lethargy, confusion, irrational behavior, and minor heart rate changes. Moderate hypothermia (86°F–93.2°F) patients exhibit rigidity, bradycardia, decreased respirations, respiratory acidosis, and hypovolemia. The blood pressure in patients with mild hypothermia is typically obtained by Doppler. In addition to decreases in peripheral arterial blood pressure, decreased renal flow leads to impaired water absorption and results in dehydration. Consequently, hematocrit increases and intravascular volume decreases. Due to increased viscosity of the blood, patients become prone to risk for myocardial infarction, stroke, pulmonary embolism, and renal failure (Samaras, Chevalley, Samaras, 2010).

Severe hypothermia, at or below 86°F, is potentially life-threatening. Symptoms include pale, cyanotic skin, fixed and dilated pupils, bradycardia, slow respiratory rate, ventricular fibrillation, or asystole. Warming is the treatment for all stages (Samaras et al., 2010).

NURSING INTERVENTIONS, MANAGEMENT, AND IMPLICATIONS

Nursing care of adults with hypothermia should initially focus on removing the patient from the cause (e.g., remove wet clothing if resent), maintaining arterial blood gases (ABGs), correcting dehydration, treating dysrhythmias, and rewarming the patient. High-flow oxygen should be provided via nonrebreather mask.

Passive or spontaneous rewarming methods include moving the patient to a warm dry place, removing wet clothing, using radiant lights, and placing warm blankets on the patient. Active surface rewarming method includes fluid or warm air-filled warming blankets or warm water emersion (98.6°F–104°F). Monitor the patient for vasodilation, which results in hypotension during the rewarming process. In severe hypothermia, alternative methods include applying heat directly to the core by using warm IV fluids (98.6°F), humidified oxygen (111.2°F), and peritoneal lavage with warm fluids (up to 113°F) while closely monitoring the patient for arrhythmias. Warming of the central trunk first to limit rewarming shock using extracorporeal circulation with rapid infuser or hemodialysis may also be done (Hoskin, Melinyshyn, Romet, & Goode, 1986; Kumar et al., 2015).

OUTCOMES

The expected outcomes of evidence-based nursing care are centered on preventing the progression of hypothermic complications and progression. The hospital use of minimally invasive rewarming for nonarrested, otherwise healthy, patients with primary hypothermia and stable vital signs has the potential to decrease morbidity and mortality. Ongoing monitoring is needed for ABG's temperature, level of consciousness, vital signs, oxygen saturation, heart rate and rhythm, electrolytes, and glucose. Active surveillance for changes in physical assessment is key in prevention progression of injury (Paal et al., 2015). Patients with moderate to severe hypothermia should have the core rewarmed before the extremities. As rewarming takes place, patients are at risk for after a further drop in core temperature. Monitoring of vital signs and gentle progression of rewarming are imperative. Gentle rewarming will avoid rewarming shock that can produce hypotension and dysrhythmias (Paal et al., 2015).

Summary

Exposure to cold is a leading cause of weather-related mortality and is responsible for approximately twice the number of deaths annually as due to exposure to heat in the United States (CDC, 2015). Prompt recognition of the signs and symptoms of hypothermia is necessary for reducing mortality. Recognition of hypothermia and intervention of symptoms include the application of evidence-based nursing rewarming guidelines. Following rewarming therapy guidelines and observing for potential systemic complications can assist the practitioner in avoiding complications.

Patients should be rewarmed by using external warming (e.g., blankets or forced heated air) for mild hypothermia and internal warming methods (e.g., body cavity lavage) for severe hypothermia. In the event of cardiac arrest, cardiopulmonary resuscitation should be performed during rewarming in accordance with published standard guidelines.

Berko J., Ingram, D., Saha, S., & Parker, J. D. (2014). Deaths attributed to heat, cold, and other weather events in the United States, 2006–2010. *National Health Statistics Report*, 76, 1–15.

Centers for Disease Control and Prevention. (2015). Hypothermia-related deaths, 2003–2013. *MMWR Weekly*, 64(6), 141–143.

Hoskin, R. W., Melinyshyn, M. J., Romet, T. T., & Goode, R. C. (1986). Bath rewarming from immersion hypothermia. *Journal of Applied Physiology*, 61, 1518–1522.

Iowa Great Lakes Water Safety Council. (2016). Cold water immersion. Retrieved from http://www.watersafety council.org/coldwaterimmersion/index.html

Jussila K., Rissanen S., Parkkola K., & Anttonen H. (2014). Evaluating cold, wind, and moisture protection of different coverings for prehospital maritime transportation—A thermal manikin and human study. *Prehospital and Disaster Medicine*, 29(6), 1–9.

Kumar, P., McDonald, G. K., Chitkara, R., Steinman, A. M., Gardiner, P. F., and Giesbrecht, G. G. (2015). Comparison of distal limb warming with fluid therapy and warm water immersion for mild hypothermia rewarming. *Wilderness and Environmental Medicine*, 26, 406–411. doi:10.1016/j.wem.2015.02.005

Lewis, S., Dirksen, S, Heitkemper, M., & Bucher, L. (2014). *Medical surgical nursing* (9th ed.). St. Louis, MO: Elsevier Mosby.

Paal, P., Gordon, L., Strapazzon, G., Brodmann Maeder, M., Putzer, G., Walpoth, B., . . . Brugger H. (2015). Accidental hypothermia—An update. The content of this review is endorsed by the International Commission for Mountain Emergency Medicine (ICAR MEDCOM). *Scandinavian Journal of Trauma, Resuscitation and Emergency Medicine*, 24(1), 111. doi:10.1186/s13049-016-0303-7

Radiant. (2016). In *The Free medical dictionary*. Retrieved from http://medical-dictionary.thefreedictionary.com/radiant+heat

Samaras, N., Chevalley, T., & Samaras, D. (2010). Older patients in the emergency department: A review. *Annals of Emergency Medicine*, 56, 261.

■ INTEGUMENTARY EMERGENCIES

Susanna Rudy

Overview

Serious, life-threatening skin disorders are rare. Presentation to the emergency department (ED) with a dermatological complaint can be frustrating for both patient and provider, particularly if there is no clear cause for the annoyance of symptoms such as rash and itching. Although most rashes are benign and self-limiting, there are serious dermatological emergencies that pose a lethal threat to health and mortality if they are not immediately differentiated or diagnosed on presentation. A delay in the identification, specialty consultation, and supportive intensive care treatment can result in a permanently debilitating or fatal outcome for the patient. A systematic approach to identification and management of some of the most common and acutely deadly rashes are reviewed.

Background

On an average, the prevalence of dermatological complaints requiring medical treatment ranges between 19% and 27%, with the majority of these cutaneous conditions being benign (Baibergenova & Shear, 2011). The epidemiology of outpatient presentation accounts for approximately 5% to 8% of these conditions. Only 3.3% present urgently to the ED and of that 94 % are discharged home after evaluation and treatment. Approximately 4% require hospital admission. Skin infections, in the form of cellulitis, account for approximately 33% of the admissions (R. A. Schwartz, McDonough, & Lee, 2013).

Of all of the types of skin rashes, there are approximately 10 that present as a predictor for potential life-threatening sequelae of pain, prolonged illness, multisystem organ failure, and, in some cases, death. The following all present with characteristic symptoms and rash that require expedient diagnoses and management: erythema multiforme major (EM), Stevens–Johnson Syndrome (SJS), toxic epidermal necrolysis (TEN), drug hypersensitivity syndrome (DHS) otherwise known as *drug rash with eosinophilia and systemic symptoms* (DRESS) syndrome, staphylococcal scalded skin syndrome (SSSS), staphylococcal/streptococcal toxic shock syndrome (TSS), *Neisseria meningitis* (meningococcemia), necrotizing fasciitis, pemphigus vulgaris (PV), vibrio, and Rocky Mountain spotted fever (RMSF). For purposes of discussion, the blistering cutaneous disorders of SJS, TENS, SJS/TENS, and DRESS are reviewed in brief.

SJS, TEN, and an overlap of SJS/TEN are severe mucocutaneous diseases thought to be extensive examples of erythema multiform (EM). They are rare and involve the loss of the epidermal layers of the skin resulting in fluid losses, potential for shock, respiratory failure, sepsis, gastrointestinal (GI) hemorrhage, and multiorgan system failure (Papadakis & McPhee, 2017; Stone & Humphries, 2011). The overall combined incidence in the worldwide population of all three is approximately two to seven per million/annually and a 1,000-fold increase in patients with HIV (R. A. Schwartz et al., 2013). TEN, SJS, and SJS/TEN are often listed together as they are all variants of the same histopathologic disease continuum differing only by severity and body surface affected. All variants are thought to be caused by an immune-mediated hypersensitivity response from specific drugs; reactions occur in 80% to 95% of cases (Pereira et al., 2007). Reactions can be delayed toward an initial exposure or rapid reexposure. This disease occurs in all age groups.

Research supports a genetic predisposition of certain individuals to hypersensitivity reactions to certain metabolite complexes formed with the breakdown of certain medications. Specific implication applies to certain antibiotics classes and drugs such as sulfa, nonsteroidal anti-inflammatory drugs (NSAIDs), anticonvulsants, and antigout medications. Other triggers of cutaneous disorders can be exposure to bacterial and viral infections, malignancy, certain vaccinations, contrast medium, and graft versus host disease (R. B. Schwartz, Sattin, & Hunt, 2013). When exposed to the triggers, certain individuals develop an immune-mediated cytotoxic reaction that results in apoptosis (cell death) of the keratinocytes in the epidermis and tissue necrosis. The diseases are hallmarked by skin peeling, separating the epidermal layer of the skin from the dermis. They are all systemic diseases that involve the integumentary, pulmonary, ophthalmic, and genitourinary systems; internal involvement results from the massive release of proinflammatory cytokines that result in epithelial sloughing (Papadakis & McPhee, 2017).

The spectral diseases are separated only by a percentage of body surface area and epidermal detachment that occurs. Features of TEN occur with or without purpura (spots). TEN with spots includes widespread purpuric macules and progression of flaccid blistering bullae, skin erosions, and painful epidermal denudation of the skin or sloughing involving the epithelium layers of the eyes, lungs, GI tract, and genitals (Papadakis & McPhee, 2017). Skin can easily be separated with gentle lateral pressure known as *Nikolsky's sign*. The course progression can occur over a period of 1 day to 3 weeks after exposure to the trigger. Total body surface area affected in TEN is more than 30% and can be as life-threatening as a severe burn (Pereira et al., 2007). The rash is central and can involve at least two mucosal sites. The active phase of blistering and skin loss occurs in 2 weeks (R. A. Schwartz et al., 2013). The cutaneous sequelae are prominent with the most

concerning involving ocular complications that can result in blindness (R. B. Schwartz et al., 2013). Patients with TEN with spots are very ill with acute skin failure and mortality rate is between 10% and 70%; primary causes of death result from septicemia and multisystem organ failure (Cohen, 2016).

SJS shares most of the same features and morphology as TEN but is differentiated from TEN in that it has less than 10% body surface area (BSA) involvement. The overlap of SJS/TEN has an affected BSA of 10% to 30% (Cohen, 2016; R. A. Schwartz et al., 2013).

DRESS syndrome is also in the same class of drug eruption (DE) life-threatening cutaneous diseases as TEN and SJS; the pathogenesis is consistent among them (Camous, Calbo, Picard, & Musette, 2012). Difficult to diagnose because of the similarities to other cutaneous diseases, as well as a delay in symptomology, DRESS is predominantly a drug-induced hypersensitivity reaction caused by the same trigger medications seen with the other spectral diseases mentioned with antiepileptic's and allopurinol being the most common. There is a strong genetic link associated with how certain populations metabolize the trigger medications that form complexes that trigger antibody formation (Camous et al., 2012). DRESS is caused by a T cell mediated response to the foreign complexes lending to the overwhelming proinflammatory response. Reactivation of the herpes virus in combination with exposure to suspected trigger drugs is specific to DRESS (Camous et al., 2012). Symptoms of DRESS appear in 2 to 6 weeks after exposure to the medications. The syndrome is characterized by a viral prodrome, high fevers, lymphadenopathy, organ involvement, hematologic abnormalities, hallmarked facial edema, skin eruptions of a morbilliform rash of more than 50% BSA. Resolution is gradual with the removal of the offending agent; typically, 6 to 9 weeks with the possibility of persistence for months with intermittent periods of remission and exacerbation (Camous et al., 2012; Papadakis & McPhee, 2017).

Clinical Aspects

ASSESSMENT

A good patient history and timely physical assessment are important to prompt treatment and management of the spectrum of life-threatening cutaneous disorders. A previous history of exposure to one of the trigger medications, a previous history or genetic predisposition to these diseases, the physical symptoms, the appearance of the affected skin, percentage involved, and time of onset can all help differentiate a diagnosis. A skin biopsy for histology and frozen section are a definitive diagnostic tools used to confirm a diagnosis.

NURSING INTERVENTIONS, MANAGEMENT, AND IMPLICATIONS

Patients with cutaneous-related problems require aggressive medical management and close monitoring. Nursing need to manage patient pain issues, fluid loss, monitoring of hemodynamics, and accurate intake and output. Patients in the early phases of blister formation affecting the mucosal areas have difficulty with eating, swallowing, and may be at risk for dehydration and poor nutrition, decreased protein intake that leads to poor wound healing. Patients also have pain and require adequate pain management. Attention to pain scores and follow-up assessments are of primary importance. Owing to the potential for skin loss, exposed skin need to be managed with dressing changes and creams; overall acuity of patients with these cutaneous diseases is higher and require more nursing time. Deterioration in respiratory, GI, and hemodynamics should be anticipated and monitored closely. Close monitoring of patient's neurological status, hemodynamics, intake and output, nutritional intake, and pain should be ongoing. Early consultation with nutrition and ophthalmology for baseline assessment should be a priority (Papadakis & McPhee, 2017; R. A. Schwartz et al., 2013).

Primary management of these dermatological emergencies involves removal of the trigger drug if the patient is still on it. It will also be noted in the patient's chart. Aggressive management includes fluid resuscitation, nutritional supplementation, and extensive wound management (Papadakis & McPhee, 2017; Stone & Humphries, 2011). Specialty care in intensive care or the burn unit is necessary to manage large cutaneous injuries, the large amounts of fluid loss, and the anticipated worsening progression of the diseases to involve the eyes, lungs, GI, and skin. The expediency of an offending drug removal and admission to intensive care improve overall prognosis. Ocular sequelae associated with these conditions can lead to blindness. Eyes should be managed with eye drops and ointments to prevent the abrasions and dry eye associated with these skin conditions. Opthalmology consult is mandatory (Papadakis & Humphries, 2017; Pereira et al., 2007; Stone & Humphries, 2011).

Pan culturing is appropriate on admission, but the administration of empiric antibiotics should be avoided because of an increased risk of resistance and no evidence of improved outcomes to support the use of empiric broad spectrum antibiotics (Pereira et al., 2007). Skin debridement may be necessary for TEN patients, and large denuded areas should be covered with allograft skin. Consideration of adjuvant treatments with intravenous immunoglobulin (IVIG), cyclosporine, plasmapheresis, tumor necrosis factor (TNF)-alpha inhibitors is a matter of clinical judgment. There is promising evidence to support the benefit of high-dosed, pulsed steroid dosing arresting disease in a shorter interval of time than without (Pereira et al., 2007). The patient should be educated on the triggers and causative mechanisms, and how to avoid them and similar classes of medications. Human leukocyte antigen (HLA) tissue typing can determine predisposition to developing life-threatening cutaneous disorders in certain patient populations and should be considered before starting therapy.

OUTCOMES

Identification and management of integumentary emergencies can be very challenging but is imperative to promote positive patient outcomes. Differentiating TEN, SJS, SSSS, and other potentially life-threatening disorders must be identified and managed appropriately. Utilizing the assessment skills and interventions discussed in this entry will assist the nurse to successfully promote positive outcomes.

Summary

Using a systematic approach to evaluating, identifying, and differentiating a presenting dermatological complaint can improve the outcome of life-threatening cutaneous rashes if identified early. The pathogenesis of apoptosis in these cutaneous diseases is rapid in onset and, once triggered, is irreversible. Timing is critical. Discontinuation of the offending medication and aggressive resuscitative management in a burn unit are essential and the overall primary predictors of overall prognosis or mortality.

Baibergenova, A., & Shear, N. H. (2011). Skin conditions that bring patients to emergency departments. *Archives of Dermatology, 147*(1), 118–120.

Camous, X., Calbo, S., Picard, D., & Musette, P. (2012). Drug reaction with eosinophilia and systemic symptoms: An update on pathogenesis. *Current Opinion in Immunology, 24*(6), 730–735.

Cohen, V. (2016). Toxic epidermal necrolysis. *Medscape.* Retrieved from http://emedicine.medscape.com/article/229698-overview

Papadakis, M. A., & McPhee, S. J. (2017). *Current medical diagnosis & treatment* (56th ed.). New York, NY: McGraw-Hill.

Pereira, F. A., Mudgil, A. V., & Rosmarin, D. M. (2007). Toxic epidermal necrolysis. *Journal of the American Academy of Dermatology, 56*(2), 181–200.

Schwartz, R. A., McDonough, P., & Lee, B. W. (2013). Toxic epidermal necrolysis. Part 1. Introduction, history, classification, clinical features, systemic manifestations, etiology, and immunopathogenesis. *Journal of American Academy of Dermatology, 69*(4), 173.e1–173.e13. doi:10.1016/j.jaad.2013.05.003

Schwartz, R. B., Sattin, R. W., & Hunt, R. C. (2013). Medical response to bombings: The application of lessons learned to a tragedy. *Disaster Medicine and Public Health Preparedness, 7*(2), 114–115.

Stone, K., & Humphries, R. (2011). *Current diagnosis & treatment: Emergency medicine* (7th ed.). New York, NY: McGraw-Hill.

■ INTRA-AORTIC BALLOON PUMP

Grant Pignatiello

Overview

With more than 70,000 annual insertions, the intra-aortic balloon pump (IABP) is the most commonly used circulatory assistive device (Parissis et al., 2016; Parissis, Soo, & Al-Alao, 2011). Positioned in the ascending aorta, the IABP uses pulsations coordinated with the patient's innate cardiac cycle to assist patients with left ventricular dysfunction by augmenting diastolic pressure, reducing systemic vascular resistance (SVR), and enhancing coronary and cerebral perfusion. Although empirical data support the benefit provided through use of the IABP, its use is not free of risk; therefore, nurses caring for patients receiving circulatory support from an IABP must possess a thorough breadth of knowledge related to cardiovascular physiology and hemodynamics, IABP functional mechanisms, and factors concerned with maintenance of patient safety and therapeutic discontinuation (Lewis, Ward, & Courtney, 2009).

Background

The first successful application of an IABP was reported in 1967 within a 45-year-old female suffering from severe cardiogenic shock after an acute myocardial infarction; subsequent testing and evaluation through the latter portion of the 20th century and mechanical/engineering developments through the early 21st century have refined the IABP as a reliable therapeutic modality for circulatory support (Parissis et al., 2016). The IABP is most commonly inserted through the femoral artery; however, it can also be inserted through the subclavian artery (Parissis et al., 2016; Raman, Loor, London, & Jolly, 2010). Ideally, the balloon, which contains a volume of 40 mL and a length ranging from 22 to 27.5 cm, should be placed such that the tip is just distal to the left subclavian branch of the aortic arch and the proximal end superior to the renal arteries.

The functionality of the IABP is contingent upon its coordination with the cardiac cycle; following counterpulsation principles, the balloon is inflated during diastole (the T-P interval of an electrocardiogram tracing) with helium gas and deflated during systole (QRS-T interval of an electrocardiogram tracing). This possesses numerous consequences for the systolic and diastolic phases of the cardiac cycle. Systolic consequences associated with IABP counterpulsation include (a) a decrease in systolic and end-diastolic blood pressure from systolic unloading by the IABP and subsequent afterload reduction and (b) decrease in left ventricular wall tension, and increased left ventricular ejection fraction and cardiac output due to afterload reduction. Diastolic consequences related to IABP counterpulsation include (a) decreased left ventricular diastolic volume secondary to enhanced ventricular unloading, (b) enhanced coronary artery perfusion due to retrograde displacement of blood pushed back through the aortic arch during diastole, (c) enhanced myocardial oxygen supply related to an increase in diastolic pressure time index and a decrease in tension time index, and (d) increased peripheral blood flow related to the increased arterial pressure from the balloon inflation resulting in an increased arterial–venous gradient (Parissis et al., 2016).

Because of the IABP's ability to reduce systemic afterload, enhance coronary perfusion, and augment diastolic pressure, it is an ideal supportive modality for clinical situations in which the patient's volume status is optimized and the patient is experiencing acute ventricular failure refractory to maximum inotropic support. Parissis et al. (2016) identify several objective clinical parameters that would indicate IABP use in the setting of acute ventricular failure: (a) cardiac index less than 1.8 L/min, (b) systolic arterial pressure less than 90 mmHg, (c) left or right atrial pressure greater than 20 mmHg, (d) urine output less than 20 mL/hr, (e)

SVR greater than 2,100 dynes, and (f) metabolic acidosis. Moreover, IABPs are used after 5% to 10% of cardiac surgeries for patients who are unable to wean from cardiopulmonary bypass and may also be indicated for myoconservation during periods of unstable angina, following acute myocardial infarctions with or without tachyarrhythmia, acute ischemic mitral incompetence, ischemic rupture of the ventricular septum, severe cardiogenic shock, and during percutaneous coronary intervention (Parissis et al., 2011, 2016).

Use of IABP is associated with decreased risk of mortality; a meta-analysis conducted by Fan et al. (2016) of 33 clinical trials containing 18,889 patients found that patients who received IABP therapy who were suffering from acute myocardial infarction were more likely to be alive 6 months later when compared to those who did not receive an IABP (odds ratio [OR]: 0.66, 95% confidence interval [CI]: 0.48–0.91, p = .010). Nevertheless, despite the IABP's effectiveness in improving patient outcomes, Krishna and Zacharowski (2009) identify several absolute and relative contraindications. Absolute contraindications to IABP placement include aortic regurgitation, aortic dissection, end-stage heart disease with no anticipated recovery, and aortic stents; whereas, the relative contraindications include uncontrolled sepsis, abdominal aortic aneurysm, tachyarrhythmia, severe peripheral vascular disease, and arterial reconstruction surgery. Moreover, use of IABP is associated with risks that must be considered for those providing nursing care to the patient.

Clinical Aspects

ASSESSMENT

Nursing care of the patient receiving IABP therapy requires skilled physical assessment and a thorough understanding of human physiology to evaluate the patient's clinical progression and for signs and symptoms of complications (Lewis et al., 2009). To maintain a global perspective on the patient's physiological status, intricate patient monitoring is necessary. Commonly, patients possess central venous catheters and intra-arterial catheters; patients may also have pulmonary artery catheters. Through this, clinicians can receive relevant clinical information in addition to vital signs on demand, such as arterial blood pressure, central venous pressure, pulmonary artery pressures, cardiac output/index, and pulmonary wedge pressures. Moreover, supportive imaging, such as radiography and echocardiography, can provide additional data

indicative of cardiac function. Furthermore, assessment of the IABP's effectiveness is evaluated by monitoring diastolic augmentation and the timing of the balloon's inflation/deflation with the patient's cardiac cycle. Moreover, as the patient's hemodynamic and cardiovascular function widely impacts other physiological processes, other indicators of cardiac function include pulmonary status (oxygenation, arterial oxygen saturation, etc.), lactate levels, renal function, and metabolic measures (Lewis et al., 2009).

In addition, IABP therapy is associated with an increased risk of specific complications. The most common complication is IABP-induced thrombocytopenia and access site bleeding (Lewis et al., 2009; Parissis et al., 2011). The IABP can cause destruction of platelets, contributing to thrombocytopenia and site bleeding. Access site bleeding should be managed by either the addition of a suture to the site or through gentle compression—excessive pressure should be avoided as it narrows the arterial lumen and may contribute to distal limb ischemia (Lewis et al., 2009). Therefore, nursing care involves regular evaluation of the insertion site for signs of bleeding and/or hematoma formation. Also, the IAPB can cause red blood cell destruction; it is not uncommon for recipients of IABPs to require intermittent blood transfusions.

Hypoperfusion of limbs and/or organ systems is another common complication of IABP therapy. Distal limb ischemia is a risk most prevalent in patients with existing peripheral vascular disease and often occurs shortly after placement of the IABP. Nursing care involves regular monitoring of extremity in neurovascular status, such as extremity temperature, color, movement, and sensation; moreover, distal pulses (dorsalis pedis and posterior tibial) should be regularly evaluated. In addition, vascular assessments should include all extremities—although unlikely, there is possibility of balloon migration and subsequent obstruction of additional vessels. Similarly, urine output should be regularly monitored—a sudden decline in urine output may indicate occlusion of the renal arteries emerging from the distal aorta. Lactate values can be monitored as an indicator of tissue perfusion (Lewis et al., 2009).

OUTCOMES

As the combination of ventilation and pharmacologic support in combination with the IABP contributes to restoration of cardiac function, IABP support should be reduced and ideally discontinued. An indication of readiness for lessening IABP support is the gradual tolerance of weaning pharmacological inotropic agents. Lessening of IABP support can be through either frequency or volume weaning. Frequency weaning involves reducing the number of assisted beats provided by the IABP; for example, full assistance by the IABP indicates a 1:1 frequency—every heartbeat is supported by IABP augmentation. Eventually, as the patient's condition improves, IABP support can be diminished to frequencies of 1:2, 1:3, and 1:4. Whereas, volume weaning involves the gradual reduction of the volume within the balloon—decreasing augmentation provided by the IABP and increasing cardiovascular workload (Lewis et al., 2009). Once the IABP is discontinued, the nurse must continue to regularly assess the access site for signs of bleeding and/or hematoma formation and distal extremity neurovascular status.

Summary

IABPs provide effective circulatory support to patients suffering acute ventricular failure by augmenting diastolic pressure, reducing afterload, and enhancing coronary artery perfusion. These patients, often critically ill, require nursing care that incorporates a proficient understanding of pathophysiology and human hemodynamics. Furthermore, nursing care requires the nurse to perform thorough physical assessments and apply such data to the patient's clinical context to anticipate and recognize signs/symptoms of complications or progress associated with IABP therapy. As mechanical circulatory devices continue to develop, the nursing discipline can anticipate the provision of more complex circulatory modalities that not only augment the diastolic phase of the cardiac cycle, but the systolic phase as well (Parissis et al., 2016).

Fan, Z.-G., Gao, X.-F., Chen, L.-W., Li, X.-B., Shao, M.-X., Ji, Q., . . . Tian, N.-L. (2016). The outcomes of intra-aortic balloon pump usage in patients with acute myocardial infarction: A comprehensive meta-analysis of 33 clinical trials and 18,889 patients. *Patient Preference and Adherence, 10,* 297–312. doi:10.2147/PPA.S101945

Krishna, M., & Zacharowski, K. (2009). Principles of intra-aortic balloon pump counterpulsation. *Continuing Education in Anaesthesia, Critical Care and Pain, 9*(1), 24–28. doi:10.1093/bjaceaccp/mkn051

Lewis, P. A., Ward, D. A., & Courtney, M. D. (2009). The intra-aortic balloon pump in heart failure management: Implications for nursing practice. *Australian Critical Care, 22*(3), 125–131. doi:10.1016/j.aucc.2009.06.005

Parissis, H., Graham, V., Lampridis, S., Lau, M., Hooks, G., & Mhandu, P. C. (2016). IABP: History-evolution-pathophysiology-indications: What we need to know. *Journal of Cardiothoracic Surgery, 11*(1), 122. doi:10.1186/s13019-016-0513-0

Parissis, H., Soo, A., & Al-Alao, B. (2011). Intra-aortic balloon pump: Literature review of risk factors related to complications of the intra-aortic balloon pump. *Journal of Cardiothoracic Surgery, 6,* 147. doi:10.1186/1749-8090-6-147

Raman, J., Loor, G., London, M., & Jolly, N. (2010). Subclavian artery access for ambulatory balloon pump insertion. *Annals of Thoracic Surgery, 90*(3), 1032–1034. doi:10.1016/j.athoracsur.2009.11.082

■ MENTAL AND BEHAVIORAL HEALTH EMERGENCIES

Lia V. Ludan

Overview

Nurses in emergency departments and critical care settings are likely to encounter individuals experiencing mental and behavioral health emergencies. Mental and behavioral health emergencies encompass a variety of psychiatric disorders that include substance abuse, depression with suicidal ideations, acute delirium, generalized or situational anxiety, and psychosis. In recent years, there has been an increase of patients presenting to the acute care and outpatient settings for care in states of a mental or behavioral health crisis. The nursing care for patients suffering from mental or behavioral health emergencies must be focused on the safety of the patient and the health care staff and should include a detailed history and physical examination, nursing care coordination, and community resources to optimize the health of the patients with a mental or behavioral health emergency.

Background

Mental health illness can affect one's mood, thinking, or feelings (National Alliance on Mental Illness, 2016). There are multiple factors that can increase one's risk for developing a behavioral health illness, such as substance abuse, chronic illness, stressful lifestyle, genetics, traumatic life events, biochemical processes, and basic brain structure. Approximately, 48 million Americans aged 18 years and older have experienced a mental or behavioral health event in a given year (National

Alliance on Mental Illness, 2016). About 10 million Americans suffer an event that is serious enough to disrupt their life's activities. Hispanic and African Americans use behavioral health resources at half the rate of Caucasian Americans, and Asian Americans use mental health services at one third the rate of Caucasian Americans (National Alliance on Mental Illness, 2016).

Individuals who have mental illness have a life expectancy decreased by 10 years. When behavioral health issues are present, it increases early mortality from other disease processes such as cardiovascular problems, diabetes, and HIV/AIDS. This can be caused by the individual's general neglect of their health, decrease in physical activity, increase in substance abuse, unhealthy eating habits, and side effects from medications. Other risk factors are low income, lower levels of education, and homelessness.

Mental illness affects youths as well as adults. One in every five youth (aged 13–18 years) undergoes a mental health event sometime during his or her life (National Alliance on Mental Illness, 2016). Half of all chronic behavioral health illness starts as early as 14 years of age, and three quarters of these issues present by the age of 24 years. An estimated 70% of youths in the justice system have at least one behavioral health issue (National Alliance on Mental Illness, 2016). About 20% of individuals have more than one behavioral health issue. Many children do not receive the services needed for their mental health illness. Researchers have calculated that approximately 50% of youths receive services for mental illness (National Alliance on Mental Illness, 2016). Of children who have died from suicidal attempts, 90% had a previous mental illness.

The elderly population is also at risk for mental illness. With the risk of cognitive decline and dementia, the elderly become more vulnerable (Yasamy, Dua, Harper, & Saxena, 2012). Loss of friends and partners can produce a feeling of loneliness, which can develop into depression. Certain chronic diseases can cause a decrease in mobility and independence, which can result in social isolation. The elderly are at risk for neglect or abuse (World Health Organization, 2012), which poses a negative influence on their psychological well-being.

When an individual suffers a serious mental illness, the individual may put his or her life on hold, meaning a loss of earnings. Each year, the American economy loses $193 billion in wages because of serious behavioral events (National Alliance on Mental Illness, 2016). According to the National Institute of Mental Health (Insel, 2015), mental disorders cost $2.5 trillion globally in 2010. The cost is projected to be $6 trillion by 2030 (National Institute of Mental Health, 2016).

According to the American College of Emergency Physicians (ACEP; 2014), psychiatric inpatient beds have decreased to less than 50,000 nationwide. This drastic decrease has forced patients to seek treatment at outpatient facilities, community resources, and other outpatient medical management groups. The outpatient facilities have been under strain because of lack of staff and budget cuts. This forces an increasing number of individuals to seek treatment at acute care settings, such as emergency rooms, for acute mental or behavioral health symptoms that require immediate nursing and medical care (ACEP, 2014).

Clinical Aspects

ASSESSMENT

One of the vital aspects of effective nursing care of a mental and behavioral health patient is obtaining a complete history and physical assessment and laboratory data. The assessment of the patient allows the nurse to identify the patient's problem and establish a relationship with the patient (Karas, 2002). The first step in the assessment process is to assess the behavior of the patient—that is, whether the patient is violent, withdrawn, overactive (manic state), or flat. If the patient is violent and can put the staff or himself or herself at risk of harm, trained security should be notified. If the patient cannot be calmed, then physical or chemical restraints may be indicated. The preferred routes of medication are: oral, intramuscular (IM), then intravenous (IV). Most clinicians start with butyrophenone, such as haloperidol, with or without a benzodiazepine such as lorazepam (ACEP, 2014). The nurse should be aware that antipsychotics are linked to prolonged QT syndrome, extrapyramidal side effects, and anticholinergic effects (ACEP, 2014). Most patients may be responsive to supportive measures alone (Karas, 2002). Placing a patient in a quiet environment, reducing noise, and ensuring a sensation of safety may promote a positive encounter. Once safety has been established, then the professional can determine whether the patient is medically or behavioral stable, and ascertain whether the patient needs oxygen, fluids, cardiac monitoring, or medications (Karas, 2002).

The first step is obtaining the client's demographics, such as age, gender, current living situation, ethnicity, and religion. Subsequently, one should determine the nature of the patient's chief complaint; this should be given in the patient's own words. This can be very different from what is reported from the ambulance personnel, family, or other witnesses. Then the nurse, should obtain the history of present illness. Questions that can be asked include: "What time was the onset of the event? What factors precipitated the event? What was the duration of the event?" (Karas, 2002). Questions regarding allergies, medications are taken daily, psychiatric history, substance abuse, and medical history should be answered. Then the nurse performs the physical examination, including taking the patient's vital signs, blood pressure, heart rate, oxygen saturation, respirations, and temperature. Performing a head-to-toe examination, inspecting the head for trauma and an ocular examination can be very helpful. Pinpoint or dilated pupils can represent the use of narcotics or other substances. Inspection of the neck and chest can be very helpful as well (Karas, 2002). Auscultation of breath sounds can reveal an indication of congestive heart failure or pneumonia. In the elderly, these disease processes can cause delirium. Adverse heart sounds can be caused by atrial fibrillation, metabolic derangements, or drug toxicities. An abdominal examination can display signs of infection, ascites, or hepatomegaly, which can cause the patient to have a change in their mental state. The nurse should inspect the skin for rashes, needle marks, diaphoresis, petechiae, or purpura (Karas, 2002).

The psychiatric examination starts with the appearance of the patient; the nurse also assesses how the patient is dressed and groomed. Subsequently, the nurse observes motor function for abnormal movement, assessing muscle tone, posture, and gait. During assessment, the nurse should note whether the patient's speech is low, fast (manic), or slow (depression) when answering questions (Zun, 2016). He or she should then inquire about suicidal ideation or violent thoughts by asking whether the patient wants to hurt himself or herself or others. The nurse should then assess the patient's insight and judgment (Zun, 2016), and whether the patient understands that there is a problem and what needs to be done to correct it. The abnormal thought process can be a key indicator for schizophrenia and psychotic disorders. The nurse should obtain a urine drug screen, alcohol testing, bedside blood glucose levels, and urine pregnancy test for all women of child bearing age (Zun, 2016). If the physical examination reveals any adverse finding, the nurse should anticipate further diagnostic testing such as medical imaging, cardiogram, and laboratory studies. Subsequently, the patient should have a psychiatric screening from a trained professional, such as a behavioral health counselor or a psychiatrist (Zun, 2016).

NURSING INTERVENTIONS, MANAGEMENT, AND IMPLICATIONS

A common nursing issue that occurs when a patient with a mental or behavioral health emergency seeks care in an ED is the delayed transfer of patients to definitive psychiatric inpatient care. Often, the prolonged boarding times in ED for patients with a mental or behavioral health emergency occur because of lack of insurance, need to transfer to an outside facility, and the lack of inpatient facility throughout the nation (ACEP, 2014). Another known issue is stigma from health care providers toward patients in states psychiatric emergency. Nurses should recognize their personal biases toward mental illness and take appropriate courses of action to prevent stigmatization of these patients (Trossman, 2011). Lastly, the majority of ED and critical care nurses lack continuing education on how to address patients with mental or behavioral health emergencies. However, nurses in these care settings should seek educational offerings to enhance the safety, manage stigma, and initiate plans of nursing care to support the needs of patients with mental or behavioral health emergencies (Trossman, 2011).

OUTCOMES

The primary outcome of nursing care for patients experiencing a mental or behavioral health emergency is safety, psychological recovery, and optimization of other acute or chronic physical conditions. This is ensured by continued assessment and close observation of the patient while in the acute care and inpatient setting. Subsequently, the nurse assesses the patient's disposition, and determines whether the patient should be discharged or become an inpatient. If the patient can be discharged from the acute care setting, the nurse should provide follow-up and community resources to the patient. He or she should ensure the patient's understanding of the follow-up instructions and how to access the community resources. Another important aspect is to educate the patient about how and when to seek care if a behavioral crisis is happening. If the patient is to be admitted the nurse must ensure that proper arrangements have been made for the transfer and set a plan for the patient's current behavioral health issue. Having an established plan helps when inpatient beds are not readily available. For the patient to have a positive outcome, care must be developed and implemented on a multidisciplinary level with evidence-based treatment plans.

Summary

Mental illness is a disease process that can be difficult to treat because it involves the consideration of many factors. When caring for a patient with mental health, nurses must keep in mind that risk factors, safety issues, and detailed assessment skills are vital in providing care to this population type. Having a complete understanding of the complex dynamics of the disease process ensure that the nurse and the patient are providing and receiving high-quality, evidence-based nursing care.

American College of Emergency Physicians. (2014). Care of the psychiatric patient in the emergency department: A review of the literature. Retrieved from https://www.acep.org/uploadedFiles/ACEP/Clinical_and_Practice_Management/Resources/Mental_Health_and_Substance_Abuse/Psychiatric%20Patient%20Care%20in%20the%20ED%202014.pdf

Insel, T. (2015). Post by former NIMH director Thomas Insel: Mental health awareness month: By the numbers. Retrieved from https://www.nimh.nih.gov/about/directors/thomas-insel/blog/2015/mental-health-awareness-month-by-the-numbers.shtml

Karas, S. (2002). Behavioral emergencies: Differentiating medical from psychiatric disease. *Emergency Medicine Practice*, 4(3), 1–20. Retrieved from http://www.ebmedicine.net/topics.php?paction=showTopic&topic_id=61

National Alliance on Mental Illness. (2016). Mental health by the numbers. Retrieved from https://www.nami.org/Learn-More/Mental-Health-By-the-Numbers

Trossman, S. (2011, April). Overcoming stigma. Retrieved from http://www.theamericannurse.org/2011/04/12/overcoming-stigma

Yasamy, M. T., Dua, T., Harper, M., & Saxena, S. (2012). *Mental health of older adults, addressing a growing concern* (pp. 4–9). Retrieved from http://www.who.int/mental_health/world-mental-health-day/WHO_paper_wmhd_2013.pdf

Zun, L. (2016). Care of psychiatric patients: The challenge to emergency physicians. *Western Journal of Emergency Medicine*, 17(2), 173–176.

■ NEUROTRAUMA

Anita Sundaresh

Overview

Neurotrauma is prevalent in adults as well as the pediatric population. It can be categorized by mechanisms of injury, clinical severity, radiological appearance, or anatomic distribution. The effects of the trauma can last from hours to days. Seat belts and helmets often protect individuals from a neurologic injury, which is the main focus of public health efforts. Migraines and strokes, common neurological disorders that affect individuals worldwide, will be discussed.

Background

Migraine is derived from the Greek word *hemicrania* (Silberstein, 2004). It is a disorder that is associated with significant neurological, gastrointestinal, as well as autonomic changes. It can be associated with episodes of headache that are pulsating in quality, unilateral or bilateral, and can be exacerbated by physical activity (Kurth & Diener, 2012). Some of the contributing factors of migraine include nonsteroidal anti-inflammatory drugs, combination analgesics, dopamine antagonists, corticosteroids, opioids, and migraine-specific medications. Migraine is a common disorder that affects about 11% of the world's total population. Females are at higher risk than males; of females, 17.6% are affected with migraines, whereas 5.7% of males are affected. Migraines are prevalent in 3% of the pediatric population aged between 2 and 7 years, increasing to 8% to 23% in children aged 11 years and older (Semenov, 2015). One's quality of life is deeply affected by migraines as they can be very debilitating. "Migraines yearly cost to employers is about US $13 billion and yearly medical costs exceed $1 million" (Silberstein, 2004, p. 381).

The World Health Organization (1978) has defined *stroke* as "a clinical syndrome, of presumed vascular origin, typified by rapidly developing signs of focal or global disturbance of cerebral functions lasting more than 24 hours or leading to death" (as cited in Intercollegiate Stroke Working Party, 2012, p. 27). Eight-five percent of strokes are due to cerebral infarction, 10% are attributed to primary hemorrhage, and 5% are caused by subarachnoid hemorrhage (SAH). Transient ischemic attack (TIA) occurs when symptoms last fewer than 24 hours. It is due to an inadequate cerebral or ocular blood supply that can result in thrombus or an embolism (Hankey & Warlow, 1994). SAH can occur with a sudden onset of headache or vomiting, and can also present with loss of consciousness. It occurs as result of a hemorrhage from a cerebral blood vessel, aneurysm, or vascular malformation.

Causes of stroke include cardioembolic, atherosclerotic, dissections, vasculitis, hypertension, and atrial fibrillation. Some of the nonmodifiable risk factors include age, gender, race, ethnicity, and genetics. Some of the modifiable risk factors include hypertension, diabetes mellitus, atrial fibrillation, and dyslipidemia, and individuals afflicted with these risk factors. Stroke is a leading cause of morbidity and results in significant financial burdens, which have been estimated at $34 billion per year for health care services, medications, and decreased days of work (Boehme, Esenwa, & Elkind, 2017).

Clinical Aspects

ASSESSMENT

The most common symptom that patients experience with a migraine is a headache. "It results from activation of meningeal and blood vessel nociceptors combines with a change in central pain modulation" (Silberstein, 2004, p. 382). Nurses need to be aware of the clinical features associated with migraines, such as the positive phenomena of migraines, which are seeing stars, spark photopsia, and complex geometric patterns (Diener & Kurth, 2012). Some of the symptoms associated with migraine headache include nausea, vomiting, photophobia, and phonophobia. Migraine stroke is suspected when aura symptoms of migraine attacks last for more than 24 hours (Diener & Kurth, 2012).

The diagnostic criteria for migraine without aura include at least five attacks, a headache that lasts for 4 to 72 hours, and a headache that results in at least two of the following characteristics: unilateral location, pulsating quality, moderate or severe intensity, and aggravation by or avoidance of routine physical activity. The following can also occur: nausea/vomiting or photophobia and phenophobia. The diagnostic criteria with aura, known as the *classic migraine*, include at least two attacks and a typical aura, hemoplegic aura, and basilar type aura. Some of the symptoms of atypical aura include visual, sensory, or speech symptoms, homogenous or bilateral visual symptoms. "Visual phenomena, which are usually benign, occurred in 1.22% of women and in 1.08% of men in a general population sample" (Silberstein, 2004, p. 384).

A nursing-related problem that can occur is when nurses are not able to identify aura that trigger migraines. Therefore, nurses should encourage patients to keep a headache diary to identify triggers that the patient experiences. The nurse should also provide patients with dietary and lifestyle approaches that can prevent headaches. Lifestyle approaches can include limiting caffeine intake, daily exercise, stress management, a low-tyramine diet, and regular sleep patterns.

The diary must include time and date of all headaches and activities that lead to migraine headaches. Nurses should anticipate medications that are used to provide relief of migraines, such as the triptans that include sumatriptan, rizatriptan, and eletriptan. Sumatriptan can provide short-acting relief, and naratriptan can be used to provide long-lasting relief. Nurses should also encourage follow-up appointments with a neurologist to discuss symptom relief, treatment, and management of migraines. Cognitive behavioral therapy and biofeedback help patients to develop management skills and ways to prevent headaches (Parker & Waltman, 2012).

Nurses should facilitate rapid diagnosis and initiation of treatment as they work together with physicians and nurse practitioners. A thorough history and neurological examination are key to identifying patients who may have suffered a stroke. Sudden numbness or weakness of face, arm, or leg, especially on one side of the body, sudden confusion, trouble speaking, severe headache, difficulty seeing, and dizziness are signs and symptoms that should warn nurses that the patient is having a stroke (Goldstein & Simel, 2005). Nurses should address the need to prevent hypertension as treating the disease reduces the risk of stroke. "The Systolic Hypertension in the Elderly Program (SHEP) study shows that treatment of isolated systolic hypertension in the elderly decreases the risk of stroke by 36%" (Gorelick et al., 1999, p.1113). Nurses must also educate stroke patients that stroke can lead to myocardial infarction (MI). The importance of adhering to oral anticoagulant agents can reduce the possibility of stroke in patients with MI. The use of anticoagulants, antiplatelet agents, and lipid-lowering agents can prevent stroke after a patient has suffered an MI. "The incidence of ischemic stroke is approximately one to two percent per year after MI. This risk is greatest in the first month after MI (31%)" (Gorelick et al., 1999, p. 1114).

Another risk factor for stroke is atrial fibrillation, which increases the risk of stroke approximately six times. It is important for health care professionals to consider the risk of stroke against the risk of hemorrhage in patients with stroke. Diabetes mellitus is another risk factor for stroke. Nurses can help patients understand the importance of taking diabetes medication or insulin therapy to control blood sugar levels. "The likelihood of stroke increased with the following acute neurological deficits: facial droop, arm drift, or a speech disturbance" (Goldstein & Simel, 2005, p. 2401) It is important for nurses to anticipate the need for neuroimaging studies to examine the extent of an injury for a patient with neurological deficits. A change is mental status needs to be reported by nurses for early intervention and treatment of care (Goldstein & Simel, 2005).

NURSING INTERVENTIONS, MANAGEMENT, AND IMPLICATIONS

It is important for nurses to be aware of effective strategies that are needed to prevent migraine and stroke in patients. Some of the risk factors for stroke include hypertension, atrial fibrillation, arterial obstruction, and hyperlipidemia. Nurses must clarify with health care professionals the parameters needed to initiate blood pressure therapy for patients with hypertension, as well as parameters to resume blood pressure therapy. "Goals for target BP level or reduction from pretreatment baseline are uncertain and should be individualized, but it is reasonable to achieve a systolic pressure <140 mmHg and a diastolic pressure <90 mmHg" (Kernan et al., 2014, p. 2170). It is also important for nurses to know the risk factors for recurrent stroke, including sleep apnea and aortic arch atherosclerosis. Therefore, it is necessary to rely on updated guidelines to manage stroke. Nurses should also be aware of patients who are diabetic as well as prediabetic to enhance the role of lifestyle modification in patient's daily lives. This will help reduce vascular problems among patients. Nurses should also help patients understand the benefit of weight loss in preventing cardiovascular risk factors that can lead to stroke. Evidence-based guidelines must be incorporated into practice to prevent stroke among patients (Kernan et al., 2014).

OUTCOMES

Nurses should facilitate rapid assessment and initiation of treatment as they work together with physicians and nurse practitioners to provide positive outcomes for patients. Education on identification of signs and symptoms of neurotrauma events is foundational in preventing initial and/or recurring events. It is also important for the nurse to provide counseling and education to the patient and family regarding medications, medication interactions, consequences of noncompliance with medications, and therapy to prevent complications and negative outcomes of the event.

Summary

Nurses must also be educated on many aspects of migraines. Migraines are worsened by physical activity and associated with cooccurring symptoms such as nausea, vomiting, and photophobia. Preventative therapy can help patients and reduce the severity of their migraine attacks (Marmura, Silberstein, & Schwedt, 2015). There is consistent evidence that individuals with migraine are approximately two times more likely to develop an ischemic stroke and vigilant nursing care should include stroke-prevention strategies to mitigate cardiovascular morbidity (Kurth & Diener, 2012, p. 3421).

Boehme, A. K., Esenwa, C., & Elkind, S. V. (2017). Stroke risk factors, genetics, and prevention. *Circulation, 120,* 472–495.

Goldstein, L. B., & Simel, D. L. (2005). Is this patient having a stroke? *Journal of the American Medical Association, 293*(19), 2391–2402. doi:10.1001/jama.293.19.2391

Gorelick, P. B., Sacco, R. L., Smith, D. B., Alberts M., Mustone-Alexander, L., Rader, D., . . . Rhew, D. C. (1999). Prevention of a first stroke: A review of guidelines and a multidisciplinary consensus statement from the National Stroke Association. *Journal of the American Medical Association, 281*(12), 1112–1120. doi:10.1001/jama.281.12.1112

Hankey, G. J., & Warlow, C. P. (1994). Transient ischemic attacks of the brain and eye. In R. J. Davenport (Ed.), *Major problems in neurology*. Philadelphia, PA: Saunders.

Intercollegiate Stroke Working Party. (2012). *National clinical guideline for stroke* (4th ed.). London, UK: Royal College of Physicians.

Kernan, W. N., Ovbiagele, B., Black, H. R., Bravata, D. M., Chimowitz, M. I., Ezekowitz, M. D., & Johnston, S. C. C. (2014). Guidelines for the prevention of stroke in patients with stroke and transient ischemic attack. *Stroke, 45*(7), 2160–2236.

Kurth, T., & Diener, H. (2006). Current views of the risk of stroke for migraine with and migraine without aura. *Current Pain and Headache Reports, 10*(3), 214–220. doi:1007/S11916-006-0048-5

Kurth, T., & Diener, H. C. (2012). Migraine and stroke. *Stroke, 43*(12), 3421–3426.

Marmura, M. J., Silberstein, S. D., & Schwedt, T. J. (2015). The acute treatment of migraine in adults: The American Headache Society Evidence Assessment of Migraine Pharmacotherapies. *Headache: The Journal of Head and Face Pain, 55*(1), 3–20.

Parker, C., & Waltman, N. (2012). Reducing the frequency and severity of migraine headaches in the workplace: Implementing evidence-based interventions. *Workplace Health & Safety, 60*(1), 12–18. doi:10.3928/21650799-20111227-02

Silberstein, S. D. (2004). Migraine pathophysiology and its clinical implications. *Cephalgia: An International Journal of Headache, 24*(Suppl. 2), 2–7.

■ OBSTETRICAL AND GYNECOLOGICAL EMERGENCY CARE

Vicki Bacidore

Overview

Patients with OB/GYN problems are frequently seen and receive treatment in emergency departments (EDs). Obstetrical emergencies not only affect the health and well-being of the mother, but also the unborn child. Gynecological emergencies affect the female reproductive system, can be life-threatening, and may have an effect on sexual function and fertility. The role of the emergency nurse is to rule out life-threatening complications associated with abnormal uterine bleeding and to obtain emergent, urgent, or routine gynecologic consultation as needed. The management of OB/GYN emergencies requires excellent assessment skills and rapid interventions.

Background

An increasing number of women, despite having a primary care provider, utilize the ED for OB/GYN-related complaints for a variety of different reasons such as access barriers, physician referrals, convenience, tradition, and the feeling that their condition warrants emergency care (Burns & Sacchetti, 2016). The most frequent OB/GYN emergencies are abnormal vaginal bleeding, miscarriage, ectopic pregnancy, acute or chronic pelvic pain, and previously undiagnosed cancer of the female genital tract and trauma (ENA, 2013).

Abnormal uterine bleeding, formerly referred to as *dysfunctional uterine bleeding*, reflects a disruption in the normal cyclic pattern of ovulatory hormonal stimulation to the endometrial lining. The most common cause of abnormal uterine bleeding during the reproductive years is abnormal pregnancy and threatened abortion, incomplete abortion, and ectopic pregnancy (Behera, 2016).

Pelvic pain is a common chief complaint and can be due to a variety of etiologies. The uterus, cervix, and adnexa all share the same visceral innervation as the lower ileum, sigmoid colon and rectum, making it difficult to distinguish pain originating from reproductive or gastrointestinal organs. Pelvic pain can be classified as acute, chronic, or cyclical (ENA, 2010) and can be of sufficient severity to cause functional disability or

lead to medical care. Nearly 4% of women are thought to have ongoing chronic pelvic pain (Davila, 2016).

Pelvic inflammatory disease (PID) is an infectious and inflammatory disorder of the upper female genital tract, including the uterus, fallopian tubes, and adjacent pelvic structures. Infection and inflammation may spread to the abdomen and surrounding hepatic structures. Typically affected is a menstruating woman aged younger than 25 years with multiple sex partners, who does not use contraception, and lives in an area with a high prevalence of sexually transmitted infections (STIs). The two most common organisms causing PID are *Neisseria gonorrheoeae* and *Chlamydia trachomatis* (Moore, 2017). A diagnosis of PID is typically based on the history and physical exam and, if untreated, can have significant long-term complications such as infertility, chronic pelvic pain, and ectopic pregnancy (ENA, 2010).

Spontaneous miscarriage is the death or expulsion of the fetus or products of conception before the age of viability and accounts for approximately 5% to 15% of all pregnancies (Gaufberg, 2017). Early pregnancy loss is primarily due to embryonic chromosomal defects and should be considered a possibility in any woman presenting to the ED with vaginal bleeding. Miscarriage after the first trimester is more likely due to advanced age, prior miscarriage, severe hypertension, endocrine dysfunction, abnormal embryologic development, or trauma (ENA, 2013).

Approximately 2% of all pregnancies in the United States are ectopic, meaning the embryo implants at a site other than the endometrium of the uterus, typically in the fallopian tube. This usually appears in the sixth week of gestation and, unless recognized, the fallopian tube will rupture, causing death of the fetus and threatening the life of the mother. The classic clinical presentation triad of ectopic pregnancy is abdominal pain, amenorrhea, and vaginal bleeding. Other signs include sudden onset of severe, unilateral pelvic pain, nausea, vomiting, dizziness, or weakness. Abdominal rigidity, involuntary guarding, evidence of shock all suggest a surgical emergency (Sepilian, 2016).

Pregnancy-induced hypertension (PIH) is described as hypertension related to pregnancy and is synonymous with preeclampsia–eclampsia, which typically occurs after the 20th week of pregnancy. Preeclampsia is the second leading cause of maternal mortality and is a multisystem condition characterized by hypertension, proteinuria, and edema. Eclampsia is a worsening of preeclampsia, is characterized by seizure activity, and has a high risk of cerebral hemorrhage, morbidity, and mortality (ENA, 2013).

Placenta previa occurs when the placenta implants in the lower uterine segment or over the cervical os, rather than its normal implantation in the upper uterine wall. As the fetus grows within the uterus, implantation may be disrupted as this area gradually thins in preparation for labor, causing painless bleeding through the cervix. *Placental abruption* is defined as the premature separation of the placenta from the uterus after the 20th week of gestation. Patients typically present with hemorrhage, uterine contractions, and fetal distress. Placental abruption is associated with high fetal and maternal morbidity and mortality and is the most common cause of fetal demise following maternal trauma (ENA, 2013).

Births in the ED are rare, but are considered high-risk deliveries. When a pregnant patient presents to the ED in labor, imminent delivery is primarily determined by crowning of the fetus and the mother's urge to push (ENA, 2013). A rapid decision is made whether or not to deliver in the ED, or, if time permits, transfer to a sterile, more desirable environment such as the labor and delivery unit. Emergency nurses must be prepared for potential delivery complications and to manage neonatal resuscitation as necessary. In the United States, there are approximately 4 million births annually, with a birth rate of 12.5 per 1,000 population (Centers for Disease Control and Prevention [CDC], 2014). The majority of these pregnancies and births are considered low risk and occur without complications. However, an increasing number of obstetrical patients do present to the ED with complications. The Emergency Nurses Association's (ENA) position statement on obstetrical patients in the ED outlines safe care in this practice setting (ENA, 2011).

Clinical Aspects

ASSESSMENT

Obtaining a thorough history is crucial to the assessment process and to all patients. Vital components of the history include chief complaint; symptom onset; pain assessment (onset, provocation, palliation, quality, radiation, severity, and timing); history of trauma; presence of vaginal discharge or bleeding; obstetrical and sexual history, including last normal menstrual period; medical/surgical history; family and social history; medications; and allergies. All females of childbearing age should be evaluated for possible pregnancy. Patients with obstetrical or gynecological emergencies can experience significant blood loss and hypovolemia. Assessment priorities should always be airway, breathing, and circulation. Focused assessment must include the patient's general appearance and vital signs, assessment of the skin, respiratory, cardiovascular, abdominal, and genitourinary systems. A complete pelvic examination should be performed. For pregnant patients, gestational age and fetal viability are determined, including the possibility of impending delivery (ENA, 2007).

Diagnostics may include laboratory studies such as a complete blood count with differential, coagulation profile, serum chemistries, urinalysis, pregnancy test, type and crossmatch with Rh factor, the Kleihauer–Betke test to assess and measure the presence of fetomaternal hemorrhage, and screening for sexually transmitted infections (STIs). Imaging studies may include pelvic or transvaginal sonography with Doppler and CT. Electronic fetal monitoring for uterine contractions and fetal heart rate may also be required (ENA, 2007).

NURSING INTERVENTIONS, MANAGEMENT, AND IMPLICATIONS

Differential diagnoses and collaborative nursing-related problems include acute pain, fluid volume deficit, ineffective tissue perfusion, fear and anxiety, risk for infection, knowledge deficit, and anticipatory grieving. Emergency nurses need to continuously assess patients for pain, bleeding amount, and mental status. Patients have the potential to decompensate quickly due to blood loss.

Nursing interventions include (a) maintaining airway, breathing, and circulation; (b) providing supplemental oxygen as indicated; (c) establishing intravenous access for the administration of fluids and medications as needed; (d) preparing for and assisting with medical procedures; (e) administering pharmacological therapy as ordered; (f) assisting with admission and/or transfer if necessary; (g) providing patient and family education, and (h) ensuring follow-up care.

OUTCOMES

The OB/GYN patient in the ED must have continuous evaluation and ongoing monitoring of pain relief, normalization of maternal and/or fetal respiratory, circulation and perfusion status, a demonstrated increase in psychological functioning, and adequate knowledge of health status. Preservation of maternal and fetal life are the primary concerns for positive outcomes.

Summary

The patient with OB/GYN problems can offer challenging opportunities for the ED nurse. Utilizing the nursing process in order to assess and prioritize care for these women is essential to assess and manage potential threats to life. Emergency nursing knowledge of how to care for common OB/GYN emergencies promotes optimal outcomes for these women and their children.

Behera, M. A. (2016). Abnormal (dysfunctional) uterine bleeding. *Medscape.* Retrieved from http://emedicine.medscape.com/article/257007-overview

Burns, J. & Sacchetti, A. (2016). Enrollment with a primary care provider does not preclude ED visits for patients with woman's health related problems. *American Journal of Emergency Medicine, 34*(2) 266–268.

Centers for Disease Control and Prevention. (2014). Births and natality. Retrieved from https://www.cdc.gov/nchs/fastats/births.htm

Davila, G. W. (2016). Gynecologic pain. *Medscape.* Retrieved from http://emedicine.medscape.com/article/270450-overview

Emergency Nurses Association. (2007). *Emergency nursing core curriculum* (6th ed.). Philadelphia, PA: Elsevier Saunders.

Emergency Nurses Association. (2010). *Sheehy's emergency nursing: Principles and practice* (6th ed.). St. Louis, MO: Elsevier Mosby.

Emergency Nurses Association. (2011). Position statement: The obstetrical patient in the emergency department. Retrieved from https://www.ena.org/SiteCollectionDocuments/Position%20Statements/OBPatientED.pdf

Emergency Nurses Association. (2013). *Sheehy's manual of emergency care* (7th ed.). St. Louis, MO: Elsevier Mosby.

Gaufberg, S. V. (2017). Early pregnancy loss in emergency medicine. *Medscape.* Retrieved from http://emedicine.medscape.com/article/795085-overview

Moore Shepherd, S. (2017). Pelvic inflammatory disease. *Medscape.* Retrieved from http://emedicine.medscape.com/article/256448-overview

Sepilian, V. P. (2016). Ectopic pregnancy. *Medscape.* Retrieved from http://emedicine.medscape.com/article/2041923-overview

■ OPHTHALMIC EMERGENCIES

Shannon M. Litten

Overview

Ophthalmic emergencies in the general population account for 2% of emergency department (ED) visits in the United States annually (Cheung et al., 2014; Sharma & Brunette, 2014). Worldwide, this number reaches 55 million and results in poor unilateral vision in 23 million people (Gardiner, 2016a). A recent review of 1,400 EDs found the vast majority of ED visits (27%) result from ocular trauma, including 73% corneal abrasions, 6% blunt eye trauma, and 5% corneal foreign body (Walker & Adhikari, 2016). In the United States, eye injuries account for 3% to 5% of all occupational injuries (Sharma & Brunette, 2014). The second most common ocular condition seen in the ED is conjunctivitis (15%), followed by glaucoma or retinal problems (6%) (Walker & Adhikari, 2016). Nurses are frequently the first health caregiver to encounter these presentations and must be prepared to obtain correct information for prompt evaluation, treatment, and consult (Sharma & Brunette, 2014).

Background

An ophthalmic emergency consists of any eye condition that requires immediate medical attention to avert vision loss or impairment (Parekh, 2016). The most common eye emergencies can be categorized into trauma, infection, and neurovascular conditions (Parekh, 2016). Top diagnoses requiring an emergent ophthalmology consult include penetrating injury, chemical injury, acute glaucoma, sudden vision loss, and orbital cellulitis (Field, Tillotson, & Whittingham, 2015).

An estimated 2.5 million traumatic eye emergencies are seen annually, including blunt or penetrating trauma and chemical burns, which threaten visual loss in up to 60,000 cases (Gardiner, 2016a; Parekh, 2016). Ocular emergencies are more prevalent in middle-aged, White men and affect as many as 80% when the emergency results from trauma (Cheung et al., 2014; Parekh, 2016; Saccomano & Ferrara, 2014). Recent literature also identifies the elderly population at higher risk for ocular emergencies, particularly when related to falls (Cheung et al., 2014). In a study conducted by Cheung et al. (2014), the most common causes of traumatic injury occurred from motor vehicle crashes (MVC), falls, and assault (17.4%, 14.4%, and 11.1%, respectively). Blunt traumatic eye injuries include trauma to the eye (ocular trauma), the orbit (periocular trauma), or both and can lead to fractures, hemorrhage, or damage to the globe (Gardiner, 2016a; Parekh, 2016). The leading traumatic injuries from MVCs or falls are open globe and orbital fractures of which open globe carries the poorest outcomes; 66.7% lead to legal blindness

(Cheung et al., 2014). However, orbital fractures are much more common than open globe injuries (45.3% vs. 6.1%) and result in 1.5% of legal blindness (Cheung et al., 2014).

Chemical injury from alkaline (lye, ammonia, fertilizers, pesticides) or acids (car batteries, bleach, and some refrigerants) can be just as detrimental to vision (Parekh, 2016; Patel, 2016; Sharma & Brunette, 2014). Alkaline destroys cell structure and leads to tissue destruction that continues until the agent is removed. Acids are less destructive due to coagulation necrosis, which precipitates tissue proteins, limiting depth of injury. Both can lead to corneal scarring (Parekh, 2016; Patel, 2016; Sharma & Brunette, 2014).

In children, corneal abrasions are the most common nonpenetrating eye injury (Saccomano & Ferrara, 2014). Although corneal abrasions affects all age groups, newborns and infants are frequently injured with an untrimmed fingernail, younger children with a toy, and adolescents during sports (Saccomano & Ferrara, 2014; Walker & Adhikari, 2016). Contact lens wearers are frequently affected from tangential impacts or foreign body debris. Other causes of corneal abrasion include dust, chemicals, sand, animal paws, and makeup brushes (Saccomano & Ferrara, 2014; Walker & Adhikari, 2016). If not treated immediately, opportunistic bacteria, virus, or fungi can infect the eye risking the development of inflammatory iritis (Walker & Adhikari, 2016).

Other causes of ocular emergency rates in Cheung et al.'s (2014) study were: infectious, 14.3%; preexisting conditions, 14%; unknown, 11.5%; and other traumatic causes, 7.5%. Ophthalmic emergencies in females were mostly a result of infectious agents or neurologic etiologies (Cheung et al., 2014). There are many causes of infectious eye conditions with varying degrees of severity. Conjunctivitis was the second most common infectious condition, affecting 15% of all eye emergencies seen in the ED and typically characterized by itchy, red eyes and discharge without visual acuity changes (Saccomano & Ferrara, 2014; Walker & Adhikari, 2016).

Although frequently viral and self-limiting, it is important to consider serious bacterial or corneal herpetic involvement that could result in vision loss without aggressive treatment (Walker & Adhikari, 2016). Common bacterial pathogens are *Staphylococcus aureus*, *Pseudomonas aeruginosa*, and *Acanthamoeba* (Parekh, 2016). Herpes zoster (HZV) and herpes simplex virus (HSV) are common viral infections. In the United States, HSV is the most common cause of corneal blindness. Fungal infections (*Fusarium* and *Candida*) are often transmitted via plants or soil and seen with agricultural workers or persons living in warm climates (Parekh, 2016). In addition to conjunctivitis, ophthalmic infections can lead to many eye conditions, such as periorbital cellulitis (infection of the eyelids), orbital cellulitis (infection of the orbital soft tissues), anterior uveitis or iritis (inflammation in anterior eye structures), keratitis (inflammation of the cornea), hordeolum (stye), endophthalmitis (inflammation in the vitreous chamber), and corneal ulcers (Parekh, 2016; Walker & Adhikari, 2016).

Neurovascular causes of ophthalmic emergencies often result from preexisting conditions such as hypertension and diabetes mellitus (Parekh, 2016). Examples include acute angle closure glaucoma, retinal detachment, and central retinal artery occlusion (CRAO) with the peak incidence between ages 50 and 70 years (Arroyo, 2016; Parekh, 2016; Sharma & Brunette, 2014; Walker & Adhikari, 2016). Acute angle closure glaucoma is precipitated by pupillary dilatation, such as from dimly lit rooms, emotional upset, or various anticholinergic or sympathomimetic medications (Sharma & Brunette, 2014). If left untreated it can lead to increased intraocular pressure, optic neuropathy, and visual loss (Walker & Adhikari, 2016). Retinal detachment can be traumatic or nontraumatic (Arroyo, 2016). Nontraumatic retinal detachment usually occurs over weeks to months with a common complaint of floaters in the visual field (Arroyo, 2016). In addition to inflammation and trauma, risk factors include myopia (nearsightedness), previous eye surgery, and family history (Arroyo, 2016; Parekh, 2016). Central retinal artery occlusion is a rare condition characterized by painless, acute visual loss that results from vascular occlusion and leads to an ischemic stroke of the retina, requiring immediate intervention (Sharma & Brunette, 2014).

Clinical Aspects

ASSESSMENT

The goal of treatment in eye emergencies is to prevent loss of function, vision, infection, and to relieve symptoms (Saccomano & Ferrara, 2014). The initial patient encounter with an ocular emergency is frequently with the nurse, who leads the triage process; the patient assessment, relevant history, and physical exam findings inform the next steps required (Field et al., 2015). Fear of blindness is terrifying to patients, therefore prompt and accurate triage is of the utmost importance (Patel, 2016). Triage includes history of the presenting complaint, past and present illnesses, current medications, allergies, previous ophthalmological history, and family history of eye problems (Field et al., 2015; Saccomano & Ferrara, 2014). Asking open-ended questions helps obtain the most accurate subjective information (Field et al., 2015). Ocular history must include vision changes; glasses or contact lens use; history of eye trauma, duration of symptoms, sudden or gradual onset; foreign body sensation; use of protective eyewear; details of any chemical injury, including immediate actions taken; excessive eye rubbing or scratching; and use of eye makeup (Saccomano & Ferrara, 2014). Visual acuity assessed by use of a Snellen chart helps inform the degree of severity as decreased visual acuity suggests severe eye emergency such as trauma, glaucoma, or iritis (Parekh, 2016; Saccomano & Ferrara, 2014). Assessing visual acuity will not be priority if the patient is seriously ill or there has been a chemical injury, in which case irrigation overrides assessment of visual acuity (Field et al., 2015; Parekh, 2016). After completing a visual acuity, the eye exam must assess for corneal transparency (smooth, clear, shiny), inflammation or redness, discharge, foreign body, rash or lesions, and extraocular movements (Parekh, 2016; Saccomano & Ferrara, 2014).

NURSING INTERVENTIONS, MANAGEMENT, AND IMPLICATIONS

At this point, the nurse will decide on the most appropriate care pathway and urgency required, such as consulting the emergency provider on duty (physician, nurse practitioner, or physician's assistant). For example, nurses can quickly and easily identify a full-thickness injury to the outer membranes of the eye, as seen in globe rupture, on visual exam alone (Patel, 2016). Another example of a complaint that is not readily obvious by traumatic etiology but can be identified by the nurse as potentially serious is acute angle closure glaucoma. These patients frequently complain of sudden-onset severe ocular pain, headache, nausea and vomiting, and vision changes such as halos or lights. Conversely, sudden painless loss of vision could indicate central retinal artery occlusion (CRAO). A painful rash around the eye that does not cross the dermatome accompanied with pain, fever, and red eye could indicate the possibility of herpes zoster ophthalmicus and the need for urgent evaluation (Patel, 2016).

Interventions that nurses can implement immediately are part of the nursing process and are directly related to positive patient outcomes. Immediate irrigation of the patient's eyes with an isotonic solution, such as normal saline or lactated Ringer's can stop the process of the chemical reaction (Field et al., 2015; Patel, 2016; Parekh, 2016). For patients with suspected globe injuries, a nursing priority is to avoid further evaluation and treatment methods that can place pressure on the globe (eyeball; Gardiner, 2016b). When indicated, pain control is essential for the well-being of the patient and should be part of nurse advocacy.

After the initial interventions have been implemented and the treatment plan determined, the nurse provides patient teaching that includes further prevention strategies, treatment plan, instructions for proper eye medication use, indications of infection, expectations, and follow-up required (Saccomano & Ferrara, 2014).

OUTCOMES

Optimal patient outcomes are best achieved with rapid recognition and early intervention (Gardiner, 2016a). One study of 11,000 eyes found 61% visual improvement when treatment was implemented early (Gardiner, 2016a). Nurses are at the forefront of early recognition for potentially vision-threatening etiologies, making their assessment skills and knowledge of eye emergencies an important part of their nursing practice.

Summary

Ophthalmic emergencies can present in many different ways, including traumatic, infectious, or neurovascular. Having a broad knowledge of these types of emergencies and their most common causes and presentations can direct care and promote positive patient outcomes (Cheung et al., 2014; Saccomano & Ferrara, 2014; Sharma & Brunette, 2014). Clinical preparation for recognition of specific signs or symptoms promotes prompt detection, triage, and treatment required, such as immediate eye irrigation for chemical injuries, pain control, or emergent ophthalmology consultation. These critical steps offer the best chance for sustaining vision and providing the best possible outcomes.

Arroyo, J. G. (2016). Retinal detachment. Retrieved from http://uptodate.com

Cheung, C. A., Rogers-Martel, M., Golas, L., Chepurny, A., Martel, J. B., Martel, J. R. (2014). Hospital-based ocular emergencies: Epidemiology, treatment, and visual outcomes. *American Journal of Emergency Medicine,* 32, 221–224.

Field, D., Tillotson, J., & Whittingham, E., (2015). *Eye emergencies: The practitioner's guide* (2nd ed.). Cumbria, UK: M&K Publishing. Retrieved from http://web.b.ebscohost .com.proxy.library.vanderbilt.edu/ehost/ebookviewer/ ebook/bmxlYmtfXzk4NTkyMF9fQU41?sid=71bac6bb -ccd2-44fd-be50-3e9a0382ac04@sessionmgr101&vid=0 &format=EB&rid=1

Gardiner, M. F. (2016a). Approach to eye injuries in the emergency department. Retrieved from http://uptodate.com

Gardiner, M. F. (2016b). Overview of eye injuries in the emergency department. Retrieved from http://uptodate.com

Patel, P. S. (2016). Top 10 eye emergencies. Retrieved from https://www.aao.org/young-ophthalmologists/yo-info/ article/top-10-eye-emergencies

Parekh, S. J. S. (2016, May). *Ophthalmic emergencies.* Lecture presented at the 8th Annual Emergency Medicine Symposium, Wayne, NJ.

Saccomano, S. J., & Ferrara, L. R. (2014). Managing corneal abrasions in primary care. *Nurse Practitioner,* 39(9), 1–6. doi:10.1097/01.NPR.0000452977.99676.cf

Sharma, R., & Brunette, D. D. (2014). Ophthalmology. In R. M. Walls (Ed.), *Rosen's emergency medicine: Concepts and clinical practice* (8th ed., pp. 909–930). Philadelphia, PA: Elsevier/Saunders.

Walker, R. A., & Adhikari, S. (2016). Eye emergencies. In J. E. Tintinalli (Ed.), *Tintinalli's emergency medicine: A comprehensive study guide* (8th ed., pp. 1543–1579). Columbus, OH: McGraw-Hill.

■ ORTHOPEDIC EMERGENCIES IN ADULTS

Cindy Kumar

Overview

Musculoskeletal injuries with hemodynamic or neurovascular compromise require emergent intervention. Orthopedic emergencies are musculoskeletal injuries that pose an imminent threat to a person's life or limb (Azmy, 2016; Williams, 2009). In orthopedic emergencies, care by the nurse should be centered around observation and assessment for blood loss; altered tissue perfusion, motor, and sensory functions to tissue distal to injury; and prevention of systemic complications secondary to a musculoskeletal injury.

Background

In the United States, approximately 77% of injury-related health care visits are for musculoskeletal complaints (Weinstein & Yelin, 2016). The leading cause of orthopedic injuries for 18- to 44-year-olds is trauma (Weinstein & Yelin, 2016), whereas falls account for the most orthopedic injuries in adults older than 44 years (Bratcher, 2014, p. 195; Weinstein & Yelin, 2016). Falls are the number one cause of injury-related deaths in those older than 72 (Bratcher, 2014).

Once discharged from the hospital, more than 50% of those older than 65 years with musculoskeletal injuries require further medical care or treatment in rehabilitation facilities (Yelin, 2016), contributing to health care cost. Orthopedic injuries are the leading cause of lost work days in people aged 18 to 64 years, thereby creating additional health care cost burden.

Any orthopedic injury has potential for serious complications; however, there are specific injuries that necessitate prompt identification and intervention. These emergencies are open-book pelvic fractures, long-bone fractures, open fractures, compartment syndrome, and amputations. Some would argue cauda equina, joint dislocations, and septic joints also as orthopedic emergencies. There are specific reasons for the heightened concern of each injury. Open-book pelvic fractures are associated with a higher mortality rate due to their higher incidence of hemodynamic instability. Femur fractures increase the risk for fat or thromboembolism. Open fractures have an increased risk for infection and often occur in the presence of concurrent injuries. Compartment syndrome can lead to neurovascular injury and loss of tissue. Amputations are associated with blood loss. Cauda equina is concerning for possible permanent loss of sensory and/or motor function. Diagnosis of these injuries is made by radiologic imaging such as plain film radiographs or computed tomography. In some cases, magnetic resonance imaging is preferred or recommended (Azmy, 2016).

There is also lack of consensus over which injuries truly qualify as emergencies. Even the most benign complaints can have the potential to become emergent (Ewen, personal communication, January 8, 2017). What is known is that one third of patients presenting to the emergency department have orthopedic injuries (Bratcher, 2014, p. 195). The most common injuries are fractures, sprains, and strains, and the extremities are the most commonly injured part of the body. Injury may involve the bone, soft tissue structures, and joint spaces. Types of injuries include "fractures, dislocations, amputations, sprains, strains, penetrating injuries, ligament tears, tendon lacerations, and neurovascular compromise" (Bratcher, 2014, p. 195). The mechanism of injury is an important aspect in the identification and management of orthopedic injuries. Mechanisms include, but are not limited to, falls, motor vehicle collisions, assaults, sports injuries, crush injuries, or blast injuries (Bratcher, 2014). "A musculoskeletal injury that potentially will lead to complications, future impairment, or loss of life or limb if not treated with appropriate expeditious care" is an orthopedic emergency (Crum, 2016).

There are many risk factors that can either contribute to the mechanism of injury or precipitate an orthopedic emergency after the fact. Examples of risk factors include weakness from a previous injury, preexisting disabilities, concurrent acute illness (i.e., infection, arthritis flare), disruption of equilibrium from infection or intoxication, and peripheral neuropathy. Some medications can predispose a patient to increased risk for injury (i.e., diuretics, sedatives, narcotics, steroids) by affecting balance, bone density, or cognition. Bone disorders, such as osteoporosis, Paget's disease, and osteogenesis imperfecta, place a patient at greater risk before, during, and after an injury. (Cerepani & Ramponi, 2016)

In the aging population, there are additional factors that increase the risk of orthopedic emergencies (Fleischman & Ma, 2016). With age, there is a loss of bone and mass; bones become more brittle. There is also a loss of vertebral body height, and age-related muscle atrophy leads to decreased strength (Cerepani & Ramponi, 2016), all of which can affect gait and can cause fatigue more easily. Degenerative changes also decrease mobility. Due to decreased strength, an elderly person may lie injured for a long period of time before help arrives. This can increase the risk for hypo/hyperthermia, dehydration and electrolyte imbalances, and rhabdomyolysis. Special consideration must be given to the pediatric population, however, that is beyond the scope of this chapter.

Clinical Aspects

ASSESSMENT

Obtaining history of present illness and past medical history is essential to nursing care of orthopedic emergencies. Mechanism of injury, determination of fall risk, previous functional status of the individual, age, and comorbidities will affect nursing care and patient outcomes. Current medications, alcohol use, and illicit drug use must be addressed. Strong assessment skills are needed for monitoring of complications in these emergencies. Skills include but are not limited to inspection, palpation, and hemodynamic monitoring. Assessment of the six Ps: pain, pallor, pressure, pulses, paresthesia,

and paralysis, must be incorporated into the nursing assessment before and after any intervention or diagnostic study. Working knowledge of anatomy and physiology is needed to support understanding of processes involved with orthopedic emergencies (Bratcher, 2014).

Blood loss is the leading cause of preventable deaths in trauma (Bratcher, 2014, p. 196). Large volumes of blood loss can occur with pelvic or longbone fractures, which can lead to hypotensive shock if left unmanaged. Pelvic fractures have an estimated blood loss potential of 2 L, whereas a femur fracture has a potential for blood loss of 1.5 L (Azmy, 2016). Blood loss may be obvious or internal. When arterial blood flow is compromised, tissue becomes ischemic. Ischemia leads to increased pain and decreased pulses. Assessment findings may include pallor, cool skin, cyanotic tissue, and prolonged capillary refill time. The nurse should anticipate the need for hemoglobin and hematocrit values.

The nurse needs to assess for concurrent injuries. For example, calcaneal fractures often have associated spinal injury/fracture (Dean, Hatch, & Pauly, 2016). Femur fractures may also have an associated posterior hip dislocation (Bratcher, 2014, p. 195). Clavicle fractures may have an associated pulmonary contusion, pneumothorax, or brachial plexus injury (Clugston, Hatch, & Taffe, 2016). The nurse should anticipate preparing the patient for additional studies, such as additional radiographic imaging, complete blood count, chemistry panel, and, in the presence of a crush injury or a patient who has been injured and stays down for a significant amount of time, a creatinine kinase and renal function should be evaluated for the presence of rhabdomyolysis or acute kidney injury.

NURSING INTERVENTIONS, MANAGEMENT, AND IMPLICATIONS

Priority nursing assessment should focus on hemodynamic and neurovascular status and the monitoring of related complications. In addition to assessment, nursing management needs to focus on the whole patient. Patient preparation for diagnostic studies and interventions, such as surgery or reductions, is the responsibility of the nurse. Documentation should include vital signs, neurovascular status, pain level, assessment findings, and responses to interventions. In the assessment, the nurse needs to include the patient's ability to understand teaching regarding splint/cast care, and signs and symptoms of complications such as infection or compartment syndrome.

Timely identification of the following potential systemic complications is crucial: nerve injury, hyperkalemia, rhabdomyolysis, and acute kidney injury. Hyperkalemia, in the presence of an orthopedic emergency, should be assessed for when there has been a resuscitative period, lengthy extraction, or a delay in transport (Bratcher, 2014). Potassium levels peak around the 12-hour mark and may be associated with tissue destruction (Bratcher, 2014, p. 198). Nerve injury can result from compression of bone from displacement or joint dislocation. Alterations in sensation and motor function can occur. The nurse should always check neurovascular status before and after any intervention. Concerning signs are paresthesia or numbness, cold skin, cyanosed tissue, and decreased or absent pulse. Crush injuries, in particular, raise concerns for severe muscle and tissue damage. Myoglobin is released into the bloodstream and when present in large amounts, can lead to kidney injury. Signs the nurse must assess for are increased muscle pain, change in sensation to affected limb, muscle weakness, and dark- or tea-colored urine (Bratcher, 2014).

OUTCOMES

Evidence-based nursing management of orthopedic emergencies is focused on restoring and/or preserving function. Close monitoring and keen observation for changes in physical assessment can reduce or prevent complications such as hypovolemic shock, compartment syndrome, venous thromboembolism or fat embolism, infection, and acute kidney injury. Expected outcomes of nursing care should concentrate on decreasing blood loss, increasing limb perfusion, minimizing tissue damage, and avoiding systemic effects (Williams, 2009).

Summary

The role of the nurse and evidence-based nursing care are key to management of orthopedic emergencies. Patient outcomes in the presence of orthopedic emergencies are dependent on ongoing assessment of hemodynamics, neurovascular status, and prompt identification of potential complications. Orthopedic emergencies truly are a matter of life or limb.

Azmy, D. A. (2016, December 30). Orthopedic emergencies. Retrieved from http://www.slideshare.net/AhmedAzmy/orthopaedic-emergencies?next_slideshow=1

Bratcher, C. M. (2014). Chapter 14: Musculoskeletal trauma. In B. B. Jacobs (Ed.), *Trauma nursing core course: Provider manual* (pp. 193–203). Des Plaines, IL: Emergency Nurses Association.

Cerepani, M. J., & Ramponi, D. R. (2007). Orthopedic emergencies. In K. S. Hoyt & J. Selfridge-Thomas (Eds.), *Emergency nursing core curriculum* (6th ed., pp. 585–603). Philadelphia, PA: Elsevier.

Clugston, J. R., Hatch, R. L., & Taffe, J. (2016). Clavicle fractures. *UpToDate.* Retrieved from https://www.uptodate.com/contents/clavicle-fractures?source=search_result&search=CLAVICLE+FRACTURE&selectedTitle=1%7E51

Crum, D. J. (2016). Orthopedic emergencies. Retrieved from http://c.ymcdn.com/sites/www.txosteo.org/resource/resmgr/imported/Orthopedic%20Emergencies%20-%20Joshua%20Crum.pdf

Dean, C., Hatch, R. L., & Pauly, K. R. (2016, August 9). Calcaneal fractures. *UpToDate.* Retrieved from https://www.uptodate.com/contents/calcaneus-fractures?source=search_result&search=calcaneal+fracture&selectedTitle=1%7E18

Fleischman, R. J., & Ma, O. (2016). Trauma in the elderly. In D. M. Cline, O. Ma, G. D. Meckler, J. Stapczynski, J. E. Tintinalli, & D. M. Yealy (Eds.), *Tintinalli's emergency medicine: A comprehensive study guide* (8th ed., pp. 1688–1691). Dallas, TX: American College of Emergency Physicians. Retrieved from http://accessemergencymedicine.mhmedical.com/content.aspx?bookid=1658&Sectionid=109445304

Weinstein, S. L., & Yelin, E. H. (2016, December 15). The burden of musculoskeletal diseases in the United States. Retrieved from http://www.boneandjointburden.org

Williams, D. S. (2009). Orthopedic emergencies. Retrieved from https://fhs.mcmaster.ca/surgery/documents/OrthopaedicEmergenciesof23Sep2009byDrDaleWilliams.pdf

Yelin, E. H. (2016, December 16). The burden of musculoskeletal diseases in the United States. Retrieved from http://www.boneandjointburden.org

■ PEDIATRIC EMERGENCIES

Rachel Tkaczyk

Overview

In 2010, the Centers for Disease Control and Prevention (CDC) database reported a total of 129.8 million emergency department visits in the United States. Of those visits, 25.5 million visits consisted of patients younger than 15 years, and an additional 20.7 million visits were patients between 15 and 24 years (Centers for Disease Control and Prevention, 2012). When it comes to the emergency room setting, there is not one universal definition as to what constitutes a "pediatric emergency." Subsequently, levels of care and the associated acuity in the emergency setting often differ among various institutions. Despite varying definitions and management techniques, the approach to identifying, assessing, and treating a pediatric emergent situation must be systematic. In order to achieve successful outcomes, the medical staff must be equipped with the knowledge to appropriately recognize and treat all pediatric emergency scenarios.

Background

Pediatric patients, who accounted for 17.4% of the emergency room visits in 2010 in the United States, present unique challenges that can ultimately hinder an emergency department's ability to provide the best possible care (Macias, 2013). Obtaining a complete history and performing a thorough assessment in the pediatric population can be accompanied by many unique challenges. Particularly in the emergency setting, the time constraint alone can elicit a sense of urgency that affects the overall quality of the patient intake and triage. This section explores several challenges that may be encountered during the evaluation and treatment of pediatric emergencies.

One identified difficulty when attempting to obtain an accurate history is the lack of an established rapport with the patients and their family. This can contribute to an incomplete, and often, inadequate extraction of critical information. Oftentimes, obtaining history is not given enough time and a therapeutic relationship is not established. This is problematic as the health history typically provides 85% of the information that is needed in order for the medical team to make a diagnosis (Reuter-Rice & Bolick, 2012). As stated previously, another barrier is the element, and possibly lack thereof, of time. In the trauma scenario, resuscitation will take precedence over the acquisition of a health history. However, it is important to realize that this does not negate the significant of the health history. Rather it is necessary to recognize the limitation and employ strategies to overcome (Reuter-Rice & Bolick, 2012).

There are several key elements of the pediatric emergent intake. While obtaining a history is clearly significant, another key element is the pediatric assessment and physical examination (Halden et al., 2014). Both components are usedin order to answer the critical questions. Is there an immediate life threat? In terms of severity, where does the patient fall? Will the patient need admission? What evidence supports the providers' differential diagnoses? In summary, the goal of assessing the pediatric patient in the emergent setting is to determine the severity of the situation and whether or not treatment is indicated. Oftentimes, this requires the initial assessment but also reassessment. When it comes

to the overall treatment of a seriously ill or injured child, the goal is to provide a systematic approach that is consistent across all institutions. The recommended model for all pediatric life-support courses consists of the general assessment, secondary assessment, and tertiary assessment (American Heart Association, 2015).

For example, in the case of a pediatric patient who presents with concern for sepsis, there are four physical exam signs that are recommended for early detection of pediatric septic shock, before hypotension occurs. They include alteration in mental status, decreased capillary refill, cold extremities, and peripheral pulse quality (Halden et al., 2014). These changes can be subtle, particularly to the provider who does not have an established baseline for a patient as a primary care provider may have had (Reuter-Rice & Bolick, 2012). Research has shown that several barriers to this practice of frequent reassessment exist and include a lack of time, increased workload, and at times a lack of nursing knowledge specific to the situation (Pretorius, Searle, & Marshall, 2014). This again reinforces the need to provide a systematic and standardized approach to assessment of the pediatric patient. With those skills, the medical team will be equipped with the tools to recognize signs of impending respiratory distress, failure, and shock. Without the ability to assess and intervene quickly, pediatric patients are at greater risk and can progress to cardiopulmonary failure that can lead to arrest (AHA, 2015).

Clinical Aspects

ASSESSMENT

In order to the meet the need for high-quality care in this population, several health care systems have integrated quality improvement methods to improve access, safety, and ultimately better the care delivered to this patient population (Macias, 2013). As discussed, one of the barriers to obtaining a thorough history from the beginning of the medical course is the lack of a developed therapeutic relationship with the patient and family. The American Academy of Pediatrics and the American College of Emergency Physicians continually recognizes the patient and family as significant decision-makers in the patient's overall care. Patient- and family-centered care is a method in health care that recognizes the essential role of the patient and family. The goal is to focus on and implement collaboration among the patient, family, and medical professionals (American Academy of Pediatrics, 2006).

NURSING INTERVENTIONS, MANAGEMENT, AND IMPLICATIONS

The American Academy of Pediatrics (AAP) and American College of Emergency Physicians have issued several recommendations to better improve the patient and medical team therapeutic relationship, which comes with its own emergency room-specific challenges. They continue to reinforce the necessity to validate a family and patient's concerns. The family member should be given the option to be present for all aspects of their child's care while in the emergency room. It is also essential that information be provided to the family during all interventions, despite their decision to be present or not (AAP, 2006).

OUTCOMES

In addition to information gathering, one of the key elements to improved outcomes in the pediatric emergency setting is early recognition and intervention. As stated previously, the sense of urgency and time constraint, increased work load, and inadequate knowledge can contribute to poor outcomes. Objective observation was recently studied in order to assess strengths and weaknesses during a pediatric resuscitation. The overall goal was to assess how well the medical providers in a pediatric emergency room adhered to cardiopulmonary resuscitation (CPR) guidelines during a resuscitation. During this study, 33 children received CPR under video recording. The results demonstrated appropriate compression rate, duration of pauses, and compression depth. It did show that there tended to be hyperventilation as well as the inability to coordinate the compression–ventilation ratio during the resuscitation. The overall recommendations included various training modalities for CPR among staff and evaluation of its effectiveness (Donoghue, 2015). This particular study is only one example of how a pediatric institution implemented a quality initiative to assess potential limitations and areas that required additional education. It demonstrates an overall approach to identify barriers to care, assess any shortcomings, and ultimately provide education to correct and improve certain practices.

Summary

The pediatric population is unique in many aspects when compared to the adult population, particularly in the emergency care setting. There are several challenges that the medical team faces, beginning from the moment the patient enters into their care and extends throughout treatment. Several strategies can be utilized in order to overcome those challenges and provide optimal care. It is of paramount importance that the medical team identifies any barriers to obtaining a thorough history and performing an in-depth assessment. Continued focus on ever-evolving education is also essential. With a consistent and systematic approach to pediatric emergency care, outcomes continue to improve.

American Academy of Pediatrics. (2006). Patient and family centered care and the role of the emergency physician providing care to a child in the emergency department. *Pediatrics, 118*(5), 2242–2244.

American Heart Association. (2015). *Pediatric advanced life support.* Elk Grove, IL: American Academy of Pediatrics.

Centers for Disease Control and Prevention. (2012). Reasons for emergency room use among U.S. children: National Health Interview Survey. Retrieved from https://www.cdc.gov/nchs/products/databriefs/db160.htm

Donoghue, A., Hsieh, T. C., Myers, S., Mak, A., Sutton, R., & Nadkarmi, V. (2015). Videographic assessment of cardiopulmonary resuscitation quality in the pediatric emergency department. *Resuscitation, 91,* 19–25. doi.10.1016/j.resuscitation.2015.03.007

Halden, F., Scoot, H. F., Donoghue, A. J., Gaieski, D. F., Marchese, R. F., & Mistry, R. D. (2014). Effectiveness of physical exam signs for early detection of critical illness in pediatric systemic inflammatory response syndrome. *BMC Emergency Medicine, 14*(24). doi:10.1186/1471-227X-14-24

Macias, C. (2013). Quality improvement in pediatric emergency medicine. *Academic Pediatrics, 13*(6), S61–S68.

Pretorius, A., Searle, J., & Marshall, B. (2014). Barriers and enablers to emergency department nurses' management of patients' pain. *Pain Management Nursing, 16*(3), 372–379. doi:10.1016/j.pmn.2014.08.015

Reuter-Rice, K. & Bolick, B. (2012). *Pediatric acute care: A guide for interprofessional practice* (1st ed.). Burlington, Ontario, Canada: Jones & Bartlett.

■ PSYCHIATRIC DISORDERS: SUICIDE, HOMICIDE, PSYCHOSIS

George Byron Peraza-Smith
Yolanda Bone

Overview

A psychiatric disorder is a syndrome characterized by a clinically significant disturbance in a person's cognition, emotional regulation, and/or behavior that reflects a dysfunction in the psychological, biological, or developmental processes underlying mental functioning (American Psychiatric Association (APA), 2009). Psychiatric disorders are accompanied with significant distress in social, occupational, or other important life activities. Suicide, homicide, and psychosis are common psychiatric disorders requiring emergency services. The Centers for Disease Control and Prevention (CDC, 2011) reported that there were an estimated 4.5 million emergency department visits nationwide with patients having a primary psychiatric disorder, accounting for 3.5% of all emergency department visits. Nursing care for psychiatric disorder emergencies is focused primarily on conducting a risk assessment, stabilizing clinical significant disturbances, and maintaining patient/staff safety.

Background

Over the past 40 years, psychiatric services for patients with psychiatric disorders have become increasingly deinstitutionalized (American College of Emergency Physicians, 2014). Services have shifted away from inpatient facilities to community-based care. Today, there are approximately 28 adult psychiatric beds per 100,000 populations with a projected need of 39 adult psychiatric beds per 100,000 populations to provide adequate services (Fuller Torrey, 2016). The resources to adequately treat psychiatric disorders in the patient with psychiatric disorders have not kept pace with the growing demand for services. This has forced patients to seek other avenues for treatment, including outpatient facilities, outpatient medical management groups, and community resources. Incarceration has become a default placement for the treatment and housing for persons with psychiatric disorders.

The insufficient numbers of psychiatric beds, inadequate funding for community-based programs, and insufficient access to treatment has caused many individuals with psychiatric disorders to utilize the emergency department for crisis management. Estimates are that the U.S. emergency departments collectively experience over 136 million patients annually (CDC, 2016) with an estimated 3% to 5% of those encounters being primarily for a psychiatric disorder (CDC, 2013, 2011). Psychiatric emergencies for suicide, homicide, and psychosis that could have been better managed and treated in the community are now overburdening emergency departments.

Suicide is the tenth leading cause of death in the United States with nearly 42,000 deaths by suicide in 2014 (CDC, 2015b). The American Foundation for Suicide Prevention (2017) categorizes suicide risk in three factors: (a) health factors (mental health condition, substance abuse disorder, chronic medical condition or pain); (b) environmental factors (overwhelming stressful life event, prolonged stressful situation, access to lethal means, exposure to another person's suicide or violence); and (c) historical factors (previous suicide attempt, family history of suicide). A visit to an emergency department may be the suicidal patient's last effort or hope for intervention. Emergency department nurses should use a comprehensive approach to suicide prevention. The nurse should ensure the patients safety, reinforce coping skills and provide the family/significant others emotional support.

Homicides by persons with mental health conditions have entered our national consciousness due to several highly publicized public shootings and murders covered in the media. Homicides in the United States accounted for 15,809 deaths in 2014 with five deaths per 100,000 populations (CDC, 2015a). Youth homicide in the United States is even more grave as the second leading cause of death among those aged 15 to 24 years and accounts for more deaths in this age group than cancer, heart disease, birth defects, influenza, diabetes and HIV combined (CDC, 2014). The emergency department nurse may be both the target of violence, as well as responsible for assessing the homicidal risk by an individual and implementing safety protocols to prevent homicides.

In a survey of more than 1,700 emergency physicians, three quarters reported seeing a patient at least once a shift requiring hospitalization for psychiatric treatment (American College of Emergency Physicians, 2016). Patients with psychosis who present to the emergency department exhibit varying clinical presentations including functional or toxic/metabolic psychosis, the behavioral side effects of medications, complications of substance abuse, and coexisting medical and psychiatric illnesses. Delirium and dementia are the most frequent nonmedication-related causes of psychosis seen in the emergency department. Caring for patients with psychosis confers special challenges because the history of these patients is often poor or unobtainable. In addition, patients with psychosis lack insight into their illness and may present with bizarre affect, agitation, and violent behavior. The emergency department nurse should ensure the safety of the patient with psychosis, manage the anxiety, identify potential causes for the psychosis, and provide the family/significant others with emotional support.

Clinical Aspects

Although it is the goal of all members of the health care team to provide improved outcome-oriented care to persons, nursing is unique in its holistic approach. Nursing views individuals, especially during crises, as a person with multiple variables influencing and driving the crisis. It is the goal of nursing to care for the patient while implementing safety measures for all involved.

ASSESSMENT

During psychiatric emergencies, such as risk of suicide and homicide and/or the psychotic patient, the person affected, family members, and care team members are at risk for injury. Assessments to evaluate risk are essential to identify problems and minimize risk to all. Nursing should use tools that assess at-risk individuals for appearance and atmosphere, behavior, communication, potential for danger, and environment (Wright & McGlen, 2012).

When assessing for appearance and atmosphere, the nurse should be observing the patient and ask himself or herself:

- How does the patient look?
- Are there signs of injury?
- Are there signs of alcohol or drugs?
- Is the patient making or averting eye contact?

With respect to behavior, how is the patient behaving? For example, is the patient guarded, engaging, fearful, angry, sad or exhibiting bizarre behavior? In addition, how does the patient communicate? Is the at-risk individual communicating at all? Does the person speaking coherently or are thoughts disorganized? Is the person responding to "voices"? Other observatory/mental questions nursing should consider are potential physical barriers such as equipment, furniture, doorways, and so on. These "barriers" have the potential to cause a dangerous environment for the at-risk individual leading to harm to self and/or others. Finally, nurses should assess the patient's environment. Where does the patient think he or she is? Does the emergency room/critical care environment affect the communication/response of the at-risk person? For the suicidal, homicidal, and/or psychotic patient,

nurses need to be conscious of the patient and staff; consequently, assessment measures do not end at the initial encounter. Rather, the assessment of the patient continues until the safety and stability of the patient are ensured.

NURSING INTERVENTIONS, MANAGEMENT, AND IMPLICATIONS

Psychiatric emergencies can cause anxiety for patients and staff alike. It is essential that emergency department nurses be aware of his or her own biases, concerns, and areas of weakness, to provide care that will ensure best outcomes. Complexities associated with at-risk patients present additional challenges to the nursing staff; consequently, causing potential delays in treatment or mismanagement of the patient experiencing a psychiatric emergency (Brosinksi & Riddle, 2015). Methods to improve upon potential anxiety measures for staff include providing education to lessen bias and improving outcomes.

OUTCOMES

Nursing interventions related to the at-risk individual involve care of the patient's physical needs, but also emotional needs. The prompt and accurate assessment skills of nursing are the most important intervention with respect to psychiatric emergencies. In addition, communication between nurse and patient is essential for patient–caregiver trust. In other words, the at-risk patient needs to feel safe, and trust within the health care relationship is necessary for the best outcome. Across health care settings, the goal of care is to improve the patient's health situation. This is challenging for the patient exercising a psychiatric emergency; however, usage of assessment tools, providing a safe environment for patient and staff, and nonthreatening communication can provide an atmosphere for which the patient's outcome will be improved and successful.

Summary

Emergency care settings are often used for nonemergent settings. However, due to many variables affecting the health care environment, such as lack of access to adequate care, patients seek care especially in emergent situations. Psychiatric emergencies, such as the suicidal, homicidal, and/or psychotic patient, seek or be brought for evaluation in an emergency department setting. Nursing staff should be attentive to assessment skills evaluating holistically the needs of the patient in crisis. Assessment should involve evaluating the safety of the at-risk patient, as well as the safety of team members. At the core of assessment is the need for nursing to engage in nonthreatening forms of communication to prevent escalation of crisis in order to assure improved outcomes.

American College of Emergency Physicians (2016). Wait times for care and hospital beds growing drastically for psychiatric emergency patients. Retrieved from http://newsroom.acep.org/2016-10-17-Waits-for-Care-and-Hospital-Beds-Growing-Dramatically-for-Psychiatric-Emergency-Patients

ACEP Emergency Medicine Practice Committee. (2014). Care of the psychiatric patient in the emergency department—A review of the literature. Retrieved from https://www.acep.org

American Foundation for Suicide Prevention. (2017). Risk factors and warning signs. Retrieved from https://afsp.org/about-suicide/risk-factors-and-warning-signs

American Psychiatric Association. (2013). *Diagnostic and statistical manual of mental disorders: DSM-5.* Arlington, VA: American Psychiatric Publishing.

Brosinski, C., & Riddell, A. (2015). Mitigating nursing biases in management of intoxicated and suicidal patients. *Journal of Emergency Nursing, 41*(4), 296–299.

Centers for Disease Control and Prevention. (2011). National hospital ambulatory medical care survey: 2010 emergency department summary tables. Retrieved from http://www.cdc.gov/nchs/data/ahcd/nhamcs_emergency/2010_ed_web_tables.pdf

Centers for Disease Control and Prevention. (2013, June). Emergency department visits by patients with mental health disorders—North Carolina, 2008–2010. *Morbidity and Mortality Weekly Report, 62*(23), 469–472.

Centers for Disease Control and Prevention. (2014). Deaths, percent of total deaths, and death rates for the 15 leading causes of death in 5-year age groups, by race and sex: United States, 2014. Retrieved from https://www.cdc.gov/nchs/data/dvs/lcwk1_2014.pdf?ncid=txtlnkusaolp00000618

Centers for Disease Control and Prevention. (2015a). Assaults or homicides. Retrieved from http://www.cdc.gov/nchs/fastats/homicide.htm

Centers for Disease Control and Prevention. (2015b). Leading causes of death. Retrieved from http://www.cdc.gov/nchs/fastats/leading-causes-of-death.htm

Centers for Disease Control and Prevention. (2016). Emergency department visits. Retrieved from http://www.cdc.gov/nchs/fastats/emergency-department.htm

Fuller Torrey, E. (2016). A dearth of psychiatric beds. Psychiatric Times. Retrieved from http://www.psychiatrictimes.com/psychiatric-emergencies/dearth-psychiatric-beds

Wright, K., & McGlen, I. (2012). Mental health emergencies: Using a structured assessment framework. *Nursing Standard, 27*(7), 48–56.

■ RESPIRATORY EMERGENCIES

Dustin Spencer

Overview

As a result of pulmonary insult or other systemic disorders, acute respiratory failure is a leading cause of emergent evaluation and treatment in the emergency department and results in a significant percentage of intensive care unit admissions (Dries, 2013). Any injury or illness that results in the inability of the respiratory system to meet the oxygenation, ventilation, or metabolic demands of the body can lead to acute respiratory failure. Acute respiratory failure from pneumonia was responsible for more than 920,000 deaths of children younger than 5 years old worldwide in 2015 (World Health Organization [WHO], 2016). Estimates of the mortality associated with acute respiratory failure approaches nearly 50% in the United States (Villar et al., 2011). Therefore, nursing care for patients with acute respiratory failure requires vigilant assessment, airway management, and urgent interventions to maintain adequate tissue respiration.

Background

Respiratory failure can result from a variety of infective, mechanical, or functional disturbances primarily within the pulmonary, neurologic, cardiovascular, or musculoskeletal system. Fundamentally, each of these cause a mismatch between the demand for oxygen and carbon dioxide exchange and the body's ability to meet these needs (Dries, 2013). In order to maintain adequate exchange of oxygen and carbon dioxide there are several requisite factors. The first factor is to ensure that there is adequate oxygen available to meet the patient's demands. The second factor is the assessment of the patient's ventilation status, in terms of adequate depth to allow for alveolar diffusion. The third factor is adequate pulmonary perfusion and impaired gas exchange. Any illness or injury that impacts one or more of these factors can lead to respiratory insufficiency and acute respiratory failure (Dries, 2013).

Although a number of chronic conditions can cause a patient to experience respiratory distress, the majority of these patients have a history of chronic obstructive pulmonary disorders (Centers for Disease Control and Prevention [CDC], n.d.). Because these patients are perpetually in a state of compensation, even typically minor illnesses can precipitate an exacerbation of their chronic condition that taxes their ability to further compensate, leading to acute respiratory failure (Dries, 2013). Although children do not typically meet criteria for a diagnosis of chronic obstructive pulmonary disorder (COPD), respiratory failure remains one of the top 10 causes of pediatric death in the United States (CDC, n.d.). The cause of death in patients with cystic fibrosis is respiratory failure in 80% of cases (Seckel, 2013).

Clinical Aspects

ASSESSMENT

Early identification of the patient with impending respiratory failure is vital to the nurse's ability to intervene and facilitate optimal outcomes. This begins with a systematic approach to the assessment process. This is most often discussed in the context of pediatric patients but applies to every patient the nurse will encounter. The assessment of patients with respiratory compromise begins as the nurse enters the patient's room. A visual inspection of the patient's condition allows the nurse to form an overall impression of the patient's appearance, circulation to the skin, and work of breathing. This general impression allows the nurse to stratify the initial urgency with which interventions need to be implemented.

Visible signs and symptoms that should signal to the nurse that emergent intervention is needed would include shallow respirations, tachypnea, bradypnea, apnea, abnormal respiratory patterns, audible breathing sounds, cyanosis, pallor, retractions, lethargy, and coma. Any of these should prompt the nurse to immediately intervene to improve oxygen ventilation and respiration while working to determine the cause of the respiratory failure. Milder symptoms in adults may be addressed less urgently; however, in children these may indicate impending collapse and should be monitored carefully.

After the initial impression, the nurse will then collect a focused history and physical exam. The nurse will be alert to items in the history that identify risk factors associated with respiratory failure such as tobacco use, occupational exposures, inhalant use, infectious disease exposure, medical history, family history of respiratory disorders. Mnemonics, such as OPQRST (onset, provocation, quality, severity, timing) or COLDSPA (character, onset, location, duration, severity, pattern and associated factors) can be beneficial in focusing the history without compromising completeness.

The focused physical exam should be done initially and then periodically throughout the course of the patient's treatment. At a minimum this should be repeated whenever there is a change in status or vital signs, after therapeutic interventions, hourly in the emergency department, and every 4 hours in the intensive care setting. The nurse should use inspection, palpation, and percussion along with auscultation to thoroughly assess the patient's respiratory system. This assessment is essential in early identification of developing or worsening respiratory distress. Although auscultation is often the hallmark assessment technique, using a combination of these techniques is required to comprehensively identify subtle changes in condition. Percussion can clue the nurse into a developing pneumothorax, hemothorax, or lung consolidation, which can be treated conservatively if addressed early and can be life-threatening if not. Palpation is often the only way to recognize subcutaneous emphysema, which may be a sign of impending fatal airway injury. Findings, especially interval changes, should be documented and addressed with the clinician(s) responsible for overseeing the patient's care.

In addition to physical and history examination, it is important to collect data on the oxygenation and perfusion status of the patient. The gold standard for assessing respiratory function is the arterial blood gas (ABG) measurement. This test quantifies the respiratory status of the patient and provides values for pH, dissolved arterial oxygen and carbon monoxide (PaO_2 and $PaCO_2$), and bicarbonate (HCO_3) in the arterial system. Other noninvasive measures of respiratory status include exhaled carbon dioxide measurement ($ETCO_2$), which is graphically represented as capnography, pulse oximetry (SpO_2), chest x-ray, or CT scan (Pierce, 2013).

NURSING INTERVENTIONS, MANAGEMENT, AND IMPLICATIONS

Management of respiratory failure focuses initially on slowing the progression of the illness rather than on correcting the underlying cause of the failure. After assisting the patient into a position that facilitates optimal air exchange, and providing airway patency through positioning or suctioning of secretions, the application of oxygen is often the first intervention (Pierce, 2013). Oxygen application often provides rapid improvement, is quick and easy to apply, easy to adjust, and can be titrated to meet the needs of the patient either through flow rate or delivery device selection. Depending on the patient's past medical history, age, and diagnosis, the oxygen level can be titrated to facilitate an SpO_2 target of as low as 90% and as high as 98% (Dries, 2013).

A number of medication classes are used to correct respiratory symptoms. Inhaled beta agonists are used in almost every case of respiratory distress associated with obstructive illness to facilitate bronchial smooth muscle relaxation. Anticholinergic agents are used in conjunction with the beta-agonists to facilitate long-term relief. There is significant data supporting the use of corticosteroids to reduce the associated inflammation in these patients as well. Antibiotic medications are used to treat infective causes using the clinician knowledge of the national, regional, and local infectious disease prevalence data (Dries, 2013).

Cardiovascular causes of respiratory failure typically are those associated with low-volume states or emboli. Treatment for these conditions remains focused on correcting the underlying cause(s). Vascular volume replacement with crystalloid solutions, blood and blood products, and vasoactive medications can correct absolute and relative low-volume states. Thrombolytic medications can be used to correct pulmonary and/or cardiac thrombosis and emboli, which are impeding the delivery of blood to the pulmonary tissues and therefore limiting alveolar gas exchange (Seckel, 2013).

Noninvasive positive pressure ventilation (NPPV) devices are used to assist patients who are in nontraumatic respiratory distress and prevent their further decline to respiratory failure. These devices deliver continuous positive pressure to the airway in a cyclical fashion allowing for inspiration and exhalation while limiting the collapse of the distal alveoli. This is a significant cause of respiratory failure in patients with COPD. Continuous pressure facilitates the movement of fluid across the alveolar membranes in pulmonary edema secondary to congestive heart failure (CHF) and other conditions (Goodacre et al., 2014).

Nurses work within the team to facilitate or perform endotracheal intubation when other measures have failed to prevent further decline or are contraindicated. Once the decision to intubate has been made, it will be vital for the nurse to be prepared to assist with not only the intubation but also with rescue airway techniques that may become necessary if complications arise. Immediately after the patient has been intubated, the nurse ensures the placement of the tube within the trachea through combination of lung assessments and chest x-ray, along with colorimetric confirmation devices and/or $ETCO_2$ measurement. Documentation

of the tube size, depth, and confirmation techniques are required as they are useful during reassessments.

OUTCOMES

The inability to maintain adequate oxygenation can be a significantly frightening and anxiety-inducing state for the patient. It is important for the care team to recognize this potential complication and minimize its impact. Another potential complication that intubated patients are at risk for is that of ventilator-associated pneumonia. Each facility has prevention protocols in place that the nurse needs to follow so that the patient's risk is minimized.

Summary

Acute respiratory failure is a common condition treated in the emergent and inpatient setting. Using a systematic approach to the identification and treatment of these conditions is effective in minimizing the cascade of complications that can lead to mortality and morbidity. The main focus must always remain on correcting this underlying problem and restoring the body's ability to maintain homeostasis while addressing emergent findings.

Centers for Disease Control and Prevention. (n.d.). 10 leading causes of death by age group, United States 2014. Retrieved from https://www.cdc.gov/injury/images/lc-charts/leading_causes_of_death_age_group_2014_1050w760h.gif

Dries, D. (2013). *Fundamental critical care support*. Mount Prospect, IL: Society of Critical Care Medicine.

Goodacre, S., Stevens, J., Pandor, A., Poku, E., Ren, S., Cantrell, A., . . . Plaisance, P. (2014). Prehospital noninvasive ventilation for acute respiratory failure: systematic review, network meta-analysis, and individual patient data meta-analysis. *Academy of Emergency Medicine, 21*, 960–970.

Pierce, L. (2013). Ventilatory assistance. In M. Sole, D. Klein, & M. Moseley (Eds.), *Introduction to critical care nursing* (6th ed., pp. 170–219). St. Louis, MO: Elsevier.

Seckel, M. (2013). Acute respiratory failure. In M. Sole, D. Klein, & M. Moseley (Eds.), *Introduction to critical care nursing* (6th ed., pp. 400–431). St. Louis, MO: Elsevier.

Villar, J., Blanco, J., Santos-Bouza, A., Blanch, L., Ambros, A., Gandia, F., . . . Kacmarek, R. (2011, December). The ALIEN study: Incidence and outcome of acute respiratory distress syndrome in the are of lung protective ventilation. *Journal of Intensive Care Medicine, 37*(12), 1932–1941.

World Health Organization. (2016). Media centre: Pneumonia. Retrieved from http://www.who.int/mediacentre/factsheets/fs331/en

■ RETURN OF SPONTANEOUS CIRCULATION WITH HYPOTHERMIA INITIATION

Laura Stark Bai

Overview

Therapeutic hypothermia, also referred to as *targeted temperature management (TTM)*, is the intentional reduction of a patient's body temperature after return of spontaneous circulation (ROSC) after cardiac arrest (Deckard & Elbright, 2011). Although survival rates from cardiac arrest vary based on cause of arrest, setting of arrest (within or outside of a hospital), and response by bystanders or medically trained personnel, studies show that therapeutic hypothermia helps to improve survival and protect neurological function in patients with ROSC. Nursing care of patients receiving therapeutic hypothermia after ROSC is complex and requires an intensive care setting in order to manage these patients safely and effectively for optimal outcomes.

Background

More than 326,000 adult cardiac arrests and over 6,300 pediatric cardiac arrests were evaluated by emergency medical services (EMS) outside of a hospital setting in America in 2014 (Sidhu, Schulman, & McEvoy, 2016). The average survival rate to hospital discharge for these arrests was 10.6% for adults and 7.3% for pediatrics and, of these survivors, only 8.3% of adults had good neurologic function (Newman, 2014). Therapeutic hypothermia after ROSC is consistently shown to improve survival rates and outcomes for these patients.

The concept of lowering body temperature was first explored by Dr. James Currie in the 1700s. However, its use in cardiac arrest was first presented in the 1930s with the first study being published in 1958, which created a foundation for this neuroprotective treatment (Sidhu et al., 2016). In 2002, two studies were published which established that therapeutic hypothermia improves neurological outcomes and should be a standard of care in patients with ROSC after cardiac arrest due to ventricular arrhythmias, and a viable option for patients with ROSC after arrest from a nonshockable rhythm (Scirica, 2013).

The guidelines from the American Heart Association (2015) regarding TTM in postcardiac arrest care recommend that "all comatose (i.e., lacking meaningful response to verbal commands) adult patients with ROSC after cardiac arrest should have TTM, with a target temperature between 32 degrees Celsius and 36 degrees Celsius selected and achieved, then maintained constantly for at least 24 hours" (p. 15). This is an increase in targeted temperature range from the previous guideline, which was 32°C to 34°C for 12 to 24 hours. Recent studies show that there are similar outcomes for patients who are cooled to 36°C and 33°C, so clinicians can make decisions based on preference or other considerations.

There are three physiologic processes that contribute toward neurologic injury after cardiac arrest. Briefly, these phases are initial lack of tissue profusion leading to cellular death, cerebral edema, and disruption of the blood–brain barrier; injury from reprofusion with production of free radicals; and an inflammatory response, which further worsens cellular injury (Sidhu et al., 2016). Therapeutic hypothermia is effective in preventing or reducing neurologic injury by preventing or counteracting these processes. It works by stabilizing the blood–brain barrier, suppressing inflammation to reduce cerebral edema, and decreasing the brain's need for oxygen by reducing cerebral metabolism (Deckard & Ebright, 2011).

Prognosis following ROSC after cardiac arrest remains a challenge, as a majority of patients expire due to neurologic complications (Scirica, 2013). Although study results vary, the benefits of therapeutic hypothermia for patients who achieved ROSC after cardiac arrest from a shockable rhythm (ventricular tachycardia or ventricular fibrillation) are evident in the literature. It is consistently shown that there is a reduction in short-term mortality and neurologic issues in patients who receive therapeutic hypothermia. However, the evidence is still conflicting for long-term benefits of therapeutic hypothermia and for patients who receive therapeutic hypothermia after ROSC from nonshockable rhythms.

Clinical Aspects

ASSESSMENT

The care of patients undergoing therapeutic hypothermia is complex and requires intensive monitoring by nurses to assess for complications of this treatment. Nurses must closely monitor vital signs to assess for proper control over body temperature during initial cooling, the first 24 hours, and after rewarming.

Electrolyte levels must also be monitored to assess for fluid and electrolyte shifts that may lead to arrhythmias. Cardiac monitoring is also important for this reason. Glucose levels must be closely checked for hyperglycemia, since therapeutic hypothermia may cause insulin resistance. Regular neurologic assessments are challenging, but are required to assess for level of sedation to control shivering and prevent rewarming. Skin integrity should be assessed regularly for breakdown. Nurses must also closely monitor for bleeding and coagulation levels, as hypothermia can lead to platelet dysfunction. Finally, nurses must closely monitor and titrate intravenous medications as needed to meet therapeutic ranges, such as vasopressors, antiarrhythmics, electrolyte replacement therapies, fluids, and insulin.

NURSING INTERVENTIONS, MANAGEMENT, AND IMPLICATIONS

Patients are at risk for multiple complications due to therapeutic hypothermia. Because this treatment suppresses the body's inflammatory response, patients are at increased risk for infection. Vigilant observation of vital signs, hand hygiene, and proper aseptic technique will help to reduce the incidence of infection. These patients are also susceptible to ventilator-acquired pneumonia due to decreased functioning of respiratory cilia and gastric hypomotility. Oral care, suctioning, and elevating the head of bed above 30° will help reduce incidence. Preventative measures should also be taken to avoid skin breakdown, such as repositioning and use of barrier products, as hypothermia may lead to vasoconstriction and reduced blood flow. Patients are at risk for bleeding due to platelet dysfunction and may require transfusion.

There are three phases of therapeutic hypothermia during which core body temperature should be closely monitored. First, the induction phase aims to quickly lower the patient's core body temperature to 32°C to 36°C through several modalities, including ice packs, noninvasive cooling devices, infusion of cooled fluids, or iced lavage. During this time, sedation and neuromuscular blockade are initiated to prevent shivering (which would cause rewarming). Next is the maintenance phase, in which the target body temperature is maintained for approximately 24 hours through use of the previously discussed cooling techniques. The rewarming phase is the final phase, during which the core body temperature is slowly increased at a rate of 0.15°C to 0.5°C per hour. This is done slowly to prevent electrolyte shifts that would cause life-threatening arrhythmias. During these three phases, nurses have the vital role of monitoring the patient's body temperature and assessing for and preventing complications.

Although therapeutic hypothermia has strong support from the research in use for patients with ROSC after cardiac arrest, this technique is only utilized 2% to 6% of the time (Sidhu et al., 2016). Consistent use of therapeutic hypothermia in patients with ROSC after cardiac arrest caused by shockable rhythms can improve neurologic functioning and short-term outcomes.

OUTCOMES

The expected outcome of evidence-based nursing care in patients receiving therapeutic hypothermia after ROSC following cardiac arrest is improved neurologic functioning and short-term outcomes from patients who had a shockable rhythm. Quick action to begin cooling after ROSC with close monitoring of vital signs, cardiac rhythm, and electrolyte levels by the nurse is a vital part of this process. Prevention of skin breakdown, bleeding, ventilator-acquired pneumonia, and bloodstream infections is also vital in the success of this treatment. Studies confirm that when this treatment is used according to the American Heart Association guidelines, there will be an improvement in mortality rates and neurologic outcomes.

Summary

Therapeutic hypothermia is the standard treatment for patients with ROSC after cardiac arrest caused by a shockable rhythm. When implemented correctly immediately after ROSC, for over 50 years studies have shown that this medical treatment improves short-term outcomes by decreasing mortality and reducing neurologic damage. Nurses play a crucial role in the success of this process through close patient monitoring, prevention and treatment of complications, and detection of alterations in patient status. Research on the effect of this treatment in patients with cardiac arrest caused by nonshockable rhythm is required.

American Heart Association. (2015). Highlights of the 2015 American Heart Association guidelines update for CPR and ECC. Retrieved from https://eccguidelines.heart. org/wp-content/uploads/2015/10/2015-AHA-Guidelines -Highlights-English.pdf

Deckard, M. E., & Ebright, P. R. (2011). Therapeutic hypothermia after cardiac arrest: What, why, who, and how.

American Nurse Today, 6(7). Retrieved from https://www.americannursetoday.com/therapeutic-hypothermia-after-cardiac-arrest-what-why-who-and-how

Newman, M. (2014). *AHA releases 2015 heart and stroke statistics*. Wexford, PA: Sudden Cardiac Arrest Foundation.

Scirica, B. (2013). Therapeutic hypothermia after cardiac arrest. *Circulation, 127*, 244–250.

Sidhu, S. S., Schulman, S. P., & McEvoy, J. W. (2016). Therapeutic hypothermia after cardiac arrest. *Current Treatment Options in Cardiovascular Medicine, 18*(5), 30.

■ SEIZURES

Eric Roberts

Overview

A seizure is an event during which neurons of the brain discharge in an abnormal fashion causing overstimulation and involuntary change in body movement, sensation, awareness, or behavior (Kornegay, 2016). The location and the number of neurons involved produce various clinical presentations. Morbidity, mortality, quality of life, and treatment modalities vary depending on the etiology, duration, and recurrence of seizures. A classification system helps individualize the approach used to evaluate and treat seizures.

Background

Seizures are classified as provoked when a precipitating event occurs within 7 days of seizure activity such as traumatic brain injury, tumors, metabolic disorders, electrolyte disturbance, withdrawal syndromes, and illness such as meningitis or encephalitis. Primary seizures are unprovoked and when recurrent are defined as epilepsy (Kornegay, 2016). Status epilepticus is an active seizure that lasts more than 5 minutes or, when seizures are consecutive, during which the patient does not regain consciousness. Refractory status epliepticus is a persistent seizure despite intravenous (IV) administration of two antiepileptic drugs (AEDs; Kornegay, 2016).

Focal, or partial, seizures are limited to a single hemisphere of the brain. These may have motor, sensory, autonomic symptoms, or produce hallucinations depending on location of the brain affected (Institute of Medicine [IOM], 2012). Simple focal seizures occur without impaired consciousness. Mentation is not affected and may be preceded by an aura (Kornegay, 2016). Complex partial seizures present with altered consciousness and may be associated with sensations of fear, paranoia, depression, elation, or ecstasy (Kornegay, 2016). These may be confused with psychological disorders.

Generalized seizures originate from both hemispheres of the brain and may or may not be subtle (IOM, 2012). They may present with isolated tonic contraction or stiffening of the body, clonic or rhythmic contractions, or atonic state with total loss of muscle tone (IOM, 2012). A tonic–clonic seizure is a severe type of seizure that starts with sudden loss of consciousness. Distinct tonic and clonic phases follow, with a postictal period of confusion. These patients will stop breathing during seizure activity and may experience anoxia, aspiration, or physical injury. Absence seizures are a type of generalized seizure with general, brief lapses in awareness typically lasting less than 10 seconds. Atypical presentations may last longer (IOM, 2012). Myoclonic seizures are characterized by sudden and brief jerking contractions involving any group of muscles and may resemble tremors (IOM, 2012).

It is estimated that 5.1 million people in the United States were diagnosed in 2013 with a seizure disorder. This represents 1.8% of the adult population and 1% of children (Centers for Disease Control and Prevention [CDC], 2016). Between 50,000 and 150,000 of these individuals experienced an episode of status epilepticus with resulting mortality rates of less than 3% in children, but as high as 30% in adults (Glauser et al., 2016). The cost associated with seizures includes $15.5 billion annually in direct medical expenses and additional indirect costs such as community services, loss in quality of life, and productivity (CDC, 2016). Epilepsy is responsive to treatment in an estimated 60% to 70% of cases; however, many people do not have access to treatment (IOM, 2012). A higher overall prevalence of epilepsy and incidence of persistent seizures has been demonstrated in patients with lower socioeconomic status (IOM, 2012).

The impact of epilepsy extends beyond the physical seizure activity. There may be significant impact to the quality of life, including limitations on daily activities, loss of the ability to drive, a social stigma affecting personal interactions, questions about living independently, ability to have children, as well as uncertainty about social and employment situations (IOM, 2012). Medication side effects are often a concern for patients as they may cause cognitive problems, impact energy levels, school performance, motor skill coordination, and impaired sexual function (IOM, 2012). Therefore, management goals for patients with epilepsy include preventing seizures in people at risk, eliminating side effects of treatments, and helping people with epilepsy achieve a high quality of life (IOM, 2012).

Clinical Aspects

ASSESSMENT

Assessment should include a detailed history. If the patient has a known seizure disorder, inquire about recent change in medication dose. Ask whether the patient is out of or stopped taking medicines because of adverse effects. Question sleep deprivation, increase in strenuous activity, recent infection, alcohol or substance abuse, and illness that may lead to electrolyte imbalance. These may precipitate seizure activity (Kornegay, 2016). A physical exam should focus on patency of the airway, adequacy of breathing, signs of hypoxia, and adventitious lung sounds suggestive of pulmonary aspiration. Inspect for signs of injury that may have occurred during the seizure such as tongue biting and shoulder injuries. A full neurologic examination and subsequent serial exams are important in evaluating for status epilepticus (Kornegay, 2016).

NURSING INTERVENTIONS, MANAGEMENT, AND IMPLICATIONS

Interventions should address both acute and chronic needs of the patient. There are currently three generations of AEDs that focus on controlling seizure recurrence of chronic disease by decreasing brain excitation (IOM, 2012). The older generations have been associated with increased side effects. However, newer medications may come at a higher cost and be less accessible to some patients. Particular consideration should be given to women of childbearing age, as many AEDs have been associated with a risk of neurodevelopmental impairments to the unborn child (IOM, 2012).

Sudden unexpected death in epilepsy (SUDEP) has been attributed to respiratory disturbances surrounding the acute seizure (Kennedy & Seyal, 2015). Brief seizures lasting fewer than 5 minutes carry the least risk of hypoxia and should receive supportive care. Maintain the airway, apply supplemental oxygen, monitor heart rhythm with EKG monitor, consider a toxicology screen, and check blood glucose levels (Glauser et al., 2016). Status epliepticus carries a high risk of hypoxia and requires IV medication in an attempt to stop seizure activity. Benzodizepines are the initial therapy of choice (Glauser, 2016). Refractory status epilepticus should be managed with IV doses of fosphenytoin, valproic acid, or levetriacetam (Glauser, 2016). For refractory seizures that last more than 40 minutes, an anesthesiologist should be contacted for administration of thiopental, pentobarbital, or propofol (Glauser, 2016).

It is important to educate the patients and their families about seizure triggers, safety concerns, and available community resources. Topics include environmental or lifestyle factors that may precipitate seizure activity such as lack of sleep, flashing lights, high fever, or excessive alcohol consumption (IOM, 2012). Patients need to understand that concurrent medications may alter AED levels or lower the seizure threshold such as antihistamines, stimulants, tramadol, and certain antibiotics (IOM, 2012). Teach patients that physical activities may place them and others at risk for injury if they experience a seizure while biking, skiing, driving, climbing, swimming, or even bathing (IOM, 2012). Patients should be familiar with community resources such as self-management programs, counseling, school-related support, and transportation services. Patients may not be permitted to operate a motor vehicle until well controlled. This education may improve quality of life.

OUTCOMES

Because of medication side effects, noncompliance concerns, and refractory seizures, many alternative treatment modalities have been considered to treat seizures with varying degree of empirical support and clinical outcomes. There is reliable evidence to suggest that ketogenic diets, vagal nerve stimulators, and surgical interventions may reduce seizure activity in in select populations (Martin, Jackson, & Cooper, 2016; Panebianco, Rigby, Westion, & Marson, 2015; West et al., 2015). There is weak evidence to suggest that yoga, transcranial magnetic stimulation, and deep brain stimulation may have positive effects of reducing seizure activity (Chen, Spencer, Weston, & Nolan, 2016; Panebianco, Sridharan, & Ramarathnam, 2015; Sprengers, Vonck, Carrette, Marson, & Boon, 2014). Modalities that have potential application but lack empirical support and require further study include the use of melatonin, acupuncture, and cannabis (Brigo, Igwe, & Del Felice, 2016; Cheuk & Wong, 2014; Gloss & Vickrey, 2014). Applying evidence-based practice may help guide treatment plans for individuals who struggle to manage their chronic disease.

Summary

Seizures may present with a wide range of physical manifestations. A key to evaluating seizures is soliciting a detailed health history. Seizure management should focus on supportive care during self-limiting seizures, strategies to stop active seizures in status epilepeticus, and mechanisms for preventing recurrence in chronic seizure disorders. Treatment is often effective, but must be individualized to meet the unique needs of the patient, while maintaining focus on safety and quality of life.

Brigo, F., Igwe, S., Del Felice, A. (2016). Melatonin as add-on treatment for epilepsy. *Cochrane Database of Systematic Reviews, 2016*(8). doi:10.1002/14615858. CD006967

Centers for Disease Control and Prevention. (2016). Epilepsy fast facts. Retrieved from https://www.cdc.gov/epilepsy/basics/fast-facts.htm

Chen, R., Spencer, D., Weston, J., & Nolan, S. (2016). Transcranial magnetic stimulation for the treatment of epilepsy. *Cochrane Database of Systematic Reviews, 2016*(8). doi:10.1002/14615858.CD011025

Cheuk, D., & Wong, V. (2014). Accupuncture for epilepsy. *Cochrane Database of Systematic Reviews, 2014*(5). doi:10.1002/14615858.CD005062

Gloss, D., & Vickrey, B. (2014). Cannabinoids for epilepsy. *Cochrane Database of Systematic Reviews, 2014*(3). doi:10.1002/14651858.CD009270

Glauser, T., Shinnar, S., Gloss, D., Alldredge, B., Arya, R., Bainbridge, J., . . . Treiman, D. (2016). Evidence-based guideline: Treatment of convulsive status epilpticus in children and adults: Report of the Guideline Committee of the American Epilepsy Society. *Epilepsy Currents, 16*(1), 48–61.

Institute of Medicine. (2012). *Epilepsy across the spectrum: Promoting health and understanding.* Washington, DC: National Academies Press.

Kennedy, J., & Seyal, M. (2015). Respiratory pathophysiology with seizures and implications for sudden unexpected death in epilepsy. *Journal of Clinical Neurophysiology, 32*, 10–13.

Kornegay, J. (2016). Seizures. In J. Tintinalli (Ed.), *Tintinalli's emergency medicine: A comprehensive study guide* (8th ed., pp. 1173–1178). New York, NY: McGraw-Hill.

Martin, K., Jackson, C., & Cooper, P. (2016). Ketogenic diet and other dietary treatments for epilepsy. *Cochrane Database of Systematic Reviews, 2016*(2). doi: 10.1002/14651858.CD001903

Panebianco, M., Sridharan, K., & Ramarathnam, S. (2015). Yoga for epilepsy. *Cochrane Database of Systematic Reviews, 2015*(5). doi:10.1002/14651858.CD001524

Panebianco, M., Rigby, A., Weston, J., & Marson, A. (2015). Vagus nerve stimulation for partial seizures. *Cochrane Database of Systematic Reviews, 2015*(4). doi:10.1002/14615858.CD002896

Sprengers, M., Vonck, K., Carrette, E., Marson, A., & Boon, P. (2014). Deep brain stimulation for epilepsy. *Cochrane Database of Systematic Reviews, 2014*(6). doi:10.1002/14615858.CD008497

West, S., Nolan, S., Cotton, J., Gandhi, S., Weston, J., Sudan, A., . . . Newton, R. (2015). Surgery for epilepsy. *Cochrane Database of Systematic Reviews, 2015*(7). doi:10.1002/14615858.CD010541

■ SEPSIS

Ronald L. Hickman, Jr.

Overview

Sepsis is a life-threatening bloodstream infection in which an infectious pathogen overwhelms the host's immune system and an injurious systemic inflammatory response results in a chain of events that include tissue injury, end-organ failure, and death (Singer et al., 2016). Adults with sepsis can manifest physiologic derangements in cellular metabolism, hemostasis, fluid and acid–base balance, and hemodynamic stability that can rapidly worsen without exposure to effective nursing and pharmacologic interventions (De Backer, Orbegozo Cortes, Donadello, & Vincent, 2014). Nursing care for adults with sepsis is focused on the early recognition of the deleterious effects of the systemic inflammatory response and the delivery of nursing interventions that optimize the effectiveness of an individual's immune system.

Background

According to the Centers for Disease Control and Prevention, sepsis affects more than 700,000 Americans per year and the projected annual incidence rate is estimated to steadily increase with the growing prevalence of older Americans (older than 65 years; Hall, Williams, Defrances, & Golosinkiy, 2011; Mayr, Yende, & Angus, 2014). In 2013, the clinical management of hospitalized adults with sepsis accounted for nearly $24 billion of annual health care costs, which makes sepsis one of the most costly life-threatening conditions in the United States (Torio & Moore, 2016). The clinical management of an adult with sepsis has shifted from the intensive care unit and recent studies indicate that more than 50% of adults with sepsis receive care outside of the intensive care unit (Mayr et al., 2014). Despite the ability to provide sepsis care outside of the intensive care unit, adults with a diagnosis of septic shock have a 40% to 70% likelihood of a sepsis-related death and those diagnosed with severe sepsis have between a 25% and 30% chance of a sepsis-related death while hospitalized (Gauer, 2013).

Although sepsis can affect adults across the life span and occur after an infection of any tissue, there are several known risk factors that predispose adults to sepsis. The most widely accepted risk factors that enhance an individual's susceptibility to sepsis are advanced age (greater than 65 years), immune system compromise (individuals with HIV infection, transplant recipients), comorbid conditions (diabetes mellitus, high blood pressure, and obesity), recent surgical procedures, and presence of indwelling catheters (Gauer, 2013; Petäjä, 2011). In addition, there is emerging evidence that sepsis disproportionately affects males; African Americans and Hispanics; and individuals who use tobacco, consume alcohol, and have nutrient-deficient diets (Mayr et al., 2014; Petäjä, 2011). It is suspected that disparities in sepsis outcomes are the result of complex interactions among the known risk factors, as well as social determinants of health and characteristics of health care organizations (Petäjä, 2011).

Diagnosis of sepsis is predicated on the presence of an infection and a minimum of two of the following indicators of systemic inflammatory response syndrome: body temperature (less than 96.8°F or greater than 100.4°F), heart rate greater than 90 beats/min, hyperventilation (respiratory rate greater than 20 breaths per minute), arterial partial pressure carbon dioxide (less than 32 mmHg [normal 35–45 mmHg]), and leukocyte count (less than 4,000/mm³ or greater than 12,000/mm³ [normal: 5,000–10,000/mm³]; Gauer, 2013).

In approximately 80% of adults with sepsis, the common sites of the localized infections are respiratory, genitourinary, gastrointestinal, and integumentary systems. Sepsis is the result of a host's exposure to an infectious pathogen, most commonly a bacterium (*Pseudomonas aeruginosa*, *Escherichia coli*, or *Staphylococcus aureus*) that overwhelms the host's local immune defenses and incites a systemic inflammatory response. Consequently, the pathogen enters into the host's bloodstream and proinflammatory mediators (interleukin [IL]-1, IL-6, and tumor necrosis factor [TNF]-) are released to recruit macrophages and lymphocytes to aid neutralization of the pathogen

(Gauer, 2013). However, the persistent release of proinflammatory mediators by macrophages provokes inflammation-induced tissue damage, associated hypoperfusion, and microemboli formation. Without intervention, the persistent release of proinflammatory mediators will facilitate the progression of sepsis toward *severe sepsis*, a state of diffuse tissue hypoxia and end-organ dysfunction, and *septic shock*, a state of cellular necrosis, impaired hemostasis, multiple end-organ failure, and hemodynamic instability due to hypovolemia.

Clinical Aspects

ASSESSMENT

A fundamental component of effective nursing care is an accurate record of the individual's history, physical assessment findings, and laboratory data. When obtaining a history from an adult suspected of having sepsis, the individual's age, onset of symptoms, functional status, comorbid conditions (immunosuppression, diabetes mellitus, HIV, chronic kidney disease), recent surgical or diagnostic procedures, and medications (glucocorticoids, chemotherapeutics, or antibiotics) should be documented and used to determine the individual's sepsis risk. The physical assessment should focus on changes in the following body systems: cardiovascular system (blood pressure, pulse pressure, heart rate, volume status, and cardiac output), respiratory system (tachypnea, oxygen saturation, diminished breath sounds, acid–base disturbance [metabolic acidosis in septic shock], and consolidation of the lungs on chest radiograph), renal system (oliguria with fluid intake, increased serum creatinine, and hypovolemia with edema), neurologic system (abnormal body temperature, altered mental status, and change in affect), and integumentary system (pallor, cyanosis, petechiae, or ecchymosis). Together, an accurate history and vigilant monitoring of changes in the individual's condition can result in the well-timed initiation of nursing care that can positively influence an individual's sepsis-related outcomes.

There is not a single laboratory test that confirms presence of sepsis or septic shock. To confirm the presence of an infection, cultures of the blood, urine, sputum, and any drainage should be collected to identify the causative pathogen. However, for more than one half of adults with sepsis, blood cultures are negative. In addition, assessment of the leukocyte count and differential profile of the leukocytes, thrombocyte count, hematocrit and hemoglobin levels, activated protein C levels, D-dimer levels, cytokine (IL-6) levels, chest radiographs, and arterial blood gases should be monitored (Gauer, 2013). Changes in the physical assessment findings, laboratory tests, and diagnostic data are indicative of sepsis recovery or progression.

NURSING INTERVENTIONS, MANAGEMENT, AND OUTCOMES

Nursing care of the adult with sepsis should principally focus on the prevention of the progression of sepsis to septic shock. Priority nursing-related problems include maintenance of adequate ventilation and perfusion to promote tissue respiration, fluid resuscitation to address volume contraction, identification of the causative pathogen and administration of pathogen-specific antibiotic therapy, pressure ulcer prophylaxis, and the provision of psychological support to the patient and family system.

OUTCOMES

The expected outcomes of evidence-based nursing care are centered on preventing the progression of sepsis to septic shock. Active surveillance for changes in physical assessment findings and laboratory testing can provide evidence of recovery or progression of sepsis that can alter the clinical trajectory of the adult with sepsis. Recent studies confirm that routine screening of high-risk adults for sepsis has resulted in the early identification and initiation of empiric antibiotic therapy that attenuated the injurious effects associated with a systemic inflammatory response. The implementation of fluid resuscitation bundles, supplemental oxygen or mechanical ventilation, inotropic or vasopressor drug therapy, and hemodynamic monitoring have been shown to improve tissue perfusion and maintain adequate cellular respiration (Gauer, 2013). The expected outcomes of effective nursing care should attenuate the effects of the systemic inflammatory response associated with sepsis and prevent end-organ dysfunction related to severe sepsis or septic shock.

Summary

Adults diagnosed with sepsis can progress rapidly from sepsis to septic shock in a matter of hours if they do not receive appropriate nursing care and pharmacotherapy. Early recognition of sepsis and initiation of evidence-based nursing care and pharmacologic therapy are crucial to derailing the vicious chain of events associated with sepsis in adults.

De Backer, D., Orbegozo Cortes, D., Donadello, K., & Vincent, J. L. (2014). Pathophysiology of microcirculatory dysfunction and the pathogenesis of septic shock. *Virulence*, 5(1), 73–79. doi:10.4161/viru.26482

Gauer, R. L. (2013). Early recognition and management of sepsis in adults: The first six hours. *American Family Physician*, 88(1), 44–53.

Hall, M., Williams, S., Defrances, C., & Golosinkiy, A. (2011). Inpatient care for septicemia or sepsis: A challenge for patients and hospitals. *NCHS Data Brief*, 62, 1–8.

Mayr, F. B., Yende, S., & Angus, D. C. (2014). Epidemiology of severe sepsis. *Virulence*, 5(1), 4–11. doi:10.4161/viru.27372

Petäjä, J. (2011). Inflammation and coagulation. An overview. *Thrombosis Research*, 127, S34–S37. doi:10.1016/S0049-3848(10)70153-5

Singer, M., Deutschman, C. S., Seymour, C., Shankar-Hari, M., Annane, D., Bauer, M., . . . Angus, D.C. (2016). The third international consensus definitions for sepsis and septic shock (sepsis-3). *Journal of the American Medical Association*, 315(8), 801–810. doi:10.1001/jama.2016.0287

Torio, C., & Moore, B. (2016, May). *National inpatient hospital costs: The most expensive condition by payer, 2013* (HCUP Statistical Brief No. 5). Rockville, MD: Agency for Healthcare Research and Quality.

■ SEXUAL ASSAULT

Patricia M. Speck
Diana K. Faugno
Rachell A. Ekroos
Melanie Gibbons Hallman
Sallie J. Shipman
Martha B. Dodd
Qiana A. Johnson
Stacey A. Mitchell

Overview

"Rape is a legal term . . . [referring] to any penetration of a body orifice (mouth, vagina, or anus) involving force or the threat of force or incapacity (i.e., associated with young or old age, cognitive or physical disability, or drug or alcohol intoxication) and non-consent" (Linden, 2011, p. 834). Sexual assault and rape are violent intrusions toward an individual or group of individuals (usually female) that are intentional and harmful, perpetrated by individuals or groups with preferential paraphilias toward victims and type of sexual offense, but variable with multiple modus operandi (Lasher, McGrath, & Cumming, 2014). Rape is also a weapon of war (United Nations News Centre, 2017). Effects of rape have lifelong consequences for the victim that deny the person quality of life, and place the victim(s) at increased risk of "unwanted pregnancy, sexually transmitted infections, sleep and eating disorders, and other emotional and physical problems" (Kruttschnitt, Kalsbeek, & House, 2014, para 2). In ancient times, virginity or chastity had value as property, hence laws were enacted that paid the owner for damage or access to (consortium) property (family or husband), but these laws also punish the victim for adultery (Conley, 2014). The social construct that places value on virginity persists in trafficking slaves today (Joffres et al., 2008; McAlpine, Hossain, & Zimmerman, 2016). In the United States, persons charged with sexual crimes publicly support their acts with justifications for forcing sex on another; misperceptions of victim behavior, including alcohol consumption; and numbers of contacts with the victim (Abbey & Jacques-Tiura, 2011; Wegner, Abbey, Pierce, Pegram, & Woerner, 2015). When alcohol exposure includes justification for force or opportunity (victim did not say "no"), or when the rapist lacks insight about the victim's view of the event, the rapist is likely to repeat the behavior (Abbey, 2011; Wegner et al., 2015). When rapists are publicly charged with a crime, their marginal logic may blame the victim, say it was consensual, or that the suspect cries "foul" because there was no "intent" to harm, which is a new defense for crimes. Understanding the victim's reactions, and the rapist's proclivity toward a specific victim, helps nursing communities plan evidence-based prevention programs, interventions, and mitigation strategies for improving a patient's predictable negative health outcomes.

Background

Sexual assault is a life-altering event, undermining an individual's confidence and perception of safety. For many, the acute traumatic reaction and allostatic load are the beginning of diminished physical and mental health (McEwen, 1998; McEwen & Seeman, 1999; Schafran, 1996; Stein et al., 2004). To date, for those surviving the rape, posttraumatic stress disorder is a primary outcome (Jaycox, Zoellner, & Foa, 2002; Krakow

et al., 2002; Zoellner, Goodwin, & Foa, 2000). For others, exposure to violence and rape increase somatic symptoms of anxiety and mood disorders in which their behavior increases the risk of sexually transmitted diseases and requests for therapeutic abortion (Tinglof, Hogberg, Lundell, & Svanberg, 2015). Although medication is available to minimize symptoms of anxiety and other mood disorders, the side effects of the medication, the person's age or gender, and having to pay for the medication may prevent many from completing the regimen, which is an opportunity for registered nurse anticipatory guidance intervention (Bogoch et al., 2014; Krause et al., 2014).

The Centers for Disease Control and Prevention is a leader in understanding sexual violence. The current understanding about sexual violence is divided into the following types:

- Completed or attempted forced penetration of a victim
- Completed or attempted alcohol/drug-facilitated penetration of a victim
- Completed or attempted forced acts in which a victim is made to penetrate a perpetrator or someone else
- Completed or attempted alcohol/drug-facilitated acts in which a victim is made to penetrate a perpetrator or someone else
- Nonphysically forced penetration that occurs after a person is pressured verbally or through intimidation or misuse of authority to consent or acquiesce
- Unwanted sexual contact
- Does not include physical contact of a sexual nature between the perpetrator and the victim; this occurs against a person without his or her consent, or against a person who is unable to consent or refuse (Basile et al., 2016, para 1)

The incidence of sexual assault and rape types in populations varies according to family dynamics, culture, and community tolerance for violence, but the primary reason for inconsistencies between statistical reports is that victims do not report (DuMont, Miller, & Myhr, 2003). One reason victims do not report is they do not know whether their experiences meet the legal definition of rape or sexual assault. They self-blame, have guilt, shame, and embarrassment, which leads to the desire to keep the assault a private matter, fearing humiliation or complicity, fear of not being believed, and lack of trust in the criminal justice system (Boykins & Mynatt, 2007; Darnell et al., 2015;

DuMont et al., 2003). Even if victims did report, the definition of rape and combining sexual crimes with other types of crimes (Kruttschnitt et al., 2014) diminishes accuracy of data. Strikingly, 37.4% of females reported their first rape occurred between the ages of 18 and 24 years (Black et al., 2011) and 12.3% of female rape victims and 27.8% of male rape victims were first raped when they were age 10 or younger (National Center for Injury Prevention and Control Division of Violence Prevention, 2012). Individuals committing sexual offenses rarely do so spontaneously and there is a significant level of planning that leads up to the offense (Lasher et al., 2014; Mitchell, Angelone, Kohlberger, & Hirschman, 2009; Terry & Freilich, 2012). Grooming is a process by which an offender draws a victim into a relationship that becomes sexual and is maintained in secrecy by using authority and supervision to delay and sustain the deception (Terry & Freilich, 2012). The outcomes of long-term predatory sexual violence promote victim risk for subsequent rape (Sadler, Booth, Mengeling, & Doebbeling, 2004) and risk behaviors (early sexual activity, sexually transmitted infections, smoking, drug and alcohol abuse, obesity, etc.), subsequent poor health (e.g., hypertension, diabetes, heart disease, stroke, and lung disease), and ultimately early death by as much as 20 years (Acierno, Resnick, Flood, & Holmes, 2003; Adams et al., 2016; Anda et al., 2009; Armstrong, 1997; R. B. Baker, 2006; Campbell, Sefl, & Ahrens, 2004; Draucker, 1999; Hillis et al., 2004; Zinzow et al., 2012). Understanding rape incidence, particularly against children, and offender methods provides nurses opportunity to screen and identify patients early, mitigating the impact by using trauma-informed and patient-centered care in all nursing settings.

In some cases, there are instances in which sexual violence results in death, particularly in domestic violence. Violent behavior during a sexual assault may escalate and the victim may be killed; older victims with frail health are at higher risk of death (Safarik, Jarvis, & Nussbaum, 2002). In 1997, male-perpetrated domestic violence caused 1,830 deaths, in which 73% of victims were women (Gilliland, Spence, & Spence, 2000). Blaming the victim is a frequent reaction to persons with trauma sequelae and manifests in a variety of negative behaviors by health care system providers (Marantz, 1990) and criminal justice responders (Venema, 2016). Questions about violent experiences *in all care settings* provide nurses the opportunity to mitigate lethal outcomes.

Clinical Aspects

ASSESSMENT

Rarely does sexual assault create visible injury requiring treatment in urgent or emergent settings (Gaffney, 2003; Jones, Rossman, Diegel, Van Order, & Wynn, 2009; Jones, Rossman, Wynn, Dunnuck, & Schwartz, 2003). The offender's modus operandi and paraphilias influence offender's choice to injure (Lasher et al., 2014), but victim responses to the capture and awareness of situation always mitigate injury, which may include the inability to act or address a threat, which is involuntary associated with postevent anxiety and posttraumatic stress disorder (PTSD; Abrams, Carleton, Taylor, & Asmundson, 2009), or surrender, which is a voluntary decision to not resist and stay alive, but not well studied (Speck, Ropero-Miller, & McCullough, 2010). Regardless, victim response is influenced by alcohol and drug use (Anderson, Flynn, & Pilgrim, 2017) as well as previous trauma reactions. Nurses are the key to providing trauma-informed and patient-centered care to support reporting victims, explaining processes, and facilitating a coordinated community response.

To date, there is no consistent education about sexual assault across curricula in basic RN or graduate programs, or the health (mental and physical), or legal outcomes following rape or sexual assault, or about the expected toll of the vicarious trauma experience from caring for victims of crimes. For RNs wanting to care for victims of sexual assault, there is education offered by the International Association of Forensic Nurses (IAFN), translated into a 40-hour training seminar for the sexual assault nurse examiner (SANE)—adolescent and adult role (International Association of Forensic Nurses, 2015). Other organizations offer continuing-education units in training to meet state board of nursing rules or regulations (Maryland Board of Nursing, n.d.; Texas Board of Nursing, 2013). Many RNs return to schools offering graduate education hours toward certificates or graduate/doctoral degrees, where online-blended graduate programs require face-to-face clinical practicums for competency demonstrations (J. Baker et al., 2016; Metcalfe, Hall, & Carpenter, 2007). Advanced Forensic Nursing Board Certification requires significant advanced forensic nursing practice hours and continuing education (American Nurses Credentialing Center, n.d.).

In a trauma-informed care environment, each patient should be screened for a history of violence and sexual assault. However, in the acute assessment of a patient with a suspicion or complaint of rape or sexual assault, the coordinated community response includes a sexual assault response team (SART) with members having unique roles and role limitations. There are tools in the literature to guide the focus on the type of assault and the developmental age, and this may include the age of the first assault, the relationship of the assailant(s), and what the patients think the impact is on their lives (Basile, Hertz, & Back, 2007). The screening tools provide the nurse insight into the patient's vulnerabilities, including risk behaviors. In addition, when there is therapeutic screening, this is the best hope for patient engagement in the health care system. The RN implements the nursing role as a gatherer of health and medical information, including medical history and conditions or what is seen and heard, objectively documenting injury, treatments, and recommendations and referrals. The nurse uses the nursing process to ensure comfort and care and forensic science to avoid contamination during sample collection, which is used to further assess the patients, their responses to the intervention, and their needs. The RN who is SANE-trained is answerable to the board of nursing under the RN licensed authority, and never becomes a law enforcement investigator (evidence collector). Samples, as well as nursing assessment documentation, are useful to the prosecution (or not), when helping either law enforcement or prosecution introduces significant RN bias and undermines the comprehensive scope and standards of the forensic nurse role in sexual assault care.

OUTCOMES

Victims of rape and sexual assault experience risk of transmission of sexually transmitted diseases, in which follow-up with sexual assault victims is poor (Ackerman, Sugar, Fine, & Eckert, 2006; Boykins & Mynatt, 2007; Parekh & Brown, 2003). Therefore, the recommendation is *treatment at point of care* by the nurse, which includes "an empiric antimicrobial regimen for chlamydia, gonorrhea, and trichomonas; emergency contraception...; post-exposure hepatitis B vaccination...; HPV vaccination is recommended for female survivors aged 9–26 years and male survivors aged 9–21 years; [and] recommendations for HIV PEP are individualized according to risk" (Centers for Disease Control and Prevention, 2017, section 3). With newer technology, nurses have opportunity to improve victim follow-up with health care systems.

Summary

Sexual assault is an intentional trauma that alters the victim's biophysiology. When one in four women and one in six men are victims of sexual assault and rape, many before age 18, it is likely that nurses will care for patients with a sexual assault history. When systems lack preparation for care of rape victims seeking treatment, the system becomes the problem and results in failed justice; the failure occurs not only in meeting the needs of the patient, but also in meeting the needs of the community at large. The libelous burden on the health system occurs when systems deny or delay treatment, when there are untoward outcomes contributing to increasing risk for mental and physical health sequelae. Eventually, these patients become high users of the systems, which began when their needs went unmet after victimization.

The SANE responds to the acute victim of sexual assault. This role, in existence since 1973 in Memphis, Tennessee, expanded in the 1990s with the advent of IAFN and its membership of mainly SANEs. The growing trend is to offer comprehensive graduate education in forensic nursing and accomplish this with integration of forensic nursing exemplars in concept-based basic and advanced nursing curricula with simulation (for instance, intentional injury as a concept in an acute care nurse practitioner curriculum). Colleges and schools now offer graduate and doctoral practice and research degrees, with paths in the specialty of forensic nursing, which guarantees an ample supply of expert forensic nurse leaders able to navigate complex medical–forensic patient presentations in a variety of hospital, community, and entrepreneurial systems.

Abbey, A. (2011). Alcohol's role in sexual violence perpetration: Theoretical explanations, existing evidence and future directions. *Drug and Alcohol Review*, 30(5), 481–489. doi:10.1111/j.1465-3362.2011.00296.x

Abbey, A., & Jacques-Tiura, A. J. (2011). Sexual assault perpetrators' tactics: Associations with their personal characteristics and aspects of the incident. *Journal of Interpersonal Violence*, 26(14), 2866–2889. doi:10.1177/0886260510390955

Abrams, M. P., Carleton, R. N., Taylor, S., & Asmundson, G. J. (2009). Human tonic immobility: Measurement and correlates. *Depression and Anxiety*, 26(6), 550–556. doi:10.1002/da.20462

Acierno, R., Resnick, H. S., Flood, A., & Holmes, M. (2003). An acute post-rape intervention to prevent substance use and abuse. *Addictive Behaviors*, 28(9), 1701–1715.

Ackerman, D. R., Sugar, N. F., Fine, D. N., & Eckert, L. O. (2006). Sexual assault victims: Factors associated with follow-up care. *American Journal of Obstetrics and Gynecology*, *194*(6), 1653–1659. doi:10.1016/j.ajog.2006.03.014

Adams, Z. W., Moreland, A., Cohen, J. R., Lee, R. C., Hanson, R. F., Danielson, C. K., . . . Briggs, E. C. (2016). Polyvictimization: Latent profiles and mental health outcomes in a clinical sample of adolescents. *Psychology of Violence*, *6*(1), 145–155. doi:10.1037/a0039713

American Nurses Credentialing Center. (n.d.). Advanced forensic nursing certification eligibility criteria. Retrieved from http://www.nursecredentialing.org/AdvForensicNursing-Eligibility.aspx

Anda, R. F., Dong, M., Brown, D. W., Felitti, V. J., Giles, W. H., Perry, B. D., . . . Dube, S. R. (2009). The relationship of adverse childhood experiences to a history of premature death of family members. *BMC Public Health*, *9*(106). Retrieved from http://www.biomedcentral.com/1471-2458/9/106

Anderson, L. J., Flynn, A., & Pilgrim, J. L. (2017). A global epidemiological perspective on the toxicology of drug-facilitated sexual assault: A systematic review. *Journal of Forensic and Legal Medicine*, *47*, 46–54. doi:10.1016/j.jflm.2017.02.005

Armstrong, R. (1997). Sexual assault: Clinical issues. When drugs are used for rape. *Journal of Emergency Nursing*, *23*(4), 378–381.

Baker, J., Kelly, P. J., Carlson, K., Colbert, S., Cordle, C., & Witt, J. S. (2016). SANE-A-PALOOZA: Logistical development and implementation of a clinical immersion course for sexual assault nurse examiners. *Journal of Forensic Nursing*, *12*(4), 176–182. doi:10.1097/jfn.0000000000000133

Baker, R. B. (2006). Genital injuries in adolescents after rape. Retrieved from http://search.ebscohost.com/login.aspx?direct=true&db=rzh&AN=109847295&site=ehost-live

Basile, K. C., DeGue, S., Jones, K., Freire, K., Dills, J., Smith, S. G., & Raiford, J. L. (2016). *STOP SV: A technical package to prevent sexual violence*. Atlanta, GA: Centers for Disease Control and Prevention, National Center for Injury Prevention and Control. Retrieved from https://www.cdc.gov/violenceprevention/sexualviolence/definitions.html

Basile, K. C., Hertz, M. F., & Back, S. E. (2007). *Intimate partner violence and sexual violence victimization assessment instruments for use in healthcare settings: Version 1*. Atlanta, GA: Centers for Disease Control and Prevention, National Center for Injury Prevention and Control. Retrieved from https://www.cdc.gov/violenceprevention/pdf/ipv/ipvandsvscreening.pdf

Black, M. C., Basile, K. C., Breiding, M. J., Smith, S. G., Walters, M. L., Merrick, M. T., . . . Stevens, M. R. (2011). *The National Intimate Partner and Sexual Violence Survey (NISVS): 2010 summary report*. Atlanta, GA: National Center for Injury Prevention and Control, Centers for Disease Control and Prevention.

Bogoch, I. I., Scully, E. P., Zachary, K. C., Yawetz, S., Mayer, K. H., Bell, C. M., & Andrews, J. R. (2014). Patient attrition between the emergency department and clinic among individuals presenting for HIV nonoccupational postexposure prophylaxis. *Clinical Infectious Diseases*, *58*(11), 1618–1624. doi:10.1093/cid/ciu118

Boykins, A. D., & Mynatt, S. (2007). Assault history and follow-up contact of women survivors of recent sexual assault. *Issues in Mental Health Nursing*, *28*(8), 867–881. doi:10.1080/01612840701493394

Campbell, R., Sefl, T., & Ahrens, C. E. (2004). The impact of rape on women's sexual health risk behaviors. *Health Psychology*, *23*(1), 67–74. doi:10.1037/0278-6133.23.1.67

Centers for Disease Control and Prevention. (2017). 2015 sexually transmitted diseases treatment guidelines: Sexual assault and abuse and STDs: Adolescents and adults. Retrieved from https://www.cdc.gov/std/tg2015/sexual-assault.htm

Conley, C. A. (2014). *Sexual violence in historical perspective*. In R. Gartner, B. McCarthy, & C. A. Conley (Eds.), *The Oxford handbook of gender, sex, and crime*. New York, NY: Oxford University Press. Retrieved from http://www.oxfordhandbooks.com/view/10.1093/oxfordhb/9780199838707.001.0001/oxfordhb-9780199838707-e-012

Darnell, D., Peterson, R., Berliner, L., Stewart, T., Russo, J., Whiteside, L., & Zatzick, D. (2015). Factors associated with follow-up attendance among rape victims seen in acute medical care. *Psychiatry*, *78*(1), 89–101. doi:10.1080/00332747.2015.1015901

Draucker, C. B. (1999). The psychotherapeutic needs of women who have been sexually assaulted. *Perspectives in Psychiatric Care*, *35*(1), 18–28.

DuMont, J., Miller, K. D., & Myhr, T. L. (2003). The role of "real rape" and "real victim" stereotypes in the police reporting practices of sexually assaulted women. *Violence Against Women*, *9*(4), 466–486.

Gaffney, D. (Ed.). (2003). *Genital injury and sexual assault*. St. Louis, MO: G. W. Medical.

Gilliland, M. G., Spence, P. R., & Spence, R. L. (2000). Lethal domestic violence in eastern North Carolina. *North Carolina Medical Journal*, *61*(5), 287–290.

Hillis, S. D., Anda, R. F., Dube, S. R., Felitti, V. J., Marchbanks, P. A., & Marks, J. S. (2004). The association between adverse childhood experiences and adolescent pregnancy, long-term psychosocial consequences, and fetal death. *Pediatrics*, *113*(2), 320–327.

International Association of Forensic Nurses. (2015). *Sexual assault nurse examiner adult/adolescent and pediatric education*. Arnold, MD: Forensics Nurses.

Jaycox, L. H., Zoellner, L., & Foa, E. B. (2002). Cognitive-behavior therapy for PTSD in rape survivors. *Journal of Clinical Psychology*, *58*(8), 891–906. doi:10.1002/jclp.10065

Joffres, C., Mills, E., Joffres, M., Khanna, T., Walia, H., & Grund, D. (2008). Sexual slavery without borders: Trafficking for commercial sexual exploitation in

India. *International Journal for Equity in Health*, 7, 22. doi:10.1186/1475-9276-7-22

Jones, J. S., Rossman, L., Diegel, R., Van Order, P., & Wynn, B. N. (2009). Sexual assault in postmenopausal women: Epidemiology and patterns of genital injury. *American Journal of Emergency Medicine*, 27(8), 922–929. doi:10.1016/j.ajem.2008.07.010

Jones, J. S., Rossman, L., Wynn, B. N., Dunnuck, C., & Schwartz, N. (2003). Comparative analysis of adult versus adolescent sexual assault: Epidemiology and patterns of anogenital injury. *Academic Emergency Medicine*, 10(8), 872–877.

Krakow, B., Schrader, R., Tandberg, D., Hollifield, M., Koss, M. P., Yau, C. L., & Cheng, D. T. (2002). Nightmare frequency in sexual assault survivors with PTSD. *Journal of Anxiety Disorders*, 16(2), 175–190.

Krause, K. H., Lewis-O'Connor, A., Berger, A., Votto, T., Yawetz, S., Pallin, D. J., & Baden, L. R. (2014). Current practice of HIV postexposure prophylaxis treatment for sexual assault patients in an emergency department. *Women's Health Issues*, 24(4), e407–e412. doi:10.1016/j.whi.2014.04.003

Kruttschnitt, C., Kalsbeek, W. D., House, C. C. & Panel on Measuring Rape and Sexual Assault in Bureau of Justice Statistics Household Surveys. (2014). *Estimating the incidence of rape and sexual assault*. Washington, DC: National Academies Press.

Lasher, M. P., McGrath, R. J., & Cumming, G. F. (2014). Sex offender modus operandi stability and relationship with actuarial risk assessment. *Journal of Interpersonal Violence*, 30(6), 911–927. doi:10.1177/0886260514539757

Linden, J. A. (2011). Clinical practice. Care of the adult patient after sexual assault. *New England Journal of Medicine*, 365(9), 834–841. doi:10.1056/NEJMcp 1102869

Marantz, P. R. (1990). Blaming the victim: The negative consequence of preventive medicine. *American Journal of Public Health*, 80(10), 1186–1187.

Maryland Board of Nursing. (n.d.). Forensic nurse examiner. Retrieved from http://mbon.maryland.gov/Pages/forensic-nurse-examiner.aspx

McAlpine, A., Hossain, M., & Zimmerman, C. (2016). Sex trafficking and sexual exploitation in settings affected by armed conflicts in Africa, Asia and the Middle East: Systematic review. *BMC International Health and Human Rights*, 16(1), 34. doi:10.1186/s12914-016-0107-x

McEwen, B. S. (1998). Stress, adaptation, and disease: Allostasis and allostatic load. *Annals of the New York Academy of Sciences*, 840, 33–44. doi:10.1111/j.1749-6632.1998.5b09546.x

McEwen, B. S., & Seeman, T. (1999). Protective and damaging effects of mediators of stress. Elaborating and testing the concepts of allostasis and allostatic load. *Annals of the New York Academy of Sciences*, 896, 30–47.

Metcalfe, S. E., Hall, V. P., & Carpenter, A. (2007). Promoting collaboration in nursing education: The development of a regional simulation laboratory. *Journal of Professional Nursing*, 23(3), 180–183. doi:10.1016/j.profnurs.2007.01.017

Mitchell, D., Angelone, D. J., Kohlberger, B., & Hirschman, R. (2009). Effects of offender motivation, victim gender, and participant gender on perceptions of rape victims and offenders. *Journal of Interpersonal Violence*, 24(9), 1564–1578. doi:10.1177/0886260508323662

National Center for Injury Prevention and Control Division of Violence Prevention. (2012). Sexual violence: Facts at a glance. Retrieved from https://www.cdc.gov/violenceprevention/pdf/sv-datasheet-a.pdf

Parekh, V., & Brown, C. B. (2003). Follow up of patients who have been recently sexually assaulted. *Sexually Transmitted Infections*, 79(4), 349.

Sadler, A. G., Booth, B. M., Mengeling, M. A., & Doebbeling, B. N. (2004). Life span and repeated violence against women during military service: Effects on health status and outpatient utilization. *Journal of Women's Health*, 13(7), 799–811.

Safarik, M. E., Jarvis, J. P., & Nussbaum, K. E. (2002). Sexual homicide of elderly females: Linking offender characteristics to victim and crime scene attributes. *Journal of Interpersonal Violence*, 17(5), 500–525. doi:10.1177/0886260502017005002

Schafran, L. H. (1996). Topics for our times: Rape is a major public health issue. *American Journal of Public Health*, 86(1), 15–17.

Speck, P. M., Ropero-Miller, J. R., & McCullough, T. (2010). *An overview of DFSA SANE/SAFE/SART Protocol 1: Surrendered rape defined* [Webinar slide 14]. Research Triangle Park, NC: Research Triangle Institute and Department of Justice Office of Victims of Crime.

Stein, M. B., Lang, A. J., Laffaye, C., Satz, L. E., Lenox, R. J., & Dresselhaus, T. R. (2004). Relationship of sexual assault history to somatic symptoms and health anxiety in women. *General Hospital Psychiatry*, 26(3), 178–183. doi:10.1016/j.genhosppsych.2003.11.003

Terry, K. J., & Freilich, J. D. (2012). Understanding child sexual abuse by Catholic priests from a situational perspective. *Journal of Child Sexual Abuse*, 21(4), 437–455. doi:10.1080/10538712.2012.693579

Texas Board of Nursing. (2013). Education—Continuing nursing education & competency. Retrieved from https://www.bon.texas.gov/education_continuing_education.asp

Tinglof, S., Hogberg, U., Lundell, I. W., & Svanberg, A. S. (2015). Exposure to violence among women with unwanted pregnancies and the association with posttraumatic stress disorder, symptoms of anxiety and depression. *Sexual & Reproductive Healthcare*, 6(2), 50–53. doi:10.1016/j.srhc.2014.08.003

United Nations News Centre. (2017). Perpetrators, not victims, should be shamed for conflict-related sexual violence—UN report [Press release]. Retrieved from http://www.un.org/apps/news/story.asp?NewsID=56675#.WSHynmjyuMp

Venema, R. M. (2016). Making judgments: How blame mediates the influence of rape myth acceptance in police response to sexual assault. *Journal of Interpersonal Violence.* doi:10.1177/0886260516662437

Wegner, R., Abbey, A., Pierce, J., Pegram, S. E., & Woerner, J. (2015). Sexual assault perpetrators' justifications for their actions: Relationships to rape supportive attitudes, incident characteristics, and future perpetration. *Violence Against Women, 21*(8), 1018–1037. doi:10.1177/1077801215589380

Zinzow, H. M., Resnick, H. S., McCauley, J. L., Amstadter, A. B., Ruggiero, K. J., & Kilpatrick, D. G. (2012). Prevalence and risk of psychiatric disorders as a function of variant rape histories: Results from a national survey of women. *Social Psychiatry and Psychiatric Epidemiology, 47*(6), 893–902. doi:10.1007/s00127-011-0397-1

Zoellner, L. A., Goodwin, M. L., & Foa, E. B. (2000). PTSD severity and health perceptions in female victims of sexual assault. *Journal of Traumatic Stress, 13*(4), 635–649. doi:10.1023/a:1007810200460

■ SHOCK AND MULTIPLE ORGAN DYSFUNCTION SYNDROME

Jennifer Wilbeck

Overview

Most often shock is a secondary set of physiological processes resulting from a primary insult or injury. As such, emergency department (ED) and critical care nurses may encounter patients both at risk for, or are experiencing shock with multiple organ dysfunction. Early recognition, combined with targeted supportive therapies, is essential to restoration of the patient's health and prevention of end-stage organ dysfunction. Without prompt and aggressive interventions, shock and multiple organ dysfunction syndrome (MODS) lead to death.

Background

Shock is an acute, generalized process of inadequate tissue perfusion resulting in cellular, metabolic, and hemodynamic alterations (Carlson & Fitzsimmons, 2014). Imbalances of cellular oxygen supply and demand occur for a variety of reasons, and are classified into four broad types of shock: hypovolemic, obstructive, cardiogenic, and distributive (Carlson & Fitzsimmons, 2014; Shapiro & Fischer, 2015).

Hypovolemic shock results from the loss or redistribution of volume (blood, plasma, or other body fluids) leading to decreased intravascular volume. Etiologies may include acute blood loss or ongoing hemorrhage, gastrointestinal (GI) losses such as vomiting and diarrhea, burns, polyuria, excess pharmaceutical diuresis, or insensible losses. The loss of vascular volume leads to inadequate preload, followed by decreased diastolic filling and ultimately a decreased cardiac output.

Obstructive shock occurs secondary to mechanical obstruction that decreases ventricular filling and/or emptying, ultimately resulting in decreases in cardiac output, tissue perfusion, and oxygen delivery. Causes of obstructive shock include cardiac tamponade, tension pneumothorax, vena cava compression or thrombus, atrial mass or thrombus, and pulmonary embolism.

Cardiogenic shock occurs when the heart fails as a pump; decreased contractility leads to decreased stroke volume, cardiac output, and blood pressure, resulting in decreased tissue perfusion. Common causes of cardiogenic shock include myocardial infarction, heart failure exacerbations, dysrhythmias, and left ventricular outflow tract obstructions.

Distributive shock results in massive vasodilation and loss of vasomotor tone from three etiologies: anaphylactic (allergic-mediated), septic (infectious etiology), and neurogenic shock. Anaphylactic and septic shock are also associated with increased capillary permeability. Spinal cord injuries above the T4 level may result in sympathetic pathway damage and lead to decreased sympathetic tone to innervated organs distal to the level of the injury, leaving them stimulated by parasympathetic tone and causing bradycardia, massive vasodilatation, and inability to regulate body temperature. As a general rule, the higher the injury, the more severe the symptoms.

Regardless of the type of shock, resulting cellular hypoxia and subsequent vital organ dysfunction progress across a continuum of decline. The four stages of shock progression are initial, compensatory, progressive (or uncompensated), and refractory (Carlson & Fitzsimmons, 2014). Left untreated, shock ultimately leads to the development of multiple organ dysfunction and/or failure. MODS is the failure of more than one organ system in acutely ill patients, which requires intervention to maintain homeostasis (Carlson & Fitzsimmons, 2014; Kaml & Davis, 2016) and its severity can be measured by any of three standardized scoring systems (Frohlich et al., 2016).

Clinical Aspects

ASSESSMENT

Although the underlying processes are the same, the development, compensation, and timing of progression may vary based on a patient's age, prior health, initial insult, and treatment. Within the geriatric population, shock progression is rapid due to reduced compensatory mechanisms and preexisting comorbidities. Changes of decreased cardiac output and perhaps slight anxiety that are seen with initial shock are discrete; clinical signs and symptoms do not appear until the intravascular volume is reduced by greater than 15%. Compensated shock may be easily overlooked as the clinical presentation is relatively stable due to compensatory mechanisms from the renin–angiotensin–aldosterone system and stimulation of the central nervous system resulting in peripheral vasoconstriction, sodium reabsorption, and water retention. Early signs and symptoms of shock include tachycardia, borderline hypotension, tachypnea, nausea, oliguria, hyperglycemia, and extremities that are cool to the touch. During compensated shock, rapid correction of underlying etiologies increases the likelihood of minimal residual effects.

If not corrected, progressive (or uncompensated shock) develops with rapid patient deterioration and ensuing failure of compensatory mechanisms, which results in cellular hypoxia. Decreased cellular perfusion exacerbates anaerobic metabolism processes due to the lack of oxygen delivery to distal tissues, which can be indirectly measured by serum lactate levels. Anaerobic metabolism produces metabolic acidosis, resulting in hyperkalemia, cellular death, and both generalized and interstitial edema (including pulmonary edema). Increased vascular permeability and vasodilation also occur at this stage. Clinically, the nurse may identify the following findings in uncompensated shock: altered mentation/decreased responsiveness, tachycardia and arrhythmias, weak thready pulses and delayed capillary refill, hypoxia, absent or hypoactive bowel sounds, oliguria/anuria, hypoglycemia, and cold extremities. If not corrected at this point, refractory shock that is unresponsive to treatment and irreversible will ensue.

MODS then develops as individual organ systems die from tissue ischemia. MODS represents a complex physiologic process wherein uncontrolled inflammatory responses, in conjunction with changes of the vascular endothelium, immune function, metabolism and circulatory system, become a self-perpetuating process that leads to organ dysfunction and failure. Mortality rates increase with the number of failed organ systems; for patients with failure of two or more organs, estimated mortality rate is 54% (Carlson & Fitzsimmons, 2014).

Although shock presentations vary, shock should be suspected in patients with a mean arterial pressure (MAP) less than 60 mmHg, or in the presence of tissue hypoperfusion. Elevated lactic acid levels serve as a surrogate marker. Both physical assessments and diagnostic testing seek to identify the underlying etiology of shock and MODS. Standardized diagnostic criteria are available for each of these processes (Kaml & Davis, 2016; Vogel et al., 2016).

NURSING INTERVENTIONS, MANAGEMENT, AND IMPLICATIONS

Progression of shock through stages to the point of MODS allows ongoing opportunities to identify and intervene to halt further deterioration. Regardless of where the patient falls within the continuum of shock and/or MODS, goals of management are to provide supportive therapy to affected body systems while identifying, managing, and treating the initial source. This is accomplished by optimizing oxygen delivery and tissue perfusion, establishment of intravenous (IV) access, preferably central access, volume resuscitation, and vasopressor support. As adequate oxygenation requires a secure and patent airway, supplemental oxygen and mechanical ventilation are often required. Appropriate volume resuscitation may be achieved using crystalloid boluses with continuous fluid infusion and, if appropriate, blood product administration. Vasopressors are utilized once any volume deficits are replaced. Ultrasound evaluation of inferior vena cava (IVC) responsiveness, echocardiogram and central venous pressure (CVP) measurements provide diagnostic options and ability to evaluate treatment efficacy.

Targeted treatments for shock states may be added to the mainstay treatment noted previously:

- Hypovolemic shock requires targeted volume resuscitation to replace lost fluids (and/or blood). Bleeding or GI losses to vomiting or diarrhea must also be resolved.

- Treatment of obstructive shock requires resolution of the underlying structural occlusion.

- For cardiogenic shock due to myocardial infarction (MI), restoration of coronary artery perfusion and anticoagulation are needed. If due to heart failure, inotropic support, afterload reduction, and diuresis are utilized. Antiarrhythmic drugs and/or defibrillation are indicated for dysrhythmias.

- Neurogenic shock requires spinal stabilization, emergency neurosurgery consult, and surgical decompression. Vasopressors are used to provide chronotropic and blood pressure support. Activities that trigger vagal responses must be avoided.

- Anaphylactic shock requires aggressive airway management, adrenergic agonists, H1 & H2 receptor antagonists, bronchodilators, corticosteroids, and often vasopressors.

- Septic shock treatment follows the Surviving Sepsis Campaign clinical guidelines, which outline the timed treatment goals, including early antibiotics for infectious etiology in addition to fluid replacement and vasopressors (Dellinger et al., 2013).

OUTCOMES

Promoting positive outcomes can be achieved through a detailed nursing health history and physical examination identifying risk factors, mechanisms, and early signs of shock and multiple organ dysfunction. Nurses must understand the normal physiology and pathophysiology of these disorders to prevent complications. Working as a team with other health professionals and providers is important to ensure high-quality care in these patients as well as any others.

Summary

Shock states are dynamic; nurses must stay vigilant and utilize a collaborative team for the required complex care to ensure best outcomes. Regardless of the advances in care, basic ABCs (airway, breathing, and circulation) remain the mainstay of treatment. Optimal patient outcomes are recognized with early recognition of shock and aggressive intervention.

Carlson, B. & Fitzsimmons, L. (2014). Shock, sepsis, and multiple organ dysfunction syndrome. In L. D. Urden, K. M. Stacy, & M. E. Lough (Eds.), *Critical care nursing* (7th ed., pp. 887–925). St. Louis, MO: Elsevier.

Dellinger, R. P., Levy, M. M., Rhodes, A., Annane, D., Gerlach, H., Opal, S. M., . . . Moreno, R. (2013). Surviving sepsis campaign: International guidelines for management of severe sepsis and septic shock, 2012. *Intensive Care Medicine, 39,* 165–228.

Frohlich, M., Wafaisade, A., Mansuri, A., Koenen, P., Probst, C., Maegele, M., . . . Sakka, S. (2016). Which score should be used for posttraumatic multiple organ failure?—Comparison of the MODS, Denver, and SOFA Scores. *Scandainavian Journal of Trauma, Resuscitation & Emergency Medicine, 24,* 130. doi:10.1186/s13049-016-0321-5

Kaml, G. J., & Davis, K. A. (2016). Surgical critical care for the patient with sepsis and multiple organ dysfunction. *Anesthesiology Clinics, 34,* 681–696.

Shapiro, N., & Fischer, C. M. (2015). Shock. In J. J. Schaider, R. M. Barkin, S. R. Hayden, R. E. Wolfe, A. Z. Barkin, P. Shayne, & P. Rosen (Eds.), *Rosen & Barkin's 5-minute emergency medicine consult* (pp. 1026–1027). Philadelphia, PA: Wolters Kluwer.

Vogel, J. A., Newgard, C. D., Holmes, J. F., Diercks, D. B., Arens, A. M., Boatright, D. H., . . . Haukoos, J. S. (2016). Validation of the Denver emergency department trauma organ failure score to predict post-injury multiple organ failure. *Journal of the American College of Surgeons, 222,* 73–82.

■ SOLID ORGAN TRANSPLANTATION

Marcia Johansson

Overview

Solid organ transplantation has become widely accepted as a treatment for end-stage organ failure. With the use of immunosuppressive medications, the organs that can now be transplanted have expanded and include liver, kidney, pancreas, small bowel, and thoracic organs. All organs remain in short supply with increased waiting times for potential recipients (HRSA, 2017). Despite the many advances in treatment, appropriate critical care management is required to support prompt graft recovery and prevent systemic complications. Immunosuppressive medications, graft rejection (acute and chronic), and specific long-term complications have a direct effect on morbidity and mortality for the organ and recipient, and will be the focus of this chapter.

Background

There is no single consensus definition that can be applied to all organ transplants but each organ has specific criterion. The overall clinical problems in solid organ transplant are availability of organs and the prevention of complications and rejection. Despite advances in medicine and knowledge as well as increased awareness of organ donation and transplantation, there continues to be a gap between supply and demand. More progress is necessary to ensure that all individuals with end-stage organ failure have a chance to receive a transplant (Health Resources and Services Administration [HRSA], 2017).

According to the Organ Procurement Transplant Network (OPTN) current statistics, there are 118,278 people on the list in need of a lifesaving organ transplant. Of those, 75,857 people are active candidates on the waiting list. In the first quarter of 2017, 5,367 organ transplants were performed. There were only 2,554 donors during that same time period (HRSA, 2017). Living-related organ transplants continue to increase for both kidney and partial liver transplant.

Evaluation of an individual for organ transplant includes identifying the cause of organ failure, comorbid conditions, social and financial support, treatment before transplant, specific laboratory values that support organ failure, human leukocyte antigen (HLA) typing, ABO compatibility with the donor, and immune response testing to the proposed donors. For orthotopic liver transplant patients (OLT), calculation of the Model for End-Stage Liver Disease (MELD) scores is necessary. The range is from 6 (less ill) to 40 (gravely ill; Klein & Miller, 2014). The individual score establishes the severity of illness and is useful in determining the urgency of an individual's need to receive a liver transplant.

There have been significant strides in overcoming immunologic barriers through the use of desensitization techniques. The pretransplant evaluation identifies opportunities to assess the risks for common posttransplant infections and to develop individualized preventive strategies.

Cardiovascular morbidity and mortality complicate the progress of a significant proportion of renal transplant recipients and have an increased prevalence among recipients of other solid organ transplants. Early transplant complications include infection and rejection. Long-term risk factors include metabolic and cardiovascular disease, which pose the most serious risk factors impacting patient survival. Significant advances in immunosuppressive therapy have prolonged the allograft and patient survival in solid organ transplant.

Clinical Aspects

ASSESSMENT

Assessment and care of the transplant patient in the immediate postoperative period is organ specific and is also dependent on the patient's preoperative clinical status and comorbidities. Determination of postoperative disposition of the patient is based on the surgeon preference, hospital protocols, and intraoperative concerns of both the surgeon and anesthesiologist.

Evaluation and care of the OLT patient is the most complex. These patients are usually admitted to the intensive care unit (ICU) for at least 24 hours. Assessment begins with the handoff of the operating room (OR) team to the bedside nurse. Hemodynamic bedside monitoring includes electrocardiogram tracing, continuous blood pressure via arterial line, and continuous cardiac output monitoring. Depending on the length of the surgical procedure, OLT patients usually remain intubated for the first 4 to 6 hours and are then weaned off the ventilator and extubated.

NURSING INTERVENTIONS, MANAGEMENT, AND IMPLICATIONS

The initial evaluation of all posttransplant patients includes monitoring electrolytes, blood count, coagulation panel, and urine output. For OLT patients, it is vital to evaluate liver function tests that include total bilirubin, aspartate transaminase (AST), gamma-glutamyltransferase (GGT), alkaline phosphatase, and surgical drain output (Klein & Miller, 2014). Surgical drains are placed in strategic areas and if there is an anastomosis leak or bleeding, it is usually visible in the drain. Elevation in transaminases can indicate acute rejection or graft thrombosis. Renal orthotopic kidney transplantation (OKT) and pancreatic transplants do not always require admission to the ICU; however, monitoring is similar and is based on the organ transplanted. OKT patients require focused attention to electrolytes, blood urea nitrogen (BUN), creatinine, and urine output. A decreased urine output can indicate graft dysfunction or dehydration. Pancreas transplant patients require focused attention to blood glucose, amylase, lipase, hemoglobin A1c (HbA1c), and C-peptide levels. Elevations in blood glucose are indicative of graft dysfunction. These are all indicators specific to graft function and patients will need ongoing surveillance throughout their hospital stay as well as during follow-up clinic visits. All transplants require routine postoperative care, including monitoring of the surgical site for integrity and infection, early ambulation, aggressive pulmonary hygiene to prevent respiratory complications, and instruction regarding medication use and compliance, signs of rejection, and postoperative protocols.

Immunosuppression is the mainstay of organ transplantation. Immunosuppressive medications are used to prevent acute and chronic rejection and are normally continued for the life of the functioning transplant. Many variables are considered in the choice of the drug and dose as well as monitoring of the level. Guidelines for dosing for each specific organ are different. OLT patients may need a lower dose of immunosuppression based on the blood levels than an OKT patient who is experiencing acute rejection. The guidelines are national but have been modified to make them center specific.

Glucocorticoids, such as prednisone, have both immunosuppressive and anti-inflammatory properties. Side effects are well known and are associated with increased morbidity for the patient.

Antiproliferative agents include azathioprine and mycophenolic acid also known as *mycophenolate mofetil*, inhibit the steps in de novo purine synthesis (Klein & Miller, 2014, p. 609). Side effects include gastrointestinal disturbances, such as nausea, diarrhea and abdominal pain, as well as hematologic disturbances such as leukopenia and thrombocytopenia. Assessing white blood cell (WBC) and platelet counts is extremely important for any patient receiving these medications.

Mammalian target of rapamycin (mTOR) inhibitors include sirolimus and everolimus. They inhibit the activation of a regulatory kinase and prohibit T-cell progression. Side effects include hyperlipidemia, proteinuria, and difficulty with wound healing. These medications should not be used in moderate to severe kidney disease, hepatic artery thrombosis and immediately postoperative due to poor wound healing.

Calcineurin inhibitors include cyclosporin and tacrolimus. The mechanism of action is inhibition of T-lymphocyte activation and proliferation. Both calcineurin inhibitors are nephrotoxic, but cyclosporin is less neurotoxic and diabetogenic than tacrolimus. There is a narrow therapeutic window and doses are adjusted based on blood levels (Klein & Miller, 2014).

Biologic agents include polyclonal antibodies (ATGAM [lymphocyte immune globulin] and thymoglobulin) and monoclonal antibodies (daclizumab and basiliximab). These drugs can be utilized at the time of transplantation to promote engraftment and as a subsequent treatment for acute rejection. Thymoglobulin is given to reduce the damage that can occur during the storage and transplant procedure. The long-term risk of malignancy remains a concern with these agents (Klein & Miller, 2014).

OUTCOMES

Infection prophylaxis includes keeping current with immunization schedules and prophylactic antibiotics to prevent opportunistic infections, such as cytomegalovirus (CMV) infections, herpes simplex virus (HSV) infections, systemic fungal infections, respiratory, and urinary tract infections. The key to preventing infections and rejection episodes includes early recognition of symptoms, close monitoring of laboratory values, and basic infection-control principles like handwashing to promote positive health care outcomes.

Summary

Prolonged allograft survival, decreased morbidity from comorbid conditions, decreased medication side effects, and decreased mortality remain the goals for posttransplant care. Education of the patient and family, vigilance with nursing care, open communication with the medical team, and attention to laboratory values produce early interventions and promote the best outcomes for a transplant program. Research is ongoing to improve the care of the transplant patient and formulation of new targets for future research to deal with this ever-increasing population of high-risk patients remains a priority for the "transplant team," which includes nurses, advanced practice providers, and physicians.

Health Resources and Services Administration. (2017). Organ procurement & transplantation network [Data file]. Retrieved from https://optn.transplant.hrsa.gov

Klein, C. L., & Miller, B. W. (2014). *The Washington manual of medical therapeutics* (34th ed.). Philadelphia, PA: Wolters Kluwer/Lippincott Williams & Wilkins.

■ SPINAL CORD INJURY

Lamon Norton
Melanie Gibbons Hallman

Overview

Spinal cord injuries (SCIs) arise from both traumatic and nontraumatic origins. Spinal injuries incurred from trauma include motor vehicle crashes; sports injuries; blast injuries; acts of violence, including stabbing and gunshot wounds; and falls. Common causes of nontraumatic SCIs include tumors, birth defects, infection, and neurodegenerative diseases. It has been estimated that as many as 337,000 patients are currently living with SCIs (National Spinal Cord Injury Statistical Center [NSCISC], 2015). SCIs may present acutely and resolve with time and treatment; but many persist, becoming chronic conditions requiring ongoing care. Nurses play an imperative role in triage and management of SCIs. Urgent identification of acute spinal injury and potential physical or structural instability are crucial to achieving quality patient outcomes. Nurses provide essential clinical care by conducting strategic triage activities that include acquisition of pertinent history, focused physical assessment, initiation of definitive care, and early prevention of complications. Evidence-based education for patients diagnosed with SCIs, including known or potential sequelae, is paramount and a key responsibility of nurses.

Background

SCIs are often permanent and debilitating. Treatment is largely palliative. National incidence of SCI estimations range between 12,000 and 20,000 new cases per year (Ma, Chan, & Carruthers, 2014). Motor vehicles accidents are the source of SCIs in the majority of cases nationwide; and over 80% of patients sustaining injury are male. Risk-taking behaviors and heavy involvement in sporting pursuits impact the incidence with regard to age and gender. Falls are the primary cause of SCIs affecting the elder population. In a study conducted by Crutcher, Ugiliweneza, Hodes, Kong, and Boakye (2014), the presence of alcohol was noted in 20% of all SCI cases regardless of age and was associated with increased hospital complications and morbidity. SCIs range from simple cord contusions with minimal symptomology, to complete transaction of the cord with potential for physiologic instability.

Long-term management of SCI is costly to patients, the health care system, and society in general. These costs are not only reflected in monetary losses, but also in potential loss of contribution to family and community dynamics. The estimated average expense for a young person who sustains complete quadriplegic injury exceeds $4.5 million (NSCISC, 2015). Financial impact is dependent on the severity of injury and disability that is sustained (Ma et al., 2015). Typically, the higher the level of injury is anatomically located within the spine, the more intense the requirement for physical support of activities of daily living will be. Patients may be relatively independent if the injury is at the level of the first thoracic vertebra or lower. Higher cervical injury necessitates more dependency and support for daily life. National education initiatives and prevention programs, such as vehicle restraint use, firearms safety, and sports injury safety, are designed to be preemptive deterrents to traumatic SCI. These strategies have proven to be successful in reducing preventable spine trauma.

Mechanisms of injury for patients seeking care in emergency departments typically include trauma related to accidents, athletics, and violence. Acute complications of chronic SCIs are another reason that patients require emergency services care. Acute SCIs have both a primary and secondary component. A primary injury is the initial injury to the cord and/or spinal column. The secondary injury is caused by bleeding, swelling, and ischemia. The majority of cord injuries are cervical, with the fewest injuries being thoracic-level injuries. Approximately 20% of traumatic cervical injuries results in complete quadriplegia. Common SCI complications consist of autonomic dysreflexia, bladder infection, respiratory dysfunction, and problematic sequelae related to sensory loss (Hagan, 2015; Silva, Sousa, Reis, & Salgado, 2014).

Clinical Aspects

ASSESSMENT

Rapid baseline clinical assessment coupled with expeditious verbal and written communication that documents evolving physical improvement or deterioration are key components to providing safe and effective care for patients presenting with SCIs. Until now, communicating changes specific to SCIs has been historically problematic; likely due to the absence of validated tools for such an assessment (Battistuzzo et al., 2016). Obtaining a clear history of the mechanism of injury is important to determining potential unappreciated injuries. It is crucial to monitor temperature, blood pressure, ventilation, and other real or potential complications when caring for a spinal cord–injured patient. Interventions to prevent infection and monitoring for early indications of infection are also important. Providing support to SCI patients in acute psychosocial distress is paramount to future psychosocial outcomes. Secondary cord injuries can precipitate worsening symptoms rapidly or over a period of weeks (Silva et al., 2014).

NURSING INTERVENTIONS, MANAGEMENT, AND IMPLICATIONS

Stabilization of the spinal column and cord is one of the highest patient care priorities if not already accomplished before triage. The only treatments currently available for SCI are stabilization and/or decompression of the spinal cord by either surgical or pharmacologic means. Neither of these interventions have been conclusively determined to be more preferential than the other. Methylprednisolone is the most commonly prescribed medication for acute SCIs in clinical practice, but this corticosteroid therapy is also highly controversial (Silva et al., 2014). There are multiple drug studies in progress to investigate the effects of medications, such as naloxone, monosialotetrahexosylganglioside (GM-1), minocycline, and thyrotropin-releasing hormone (TRH), on SCI treatment outcomes.

Serial recording of assessments, occurring hourly at a minimum during the acute phase, and additional assessments if deterioration is suspected, or the patient has been moved substantially (i.e., transported, rolled) are imperative to patient safety. Close scrutiny of vital signs is crucial since symptoms of autonomic dysreflexia are common in SCIs and can be fatal. Severe respiratory complications, such as atelectasis, pneumonia, and respiratory failure, are evidenced in 67% of acute SCI patients (Hagan, 2015). Pulmonary toileting and bronchodilator administration are common orders requiring nursing intervention for SCI patients. The goal of these interventions is to prevent respiratory insufficiency or failure. Cardiovascular assessment is necessary as the spinal cord-injured patient is predisposed to hypotension. The nurse should anticipate managing hypotension with volume resuscitation and administration of vasopressors. Increased predisposition to thromboembolism due to venous stasis and physical inactivity is also a concern for these patients. Deep vein thrombosis (DVT) prophylaxis measures should be anticipated. Bradycardia is sometimes present in the acute phase, but most patients adapt over time. Poikilothermia is more commonly noted with cervical level injuries and complete motor loss injuries (Hagan, 2015). Monitor and adjust environmental temperature as needed to stabilize core temperatures. Core temperature measurement may be accomplished by obtaining rectal temperatures unless continuous core temperature monitoring has been instituted. Bladder decompression is necessary to prevent urinary retention, thus requiring early Foley catheter insertion during the acute phase. Abdominal assessment for distention, and bowel elimination monitoring are necessary to detect development of an ileus or constipation. Distention of the bladder or bowel may result in acute autonomic dysreflexia. Frequent range-of-motion exercises and antispasmodic administration help to prevent contractures. Dermatologic problems associated with skin breakdown may be prevented by providing frequent, thorough skin care and assessment. Repositioning every 2 hours, weight shifting every 30 minutes whenever the patient is upright; and paying particular attention to bony prominences and areas beneath splints or braces are imperative to skin protection (Hagan, 2015). Psychological stress, depression, and anxiety are all commonly associated with this stressful life event. Current life situations, including social stability, employment status, social and family support availability, and financial security, are variables that warrant consideration while evaluating the level of stress response in individual patients. Facilitating therapeutic engagements that include all members of the patient's professional team may prove to assist the patients in their psychological rehabilitation (Hagan, 2015).

Autonomic dysreflexia (AD) or hyperreflexia is a medical emergency and one that is not uncommon in SCIs at the level of T6 and higher. It is a serious complication affecting both acute and long-term spinal cord-injured patients. Complications of this phenomena include stroke, seizures, myocardial infarction, and possible death (Hagan, 2015; Wan & Krassioukov, 2014). Autonomic dysreflexia causes a sudden onset of blood pressure elevation. In the setting of a spinal cord-injured patient and the typically lower normal blood pressure to which they adapt, it is important to consider AD even in the case of a "normal" blood pressure. This response may provide early evidence of an underlying instigating problem. Comparing an elevation in blood pressure to a patient's typical baseline blood pressure is the best method to identify early onset of AD. The clinical syndrome of AD is precipitated by a stimulus lower than the level of cord injury. Overfull bladder, constipation, pressure sores, other musculoskeletal injuries, tight clothing or device pressure, and sexual stimulation are all examples of possible precipitating circumstances.

OUTCOMES

It is not common for a patient with acute SCI to have concomitant injuries that require urgent attention. If not addressed, these injuries may have synergistic negative impact on ultimate rehabilitation. Traumatic brain injury, extremity fractures, and pneumohemothorax are often companion injuries of SCI. Timely interventions and expedited transfer to a specialty medical center are associated with better long-term outcomes for the patients (Hagan, 2015).

Summary

Patients sustaining SCIs are common presentations in emergency departments. Nurses play a vital role in close assessment with particular attention to early identification of potential complications, care, and treatment for these patients. Providing skillful nursing interventions with caring compassion creates optimal conditions for the transitional life experience for SCI patients.

Battistuzzo, C., Smith, K., Skeers, P., Armstrong, A., Clark, J., Agostinello, J., . . . Batchelor, P. (2016). Early rapid neurological assessment for acute spinal cord injury trials. *Journal of Neurotrauma, 33*(21), 1936–1945.

Crutcher, C., Ugiliweneza, B., Hodes, J., Kong, M., & Boakye, M. (2014). Alcohol intoxication and its effect on spinal cord injury outcomes. *Journal of Neurotrauma, 31*(9), 798–802.

Hagan, E. (2015). Acute complications of spinal cord injuries. *World Journal of Orthopedics, 18*(6), 17–23.

Ma, V., Chan, L., & Carruthers, K. (2014). Incidence, prevalence, costs, and impact on disability of common conditions requiring rehabilitation in the United States: Stroke, spinal cord injury, traumatic brain injury, multiple sclerosis, osteoarthritis, rheumatoid arthritis, limb loss, and back pain. *Archives of Physical Medicine and Rehabilitation, 95*, 986–995.

National Spinal Cord Injury Statistical Center. (2015). *Facts and figures at a glance*. Birmingham, AL: National Spinal Cord Injury Statistical Center, University of Alabama at Birmingham.

Silva, N., Sousa, N., Reis, R., & Salgado, A. (2014). From basics to clinical: A comprehensive review on spinal cord injury. *Progress in Neurobiology, 114*, 25–57.

Wan, D., & Krassioukov, A. (2014). Life-threatening outcomes associated with autonomic dysreflexia: A clinical review. *Journal of Spinal Cord Medicine, 37*(1), 2–10.

■ SUBSTANCE USE DISORDERS AND TOXICOLOGICAL AGENTS

Al Rundio

Overview

The purpose of this entry is to discuss the major substances of abuse, common street names of substances that are abused, and the most prevailing clinical effects. Common toxidromes encountered in emergency situations are also described.

Background

Substance use disorders have been a problem in the U.S. society for some time now. Under President Richard Nixon the Controlled Substances Act of 1970 was enacted, which established the Drug Enforcement Agency (DEA), as an attempt to control substance abuse in the United States (Van Dusen & Spies, 2007). Despite such efforts, the problem continues to grow at an alarming rate.

The United States is dealing with an opiate epidemic. Provider prescribing of opiates for pain control is one of the major factors that contributes to this epidemic. Pain as the fifth vital sign and accrediting bodies' focus on pain control is now being questioned (Rundio, 2013).

The use of benzodiazepines has also increased and many substance users abuse benzodiazepines along with opiates. This synergistic effect is most pronounced on the respiratory system most often causing respiratory depression with resultant cardiac arrest and death.

It has been estimated that the total economic cost of substance use disorders (alcohol, tobacco, and illicit drugs) in the United States exceeds $700 billion annually (National Institute of Drug Abuse [NIDA], 2017). This dollar amount is inclusive of costs related to crime, lost work productivity, and the cost of health care.

The anxiolytic class of substances is becoming more popular among young adults. Alcohol falls in this class as well as benzodiazepines, barbiturates, rohypnol, and GHB (gamma hydroxybutyrate). The common names for these substances include *beer, wine, distilled spirits, Xanax, Valium, roofies*, and *Liquid X*. These substances can be ingested or snorted. The effects from the use of these substances include disorientation, poor coordination, slurred speech, headache, nausea, vomiting, diarrhea, decreased mental alertness, miosis, hyporeflexia, decreased bowel sounds, hypothermia, hypotension, bradycardia, respiratory depression, and unconsciousness.

The opiate class of drugs are derived directly from the opium poppy and also can be semisynthetic or synthetic in nature. The drugs in this class are morphine and codeine. The semisynthetic opioids are heroin (diacetylmorphine), hydromorphone (Dilaudid), oxycodone (Percocet, OxyContin) and hydrocodone (Loricet, Vicodin). The synthetic opioids are methadone, fentanyl, meperidine (Demerol), and propoxyphene (Darvocet). Common street names for these drugs are *junk, H, dope, smack, chiba, tar, brown sugar, chiva, white horse, skag, dragon*, and *white*. These drugs are primarily used via nasal insufflation and direct intravenous injection.

Medically, they are used as pain killers with the exception of heroin. The drugs block pain and produce euphoria. They are highly addictive.

The effects of use of these drugs include decreased mental alertness, miosis, hyporeflexia, hypothermia, hypotension, bradycardia, decreased bowel sounds, respiratory depression, and death.

Overdoses may result from variability in the potency of the heroin purchased on the street, rapid loss of tolerance after abstinence, and concurrent use of other central nervous system depressants, for example, heroin is now being laced with fentanyl, which is responsible for many deaths.

The stimulant class of drugs includes cocaine, crack cocaine, amphetamines, methamphetamine, and MDMA (methylene dioxymethamphetamine). Common names are *coke, blow, crack, rock, speed, uppers, cross tops, ectasy, XTC, X, club drug, rolls, love drug*, and *Adam*. These drugs can be snorted, smoked, injected, or ingested.

The effects of use of these drugs are alertness, a false sense of power, tachycardia, elevated blood pressure (BP), itchy skin, compulsive tooth grinding, tachycardia, weight loss, hallucinations, nausea, insomnia, and an elevated body temperature.

The common names for tetrahydrocannabinol (THC) or cannabis is marijuana or hashish. Street names include *weed, pot, grass, bud, joints, bong hits, hash*, and *hash oil*. This class of drugs is usually smoked. The effects of use of cannabis include poor concentration, short-term memory loss, anxiety, and increased appetite. Although many individuals feel that THC should be legalized for use, it causes profound effects most noted on the adolescent brain. This class of drugs is often used by adolescents as well as others in society.

One of the more common toxidromes are the anticholinergics (antimuscarinics). This class of drugs include antihistamines, antiparkinsonian agents, antipsychotics, tricycle antidepressants, mydriatics, antispasmodics, and plants with atropine, for example, *Datura stramonium* (malpitte).

These drugs are primarily ingested. The effects of use of these substances include delirium, dilated pupils, seizures, elevated temperature, tachycardia, urinary retention, decreased bowel movements, dry skin, flushed skin, myclonus, cardiac dysrhythmias (van Hoving, Veale, & Müller, 2011).

The other common toxidromes are the cholinergics (muscarinic and nicotine receptor stimulation). Common agents are organophosphate and carbamate pesticides (e.g., household, garden, and farm insecticides). These drugs are primarily ingested. The effects include confusion, central nervous system (CNS) depression, miosis, seizures, muscle fasiculations, muscle weakness (including respiratory muscles), diaphoresis, salivation, lacrimation, bronchorrhoea, and pulmonary edema (Hoving et al., 2011).

Clinical Aspects

ASSESSMENT

Assessment of substance use disorders follows general assessment guidelines for nursing with additional key components. These components include obtaining an accurate history on the type of substance used, the method of use, the frequency of use, and the last time used. It is also important to assess whether the patient is sharing needles and other paraphernalia as such behaviors may lead to other types of illnesses such as HIV, hepatitis A, B, and C. As substance abusers also present with other comorbidities (psychological and/or medical) assessing for such comorbidities is critical. Many substance abusers have an underlying depression and may be suicidal. Assessment of suicide ideation and plan are necessary in the initial assessment and ongoing assessments.

NURSING INTERVENTIONS, MANAGEMENT, AND IMPLICATIONS

Nursing must complete accurate and timely ongoing assessment especially when one is in the detoxification stage of treatment. Accurately recording vital signs with specific attention to alertness and respirations is essential. Use of clinical withdrawal scales, such as the COWS (Clinical Opiate Withdrawal Scale) for opiates and the CIWA (Clinical Institute Withdrawal Alcohol Scale) for alcohol and benzodiazepines is necessary. These scales rate objective criteria for how symptomatic a patient is. The administering of detoxification medications is based on defined parameters from these scales and approved by the treatment facility's medical staff.

Benzodiazepines are generally prescribed for detoxification from alcohol and benzodiazepines. Such medications include Librium, Ativan, Serax, or Valium. Buprenorphine or a combination of buprenorphine with naloxone (Suboxone) is used for opiate withdrawal. Naloxone is administered for opiate overdose situations. Cannabis (THC) and the stimulant class of drugs generally do not require specific detoxification medications.

OUTCOMES

The ability of the nurse to not only identify persons potentially or actually abusing substances but also have an understanding of the effects the substances have on the body is beneficial for assisting the patient to be successful with interventions and rehabilitation. It can be difficult to manage a person using substances that can be lethal and toxic but the nurse needs to do his or her best to assist the patient through the process. Advocating for patients through interdisciplinary team approached care is optimal for positive patient outcomes.

Summary

The goal of treatment is to have the patient detox safely and engage in other necessary treatment modalities such as individual and group counseling, psychotherapy and attendance at 12-step meetings. As substance use disorders are considered chronic illnesses, monitoring the patient's recovery for long-term maintenance of sobriety is necessary. Recovery systems of care must be implemented.

National Institute of Drug Abuse. (2017). Trends and statistics. Retrieved from https://www.drugabuse.gov/related-topics/trends-statistics.

Van Dusen, V., & Spies, A. R. (2007). An overview and update of the controlled substances act of 1970. *Pharmacy Times.* Retrieved from http://www.pharmacytimes.com/publications/issue/2007/2007-02/2007-02-6309

van Hoving, D. J., Veale, D. J. H. & Müller, G. F. (2011). Clinical review: Emergency management of acute poisoning. *African Journal of Emergency Medicine, 1*(2), 69–78.

■ THORACIC AORTIC ANEURYSM

Megan M. Shifrin
Ronald L. Hickman, Jr.

Overview

Thoracic aortic aneurysms (TAAs) remain one of the most life-threatening conditions in adult patients with atherosclerosis. Prompt preoperative diagnosis of expanding or ruptured aortic aneurysms is critical to improving patient morbidity and mortality. High-quality nursing care across the perioperative continuum is critical to ensure optimal outcomes in patients living with a TAA.

Background

Aortic aneurysms have been traditionally defined as permanent, localized dilation of at least 50% of the expected diameter of the aortic artery (Abraha, Romagnoli, Montedori, & Cirocchi, 2016). However, several organizations have favored using objective numerical measurements to standardize criteria for evaluation and intervention (Erbel et al., 2014; Hiratzka et al., 2010). Aortic aneurysms can be broadly divided into two separate categories based on location: TAA and abdominal aortic aneurysm (AAA). Major morbidity and mortality associated with both TAAs and AAAs stems from aortic dissection and aortic rupture (Abraha et al., 2016; Erbel et al., 2014; Hiratzka et al., 2010; Vapnik et al., 2016).

TAAs are typically associated medial degeneration along with a host of acute and chronic conditions that affect the integrity of the vessel wall of the thoracic aorta. Medial degeneration is an inflammatory process that results in the production of free oxygen radicals and proinflammatory cytokines that contribute to the degradation of proteins and smooth muscle apoptosis. The end result of medial degeneration is the loss of the medial elastic lamellae and thinning of the tunica media of the aortic arterial wall. These pathophysiologic alterations in the integrity of the ascending aortic arterial wall make the affected area susceptible to the wall strain due to the velocity and hydrostatic pressure of the blood flowing through the thoracic aorta. Chronic hypertension creates higher than normal mechanical and shear forces that contribute to the weakening of the thoracic aortic vessel wall. In addition to medial degeneration and chronic hypertension, other processes that weaken and cause damage to the vessel are atherosclerosis of the thoracic aortic vessel, infections (e.g., syphilis), collagen disorders (e.g., Marfan syndrome), and traumatic injury to the chest. There is also emerging evidence of the gene polymorphisms that enhance an individual's susceptibility to the development of a TAA.

TAAs encompass aneurysms that occur in the ascending aorta, aortic arch, and descending aorta to the level of the diaphragm. Risk factors for TAAs include hypertension, Marfan syndrome, bicuspid aortic valve, genetic predisposition, and atherosclerosis (Abraha et al., 2016). TAAs have an incidence of 10.4 per 100,000 (Abraha et al., 2016). Patients with a TAA diameter greater than 50 mm who also have preexisting risk factors and a rapid aneurysmal expansion should be considered for surgical intervention (Erbel et al., 2014; Hiratzka et al., 2010). The reported 5-year mortality risk for patients with

TAAs greater than 60 mm ranges from 38% to 64%. However, once a TAA has ruptured, reported mortality rates have been reported as high as 97% (Abraha et al., 2016). Acutely symptomatic patients with a history of TAA should undergo expedited radiographic imaging to assess the need for emergent surgical intervention to lower their morbidity and mortality risk.

Clinical Aspects

ASSESSMENT

Patients who present with a TAA should be carefully assessed for neurovascular, cardiac, and pulmonary complications. In particular, the nurse should assess for the presence or absence of pain or chest pressure. From a neurovascular standpoint, patients with a TAA are at a risk for neuralgic pain and ipsilateral dilation of the pain, which may result in nerve compression. In addition, patients may experience dyspnea, cough, hoarseness, and dysphagia due to aneurysmal compression on the laryngeal nerve and esophagus, or displacement of the trachea, which should be assessed. Given the pathophysiology of the TAA, nurses should assess for blood pressure variations between arms and dilated superficial veins of the chest wall, which are indicators of compromised systemic circulation.

There are several diagnostic tests that can help the nurse and the health care team inform the care of the patient with a TAA. An initial workup for a patient suspected to have a TAA may include chest radiographs, which indicate calcification of the affected aorta and establish the presence of an aneurysm. A CT scan or magnetic resonance angiography (MRA) are often used to monitor the size of the aneurysm and evaluate the arterial circulation, respectively.

NURSING INTERVENTIONS, MANAGEMENT, AND IMPLICATIONS

Patients who have a TAA are at high risk for developing neurovascular complications in the postoperative period. Maintaining meticulous care of patients with lumbar drains and maintaining hemodynamic goals may help prevent neurovascular complications. For patients with a TAA repair, neurological status and extremity sensation, movement, and strength should be assessed hourly in the immediate postoperative period (Cronenwett & Johnston, 2014). Change in a patient's neurological exam, paresthesia, or paralysis may be indicative of a compromise in vascular perfusion. Immediate

notification of the vascular surgical team is warranted in these circumstances (Cronenwett & Johnston, 2014).

Patients with a TAA frequently vacillate between hypotensive to hypertensive states, and thus, should be monitored closely. Patients with hypotension tend to be at higher risk for end-organ ischemia and vascular occlusion. Volume resuscitation with crystalloid intravenous fluids combined intravenous vasopressors remains a mainstay of treatment (Chen & Crozier, 2014; Cronenwett & Johnston, 2014). For patients with hypertension, intravenous beta-1 agonists and calcium channel blockers may be administered. If a patient is also at high risk for developing a postoperative myocardial infarction or has objective findings indicative of an evolving myocardial infarction, nitrates may also be considered for hypertensive management (Chen & Crozier, 2014; Cronenwett & Johnston, 2014).

Following either open or endovascular repair of a TAA, acute blood loss anemia and coagulopathy are common. Potential coagulopathies should be quickly evaluated by assessing a patient's prothrombin time (PT)/international normalized ratio (INR), activated partial thromboplastin time (aPTT), fibrinogen, platelet count, and platelet function; the administration of products, such as fresh frozen plasma, cryoprecipitate, and pooled platelets, should also be considered (Cronenwett & Johnston, 2014). Packed red blood cells should be administered to patients with a hemoglobin level less than 7 mg/dL who also have signs and symptoms of hemodynamic instability and/or ischemia. Noncoagulopathic causes of acute postoperative anemia include bleeding from the surgical anastomosis site or endovascular leak. Ongoing postoperative bleeding that is not associated with coagulopathy may warrant surgical reexploration (Cronenwett & Johnston, 2014).

In preoperative care settings, the nurses should prioritize their neurovascular, cardiac, and respiratory assessments of patients with acute symptoms of a TAA. Specifically, nurses should monitor for signs and symptoms of worsening chest pain, paresthesia, stroke, dyspnea, and cardiac tamponade. Frequent monitoring of neurologic status, blood pressure, peripheral pulses, respiratory rate, pulse oximetry, and capillary refill is recommended and changes reported.

OUTCOMES

For patients who require a surgical intervention for a repair of a TAA, the nurse should continue to be vigilant in the assessment of the patient's neurovascular, cardiac, and respiratory status. During the immediate postoperative period, monitoring for signs of blood loss and anemia (e.g., hypotension, tachycardia, urine output, and pallor) is recommended. Similar to other populations of surgical patients, the nurse should aim to provide adequate pain management, assess for signs of surgical site infection, and administer prescribed antibiotics in a timely fashion to optimize the patient's postoperative outcomes.

Summary

Expanding and ruptured TAAs are associated with extensive morbidity and mortality. However, prompt diagnosis, surgical and endovascular management, and vigilant critical care nursing management can improve patient outcomes. Ongoing cardiovascular, neurological, and abdominal assessments are of particular importance given the postoperative complications that may occur. Hemodynamic management, coagulopathy evaluation and correction, and volume resuscitation are also mainstays of effective postoperative treatment.

Abraha, I., Romagnoli, C., Montedori, A., & Cirocchi, R. (2016). Thoracic stent graft versus surgery for thoracic aneurysm. *Cochrane Database of Systematic Reviews*, *2016*(6). doi:10.1002/14651858.CD006796 .pub4

Chen, T., & Crozier, J. A. (2014). Endovascular repair of thoracic aortic pathologies: Postoperative nursing implications. *Journal of Vascular Nursing*, *32*(2), 63–69. doi:10.1016/j.jvn.2013.07.001

Cronenwett, J. L., & Johnston, K. W. (2014). *Rutherford's vascular surgery* (8th ed.). Philadelphia, PA: Elsevier Saunders.

Erbel, R., Aboyans, V., Boileau, C., Bossone, E., Di Bartolomeo, R., Eggebrecht, H., . . . Vlachopoulos, C. (2014). 2014 ESC guidelines on the diagnosis and treatment of aortic diseases. *European Heart Journal*, *35*(41), 2873–2926. doi:10.1093/eurheartj/ehu281

Hiratzka, L. F., Bakris, G. L., Beckman, J. A., Bersin, R. M., Carr, V. F., Casey, D. E., . . . Williams, D. M. (2010). 2010 ACCF/AHA/AATS/ACR/ASA/SCA/SCAI/SIR/STS/SVM guidelines for the diagnosis and management of patients with thoracic aortic disease: Executive summary. *Journal of the American College of Cardiology*, *55*(14), 1509–1544. doi:10.1016/j.jacc.2010.02.010

Vapnik, J. S., Kim, J. B., Isselbacher, E. M., Ghoshhajra, B. B., Cheng, Y., Sundt, T. M., . . . Lindsay, M. E. (2016). Characteristics and outcomes of ascending versus descending thoracic aortic aneurysms. *American Journal of Cardiology*, *117*(10), 1683–1690. doi:10.1016/ j.amjcard.2016.02.048

■ THROMBOCYTOPENIA IN ADULTS

Khoa (Joey) Dang

Overview

Thrombocytopenia is a common and potentially life-threatening condition in which there is a decrease in platelet count within the circulating blood volume. Adults can develop thrombocytopenia from various causes, including bone marrow suppression from radiation or chemotherapy, liver failure, disseminated intravascular coagulation, bacterial or viral infections, autoimmune disorders, and various medication effects (Chavan, Chauhan, Joshi, Ojha, & Bhat, 2014; Hunt, 2014).

Background

Thrombocytopenia is identified as a platelet count below the lower limit of normal of 150,000/μL (normal range 150,000–450,000/μL), based on most laboratory standards (Sekhon & Roy, 2006). Platelets are developed from the fragmentation of megakaryocytes and circulate in the blood for a week to 10 days. Thrombocytopenia can be caused from various conditions and can be associated with different degrees of risk from life-threatening bleeding to no risk of complications.

Thrombocytopenia can result from pathophysiologic mechanisms of platelet destruction and consumption, bone marrow disease, dilutional processes, and splenic disorders. Patients who present without symptoms are more likely to have immune thrombocytopenia, also known as *idiopathic thrombocytopenic purpura (ITP)*. However, patients who are acutely ill with symptoms of thrombocytopenia typically have multisystem involvement with etiologies of infection/sepsis, nutritional deficiencies, autoimmune disease, drug-induced thrombocytopenia (such as in heparin-induced thrombocytopenia) or platelet destruction.

In children with thrombocytopenia, the causes can generally be categorized by either platelet-destructive mechanisms or by decreased production of platelets. Platelet-destruction disorders include immune-mediated destruction (such as immune thrombocytopenia), platelet activation and consumption (such as in disseminated intravascular coagulation and thrombotic thrombocytopenic purpura), drug-induced thrombocytopenia, mechanical destruction (from the use of extracorporeal therapies), and sequestration and trapping (such as with hypersplenism). Thrombocytopenia caused from decreased platelet production can occur with infection (usually from suppression of bone marrow or immune mediated process), bone marrow disorders, deficiencies from poor nutrition, and genetic conditions.

The prevalence of thrombocytopenia is determined based on the underlying etiology causing the low platelet count. The most recent estimates of ITP show a prevalence exceeding incidence and that ITP affects all ages, with approximately eight per 100,000 cases in children and 12 in 100,000 in adults (Terrell et al., 2008). With drug-induced immune thrombocytopenia, the estimated incidence is 10 cases per million population per year and accounts for approximately 20% to 25% (when combined with ITP and TTP) of all blood disorders (Kam & Alexander, 2014). Thrombocytopenia occurrence in pregnancy is common with many etiologies and not always clinically relevant. The most common cause of thrombocytopenia during pregnancy, with rates as high as 5% of all pregnant women, is gestational thrombocytopenia (Kasai et al., 2015).

Bleeding risk is the main concern with patients who have thrombocytopenia and spontaneous hemorrhage is considered when other factors exist, such as previous history of bleeding, other coagulopathies, and platelet-function defects. Although there are no evidence-based recommendations on what is considered a safe platelet count, clinical judgment and history of prior bleeding should be evaluated to determine bleeding risk. There appears to be no correlation between the risk of spontaneous bleeding and specific platelet counts.

Clinical Aspects

ASSESSMENT

A thorough patient history is crucial in determining other conditions that may explain thrombocytopenia in both inpatient and outpatient settings. Individualized, patient-centered nursing care begins with obtaining a complete history, performing a full physical assessment/exam, and evaluating pertinent laboratory data. The history data should be obtained from sources, including the patient, other medical records, family members of the patient, and other clinicians who have cared for the patient. Important historical data helpful in managing the patient include prior platelet counts, history of bleeding or blood dyscrasias, infectious exposures (viral, bacterial, rickettsial) or recent travel to endemic areas, dietary practices, medication exposures (such as heparin, aspirin, anticoagulants, sulfa-containing medications, etc.), family history of bleeding disorders or thrombocytopenia, and other medical conditions (such as autoimmune disorders, rheumatological diseases, malignancies, blood transfusions, etc.). A thorough physical exam can provide important information on potential causes of the thrombocytopenia (such as hepatomegaly and lymphadenopathy) and should be focused on identifying signs of bleeding. Bleeding-related changes in the skin and other sites of bleeding include purpura (bleeding into skin), petechiae, or ecchymosis. Marking the skin bleeding by circumscribing the area is helpful to assess and document the extent of bleeding and determine the persistence or worsening of thrombocytopenia. The liver, spleen, and lymph nodes should be palpated for enlargement and pain; these signs can denote a specific etiology of thrombocytopenia. Additional physical assessments in the following areas can evaluate new-onset or worsening of bleeding: cardiovascular (hypotension, tachycardia, dizziness or epistaxis), pulmonary (tachypnea, hemoptysis or respiratory distress), gastrointestinal (hematemesis, abdominal discomfort or distension, rectal bleeding), genitourinary (vaginal or urethral bleeding), and neurological (headache, changes in vision, altered level of consciousness). The full nursing assessment/exam must be performed every shift with focused bleeding risk assessments throughout the shift to determine worsening physical status and to evaluate any new onset of bleeding.

Laboratory monitoring of a complete blood count (CBC) with an emphasis on the platelet count, hemoglobin and hematocrit, and white blood count (WBC) is important to determine bleeding risks, severity of acute bleeding, acute infections, and the possibility of systemic disorders. Blood crossmatch and typing are recommended if a blood transfusion is anticipated in the setting of severe anemia secondary to acute blood loss. Testing of urine, stool, and emesis for occult blood is advised to evaluate for systemic bleeding from thrombocytopenia.

NURSING INTERVENTIONS, MANAGEMENT, AND IMPLICATIONS

The nursing care of a patient with thrombocytopenia should be focused on decreasing the risk of bleeding and reducing complications of active bleeding. Additional responsibilities should include managing underlying conditions attributed to thrombocytopenia and providing support to the systems affected by thrombocytopenia.

The nursing care interventions are aimed at decreasing bleeding complications of thrombocytopenia. Performing physical assessments and reassessments at regular intervals allows for early identification of hemorrhaging and alerts providers to initiate appropriate medical management. Other interventions to prevent complications include avoiding medications that worsen bleeding (such as anticoagulants), avoiding certain routes of medication administration (such as intramuscular injections and suppositories), using stool softeners or laxatives to prevent constipation, applying direct pressure to venipuncture sites for at least 5 minutes or until the bleeding ceases, avoiding unnecessary suctioning (oral, nasotracheal, and endotracheal), preventing falls by ambulatory patients, and administering blood products (such as platelets, packed red blood cells, and fresh frozen plasma) as prescribed (Winkeljohn, 2013).

OUTCOMES

A nursing evaluation for risk of bleeding from activity should be also be included in the nursing interventions. Health education and patient teaching should address signs and symptoms of disease exacerbation, medication therapy, activity restrictions (if applicable), diet selection that does not contribute to platelet reduction, and routine monitoring of platelet count. Careful evaluation, interventions, and education promote positive outcomes in these patients.

Summary

Nursing care for thrombocytopenia should coordinate medical management with nursing interventions to decrease morbidity and mortality. General management principles apply to all patients with thrombocytopenia, regardless of etiology: activity restrictions in moderate to severe thrombocytopenia (less than 50,000/μL), antiplatelet medication avoidance, avoiding invasive procedures if platelet count is low, and management of bleeding. Nursing management of thrombocytopenia

requires performing accurate assessment and evaluation of severity of disease, developing nursing care objectives, implementing timely treatment strategies and nursing interventions, and ongoing appraisal and revision of nursing care goals.

Chavan, P., Chauhan, B., Joshi, A., Ojha, S., & Bhat, V. (2014). Differential diagnosis of thrombocytopenia in hematopoietic stem cell transplant patients. *Journal of Hematology & Thromboembolic Diseases, 2,* 168. doi:10.4172/2329–8790.1000168

Hunt, B. J. (2014). Bleeding and coagulopathies in critical care. *New England Journal of Medicine, 370*(22), 2153. doi:10.1056/NEJMc1403768

Kam, T., & Alexander, M. (2014). Drug-induced immune thrombocytopenia. *Journal of Pharmacy Practice, 27*(5), 430–439. doi:10.1177/0897190014546099

Kasai, J., Aoki, S., Kamiya, N., Hasegawa, Y., Kurasawa, K., Takahashi, T., & Hirahara, F. (2015). Clinical features of gestational thrombocytopenia difficult to differentiate from immune thrombocytopenia diagnosed during pregnancy. *Journal of Obstetrics and Gynaecology Research, 41*(1), 44–49. doi:10.1111/jog.12496

Sekhon, S. S., & Roy, V. (2006). Thrombocytopenia in adults: A practical approach to evaluation and management. *Southern Medical Journal, 99*(5), 491–498; quiz 499. doi:10.1097/01.smj.0000209275.75045.d4

Terrell, D., Beebe, L. A., George, J., Neas, B. R., Vesely, S. K., & Segal, J. (2008). The prevalence of immune thrombocytopenic purpura (ITP). *Blood, 112*(11), 1277–1277.

Winkeljohn, D. (2013). Diagnosis, treatment, and management of immune thrombocytopenia. *Clinical Journal of Oncology Nursing, 17*(6), 664–666. doi:10.1188/13.CJON.664-666

■ THYROID CRISIS

Cynthia Ann Leaver

Overview

Thyroid crisis, also known as *thyrotoxic crisis, thyroid storm,* or *hyperthyroid storm,* is an acute, life-threatening exacerbation of thyrotoxicosis (De Groot & Bartalena, 2015; Ross et al., 2016). Thyroid crisis occurs in the presence of thyrotoxicosis, in which an individual's ability to maintain adequate metabolic, thermoregulatory, and cardiovascular compensatory mechanism is surpassed (Warnock, Cooper, & Burch, 2014). Thyroid crisis ranks as one of the most critical endocrine emergencies and requires immediate recognition and steadfast commitment to an aggressive, therapeutic, and multifaceted intervention to prevent the high morbidity and mortality associated with the disorder (Angell et al., 2015; Ross et al., 2016; Warnock et al., 2014). It is noteworthy that the American Thyroid Association recommends the diagnosis of thyroid storm as a clinical diagnosis that is augmented by the use of sensitive empiric diagnostic systems (Burch-Wartofsky Point Scale [BWPS] or the Japanese Thyroid Association criteria). Nursing care of the patient with thyroid crisis requires rapid assessment and intervention for multisystem decompensation (Ross et al., 2016).

Background

Thyroid crisis is one on the most critical endocrine emergencies; incidence for patients hospitalized for thyrotoxicosis, progressing to thyroid crisis, is identified to be less than 10% (Warnock et al., 2014). However, the mortality rate due to thyroid crisis ranges from 8% to 25% (De Leo, Lee, & Braverman, 2016; Ross et al., 2016). An apparent trigger of thyroid crisis can be identified in up to 70% of cases (De Leo et al., 2016). In the past, thyroid crisis most frequently occurred after surgery for thyrotoxicosis. Today, with earlier diagnosis and treatment of thyrotoxicosis, and improvement in pre- and postoperative medical management, postoperative thyroid crisis is now a rare occurrence (De Groot & Bartalena, 2015). Currently, the most common underlying cause of thyrotoxicosis progression to thyroid crisis is Graves' disease (80%), and it is notable that Graves' disease occurs most frequently in young women, but can occur in either gender and any age group (Carroll & Matfin, 2010).

Thyroid crisis represents the extreme manifestations of thyrotoxicosis, in which factors have provoked progression on the thyrotoxic continuum (De Groot & Bartalena, 2015; Warnock et al., 2014). The spectrum of thyrotoxicosis ranges from asymptomatic, subclinical, to life-threatening thyroid crisis. *Hyperthyroidism* refers to disorders that result from overproduction of hormone from the thyroid gland, *thyrotoxicosis* refers to any case of excessive thyroid hormone concentration, and *thyroid crisis* is the severely thyrotoxic patient with systemic decompensation. The factors impacting thyrotoxicity include age, comorbidities, rapid onset of hormone excess, and presence or absence of precipitating event (Warnock et al., 2014). Therefore, management of thyroid storm is broadly divided into therapy directed against thyroid hormone secretion, synthesis, and action at the tissue level; reversal of systemic decompensation, and treatment of the precipitating event (Ross et al., 2016).

Normal thyroid function is maintained by endocrine interactions among the hypothalamus, anterior pituitary, and thyroid gland (Carroll & Matfin, 2010). Iodide is transported across the basement membrane of the thyroid cells by an intrinsic membrane protein (Na/I symporter). Then, at the apical boarder, a second iodide transport protein (pendirin) moves iodide into the colloid, where iodide is involved in hormonogenesis of thyroxine (T4) and triiodothyronine (T3). Thyroxine (T4) is the major thyroid hormone secreted into the circulation. Circulating thyroid hormone consists of 90% T4, and 10% T3. (Carroll & Matfin, 2010). There is evidence that T4 is converted to T3 before it can act physiologically, therefore making T3 the active form of circulating thyroid hormone.

The precise pathogenesis of thyroid crisis is still poorly understood (De Leo et al., 2016). One hypothesis to explain the pathogenesis of thyroid crisis is an increase in the amount of free thyroid hormones. One study found mean T4 concentration was higher in subjects with thyroid crisis, whereas the total T4 concentration was similar in both study groups (De Groot & Bartalena, 2015). Another theory that may explain the pathogenesis of thyroid crisis is a possible increase in target cell beta-adrenergic receptor density or postreceptor modification in signaling pathways (Nayak & Burman, 2006).

Ross et al. (2016) identified general impetuses for thyrotoxicosis to be excessive thyroid stimulation by trophic factors; thyroid hormone synthesis and secretion, leading to autonomous release of excess thyroid hormone; thyroid stores of performed hormone are passively released in excessive amounts owing to autoimmune, infectious, chemical, or mechanical insult; or exposure to extrathyroidal sources of thyroid hormone, which may be either endogenous (struma ovarii, metastatic differentiated thyroid cancer) or exogenous (factitious thyrotoxicosis). Consequently, thyrotoxicosis provoked by age, comorbidities, rapid onset of hormone excess, and presence or absence of precipitating event may lead to thyroid crisis (Carroll & Matfin, 2010; Warnock et al., 2014).

Clinical Aspects

ASSESSMENT

The important clinical point in effective nursing care of a patient considered for potential thyroid crisis is to assess and treat in an active, preemptory fashion when possible. The distinction between severe thyrotoxicosis and thyroid crisis is a matter of clinical judgment.

Nursing care of thyroid crisis is to include history, physical assessment, and laboratory data. Accurate history of an individual who is suspected to have thyroid crisis must include query into any condition predisposing the individual to risk of thyrotoxicosis and reported for medical treatment.

The physical assessment should focus on general organ decompensation and changes in the following body systems should include fever 102.2°F or higher; respiratory system (tachypnea greater than 20 breaths/minute, breath sounds reveal signs and symptoms consistent with congestive heart failure to include bibasilar rales and crackles); cardiovascular system (systolic hypertension or hypotension; tachycardia and disproportionate to the degree of fever; bounding pulses, systolic murmur, widening pulse or weak thready pulses; peripheral edema); neurologic system (agitation, delirium, psychosis, tremors, seizures, extreme lethargy, or coma); gastrointestinal system (increase in bowel sounds, diarrhea, nausea/vomiting, or abdominal pain, and possible jaundice); and endocrine system (enlarged or nodular thyroid). Assessment of diagnostic data is to be followed astutely for indications of progression or recovery of thyroid crises.

NURSING INTERVENTIONS, MANAGEMENT, AND IMPLICATIONS

Nursing care of the patient with possible thyroid crisis should principally focus on management of the ABCDEs (i.e., airway, breathing, circulation; disability, i.e., level of consciousness; and examination). Priority nursing-related issues include decreased cardiac output related to increased cardiac work secondary to increased adrenergic activity and deficient fluid volume secondary to increased metabolism and diaphoresis.

Nursing management of the patient with thyroid crisis consists of dextrose-containing intravenous fluids as ordered to correct fluid and glucose deficits, assessment for heart failure or pulmonary edema, dopamine may be used to support blood pressure, and supplemental oxygen as ordered to help meet increased metabolic demands.

Once the patient is hemodynamically stable, nursing management comprises pulmonary hygiene to reduce pulmonary complications. If the patient is in heart failure, typical pharmacologic agents for treatment of heart failure may also be indicated. Nursing management must include strategies to reduce oxygen demands by decreasing anxiety, reduce fever, decrease pain, and limit visitors if necessary. Nursing care must anticipate aggressive treatment of precipitating factors and institute pressure ulcer strategies.

OUTCOMES

The expected outcomes of evidence-based nursing care are focused on preventing progression of thyroid crisis. Nursing outcome criteria include continuous monitoring of oxygen saturation with pulse oximetry, lung sounds clear to auscultation, level of consciousness, peripheral pulses palpable and presence of peripheral edema, continuous EKG monitoring for dysthymias or heart rate greater than 140 beats/minute that can adversely affect cardiac output, life-threatening dysrhythmias, ST segment changes indicative of myocardial ischemia, continuous monitoring of pulmonary artery pressure, urine output 30 mL/hr, fluid volume status with hourly urine output and determination of fluid balance every 8 hours, and serial ABGs for hypoxemia and acid–base imbalance.

Summary

Thyroid crisis, also known as *thyrotoxic crisis, thyroid storm*, or *hyperthyroid storm*, is a life-threatening exacerbation of thyrotoxicosis, in the presence of a precipitating factor, and results when an individual's ability to maintain adequate metabolic, thermoregulatory, and cardiovascular compensatory mechanism is surpassed. Immediate recognition and aggressive, therapeutic, and multifaceted intervention to prevent the high morbidity and mortality associated with the disorder are required. Nursing care of patients with thyroid crisis is principally focused on management of ABCDEs, with vigilant assessment for factor precipitating the thyroid crisis.

Angell, T., Lehner, M. G., Nguyen, C. T., Salvato, V. L., Nicoloff, J. T., & LoPtesti, J. S. (2015). Clinical features and hospital outcomes in thyroid storm: A retrospective cohort study. *Journal of Clinical Endocrinology and Metabolism, 100*(2), 451–459. doi:10.1210/jc.2014-2850

Carroll, R., & Matfin, G. (2010). Endocrine and metabolic emergencies: Thyroid storm. *Therapeutic Advances in Endocrinology and Metabolism, 1*(3), 139–145. doi:10.1177/2042018810382481

De Groot L. J., & Bartalena L. (2015). Thyroid storm. In L. J. De Groot, G. Chrousos, K. Dungan, K. R. Feingold, A. Grossman, J. M. Hershman, . . . A. Vinik (Eds.), *Endotext* [Online]. South Dartmouth, MA: MDText. Retrieved from https://www.ncbi.nlm.nih.gov/books/NBK278927

De Leo, S., Lee, S. Y., & Braverman, L. E. (2016). Hyperthy-roidism. *Lancet*, 27(388), 906–918. doi:10.1016/S0140 -6736(16)00278-6

Nayak, B., & Burnam, K. (2006). Thyrotoxicosis and thyroid storm. *Endocrinology and Metabolism Clinics of North America*, 35, 663–686. doi:10.1016/j.ecl.2006.09.008

Ross, D. S., Burch, H. B., Cooper, M., Greenlee, C., Laurberg, P., Mala, A. L., . . . Walter, M. A. (2016). 2016 American thyroid association guidelines for diagnosis and man-agement of hyperthyroidism and other causes of thy-rotoxicosis. *Thyroid*, 26(10), 1343–1422. doi:10.1089/ thy.2016.0229

Warnock, A. L., Cooper, D. S., & Burch, H.B. (2014). Life-threatening thyrotoxicosis: Thyroid storm and adverse effects of antithyroid drugs. In G. Matfin (Ed.), *Endocrine and metabolic medical emergencies: Thyroid disorders* (pp. 110–126). Washington, DC: Endocrine Society/ Endocrine Press. Retrieved from http://press.endocrine .org/doi/pdf/10.1210/EME.9781936704811.ch11

■ TRAUMATIC BRAIN INJURY

Elizabeth Wirth-Tomaszewski

Overview

Traumatic brain injury (TBI) is the leading cause of trauma-related death and disability worldwide, affecting both adult and pediatric populations sig-nificantly. The incidence in the United States is esti-mated at 1.36 million cases with 52,000 deaths, as well as 275,000 hospitalizations annually (Centers for Disease Control and Prevention [CDC], 2016). Worldwide, TBI remains the leading cause of morbid-ity and mortality in those aged younger than 45 years (Andersen, Gazmuri, Marin, Regueira, & Rovegno, 2015). TBI encompasses a wide variety of conditions, ranging from mild to life-threatening, and can best be described as an alteration in brain function and/or structure due to external forces such as blunt or pen-etrating trauma or acceleration/deceleration forces (White & Venkatesh, 2016). Many types of TBI exist, such as concussions, hemorrhages, axonal injuries, and skull fractures, to name a few. These injuries may further be designated as acute, subacute, chronic, or acute on chronic. TBIs also include primary and secondary injury classifications. Nursing implica-tions include the assessment, identification of nursing problems, interventions, evaluation, and prevention of these injuries.

Background

TBIs are defined as a pathological alteration in the func-tion or structure of the brain by way of external forces. These forces can cause friction of the tissue, tearing of the vessels, or axonal injuries at the cellular level that cause impairment of function. Initial injuries are capa-ble of causing secondary injuries, usually due to cerebral edema, increased intracranial pressure (ICP; intracranial hypertension), oxidative stress, excitotoxicity, and sei-zures. Performing a thorough assessment and perform-ing appropriate intervention, the incidence of secondary brain injuries can be reduced (Andersen et al., 2015).

PREVALENCE OF TBI VARIES BY AGE

Children younger than 4 years of age, adolescents between 15 and 19 years of age, and adults older than the age of 65 years are most often diagnosed with TBI. Children under 14 years of age constitute approximately half of a million emergency department visits annually. Those aged 75 years and older are most likely to incur TBI-related hospitalization and death. TBI is a contributing factor to one third of all injury-related deaths in the United States. Mild TBIs constitute a majority of the reported injuries, with no available data on those who suffer mild TBI and do not seek care. TBI is a costly public health issue, total-ing approximately $60 billion per year when accounting for the direct and indirect costs (CDC, 2016).

Mild TBIs, such as concussions, are most prominent and are responsible for 80% of all TBIs. The leading cause of severe TBI is motor vehicle collisions, accounting for 30% to 50% of head injuries, with males aged 15 to 24 years being the demographic most affected. Other risk fac-tors include participation in contact sports, falls, advanced age (due to polypharmacy and sensory losses related to age), and failure to use safety devices, such as helmets, seat belts, and handrails (Garton & Lehmann, 2015). The structural pathology in TBI includes primary and second-ary causes, as well as Monro–Kellie hypothesis (equilib-rium of pressure and volume of brain structures inside the skull), and Cushing's triad phenomena (irregular respira-tions, bradycardia, and widening pulse pressure).

Primary TBIs include skull fractures, hemorrhages, contusions, and diffuse axonal injury (DAI). Due to the extreme forces required, there exists high suspicion for concomitant cervical spine injury, and care should be taken to immobilize the spine. Skull fractures may require surgery to repair, or may be medically managed by observation. Hemorrhages are treated differently, depending on type and severity. Epidural hemorrhages are arterial in nature, usually arising from a torn temporal artery and usually require surgical intervention. Subdural hemorrhages are venous in origin, and may require evacuation if there is significant mass effect or deficits noted. Traumatic subarachnoid hemorrhages may require an external ventricular drain (EVD) to be placed to monitor bleeding and ICP. Contusions and DAI are medically monitored (Garton & Lehmann, 2015).

SECONDARY TBI

Secondary TBI includes cytotoxic and/or vasogenic cerebral edema, cellular ischemic injury, and loss of cerebral blood flow regulation, which occurs in response to the primary brain injury. Mechanisms include apoptosis, calcium-dependent cascades, and oxidative stress creating damage at the cellular level. Prevention of hypoperfusion of the brain and increased metabolic demands are key to limiting secondary brain injuries (Andersen et al., 2015; Garton & Lehmann, 2015).

ICP is the result of three components within the skull: the brain tissue, cerebrospinal fluid, and blood. The brain is able to compensate for a small amount of tissue swelling, with displacement of the cerebrospinal fluid (CSF) and blood. When the brain tissue becomes compressed related to its own edema or mass effect from hematomas, blood supply is reduced leading to cerebral hypoperfusion and secondary brain injury. Untreated, this may lead to herniation through foramen magnum (tonsillar herniation) or skull fractures (Garton & Lehmann, 2015).

The constellation of symptoms that many times accompanies herniation is known as *Cushing's triad*. This includes bradycardia, hypertension, and respiratory irregularities. If the patient is intubated and on mechanical ventilation, many times the respiratory pattern goes unnoticed. The presence of Cushing's triad is ominous, and requires immediate attention by the neurosurgical provider. In severe cases of TBI with high ICPs and danger of herniation, decompressive craniectomy (removal of skull bone flap) may be required to allow expansion of the tissue in an effort to preserve life (Garton & Lehmann, 2015).

Clinical Aspects

ASSESSMENT

Obtaining an accurate history of the injury is important, as injury patterns may be identified. For instance,

epidural hemorrhages are suspected when there is an initial loss of consciousness, a period of lucidity, and then loss of consciousness once again. Amnesia, nausea, vomiting, headache, vertigo, nuchal rigidity, and vision disturbances are examples of significant findings in those with TBI (Garton & Lehmann, 2015).

In terms of physical assessment, frequent serial neurological exams are key in those diagnosed with TBI. Consistency of those exams between providers is extremely important, and should be performed with both receiving and departing providers present to ensure continuity in method and examination findings. Components of the assessment should include airway patency, adequacy of breathing, blood pressure monitoring parameters, Glasgow Coma Scale scoring, protective reflexes (cough, gag, corneal), pupillary size, equality and reaction, level of consciousness, as well as any focal deficits identified. Changes in exam should promptly be reported to the attending provider or neurosurgeon. Any impairment in airway patency (including loss of gag or cough reflex), ventilation, and/or depression in level of consciousness with a Glasgow Coma Scale score less than 8 requires emergency intervention for airway protection and mechanical ventilation (Garton & Lehmann, 2015).

Nursing problems associated with TBI include alteration in tissue perfusion, potential for alteration in airway patency, potential for seizures, potential for infection (related to monitoring/drainage devices), malnutrition, alteration in skin integrity related to immobility, and alteration in mental status related to acute TBI.

NURSING INTERVENTIONS, MANAGEMENT, AND IMPLICATIONS

Nursing interventions for TBI center on supportive care, prevention of secondary brain injuries, and restoration of homeostasis. For those diagnosed with mild TBI, serial neurological exams may be required for the first few days, with neurology follow-up. In moderate TBI, serial exams and cardiovascular monitoring may be required for close observation. In severe TBI, serial exams and cardiovascular monitoring are required, along with other possible modalities. Intracranial monitoring may be initiated by neurosurgery to facilitate monitoring of cerebral perfusion pressures (CPP) or EVDs employed to monitor and treat elevated ICPs by way of removal of CSF through a conduit placed in the ventricle. EEG may be used if seizures are suspected. Seizure precautions should be instituted by nursing, and antiepileptic drugs may be ordered by neurology on a prophylactic basis (Carney et al., 2016).

Maintenance of normal ventilation is essential in patients mechanically ventilated with severe TBI. Ventilation strategies are aimed at maintaining a normal level of carbon dioxide (CO_2; 35–45 mmHg). Lower CO_2 levels cause cerebral perfusion and ischemia, and higher CO_2 levels cause vasoconstriction and increased ICP.

Temperature-targeted therapy (therapeutic hypothermia) may be instituted to decrease metabolic demands and reduce cytotoxic events associated with cerebral edema. This type of therapy requires the critical care environment and is reserved for those with severe TBI. These patients are intubated, mechanically ventilated, and may require vasopressors to support a blood pressure sufficient enough to maintain cerebral perfusion (Andersen et al., 2015; Carney et al., 2016).

Cerebral edema may also be treated with hyperosmolar therapy in the form of mannitol or hypertonic saline. Both modalities employ osmolar pull to reduce edema in the brain by increasing the osmolality of the serum to pull fluid from this tissue. Mannitol has an additional diuretic component, which can ultimately affect blood pressure and reduce CPP. Hypertonic (3%) saline has been employed for the same osmotic effect, without diuretic properties (Carney et al., 2016).

Central diabetes insipidus is a condition related to antidiuretic hormone deficiency, characterized with large amounts of dilute urine output with low-specific gravity, and high serum osmolality is noted. This condition leads to hypernatremia, and is the body's attempt at hyperosmolar treatment. Desmopressin acetate may be required to control this phenomenon (Fitzgerald, 2017).

OUTCOMES

Goals of therapy include stabilization of primary injury, minimization of secondary injury, and return of homeostasis. Targets should include protecting airway patency and optimal ventilation, minimizing metabolic demands, providing nutrition support, and seizure precautions/prophylaxis. Measureable outcomes include maintaining a mean arterial pressure sufficient to provide cerebral perfusion (CPP = 60–70 mmHg), measureable with monitoring devices such as intracranial bolts or EVDs. ICPs should ideally be maintained at 0 to 10 mmHg. Normoglycemia, fever prevention, and normocarbia are also measureable outcomes that benefit those diagnosed with TBI (Carney et al., 2016).

Prevention is the most valuable of all interventions. Nurses are at the forefront of public health, and are in a position to provide assessment and education to those identified at risk. Nurses should encourage the use of concussion guidelines in sports, promote the use of helmets and other safety devices, and assist in the provision of home safety, medication reconciliation, and sensory screening for elders.

Summary

TBI is a prevalent world health issue and carries significant financial cost, as well as the morbidity and mortality associated with head injuries in many demographics. The long-term sequelae of TBI can last a lifetime, and prevention is the key. The utilization of safety devices and established guidelines in contact sports should be encouraged for all age groups.

TBI can be characterized as primary or secondary, by the acuity, and also by severity. Concussions, contusion, hemorrhages, and cellular injuries are some examples. Maintenance of cerebral perfusion and prevention of secondary injury are paramount in those with TBI. The goals of care are supportive and restorative, with guidelines in place by the Brain Trauma Foundation to guide providers in the care of these very complex patients. An ever-expanding wealth of knowledge is being gained in the area of TBI, and updates to these guidelines occur regularly.

Andersen, M., Gazmuri, J. T., Marin, A., Regueira, T., & Rovegno, M. (2015). Therapeutic hypothermia for acute brain injuries. *Scandinavian Journal of Trauma, Resuscitation, and Emergency Medicine, 23*(42), 1. doi:10.1186/s13049-015-0121-3

Carney, N., Totten, A. M., O'Reilly, C., Ullman, J. S., Hawryluk, G. W. J., Bell, M. J., . . . Ghajar, J. (2016). *Guidelines for management of traumatic brain injury* (4th ed.). Retrieved from https://braintrauma.org/uploads/03/12/Guidelines_for_Management_of_Severe_TBI_4th_Edition.pdf

Centers for Disease Control and Prevention. (2016). Get the stats of traumatic brain injury in the United States. Retrieved from https://www.cdc.gov/traumaticbrain injury/pdf/BlueBook_factsheet-a.pdf

Fitzgerald, P. A. (2017). Endocrine disorders. In M. A. Papadakis & S. J. McPhee (Eds.), *Current medical diagnosis and treatment* (56th ed., pp. 1113–1114). New York, NY: McGraw-Hill.

Garton, H., & Lehmann, E. (2015). Neurosurgery. In G. M. Doherty (Ed.), *Current diagnosis and treatment: Surgery* (14th ed., pp. 863–874). New York, NY: McGraw-Hill.

White, H., & Venkatesh, B. (2016). Traumatic brain injury. In W. Kolka, M. Smith, & G. Citerio (Eds.), *Oxford textbook of neuro critical care* (p. 210). Oxford, UK: Oxford University Press.

■ TRAUMATIC INJURY

Dustin Spencer

Overview

Traumatic injury is a significant cause of morbidity and mortality for people worldwide. Trauma is a frequent cause for patients across the life span to receive medical treatment in the outpatient, emergency, or inpatient setting. The sudden application of external force to tissues, whether intentional or unintentionally inflicted, results in traumatic injuries (American College of Surgeons Committee on Trauma, 2012). These injuries can range from relatively minor cutaneous contusions and abrasion to immediately life-threatening internal organ damage. Because of this, a deliberate and systematic approach to the trauma patient is required to identify injuries early in the treatment of the patient so that they can be addressed with the goal of achieving optimal short- and long-term outcomes (American College of Surgeons Committee on Trauma, 2012). This approach is applied across the trauma continuum: from public health prevention efforts to the prehospital phase through initial resuscitation, hospital admission, discharge, and postdischarge follow-up.

Background

Traumatic injury is a leading cause of disability worldwide. Globally, nearly 970 million people required some sort of medical attention due to a traumatic injury in 2013, of these nearly 5 million people died from their injuries (Haagsma et al., 2015). In the United States, unintentional injury remains the number one cause of death in the 1- to 44-year-old age group and is in the top 10 for every other age group (Centers for Disease Control and Prevention, n.d.). Of the nearly 27 million people treated in the emergency department for traumatic injuries in 2014, approximately 10% were hospitalized, leading to a total medical cost of over $80 million and work loss costs of over $150 million (CDC, 2017). Annually nearly 10 million people in the United States suffer disabling injuries and of these 3 million will experience some sort of permanent disability. In the United States, traumatic injuries cost upwards of $400 billion annually (CDC, 2017).

Common mechanisms of injury include motor vehicle collisions, falls, firearms, and burns. Of these, falls are the most common with approximately 9 million falls annually. Serious injury can result from falling from even relatively low-level heights, especially in the very young and very old. Motor vehicle injuries are the second most common and result in over 36,000 deaths per year (CDC, 2017). These deaths are predominately related to blunt trauma of the thorax, abdomen, pelvis, and head. These injuries can present as obvious initially or delayed by hours or days (American College of Surgeons Committee on Trauma, 2012).

Due to a direct blow, concussive transfer of energy, or the forces of inertia contribute to internal injuries that may not be notable without radiographic imaging or ultrasonography. Blunt trauma to the thorax can result in injury to great vessels leading to hemothorax and/or cardiac tamponade. Injury to the pulmonary tissue can lead to pulmonary contusion, pneumothorax, or tension pneumothorax (American College of Surgeons Committee on Trauma, 2012). Blunt trauma to the abdomen and pelvis can result in injury to the hollow organs (urinary bladder, stomach, intestines), solids organs (liver, spleen, kidneys, pancreas), genitourinary tract, diaphragm, aorta, or bony pelvis.

Traumatic injury to the musculoskeletal system occurs in far greater frequency than either thoracic or abdominal trauma. Although these injuries typically are less likely to be fatal, they can lead to significant disability and morbidity if potential sequelae are not prevented and identified early. A single-closed femur fracture can lead to significant blood loss and put the patient at risk for developing a fat embolus, both of which are potentially fatal conditions. An open fracture of any bone creates the potential for potentially serious infection to develop (American College of Surgeons Committee on Trauma, 2012). Injured muscle tissue can lead to an overwhelming demand on the kidneys, causing rhabdomyolysis. Penetrating trauma from a stab wound, impaled object, or a projectile, such as shrapnel or a bullet, results in similar injuries to these systems but with an added component of unpredictability associated with the movement of the penetrating object once it enters the cavity and travels to nearby cavities and organs (American College of Surgeons Committee on Trauma, 2012).

Clinical Aspects

ASSESSMENT

Each of these potential injuries has a unique presentation and associated interventions that are necessary to facilitate immediate, short-term and long-term survivability and limit disability. The single most important intervention is the application of a systematic process for assessment and management of the trauma patient. This process begins in the prehospital setting and follows the patient through the hospital stay until discharge. For this reason, trauma patients are best cared for in hospitals designated as trauma treatment centers. These facilities have verified that they have the specialized services, staff education, and follow-up procedures in place to achieve the best possible outcomes for trauma patients.

Early recognition of these injuries is paramount to determining the treatment priorities that are unique to the presenting case. The American College of Surgeons Committee on Trauma (2012) recommends an initial assessment and management phase followed by a secondary survey and management phase. During the initial assessment and management phase, the nurse should focus on the assessment and management of life-threatening compromise of a patient's airway, breathing, circulation, disability, and environment. In this order deficits are identified and corrected before moving to the next assessment. Only after airway, breathing and circulation have been stabilized can the secondary survey begin to help identify radiographic studies, laboratory studies, and diagnostic or treatment interventions that are necessary to further stabilize the patient before transfer to definitive care (American College of Surgeons Committee on Trauma, 2012).

During the secondary survey, assessment of the trauma patient's abdomen, thorax, and musculoskeletal system consists of the common skills of inspection, auscultation, and palpation. Inspection and palpation of the entire patient from head to toe allow the nurse to find occult injuries that may not be evident otherwise. These findings assist in the identification of further diagnostic testing considerations.

NURSING INTERVENTIONS, MANAGEMENT, AND IMPLICATIONS

The nursing focus during the care of trauma patients should be three pronged. First nurses should ensure that there are no subtle or overt changes in the patient's condition (vital signs, pain level, perfusion status, bowel sounds, etc.) that could indicate a change in hemodynamic stability. As noted earlier, trauma patients can have multisystem injuries, some of which may not present for a significant amount of time after the initial insult (American College of Surgeons Committee on Trauma, 2012). An astute nurse should be aware

of these potentials and recognize these early signs. The second focus is on prevention of further injury. Trauma patients are often a fall risk at baseline and once given pain medications this risk increases. Many of these patients are admitted to the nursing unit following surgical procedures and as such they are prone to confusion and potentially may be unsteady on their feet. The third focus of the nurse should be on ensuring that an adequate postdischarge rehabilitation plan is in place. This should include not just follow-up with the appropriate medical and rehabilitation specialist, but also resources for nutritional support, psychosocial support, environmental accommodations, and prevention of further injury (Worsowicz, Hwang, & Dawson, 2015).

OUTCOMES

The care of trauma patients is focused on facilitating survival with the least amount of residual disability. To meet these outcomes, trauma systems have dedicated resources to creating an infrastructure that supports the training, treatment, evaluation, and follow-up of patients who experience traumatic injuries (American College of Surgeons Committee on Trauma, 2012). Using a centralized data-collection tool, data are collected on trauma patients across the trauma continuum. This data is used to establish the evidence-based practice guidelines necessary for greater achievement of these outcome goals (American College of Surgeon, 2017).

Summary

Nurses across the trauma continuum have a direct impact on the outcomes their patients achieve. Using a systematic approach, the health care team can achieve the highest quality, evidence-based care for patients who have experienced a traumatic injury. This approach is based on an extensive analysis of the available data and designed to rapidly identify and proficiently intervene to address the apparent and occult injuries resulting from the traumatic event.

American College of Surgeons. (2017). National trauma data bank (NTDB). Retrieved from https://www.facs .org/quality-programs/trauma/ntdb

American College of Surgeons Committee on Trauma. (2012). *Advanced trauma life support* (9th ed.). Chicago, IL: Author.

Centers for Disease Control and Prevention. (n.d.). 10 leading causes of death by age group, United States 2014. Retrieved from https://www.cdc.gov/injury/images/lc-charts/leading_ causes_of_death_age_group_2014_1050w760h.gif

Centers for Disease Control and Prevention. (2017). Welcome to WISQARS: Cost of injury data. Retrieved from https://wisqars.cdc.gov:8443/costT

Haagsma, J., Graetz, N., Bolliger, I., Naghavi, M., Higashi, H., Mullany, E., . . . Vos, T. (2015). The global burden of injury: Incidence, mortality, disability-adjusted life years and time trends from the Global Burden of Disease study 2013. *Injury Prevention*, 22(1), 3–18.

Worsowicz, G., Hwang, S., & Dawson, P. (2015). Trauma Rehabilitation. In I. Maitin & E. Cruz (Eds.), *Current diagnosis & treatment*. New York, NY: McGraw-Hill.

■ UROLOGIC EMERGENCIES

Kelley Toffoli

Overview

Several urologic conditions warrant prompt diagnosis and treatment. Urinary tract infection, pyelonephritis, renal calculi, acute urinary retention, acute kidney injury, and testicular torsion necessitate emergent treatment. This section provides a meaningful overview of these urologic disorders that may manifest as a urological emergency.

Urinary Tract Infection

Background

Urinary tract infection (UTI) is a common urologic problem. In the United States, UTI is one of the most prevalent infections (Lingenfelter et al., 2016). UTIs occur throughout all age groups. UTI occurs more often in females than in males. It is estimated that 50% of females will experience at least one UTI in their lifetime (Barber, Norton, Spivak, & Mulvey, 2013).

Clinical Aspects

A UTI is defined as microbial infiltration of an otherwise sterile urinary tract (Barber et al., 2013). UTI can occur within the urethra, bladder, ureters, and kidney. *Escherichia coli* is the most common bacterial cause of UTI, estimated to be responsible for infection 54% to 90% of the time (Traisman, 2016). A UTI is considered to be complicated in patients with pregnancy, neurogenic dysfunction, bladder outlet obstruction, obstructive uropathy, bladder catheterization, urologic instrumentation, indwelling stent, urinary tract surgery, chemotherapy, radiation injury, renal impairment, diabetes, and immunodeficiency (Tonolini & Ippolito, 2016).

ASSESSMENT

Diagnosis of UTI should be based on clinical symptoms and confirmed by positive urine microscopy and culture (Schulz, Hoffman, Pothof, & Fox, 2016). Clinical symptoms of UTI may include acute dysuria or burning with urination, fever, urinary urgency, urinary frequency, urinary incontinence, suprapubic pain, gross hematuria or obvious blood in the urine, costovertebral angle tenderness or flank pain, shaking, chills, change in mental status, or change in functional status (Eke-Usim, Rogers, Gibson, Crnich, & Mody, 2016). UTI diagnosis is made from a midstream clean-catch urine specimen, urinary catheter specimen, or urine specimen from suprapubic aspiration. A quality urine specimen has fewer than five epithelial cells in urinalysis (Schulz et al., 2016). Diagnosis of UTI should be made in patients with elevated urine nitrate, and/or elevated leukocyte esterase with greater than five white blood cells in the presence of clinical signs and symptoms of UTI.

Pyelonephritis

Background

Acute pyelonephritis is less common than acute cystitis or infection of the bladder. Pyelonephritis can occur in all individuals of all ages. The estimated annual incidence per 10,000 people is 27.6 cases in the United States (Neumann & Moore, 2014). Pyelonephritis is more common in women. Women are approximately five times more likely than men to be hospitalized with acute pyelonephritis (Neumann & Moore, 2014).

Clinical Aspects

Acute pyelonephritis, or upper UTI, is caused by bacterial infiltration of the renal pelvis and sometimes the renal parenchyma. Pyelonephritis is potentially an organ-threatening and life-threatening infection. Infection can be a result of an infection of the bladder or lower urinary tract, and sometimes from infection of the bloodstream. Most cases of pyelonephritis are caused by a gram-negative bacterial infection, usually *Escherichia coli*, but like UTI, may be caused by other organisms (Neumann & Moore, 2014).

Mortality with pyelonephritis is greater in those individuals older than 65 years, with concomitant septic shock, those who are immobilized or bedridden, and those with immunosuppression. Individuals with pyelonephritis who have underlying renal disease, diabetes mellitus, and/or immunosuppression may have a poor prognosis (Neumann & Moore, 2014).

ASSESSMENT

Acute pyelonephritis is defined by the following criteria: fever (temperature greater than 100.4°F or 38.0°C), or a history of chills within 24 hours of initial presentation, and at least one symptom associated with a UTI (i.e., dysuria, frequency, urgency, perineal pain, flank pain, or tenderness of the costovertebral angle), and a positive UTI based on a urinalysis (Park et al., 2016). Renal ultrasound or CT scan may be utilized to assess for the presence of pyelonephritis and affected structures.

Renal Calculi

Background

A renal calculus, or nephrolithiasis, can occur in individuals across the life span. Ingimarsson, Krambeck, and Pais (2016) found that nephrolithiasis affects approximately 10% of adults. Male gender, Caucasian race, lower socioeconomic status, obesity, diabetes, and gout have been associated with a higher incidence of nephrolithiasis (Ingimarsson et al., 2016).

Clinical Aspects

Renal calculi are usually composed of salts, commonly calcium and urate. Dietary intake, endocrine factors, and malabsorptive intestinal disorders, such as ulcerative colitis, pancreatitis, and short gut syndromes, have all been associated with the development of renal calculi (Ingimarsson et al., 2016). Renal calculi can be found throughout the urinary tract. Renal calculi can cause ureteral scar, ureteral stricture, and obstruction of the urinary tract (Ingimarsson et al., 2016). Hydronephrosis, or fluid within or surrounding the kidney, is a complication associated with obstructive renal calculi. Sepsis is a severe complication of nephrolithiasis.

ASSESSMENT

Renal calculi present in the ureter are often painful, leading to a condition known as *renal colic*. Pressure in the ureter stimulates nerve endings in the urothelium to spasm, which causes a colicky pain, thus the term *renal colic* is used to describe this phenomenon (Ingimarsson et al., 2016). Individuals may present with pain in the flank region, also known as the *costovertebral angle region*, or pain in the abdomen and/or nausea and vomiting (Ingimarsson et al., 2016). Hematuria, gross or microscopic, may be present in the urine. Absence of hematuria does not exclude the presence of renal calculi; hematuria is only accurate for predicting renal calculi 62% of the time (Ingimarsson et al., 2016). Individuals with renal calculi and renal colic may or may not have associated UTI.

Acute Urinary Retention

Background

Acute urinary retention (AUR) is typically found in men older than 60 years of age (Sliwinski, D'Arcy, Sultana, & Lawrentschuk, 2016). AUR can also occur in women and children. The overall AUR incidence in the general male population varies between 2.2 and 8.5 of 1,000 man-years without known risk factors or previous history of AUR (Oelke, Speakman, Desgrandchamps, & Mamoulakis, 2015).

Clinical Aspects

AUR is a urologic emergency. AUR is most commonly a result of benign prostatic hyperplasia (BPH) in men (Sliwinski et al., 2016). AUR in men and women can be caused by renal calculi or other obstructive pathology. AUR in children is uncommon, but can be a result of constipation.

ASSESSMENT

AUR is characterized by the painful inability to void. Pain or discomfort and bloating in the lower abdomen along with a painful urgent feeling of need to urinate are common symptoms of AUR.

Acute Kidney Injury

Background

Acute kidney injury (AKI) is characterized by an abrupt decline in renal function. AKI can affect individuals of all ages. AKI was previously referred to as *acute renal failure*. AKI is associated with a great risk for morbidity and mortality (Yang, Zhang, Wu, Zou, & Du, 2014).

Clinical Aspects

An intact renal system is essential in order to maintain homeostasis. The renal system regulates the body's fluid volume, maintains electrolyte balance, and excretes toxic metabolic agents through glomerular filtration, tubular reabsorption, and tubular secretion via the formation and excretion of urine (Yang et al., 2014).

AKI is most often due to infection, obstruction, renal ischemia, and/or nephrotoxic drugs (Yang et al., 2014). AKI has clinical manifestations ranging from a small elevation in serum creatinine levels to anuric renal failure (Yang et al., 2014). AKI is classified into three groups: prerenal, renal, and postrenal. Recovery of AKI is based on improvement of renal function measured by serum creatinine levels and urine output.

ASSESSMENT

Clinical presentation of AKI may be retention of fluid or swelling. Individuals may report decreased urine output. Symptoms of electrolyte imbalance associated with AKI may include nausea, vomiting, muscle aches, fatigue, seizure, tachycardia, irregular heartbeat, diarrhea, and/or constipation.

Testicular Torsion

Background

Testicular torsion (TT) is one of the most common urologic emergencies. It is estimated that one in 1,500 males under the age of 18 years will suffer from TT (Afsarlar et al., 2016). TT is most common in neonates, children, and adolescents. Those at greatest risk for TT are African American, of younger age (12–18 years), and lacking private insurance (American Urological Association, 2016). Rate of testis loss with TT has been estimated to be as high as 42% (Afsarlar et al., 2016).

Clinical Aspects

In TT, the spermatic cord is twisted, which can cause decreased blood supply to the testis. Scrotal ultrasound

(US) is highly sensitive in the diagnosis of TT, reported to be over 90% sensitive (Yagil et al., 2010). Early presentation, accurate diagnosis, and prompt treatment are essential for the best outcome. TT can lead to infarction of the testicle, loss of testicle, infertility, infection, and cosmetic deformity.

ASSESSMENT

Individuals with TT often present with severe sudden onset of testicular pain and/or pain in the abdomen, nausea or vomiting, high-rising testicle, and sometimes swelling of the scrotum. Individuals may have a diminished cremasteric reflex. Assessment of positive Prehn's sign is indicative of TT. Prehn's sign is relief of pain with elevation of the scrotum. Emergent manual detorsion may be indicated.

NURSING INTERVENTIONS, MANAGEMENT, AND IMPLICATIONS

It is essential for nurses to understand and recognize various serious urologic conditions. Nursing education and guidance related to prevention of infection are essential. Regular voiding and stooling, perineal hygiene, use of probiotics, polyethylene glycol as needed for constipation, regular physical activity, increased intake of oral fluids, consumption of fresh or dried cranberries, prevention of perineal irritation, avoiding tight clothing, avoiding bubble bath, avoiding pools, encouraging the use of condoms, encouraging voiding after sexual intercourse, and the use of oxybutynin for bladder spasticity may reduce incidence of UTI (Traisman, 2016).

If obstructive uropathy is present, nursing must implement measures to relieve obstruction as quickly as possible to prevent AKI. In the case of urinary obstruction, placement of an indwelling urinary catheter may be need. Nursing should carefully consider need before placing an indwelling urinary catheter. Catheter-acquired urinary tract infection (CAUTI) is one of the most common preventable health care-associated infections (Flanders, 2014).

OUTCOMES

Treatment of urologic infection is essential. Prompt identification of the offending bacterial pathogen and antimicrobial susceptibility testing via urine culture for effective treatment may limit complications. Complications may include renal abscess, renal impairment, and septic shock (Neumann & Moore, 2014).

Individuals with tachycardia and hypotension may indicate more severe diseases such AKI and/or sepsis.

Nursing care related to urologic emergencies includes management of pain, management of electrolyte imbalances, acidosis, focus on restoring renal profusion and fluid balance, providing nutritional support, avoiding nephrotoxic drugs, and providing necessary pharmacological intervention if appropriate. Individuals may need to be prepared for renal dialysis in severe cases.

Summary

Nurses are challenged to provide the most effective, evidence-based care in order to treat and limit the progression and severity of urologic disease. Early presentation, accurate diagnosis, and prompt treatment are essential for the best patient-centered outcomes.

Afsarlar, C., Ryan, S., Donel, E., Baccam, T., Jones, B., Chandwani, B., . . . Chester, K. (2016). Standardized process to improve patient flow from the emergency room to the operating room for pediatric patients with testicular torsion. *Journal of Pediatric Urology, 12*(4), 233.e1–233.e4.

American Urological Association. (2016). Acute scrotum. Retrieved from https://www.auanet.org/education/acute-scrotum.cfm

Barber, A., Norton, P., Spivak, A., & Mulvey M. (2013). Urinary tract infections: Current and emerging management strategies. *Clinical Infectious Diseases, 57*(5), 719–724.

Eke-Usim, A., Rogers, M., Gibson, K., Crnich, C., & Mody, L. (2016). Constitutional symptoms trigger diagnostic testing before antibiotic prescribing in high-risk nursing home residents. *Journal of the American Geriatrics Society, 64*(10), 1975–1980.

Flanders, K. (2014). Rounding to reduce CAUTI. *Nursing Management, 45*(11), 21–23.

Ingimarsson, J., Krambeck, A., & Pais, V. (2016). Diagnosis and management of nephrolithiasis. *Surgical Clinics of North America, 96*(3), 517–532.

Lingenfelter, E., Drapkin, Z., Fritz, K., Youngquist, S., Madsen, T., & Fix, M. (2016). ED pharmacist monitoring of provider antibiotic selection aids appropriate treatment for outpatient UTI. *American Journal of Emergency Medicine, 34*(8), 1600–1603.

Neumann, I., & Moore, P. (2014). Clinical evidence: Pyelonephritis in non-pregnant women. *BMJ Clinical Evidence, 807.* Retrieved from https://www.ncbi.nlm.nih.gov/pmc/articles/PMC4220693

Oelke, M., Speakman, M., Desgrandchamps, F., & Mamoulakis, C. (2015). Acute urinary retention rates in the general male population and in adult men with lower urinary tract symptoms participating in pharmacotherapy trails: A literature review. *Urology, 86*(4), 654–665.

Park, S., Oh, W., Kim, Y., Yeom, J., Choi, H., Kwak, Y., . . . Kim, B. (2016). Health care-associated acute pyelonephritis is associated with inappropriate empiric antibiotic therapy in the ED. *American Journal of Emergency Medicine, 34*(8), 1415–1420.

Schulz, L., Hoffman, R., Pothof, J., & Fox, B. (2016). Top ten myths regarding the diagnosis and treatment of urinary tract infections. *Journal of Emergency Medicine, 51*(1), 25–30.

Sliwinski, A., D'Arcy, F., Sultana, R., & Lawrentschuk, N. (2016). Acute urinary retention and the difficult catheterization: Current emergency management. *European Journal of Emergency Medicine, 23*(2), 80–88.

Tonolini, M., & Ippolito, S. (2016). Cross-sectional imaging of complicated urinary infections affecting the lower tract and male genital organs. *Insights into Imaging, 7*(5), 689–711.

Traisman, E. (2016). Clinical management of urinary tract infections. *Pediatric Annals, 45*(5), e108–e111.

Yagil, Y., Naroditsky, I., Milhem, J., Leiba, R., Leiderman, M., Badaan, S., & Gaitini, D. (2010). Role of Doppler ultrasonography in the triage of acute scrotum in the emergency department. *Journal of Ultrasound Medicine, 29*(1), 11–21.

Yang, F., Zhang, L., Wu, H., Zou, H., & Du, Y. (2014). Clinical analysis of cause, treatment and prognosis in acute kidney injury patients. *PLOS ONE.* doi:10.1371/journal.pone.0085214

■ VENTILATOR-ASSOCIATED PNEUMONIA

Nancy Jaskowak Cresse

Overview

Pneumonia is an infection in the lungs that can vary from mild to severe. Caused by bacteria, viruses, or fungi, pneumonia can be acquired in the community, or associated with contact with the health care system (Centers for Disease Control and Prevention [CDC], 2017). Health care-associated conditions are also referred to as *nosocomial.* The most serious of health care-associated infections is ventilator-associated pneumonia (VAP), impacting patient mortality, ventilator days, and costs (CDC, 2017; Lim et al., 2015). As science is evolving the current definition and reportable event protocol to improve sensitivity and specificity of VAP, the focus of nursing care is on reduction of incidence, and prevention of VAP through the use of a set of interventions called a *care bundle* that reduces the incidence of VAP thereby reducing patient length of stay, cost, and mortality (Alcan, Kormaz, & Uyar, 2016; CDC, 2017).

Background

VAP is a lung infection that develops in a person who is on a ventilator. A ventilator is a machine that helps a patient breathe by giving breaths, providing oxygen, and it can administer a varying depth of each breath. To accomplish patient oxygenation, a tube is placed in the patient's nose or mouth (endotracheal), or through a hole that is placed in the front of the patient's neck (tracheostomy; CDC, 2017).

Mechanical ventilation is a necessary, life-sustaining therapy for many patients with critical injury or illness. Ventilated patients are a vulnerable population at increased risk for complications, poor outcomes, and death. Complications of receiving mechanical ventilation include VAP, acute respiratory distress syndrome (ARDS), pulmonary embolism, and pulmonary edema. If a patient were to develop a complication, it can lead to additional time on the ventilator, longer stays in intensive care and the hospital, increased costs, and increased risk of disability and death (CDC, 2017). National surveillance and data collection before 2013 was limited to VAP and the incidence ranged from 0.0 to 4.4 per 1,000 ventilator days in medical–surgical intensive care units (ICUs) in the United States, and in developing countries it ranged from 10 to 41.7 cases per 1,000 ventilator days (CDC, 2017; Lim et al., 2015). Between 10% and 20% of patients receive mechanical ventilation for a duration more than 48 hours develop VAP (Speck et al., 2016). In 2013, the CDC proposed new surveillance categories capturing ventilator-associated events (VAE), infectious ventilator-associated events (IVAC), and then possible ventilator-associated pneumonia (PVAP; CDC, 2017; Nair & Niederman, 2015). It is not certain that these newer surveillance designations, although broader in scope, will support the efficacy of the care bundles for VAP (Nair & Neiderman, 2015; O'Horo et al., 2016).

Although there is no standard definition, VAP has been defined as a lower respiratory tract infection developed after 48 hours of intubation with mechanical ventilation, or within 48 hours after disconnecting the ventilator (CDC, 2017; Lim et al., 2015). Clinically, VAP can be divided into early onset (less than 5 days) or late onset (longer than 5 days after hospitalization), but some studies vary that parameter (Nair & Niederman, 2015). And although there were practice guidelines used to prevent VAP, several studies from

1999 to 2009 identified approximately 50% of patients received evidence-based care (Alcan et al., 2016). For this reason, the Institute for Healthcare Improvement (IHI) introduced a care bundle, a set of evidence-based practices that, when executed together, improves the patient recovery process and outcomes better than when implemented separately (Alcan et al., 2016).

Clinical Aspects

ASSESSMENT

A critical component of nursing care is accurate assessment and documentation. Identifying a patient who requires increased oxygen concentrations from the ventilator, or increased positive pressure from the ventilator to deliver the oxygen (as in use of positive end-expiratory pressure [PEEP]) is a primary function of the nurse in acute care and is pivotal in identifying early VAE. Monitoring patient temperature to identify a temperature above 38°C, as well as documenting increased frequency of suctioning and/or change in the purulent appearance of endotracheal or tracheal secretions will capture the data consistent with VAE or IVAE.

NURSING INTERVENTIONS, MANAGEMENT, AND IMPLICATIONS

Nursing care of the adult on a ventilator or who has recently been on a ventilator and who is at risk for VAP should center around maintaining patent airway and adequate patient oxygenation. Caring for the patient holistically, using priority nursing-related problems/diagnoses includes maintaining adequate ventilation (ineffective airway clearance, ineffective breathing pattern), noting imbalanced nutrition, immobility, hyperthermia, risk for infection, risk of fluid volume deficit, and disturbed sleep pattern.

The commonly used ventilator bundle developed by the IHI identifies five elements to reduce the rate of VAP. These measures include (a) head of the bed (HOB) elevation 30° to 45°, (b) daily sedation vacation and patient assessment for readiness to wean, (c) peptic ulcer disease prevention, (d) deep vein thrombosis prophylaxis, and (e) daily oral care with chlorhexidine (Lim et al., 2015). In addition to the HOB elevation, and daily oral care by nursing, several other elements have evidence-based support to include in a *customized* bundle of care interventions, including hand hygiene before and after patient contact and endotracheal tube cuff pressure monitoring (greater than 20–25 cm H_2O; Alcan et al., 2016; Lim et al., 2015). Standardizing nursing interventions also has a positive impact on VAP rates, such as oral cavity secretion clearance before changing position or supination (every 2–4 hours), and oral care with chlorhexidine every 8 hours.

OUTCOMES

Ventilator care bundle implementation in clinical practice has exposed barriers, and compliance in some centers remain modest (Nair & Niederman, 2015). Lim et al. (2015) identified keys to success in care bundle implementation and nurse efficacy through the development and use of nursing checklists, staff education, posters, and standardizing interventions that will contribute to a reduction in VAP rates. It was also noted that nurse compliance rates in applying the ventilator care bundle improved when staff is observed and compliance is recorded (Alcan et al., 2016).

Efforts to continually improve clinical care quality and patient safety are important, as is clinician involvement and buy-in (Speck et al., 2016). Obtaining clinician input on what interventions to include, and the supporting processes necessary for the implementation, increases the likelihood that caregivers and providers adhere to the intervention bundle.

Summary

VAP is the most common and serious type of health care infection in the ICU, and is associated with significant mortality, morbidity, and cost. Ventilator care bundles include nursing care interventions that have shown to reduce the incidence of VAP. New knowledge supports customizing the care bundle to maximize the effect of reducing incidence of VAP and improving patient outcomes.

Alcans, A. O., Korkmaz, F. D., & Uyar, M. (2016). Prevention of ventilator-associated pneumonia: Use of the care bundle approach. *American Journal of Infection Control, 44,* 173–176. doi:10.1016/j.ajic.2016.04.237

Centers for Disease Control and Prevention. (2017). *Ventilator-associated event (VAE)* (pp. 1–44). Retrieved from https://www.cdc.gov/nhsn/pdfs/pscmanual/10-vae_final.pdf

Lim, K. P., Kuo, S. W., Ko, W. J., Sheng, W. H., Chang, Y. Y., Hong, M. C., . . . Chang, S. C. (2015). Efficacy of ventilator-associated pneumonia care bundle for prevention of ventilator-associated pneumonia in the surgical intensive care units of a medical center. *Journal of Microbiology, Immunology and Infection, 48,* 316–321. doi:10.1016/j.jmii.2013.09.007

Nair, G. B., & Niederman, M. S. (2015). Ventilator-associated pneumonia: Present understanding and ongoing debate. *Intensive Care Medicine, 41,* 34–48. doi:10.1007/s00134-3564-5

O'Horo, J. C., Lan, H., Thongprayoon, C., Schenck, L., Ahmed, A., & Dziadzko, M. (2016). "Bundle" practices and ventilator-associated events: Not enough. *Infection Control & Hospital Epidemiology, 37*(12), 1453–1457. doi:10.1017/ice.2016.207

Speck, K., Rawat, N., Weiner, N. C., Tujuba, H. G., Farley, D., & Berenholtz, S. (2016). A systematic approach for developing a ventilator-associated pneumonia prevention bundle. *American Journal of Infection Control, 44,* 652–656. doi:10.1016/j.ajic.2015.12.020

■ VENTRICULAR ASSIST DEVICES

S. Brian Widmar

Overview

A ventricular assist device (VAD) is a mechanical pump that is surgically implanted and assists the failing ventricle by increasing cardiac output (Chmielinski & Koons, 2017). The VAD is most often used to support the failing left ventricle (LVAD), but the right ventricle (RVAD) or both ventricles (BIVAD) can also be supported. The LVAD can be used as a bridge to transplantation (BTT), supporting the patient until a heart transplant is received, or as destination therapy (DT), supporting the patient as a permanent therapy for heart failure (Chmielinski & Koons, 2017; O'Shea, 2012). In addition, the LVAD can be used as a bridge to decision, when ventricular support is required before a determination of eligibility for transplant can be made, or as a bridge to recovery, in which the LVAD supports the patient while the heart recovers from injury and can eventually be removed, or explanted, as myocardial function recovers (Chmielinski & Koons, 2017).

Background

Approximately 6.5 million Americans are living with heart failure, and 960,000 new heart failure cases are diagnosed annually (Writing Group Members et al., 2016). Heart failure is a progressive and chronic condition, and is categorized in stages, by both the severity of presenting signs and symptoms and by the goal-directed therapies aimed at relieving them (Hunt et al., 2001a). Stage D heart failure is seen in patients with advanced structural heart disease who have symptoms of heart failure at rest or refractory to optimized medical therapy, and these patients require specialized treatments or interventions in order to survive (Hunt et al., 2001b). Interventions for patients with stage D heart failure include optimized and maximal medical therapies, continuous intravenous (IV) inotropes, heart transplantation, mechanical circulatory support device therapy, or palliative or hospice care (Fang et al., 2015).

Limited data are available regarding stage D heart failure, but despite advances in medical management and technology, prognosis for end-stage heart failure patients remains poor. From 1987 until 2012, 40,253 people were waiting for heart transplant, whereas only 26,943 received a transplant, which highlights the clinical impact of VADs as a strategy to prolong the life of patients living with end-stage heart failure (Writing Group Members et al., 2016). In the Randomized Evaluation of Mechanical Assistance for the Treatment of Congestive Heart Failure (REMATCH) trial, end-stage heart failure patients who were managed medically had a 75% mortality rate at 1 year (Fang et al., 2015; Rose et al., 2001). From 2006 until 2016, the Interagency Registry for Mechanically Assisted Circulatory Support (INTERMACS) database reports a total of 19,013 VAD implants, with 2,480 VAD implants in 2016 alone; survival at 1 year was 80%, and 70% at 2 years (INTERMACS, 2017). Patients receiving VAD support have reported an improvement in quality of life (Grady et al., 2004; Maciver & Ross, 2012). VAD therapy has not proven to be a cost-effective solution compared to heart transplantation, possibly due to issues such as equipment costs, hospital length of stay, and hospital readmissions. The most commonly reported causes of hospital readmissions include device malfunction, cardiac arrhythmia, infection, gastrointestinal (GI) bleeding, and stroke (Writing Group Members et al., 2016).

VADs vary by type of support offered (LVAD, RVAD, BIVAD), by anatomical position (internal or "intracorporeal"; external or "extracorporeal"), and by the duration of time support can be maintained. Some devices are designed to provide temporary support, permitting recovery from cardiogenic shock or from high-risk cardiac surgery, whereas others offer a longer duration of support, such as a bridge to transplant or as a destination therapy (Chilcott & Hazard, 2017). Examples of long-term or durable VADs include the Heartmate II, the HeartWare HVAD, and the Thoratec paracorporeal VAD. Short-term support VADs include intra-aortic balloon pumps (IABPs), Tandem Heart, Impella, CentriMag, Maquet, and Medtronic VADs (Chilcott & Hazard,

2017). The IABP, Tandem Heart, and Impella devices can be placed percutaneously (Hollenberg & Parrillo, 2014). In addition, VADs can be further categorized by the type of flow generated by the device. Pulsatile-flow VADs generate a pulsation of blood through sequential filling and emptying, similar to normal cardiac function. Continuous-flow VADs deliver a continuous flow of blood throughout systole and diastole; these include axial and centrifugal flow pumps (Chilcott & Hazard, 2017; O'Shea, 2012). One important variant of continuous flow pumps is that patients with continuous flow devices have lower systolic blood pressures and elevated diastolic pressures, resulting in a greatly diminished pulse pressure. At normal settings, the patient with a continuous-flow VAD may not have a palpable pulse (Chilcott & Hazard, 2017; O'Shea, 2012).

Clinical Aspects

Immediate postoperative monitoring and care is similar despite the type of VAD implanted (Grady & Shinn, 2008). VADs are preload sensitive, and pump flow relies on adequate filling of the pump chamber. Vital signs, fluid volume status, pump settings and function, anticoagulation, maintaining adequate end-organ perfusion, and reducing risk of infection are all important considerations in the postoperative setting (Chilcott & Hazard, 2017).

ASSESSMENT

Close monitoring for cardiac arrhythmias is important, and any arrhythmias should be promptly reported. VAD patients are at high risk for atrial and ventricular arrhythmias. Alterations in cardiac rate and rhythm can decrease cardiac and pump filling, ultimately reducing pump flow (Chmielinski & Koons, 2017). Blood pressure should be closely monitored, as hypertension can increase resistance to pump flow (Chilcott & Hazard, 2017). Mean arterial pressure (MAP) between 70 and 80 mmHg should be maintained to ensure adequate end-organ perfusion while decreasing resistance to pump flow. Due to the very narrow pulse pressure noted in continuous-flow VADs, noninvasive blood pressure cuff monitoring can prove especially difficult; blood pressure measurements may be obtained using Doppler (Chmielinski & Koons, 2017; O'Shea, 2012). Secondary organ dysfunction may occur due to hypoperfusion during surgery. In addition to maintaining an acceptable MAP between 70 and 80 mmHg, close monitoring of urine output, blood urea nitrogen (BUN) and creatinine, as well as liver function test (LFT) is important in identifying hepatic or renal dysfunction postoperatively (Chilcott & Hazard, 2017).

NURSING INTERVENTIONS, MANAGEMENT, AND IMPLICATIONS

VAD pump settings should be confirmed with the physician or provider. Continuous-flow VADs have one setting that is ordered by the provider: the pump speed, which is noted on the VAD device as revolutions per minute (RPM). Blood flow through the pump and pump power are approximations: Pump power is the amount of energy needed to generate the set RPM, and flow is calculated from pump speed and power (Chilcott & Hazard, 2017).

Close monitoring of clotting times and anticoagulation therapy is crucial to the prevention of complications related to bleeding or thromboembolism, both of which are known adverse events after VAD implantation (Chmielinski & Koons, 2017). All VAD pumps include an artificial chamber that comes into direct contact with the patient's blood, increasing the potential for thrombus formation. Ischemic strokes occur in roughly 8% to 10% of VAD patients, most commonly due to pump thrombosis or subtherapeutic anticoagulation. Hemorrhagic strokes may occur from a previous ischemic stroke, from supratherapeutic anticoagulation, or infection (Chmielinski & Koons, 2017). In the absence of postoperative bleeding, the International Society for Heart and Lung Transplantation supports an international normalized ratio (INR) of 2.0 to 3.0 in continuous-flow VAD devices (Chilcott & Hazard, 2017). GI bleeding is another known adverse effect in VAD patients, and may be due to anticoagulation therapy, or the development of acquired von Willebrand disease, or GI tract angiodysplasia, both of which are thought to be due to the decreased pulsatility seen in continuous-flow VAD devices (Chmielinski & Koons, 2017). Melena, or frank blood from stools, should be reported, as anticoagulation reversal and blood volume replacement could be required (Chilcott & Hazard, 2017; Chmielinski & Koons, 2017).

Postoperative infection is one of the more common complications of VAD therapy and can develop at multiple sites, including the VAD driveline exit site, pump pocket, sternal incision, invasive lines, or bloodstream (O'Shea, 2012). Nurses must closely follow VAD program protocols for site care and immobilization of the VAD exit site as well as site care of invasive lines, and antibiotic prophylaxis must be given to reduce the risk of surgical wound infections (Druss, Rohrbaugh, Levinson, & Rosenheck, 2001; O'Shea, 2012). Timely extubation and pulmonary hygiene; removal of vascular access catheters, indwelling urinary catheters, and chest tube drains as soon as clinically appropriate; and early mobilization are essential to reducing postoperative infection risk (Chilcott & Hazard, 2017; O'Shea, 2012).

OUTCOMES

VAD device malfunction is rare, but is possible. Health care providers caring for VAD patients must understand the critical alarms associated with the specific device supporting the patient. In the event of VAD alarms, the patient's VAD coordinator or physician should be notified immediately (Chmielinski & Koons, 2017). Critical alarms are due to either pump failure, low power, or controller failure (Chmielinski & Koons, 2017). Patients and their caregivers are instructed to carry spare power sources, such as additional batteries, and a spare device controller that is programmed to the same settings the primary controller is set to (O'Shea, 2012). In the event of a critical alarm, nurses should assess the patient, and then the connection from the driveline, controller, and VAD power source. The VAD coordinator or provider should be contacted immediately to assist if correct connections do not alleviate critical alarms, or if controller exchange is required (Chmielinski & Koons, 2017; O'Shea, 2012). In the event of patient arrest, device malfunction should be suspected and the cardiac surgeon, VAD coordinator, and cardiologist should be notified immediately. Advanced cardiac life support protocols should be followed, but the care team must be aware of the risk of internal bleeding from cardiopulmonary resuscitation (CPR) should dislodgement of the device occur (Chmielinski & Koons, 2017). VAD centers have protocols in place for responding to VAD patient arrest situations, and CPR is generally avoided (Lala & Mehra, 2013).

Summary

VADs are indicated for patients in stage D heart failure as either a BTT; bridge to decision; bridge to recovery; or as a chronic, destination therapy for heart failure. VADs may provide short-term or long-term support, depending upon the clinical indication for therapy. VADs can support the failing left ventricle, a failing right ventricle, or can provide biventricular support. VADs may be pulsatile- or continuous-flow devices; in continuous-flow devices, a pulse may not be palpable. Due to numerous types of VADs used, nurses should understand the type of device used and its settings. Monitoring of heart rate and blood pressure, filling pressures, pump settings and function, and anticoagulation are crucial to maintaining adequate MAP for end-organ perfusion and reducing the likelihood of device-related adverse events. Nurses should closely follow hospital protocols for device wound-site care, and monitor and report any signs of infection. Lastly, nurses must be aware of potential device-related complications, and signs and symptoms of device malfunction and should seek assistance immediately should a critical alarm or patient arrest situation occur.

Chilcott, S. R., & Hazard, L. (2017). Mechanical circulatory support. In S. Cupples, S. Lerret, V. McCalmont, & L. Ohler (Eds.), *Core curriculum for transplant nurses* (pp. 414–452). Philadelphia, PA: Mosby.

Chmielinski, A., & Koons, B. (2017). Nursing care for the patient with a left ventricular assist device. *Nursing, 47*(5), 34–40. doi:10.1097/01.NURSE.0000515503.80037.07

Druss, B. G., Rohrbaugh, R. M., Levinson, C. M., & Rosenheck, R. A. (2001). Integrated medical care for patients with serious psychiatric illness: A randomized trial. *Archives of General Psychiatry, 58*(9), 861–868.

Fang, J. C., Ewald, G. A., Allen, L. A., Butler, J., Westlake Canary, C. A., & Colvin-Adams, M. (2015). Advanced (stage D) heart failure: A statement from the Heart Failure Society of America Guidelines Committee. *Journal of Cardiac Failure, 21*(6), 519–534. doi:10.1016/j.cardfail.2015.04.013

Grady, K. L., Meyer, P. M., Dressler, D., Mattea, A., Chillcott, S., Loo, A., . . . Piccione, W. (2004). Longitudinal change in quality of life and impact on survival after left ventricular assist device implantation. *Annals of Thoracic Surgery, 77*(4), 1321–1327. doi:10.1016/j.athoracsur.2003.09.089

Grady, K. L., & Shinn, J. A. (2008). Care of patients with circulatory assist devices. In D. K. Moser & B. Riegel (Eds.), *Cardiac nursing: A companion to Braunwald's heart disease* (pp. 977–997). St. Louis, MO: Saunders.

Hollenberg, S. M., & Parrillo, J. E. (2014). Cardiogenic shock. In J. E. Parrillo & R. P. Dellinger (Eds.), *Critical care medicine: Principles of diagnosis and management in the adult* (4th ed., pp. 325–337). Philadelphia, PA: Elsevier.

Hunt, S. A., Baker, D. W., Chin, M. H., Cinquegrani, M. P., Feldman, A. M., & Francis, G. S., . . . Smith, S. C. (2001a). ACC/AHA guidelines for the evaluation and management of chronic heart failure in the adult: Executive summary. A report of the American College of Cardiology/American Heart Association Task Force on Practice Guidelines (Committee to Revise the 1995 Guidelines for the Evaluation and Management of Heart Failure): Developed in collaboration with the International Society for Heart and Lung Transplantation; endorsed by the Heart Failure Society of America. *Circulation, 104*(24), 2996–3007.

Hunt, S. A., Baker, D. W., Chin, M. H., Cinquegrani, M. P., Feldman, A. M., Francis, G. S., . . . American College of Cardiology/American Heart Association. (2001b). ACC/AHA guidelines for the evaluation and management of chronic heart failure in the adult: Executive summary. A report of the American College of Cardiology/American Heart Association Task Force on Practice Guidelines (Committee to Revise the 1995 Guidelines for the Evaluation and Management of Heart Failure). *Journal of the American College of Cardiology, 38*(7), 2101–2113.

Interagency Registry for Mechanically Assisted Circulatory Support. (2017). Public statistical reports. Retrieved from https://www.uab.edu/medicine/intermacs/reports/public-statistical-reports

Lala, A., & Mehra, M. R. (2013). Durable mechanical circulatory support in advanced heart failure: A critical care cardiology perspective. *Cardiology Clinics, 31*(4), 581–593; viii–ix. doi:10.1016/j.ccl.2013.07.003

Maciver, J., & Ross, H. J. (2012). Quality of life and left ventricular assist device support. *Circulation, 126*(7), 866–874. doi:10.1161/CIRCULATIONAHA.111.040279

O'Shea, G. (2012). Ventricular assist devices: What intensive care unit nurses need to know about postoperative management. *AACN Advanced Critical Care, 23*(1), 69–83; quiz 84-65. doi:10.1097/NCI.0b013e318240aaa9

Rose, E. A., Gelijns, A. C., Moskowitz, A. J., Heitjan, D. F., Stevenson, L. W., Dembitsky, W.; Randomized Evaluation of Mechanical Assistance for the Treatment of Congestive Heart Failure Study Group. (2001). Long-term use of a left ventricular assist device for end-stage heart failure. *New England Journal of Medicine, 345*(20), 1435–1443. doi:10.1056/NEJMoa012175

Writing Group Members, Mozaffarian, D., Benjamin, E. J., Go, A. S., Arnett, D. K., Blaha, M. J., . . . Stroke Statistics Subcommittee. (2016). Heart disease and stroke statistics—2016 update: A report from the American Heart Association. *Circulation, 133*(4), e38–360. doi:10.1161/CIR.0000000000000350

■ THE VIOLENT PATIENT

Janet E. Reilly
Michael Wichowski

Overview

Direct patient-care providers, like nurses, are often the victims of violence, especially in the emergency department (ED) and critical care settings. The occurrence of workplace violence in health care settings is four times higher than the reported rates across non-health care sectors of the industry (Occupational Safety and Health Administration [OSHA], 2015b), and is often under reported by nurses. Workplace violence, classified as type II: customer/client violence, occurs when patients act violently toward health care workers, and is the most common type of workplace violence in health care settings (Centers for Disease Control and Prevention [CDC], n.d.). Workplace violence comes in many forms (e.g., physical assaults, threatening behavior, verbal abuse, and sexual harassment) and occurs on a spectrum from verbal statements that result in minor physical or psychological harm to physical assaults resulting in life-threatening injuries. Nurses need to be aware of precipitating factors of workplace violence, type II, as well as be able to accurately assess, prevent, and implement effective, evidence-based strategies that maximize safety for themselves, patients, and others.

Background

Violence within health care settings like the ED is escalating, with the number of violent acts against nurses and nursing assistants doubling between 2012 and 2014 (Gomaa et al., 2015). Violent behavior is often associated with patients who experience mental health crises, like substance abuse or extreme stress, both of which are increasing to almost epidemic levels. In 2014, over 20 million adults in the United States had substance abuse issues; half of these people also have underlying psychological disorders (U.S. Department of Health and Human Services, 2015). More psychological disorders continue to be identified, resulting in greater than one in six Americans being prescribed a psychiatric medication to optimize mental health (Moore & Mattison, 2016). Changes in the economy since 2008 have led to increased stress and negative health outcomes in individuals, as well as less funding for inpatient and outpatient mental health treatment nationwide (Mucci, Giorgi, Roncaioli, Perez, & Arcangeli, 2016; Nesper, Morris, Scher, & Holmes, 2016). These factors, plus the inherent stress from crowded environments and highly charged emotional and life-threatening situations that occur in intensive care units and EDs, can easily trigger a patient to become violent.

There are obvious legal consequences for violent patients, 37 out of 50 states have legislation (e.g.,

felony charges) for perpetrators of type II violence in health care settings (Jacobson, 2014). Type II violence compromises nurse safety, increases risk of injury, and decreases job satisfaction, which can lead to higher nurse turnover, nursing shortages, and a subsequent lower quality of nursing care. Financially speaking, health care systems can spend between $27,000 and $103,000 to replace a nurse (OSHA, 2015a). Recognizing and preventing violence in health care is key and nurses play a critical role in prevention. Furthermore, workplace violence in health care settings has significant impact on the nursing workforce, the financial status of health care systems, and state legislation and judicial processes have been instituted in most states to mitigate the negative consequences of workplace violence.

Clinical Aspects

ASSESSMENT

Nursing assessment, an essential step in the nursing process, should include situational awareness of the patient and environment for potential violence as well as physical and psychosocial evaluations of patients. Using situational awareness, nurses focus on everything happening around them; assess the situation; and identify abnormal data and unsafe conditions (Solon & Kratz, 2016). Nurses need to assess the clinical environment for unsafe practices or weapons, or objects that could be used to harm others in order to prevent type II violence. For example, some exam and patient rooms are arranged with the patient situated between where the nurse works and the door, which blocks a safe exit route for the health care worker, if violence erupts.

Nurses should also carefully assess the patients for risk factors and behaviors that could potentially lead to violence. Research indicates patients who act violently often have one or more of these common traits: male gender, aged 26 to 35 years; a history of violence; high-level stress or loss of control in the current situation; agitation or aggression; homelessness or unemployment; and low socioeconomic status (Arnetz et al., 2015; Tishler, Reiss, & Dundas, 2013; Villaire, 1995). Assessment of individual patients and their physical and psychological status is also critical. Many disorders can precipitate patient violence, particularly diseases of the brain causing cognitive impairment (e.g., dementia, intellectual disability); endocrine disorders (e.g., hyperthyroidism or hyperglycemia);

diseases leading to oxygen deprivation to the brain, or hypoxia (e.g., seizures, chronic obstructive pulmonary disease [COPD], or carbon monoxide poisoning); head trauma; and infections (e.g., sepsis, HIV/AIDs, encephalitis, meningitis, etc.). Patients with a history of or current mental health/psychiatric disorders are also at risk for committing type II violence. Substance abuse, whether from alcohol, prescribed, or illegal substances, also puts patients at risk of acting violently. Violence can also be a result of adverse effects or polypharmacy from certain prescribed medications, such as antipsychotics, antidepressants, amphetamines, benzodiazepines, tobacco-cessation aides (i.e., varenicline), antimalarials (i.e., mefloquine), anticonvulsants, and sedatives (i.e., zolpidem), which have shown to enhance aggression or violent acts among individuals prescribed these medications in various combinations (Arnetz et al., 2015; Tishler, Reiss, & Dundas, 2013; Villaire, 1995).

In addition, nurses should be alert to and assess for patient behaviors that may indicate escalation in aggression or violence, such as pacing or restlessness; increasingly loud or rapid speech; insistence or demanding behavior; threats; use of profanity; intimidating or overly sexual language; clenched fists, throwing, or punching objects; or accusing health care workers of conspiracy (OSHA, n.d.; Tishler et al., 2013). Situations that often incite type II violence include patients who demand discharge against medical advice, patients undergoing painful procedures or transfers, patient transitions in care and use of patient restraints (Arnetz, et al., 2015).

NURSING INTERVENTIONS, MANAGEMENT AND IMPLICATIONS

Appropriate interventions and evaluation of their effectiveness are the next steps in the nursing process with the violent patient. Therapeutic communication can help patients feel understood, and, when coupled with patience while teaching/explaining, can empower patients with better understanding. Simple interventions that address basic patient needs (i.e., offering food to a hungry or homeless patient) are other ways nurses can intervene to prevent patient violence. Utilizing proper nursing technique in procedures and creative interventions, like numbing cream or ice applied to the site before needle injections, can help decrease and manage pain associated with patient care and diffuse violence. When physical or chemical restraints (antipsychotics, benzodiazepines, etc.) are ordered, clear documentation of the indication for use and assessment at regular intervals of vital signs, neurological and extremity

checks, Glasgow Coma Scale, and/or sedation scale scores should be frequently assessed as indicators of agitation and therapeutic response. Nurses must never use patient restraints as punishment, and restraints must be discontinued as soon as the threat of violence has ended. Nurses need to be constantly aware of potential violence. If a situation does become violent and a nurse feels unsafe, every effort should be made by the nurse to leave the situation. In the event that an unsafe or violent situation has occurred, nurses should be offered debriefing and counseling to deal with the recent event and prepare better for future experiences (Tishler et al., 2013; Villaire, 1995).

OUTCOMES

Prevention and reduction of violence in heath care is the desired outcome. This can be achieved in many ways by nurses, but health system support and resources, like the appropriate use of security guards and video monitoring, are also needed. Other methods used to prevent and reduce violence include (a) active safety and health committees that can create nurses' awareness and sensitivity to violence and (b) the establishment of open and trusting health care work cultures that support and encourage the report of type II violence. Violence prevention programs are an upcoming trend in health care that also promote quality of care and safety for patients and nurses. Regular rehearsal and adoption of violence-prevention programs, like the OSHA (2015a) *Guidelines for Prevention Workplace Violence for Healthcare and Social Service Workers*, should be mandated for hospitals, as well as violence-reporting policies put in place to enact a cultural shift that type II violence in health care settings is unacceptable.

Summary

Violent acts committed by patients have been escalating in health care, particularly in the ED and critical care due to multiple intrapersonal and social factors. Prevention of violence is key and depends on effective use of accurate assessment and effective nursing interventions with patients who are at risk for violence. In addition to prevention, nurses need to be constantly aware of potential threats. Accurate assessment can identify patients with potential for violence and possibly prevent such acts. A systematic approach to antiviolence by nurses and health care organizations for violence prevention, management, and evaluation is needed. Although all violent acts cannot be prevented, with proper training, assessment, and system resources, they can be decreased.

Arnetz J., Hamblin L., Essenmacher L., Upfal M., Ager J., & Luborsky, M. (2015). Understanding patient-to-worker violence in hospitals: A qualitative analysis of documented incident reports. *Journal of Advanced Nursing, 71*(2), 338–348.

Centers for Disease Control and Prevention. (n.d.). Workplace safety and health: Workplace violence course. Retrieved from https://wwwn.cdc.gov/wpvhc/Course .aspx/Slide/Unit1_5

Gomaa, A. E., Tapp, L. C., Luckhaupt, S. E., Vanoli, K., Sarmiento, R. F., Raudabaugh, W. M., . . . Sprigg, S. M. (2015, April 24). Occupational traumatic injuries among workers in health care facilities—United States 2012–2014. *Morbidity and Mortality Weekly Report.* Retrieved from https://www.cdc.gov/mmwr/preview/ mmwrhtml/mm6415a2.htm

Jacobson, R. (2014, December 31). Hospital administrations and the judicial system do little to prevent assaults against nurses and other caregivers by patients. *Scientific American.* Retrieved from https://www.scientific american.com/article/epidemic-of-violence-against -health-care-workers-plagues-hospitals

Moore, T., & Mattison, D. (2016). Adult utilizations of psychiatric drugs and differences by sex, age, and race. *JAMA Internal Medicine.* doi:10.1001/jamain ternmed.2016.7507

Mucci, N., Girogi, G., Roncaioli, M., Perez, F., & Arcangeli, G. (2016). The correlation between stress and economic crisis: A systematic review. *Neuropsychiatric Disease and Treatment, 12,* 983–993. doi:10.2147/NDT.S98525

Nesper, A. C., Morris, B. A., Scher, L. M., & Holmes, J. F. (2016). Effect of decreasing county mental health services on the emergency department. *Health Policy/Brief Report, 67*(4), 525–530.

Occupational Safety and Health Administration. (n.d.). ICU: Workplace violence. Retrieved from https://www.osha.gov/SLTC/etools/hospital/icu/icu .html#WorkplaceViolence

Occupational Safety and Health Administration. (2015a). *Guidelines for prevention of workplace violence for healthcare and social service workers* (OSHA Report No. 3148-04R 2015). Washington, DC: U.S. Department of Labor.

Occupational Safety and Health Administration. (2015b). Workplace violence in healthcare: Understanding the challenge. Retrieved from: https://www.osha.gov/ Publications/OSHA3826.pdf

Solon, R., & Kratz, R. (2016). How mindfulness and situational awareness training help workers. *Benefits Magazine, 53*(3), 30.

Tishler, C., Reiss, N., & Dundas, J. (2013). The assessment and management of the violent patient in critical hospital settings. *General Hospital Psychiatry, 35,* 181–185.

U.S. Department of Health and Human Services. (2015). Substance Abuse and Mental Health Services Administration: Results from the 2014 National Survey on Drug Use and Health: Mental Health Findings, NSDUH Series H-50 (HHS Publication No. [SMA] 15-4927). Retrieved from http://www.samhsa.gov/data/ sites/default/files/NSDUH-FRR1-2014/NSDUH-FRR1 -2014.pdf

Villaire, M. (1995). Peter De Blieux, MD: Violence: Living with the growing shadow. *Critical Care Nurses, 15*(5), 80–87.

Geriatric Nursing

Older patients may have health experiences that are unique and that require a specialized approach to their nursing care. Older adults (i.e., people older than 65 years) account for 14.5% of the U.S. population at the time of this publication, and this percentage is projected to increase to 16.9% by 2020 and to 22% by 2050 (Administration for Community Living, 2016). The oldest U.S. citizens (i.e., the number of people older than 85 years) were recently estimated to represent 1.9% of the U.S. population (Administration for Community Living, 2016), and this oldest segment of the U.S. population will increase to 4.5% by 2050 (Administration for Community Living, 2017; Colby & Ortman, 2014). As elucidated in one of the entries, frailty, the risk for frailty—and thus, the vulnerability for adverse health outcomes—increases in the oldest patients. More information profiling this population is available through the references provided in this introduction.

The entries in this section are arranged alphabetically by topic. The topics that are included in this section address the principles for older adults' care, including content that helps nurses to distinguish age-related changes from the pathogenesis of disease processes. In addition, entries are included that will enable nurses to understand why aging in place seems to be desirable for older people, why care for the caregiver and assessment of the caregiving situation is essential, why physical activity is important for maintaining function and preventing chronic disease, and why functional assessment is a cornerstone of nursing care for older adults. Nurses' advocacy for older patients is supported by content in the entry on elder neglect, abuse, and exploitation. Also, nurses' role in helping older adults to safely manage medications is supported through entries on medication reconciliation, age-related pharmacokinetic changes, and polypharmacy. In addition to common problems, such as polypharmacy, this section includes vital information about common syndromes that are also largely preventable, with practical assessment and intervention strategies to manage conditions that may be commonly experienced by older adults. The topics include falls, delirium, pain, sleep problems, infection, malnutrition, urinary incontinence, decubiti/pressure-related injury, and dementia. We encourage readers to explore topics thoroughly through the references that are provided in each entry.

Administration for Community Living. (2016). *Aging statistics*. Retrieved from https://aoa.acl.gov/Aging_Statistics/Index.aspx

Administration for Community Living. (2017). *A profile of older Americans: 2016*. Washington, DC: U.S. Department of Health and Human Services. Retrieved from https://aoa.acl.gov/aging_statistics/profile/index.aspx

Colby, S. L., & Ortman, J. M. (2014). *An aging nation: The older population in the United States. Populations and projections*. Washington, DC: U.S. Census Bureau. Retrieved from https://www.census.gov/prod/2014pubs/p25-1140.pdf

- ■ Age-Related Changes *Evanne Juratovac*
- ■ Aging in Place *Evanne Juratovac*
- ■ Caregivers *Evanne Juratovac*
- ■ Delirium *Evanne Juratovac*
- ■ Dementia *Lori Constantine*
- ■ Elder Abuse, Neglect, and Exploitation *Sharon Ward-Miller*
- ■ Falls *Uvannie Enriquez Castro*
- ■ Frailty *Nirmala Lekhak and Evanne Juratovac*
- ■ Infection *Irena L. Kenneley*
- ■ Medication Reconciliation *Mary Jo Krivanek and Mary A. Dolansky*
- ■ Nutrition *Marianna K. Sunderlin*
- ■ Persistent Pain *Felvic Adriatico Javier*
- ■ Pharmacokinetic Changes *Carli A. Carnish*
- ■ Physical Activity *Michelle Borland*
- ■ Polypharmacy *Maria A. Mendoza*
- ■ Pressure Injury *Monica Cabrera, Lisa Torrieri, and Ekta Vohra*
- ■ Sleep Disorders *Kerry Mastrangelo and Mary T. Quinn Griffin*
- ■ Urinary Incontinence *Felvic Adriatico Javier*

■ AGE-RELATED CHANGES

Evanne Juratovac

Overview

A major challenge in the health sciences is understanding what is considered the normal aging process, thus, a challenge for nursing care of older adults is sorting out changes in health and function that may be considered to be a physical age-related process, versus a trend in a person's health and function that is related to a pathophysiological process (i.e., disease). This entry provides examples of physical age-related changes (i.e., attributed to the aging process), to help nurses recognize when a symptom experience is erroneously attributed to the "aging process" when it may, in fact, be the pathogenesis of a disease. Psychosocial aging experiences (e.g., growth and development, coping, support systems) are not covered in this entry.

Background

To call a sign or symptom an age-related change, the observed change would logically be observable in nearly every person, at nearly the same rate in the population, with nearly the same clinical presentation, eventually. Accurate use of terminology related to human aging is an important starting place: *Senescence* simply means "old," and may refer to the process of aging via problems with cell division and growth; *gerontology* is the study of human aging and the experience(s) of being old; and *geriatric* refers to the diseases and disorders commonly observed in caring for older patients. It is also important to establish that *age-associated* (i.e., a condition that may be more common in late life) does not mean age-caused.

Elderly patients are a heterogenous population. Because of their varied presentation of health and illness, elderly patients may present with "*atypical* presentation" of the signs and symptoms of disease, or with cooccurring signs and symptoms that mask or mimic each other. Advanced age is very commonly identified as a risk factor for the development of conditions/disorders that sometimes are called age-associated disorders (i.e., disease processes such as osteoporosis, arthritis, macular degeneration, hypertension). Fatigue and acute confusion are two examples of atypical presentation of illness, such as hypoperfusion and infection, respectively, and neither are expected to be "normal" age-related changes.

Biological explanations for what causes human aging usually highlight a distinction between stochastic (error, exposure, random, oxidative stress) causes and nonstochastic (biological clock, neuroendocrine, immunological, telomere shortening) causes. Within the last decade, more literature has described the implications of random accumulation of errors and toxins and deposits as a kind of damage that manifests in aging events. Particularly, apoptosis (cellular death that occurs naturally throughout life) plus the body's reparative attempt to fight DNA damage to fight oxidative stress and an accumulation of error seems to evoke a compensatory, proinflammatory cytokine response (Xu & Kirkland, 2017). This evolving response of the body through inflammation might be implicated in changes that are eventually observable in the structure of the heart and vessels, and even in musculoskeletal, neurosensory, integument, and immune system function. Also, the mechanisms by which adult cells replace themselves are not consistent across body systems and types of structures, apparently, as gastrointestinal and integumentary cells that more rapidly have to replace themselves may have more (protective) telomerase activity to protect against DNA errors, while also combating oxidative stress and mitochondria malfunction (Sousa-Victor, Neves, & Jasper, 2017).

Several background sources, such as textbooks, recount the structural and functional changes that are most apparent and may even be daringly considered "inherent" in the aging process (Boltz, Capezuti, Fulmer, & Zwicker, 2016; Fillit, Rockwood, & Young, 2017; Mauk, 2017), so they are not enumerated here. Recent increases in understanding of human senescence build on earlier conceptualizations of an inflammation–aging connection or inflammaging (Hunt, Walsh, Voegeli, & Roberts, 2010; Sousa-Victor et al., 2017), and of a threshold at which the body's homeostatic mechanisms become overwhelmed and the trend is toward homeostenosis (Taffet, 2016). These processes would most likely overwhelm the homeostatic functions of the oldest (above 85 years of age) patients.

Clinical Aspects

ASSESSMENT

In assessing an elderly patient for changes that are typically seen in older patients, it may be a useful focus to consider, "How does the age-related change put the older patient at risk for the development of other problems and disorders?" Several examples follow.

■ Changes to the heart and blood vessels mean that age is a risk factor for high blood pressure: that is, increased peripheral resistance may increase the risk for developing essential hypertension.

■ Changes to vision and tactile sensation may mean that reduced visual acuity and accommodation and the potential for reduced foot sensation combine to increase the risk for falls.

■ Changes to pulmonary function and gas exchange, coupled with electrical and baroreceptor changes in the cardiovascular system may mean that age is a risk factor for decompensation in the presence of sudden increased cardiac workload, either in exercise or in stressful situations.

■ Changes to the integument, including reduced subcutaneous fat, increased fragility of capillaries, decrease in the interface between the dermis and epidermis, decreased sebaceous gland production increases the risk for pressure-related injury and thermoregulation problems.

■ Changes in smooth muscle may increase the potential for incomplete bladder emptying and insufficient esophageal sphincter closure, which can increase the risk for bacteremia and urge-related incontinence and gastroesophageal reflux, respectively.

■ Changes in the immune system (immunosenescence) and a decreased likelihood that the older adult shows a robust febrile response to an infectious process may increase the risk for the older adult's body to mount a defense against infectious and abberant/cancerous cells, as well as increasing the risk for an autoimmune response against the body's own cells.

■ Changes in the amount of total body water, gastric emptying, lean-to-fat body mass ratio, hepatic enzymes, and glomerular filtration have resultant changes in pharmacokinetic (liberation, absorption, distribution, metabolism, excretion) function that likely increase the risk for toxicity and adverse medication reactions.

Several multisystem, multicause "geriatric syndromes" exist, and the principle that guides assessment is to recognize that these following conditions are never "normal" aging changes, and they include falls, confusion, pressure injury, eating and sleeping problems, and incontinence. A simple screening instrument to use in screening for these geriatric syndromes in clinical areas is the SPICES (sleep disorders, problems with eating or feeding, incontinence, confusion, evidence of falls, skin breakdown) mnemonic (Fulmer, 2007). Polypharmacy and pain should also be included in a list of conditions or patient experiences that should never be passed off as expected, age-related experiences. Recent-onset confusion and incontinence are never "normal" and may need an aggressive quest to determine the cause(s) in the individual and in the environment in order to reverse the conditions.

NURSING INTERVENTIONS, MANAGEMENT, AND IMPLICATIONS

Patient and family education should include teaching about examples of what to expect as you grow older. Patients and families, in particular, can be taught to recognize signs that something is an abnormal change in status that is not a "normal" part of the aging process, such as sudden-onset confusion, unexplained tiredness or weakness, or shortness of breath at rest.

Preventing delay in recognition of problems is essential. Nursing interventions are appropriately aimed at preventing excess morbidity and mortality in the oldest of patients.

OUTCOMES

Transitions in care, such as discharge, may be the ideal time for the team to reaffirm the patient's baseline and to review signs and symptoms of disease so that all providers in the handoff—including patients' family caregivers—are aware of the patient's function (Hirschman, Shaid, McCauley, Pauly, & Naylor, 2015). Ideal outcomes for patients and health care providers include promoting the shortest possible length of stay in an unfamiliar setting (such as the acute care hospital), preventing errors related to medications and treatments, increasing patient and family satisfaction with the discharge plan, reducing the need for rehospitalization, or emergency care related to errors or exacerbation of condition (Hirschman et al., 2015). An ultimate and paramount outcome is restoration of the older patient to his or her healthy baseline.

Summary

As the size of the older adult population rapidly grows, both nationally and globally, it is important for nurses to rely on their knowledge of expected age-related changes to improve nursing assessment and interventions with older people and their families. Knowledge of how to distinguish an age-related change from the beginning of a pathological (not age-related) process, early in its pathophysiology is important. Furthermore, knowing how an age-related change increases the risk for developing acute and chronic health conditions has implications for preventive care when younger. Finally, knowing that some presentations of illness may be erroneously assumed to be part of a "normal" aging process (i.e., confusion) can be lifesaving for patients and families.

Boltz, M., Capezuti, E., Fulmer, T. T., & Zwicker, D. (2016). *Evidence-based geriatric protocols for best practice* (5th ed.). New York, NY: Springer Publishing.

Fillit, H. M., Rockwood, K., & Young, J. B. (2017). *Brocklehurst's textbook of geriatric medicine and gerontology* (8th ed.). Philadelphia, PA: Elsevier.

Fulmer, T. (2007). Fulmer SPICES. *American Journal of Nursing, 107*(10), 40–48.

Hirschman, K. B., Shaid, E., McCauley, K., Pauly, M. V., & Naylor, M. D. (2015). Continuity of care: The transitional care model. *Online Journal of Issues in Nursing, 20*(3), 1.

Hunt, K. J., Walsh, B. M., Voegeli, D., & Roberts, H. C. (2010). Inflammation in aging part 1: physiology and immunological mechanisms. *Biological Research for Nursing, 11*(3), 245–252. doi:10.1177/1099800409352237

Mauk, S. (2017). *Gerontological nursing: Competencies for care* (4th ed.). Boston, MA: Jones & Bartlett.

Sousa-Victor, P., Neves, J., & Jasper, H. (2017). Theories of stem cell aging. In V. L. Bengtson & R. A. Settersten (Eds.), *Handbook of theories of aging* (pp. 153–172). New York, NY: Springer Publishing.

Taffet, G. E. (2016). Normal aging. Retrieved from https://www.uptodate.com/contents/normal-aging

Xu, M., & Kirkland, J. L. (2017). Inflammation and aging. In V. L. Bengtson & R. A. Settersten (Eds.), *Handbook of theories of aging* (pp. 137–152). New York, NY: Springer Publishing.

■ AGING IN PLACE

Evanne Juratovac

Overview

Many older adults manage their health conditions in the community, either independently, or with the help of their family. When nurses care for older adults in acute and subacute care settings, they must understand the function and care needs of the older patient, in order to help the patient to return safely to the community. The phrase aging in place describes a preference for the place in which long-term services and supports (LTSS) are provided: Care for everyday physical needs, and for health maintenance or home maintenance needs, is provided in the home, wherein the goal of the aging person and the health care system is to live in the community for as long as possible (Administration for Community Living, 2017a; Partners for Livable Communities, 2017). This entry provides assessment and intervention recommendations for nurses to promote aging in place for their older patients.

Background

The majority of older people in the United States live in the community, according to the most recent national profile of older adults (Administration for Community Living, 2016). Several phrases have emerged over the past two decades to describe a trend in the United States and worldwide, including *successful aging* and *elder-friendly communities* (Community Research Partners, 2006) in the United States, and most recent, a *livable community* promotes the idea that if the community is elder-friendly, some of the accommodations are friendly for other citizens to benefit. These include physical barrier reduction (in the form of crosswalks and curbcuts), signage, and opportunities for intergenerational programming (Partners for Livable Communities, 2017). To age in place means to safely stay in one's own home setting, regardless of financial or functional status; and thus, to stay within a community that provides for older people's safety and maximizes their function (Centers for Disease Control and Prevention [CDC], 2016). To age in place, this also means that older persons do not need to move to particular care settings as their care needs change—instead, instrumental supports are brought into the home setting—and the benefit is that they remain as engaged (i.e., socially connected) as possible in their community of choice (Partners for Livable Communities, 2017).

This goal of supporting aging in place has become integrated into policy discussions about older adult care to the extent that the U.S. government website dedicated to the Administration for Community Living (i.e., acl.gov) directly presents information regarding safety, health care financing, and instrumental support services for older adults and their families (Administration for Community Living, 2017a). According to the American Association of Colleges of Nursing (AACN) and Quality and Safety Education for Nurses (QSEN) competency standards, nurses must provide care to older patients and families—across settings—that demonstrates gerontological nursing knowledge and skill to address age-related changes, functional assessment, environmental and interpersonal safety, injury prevention, and care transition needs (AACN, 2010); and, quality and safe care for older adults also includes assessing the environment of care and assisting with transitions in care (Cronenwett et al., 2007).

Clinical Aspects

ASSESSMENT

In order to provide for services and supports that promote aging in place, the nurse needs to have a solid foundation in functional assessment knowledge and skills. Two fundamental assessment tools to measure functional ability are the "Katz Index of Activities of Daily Living" (ADL; Katz, Downs, Cash, & Grotz, 1970), which is used to assess the ability of the older adult to independently provide for his or her personal care needs, and the Lawton "Instrumental Activities of Daily Living" (IADL) scale (Lawton & Brody, 1969), which is used to assess the ability of the older adult to independently manage health maintenance and home maintenance tasks and responsibilities. Examples of ADL include bathing, dressing, and eating, whereas examples of IADL include laundry, medication management, arranging transportation, and meal preparation. To promote aging in place, interpret ADL and IADL findings as follows: A lower score on a person's ADL scale means that he or she may need assistance with direct personal care; and a lower score on a person's IADL scale means that he or she may need assistance with maintaining the home, or in getting around the neighborhood, or in procuring medications and groceries. To promote safe and sound care, including the discharge plan, the nurse's health care agency should incorporate similar ADL and IADL assessment content into the documentation system.

NURSING INTERVENTIONS, MANAGEMENT, AND IMPLICATIONS

Knowledge of community services and supports (i.e., LTSS) in the patient's community may be enhanced by partnering with the "Area Agency on Aging" in the vicinity of the health care organization (Administration for Community Living, 2017a). Several ideas for community-based interventions based on the region in which the nurse practices may be found through the Administration for Community Living's "Community Innovations for Aging in Place" (CIAP) resources (Administration for Community Living, 2017b). Provisions in the U.S. Older Americans Act explain how guidelines and funding direct local social services agencies in the community to review benefit eligibility and support needs of the patients and their families; provide evidence-based health education to promote self-management; support care coordination in the community; address IADL needs, such as nutrition (e.g., deliver home-delivered meals) and transportation (i.e., to take older people to health care appointments, senior center programming, and other community-engagement activities); ensure safe housing and utilities (e.g., heating assistance, chores); and protect against harm, such as elder abuse and exploitation (Administration for Community Living, 2017a).

Some of the provisions of nationally supported services in the United States are related to the outcomes of successful aging initiative projects that demonstrated in landmark reports what constituted an elder-friendly community in the first part of the 21st century: Findings led to cooperative transportation, social programming, and health care services in communities to (a) meet people's basic needs, (b) optimize physical and mental well-being, (c) encourage social engagement in the community, and maximize function and independence for older people and others who may have disability (Community Research Partners, 2006). More recent, elder-friendly, aging-in-place discussions are informing broader conversations about the livability of the community for all (Partners for Livable Communities, 2017).

OUTCOMES

A few decades into the evolution of the language about aging in a safe, supportive community, it seems that much of the published work that inform nurses who are intent on promoting the health and well-being of older adults can be found outside of nursing and health-related literature. Governmental and nongovernmental policy groups have published suggestions for ways that communities can promote aging in place, but it should be understood that some recommendations may not meet the needs of the diverse neighborhoods in which older adults chose to remain. The effectiveness of aging in place has been examined, and two suggested benefits of interventions to promote aging in place are cost savings and preventing mortality (Jutkowitz, Gitlin, Pizzi, Lee, & Dennis, 2012).

Summary

Perhaps the goal is for all citizens of a community, at any age, is to age in place. Aging in place is promoted when transitions within and back to the community are made based on a firm foundation of functional assessment. Furthermore, nurses' knowledge and skill in making referrals to community supports and services (LTSS) promotes older patients' ability to live well, to engage, and to thrive in their preferred place.

Administration for Community Living. (2016). *Aging statistics.* Retrieved from https://aoa.acl.gov/Aging_Statistics/Index.aspx

Administration for Community Living. (2017a). *A profile of older Americans: 2016.* Washington, DC: U.S. Department of Health and Human Services. Retrieved from https://www.acl.gov/sites/default/files/Aging%20and%20Disability%20in%20America/2016-Profile.pdf

Administration for Community Living. (2017b). *Community innovations for aging in place.* Washington, DC: U.S. Department of Health and Human Services. Retrieved from https://www.acl.gov/node/495

American Association of Colleges of Nursing. (2010). *Recommended baccalaureate competencies and curricular guidelines for the nursing care of older adults.* Washington, DC: Author.

Centers for Disease Control and Prevention. (2016). *Healthy aging & the built environment.* Atlanta, GA: Author.

Community Research Partners. (2006). *The Cleveland Foundation successful aging initiative final evaluation report.* Columbus, OH: Author. Retrieved from http://www.communityresearchpartners.org/wp-content/uploads/Reports/strategic-aging-initiative/tcf_aging_report.pdf

Cronenwett, L., Sherwood, G., Barnsteiner, J., Disch, J., Johnson, J., Mitchell, P., . . . Warren, J. (2007). Quality and safety education for nurses. *Nursing Outlook,* 55(3), 122–131. doi:10.1016/j.outlook.2007.02.006

Jutkowitz, E., Gitlin, L. N., Pizzi, L. T., Lee, E., & Dennis, M. P. (2012). Cost effectiveness of a home-based intervention that helps functionally vulnerable older adults age in place at home. *Journal of Aging Research, 2012,* 680265. doi:10.1155/2012/680265

Katz, S., Downs, T. D., Cash, H. R., & Grotz, R. C. (1970). Progress in development of the index of ADL. *The Gerontologist, 10*(1), 20–30.

Lawton, M. P., & Brody, E. M. (1969). Assessment of older people: self-maintaining and instrumental activities of daily living. *The Gerontologist, 9*(3), 179–186.

Partners for Livable Communities. (2017). *Aging in place initiative*. Washington, DC: Author. Retrieved from http://livable.org/program-areas/livable-communities -for-all-ages-a-aging-in-place/programs

■ CAREGIVERS

Evanne Juratovac

Overview

Although many older adults do not require assistance for their daily functioning, nurses will care for older adults who require assistance from another person, either temporarily or long term. When care is needed, most long-term services and supports (LTSS) for health and function are provided by family caregivers rather than, or in addition to, agency-based caregivers. Family caregivers are immediate family members, partners, or kin (a close, though not immediate-family relation) who provide some form of care for everyday physical needs and/or remote or in-person supervision, either because of a physical, cognitive, or behavioral condition (Family Caregiver Alliance [FCA], 2014; National Alliance for Caregiving [NAC], 2016; Schulz & Eden, 2016), or for a related situation, such as a transition in care. This entry provides support for the nurse's role in family caregiver assessment and intervention as an integral part of elder care.

Background

When older adults require care, most care is unpaid, provided by family or kin. Sometimes the caregiving situation is specified according to the condition or needs of the elder, such as dementia caregiving or cancer caregiving. Often the care is directly related to activities of daily living and to manage chronic health conditions (NAC & AARP, 2015). Quality and safe care for older adults, as described in the Quality and Safety Education for Nurses (QSEN) competencies (Cronenwett et al., 2007), includes assessing the environment of care and communicating with the family as part of the health care delivery team. Quality and safe care is thus maximized when the nurse demonstrates specific competencies in assessing the family caregiver and caregiving situation (American Association of Colleges of Nursing [AACN], 2010; Cronenwett et al., 2007), as family-centered care is inherent in patient-centered care.

Several reports describe the family caregiving workforce in the United States. Recently, national survey estimates suggest that nearly 45 million family caregivers care for adults older than 50 years; however, many adults who require care are aged 80 years and much older, and many of the caregivers are in their later decades of life as well (NAC & AARP, 2015). Family caregivers' time and effort is expended in providing this unpaid care, yet they are also balancing that caregiving workload and effort along with their other relationships, roles, and responsibilities (Juratovac, Morris, Zauszniewski, & Wykle, 2012). This unpaid elder care is not without cost to the caregiver—cost that manifests in poor health. A growing literature has documented the health risks associated with family-provided care for the family caregiver. A landmark report documents risk that is due to the protracted exposure to the stressors and strains associated with the care, and possible neglect of one's own regular health-promotion activities: The exposure seems to ultimately result in disability and disease (NAC & Evercare, 2006). This means that family caregivers who are having difficulty with their health and functioning may be compromised in their role to provide care to vulnerable older adults in need of that care.

Clinical Aspects

Although many positive aspects of older adult caregiving are reported by family caregivers, the risks for problems with the caregiver's health are a call to action for agency-based caregivers to partner with family caregivers. National advocacy organizations have called for family caregiver assessment to be incorporated across care settings (FCA, 2016). Baccalaureate-prepared nurses are expected to demonstrate competency in partnering with families to assess the function of the patient and safety of the caregiving situation, particularly during transitions in care (AACN, 2010). Caregiver assessment and caregiver education are recommended gerontological nursing activities across practice settings.

The complexity and intensity of care that family caregivers provide has been documented in an important national report in which families report managing very technical procedures commonly considered formal nursing care tasks, including administering intravenous medication, providing for safe mobility, and performing wound care (AARP & United Hospital Fund [UHF], 2012). Thus, though family caregivers are sometimes called "informal" caregivers to contrast with "formal" (agency-based) caregivers, this can be a misnomer, as their care may actually be very formal in nature. Nurses are in a unique position to educate and support families who provide care that requires a high level of knowledge and skills.

ASSESSMENT

Partnering with families to meet the function and care needs of the older adult is already a nursing role expectation across settings of care. Caregiver assessment is inclusive of the recipient of care, the caregiver, the broader caregiving situation, and specific caregiving needs (FCA, 2016). Thus, assessing the functioning of the elder includes assessing the family caregiver. It is important for the nurse to understand whether the workload is stable, or whether there are new or changing responsibilities and to recognize that it may not just be the workload that is problematic, but the outpouring of mental and physical effort and time needed to accomplish the tasks and responsibilities of that workload (Juratovac et al., 2012). Assessing for the effects of caregiving on the family caregiver has become strongly recommended within the last decade. Because high-strain caregiving has been associated with the disproportionate distress—particularly in the form of depressive symptoms—in family caregivers (NAC & Evercare, 2006), assessing the caregiver is vital. Assessing the caregiving *situation* is also important because high-stress situations involving the caregiver and the elderly person requiring the care are known risks for elder neglect, abuse (verbal, emotional, and physical), and abandonment (Schulz & Eden, 2016). It is proposed here that, similar to the QSEN competencies (Cronenwett et al., 2007), the nurse should assess the family caregiver's knowledge, skills, and attitude about their caregiving responsibilities.

Some caregiving instruments may be better suited for research purposes, rather than clinical purposes. To consider whether an instrument is suitable for use in clinical settings, consider the purpose of the assessment. For example, assessment of the care recipient's functional abilities, the positive and negative aspects affecting the well-being of the family caregiver, the knowledge and skills of the family caregiver, the effects of caregiving on the caregiver (including physical and financial/work strain), resources that a caregiver could use (FCA, 2014) guide selection of an assessment strategy. Some assessment strategies, such as Tailored Caregiver Assessment and Referral (TCARE), as described in an evidence-based collection of caregiving assessments (Rosalynn Carter Institute for Caregiving [RCI], 2012), includes caregiver assessment plus decision paths, to refer the caregiver to resources based on the findings of the assessment.

NURSING INTERVENTIONS, MANAGEMENT, AND IMPLICATIONS

Assessing the caregiver and the caregiving situation guides the nurse toward educational interventions and resources that might help to support the family caregiving situation. Many evidence-based interventions are described to help caregivers manage the health conditions and behaviors of the older adult, and/or to manage their reaction to the caregiving situation (FCA, 2014; RCI, 2012). Caregivers can be taught specific skills, such as wound care, medication management, falls prevention, and behavioral care. For example, when surveyed, families have reported that more knowledge and skills help them to manage wound care and medications in the home, further reporting that the majority of the training that they received was provided by health care providers such as acute, outpatient, and home care nurses (AARP & UHF, 2012).

It is also important to have a working knowledge of resources in the community (FCA, 2014), in order to recommend services that are appropriate to the person's situation, for example, emotional support related to a diagnosis, such as dementia, or practical support related to a functional need, such as transportation.

OUTCOMES

Elder care is complex, costly care. Measuring the outcomes of family caregiving for patients with chronic medical conditions, such as with the Bakas Caregiving Outcomes Scale, may reveal risky issues facing the family caregiver (Bakas, 2014) and older patient. Family-provided care may prevent costly formal care: In a landmark national survey focused on the complexity of family-provided care, the majority of families who performed more than five "nursing" tasks at home reported that their care prevented institutionalization of the recipient of care (AARP & UHF, 2012), which represents cost-saving. And perhaps, quality and satisfaction data may reveal caregiving situational needs that can be the focus of family-centered care.

Summary

With the increasing age of the population in the United States, the need for family caregivers for older adults who require care will certainly grow. Consistent with the AACN competencies for older adult care and the QSEN competencies, nurses must know how to (a) assess the caregiving situation, (b) promote family caregivers' health and functioning, (c) reduce quality and safety risks related to transitions in care, and (d) reduce the likelihood of geriatric care problems that may be related to family caregiver knowledge and skills. Thus, caring for the older patient and the family caregiver *together* is an appropriate approach to quality care.

American Association of Colleges of Nursing. (2010). *Recommended baccalaureate competencies and curricular guidelines for the nursing care of older adults.* Washington, DC: Author.

American Association of Retired Persons & United Hospital Fund. (2012). *Home alone: Family caregivers providing complex chronic care.* Washington, DC: AARP.

Bakas, T. (2014). Bakas caregiving outcomes scale. In A. C. Michalos (Ed.), *Encyclopedia of quality of life and well-being research* (pp. 319–321). New York, NY: Springer Publishing. doi:10.1007/978-94-007-0753-5

Cronenwett, L., Sherwood, G., Barnsteiner, J., Disch, J., Johnson, J., Mitchell, P.,...Warren, J. (2007). Quality and safety education for nurses. *Nursing Outlook, 55*(3), 122–131. doi:10.1016/j.outlook.2007.02.006

Family Caregiver Alliance. (2014). *Caregivers count too! Examples of caregiver assessment tools* (Section four). San Francisco, CA: Author. Retrieved from https://www.caregiver.org/caregivers-count-too-s4 -assessment-tool-examples

Juratovac, E., Morris, D. L., Zauszniewski, J. A., & Wykle, M. L. (2012). Effort, workload, and depressive symptoms in family caregivers of older adults: conceptualizing and testing a work-health relationship. *Research and Theory for Nursing Practice, 26*(2), 74–94.

National Alliance for Caregiving & American Association of Retired Persons. (2015). *Caregiving in the U.S.* Washington, DC: National Alliance for Caregiving.

National Alliance for Caregiving & Evercare. (2006). *Caregivers in decline: A close-up look at the risks of caring for a loved one.* Bethesda, MD: Author.

Rosalynn Carter Institute for Caregiving. (2012). Caregiver assessment. Retrieved from http://www.rosalynncarter .org/caregiver_assessment

Schulz, R., & Eden, J. (2016). *Families caring for an aging America.* Washington, DC: National Academies Press.

■ DELIRIUM

Evanne Juratovac

Overview

Delirium is a multisystem syndrome that presents in patients across the life span and across health care settings. According to the *Diagnostic and Statistical Manual of Mental Disorders* (5th ed., *DSM-5*;

American Psychiatric Association [APA], 2013), delirium is an acquired cognitive deficit for which there may exist multiple etiologies. Delirium is defined by its hallmark features: problems with attention and awareness, which has a sudden onset and fluctuating course; its prevalence is highest among hospitalized elderly patients (APA, 2013). This entry describes risk factors for delirium as a form of reversible confusion, provides assessment strategies to identify the cause(s) of delirium, and suggests interventions to minimize the excess morbidity from and/or reverse the cause(s) of delirium.

Background

Delirium is classified as a neurocognitive disorder (NCD) in the *DSM-5*, and is recognized as a syndrome of disturbed attention and orientation, which develops relatively suddenly as a notable change from the person's baseline, and presents with difficulty sustaining attention over a fluctuating course (APA, 2013). It is important to note that no firm pathophysiological process has been identified (Davis et al., 2013), yet well before the patient manifests behavioral signs of delirium, some metabolic process and physiological stress response has likely begun.

Caution has been recommended in estimating the prevalence of delirium based on the care setting or the patient's diagnosis, as numbers can vary according to how the word delirium is operationalized, and based on the diagnostic categorization system that is used (Davis et al., 2013). A particular problem in estimating the prevalence of delirium is that delirium is colloquially described according to the presumed pathology of the patient, such as *altered* mental status, or defined by the setting of care, such as ICU *psychosis*. The many terms and provisional diagnoses found in patients' records, and in families' explanations of patients' history, may obscure whether patients have a history of delirium. Although the prevalence of delirium in the older population is uncertain, what is certain is that delirium is life-threatening; thus, recognizing and reversing delirium is lifesaving.

Risk factors for delirium are both intrinsic and extrinsic. Note that risk factors for older patients include a history of delirium and advanced age, which is why it is important to document the older patient's history of delirium, using consistent terminology. Other intrinsic risk factors may include the presence of other chronic medical disorders (particularly, a pre-existing NCD such as dementia), sleep disturbance, sensory/perceptual deficits (e.g., hearing, vision), poor nutrition, substance-related and adverse medication effects, infection, dehydration, hypoxia, pain, trauma, and perhaps the absence of familiar surroundings or caregivers. Causes of delirium may be related to these risk factors and include medical disorders that can affect hydration status, oxygenation, and perfusion. Additional risk factors are extrinsic, including procedures and characteristics of the environment. Extrinsic risk factors include light, noise, clutter, medications, anesthesia, extended stay in the emergency department or intensive care unit, and invasive equipment and procedures. Causes of delirium may be related to the interventions used for the medical disorders being treated (procedures such as catheterization and intubation). It is important to remember that delirium is understood to be a disturbance in physical and behavioral functioning that tends not to reverse without intervention.

Clinical Aspects

ASSESSMENT

Assessment instruments for detecting delirium in a clinical setting should minimally include the aforementioned hallmark features of delirium. Because a patient who is experiencing delirium has impaired awareness, self-report by the patient is never reliable and early recognition by another person is imperative (Juratovac & Lange, 2015). In addition to careful documentation of a patient's past history of delirium, interviewing a person familiar with the patient's baseline is essential. Delirium can be hyperactive, hypoactive, or mixed: Because the hypoactive subtype is more difficult to notice, it is easier to miss, and is associated with a greater risk for mortality than the hyperactive subtype (APA, 2013). Current clinical practice guidelines and diagnostic criteria could still miss a lot of delirium: If a patient's presentation does not meet criteria for a full-blown episode of delirium, then could the health care team be missing clinically significant subsyndromal delirium?

The Confusion Assessment Method (CAM) is a brief, easy-to-administer instrument used to screen for delirium in clinical areas to identify the core features of delirium: The patient must have an acute onset and a fluctuating course and shows signs of disorganized thought and/or altered consciousness (Inouye et al., 1990). The Family CAM (FAM-CAM) is the CAM that is appropriate for interviewing family members (Hospital Elder Life Program, 2017; Steis et al., 2012). The FAM-CAM is essential for empowering family caregivers, who know a patient's baseline, to recognize and

report characteristics of delirium to nurses and other members of the team (Juratovac & Lange, 2015). It may be possible for nurses to quickly screen the older patient for delirium using as few as two items (Fick et al., 2015).

When a patient already has dementia—a high risk for delirium—unfortunately the onset of delirium can be misinterpreted as being part of the person's dementia. Worse, delirium can be misinterpreted as the person's underlying dementia suddenly worsening. It is proposed here that dementia does not suddenly worsen. An updated, computerized algorithm specifically guides the assessment of delirium that is superimposed on dementia (Fick, Steis, Mion, & Walls, 2011). Such an addition to electronic charting and decision support systems would help health care providers to recognize delirium as an episode of acute confusion that is beyond the patient's baseline (i.e., pre-existing) NCD and is amenable to intervention.

NURSING INTERVENTIONS, MANAGEMENT, AND IMPLICATIONS

Delirium interventions are documented elsewhere in practice guidelines for long-term care and intensive care settings. The following general intervention suggestions can be implemented in acute care, long-term care, and home care settings: wherever older adults receive nursing care. The well-accepted primary treatment strategy is to identify and eliminate the cause(s) of the present episode, because prevention of further morbidity and mortality is of the utmost importance. Therefore, nursing intervention is aimed at recognizing the causes of the current episode of delirium and implementing interventions to quickly reverse the causes. Knowing the common risk factors and common presenting features (i.e., inattention) enables nurses to recognize and reverse possible systemic and environmental causes of the outward behavioral change; accurate documentation is essential (Juratovac & Lange, 2015). The following are some examples of how the intervention can be implemented based on the suspected causes, both pharmacological and nonpharmacological/environmental.

Pharmacological

It is not clear whether traditional (e.g., haloperidol) and second-generation (e.g., quetiapine) antipsychotic medications are better than placebo for reducing the length or severity of a delirium episode, but approaches that reduce the adverse effects of anesthesia and procedure-related sedation may be helpful (Friedman, Soleimani, McGonigle, Egol, & Silverstein, 2014). If potentially inappropriate medications have been used and the patient has had an adverse medication reaction, the American Geriatrics Society's (AGS) most recent criteria (AGS, 2015) may provide support for the interprofessional team to choose lower risk medications.

Nonpharmacological

For example, if hypoxia and fluid/electrolyte imbalances are noted, they need to be corrected (reversed); if the patient seems overstimulated from excess environmental noise, the noise needs to be reduced, and if an infectious process is confirmed, the infection(s) need to be treated. Nurses can also reverse the causes of delirium by addressing sleep–wake disturbances, treating pain and promoting comfort, and preventing injury resulting from a patient's reduced awareness (e.g., falls prevention interventions). For problems related to disorientation, minimizing changes to the environment and maintaining consistent staff may be helpful. Simple, one-step instructions may improve comprehension. Sometimes the simplest solution may be to make sure that the older patient who needs glasses or hearing aids for improving communication and sensory perception is wearing them. Overall, the nonpharmacological approaches have been recommended as best practice to prevent and to minimize the duration of delirium (Martinez, Tobar, & Hill, 2015).

OUTCOMES

Delirium is largely reversible, and delirium can be deadly. For improving the outcomes of care for patients with delirium, nurses should regularly reassess the severity of the episode of delirium with a delirium instrument; regularly assess cognitive function; document the hallmark features (or their resolution); review vital signs and biometric data (including laboratory test results); compare pain, fall, and injury risk assessment findings to the patient's baseline, if known; and work with the interprofessional team, including family members' participation in care and planning, to reduce the length of stay in an unfamiliar environment.

Summary

Because a history of delirium is a risk factor for developing delirium and for adverse outcomes such as complicated recovery and even mortality, nurses are in a key position to accurately document delirium history and presenting features. Nurses are also in a key position to implement interventions in the environment to reduce the impact of the current episode of delirium. Families remain essential partners in recognizing and reversing delirium in older patients.

American Geriatrics Society. (2015). Updated Beers criteria for potentially inappropriate medication use in older adults. *Journal of the American Geriatrics Society, 63*(11), 2227–2246.

American Psychiatric Association. (2013). *Diagnostic and statistical manual of mental disorders* (5th ed.). Arlington, VA: America Psychiatric Publishing.

Davis, D. H., Kreisel, S. H., Muniz Terrera, G., Hall, A. J., Morandi, A., Boustani, M.,…Brayne, C. (2013). The epidemiology of delirium: Challenges and opportunities for population studies. *American Journal of Geriatric Psychiatry, 21*(12), 1173–1189. doi:10.1016/j.jagp.2013.04.007

Fick, D. M., Inouye, S. K., Guess, J., Ngo, L. H., Jones, R. N., Saczynski, J. S., & Marcantonio, E. R. (2015). Preliminary development of an ultrabrief two-item bedside test for delirium. *Journal of Hospital Medicine, 10*(10), 645–650. doi:10.1002/jhm.2418

Fick, D. M., Steis, M. R., Mion, L. C., & Walls, J. L. (2011). Computerized decision support for delirium superimposed on dementia in older adults. *Journal of Gerontological Nursing, 37*(4), 39–47. doi:10.3928/00989134-20100930-01

Friedman, J. I., Soleimani, L., McGonigle, D. P., Egol, C., & Silverstein, J. H. (2014). Pharmacological treatments of non-substance-withdrawal delirium: A systematic review of prospective trials. *American Journal of Psychiatry, 171*(2), 151–159. doi:10.1176/appi.ajp.2013.13040458

Hospital Elder Life Program. (2017). The FAM-CAM. Retrieved from https://www.hospitalelderlifeprogram.org

Inouye, S. K., van Dyck, C. H., Alessi, C. A., Balkin, S., Siegal, A. P., & Horwitz, R. I. (1990). Clarifying confusion: The confusion assessment method. A new method for detection of delirium. *Annals of Internal Medicine, 113*(12), 941–948.

Juratovac, E., & Lange, A. T. (2015, February). *Teaching nursing students to teach families: Using service learning to increase delirium knowledge in family caregivers of older adults.* Paper presented at the Association for Gerontology in Higher Education's 41st Annual Meeting and Educational Leadership Conference, Nashville, TN.

Martinez, F., Tobar, C., & Hill, N. (2015). Preventing delirium: Should non-pharmacological, multicomponent interventions be used? A systematic review and meta-analysis of the literature. *Age and Ageing, 44*(2), 196–204. doi:10.1093/ageing/afu173

Steis, M. R., Evans, L., Hirschman, K. B., Hanlon, A., Fick, D. M., Flanagan, N., & Inouye, S. K. (2012). Screening for delirium using family caregivers: Convergent validity of the Family Confusion Assessment Method and interviewer-rated Confusion Assessment Method. *Journal of the American Geriatrics Society, 60*(11), 2121–2126. doi:10.1111/j.1532-5415.2012.04200.x

■ DEMENTIA

Lori Constantine

Overview

Dementia is a cluster of symptoms, chronic and progressive in nature, that affects a person's memory, behavior, cognition, and functional status (Alzheimer's Association, 2016). Dementia has been recognized by the World Health Organization (WHO) as a public health priority and as a significant cause of disability and loss of independence (WHO, 2016). Dementia not only affects the patient, but also places significant financial, emotional, social, and physical burdens on caregivers and families. Expert nursing care is required when caring for the older adult with dementia. Focused cognitive and physical examinations coupled with a thorough patient history allow for problem recognition and implementation of appropriate care interventions. Outcomes of care are guided by stage of dementia and focused on maintaining function, independence, and safety, while preventing complications.

Background

The hallmarks of a dementia diagnosis are usually identified by the patient or family. Evidence of significant cognitive decline from a previous level of functional performance in at least one cognitive domain is required for diagnosis. These cognitive domains include learning and memory, language, executive function, complex attention, perceptual–motor capabilities, and social cognition. Cognitive deficits must also be severe enough to interfere with independence in completing instrumental activities of daily living. Finally, delirium or other mental disorders, such as major depressive disorder or schizophrenia, must be ruled out (American Psychiatric Association, 2013).

Dementia is an umbrella term that encompasses a range of cognitive impairments. Alzheimer's disease (AD) is the most prevalent cause of dementia, and accounts for approximately 50% to 75% of all dementias. Vascular dementias account for 20% to 30% of

dementias. Other less common causes of dementia include dementia with Lewy bodies, accounting for 10% to 25% and frontotemporal dementia, accounting for 10% to 15% of dementias. Still, there are mixed forms of dementia that are less common and include a combination of one or more dementia types. Early-onset dementia is diagnosed usually around age 30 to 50 years, and affects about 5% of the 5 million persons diagnosed with Alzheimer-type dementia (Alzheimer's Association, 2016). Dementia should not be confused with mild neurocognitive disorder, also known as *mild cognitive impairment (MCI)*. MCI does not affect the person enough to interrupt daily activities. However, MCI is a risk factor for later development of dementia (Alzheimer's Association, 2016; American Psychiatric Association, 2013).

Nonmodifiable risk factors for dementia include age, family history, and being a carrier of the *APOE4* gene. Age is the greatest of these risk factors. Although family history of dementia does not guarantee development of the disease, persons with first-degree relatives with the disease are more likely to develop dementia. Modifiable risk factors for dementia include sedentary lifestyle and other cardiovascular risk factors, such as smoking, hypertension, diabetes, and obesity. People with more years of formal education may have increased cognitive reserve, allowing better adaption to pathological brain changes. In addition, remaining socially and cognitively stimulated throughout the life span has been shown to reduce the risks of developing dementia (Alzheimer's Association, 2016).

Although dementia mainly affects older adults, it is not considered a normal part of the aging process. Yet, it is quite prevalent. Currently, one in three older adults in the United States dies with a history of Alzheimer's or another dementia (Alzheimer's Association, 2016). The incidence of dementia is rising. The rise is predominant in lower- to middle-income countries due to low average educational level and rising vascular risk factors (Rizzi, Rosset, & Roriz-Cruz, 2014). Alternatively, the age-specific incidence of dementia is declining in high-income countries (Jones & Greene, 2016). This is attributed to increased education and wealth, and better control of vascular risk factors (Jones & Greene, 2016; Satizabal, 2016).

Dementia significantly impacts medical costs and weighs heavily on families and caregivers. Worldwide monetary costs of dementia are estimated to be approximately $818 billion in 2015 and expected to reach $1 trillion by 2018 (Wimo et al., 2017). In addition to monetary costs, the emotional and financial pressures of caring for loved ones with dementia can be overwhelming. In the United States, greater than 80% of care is provided by unpaid caregivers (Friedman, Shih, Langa, & Hurd, 2015), who are at risk of experiencing significant employment and health consequences associated with the caregiving role (Alzheimer's Association, 2016).

Clinical Aspects

ASSESSMENT

Persons with dementia experience symptoms that can be elicited by a thorough assessment. The nurse assessing the patients with dementia should ask about the person's daily memory, ability to concentrate or organize, use of language, visuospatial skills, and orientation. Persons with dementia will likely have difficulty recalling recent events, making decisions, solving problems, or executing sequential tasks such as planning a meal or dressing for the day. They may also experience difficulty attending to conversations or finding the correct words to convey thoughts. Persons with dementia may have trouble with depth perception, leading to difficulty using stairs and confusion about their location or what day it is. Furthermore, they may experience mood changes, becoming frustrated, anxious, or even apathetic. Finally, hallucinations and delusions may occur. Recognition of these symptoms should prompt a formal screening evaluation: The Mini-Cog (Borson, Scanlan, Chen, & Ganguli, 2003) can be useful in documenting the person's cognition and identifying patients for expert follow up. Neuroimaging may reveal characteristics specific to dementia and rule out other causes of cognitive dysfunction (Alzheimer's Association, 2016).

NURSING INTERVENTIONS, MANAGEMENT, AND IMPLICATIONS

There is no cure for dementia, and in time it is fatal (Alzheimer's Association, 2016). The pace at which symptoms progress and cognitive function declines is individual. Eventually, the person with dementia will likely experience weight loss, weakness, and sleep disturbances. He or she may fail to recognize loved ones, become incontinent of bowel and bladder, and lose the ability to move or eat independently. In addition, he or she will become more vulnerable to decubitus ulcers and infections. In fact, pneumonia is a frequent cause of death in persons with advanced disease due to the inability to swallow properly and clear airway secretions (Alzheimer's Association, 2016).

OUTCOMES

Nursing care of the person with dementia should focus on maintaining function and independence, preventing complications, and keeping the patient safe. Assistance with activities of daily living will eventually be required. Prevention of complications, such as aspiration pneumonia, decubitus ulcers, falls, and wandering, is paramount. Careful conversations with persons with dementia and their families or loved ones regarding advance care planning can prevent unwanted treatments as the disease progresses. Finally, pharmacological therapies may be beneficial in improving cognitive symptoms, but do not cure the disease. Acetylcholinesterase inhibitors and memantine have been shown to help with memory, motivation, and concentration in activities of daily living, although these do not prevent or alter pathological brain changes associated with the disease (Alzheimer's Association, 2016; Dodd, Cheston, & Ivanecka, 2015).

Summary

Expected outcomes of care for persons with dementia include supporting function, preventing complications, and supporting the caregiver. Preventing complications, careful coordination of care, participation in social activities, and support groups for caregivers are helpful in managing the care of persons with dementia. Future research aimed at diagnosing, preventing, and treating the dementia and implementation of greater support systems for caregivers should be undertaken.

Alzheimer's Association. (2016). Alzheimer's Association report: 2016 Alzheimer's disease facts and figures. *Alzheimer's and Dementia: The Journal of the Alzheimer's Association, 12,* 459–509.

American Psychiatric Association. (2013). *Diagnostic and statistical manual of mental disorders* (5th ed.). Arlington, VA: American Psychiatric Publishing.

Borson, S., Scanlan, J. M., Chen, P., & Ganguli, M. (2003). The Mini-Cog as a screen for dementia: Validation in a population-based sample. *Journal of the American Geriatrics Society, 51*(10), 1451–1454.

Dodd, E., Cheston, R., & Ivanecka, A. (2015). The assessment of dementia in primary care. *Journal of Psychiatric and Mental Health Nursing, 22*(9), 731–737. doi:10.1111/jpm.12250

Friedman, E. M., Shih, R. A., Langa, K. M., & Hurd, M. D. (2015). U.S. prevalence and predictors of informal caregiving for dementia. *Health Affairs, 34*(10), 1637–1641. doi:10.1377/hlthaff.2015.0510

Jones, D. S., & Greene, J. A. (2016). Is dementia in decline? Historical trends and future trajectories. *New England Journal of Medicine, 374*(6), 507–509. doi:10.1056/NEJMp1514434

Rizzi, L., Rosset, I., & Roriz-Cruz, M. (2014). Global epidemiology of dementia: Alzheimer's and vascular types. *BioMed Research International, 2014*, 908915. doi:10.1155/2014/908915

Satizabal, C. L., Beiser, A. S., Chouraki, V., Chêne, G., Dufouil, C., & Seshadri, S. (2016). Incidence of dementia over three decades in the Framingham Heart Study. *New England Journal of Medicine, 374*(6), 523–532. doi:10.1056/NEJMoa1504327

Wimo, A., Guerchet, M., Ali, G. C., Wu, Y. T., Prina, A. M., Winblad, B.,…Prince, M. (2017). The worldwide costs of dementia 2015 and comparisons with 2010. *Alzheimer's & Dementia: The Journal of the Alzheimer's Association, 13*(1), 1–7. doi:10.1016/j.jalz.2016.07.150

World Health Organization. (2016). Dementia: Fact sheet. Retrieved from http://www.who.int/mediacentre/factsheets/fs362/en/

■ ELDER ABUSE, NEGLECT, AND EXPLOITATION

Sharon Ward-Miller

Overview

Elder abuse as a global phenomenon is increasing each year and has been described to be at epidemic proportions by researchers. The global population of people aged 60 years and older will be more than double by the year 2050. In 2015, there were 900 million people older than 60 years of age. By 2050, this number will increase to 2 billion older adults. Experts report that data about prevalence lags at least 20 years behind that of child abuse and domestic violence research. According to the National Center on Elder Abuse (NCEA), there is no one definition of elder abuse that is accepted by all involved disciplines (NCEA, 2016). Lack of awareness of signs of elder abuse and inadequate education may also contribute to underreporting of the incidence by professionals, families, and victims. There is consensus by experts that there is an urgent need for more research that is systematic and coordinated, which involves policy makers, researchers and funders (Connolly, Brandl, & Breckman, 2014).

Background

The World Health Organization (WHO) defines elder abuse as

A single or repeated act, or lack of appropriate action, occurring within any relationship where there is an expectation of trust, which causes harm or distress to an older person. This type of violence constitutes a violation of human rights and includes physical, sexual, psychological, emotional, financial, and material abuse; abandonment; neglect; and serious loss of dignity and respect. (WHO, 2016, para 1)

It is estimated that one in 10 older adults are victims of abuse each month but only one in 24 incidents are reported. The rates of abuse for those living in institutions is believed to be higher than those living in the community. The most common type of elder abuse is difficult to determine due to several factors: numerous operational definitions, research methods and samples, and administrative data. It has been reported by researchers that victims of elder abuse may experience more than one type of abuse at any given time, making accurate data more difficult to obtain. For example, victims may report financial exploitation but not physical abuse for fear of retaliation by the abuser. The Centers for Disease Control and Prevention has identified a four-step approach to addressing this serious public health problem, which includes defining the problem, identifying the risk and protective factors, developing prevention strategies, and widespread adoption of these strategies (National Center for Injury Prevention and Control, 2016). The consequences for the older adult who is abused and neglected contribute significantly to a decrease in quality of life. The experience of physical trauma, reduced self-worth and dignity, and a lost sense of safety and security may lead to an increased risk of early death. The economic impact of additional health care interventions, including hospitalizations, lost productivity, and law enforcement activities, also contribute to the significance of this health and societal problem. There has been an increase in efforts to develop screening tools and algorithms to identify early-warning signs, but no one tool has proven most effective in decreasing the incidence of elder abuse. Early signs of abuse and neglect are often missed by health professionals, due to lack of adequate training. The older adult may not self-report due to cognitive or physical inability, fear of retaliation, or reluctance to report the abuser.

Educating nurses and other health professionals in detection of early-warning signs of abuse and neglect as well as in the use of available screening tools and algorithms, continues to be recognized as a key factor in maximizing prevention efforts.

Clinical Aspects

ASSESSMENT

While providing care to older adults, the nurse has many opportunities to interact with the older adult and, when available, the family thereby learning the living arrangements. Establishing a trusting relationship with the individual will facilitate engagement in a comprehensive assessment of all health care needs and alert the nurse to possible early signs and symptoms of elder abuse and neglect. The nurse and other health professionals must ensure the privacy and confidentiality of the older adult to the extent possible unless legally obligated to act to maintain the individual's safety. The nurse and other health professionals must consider the individuals' rights to be included in decisions about care and lifestyle.

Research has identified key factors that place an older person at increased risk of becoming a victim of elder abuse. They include low social support, low income or poverty, functional impairment and poor physical health, symptoms of dementia, female gender and living with many household members. Specifically associated with financial exploitation are the identified key factors, nonuse of social services, need for assistance with activities of daily living, poor self-rated health, no spouse/partner, African American race, and lower age (Peterson et al., 2014). The abusers are described as predominantly adult children or spouses, more likely to be male. They may be experiencing increased stress related to financial problems, unemployment, and past or present substance abuse. Mental and physical problems, social isolation, and possible encounters with the police may be additional factors for the abuser (Lachs & Pillemer, 2015). Recognizing the early-warning signs of elder abuse and acting to prevent further abuse are critical steps toward decreasing its impact on the individual and society. The following are identified as the most common types of abuse and neglect:

Physical abuse is defined as infliction of pain or injury on the older adult. This may present as bruises, pressure marks, broken bones, abrasions, and burns.

Sexual abuse is defined as touching, fondling, intercourse, or any other sexual activity when the older adult is unable to understand, unwilling to consent, threatened, or physically forced.

Emotional abuse is defined as verbal assaults, threats of abuse, harassment, or intimidation, belittling,

and use of power to control the individual. Behaviors associated with emotional abuse may include unexplained withdrawal from regular activities, depression, change in alertness, increase in tension, and arguments with caregiver and older adult.

Neglect is defined as the caregiver's withholding of food, clothing, shelter, or medical care. Physical signs may include bedsores, poor hygiene, unexpected weight loss, and unmet medical needs.

Financial exploitation is defined as another person withholding or misusing the resources of the older adult. A sudden change in the financial status of the older adult may be an indication of financial exploitation.

NURSING INTERVENTIONS, MANAGEMENT, AND IMPLICATIONS

A plan of care must be developed in collaboration with the individual, the family when possible, and other health care providers, that addresses education and support for the older adult and family, provides resources and referrals as needed as part of a safety plan (Registered Nurse Association of Ontario [RNAO], 2014).

OUTCOMES

If the older adult is willing to accept the intervention, the following steps are put into action: a safety plan is implemented, emergency information is provided, the older adult is educated, goals for ongoing care are developed, the causes of abuse are alleviated, the older adult and family are referred for services, and follow-up is arranged. If the older adult lacks capacity to decide about an intervention, the Adult Protective Services role may include financial management, guardianship, or court proceedings to protect the individual from ongoing abuse and/ or neglect (Hoover & Polson, 2014).

Summary

Four strategies have been identified as interventions in preventing elder abuse and neglect: psychoeducation for professionals and older adults; multidisciplinary case management programs; legal intervention with police involvement; and psychological interventions, including home visits (Fearing, Sheppard, McDonald, Beaulieu, & Hitzig, 2017). The Elder Abuse Suspicion Index (EASI) screening tool includes an algorithm for determining specific interventions. Positive findings of abuse and neglect direct the professional to first assess for safety. Is there immediate danger? If yes, it is recommended that Adult Protective Services be contacted and a referral initiated. Efforts to address the complex needs of the abused older adult require improved early detection and reporting mechanisms; educational programs for health professionals, individuals and families, and law enforcement personnel; as well as ongoing research studies that will impact the incidence and prevalence of burgeoning health and societal epidemic.

Connolly, M. T., Brandl, B., & Breckman, R. (2014). *The elder justice roadmap: A stakeholder initiative to respond to an emerging health, justice, financial and social crisis.* Philadelphia, PA: U.S Department of Justice, Department of Health and Human Services.

Fearing, G., Sheppard, C. L., McDonald, L., Beaulieu, M., & Hitzig, S. L. (2017). A systematic review on community-based interventions for elder abuse and neglect. *Journal of Elder Abuse & Neglect, 29*(2–3), 1–27. doi:10.1080/08946566.2017.1308286

Hoover, R. M., & Polson, M. (2014). Detecting elder abuse and neglect: Assessment and intervention. *American Family Physician, 89*(6), 453–460.

Lachs, M., & Pillemer, K. (2015). Elder abuse. *New England Journal of Medicine, 373,* 1947–1956. doi:10.1056/NEJMra1404688

National Center for Injury Prevention and Control. (2016). Understanding elder abuse: Fact sheet. Retrieved from https://www.cdc.gov/violenceprevention/pdf/em-factsheet-a.pdf

National Center on Elder Abuse. (2016). What is elder abuse? Retrieved from https://ncea.acl.gov

Peterson, J., Burnes, D., Caccamise, P., Mason, A., Henderson, C., Wells, M., & Lachs, M. (2014). Financial exploitation of older adults: A population-based prevalence study. *Journal of General Internal Medicine, 29*(12), 1615–1623. doi:10.1007/s11606-014-2946-2

Registered Nurse Association of Ontario. (2014). Preventing and addressing abuse and neglect of older adults: Person-centered, collaborative, system-wide approaches (Best Practice Guideline). Retrieved from http://RNAO.ca

World Health Organization. (2016). Elder abuse [Press release]. Retrieved from http://www.who.int/mediacentre/factsheets

■ FALLS

Uvannie Enriquez Castro

Overview

Falls are the leading cause of morbidity and mortality in the elderly. In 2015, more than 60% of adults aged 65 years and older died of fall-related deaths. The direct medical cost relating to nonfatal falls was estimated to be over $31 billion in 2015, whereas the direct medical costs of fatal falls was $637.2 million (Burns, Stevens, & Lee, 2016). The risks of falling increase exponentially with age. With the aging population projected to increase 55% by 2030, the call to action is louder than ever (Bergen, Stevens, & Burns, 2016).

Background

A fall is defined as an event that results in a person coming to rest inadvertently on the ground or floor or other lower level. The etiology of falls among the elderly is multifactorial. Only 15% of cases clearly identified the cause of a fall (Barban et al., 2017). The World Health Organization (WHO) identified risk factors of elderly falls, classified into four main categories: biological, behavioral, environmental, and socioeconomic. Each risk factor does not cause a fall by itself, rather the interaction of more than one precipitates an elderly fall.

The biological risk factors pertain to the physical, sensory, and cognitive decline associated with aging, compounded by comorbidities common among this age group. Most notable risk factors include impaired balance and gait, loss of muscle mass and strength, impaired vision, incontinence, and disorientation. Pain is an important factor to consider. Pain limits range of motion. Inactivity reduces gait fluency and further increases pain. In a study by Talarska et al. (2017), pain doubled the risk of falls in their study group. Demographic factors, such as gender, play a role as well. Older women are more prone to falling. However, their male counterparts are more likely to die of fall-related injuries due to a higher level of risk-taking behavior and delayed tendency to seek medical attention.

Behavioral risk factors include fear of falling, which results in inappropriate cautious gait, polypharmacy, lack of social activity, and risk-taking behaviors, such as poor body mechanics and refusal to use assistive devices (canes, walker, etc.).

Falls are reported in 30% to 40% of elderly living in the community and 50% living in nursing homes (Barban et al., 2017). Common environmental risk factors are multiple obstacles, poor lighting, long hallways that render public spaces, such as restrooms and sitting rooms, inaccessible.

There is a direct correlation between socioeconomic factors and the risk of falling among the elderly. Low socioeconomic status translates to general poor health choices, substance abuse, poor housing conditions, poor diet, poor weight management, and lack of access to health care services geared toward disease prevention and/or management of chronic illness.

History of previous falls is telling. In 2014, 28.7% of older adults reported falling at least once in the preceding 12 months (Bergen et al., 2016). Postfall syndrome is characterized by fear of falling, which results in inappropriate cautious gait and an increased risk for successive falls.

Clinical Aspects

ASSESSMENT

Most of the risk factors that predispose an elder to fall are modifiable. Preventing falls is therefore paramount. The Centers for Medicare & Medicaid Services (CMS) incentivized falls prevention efforts through two quality measures: Falls Risk Assessment and Falls Plan of Care. Precise identification of falls risk is achieved through a standardized, validated falls risk assessment tool. The Joint Commission identified that the Morse Fall Scale or Hendrich II Fall Risk Model integrated within the electronic medical record are examples of effective tools for assessing falls. Assessing for history of previous falls may reveal underlying factors that remain unresolved and therefore continue to put an elderly patient at risk. Physical examinations may include visual acuity check, cognitive screen, assessment of functional abilities, feet and footwear assessment, use of mobility aids, and medication review. Continuous assessment is necessary to detect any changes in condition that may predispose an elderly person to fall.

NURSING INTERVENTIONS, MANAGEMENT, AND IMPLICATIONS

The best approach to preventing falls is to customize care plans based on individual risk assessments. Intervention bundles are tailored for low, moderate, and high risk. Measures that address falls may include patient education on the incidence of falls among the elderly. This promotes heightened awareness resulting in better health-seeking behaviors. Furthermore, enlisting participation of the patient and his or her support system in carrying out the care plan will ensure sustained results. Exercise to optimize musculoskeletal functioning is another strategy. Motor training for strength and balance is currently the most effective intervention to prevent falls (Barban et al., 2017).

Nutritional supplementation of calcium, vitamin D, and protein may be helpful to prevent osteoporosis and sarcopenia (Daly, 2017). Review of medications, including modification of regimen, adequate disease management, vision improvement, and elimination of podiatric issues, may also help prevent falls.

The nursing implication on hourly rounding cannot be overstated in preventing falls. These scheduled rounds preemptively address the 4Ps of patient care: pain, personal needs, position (to preserve skin integrity), and placement of patient's essential belongings within reach (Agency for Healthcare Research and Quality, 2013). Modifying the environment for patient safety, such as removing clutter, removing unstable furniture, providing adequate lighting, and inspecting assistive devices for repair, may also be accomplished during hourly rounding.

OUTCOMES

Preventing falls, and the excess morbidity and mortality associated with falls, is paramount. As fall risk factors are multifactorial, prevention is also multidisciplinary. Communication of risk level and plan of care within the care team is crucial. Postfall huddles are critical in preventing future falls from an organizational perspective.

Summary

Elderly falls are a public health issue. The associated costs of hospitalization, emergency department (ED) visits, rehabilitation, outpatient visits, and extended home health services are indisputable. Although the risk of falling increases with age, falls and their sequelae do not have to be a normal aspect of aging. With thoughtful nursing assessment and tailored evidence-based interventions, the upward trajectory of disability and reduced quality of life can be curtailed.

Agency for Healthcare Research and Quality. (2013). Preventing falls in hospitals: Which fall prevention practices do you want to use? Retrieved from http://www .ahrq.gov/professionals/systems/hospital/fallpxtoolkit/ fallpxtk3.html

Barban, F., Annicchiarico, R., Melideo, M., Federici, A., Lombardi, M. G., Giuli, S., & Caltagirone, C. (2017). Reducing fall risk with combined motor and cognitive training in elderly fallers. *Brain Sciences, 7*(2), 19. doi:10.3390/brainsci7020019

Bergen, G., Stevens, M. R., & Burns, E. R. (2016). Falls and fall injuries among adults aged ≥ 65 years—United States, 2014. *Morbidity and Mortality Weekly Report, 65*(37), 993–998. doi:10.15585/mmwr.mm6537a2

Burns, E. R., Stevens, J. A., & Lee, R. (2016). The direct costs of fatal and non-fatal falls among older adults—United States. *Journal of Safety Research*, *58*, 99–103. doi:10.1016/j.jsr.2016.05.001

Daly, R. M. (2017). Exercise and nutritional approaches to prevent frail bones, falls and fractures: An update. *Climacteric: The Journal of the International Menopause Society*, *20*(2), 119–124. doi:10.1080/13697137.2017.1286890

Schoene, D., Valenzuela, T., Lord, S. R., & de Bruin, E. D. (2014). The effect of interactive cognitive-motor training in reducing fall risk in older people: A systematic review. *BioMed Central Geriatrics*, *14*, 107. doi:10.1186/1471-2318-14-107

Talarska, D., Strugała, M., Szewczyczak, M., Tobis, S., Michalak, M., Wróblewska, I., & Wieczorowska-Tobis, K. (2017). Is independence of older adults safe considering the risk of falls? *BioMed Central Geriatrics*, *17*, 66. doi:10.1186/s12877-017-0461-0

■ FRAILTY

Nirmala Lekhak
Evanne Juratovac

Overview

Frailty is a physiologic state characterized by increased susceptibility to stressors leading to negative outcomes such as disability, falls, delirium, institutionalization, and mortality (Wallington, 2016). With a growing aging population, frailty is likely to become one of the major health issues facing our society. Appropriate diet and exercise have been found to lower the risk of frailty and/or its adverse outcomes (Ward & Reuben, 2016). It is important for nurses to understand the complexity and signs of frailty to provide proper individualized care to their frail patients.

Background

Frailty has been defined as "a biologic syndrome of decreased reserve and resistance to stressors, resulting from cumulative declines across multiple physiologic systems, causing vulnerability to adverse outcomes" (Fried et al., 2001, p. M146). According to the National Health and Aging Trend longitudinal study, 15% of older adults living in the United States are considered frail (Bandeen-Roche et al., 2015). The risk of frailty increases by 9% at ages 65 to 69 years and by 38% among those 90 years and older (Bandeen-Roche et al., 2015). The older adults living in long-term care settings are at higher risk of frailty than the general aging population (Bandeen-Roche et al., 2015). Although frailty is highly prevalent among older adults, it is not a consequence of aging (Wallington, 2016). Two thirds of older adults living outside of nursing homes are not frail (Bandeen-Roche et al., 2015). It is important to recognize that frailty differs from disability (Fried et al., 2001). Disability is limitation in an individual's functional ability to perform daily activities. Frailty, however, is a lack of physiologic reserve, which results into homeostasis imbalance. Presence of disability and/or multimorbidity can increase the risk of frailty; however, frailty can occur without these conditions (Fried et al., 2001).

Frailty is a dynamic process, which often worsens over time with lack of proper and timely interventions (Wallington, 2016). Frailty is particularly problematic because it involves multiple interrelated organ systems such as nervous, endocrine, immune, and/or skeletal systems. Frailty becomes evident when there is a critical decline in "physiological reserve in the respiratory, cardiovascular, renal, and haemopoietic and clotting systems" (Clegg, Young, Iliffe, Rikkert, & Rockwood, 2013, p. 753). This increases the vulnerability of older adults to adverse outcomes (e.g., hospitalization, delirium, disability) when exposed to stressors (e.g., infection, surgery, new drug treatment; Clegg et al., 2013). Therefore, unmanaged frailty increases the risk of disability, falls, delirium, hospital admission, institutionalization, and death (Wallington, 2016).

There are multiple factors associated with frailty. Along with older age, being female gender, belonging to a racial minority; and having lower income, less education, poorer health, disability, and multimorbidity makes one vulnerable to frailty and its ensuing consequences (Bandeen-Roche et al., 2015). Frailty is also shown to have positive association with cognitive decline/impairment and depression (Fried et al., 2001). Lifestyle factors, such as proper diet and physical activities, may reduce the risk of frailty and associated adverse outcomes (Ward & Reuben, 2016).

Clinical Aspects

ASSESSMENT

Evidence of frailty should initiate proper assessment and care planning toward improving health outcomes and lowering preventable damage (Regional Health Council, 2015). Nurses are critical in identifying frailty and preventing associated adverse outcomes.

All health care providers are recommended to assess for frailty while caring for older adults aged 75 years and older (Regional Health Council, 2015). Two models to define frailty and its risk have been recommended: phenotype and cumulative deficit models. Most of the clinical guidelines for frailty assessment are based on the frailty phenotype introduced by Fried and colleagues (2001). Frailty is established when the older patients show three or more of the following symptoms: greater than 5% unintentional weight loss in last 12 months, lack of energy (self-report of exhaustion), loss of muscle mass and strength (grip strength 20% lower than baseline), unbalanced and slow gait (e.g., score of less than 3 in short physical performance battery-gait test), and inactivity or reduced weekly frequency of physical activity (Fried et al., 2001; Regional Health Council, 2015). Presence of one or two of these symptoms may indicate prefrailty (Fried et al., 2001). Rockwood and colleagues (2005) defined frailty as a "syndrome" or a collection of predetermined deficits (i.e., changes in everyday activities, sleep problem, memory changes, loss of hearing, chronic illness) as listed in the 70-item Canadian Study of Health and Aging (CSHA) Clinical Frailty Scale. An increase in the number of predetermined deficits for an individual quantifies his or her likelihood to be frail (Wallington, 2016). Out of seven markers identified (deficits in physical strength, physical activity, mobility, energy, mood, nutrition, and cognition), problems with physical strength is suggested to possibly have the greatest influence on functional disability in elderly people (Sourial et al., 2012).

Confirmation of frailty in older adults requires assessment by a group of multiprofessional health care providers (including nurses) of their ability to perform instrumental activities of daily living (IADLs), clinical status, cognitive function and mental status, and pharmacological treatments. It is also important to assess for socioeconomic conditions and environment, cultural values, and need and preferences of the patients to provide individualized and effective care (Regional Health Council, 2015).

NURSING INTERVENTIONS, MANAGEMENT, AND IMPLICATIONS

As mentioned, frailty is a dynamic process. Therefore, there should be continuous effort to overcome deficits leading to frailty by providing resources to improve stability (Rockwood et al., 2005). Nurses play a vital role in providing these resources to patients experiencing frailty.

Depending on the need of the patients, nurses should work with occupational and physical therapists to build physical strength to improve gait and muscle strength. Slow movement exercises, such as Tai Chi, yoga, and meditation, have been shown to improve gait and balance (Rogers, 2016). Proper diet and nutritional supplements are critical during frailty to fight against weight loss, weakness, and fatigue (Regional Health Council, 2015). Nurses should pay special attention to the oral hygiene of their frail patients. Personal resources, such as positive attitude and resiliency, and social support help facilitate the balance between frailty and stability. Environmental modifications at home, such as grip bars in the bathroom, rails along the bed, and a nonskid mat near the bed, are helpful measures to prevent adverse outcomes (e.g., fall and hospitalization). Therefore, individualized care plans include multiple management and prevention techniques when caring for persons with frailty. Involving family caregivers in care planning and education is recommended. Frailty increases the risk of cognitive decline and mortality. Thus, nurses should encourage advance-care planning to their frail patients when appropriate (Ward & Reuben, 2016).

OUTCOMES

Proper comprehensive geriatric nursing assessment and intervention can provide older adults with autonomy to perform their daily activities and safety from unintended consequences such as fall, rehospitalization, institutionalization, disability, and premature death.

Summary

Frailty is a multisystem condition. Therefore, our health care system, which is focused in a single system/disease, is insufficient in assessing and treating frailty. It is important that nurses are well trained in assessing and managing frailty holistically, and work in a team with other health care professionals to care for frail patients. Frail elderly people require considerable care and environmental support across the continuum of care. Thus, nurses in the community need expertise in recognizing and managing frailty in post-acute and community-based care settings.

Bandeen-Roche, K., Seplaki, C. L., Huang, J., Buta, B., Kalyani, R. R., Varadhan, R.,...Kasper, J. D. (2015). Frailty in older adults: A Nationally Representative Profile in the United States. *Journals of Gerontology: Series A, 70*(11), 1427–1434. doi:10.1093/gerona/glv133

Clegg, A., Young, J., Iliffe, S., Rikkert, M. O., & Rockwood, K. (2013). Frailty in elderly people. *Lancet, 381*(9868), 752–762. doi:10.1016/S0140-6736(12)62167-9

Fried, L. P., Tangen, C. M., Walston, J., Newman, A. B., Hirsch, C., Gottdiener, J.,...McBurnie, M. A. (2001). Frailty in older adults: Evidence for a phenotype. *Journals of Gerontology: Series A, 56*(3), M146–M157.

Regional Health Council. (2015). *Frailty in elderly people.* Florence, Italy: Regione Toscana, Consiglio Sanitario Regionale. Retrieved from https://www.guideline.gov

Rockwood, K., Song, X., MacKnight, C., Bergman, H., Hogan, D. B., McDowell, I., & Mitnitski, A. (2005). A global clinical measure of fitness and frailty in elderly people. *Canadian Medical Association Journal, 173*(5), 489–495.

Rogers, C. E. (2016). Tai Chi to promote balance training. In B. Resnick & M. Boltz (Eds.), *Annual review of gerontology and geriatrics* (Vol. 36, pp. 229–249). New York, NY: Springer Publishing.

Sourial, N., Bergman, H., Karunananthan, S., Wolfson, C., Guralnik, J., Payette, H.,...Beland, F. (2012). Contribution of frailty markers in explaining differences among individuals in five samples of older persons. *Journals of Gerontology: Series A, 67*(11), 1197–1204.

Wallington, S. L. (2016). Frailty: A term with many meanings and a growing priority for community nurses. *British Journal of Community Nursing, 21*(8), 385–389.

Ward, K. T., & Reuben, D. B. (2016). Comprehensive geriatric assessment. *UpToDate.* Retrieved from http://www.uptodate.com/contents/3009

■ INFECTION

Irena L. Kenneley

Overview

Infectious diseases are a frequent cause of morbidity and mortality in older adults. Numerous infectious diseases are more serious and have more drastic consequences for the elderly than for people of other ages. Signs and symptoms of infection may be different in older adults, causing a delay in diagnosis. In addition, waning immune system function, decreased vaccine response, thinning skin, glandular secretion reduction, and comorbid illnesses heighten the risk of infectious diseases in older adults (Schneider, 2014).

Background

Infection is the primary cause of death in one third of individuals aged 65 years and older and is a contributing cause of death for many others. Infection also has a marked impact on morbidity in older adults, exacerbating underlying illnesses and initiating functional decline (Francis & Lahaie, 2012). There are a number of factors that increase the risk of infection in older adults when compared to younger adults. The relationships among these risk factors, whether they are comorbidities, declining immunity, or age itself, may be very complex. Malnutrition in conjunction with a stressful incident may increase the risk of infection in this population. The many risk factors and the complexity involved make it difficult to determine the attributable risk of any one characteristic. Also, any risk factor in isolation cannot be considered "the cause" of infectious risk in the older adult.

However, the following well-recognized features associated with advanced age clearly do increase risk for clinical infection in the older adult (Francis & Lahaie, 2012):

Comorbidity. The increased incidence of infection is likely a direct result of common comorbid conditions (e.g., diabetes, renal failure, chronic pulmonary disease, edema, immobility).

Immunity. Immune senescence is not merely a global state of reduced immunity, but an impairment of immune responses at multiple levels. Components activated in the inflammatory response can be measured, such as elevated C-reactive protein and interleukin-6 (IL-6) blood levels, and cellular activation of nuclear factor-kappa B (NF-κB). However, other innate immune responses (e.g., natural killer [NK] cell activity) are frequently reduced in older adults, and recent data suggest polymorphonuclear neutrophil (PMN) function may also be impaired with reduced microbial phagocytosis and killing (Jeyapalan & Sedivy, 2008).

Nutrition. Nutritional status is linked to delayed wound healing, pressure ulcer formation, community-acquired pneumonia (CAP), and increased risk of health care-associated infections.

Social and Environmental Factors. Population-based studies reveal that lower income is associated with higher rates of CAP and invasive pneumococcal infections among elderly individuals.

Clinical Aspects

ASSESSMENT

Infectious diseases frequently present with atypical features in older adults. Serious infections may be indicated by nonspecific declines in functional or mental status, or anorexia with decreased oral intake. Underlying illness (e.g., congestive heart failure [CHF] or diabetes) may be exacerbated, leading the elderly patient to seek medical attention (Montoya & Moody, 2011).

Fever is the most common sign that triggers the clinician to look for infection, but is often absent in the elderly patient. Several studies show that frail elderly individuals have lower mean baseline body temperatures than the currently accepted normal of 98.6°F (37°C). The decline in basal temperature and reduced response to inflammatory stimuli make it less likely that a frail, older adult will achieve a body temperature commonly recognized as fever. It has been suggested that fever in frail older adults should be defined as (a) persistent elevation of body temperature of at least 2°F (1.1°C) over baseline values, or (b) oral temperatures of 99°F (37.2°C) or greater on repeated measures, or (c) rectal temperatures of 99.5°F (37.5°C) or greater on repeated measures. The sensitivity of detecting fever and infection in the nursing home setting has been improved using this definition, and reasonable specificity maintained (Montoya & Moody, 2011). The importance of a "normal" or reduced temperature even in the presence of significant infection cannot be overemphasized. A diminished febrile response often leads to delayed diagnosis and is an indicator of a poor prognosis (Montoya & Moody, 2011).

Cognitive impairment also heavily contributes to the difficulty in diagnosing infection in the elderly. Older adults are often unable to communicate symptoms and clinicians should be mindful in pursuing objective assessments (e.g., laboratory and radiologic evaluations) in cognitively impaired elderly with changes in functional status.

The following infections are those most commonly encountered in the older adult population.

Bacterial Pneumonia. Respiratory infections are a leading cause of illness and death for older adults, both community acquired and health care associated (Montoya & Moody, 2011; Wohl, 2009). The risk for pneumonia is greater in older adults due to declined pulmonary function, reduced cough reflex, diminished mucociliary action, and limited lung capacity. The aspiration of secretions is a chief cause of pneumonia for elderly patients.

Urinary Tract Infections. Urinary tract infections (UTIs) in older adults living in the community are the second most commonly diagnosed infection. Among older adults living in long-term care facilities, UTIs are the most frequently documented infection (Montoya & Moody, 2011). UTIs are often incorrectly diagnosed and overtreated. The prevalence of asymptomatic bacteriuria, which does not always require treatment, and atypical presentations in the older adult (i.e., delirium) make the diagnosis of UTI challenging in this population (Montoya & Moody, 2011).

Clostridium difficile *Infection.* The incidence of *C. difficile* infections (CDIs) is increasing. CDI is a common and sometimes fatal health-care-associated infection (HAI), with the greatest impact being felt in those older than 65 years. More than 90% of deaths from CDI have occurred in this population (CDC, 2012). CDI may occur in health care settings where antibiotics are prescribed, in long-term care facilities, or within the community. For older adults, antibiotic exposure and inpatient or long-term care facility stays increase their risk of CDI.

Herpes Zoster. Herpes zoster, often referred to as shingles, results from a reactivation of the virus that causes chicken pox—that is, the varicella zoster virus. Diminished immune function, drugs, and illness can trigger the latent virus to reactivate. Prevention of herpes zoster with the new U.S. Food and Drug Administration-approved zoster vaccine is possible.

Influenza. In elderly adults, influenza may present atypically with a less pronounced infection. For the older adult, whether vaccinated or unvaccinated, influenza causes high morbidity and mortality. In 2010, influenza and pneumonia were the ninth leading cause of death. In addition, the number of elderly hospitalizations associated with influenza have increased over the past two decades. The Centers for Disease Control and Prevention (CDC) estimates that 60% of the seasonal influenza hospitalizations and 90% of the seasonal influenza deaths each year occur in older adults (CDC, 2013).

Pulmonary Tuberculosis. Several age-associated changes in older adults predispose reactivation of latent tuberculosis infection (LTBI). Although (TB) cases and deaths have decreased in the United States, individuals aged 65 years and older continue to have the highest rates.

Infections From Indwelling Medical Devices. The use and abuse of invasive devices, such as urinary catheters and central lines, greatly increases the risk for infection. Devices provide a pathway or portal of entry for microorganisms to enter the body or act as inanimate surface where pathogens are protected from the immune system.

NURSING INTERVENTIONS, MANAGEMENT, AND IMPLICATIONS

A primary prevention strategy is that of immunization. The recommended immunizations for adults older than 65 years are intended to decrease infection-related morbidity and to decrease mortality. Nurses should take note that the immune response from vaccinations for older adults may be less than the response in younger adults (The Association for Professionals in Infection Control and Epidemiology [APIC], 2015; Nettina, 2014).

Nurses are central members of a multidisciplinary team. As leaders in patient safety, infection prevention strategies must be instituted. These strategies include handwashing, aseptic technique, cleaning and disinfection, standard and transmission-based precautions, patient education, use of safety devices, removal of invasive devices as soon as possible, and use of bundle strategies for infection prevention (e.g., ventilator and central line insertion bundles).

Many nurses struggle with the decision to stay away from work because they know their presence will be missed by peers and patients. However, communicable diseases have been transmitted to patients who are under the care of health care workers who report to work when they are ill. Patient safety comes first and this means that if a nurse or staff member has active symptoms of infection, such as fever, cough, sore throat, and gastrointestinal disease, the individual should *not* report to work.

OUTCOMES

Older adults do not typically present according to some team members' knowledge of the "typical" infectious illness. Nurses are in a key position to educate other members of the team, based on knowledge of the principles of immunosenescence as described in this entry. Increased training and surveillance in clinical care settings has the potential to greatly reduce the excess morbidity and mortality associated with infection in older patients.

Summary

Knowledge and understanding of the process of aging will assist the nurse in identifying age-associated changes that contribute to the increased risk of infection and infection prevention strategies. Infection control programs for the older adult in all health care delivery settings should address surveillance for infections

and antimicrobial resistance, outbreak investigation and control plan for epidemics, isolation precautions, hand hygiene, staff education, and employee and resident health programs.

The Association for Professionals in Infection Control and Epidemiology. (2015). *APIC text of infection control and epidemiology.* Washington, DC: Author.

Centers for Disease Control and Prevention. (2012). Vital signs: Preventing *Clostridium difficile* infections. *Morbidity and Mortality Weekly Report, 61*(9), 157–162.

Centers for Disease Control and Prevention. (2013). CDC influenza update for geriatricians and other clinicians caring for people 65 and older. CDC website. Retrieved from http://www.cdc.gov/vaccines/vpd-vac/shingles/vacc-need-know.htm

Francis, D. C., & Lahaie, J. (2012). The nurse's role in preventing harm. In M. Boltz, E. Capezuti, T. Fulmer, & D. Zwicker (Eds.), *Evidence-based geriatric nursing protocols for best practice* (4th ed., pp. 220–228). New York, NY: Springer Publishing.

Jeyapalan, J. C., & Sedivy, J. M. (2008). Cellular senescence and organismal aging. *Mechanisms of Ageing and Development, 129*(7–8), 467–474. doi:10.1016/j.mad.2008.04.001

Korniewicz, D. M. (2014). *Infection control for advanced practice professionals.* Lancaster, UK: DEStech Publications.

Montoya, A., & Mody, L. (2011). Common infections in nursing homes: A review of current issues and challenges. *Aging Health, 7*(6), 889–899. doi:10.2217/AHE.11.80

Nettina, S. M. (2014). Care of the older or disabled adult. In S. M. Nettina (Ed.), *The Lippincott manual of nursing practice* (10th ed., pp. 163–195). Philadelphia, PA: Lippincott Williams & Wilkins.

Schneider, M. J. (2014). Public health and the aging population. In M. J. Schneider (Ed.), *Introduction to public health* (4th ed., pp. 495–518). Sudbury, MA: Jones & Bartlett.

Wohl, D. A. (2009). Serious infections in the elderly. In C. Arensen, J. Busby-Whitehead, K. Brummel-Smith, J. G. O'Brien, M. H. Palmer, & W. Reichel (Eds.), *Reichel's care of the elderly: clinical aspects of aging* (6th ed., pp. 241–249). New York, NY: Cambridge University Press.

■ MEDICATION RECONCILIATION

Mary Jo Krivanek
Mary A. Dolansky

Overview

Medication errors cause at least one death every day and injure approximately 1.3 million people annually in the United States (U.S. Food and Drug Administration

[FDA], 2016). The Institute for Healthcare Improvement (2017) states that preventing harm from medications, or adverse drug events (ADEs), remains a top patient safety priority not only in hospitals but also across the continuum of care for patients. The Joint Commission (2017) defines the process of medication reconciliation as when a clinician compares the medications a patient should be using (and is actually using) to the new medications that are ordered for the patient and resolves the discrepancies. Nursing is often involved in obtaining information on the medications the patient is currently taking on admission to the hospital or outpatient setting. This list is very useful to those who manage medications. The Joint Commission (2017) explains that when it is difficult to obtain a complete list of current medications, that a good faith effort should occur to obtain this information from the patient and/or other sources.

Background

In 2006, the Institute of Medicine reported that the average hospitalized patient is subject to at least one medication error per day. More than 40% of medication errors are believed to result from inadequate reconciliation in handoffs during admission, transfer, and discharge of patients (Hughes, 2008). More recent, the Agency for Healthcare Research and Quality (AHRQ; 2012) reported that the occurrence of unintended medication discrepancies ranges from 30% to 70%, and medication reconciliation can be an effective intervention detecting and averting up to 85% of medication discrepancies (AHRQ, 2012; Michaelsen, McCague, Bradley, & Sahm, 2015). Medication reconciliation has been reported to reduce medication errors by 24% to 43% (Mueller, Sponsler, Kripalani, & Schnipper, 2012).

According to the FDA (2016), medication errors can occur anywhere in the distribution system: (a) prescribing, (b) repackaging, (c) dispensing, (d) administering, or (e) monitoring. The FDA (2016) also lists common causes of such errors to include (a) poor communication; (b) ambiguities in product names, directions for use, medical abbreviations or writing; (c) poor procedures or techniques; or (d) patient misuse because of poor understanding of the directions for use of the medication. The FDA (2016) states that in addition, job stress, lack of product knowledge or training, or similar labeling or packaging of a medication may be the cause of, or contribute to, an actual or potential error.

The Joint Commission (2017) recognizes that organizations face challenges with medication reconciliation. The best medication reconciliation requires a complete understanding of what the patient was prescribed and what medications the patient is actually taking. The comparison addresses duplications, omissions, interactions, and the need to continue currently prescribed medications. As health care evolves with the adoption of more sophisticated systems (such as centralized databases for prescribing and collecting medication information), the effectiveness of these processes will grow (The Joint Commission, 2017).

The types of information that clinicians use to reconcile the medications include the medication name, dose, frequency, route, and purpose (The Joint Commission, 2017). The information should be obtained when the patient is admitted to the hospital or an outpatient setting. The medications that are taken at scheduled times and those that are taken on an as-needed basis should be included (The Joint Commission, 2017). The medication list should also include herbals, vitamins, nutritional supplements, over-the-counter drugs, vaccines, diagnostic and contrast agents, radioactive medications, parenteral nutrition, blood derivatives, and intravenous solutions (Hughes, 2008).

Hughes (2008) relays that the steps in medication reconciliation are seemingly straightforward. For a newly hospitalized patient, the steps include (a) obtaining and verifying the patient's medication history, (b) documenting the patient's medication history, and (c) creating a medication administration record. At discharge, the steps include (a) determining the postdischarge medication regimen, (b) developing discharge instructions for the patient for home medications, (c) educating the patient, and (d) transmitting the medication list to the follow-up physician(s). For patients in ambulatory settings, the main steps include documenting a complete list of the current medications and then updating the list whenever medications are added or changed.

Clinical Aspects

ASSESSMENT

The Medications at Transitions and Clinical Handoffs (MATCH) Toolkit for Medication Reconciliation (AHRQ, 2012) helps to facilitate a review and improvement of current medication practices to strengthen the process with the result of improved patient safety. The toolkit promotes a successful approach to medication management and reconciliation that emphasizes the importance of standardization of the process for doctors, nurses, and pharmacists. According to AHRQ (2012), standardizing the process for collecting a patient's home medication lists ensures that the most accurate medication history is documented for each patient, that all inpatient and home medications are reconciled, and that the information is accessible to the patient's entire health care team.

NURSING INTERVENTIONS, MANAGEMENT, AND IMPLICATIONS

Nurses collect a list of all current medications on admission and verify the list with the patient or significant other if the patient is unable to participate. Nursing staff place the medication list in the electronic health record or in a predetermined, visible location in the patient's chart. Nursing staff should consult with a pharmacist as needed throughout the medication reconciliation process. Nurses should use caution when transferring a patient between care units or facilities, and when discharging patients by reconciling medications at the time of admission, during transfers, and at discharge. Nursing staff must reconcile any medication discrepancies following established time frames that have been determined by the facility.

OUTCOMES

When nurses teach a patient about medications, nurses give the patient the knowledge and skills needed to take medications correctly and maintain his or her health. Nurses must ensure that discharge planning begins at admission and establish what the patient already knows about the medication and what level of ability the patient has to self-manage. The medication reconciliation needs to include prescriptions from all providers and any over-the-counter medication or herbal remedies. A new requirement in The Joint Commission's (2017) National Patient Safety Goals (NPSG) addresses the patient's role in medication safety. It requires organizations to inform the patient about the importance of maintaining updated medication information.

Summary

According to Hughes (2008), the process of gathering, organizing, and communicating medication information across the continuum of care is not straightforward

and varies from one health care facility to another. There is a tremendous amount of variation in the process for gathering a patient's medication history. Also, there are at least three disciplines generally involved in the process—medicine, pharmacy, and nursing—with little agreement on each profession's role and responsibility for the reconciliation process. Finally, there may be duplication of data gathering when nurses, pharmacists, and physicians take medication histories. As Hughes (2008) reports, the documentation may be done in different places in the chart, and rarely are there comparisons and resolutions of the discrepancies between the discipline-specific histories. According to Hughes (2008), there is no standardization of the process of medication reconciliation, which results in tremendous variation in the historical information gathered, sources of information used, comprehensiveness of medication orders, and how information is communicated to various providers across the continuum of care. Through the Medications At Transitions and Clinical Handoffs (MATCH) toolkit (AHRQ, 2012), a multidisciplinary team with frontline staff can contribute to process improvements for medication reconciliation. The Joint Commission's (2017) new NPSG requirement includes the patient's role in medication safety. The elements of performance in this medication NPSG are designed to help organizations reduce negative patient outcomes associated with medication discrepancies.

Agency for Healthcare Research and Quality. (2012). *Medications and Transitions and (MATCH) Toolkit for medication reconciliation* (AHRQ Publication No. 11(12)-0059). Rockville, MD: Author. Retrieved from https://www.ahrq.gov/sites/default/files/publications/files/match.pdf

Gleason, K. M., McDaniel, M. R., & Feinglass, J., Baker, D. W., Lindquist, L., Liss, D., & Noskin, G. A. (2010). Results of the Medications At Transitions and Clinical Handoffs (MATCH) Study: An analysis of medication reconciliation errors and risk factors at hospital admission. *Journal of the Society of General Internal Medicine*, 25(5), 441–447.

Hughes, R. (2008). *Patient safety and quality*. Rockville, MD: Agency for Healthcare Research and Quality.

Institute for Healthcare Improvement. (2017). Medication reconciliation to prevent adverse drug events. Retrieved from http://www.ihi.org/Topics/ADEsMedicationReconciliation/Pages/default.aspx

Institute of Medicine. (2006). *Preventing medication errors*. Washington, DC: National Academies Press.

Michaelsen, M. H., McCague, P., Bradley, C. P., & Sahm, L. J. (2015). Medication reconciliation at discharge from hospital: A systematic review of the Quantitative literature. *Pharmacy, 3*, 53–71.

Mueller, S. K., Sponsler, K. C., Kripalani, S., & Schnipper, J. L. (2012). Hospital-based medication reconciliation practices: A systematic review. *Archives of Internal Medicine, 172*(14), 1057–1069. doi:10.1001/archinternmed.2012.2246

The Joint Commission. (2017). National patient safety goals 2017. Retrieved from https://www.jointcommission.org/hap_2017_npsgs

U.S. Food and Drug Administration. (2016). Medication error reports. Retrieved from https://www.fda.gov/Drugs/DrugSafety/MedicationErrors/ucm080629.htm

■ NUTRITION

Marianna K. Sunderlin

Overview

Adequate nutrition is necessary to support optimal health at any age. Daily dietary recommendations for people 50 years of age and older, who are not physically active, are 1,600 calories for women and 2,000 calories for men according to the National Institute on Aging (NIA; 2016). This includes 2.5 cups of vegetables, 2 cups of fruit, 3 cups dairy, 6 ounces grain, and 5.5 ounces of protein. Studies show, however, that many elderly people do not meet this recommendation. One recent study (Koren-Hakim et al., 2016) of patients aged 65 years and older (*n* = 215) noted that malnutrition present on admission was 20% to 55%, based on body mass index (BMI), report of weight loss, and dietary intake. Unintentional weight loss of up to 5% may be as prevalent as 15% to 20% in the elderly population (Gaddey & Holder, 2014) and often has no readily identifiable cause.

Access to food due to cost, the ability to drive and shop, or to cook are often the problems faced by elderly people. Medications used to treat chronic conditions often cause dry mouth, diarrhea, or constipation. Elderly people are often on medically prescribed diets that limit taste and choices. In addition, physical changes of aging lead to decrease in appetite and issues with chewing, swallowing, and processing nutrients, making the elderly people vulnerable to weight loss and malnutrition.

Background

According to the American Society for Parenteral and Enteral Nutrition (ASPEN), adults at risk of malnutrition are characterized by a BMI less than 18.5, the presence of chronic disease, or unexpected weight loss greater than 5% in 1 month (ASPEN, 2017). Elderly people should be assessed for malnutrition and weight loss as this is known to increase morbidity and mortality (Koren-Hakim et al., 2016). Chronic illness, depression, and neurological impairments are often causes of unintentional weight loss of people aged 65 years and older (Geddey & Holder, 2014), leading to decreased function and quality of life. Impaired swallow related to stroke or dementia affects as many as 600,000 in the United States (Sura, Madhavan, Carnaby, & Crary, 2012) increasing risk of aspiration, pneumonia, and malnutrition. Understanding the normal changes of aging includes awareness of decreased appetite and thirst, which lessen the ability to take in adequate nutrition, and alter the enjoyment of meals. Side effects of medication often cause fatigue, nausea, or dry mouth. Although many Americans are keeping their natural teeth due to improvements in dental care, normal changes in the mouth related to aging leave the elderly population at risk of gingivitis, dental caries, candidiasis, cheilitis, and stomatitis due to decrease in blood vessels feeding the tooth enamel, thickening of tissues, dryness, and recession of the gums (Gonsalves, Wrightson, & Henry, 2008).

Clinical Aspects

ASSESSMENT

Assessment of nutritional status in elderly people commonly includes weight, BMI, dietary habits, and lab tests. Screening for malnutrition in the elderly population should be done regularly, given the high incidence of occurrence. Use of standardized tools is recommended. Some commonly used tools for nutrition assessment in the elderly population are as follows:

- Nutrition Risk Screening 2002 (NRS-2002) scores self-report of illness and dietary intake. This assessment does not include a physical exam. Scores range from 0 to 6, with a lower score indicating less nutritional risk (Koren-Hakim et al., 2016).

- Malnutrition Universal Screening Tool (MUST) scores risk of malnutrition based on BMI, unplanned weight loss percentage, and illness likely to cause a decrease in food intake. A score of 2 or more indicates risk (Koren-Hakim et al., 2016).

- Mini Nutrition Assessment (MNA) scores weight loss, BMI, appetite, mobility, stress, and cognition to determine nutritional risk. With 0 to 14 possible points, lower scores indicate an increase in nutritional risk, with 7 or below indicating malnutrition. MNA was demonstrated to be more sensitive in predicting morbidity and mortality over the NRS and MUST (Koren-Hakim et al., 2016).

■ Simplified Nutritional Appetite Questionnaire (SNAQ) is a four-question self-report assessment that predicts risk for unintentional weight loss greater than 5% due to loss of appetite (Pilgrim, Robinson, Sayer, & Roberts, 2015).

For all elderly people, regardless of the apparent risk, the following should be considered to maintain good eating habits. Impaired vision, smell, and taste may have a negative effect on appetite. The environment can be improved with bright lighting, a table cloth, colorful plates, and use of plates with a rim to keep food from being pushed off (Pilgrim et al., 2015). Utensils can be modified for ease of grasp, encouraging self-feeding. Eating is social and should not be rushed. Sharing a meal with friends can increase enjoyment of eating. Be aware when television or music is creating a distraction. Pain and toileting should also be assessed and treated in advance of a meal.

Mouth care before a meal can enhance taste and decrease problems with gingivitis or dental caries. A daily multivitamin can help decrease sores in the mouth. There are artificial saliva solutions available for dry mouth caused by medications. Frequent sips of water or use of hard sugar-free candies, and avoidance of alcohol can help to alleviate the symptoms of dry mouth. Missing teeth may require precut foods and soft items for chewing. Dentures should be well fitted and worn for meals. Dentures should be soaked in cleaning solution when not in use to prevent fungal or bacterial growth. Topical antifungals are effective treatment for candidiasis, cheilitis, and stomatitis that cause discomfort in the mouth (Gonsalves et al., 2008).

When appetite is poor, use of liquid meal supplements high in protein and calories do not usually cause satiety, allowing for increased caloric intake with or between meal times (Pilgrim et al., 2015). Cooking with butter, cream, whole milk, and eggs can increase the calorie and protein content without adding to the size of portions. Use of flavor enhancers and spices can be useful for deficits in taste, as long as they do not interfere with special diets or cause indigestion. Plan meals with a variety of foods and personal favorites as often as possible.

In people with dysphagia, thickening liquids may allow for safer swallow, but along with a pureed diet has been associated with decreased meal compliance.

According to experts (Sura et al., 2012), there is little evidence that chin tuck maneuvers improve aspiration risk, but postural adjustments continue to be standard care. Swallow maneuvers, such as supraglottic or effortful swallow as taught by a speech therapist, may provide benefit.

Nonpharmacologic methods can be used to hasten transit of food through the digestive track, avoiding constipation includes increased fluid intake and regular exercise. Fruits and vegetables (fiber) can create bulk that will help transit, but only in the presence of adequate fluids. Prunes or prune juice and consumption of coffee are simple means to prevent constipation. Use of medications to increase appetite have been shown to have short-term gains only and significant adverse effects (Gaddey & Holder, 2014).

Summary

Careful attention to the changing needs of elderly people can help alleviate many of the barriers to achieving optimal nutrition. Oral hygiene and regular dental care can prevent painful problems and enhance pleasure in eating. Although assistance with shopping, planning, and preparing meals may be needed, maintaining self-care and normalized meals can improve caloric intake. Screening for malnutrition risk should be performed at regular intervals as it can identify and reduce problems of malnutrition and unintended weight loss in the elderly.

American Society for Parenteral and Enteral Nutrition. (2017). Definitions: Malnutrition. Retrieved from http://www.nutritioncare.org/Guidelines_and_Clinical_Resources/Toolkits/Malnutrition_Toolkit/Definitions

Gaddey, H. L., & Holder, K. (2014). Unintentional weight loss in older adults. *American Family Physician, 89*(9), 718–722.

Gonsalves, W. C., Wrightson, A. S., & Henry, R. G. (2008). Common oral conditions in older persons. *American Family Physician, 78*(7), 845–852.

Koren-Hakim, T., Weiss, A., Hershkovitz, A., Otzrateni, I., Anbar, R., Gross Nevo, R. F.,...Beloosesky, Y. (2016). Comparing the adequacy of the MNA-SF, NRS-2002 and MUST nutritional tools in assessing malnutrition in hip fracture operated elderly patients. *Clinical Nutrition, 35*(5), 1053–1058. doi:10.1016/j.clnu.2015.07.014

National Institute on Aging. (2016). Eating well as you get older. *NIH Senior Health.* Retrieved from https://nihseniorhealth.gov/eatingwellasyougetolder/knowhowmuchtoeat/01.html

Pilgrim, A. L., Robinson, S. M., Sayer, A. A., & Roberts, H. C. (2015). An overview of appetite decline in older people. *Nursing Older People, 27*(5), 29–35. doi:10.7748/nop.27.5.29.e697

Sura, L., Madhavan, A., Carnaby, G., & Crary, M. A. (2012). Dysphagia in the elderly: Management and nutritional considerations. *Clinical Interventions in Aging, 7,* 287–298. doi:10.2147/CIA.S23404

■ PERSISTENT PAIN

Felvic Adriatico Javier

Overview

Persistent pain is a predominant condition among the elderly population. Persistent pain refers to a persistent unpleasant sensory and emotional experience over an extended period. Older persons are more likely to suffer from persistent pain than younger persons. Persistent pain affects one's quality of life and has an impact on activity, sleep, and psychological well-being of an older adult. Comprehensive assessment is an important aspect in developing a patient-centered nursing care plan. Health education and counseling play an important role in nursing management of persistent pain among the elderly population.

Background

Persistent pain is common among the elderly population. Persistent, noncancer pain is a diverse group of clinical entities that has two important components: the presence of pain and the persistence of the pain over an extended period. The International Association for the Study of Pain (IASP) defines pain as "an unpleasant sensory and emotional experience associated with actual or potential tissue damage, or described in terms of such damage" (Taylor, 2015, p. 3). It is further defined as pain that lasts longer than 3 to 6 months; however, some authors prefer a definition that does not use a limited time and define persistent pain as the pain that extends beyond the expected period of healing. Pain is a very common problem for older persons, with persistent pain affecting more than 50% of older persons living in the community setting, and more than 80% of nursing home residents (IASP, 2017). Pain is always subjective.

Nurses need to know that factors associated with, but not limited to, persistent pain are older age and female gender, and conditions such as arthritis, osteoarthritis, fibromyalgia, diabetic peripheral neuropathy, post-herpetic neuralgia, persistent joint pain, and sciatica. A broad literature on persistent pain suggests its adverse effects on mobility, sleep patterns, mood, quality of life, ability to perform activities of daily living (ADL) and instrumental activities of daily living (IADL), and its association with disability, depression, anxiety, loneliness, social isolation, and suicidal ideation in older people (Molton & Terrill, 2014). The relationship between pain and depression may also be cyclical, with increases in pain predicting increases in depression, and vice versa (Chou, 2007). All of these pain-related symptoms could negatively affect health-related quality of life (HRQoL; Lapane, Quilliam, Benson, Chow, & Kim, 2014). However, in the case of persistent pain, limiting activity may lead to a cycle of restriction, decreased participation, and greater disability (Jensen, Moore, Bockow, Ehde, & Engel, 2011). Older adults with severe, persistent pain are twice as likely to report difficulties in initiating sleep, in staying asleep, and with sleeping longer than usual (Chen, Hayman, Shmerling, Bean, & Leveille, 2011).

Clinical Aspects

ASSESSMENT

A thorough assessment includes medical history, imaging studies, diagnostic tests, physical examination, subjective data, and psychosocial history. Subjective data assesses the severity or intensity, location, characteristics, pain pattern, mitigating and aggravating factors. The Joint Commission's current standards require that organizations establish policies regarding pain assessment and treatment and conduct educational efforts to ensure compliance. Examples of intensity scale measurements are Numerical Pain Scale, Visual Analog Scale, Simple Descriptive Pain Scale, and Subjective Pain Intensity Rating. The modified Brief Pain Inventory appears to be useful for assessing the intensity and interference associated with pain (Lapane et al., 2014). Nurses should assess the patient's ability to perform ADL, the patient's current and previous pain coping strategies, and the patient's level of understanding about persistent pain as a basis for developing the nursing care plan. The study by Park, Engstrom, Tappen, and Ouslander (2015) suggests that ethnicity and physical and mental health are associated with pain intensity in ethnically diverse older adults. The findings highlight the important role of geriatric nurses, who provide appropriate pain assessment and treatment.

NURSING INTERVENTIONS, MANAGEMENT, AND IMPLICATIONS

Functional limitation, decreased mobility, sleep pattern disturbance, anxiety, and depression are among common related problems in persistent pain among elderly patients. These problems should be considered and addressed appropriately.

Education and counseling are based on the patient's level of understanding and should include the patient's caregiver and family. Medication teaching is needed on dosage, frequency, side effects, appropriate use of over-the-counter (OTC) medications as well as instructions on the application and care of topical pain medications. Assistance with ambulation and the use of assistive walking devices increases mobility. Pain medication should be administered as prescribed. Stress the importance of proper nutrition and the need to increase fluids to promote good bowel movement, as constipation is one of the side effects of taking opioid medications. Assist patient in adhering to the pain management treatment plan such as participating in physical therapy.

OUTCOMES

Evidence show that psychological interventions (cognitive-behavioral therapy and progressive relaxation), exercise, interdisciplinary rehabilitation, functional restoration, and spinal manipulation are effective for persistent or subacute low back pain (Chou & Huffman, 2007). A program of physical exercise is effective in relieving pain and improving certain psychological functions for older residents and offers significant improvement in physical mobility and range of motion of common painful joints (Tse, Tang, Wan, & Vong, 2014). Older adults with persistent low back pain displayed a significant improvement in measurements of pain acceptance and activities engagement after participating in the mindfulness-based meditation program. Follow-up data suggest sustained benefits from the program and sustained improvement in physical function and pain acceptance (Sorrell, 2015). Guided imagery is an approach whereby one's attention is focused on sights, sounds, music, and words to create feelings of empowerment and relaxation. Relaxation and guided imagery may be effective strategies for pain management, although most studies have not included control groups. Biofeedback training may be used as part of multidisciplinary pain management programs and generally includes relaxation training. There is a growing concern regarding the misuse/abuse of opioid medications among the elderly (Chang & Compton, 2016). Understanding how older adults take their prescription opioid drugs will increase awareness of misuse and abuse among this population, caregivers, and health care providers, as well as better identify and treat opioid drug use disorders (Taylor, 2015).

Summary

Understanding the phenomena of persistent pain is especially important among the elderly. Particular emphasis is placed on the assessment in terms of pain intensity, functional limitations, and its effect on ADL. Important nursing intervention management includes health teaching and counseling, increase in mobility, supportive measures, preventing side effects, and complications of pain medications. Psychological interventions, meditation, guided imagery, and relaxation are among the interventions that provide more current evidence of positive outcomes.

Chang, Y.-P., & Compton, P. (2016). Opioid misuse/abuse and quality persistent pain management in older adults. *Journal of Gerontological Nursing*, 42(12), 21–30. doi:10.3928/00989134-20161110-06

Chou, R., & Huffman, L. H. (2007). Nonpharmacologic therapies for acute and chronic low back pain: A review of the evidence for an American Pain Society/American College of Physicians Clinical Practice Guideline. *Annals of Internal Medicine*. Retrieved from http://annals.org/aim/article/736834/nonpharmacologic-therapies-acute-chronic-low-back-pain-review-evidence-american

International Association for the Study of Pain. (2017). *Facts on pain in older persons*. Retrieved from https://www.iasp-ain.org/files/Content/ContentFolders/GlobalYearAgainstPain2/20062007PaininOlderPersons/fspainolderpersons.pdf

Jensen, M. P., Moore, M. R., Bockow, T. B., Ehde, D. M., & Engel, J. M. (2011). Psychosocial factors and adjustment to chronic pain in persons with physical disabilities: A systematic review. *Archives of Physical Medicine Rehabilitation*, 92(1), 146–160.

Lapane, K. L., Quilliam, B. J., Benson, C., Chow, W., & Kim, M. (2014). One, two, or three? Constructs of the brief pain inventory among patients with non-cancer pain in the outpatient setting. *Journal of Pain and Symptom Management*, 47(2), 325–333. doi:10.1016/j.jpainsymman.2013.03.023

Molton, I., & Terrill, A. (2014). Overview of persistent pain in older adults. *American Psychologist*, 69(2), 197–207. doi:10.1037/a0035794

Park, J., Engstrom, G., Tappen, R., & Ouslander, J. (2015). Health-related quality of life and pain intensity among ethnically diverse community-dwelling older adults. *Pain Management Nursing*, 16(5), 733–742. doi:10.1016/j.pmn.2015.04.002

Sorrell, J. (2015). Meditation for older adults: A new look at an ancient intervention for mental health. *Journal of Psychosocial Nursing & Mental Health Services*, 53(5), 15–19. doi:10.3928/02793695-20150330-01

Taylor, D. R. (2015). Introduction to chronic pain. In D. R. Taylor (Ed.), *Managing patients with chronic pain and opioid addiction* (pp. 3–17). New York, NY: Springer.

Tse, M. M., Tang, S. K., Wan, V. T., & Vong, S. K. (2014). The effectiveness of physical exercise training in pain, mobility, and psychological well-being of older persons living in nursing homes. *Pain Management Nursing*, 15(4), 778–788. doi:10.1016/j.pmn.2013.08.003

■ PHARMACOKINETIC CHANGES

Carli A. Carnish

Overview

The older adult population of the United States (65 years and older) represented 14.5% of the population in 2014, approximately 46 million people. By the year 2040, this group is expected to comprise greater than 20% of the population, about one in every five Americans (Administration for Community Living, 2016). Longer life span and advancements in pharmacologic and diagnostic capabilities contribute to the number of older adults with an increasingly complex list of comorbidities and drug utilization. Nurses have a professional responsibility to act as patient advocates and promote safe drug administration for this unique group of individuals. A strong understanding of pharmacokinetic changes in geriatrics is imperative to maintain the safety of adults as they age by minimizing risk of adverse drug events.

These health and population changes all contribute to rising concern of polypharmacy in older adults. Ninety percent of noninstitutionalized older adults take at least one prescribed medication. The older adult seeking medical attention in a health care provider's office takes, on average, six to eight medications (Pretorius, Gataric, Swedlund, & Miller, 2013). The risk of adverse drug events is directly related to the number of medications taken. One of six hospitalizations among older adults is secondary to an adverse drug event, 50% of which are considered preventable (Pretorius et al., 2013). The vast quantity of medication utilization combined with age-related physiologic changes compound the need for nurses to understand pharmacokinetic principles unique to the older adult population. This knowledge facilitates competency in safe and effective provision of patient-centered care.

Background

The term *pharmacokinetics* broadly refers to how an individual's body processes a drug. This is the branch of pharmacology that studies the metabolism and action of drugs within the body and is subdivided into four categories: absorption, distribution, metabolism, and elimination. Throughout the aging process, the human body undergoes physiological changes that influence its ability to process drugs.

ABSORPTION

Although gastrointestinal (GI) absorption in older adults may be slower, age-related changes generally do not change the amount of drug that is absorbed. Absorption of medications through the gastrointestinal tract may be slightly slower due to age; however, decrease in medication absorption can usually be credited to medication interactions (Semla, 2011). Common examples of this include over-the-counter (OTC) preparations, such as antacids and vitamin supplements (iron, calcium, magnesium/aluminum hydroxide), that inhibit absorption of other medications such as antibiotics (e.g., fluoroquinolones and tetracyclines). This substantiates the need for comprehensive medication reconciliation, including all prescription, OTC medications, vitamin, and herbal supplements used.

DISTRIBUTION

The aging process has a more profound pharmacokinetic effect on drug distribution. Older adults tend to have a greater body fat composition compared to skeletal muscle. As a result, there is reduced fluid volume and smaller doses of hydrophilic drugs are necessary to achieve therapeutic effect. In contrast, lipophilic drugs may take higher and greater number of doses to achieve steady state and a longer time for drug clearance from the body. Reduced total protein or serum albumin secondary to inflammatory states, malnutrition, or other physiologic cause, is another common finding in older adults. The result is increased serum concentration of protein-bound medications and accumulation of free drug levels, increasing the risk for toxicity (Semla, 2011).

METABOLISM

Metabolism of drugs primarily occurs via the liver. Decrease in hepatic blood flow, hepatic size, and mass occurs during the aging process. These changes often are compounded by chronic (or acute) conditions commonly seen in the geriatric population, including congestive heart failure, hepatitis, or chronic alcohol abuse. The result is a slower metabolism and clearance of drugs from the body. Drugs are metabolized via either phase I or phase II pathways. Phase I pathways convert drugs to metabolites of lesser, equal, or greater pharmacologic effect compared to their parent drug, whereas those utilizing phase II pathways are converted to metabolites of inactive compounds. Those utilizing phase II pathways are the preferred choice for older adults because inactive metabolites will not accumulate, reducing the risk for adverse effects (Harvey, 2012).

ELIMINATION

Elimination of medications may occur through the gastrointestinal tract in bile or feces or the skin. However, most medications are elimination by the kidneys. An estimated 26 million adult Americans have chronic kidney disease and the risk of developing chronic kidney disease increases with age (National Kidney Foundation, 2017). Slowing of the glomerular filtration that results from the aging kidney results in delayed elimination and clearance of drugs from the body (Semla, 2011).

Clinical Aspects

ASSESSMENT

Nurses should complete comprehensive medication reconciliations with every patient encounter. This should include all prescription and OTC drugs in addition to any vitamin or herbal supplements taken. Nutrition assessments should be completed to ensure appropriate weight-based dosing of medications. In addition, significant weight loss or gain may alert the provider to compromising changes in patient condition.

A functional assessment of the geriatric patient or caregiver is essential to evaluate the ability to safely administer medications. Close attention should be paid to any sensory impairments, history of falls, memory loss, depression, sleep disturbances, and incontinence of the bladder or bowel. Impairment in any of these domains may impact the older adult patients' ability to adhere to the medication regimen as directed by the health care provider. Note that any new deficit or decline in function may warrant consideration of an adverse drug reaction that needs to be addressed.

The nurse should review the patient medical history to identify all existing health conditions. If, during the patient interview any new diagnoses are identified, the nurse should ascertain any pertinent laboratory, pathology, or radiology studies, in addition to current treatments being provided to the patient by other providers. There is strong likelihood that this information will impact the patient's level of risk associated with current or new medication use and overall plan of care.

Nursing assessment of patient and/or caregiver knowledge related to medication use, indications, and diagnoses should be completed for all new and existing medications. The patient and caregiver should be encouraged to ask questions. Adequate time should be allotted to avoid rushing this process to promote safe medication administration. The teach-back method has demonstrated effectiveness in patient education, improving disease knowledge, and medication adherence (Ha Dinh, Bonner, Clark, Ramsbotham, & Hines, 2016).

NURSING INTERVENTIONS, MANAGEMENT, AND IMPLICATIONS

The nurse may encounter numerous challenges associated with older adults, age-related changes, and pharmacokinetics. These problems can be categorized according to the meta-paradigm of nursing practice. Patient-related problems include knowledge deficits related to disease management, medications, or both. Other patient problems may be language barriers, lack of motivation, fatigue, mobility limitations, risk-prone health behaviors, or stress.

Patient health status, a dynamic process, is influenced by multiple factors related to the person's physical and emotional health. Depression, anxiety, and sleep disturbances may prevent patients from taking their medications as they were recommended. This can disrupt the metabolism and distribution of their other medications, increasing risk for adverse reactions. Renal and/or hepatic disease impedes drug clearance in the older adult's body and therefore medical and surgical history should be continuously reviewed and updated for disease.

Environment is influenced by psychosocial issues, including lack of familial or caregiver support, limited financial resources, transportation and communication barriers, and environmental safety. The nurse may encounter numerous problems, including adverse drug reactions, medication errors, inappropriate prescribing, polypharmacy, or problems with medication adherence. The nurse may encounter internal conflict when working with the older adult population. This may be related to personal biases, pressure related to time limitations and staffing ratios, or fatigue. The nurse must always strive to promote an open dialogue based on therapeutic communication in a nonjudgmental way. This should encourage the patient or caregiver to seek help and ask questions regarding care without apprehension.

A critical responsibility of nurses lies in their ability to effectively educate patients and caregivers on disease management and medication administration. The United States Department of Health and Human Services (2016) has estimated that approximately 12% of adults possess "proficient" health literacy. It is imperative that nurses educate the patient using appropriate terminology and evaluate learning using teach back. The nurse can employ this technique to educate the patient regarding his or her health, appropriate monitoring, and potential side effects. The nurse should emphasize any factors unique to the patient that increases his or her risk for adverse drug events.

Several clinical tools exist that are available to aid the nurse's judgment when administering medications and providing patient education. These may prove useful when acting as a patient advocate to maintain safety. The Beers List, or Beers Criteria for Potentially Inappropriate Medication Use in Older Adults, published by the American Geriatrics Society Beers (AGS) Criteria Update Expert Panel, provides a list of medications that are potentially inappropriate for use in older adults. The list of drugs was developed primarily for use as a guide to prescribers, to promote best practice when providing care to older adults (AGS Criteria Update Expert Panel, 2015). As patient advocates and health care providers, nurses should be aware of this helpful and accessible tool.

The Screening Tool of Older Persons' potentially inappropriate Prescriptions (STOPP) and Screening Tool to Alert doctors to Right Treatment (START) criteria were first introduced in 2008 (O'Mahony et al., 2015). These criteria were developed to address gaps in the Beers List and other medication screening tools for

older adults. The STOPP criteria provide a more comprehensive list of potentially inappropriate medications; however, it also lists those medications significantly associated with adverse drug reactions. The START criteria focuses on inappropriate prescribing omissions (O'Mahony et al., 2015).

Although these tools were initially developed and intended for use by medication prescribers, nurses should be aware of the tools and how to access them. It would not be unreasonable for the nurse to review medications against these lists. Concerns related to risk for or actual adverse drug reactions should be discussed with the patients, caregivers, and any appropriate health care providers. These interventions also fall under the initial step in the nursing process, assessment. Therefore, the assessment process should never be skipped or rushed. It provides the nurse and the patient and/or caregivers with valuable information that will ultimately influence the patient's overall health and safety.

OUTCOMES

The ultimate goal is comprehensive assessment of all older adult patients, their caregivers, elimination of unnecessary medications, and minimization of adverse drug reactions. Patient safety is at the core of nursing practice and always is a priority regardless of the patient population to which the nurse is providing care. Following the nursing strategies discussed will allow safe and appropriate patient-centered care. Comprehensive nursing assessments allow the nurse the opportunity to bond with the patient, establish trust and determine the patient's preferences, goals, and values (Quality and Safety Education for Nurses Institute, 2017). These findings may then be communicated to other appropriate health care providers to maintain care continuity and affirm the patient as an integral member of the health care team.

Summary

These clinical tools are only meant to be used as a guide in medication management and not to replace clinical judgment. It remains a primary responsibility of the nurse to promote and maintain patient safety. Screening provides the opportunity to identify any duplicate use, inappropriate use, or non-use of medications. The nurse often acts as a liaison between the patient and prescriber. A solid foundation in pharmacokinetics, pharmacodynamics, and physiology of aging offers the nurse a unique and invaluable role in the care of older adults.

Administration for Community Living. (2016). Aging statistics. Retrieved from https://www.acl.gov/aging -and-disability-in-america/data-and-research

American Geriatrics Society Beers Criteria Update Expert Panel. (2015). American Geriatrics Society 2015 Updated Beers Criteria for potentially inappropriate medication use in older adults. *Journal of the American Geriatrics Society, 63*, 2227–2246.

Ha Dinh, T. T., Bonner, A., Clark, R., Ramsbotham, J., & Hines, S. (2016). The effectiveness of the teach-back method on adherence and self-management in health education for people with chronic disease: A systematic review. *JBI Database of Systematic Reviews and Implementation Reports, 14*(1), 210–247. doi:10.11124/ jbisrir-2016-2296

Harvey, R. A., Clark, M. A., Finkel, R., Rey, J. A., & Whalen, K. (Eds.). (2012). Principles of drug therapy. *Pharmacology* (5th ed., pp. 1–36). Philadelphia, PA: Lippincott Williams & Wilkins.

National Kidney Foundation. (2017). About chronic kidney disease. Retrieved from https://www.kidney.org/atoz/ content/about-chronic-kidney-disease

O'Mahony, D., O'Sullivan, D., Byrne, S., O'Connor, M. N., Ryan, C., & Gallagher, P. (2015). STOPP/START criteria for potentially inappropriate prescribing in older people: Version 2. *Age and Ageing, 44*(2), 213–218. doi:10.1093/ ageing/afu145

Pretorius, R. W., Gataric, G., Swedlund, S. K., & Miller, J. R. (2013). Reducing the risk of adverse drug events in older adults. *American Family Physician, 87*(5), 331–336.

Quality and Safety Education for Nurses Institute. (2017). QSEN competencies. Retrieved from http://qsen.org/ competencies/pre-licensure-ksas/

Semla, T. P. (2011). Pharmacotherapy. In E. Flaherty & B. Resnick (Eds.), *Geriatric nursing review syllabus: A core curriculum in advanced practice geriatric nursing* (3rd ed., pp. 72–80). New York, NY: American Geriatrics Society.

U.S. Department of Health and Human Services. (2016). Quick guide to health literacy. Retrieved from https://health.gov/ communication/literacy/quickguide/factsbasic.htm

■ PHYSICAL ACTIVITY

Michelle Borland

Overview

Individuals are living longer and the elderly population makes up an unprecedented proportion of the total population. Physical activity is one of the most important things an individual can do to improve health and

prevent many health problems associated with aging (Centers for Disease Control and Prevention [CDC], 2015). The aging adult experiences a higher risk of chronic conditions and falls, which together account for 84% of all health care spending. Furthermore, lack of physical activity is either a direct cause of and/ or exacerbating factor for these conditions (Chase, 2015). More than 133 million people report at least one chronic condition and many have multiple chronic conditions (Centers for Medicare & Medicaid Services, 2016). Improving the health, function, and quality of life of older adults was included as a World Health Organization (WHO) goal in its *Healthy People 2020* project. Those adults with chronic illness have higher rates of disability, hospitalization, and polypharmacy; therefore, adding physical activity may facilitate the management of chronic illness among older adults (Chase, 2015). Improving physical activity among older adults requires an interprofessional team. The team of health care professionals, including nurses, should focus upon interventions that can have a positive influence on physical activity and can thereby contribute to improved physical and mental health for this population.

Background

Most developed countries have accepted the definition of *elderly* or older person as the chronological age of 65 years (WHO, 2017). The population of adults aged 65 years or older in 2014 was 46.3 million and is expected to more than double to 98 million by 2060 (Colby & Ortman, 2014). According to the CDC, the prevalence of inactivity increases with age. In 2014, the Behavioral Risk Factor Surveillance System reported inactivity for adults aged 65 to 74 years to be 26.9% and 35.3% for those individuals above 75 years of age (Watson et al., 2016).

As individuals age, gradual changes occur that affect physical activity. How the body ages depends on genetic and lifestyle choices. Lifestyle choices have a large impact on the aging process and are modifiable. Other changes include change in height due to physiologic changes in posture and joints, loss of muscle strength and flexibility, loss of high-frequency hearing acuity, decline in visual sharpness, loss of bone density and bone strength, loss of blood vessel elasticity, some loss of heart rate response to stress, and loss of memory efficiency (Mayo Clinic, 2015). Mayo Clinic recommends including physical activity into the daily routine to counteract changes that occur during the aging process. Physical activity increases blood flow to the whole body, prevents constipation, helps build and maintain strong bones, helps maintain a healthy weight, and lowers blood pressure (Mayo Clinic, 2015). Adding physical activity to self-management positively modifies cardiovascular risk factors, improves pain and physical function in arthritic patients, and decreases depressive symptoms (Chase, 2015). Even small increases in daily physical activities, such as walking, have many health benefits.

The ODPHP (2016) defines physical activity as any bodily movement that is produced by skeletal muscles and requires energy expenditure. Physical activity aids in the prevention of injury among elderly individuals and helps delay, prevent, and manage many chronic illnesses. Chronic disease has a negative impact upon the length and quality of life, as well as the ability for the older adult to live independently. Hypertension, diabetes mellitus, stroke, heart disease, cancer, falls, and lung disease are among those conditions that can be affected by physical activity levels (Watson et al., 2016). The U.S. Department of Health and Human Services concluded that cardiovascular, musculoskeletal, and mental health outcomes improve with physical activity (Vaz Fragoso et al., 2016).

The CDC (2015) and the WHO (2017) recommend that an elderly person get a total of 150 minutes of moderate-intensity aerobic activity every week and 2 days of muscle-strengthening exercises. Examples of aerobic activity include walking, dancing, mowing the lawn, and biking for at least 10-minute intervals. Strengthening activities include lifting weights, using resistance bands, using body weight resistance with sit-ups or push-ups, and engaging in heavier gardening activities. For those older adults with poor mobility, it is recommended that they perform physical activities 3 or more days per week (CDC, 2015; WHO, 2017).

Clinical Aspects

ASSESSMENT

Assessment is the first step in delivering care that is a vital tool in the development and guidance of care provided to the patient by the nurse. Assessing a patient's baseline status should include mobility and strength testing, as well as subjective questions regarding physical activity and fall risk assessment. When obtaining the history of physical activity from a patient, the type of activity, duration of activity, frequency of activity, and the age at which the physical activity began should be documented. The physical assessment should focus on strength testing (manual muscle testing), mobility (ambulation, get up and go test, sit-to-stand test, balance test), and fall risk (Morse, FRAT [falls risk assessment tool], Hendrich). By utilizing the health history and physical assessment for activity level, an individual plan of care can be developed by the nursing team, which would lead to positive outcomes. There is no laboratory test that measures the level of physical activity of an individual. However, thorough assessment and implementation of sound activity modification plans into the older adult's daily routine can lead to critical changes in the management of chronic conditions.

NURSING INTERVENTIONS, MANAGEMENT, AND IMPLICATIONS

Nursing care of the older adult, regarding physical activity, focuses on preventing complications of chronic illness and improving quality of life. Problems that should be given priority are identification and modification of fall risk related to mobility or decreased strength, management of constipation arising from inactivity, prevention of skin breakdown associated with immobility, improved oxygenation and circulation with movement and improved independence with ADL skills.

Nursing interventions include assessment of physical activity and muscle strength, fall risk assessment, ambulating patients, performance of range-of-motion exercises, education in appropriate activities and health benefits, identifying resources available, and facilitating physical and occupational therapy interventions. Fall risk assessment tools include the Morse Fall Scale, FRAT, and the Hendrich Fall Risk Model (CDC, 2015). Education opportunities include review of the importance and benefits of physical activity, self-monitoring and journaling, goal setting, and identification of community resources available to the individual (Chase, 2015).

OUTCOMES

Successful maintenance and improvement in physical activity levels of older adults are the expected evidence-based outcome of nursing interventions for this clinical problem. Recent studies confirm that physical activity positively modifies cardiovascular risk factors, improves pain management and physical function, and reduces mortality outcomes related to stroke and heart failure. Furthermore, physical activity has a direct impact on independence and quality of life (Chase, 2015).

Summary

The population of older adults is expected to rise to unprecedented levels by 2060. With the rise in the older population, chronic conditions, such as cardiovascular and respiratory disease, as well as falls, will also be expected to rise. Physical activity is one of the most important factors that can influence health conditions associated with aging. Nurses play a pivotal role within the interprofessional team in assessing, implementing, and educating the older adult in regard to physical activity. Improving patient quality of life and promoting independence for the elderly population can be achieved by incorporating physical activity in the older adult's plan of care.

Centers for Disease Control and Prevention. (2015). Physical activity. Retrieved from https://www.cdc.gov/physical activity/basics/older_adults/index.htm

Centers for Medicare & Medicaid Services. (2016). Quality strategy. Retrieved from https://www.cms.gov/medicare/ quality-initiatives-patient-assessment-instruments/ qualityinitiativesgeninfo/cms-quality-strategy

Chase, J. (2015). Interventions to increase physical activity among older adults: A meta-analysis. *The Gerontologist, 55*(4), 706–718. doi:10.1093/geront/gnu090

Colby, S. L., & Ortman, J. M. (2014). *Projections of the size and composition of the U.S. Population: 2014 to 2060, Current Population Reports, P25-1143.* Washington, DC: U.S. Census Bureau.

Mayo Clinic. (2015). Aging: What to expect. Retrieved from https://www.mayoclinic.org/healthylifestyle/healthy -aging/in-depth/aging/art-20046070?pg=1

Office of Disease Prevention and Health Promotion. (2016). Older adults. In *Healthy People 2020.* Washington, DC: U.S. Department of Health and Human Services. Retrieved from https://www.healthypeople.gov/2020/topics -objectives/topic/older-adults

Vaz Fragoso, C., Beavers, D., Anton, S., Liu, C., McDermott, M., Newman, A.,...Gill, T. M.; Lifestyle Interventions and Independence in Elders Investigators. (2016). Effect of structured physical activity on respiratory outcomes in sedentary elderly adults with mobility limitations. *Journal of the American Geriatrics Society, 64,* 501–509.

Watson, K. B., Carlson, S. A., Gunn, J. P., Galuska, D. A., O'Connor, A., Greenlund, K. J., & Fulton, J. E. (2016). Physical inactivity among adults aged 50 years and older—United States, 2014. *Morbidity and Mortality Weekly Report, 65,* 954–958. doi:10.15585/mmr.mm6536a3

World Health Organization. (2017). Health statistics and information systems. Retrieved from http://www.who .int/healthinfo/surveyageingdefnolder/en

■ POLYPHARMACY

Maria A. Mendoza

Overview

There is no standard definition of polypharmacy. Simplistically, it is often described as an individual taking four to five prescribed drugs simultaneously. Data from the National Health and Nutrition Examination Survey (NHANES) showed an increasing trend in the prevalence of polypharmacy (use of five or more prescription medications) over the last decade from 8.2% in 1999 to 2000 to 15% in 2011 to 2012 (Kantor, Rehm, Haas, Chan, & Giovannucci, 2015). Ensuring patient safety and improving quality of life (QOL) are major challenges in the nursing care of patients with multiple drug prescriptions.

Background

The arbitrary use of drug quantity thresholds to define polypharmacy is controversial (Payne, 2016). The prescriber generally associates the term with negative behavior with the possible consequence of underprescribing medication, especially in older adults (Cooper et al., 2015), a practice that is as detrimental as polypharmacy. To address the controversy, a report by the King's Fund, an independent charity in England to improve health care, proposed classifying polypharmacy as either appropriate or problematic (Payne, 2016). Appropriate prescribing is the responsible use of drugs to treat chronic conditions with comorbidities based on best evidence that improve quality of life (QOL) and promote patient safety. Problematic polypharmacy is the inappropriate prescribing of drugs that lack evidence of efficacy and benefit to the patient. In both scenarios, there is always a potential for adverse drug effects (ADEs), drug interactions, and poor adherence.

Although problematic polypharmacy may occur at any age, the elderly are most vulnerable for harm. Alterations in age or disease-related kidney, liver, and other bodily functions may affect the pharmacokinetics of drugs leading to increased side effects, ADEs, drug interactions, and hospitalizations. Inappropriate drug use has been implicated in falls, confusion, decreased alertness, depression, anxiety, weakness, hallucinations, loss of appetite, and elimination problems in the elderly. All these unpleasant side effects and dangerous ADEs greatly affect the QOL of the elderly person.

There are demographic and social factors that lead to polypharmacy. With the aging society, there is higher prevalence of chronic illness with comorbidities and acute exacerbations. Advances in medicine lead to discovery of many new drugs, increased knowledge of preventive medicine, and access to best evidence clinical guidelines. These factors often necessitate prescribing multiple drugs for maximum clinical benefits. For example, to maximize clinical outcomes in treating type 2 diabetes and preventing complications using the best evidence guidelines, it may be necessary to prescribe as many as 12 drugs per day (Bauer & Nauck, 2014).

Factors that predispose to polypharmacy and the adverse effects of multiple medications, including nonadherence, may be grouped into biophysiological/functional and socioeconomic/environmental categories. The biophysiological/functional factors include advanced age, frailty, cognitive impairment, chronic illness and multiple medical diagnoses, and decreased mobility and functional ability. The socioeconomic/environmental factors include taking more than five drugs per day, living alone or lacking family support, multiple hospitalizations and emergency room visits, multiple health care providers, use of multiple pharmacies, inadequate/lack of medical/drug insurance, and lack of transportation.

There are numerous screening tools to ensure appropriate drug use. The American Geriatrics Society periodically updates and publishes the *Beers Criteria for Potentially Inappropriate Medication Use in Older Adults*. This guideline is available online and provides a good reference for health care professionals to safely prescribe and assess drug therapy in the elderly. A Cochrane systematic review reported pooled data from two studies that showed improvement in the experimental group compared to a control group in the number of prescriptions among participants in the experimental group versus the control group post-intervention using Beers Criteria (Cooper et al., 2015). A criticism of the Beers Criteria is that it does not address drug-to-drug interactions, drug dosing to adjust for renal impairment, and possible duplication of drug therapy (Penge & Crome, 2013). Other tools include Screening Tool of Older Persons' potentially inappropriate Prescription (STOPP), Screening Tools to Alert doctors to Right Treatment (START), and Medication Appropriateness Index (MAI). Although all these screening tools have been found effective on reducing inappropriate prescribing, results on their effect on hospitalization, drug-related problems, and reported QOL are not consistent (Penge & Crome, 2013).

Clinical Aspects

ASSESSMENT

Patient history to identify the presence of the aforementioned risk factors should be obtained. Red flags, such as patient deterioration or lack of improvement in condition (e.g., blood pressure, blood sugar, lipid levels) despite increased drug therapy and failure to follow up for appointments, should be noted and further assessed. Physical assessment of the high-risk patient should include mental status screening, weight and height (body mass index), vital signs, nutritional status, functional status, laboratory screening to identify renal and liver functions, cardiorespiratory assessment, and other relevant screening specific to the diagnoses. A review of all medications—prescribed, over-the-counter (OTC) and herbal products—should also be done.

NURSING INTERVENTIONS, MANAGEMENT, AND IMPLICATIONS

Older patients are particularly vulnerable to polypharmacy. Thus, the following protocols and interventions are recommended.

1. **Screening protocol to address polypharmacy in primary care.** A literature review by Skinner (2015) found that a standardized, simple, screening protocol designed by the individual institutions and administered routinely may provide an effective assessment tool to prevent patient harm. This screening tool should identify high-risk patients who are elderly, taking multiple and/or high-risk medications, recently discharged from the hospital or seen by a specialist, and taking new medications. There should also be questions to determine clear indication of the drug, lowest therapeutic dose, duplication, and use of OTC drugs.

2. **Medication review and reconciliation** is the process of reviewing the medication regimen during transition of care to prevent discrepancies. It is generally a nursing or pharmacist responsibility in many institutions. Evidence on this procedure has small clinical effect on medication discrepancies at discharge (Agency for Healthcare Research and Quality, 2015). An older, single-site, small study (Blozik et al., 2010) of a nurse-led interdisciplinary team using the Beer's Criteria in a nursing home showed a reduction of number of drugs prescribed from 17.4% to 3.3% at 1-year follow-up.

3. **Patient education and teach back**, including assessment of health literacy. Numerous studies have demonstrated the effect of patient education and teach back on adherence and health outcomes (Ha Dinh, Bonner, Clark, Ramsbotham, & Hines, 2016; Skinner, 2015).

4. **Multidisciplinary care with managed coordination.** The nurse as a member of the multidisciplinary team can advocate on behalf of the patient/family by initiating a managed care referral of high-risk patients. There is evidence that coordinated care led by a nurse can decrease drug utilization and positive impact on health and functional abilities (Popejoy et al., 2015).

OUTCOMES

Outcomes to avoid, related to polypharmacy, include the potential for harm and injury related to ADEs, side effects that mask or mimic other conditions, drug–drug interactions, food–drug interactions, patient nonadherence to drug regimen, inappropriate use of prescribed drugs (e.g., self-medication, drug sharing with others), and inappropriate use of OTC drugs and herbal preparations.

Summary

Polypharmacy is a major problem that impacts on patient safety, functional status, and QOL. It is important to differentiate between appropriate and problematic polypharmacy to prevent underprescribing. The elderly are greatly affected by the adverse effects of polypharmacy because of biophysiological and socioeconomic/environmental factors. Nurses play a major role in the interdisciplinary approach to care to decrease inappropriate medications, prevent ADE, interactions, and side effects.

Agency for Healthcare Research and Quality. (2015). Patient safety primer: Medication reconciliation. Retrieved from https://psnet.ahrq.gov/primers/primer/1/medication-reconciliation

Bauer, S., & Nauck, M. A. (2014). Polypharmacy in people with Type 1 and Type 2 diabetes is justified by current guidelines—A comprehensive assessment of drug prescriptions in patients needing inpatient treatment for diabetes-associated problems. *Diabetic Medicine, 31*(9), 1078–1085. doi:10.1111/dme.12497

Blozik, E., Born, A. M., Stuck, A. E., Benninger, U., Gillmann, G., & Clough-Gorr, K. M. (2010). Reduction of inappropriate medications among older nursing-home residents: A nurse-led, pre/post-design, intervention study.

Drugs & Aging, 27(12), 1009–1017. doi:10.2165/11584770-000000000-00000

Cooper, J. A., Cadogan, C. A., Patterson, S. M., Kerse, N., Bradley, M. C., Ryan, C., & Hughes, C. M. (2015). Interventions to improve the appropriate use of polypharmacy in older people: A Cochrane systematic review. *BMJ Open, 5*(12), e009235. doi:10.1136/bmjopen-2015-009235

Ha Dinh, T. T., Bonner, A., Clark, R., Ramsbotham, J., & Hines, S. (2016). The effectiveness of the teach-back method on adherence and self-management in health education for people with chronic disease: A systematic review. *JBI Database of Systematic Reviews and Implementation Reports, 14*(1), 210–247. doi:10.11124/jbisrir-2016-2296

Kantor, E. D., Rehm, C. D., Haas, J. S., Chan, A. T., & Giovannucci, E. L. (2015). Trends in prescription drug use among adults in the United States from 1999–2012. *Journal of the American Medical Association, 314*(17), 1818–1831. doi:10.1001/jama.2015.13766

Payne, R. A. (2016). The epidemiology of polypharmacy. *Clinical Medicine, 16*(5), 465–469. doi:10.7861/clinmedicine.16-5-465

Penge, J., & Crome, P. (2013). Appropriate prescribing in older adults. *Review of Clinical Gerontology, 24*, 187–197.

Popejoy, L. L., Galambos, C., Stetzer, F., Popescu, M., Hicks, L., Khalilia, M. A.,…Marek, K. D. (2015). Comparing aging in place to home health care: Impact of nurse care coordination on utilization and costs. *Nursing Economic$, 33*(6), 306–313.

Skinner, M. (2015). A literature review: Polypharmacy protocol for primary care. *Geriatric Nursing, 36*(5), 367–371. doi:10.1016/j.gerinurse.2015.05.003

■ PRESSURE INJURY

Monica Cabrera
Lisa Torrieri
Ekta Vohra

Overview

A pressure injury is defined as localized damage to the skin and underlying soft tissue usually over a bony prominence or related to a medical or other device. The injury can present as intact skin or an open ulcer and may be painful. The injury occurs as a result of intense and/or prolonged pressure or pressure in combination with shear. The tolerance of soft tissue for pressure and shear may also be affected by microclimate, nutrition, perfusion, comorbidities, and condition of the soft tissue. Pressure injuries are staged based on the extent of tissue damage. Pressure injury stages include stages 1 to 4, unstageable, and deep tissue pressure injury. When the deepest anatomic structures of the injury can be identified numeric stages 1 to 4 are utilized. When the deepest anatomic structures cannot be identified unstageable or deep tissue pressure injury may apply (National Pressure Ulcer Advisory Panel [NPUAP], 2016).

Background

Pressure injury incidence rates vary significantly by health care settings, the largest incidence occurring in the acute care setting with a rate of up to 38%. It is estimated that each year, more than 2.5 million patients in U.S. acute care facilities develop a pressure injury and 60,000 patients die from pressure injury-related complications. In the long-term setting, pressure injury prevalence rates range from 2.2% to 23.9% and in-home care from 0% to 17%. Risk factors for the development of pressure injuries include advanced age, immobility, incontinence, neurosensory deficiencies, inadequate nutrition and hydration, impaired circulation, multiple comorbidities, and device-related skin pressure.

Pressure injuries pose a significant problem for both individuals and health care institutions. Individuals who develop pressure injuries may experience pain, decreased functionality, increased hospitalization, and, in some instances, premature mortality. Pressure injuries also increase hospital costs substantially. It is estimated that in the United States, pressure injury treatment will approach $11 billion annually, with a cost of $500 to $70,000 per individual pressure injury.

Clinical Aspects

ASSESSMENT

Stage 1 pressure injuries are defined as areas of intact nonblanchable erythema. In people with darker pigmented skin, this injury may present differently and may be more difficult to detect. These areas can present with changes in temperature, sensation, and firmness. To be classified as a stage 1 sore, discoloration is reddened, not purple or maroon.

Stage 2 pressure injuries are defined as a partial thickness skin loss with exposed dermis. It generally presents as an open ulcer with a shallow wound bed. Wound bed is pink or red without evidence of slough tissue. It can also be seen as an intact or ruptured serous-filled blister. Stage 2 pressure injuries are sometimes confused with skin tears, maceration, or incontinence-associated dermatitis. To determine the difference, it is important to assess and confirm the location of the wound.

Stage 3 pressure injuries are defined as a full thickness tissue loss with possible subcutaneous tissue presentation. Wound bed may present with yellow subcutaneous tissue, but bone and tendon are not visualized. Slough tissue can be present but it does not distort the base of the wound bed. Undermining and tunneling may be present. Depending on the location of stage 3 pressure injury, depth of wound bed may vary. In areas that are more bony (nose, heels, occiput), adipose tissue is limited and the wound bed is shallow. Although in areas of increased adipose tissue, wound depth can be greater.

Stage 4 pressure injuries are defined as full thickness tissue loss with bone, tendon, or muscle exposure. Slough or eschar may be present in the wound bed. Undermining and tunneling are commonly seen. Similar to stage 3 pressure injuries, depth of the wound bed varies by location of wound. Bone is usually exposed or palpated. When this occurs, patient can be at risk for osteomyelitis.

Unstageable pressure injuries are defined as a full thickness tissue loss, the wound is unable to be staged due to inability to visualize the base of the wound bed. The wound bed is entirely covered with either loosely adherent slough (yellow, tan, gray, or brown) tissue or fixed eschar (brown, black, or tan) tissue. In unstageable pressure injuries, stage is indeterminate due to inability to fully visualize the entire wound bed. Until the slough or eschar is removed and wound bed is visualized, wound will remain unstageable.

Deep tissue injuries (DTI) are defined as areas of intact dark purple- or maroon-colored skin. They may also present as blood-filled blisters. DTI occurs due to damage to underlying tissue. DTI may present with areas of firm, boggy, warm, or cooler areas of tissue. Similar to stage 1 pressure injuries, DTI may be difficult to detect in individuals with darker pigmented skin.

NURSING INTERVENTIONS, MANAGEMENT, AND IMPLICATIONS

A prevention program is a key factor in reducing the incidence of pressure injuries. Although prevention has been shown to be successful in decreasing incidences, involving a wound specialist is a best practice for any institution.

Best practices for prevention include inspection of skin; assessing patient's risk; and maintenance of skin health, pressure redistribution, nutrition, hydration, and patient education (Bryant & Nix, 2012).

Inspection of skin should be conducted shortly after admission. Perlustration of the skin serves as a method used to establish what is clinically present at baseline. Pressure injuries can develop within a small time frame and identifying what the skin looks like upon admission is paramount. For patients who are considered at risk, daily skin inspection is important. Should the skin be manifesting differently than baseline or not appear the same as adjacent skin, the changes should be documented. Assessment requires the interpretation and collection of information of a patient as a whole (Bryant & Nix, 2012).

Risk assessment enables the nurse to comprehend to what extent a patient is prone to pressure injuries. The Braden Scale is one of the most researched and widely utilized risk assessment tools across various institutions. Total scores range from 4 to 23 and are understood as follows: not at risk: score greater than 18, mild risk: 15–18, moderate risk: 13–14, high risk: 10–12, and very high risk: less than or equal to 9. The Braden Scale measures *six risk factors*. Those factors include *sensory perception*, described as a patient's ability to respond meaningfully to pressure-related discomfort; *moisture*, as this contributes to an increased risk for development of a pressure injury over a bony prominence; *activity*, referring to patient's ability to move; *mobility* refers to the patient's ability to change or control body position; *nutrition* measures the patient's usual food intake pattern; and *friction* (when the skin rubs on another surface) and *shear* (when friction acts with gravity). An example of shear can occur when the head of the bed has been elevated and a patient is sliding down.

According to Bryant and Nix (2012), maintaining healthy skin is a vital component of a prevention program. Interventions to maintain skin integrity include avoiding alkaline soaps, atraumatic cleansing of skin, applying moisturizer or an emollient, maintaining hydration, use of moisture barrier ointments, moving and transferring with a lift sheet, and utilizing proper equipment for patient transfers.

Sufficient nutrition and hydration are important components of a prevention program. Furthermore, malnourished patients are twice as likely to develop skin breakdown (Bryant & Nix, 2012). Patients who are at risk of a pressure injury may need a diet higher in protein with an increase in vitamins C, E, and zinc as these facilitate wound healing. Optimizing nutrition is essential for prevention and wound healing.

According to Bryant and Nix (2012), pressure distribution and offloading patients at risk comprises a large piece of prevention. Pressure redistribution occurs with the assistance of support surfaces such as a low air loss bed or chair cushions. Best practice for offloading a patient who is considered at risk is turning and positioning the patient. Proper technique for turning a patient is in a 30-degree side-lying position with a pillow between the knees. Frequency of repositioning is used to decrease the amount of time pressure is applied on tissue. Repositioning can occur every 2 hours; however, the patient's tissue tolerance, activity, mobility, and overall health are significant considerations in determining turning frequency. Other ways to offload patients from bony prominences are to use devices such as pillows and specific-heel boots.

Providing patient education on pressure injury prevention is crucial in decreasing incidence of pressure ulcers. When patients and their families understand the clinical picture of a pressure injury and methods of prevention, they, too, can become strong advocates of skin care. Knowledge is power and having the education helps decrease incidences of pressure injuries (Bryant & Nix, 2012).

Should a pressure injury develop despite preventive interventions, principles of wound management should be implemented. Controlling or eliminating causative factors, providing systemic support to reduce existing cofactors, and maintaining physiologic local wound environments are three best practices (Bryant & Nix, 2012). These areas focus on a patient holistically and address the reason for development of a pressure injury. Understanding these three principles enables the clinician to maximize comprehension and implement the most appropriate treatment.

Summary

Pressure injuries present a significant quality-of-life threat for individuals and a large economic burden for health care institutions. Prevention is the key in decreasing the incidence of pressure injuries across all health care settings. Routine skin inspection, patient risk assessment, pressure redistribution, adequate nutrition and hydration, and patient education are all key factors for pressure injury prevention. Implementation of these measures can decrease harm to individuals most at risk for the development of pressure injuries and can save health care institutions unnecessary treatment costs.

Bryant, R. A., & Nix, D. P. (2012). *Acute & chronic wounds, current management concepts* (4th ed.). St. Louis, MO: Elsevier Mosby.

National Pressure Ulcer Advisory Panel. (2016). National Pressure Ulcer Advisory Panel announces a change in terminology from pressure ulcer to pressure injury and updates the stages of the pressure injury. Retrieved from http://www.npuap.org/resources/educational-and-clinical-resources/npuap-pressure-injury-stages

■ SLEEP DISORDERS

Kerry Mastrangelo
Mary T. Quinn Griffin

Overview

Sleep-related disorders are among the most common medical complaints and are even more common among adults aged 65 years and older. The cause of impaired sleep in older adults is often difficult to diagnose as it frequently coexists with medical, psychiatric, and neurological disorders. Sleep-related disorders are major health concerns as the sequelae of impaired sleep can cause daytime sleepiness leading to cognitive difficulties, motor vehicle accidents, poor work performance, and falls in older adults. Impaired sleep is known to increase the risk of cardiovascular disease, substance abuse, and suicide (Bonnet, Burton, & Arand, 2014).

Background

Sleep disorders affect 10% to 30% of the U.S. population and generate 5 million office visits per year in the United States alone. The cost of sleep-related disorders has been estimated to $92.5 to $107.5 billion annually (Maness & Khan, 2015). According to The International Classification of Sleep Disorders (American Academy of Sleep Medicine, 2014), there are seven major categories of sleep disorders. These include insomnia, sleep-related breathing disorders, central disorders of hypersomnolence, circadian rhythm sleep–wake disorders, as well as other sleep disorders. There is evidence that sleep architecture changes as a person ages. The time to reach the first rapid eye movement (REM) cycle shortens, the amount of time spent in REM decreases, and slow-wave sleep decreases from 20% in young adulthood to 10% in the older adult (Feinsilver, 2017). The overall effect of these changes in older adults leads to complaints of difficulty falling asleep and maintaining sleep. Sleep disorder prevalence increases with age and is diagnosed more frequently in women than men. Predisposing factors to sleep disorders are age; female gender; chronic pain; and comorbidities such as thyroid disease alcoholism, shift work, stressful life events, and psychological disorders.

Clinical Aspects

ASSESSMENT

Insomnia is classified as either short term, meaning symptoms are present for less than 3 months, or long term, in which symptoms are present for more than 3 months. The diagnosis of insomnia must be made by developing a clinical picture; a sleep history is the only diagnostic evaluation to confirm diagnosis. In order to diagnose insomnia three criteria must be met, first the insomnia must occur three times a week for longer than 1 month. Second, the patient reports difficulty falling asleep, maintaining sleep, or waking up too early, the sleep difficulty occurs despite adequate opportunity and circumstances for sleep. Third, the impaired sleep produces deficits in daytime functioning (Maness & Khan, 2015). Sleep-related breathing disorders are characterized by abnormal respiration during sleep. These include obstructive sleep apnea and central sleep apnea. Obstructive sleep apnea is more common and has been associated with increased mortality in older adults. Older adults with obstructive sleep apnea have a higher risk of ischemic stroke and hypertension (Bonnet et al., 2014). The clinical manifestations are excessive daytime sleepiness, fatigue, poor concentration, headaches, snoring, and choking or gasping during sleep. A diagnosis of sleep apnea is made with polysomnography and treatment includes continuous positive air pressure (CPAP), an oral appliance, or surgery. Central disorders of hypersomnolence, such as narcolepsy, present with the primary complaint of excessive episodes of daytime sleepiness or an irrepressible need for sleep. Diagnosis is made through sleep logs and actigraphy. Circadian sleep–wake rhythm disorders are characterized by a chronic or recurrent sleep disturbance due to alteration of the circadian system. Sleep-related movement disorders, such as restless leg syndrome, are characterized by simple, stereotactic movements that disturb sleep.

The goal of ascertaining the patient history and performing the physical examination is to identify the cause of sleep disorder. History taking should include a detailed sleep history, focusing on time it takes to fall asleep, hours spent sleeping, and number of awakenings during sleep. Ask the patient about the sleep environment and sleep habits. If the patient has a sleep partner, ask the partner whether the patient snores or has breathing pauses during sleep. Question the patient about daytime symptoms, alcohol use, current life stressors, and caffeine intake. Complete a detailed medical history and a review of prescribed and over-the-counter medications the patient is taking. Always screen for depression in sleep impairment, especially in older adults. Complete a thorough physical exam and vital signs. Diagnostic testing includes complete blood count (CBC), electrolytes, thyroid-stimulating hormone (TSH), prostate-specific antigen (PSA) for men, urine drug screen, polysomnography, and actigraphy. Treatment depends on the underlying cause of the sleep impairment. Behavioral and pharmacologic therapies are available as treatment options. A trial of short-term therapy with sedatives, anxiolytics, and hypnotics may be prescribed. Anxiolytics are contraindicated in patients with sleep apnea. Hypnotics should be prescribed carefully in the older adult due to the high risk of adverse reactions, including oversedation, cognitive impairment, night wandering, and falls. Referral to a sleep disorder specialist should be considered if symptoms persist for more than 1 month (Cash & Glass, 2017).

NURSING INTERVENTIONS, MANAGEMENT, AND IMPLICATIONS

The nursing problem of disturbed sleep pattern related to difficulty falling asleep, maintaining sleep, or early awakening focuses on improvement of symptoms. Have the patient keep a 2-week sleep diary detailing time of awakening, hours slept, and time it takes to fall asleep. The sleep diary should include entries on naps during the day, daily stressors, intake of alcohol, and medications taken. Educate the patient on sleep hygiene measures, including avoiding alcohol, caffeine, large meals, and exercise before bed, going to bed each night at the same time, waking up each day at the same time, turning the television off before sleep, and avoiding daytime naps. If CPAP is required for treatment of obstructive sleep apnea, the patient must be instructed on the use and settings of the machine.

OUTCOMES

Successful treatment will result in improved sleep at night and improvement of daytime deficits. Improved sleep will also lead to overall better functioning and enhanced quality of life.

Summary

It is estimated that more than half of older adults are estimated to have some form of sleep disturbance.

Changes in sleep patterns may be associated with the normal aging process, although it is critical to distinguish these changes from pathological processes. Older adults are the largest group of people using hypnotic drugs and over-the-counter sleep remedies. Sleep disturbances are associated with a decreased quality of life. Older adults with impaired sleep are more likely to have motor vehicle accidents, experience falls, and develop medical comorbidities. Sleep disorders are a strong predictor for the development of depression, anxiety, and alcohol abuse in this population (Maness & Khan, 2015). Treatment decisions must be individualized according to the underlying etiology of the sleep disorder and the potential benefits versus the risks in this population.

American Academy of Sleep Medicine. (2014). *International classification of sleep disorders* (3rd ed.). Darien, IL: Author.

Bonnet, M. H., Burton, G. G., & Arand, D. L. (2014). Physiological and medical findings in insomnia: implications for diagnosis and care. *Sleep Medicine Reviews, 18*(2), 111–122. doi:10.1016/j.smrv.2013.02.003

Cash, J., & Glass, L. (2017). *Family practice guidelines* (4th ed.). New York, NY: Springer Publishing.

Feinsilver, S. (2017). Sleep apnea and other causes of impaired sleep in older adults. In G. Finlay (Ed.), *UpToDate.* Retrieved from https://www.uptodate.com/contents/sleep-apnea-and-other-causes-of-impaired-sleep-in-older-adults

Maness, D. L., & Khan, M. (2015). Nonpharmacologic management of chronic insomnia. *American Family Physician, 92*(12), 1058–1064.

■ URINARY INCONTINENCE

Felvic Adriatico Javier

Overview

Urinary incontinence (UI) is defined as the involuntary emission of urine (Testa, 2015), which is common among the elderly population and occurs more in women than men. It has a negative impact on the quality of life of patients and could lead to urinary tract infection or a bladder infection and for patients in nursing homes, could lead to pressure ulcers. Knowledge of UI and the nursing process appropriate for the elderly population is important in the community setting or in nursing homes and other senior facilities.

Background

UI is a condition characterized by bladder sphincter injury or neurological dysfunction that results in the loss of self-control of urination and the involuntary loss of urine. The elderly population aged 65 years and older represents the highest incidence of UI. The incidence increases with age and is mostly predominant in elderly women. Among the different types of UI, mixed UI and overflow UI are commonly seen among the elderly population. Mixed type of UI is commonly found in older women, whereas overflow UI is common among older men. UI increases morbidity, could lead to frequent urinary tract infection, bladder infection, and pressure sores. It has an impact on the patient's social life and quality of life and increases demand from caregivers and family.

UI is a predictor of higher mortality in general and particularly in the geriatric population (John, Bardini, Combescure, & Dallenbach, 2016). It seems that the functional decline of the pelvic floor muscles in the elderly is the main factor in UI (Rosa, Braz, Alves, Filha, & Moraes, 2016). Studies that reviewed incontinence associated with other factors and comorbidities included residents with stroke, dementia, cognitive and functional decline, and immobility (Roe, Flanagan, & Maden, 2015). Psychosocial factors of UI include embarrassment, social isolation and low self-esteem, stigma and taboo, depression, and dependence. Misconception is also an important psychosocial factor as incontinence has typically been seen as being a "natural" part of aging, or the outcome of treatment for prostate problems or a result of childbirth; therefore, help is not often sought. Social factors may also influence how people cope with UI. For example, women without spouses were more likely to adopt the negative coping style of acceptance–resignation related to UI, suggesting that factors such as social roles, social environment, and culture may influence these women's coping style. In the present study, elderly women patients with stress UI tend to adopt the negative coping styles of avoidance or acceptance–resignation, with the choice of coping style influenced by age, marital status, education level, and cognition level.

Clinical Aspects

ASSESSMENT

A complete history should be obtained, including medical history, diagnostic tests, physical examination, subjective data, and psychosocial history. Medical history should include documentation of medical comorbidities and surgical history (e.g., vaginal delivery, past or current treatment for an enlarged prostate gland or prostate cancer). A review of medications that could be causing or aggravating the incontinence should include documentation of the pattern of the urinary incontinence, the volume and frequency of urine passed, and the pattern of bowel elimination. Causes of the UI are urinary or kidney infection, bladder stones, excessive caffeine consumption, certain medications, and constipation (Payne, 2015).

Assessment of the patient's functional status is highly important especially in terms of mobility, transference, and capacity to go to the toilet (Rosa et al., 2016). It is also important to assess the patient's level of understanding about UI along with his or her coping style. Patient's lifestyle should be assessed, including diet and self-care practices. In the community setting, nurses should ask about the patient's urinary pattern to identify problems early on. The patient can submit a bladder diary to establish the urinary pattern.

NURSING INTERVENTIONS, MANAGEMENT, AND IMPLICATIONS

Nurses should be aware of potential or actual urinary tract infection and impaired skin integrity. The goal of care is to promote continence and prevent complications. Nursing intervention and management may differ depending on the setting of the nurse–patient encounter. Several conservative treatment strategies for UI are summarized elsewhere (Cameron, Jimbo, & Heidelbaugh, 2013). Successful nursing intervention has included bladder training and toileting programs. It is important to develop an individualized care plan. Patient's preference and a shared goal with the patient and caregiver are important to improving patient and caregiver participation and thereby care outcomes. In the community, identification of the problem or condition is an integral part of the nursing process. Promote a positive coping style by assisting the patient in promotion of continence and/or participation in prevention strategies. Health education, counseling, and collaboration with the primary care team; community or home-based organizations; and participation of the caregiver or family are vital in the implementation of the care plan. Nurses need to teach patients proper self-care, prevention strategies, and how to promote continence. It is important that nurses teach UTI patients how to do Kegel exercises to help strengthen the pelvic floor muscles. Information on correct dose timing and medication side effects is an essential part of patient teaching. Nurses should counsel patient on lifestyle changes such as avoiding caffeinated drinks. Stress the need for adequate hydration, offer or encourage fluids during the day, and limit liquids before bedtime. Timed voiding is also a nursing management consideration for patients with UI. The patient should have access to a bedside commode, bedpan, or urinal or access to the toilet with appropriate lighting. Noninvasive methods, such as toileting and use of pads, are common approaches to managing incontinence in residents in care homes. Older people and their families should be involved with decisions for their care, management of incontinence, goals, and outcomes (Roe et al., 2015). Administer medication as prescribed such as oxybutynin. Provide skin care or prevent infections.

OUTCOMES

Toileting programs, in particular prompted voiding with use of incontinence pads, are the main conservative behavioral approach used for the management of incontinence and promotion of continence in this population with evidence of effectiveness in the short term (Roe et al., 2015). Studies have shown some evidence that use of pH cleansers with or without barrier cream is beneficial compared to soap and water in relation to skin integrity and is less time-consuming to use. Ensuring adequate hydration of older residents is an important associated factor related to incontinence and an indicator of quality care. (Flanagan et al., 2014). Patients who have a higher cognitive level are more likely to adopt a positive coping style (Yu, Xu, Chen, & Liu, 2016). Flanagan and colleagues' study (2014) measured dehydration and weight of pads following "rounding," which included prompting for drinks, toileting, and pad/linen change versus usual care; the more aggressive care had positive effects on hydration and continence in nonambulatory residents. Individual toileting, use of incontinence pads, attention to hydration, skin care, and maintaining optimum mobility and exercise are also essential for this vulnerable population. Involving older people and family as partners in their care is paramount. All of which are not only indicators of quality care but also still core components of nursing practice (Roe et al., 2015).

Summary

UI is prevalent among the elderly population both in the community and in nursing homes and senior center facilities. A negative impact on patient's quality of life and potential for developing infection and skin breakdown can result from UI. Some patients may consider the condition a normal part of aging, therefore no help is sought. Thus, an assessment of urinary patterns in the older population is important so as to identify the problem early. Developing a positive coping style has been shown to improve outcomes. Timed-voiding, bladder training, Kegel exercises, use of incontinence pads, and rounding are some of the beneficial nursing interventions for this disease. Older people and their families should be involved with decisions for their care, management of incontinence, goals, and outcomes.

Cameron, A. P., Jimbo, M., & Heidelbaugh, J. J. (2013). Diagnosis and office-based treatment of urinary incontinence in adults. Part two: Treatment. *Therapeutic Advances in Urology, 5*(4), 189–200. doi:10.1177/1756287213495100

Flanagan, L., Roe, B., Jack, B., Shaw, C., Williams, K. S., Chung, A., & Barrett, J. (2014). Factors with the management of incontinence and promotion of continence in older people in care homes. *Journal of Advanced Nursing, 70*(3), 476–496. doi:10.1111/jan.12220

John, G., Bardini, C., Combescure, C., & Dallenbach, P. (2016). Urinary incontinence as a predictor of death: A systematic review and meta analysis. *PLOS ONE, 11*(7). Retrieved from http://journals.plos.org/plosone/article?id=10.1371/journal.pone.0158992

Payne, D. (2015). Selecting appropriate absorbent products to treat urinary incontinence. *British Journal of Community Nursing, 20*(11), 551–558. doi:10.12968/bjcn.2015.20.11.551

Roe, B., Flanagan, L., & Maden, M. (2015). Systematic review of systematic reviews for the management of urinary incontinence and promotion of continence using conservative behavioural approaches in older people in care homes. *Journal of Advanced Nursing, 71*(7), 1464–1483. doi:10.1111/jan.12613

Rosa, T., Braz, M., Alves, V., Filha, V., & Moraes, A., (2016). Evaluation of factors associated with urinary incontinence in elderly people in long-term care homes. *Acta Scientiarum. Health Sciences, 38*(2), 137–142.

Testa, A. (2015). Understanding urinary incontinence in adults. *Urologic Nursing, 35*(2), 82–86. Retrieved from http://www.medscape.com/viewarticle/844191

Yu, B., Xu, H., Chen, X., & Liu, L. (2016). Analysis of coping styles of elderly women patients with stress incontinence. *International Journal of Nursing Sciences, 3*(2), 153–157.

Health Systems and Health Promotion

HEALTH SYSTEMS

Today's health care environment is highly complex and dynamic. As noted in this subsection, health care systems strive to address the goals of the Institute for Healthcare Improvement's Triple Aim: to provide health care characterized by an optimal patient experience (e.g., safety, quality, and satisfaction) that addresses the health of populations as well as the individual patient, all in a cost-effective manner. Nurses are the frontline of health care and traditionally have "shouldered much of the responsibility when patient care falls short of standards" (Hughes, 2008, p. 1). However, it is now recognized that meeting standards, such as the Triple Aim, requires moving to a "balcony" perspective of health care and recognizing that system-level factors and conditions influence patient outcomes as well. This section includes entries on system-level topics that influence the practice of direct care nurses. Reciprocally, the work of direct care nurses influences the success of their health care organization.

HEALTH PROMOTION

As noted in this subsection, the top five causes of death in the United States are largely preventable. Nurses, with their emphasis on health as well as illness and a holistic view of the determinants influencing health, can play key roles in promoting health and preventing disease of individuals, groups, and populations. Nurses should use every patient encounter to seek opportunities to promote health, for example, assessing for smoking and counseling as indicated. This section includes entries on topics considered by nurses who engage in health promotion.

Hughes, R. (2008). Nurses at the "sharp end" of patient care. In R. Hughes (Ed.), *Patient safety and quality: An evidence-based handbook for nurses.* Washington, DC: Agency for Healthcare Quality & Research.

HEALTH SYSTEMS

- Advocacy *Ruth Ludwick and Margarete L. Zalon*
- Health Economics *Margarete L. Zalon and Ruth Ludwick*
- Health Policy *Ruth Ludwick and Angela Contant*
- Hospital Accreditation *Catherine S. Koppelman*
- Infection Prevention and Control *Irena L. Kenneley*
- Nursing Leadership *Catherine S. Koppelman*
- Nursing Management *Cynthia L. Danko*
- Nursing Process: Systems Approach *Shanina C. Knighton, Aniko Kukla, and Mary A. Dolansky*
- Patient Experience *Catherine S. Koppelman*
- Population Health *Deborah F. Lindell*
- Quality Improvement *Aniko Kukla, Mary A. Dolansky, and Shanina C. Knighton*
- Quality and Safety Education *Nadine M. Marchi*
- Social Determinants of Health *Rita M. Sfiligoj*
- Transitional Care Coordination *Nadine M. Marchi*

HEALTH PROMOTION

- Health Behavior *Deborah F. Lindell*
- Health Education *Rita M. Sfiligoj*
- Health Literacy *Joseph D. Perazzo*
- Self-Management *Marym M. Alaamri*
- Wellness *Elizabeth R. Click*

HEALTH SYSTEMS

■ ADVOCACY

Ruth Ludwick
Margarete L. Zalon

Overview

Advocacy is a critical but sometimes overlooked basic nursing competency required in all health care settings. There are three levels of advocacy by nurses.

Patient advocacy is often the first level of activism assumed when the topic of advocacy is raised, but in reality advocacy in nursing is a much broader concept. The second level of advocacy for nurses is populations, or patients geographically grouped or in a community, or with a defining characteristic of a disease (patients with cancer or opioid abusers) or a special age, for example, children or elderly. The third major level of advocacy by nurses is activism for the profession.

Advocacy for patients' health and well-being and the nursing profession are well documented explicitly and implicitly in two core American Nurses Association's (ANA) documents: (a) the *Nursing: Scope and Standards of Practice* (2015a) and (b) the *Code of Ethics for Nurses With Interpretative Statements* (2015b). Numerous definitions of advocacy exist, but at the root of all definitions is the idea of working to represent concern or raise awareness of an issues(s) for yourself or someone else so as to provide a solution (Tomajan, 2012).

Background

Nurses are overwhelmingly the public's most trusted professional group as evidenced by the results of Gallup polls since nurses were first included in the polls in 1999 (Norman, 2016). This trust underpins the nurses' responsibility for advocacy and the obligation to uphold that trust. In the landmark report, *The Future of Nursing: Leading Change, Advancing Health,* the Institute of Medicine (IOM; 2011) emphatically states, "All nurses must be leaders in the design, implementation, and evaluation of—as well as advocacy for—the ongoing reforms to the system that will be needed" (p. 221). In the report, examples of nurse advocacy for patients are highlighted, such as the school nurse, Mary Pappas, BSN, RN, who was the first professional to sound the alert about the outbreak of swine flu (H1N1 influenza) in the school she worked in New York City.

Individual nurses and nurse organizations have exemplified professional advocacy in response to the recent outbreaks of infectious diseases like Ebola and Zika. Areas of professional advocacy extend well beyond infectious diseases and include, but are not limited to, diverse topics such as violence against nurses, staffing, shift work, alarm fatigue, care transitions, and preventing work injuries.

Advocacy can be carried out in a variety of settings, whether advocating for patients or the nursing profession. These include point of care or work (e.g., hospital, clinic, school, or nursing program) environments and can extend to the community, state, nation, or globally.

Clinical Aspects

ASSESSMENT

Awareness is the first step in recognizing the need for advocacy. Advocacy for individual patients or populations of patients who are vulnerable may be easier to see than the advocacy needed for the profession. Patients and groups of patients considered to be vulnerable often include those who are marginalized by age extremes (children and the elderly), diseases (cancer, obesity), cognitive changes (dementia, delirium), economic status, health literacy, race, ethnicity, gender, or sexuality.

Assessment of the need for advocacy at the patient level is rooted in person-centered care (Ronnebaum & Schmer, 2015), and transferring public trust to individual trust as you work with patients and their families or a patient population. Patient advocacy assessment starts with meeting the patient and/or family or group of patients and continues through the end of the encounter. With trust and careful assessment, patients are more likely to share their backgrounds, concerns, beliefs, values, and goals thus revealing issues like their call lights going unanswered; that they do not feel safe in their home because of drugs or guns or violence; or the reason they have not been taking their medicines is that they cannot afford them. Every encounter with a nurse should allow the patient an opportunity to voice his or her vulnerability concerns.

Sometimes patient-level advocacy might involve a simple step such as obtaining a needed service for a patient. This kind of advocacy, being the guardian of an individual patient's rights, is one that the nurses most easily relate to in their daily work and can be more readily mastered as one gains experience in a specialized area of practice. However, in other instances, advocacy might require navigating an organization that is not particularly hospitable to questions raised about established processes. It is in these circumstances that the nurses need support and guidance regarding effective strategies to address the needs of vulnerable individuals. Help for this level of advocacy can come from nurse leaders who have a responsibility to foster work environments that facilitate advocacy so that nurses can take on more significant roles in leading change in health care delivery. It can also come from nursing organizations like the American Nurses Association, or a specialty nursing organization like the American Association of Critical-Care Nurses or American Psychiatric Nurses Association.

Advocacy for the profession may also include addressing concerns for those nurses who may be marginalized. Examples of nurses who may need advocacy are new graduates, those who are caretakers in their personal lives or are ill, or those who have chronic health conditions or disabilities. Professional advocacy may be assumed to be taken care of by "others" like management, or professional nursing organizations like those named earlier. These organizations offer guidelines, education, and support for advocacy and may help with broad-based advocacy issues for nurses and patients. Often nurse organizations have resources devoted to advocacy initiatives, usually at the federal level, including staffed government relation departments and materials available to the membership such as toolkits and position statements. At the state level, considerable advocacy initiatives are often undertaken by the state nurses association and advanced practice registered nurses groups that have resources devoted to advocacy efforts. Nurses can also become involved in consumer groups composed of community members, health care professionals, and other issue stakeholders.

NURSING INTERVENTIONS, MANAGEMENT, AND IMPLICATIONS

Like other expected nursing competencies, a wide array of interventions can be used to provide a solution for issues that require advocacy, whether it is a patient who does not fully understand a treatment because information has not been clearly communicated, an identified community need such as water-supply safety, a new nurse who expresses doubts about herself because of bullying, or a senator who has proposed changes to the nurse practice act in your state. Basic advocacy at all levels requires the following skills as outlined by Hatmaker and Tomajan (2015): (a) problem-solving, (b) communication, (c) influence, (d) collaboration, and (e) resource identification.

Problem solving, a basic competency, includes assessment, as discussed earlier, and then identifying and analyzing the problem, determining possible solutions, taking action(s), and evaluating the effectiveness of the advocacy.

Communication begins with trust, hearing what the issue is from the viewpoint of the person or group for whom you are advocating, and communicating the plan and how it will be carried out. Communication for advocacy can be aided by any number of formats—verbal, written, or visual—and can be traditionally delivered or electronically delivered via email or various types of social media.

Influence is the third skill needed as an advocate. The public trust patients have in registered nurses is one way to leverage their influence; our experience is another. A story from a community nurse about the lack of smoke detectors in a marginalized neighborhood illustrates how a small cost can have a big impact. Becoming involved in

shared governance at work or helping a legislator running for election are additional ways to gain influence.

Collaboration is as important in advocacy as it is when doing cardiopulmonary resuscitation. Collaboration with other nurses and often with other professionals is basic to being an effective advocate. Often overlooked is the role that the patients themselves can play in helping with advocacy; not only in telling their stories but in obtaining solutions to their problems. Hence, the emphasis is on patient-centered care. Patients can be and should be members of teams when a problem is analyzed and solutions postulated.

Given the complex nature of advocacy and the health care delivery system, advocacy beyond the individual level should include being part of an organized group. The strength of these organizations lies in their ability to represent large numbers of nurses. Therefore, to meet nursing's obligation to society, it is incumbent on nurses to be actively engaged in the advocacy efforts of larger groups in order to achieve the broader goals of society. Not only do the organizations need numbers of nurses to achieve their advocacy goals, the nurses need the organizations—the relationship is reciprocal. Involvement in professional organizations is associated with engaging in political activism (Kung & Rudner Lugo, 2015).

Finally, resource identification is necessary for effective advocacy. A starting point for resources is to review peer-reviewed literature and guidelines and standards from nursing's professional associations as well as accrediting body and government data repositories.

OUTCOMES

The desired outcome for the profession of nursing is that nurses understand their role in relation to advocacy at the individual level, as members of their communities, and as leaders in advancing the profession and promoting health. When more nurses are involved in advocacy efforts, it enhances society's goal of providing health care for all. Because nurses have a unique perspective, it is essential that more nurses become involved in leadership roles in health care organizations and their communities.

Summary

Advocacy is a basic competency of nursing outlined in the ANA's professional documents and is a function that is needed for an effective health care system. The IOM has identified the clear role of nursing in advocacy. Nurses often act as advocates at the point of care for the individual patient but do not always accept their responsibility for professional advocacy for the society as a whole. The competencies of the problem solving, communication, influence, collaboration, and resource identification are not unique to advocacy but are skills that nurses learn in their education and practice every day at work. Working with others and in organizations is a key strategy that can extend nurses' leadership roles in advocacy to promote health and advance the profession.

American Nurses Association. (2015a). *The code of ethics for nurses with interpretive statements*. Silver Spring, MD: Nursesbooks.org.

American Nurses Association. (2015b). *Nursing: Scope and standards of practice* (3rd ed.). Silver Spring, MD: Nursesbooks.org.

Hatmaker, D. D., & Tomajan K. (2015). Advocating for nurses and for health. In R. Patton, M. Zalon, & R. Ludwick (Eds.), *Nurses making policy: From bedside to boardroom* (pp. 41–76). New York, NY: Springer Publishing.

Institute of Medicine. (2011). *The future of nursing: Leading change, advancing health*. Washington, DC: National Academies Press. Retrieved from http://books.nap.edu/openbook.php?record_id=12956&page=R1

Kung, Y. M., & Rudner Lugo, N. (2015). Political advocacy and practice barriers a survey of Florida APRNs. *Journal of the American Association of Nurse Practitioners*, 27(3), 145–151.

Norman, J. (2016). Americans rate healthcare providers high on honesty, ethics. Retrieved from http://www.gallup.com/poll/200057/americans-rate-healthcare-providers-high-honesty-ethics.aspx?g_source=Social%20Issues&g_medium=lead&g_campaign=tiles

Ronnebaum, E., & Schmer, C. (2015). Patient advocacy and the Affordable Care Act: The growing need for nurses to be culturally aware. *Open Journal of Nursing*, 2015, 5, 237–245. doi:10.4236/ojn.2015.53028

Tomajan, K. (2012) Advocating for nurses and nursing. *Online Journal of Issues in Nursing*, 17(1), 4. Retrieved from http://nursingworld.org/MainMenuCategories/ANAMarketplace/ANAPeriodicals/OJIN/TableofContents/Vol-17-2012/No1-Jan-2012/Advocating-for-Nurses.html

■ HEALTH ECONOMICS

Margarete L. Zalon
Ruth Ludwick

Overview

With health care spending in the United States reaching $3.2 trillion in 2015 and 17.8% of the gross domestic product (Centers for Medicare & Medicaid Services [CMS], 2016), the field of health economics has become increasingly important for health care policy. Health economics, a field that has developed over the past 50 years, applies the principles of economics to health care problems and the financing and delivery of health care services. It has to do with how health care services are produced, distributed and consumed (Rambur, 2015). Health care economics is concerned with the costs, efficiency, and effectiveness of treatments; the impact of behavior; and the value placed on various aspects of health care.

It is important for nurses to understand health care economics because the resources for providing health care services are limited and there may be compelling, competing interests and demands for those resources. Health economics can be examined from the macro level; at the large system level, or population health perspective; or at the micro level, which involves the examination of a specific health care intervention.

It is important for nurses in all roles to understand how economics influences decisions made about health care for individual patients, health care organizations, and governmental policies. As resources for the delivery of health care are limited, understanding the complex, dynamic interplay of economic forces influencing health care can help nurses to strategize and implement solutions that are cost-effective while improving the care quality. The inclusion of economic analyses with the examination of nursing care outcomes strengthens the scientific foundation for nursing and has the potential to advance policy that supports professional practice. Economic evaluation is just one aspect of the complex decision making necessary for changing and making health policy at all levels.

Background

Health economics not only encompasses evaluations of specific intervention or groups of interventions performed by nurses, other health care professionals, and teams of professionals, but it also includes evaluations of health policies and their broad societal, economic impact. These evaluations may be conducted by traditional researchers in universities and health care organizations, as well as government agencies at the local, state, and federal level, as well as by private organizations. For example, the federal Office of Management and Budget is charged with the analysis of the financial impact of regulations. Other agencies, such as the CMS, conduct analyses of the financial impact of their programs. The Kaiser Family Foundation, Robert Wood Johnson Foundation, and other private groups are additional sources of economic evaluation of broad health care policies on the national level.

Clinical Aspects

ASSESSMENT

Nursing and nursing care are a significant part of every system of health care finance and the production of health. Nurses recognize that the value of nursing is directly related to the demonstrated impact on outcomes. Thus, nurses are assessing the costs associated with providing an intervention, the impact on outcomes, and the costs incurred related to those outcomes. The number of projects that demonstrate the economic value of nursing care is growing and includes numerous diverse approaches such as (a) the use of evidence-based practice (EBP) to refine and improve nursing-controlled outcomes, (b) comparative analyses of care outcomes provided by advanced practice registered nurses (APRNs) to physician care, (c) examination of the impact of nurse staffing on patient outcomes like morbidity and mortality, and (d) scrutiny of the financial impact of strategies to reduce workplace injuries.

Economic evaluations of interventions examine their costs as well as their effects in monetary units, clinical impact, and/or patient preferences (e.g., quality of life). These may include (a) cost–benefit analysis (monetary benefits are summed and then subtracted from product/service costs), (b) cost-effectiveness analysis (relative costs versus outcomes measured in the same units), (c) cost-effectiveness ratio (proportion of both total benefits conveyed in both money and benefit), (d) cost-utility analysis (variation of cost-effectiveness that weighs services/outcomes to an individual(s) quality of life), and (e) cost-consequence analysis (matrix of alternatives, costs, and consequences). Other strategies that may be used include cost avoidance (slowing the rate of cost increases or future costs) and examining the return on investment (ROI; evaluating the efficiency of an investment as if it were a new service).

NURSING INTERVENTIONS, MANAGEMENT, AND IMPLICATIONS

Nursing interventions can be at the micro level and be as simple as using good stewardship of materials and

preventing waste. Interventions can be examined from a macro view using EBP, economic analyses, impact on pay-for-performance, effective nursing workforce use, and helping patients make informed decisions about health care services. Evaluations of nursing interventions depend on high-quality data collected before and after their implementation. These economic evaluations can be done to assess an individual intervention, delivery of complex care (e.g., preventing readmission of patients with heart failure), or to evaluate at a system level.

Examples of widely adopted EBP at the individual intervention level are efforts to reduce central-line associated blood stream infections (CLABSIs) and catheter-associated urinary tract infections (CAUTIs). CLABSIs were reduced by 80% over a 15-year period (Wise et al., 2013). Similarly, reduction in CAUTIs has been linked to the adoption of evidence-based preventive practices (Saint et al., 2013).

Economic analyses can support policy decision making, which may or may not result in policy change, as illustrated in the following examples. In the acute care arena, more than 15 years of published data show the link between hospital nurse staffing to patient care outcomes, including mortality, readmissions, nosocomial infections, and falls. Recently, cost comparisons have been made across settings to examine the value of care, which takes into consideration both outcomes and costs. In comparing the outcomes for patients at hospitals recognized for having a good nursing work environment and those without such recognition, the hospitals with better work environments had a lower 30-day mortality and similar costs per patient (Silber et al., 2016). Similarly, economic analyses in nursing home settings indicate that longer tenure of registered nurses is associated with lower costs, indicating the value of retaining a more experienced registered nurse workforce in this setting (Uchida-Nakakoji, Stone, Schmitt, Phibbs, & Wang, 2016).

A clear financial impact of nursing interventions is illustrated with a comprehensive examination of the cost and benefits of school nursing in Massachusetts, which is increasingly important as school districts seek to cut delivery of health services. Wang et al. (2014) demonstrated that school nursing services cost $79 million, but saved $28.1 million in parent productivity loss, $20 million in medical care costs, and $129.1 million in teachers' productivity losses.

The 2005 Deficit Reduction Act, along with the Affordable Care Act, provides other opportunities to demonstrate the value of clinical nursing interventions with the creation of pay-for-performance programs. Value-based purchasing links payment to hospitals for their actual performance on quality measures, including a patient survey, the Hospital Consumer Assessment of Healthcare Providers and Systems (HCAHPS); the Hospital Readmission Reduction Program that examines hospital readmissions in 30 days for heart attack, heart failure, and pneumonia; and the Hospital-Acquired Condition (HAC) Payment Reduction Program. This data is not only publicly reported, but hospitals with deficits in all three areas are likely to experience greater difficulty in meeting their operating expenses because of lowered reimbursement rates.

Another approach to cost saving is focused on strategic use of the health care workforce. In primary care settings, the roles of RNs are typically related to patient triage. However, they can be more effectively used in caring for high-cost patients with chronic illness, complex health care needs, and those who require transitional care by focusing on the use of standing orders, care coordination, telehealth, patient education, and health coaching (Josiah Macy Jr. Foundation, 2016). Realizing the potential of RNs in primary care settings requires removing financial barriers under the traditional fee-for-service payment model by increasing the number of billable services, adoption of new payment models, and reducing the use of services (Macy, 2016).

Major initiatives are underway to harness the power of patient engagement, involving patients in their care to not only improve health outcomes but to reduce costs as well. One example of a concerted effort is the Choosing Wisely program of the ABIM Foundation. This program has encouraged professional societies in medicine and other health care disciplines to identify practices that should be discussed between the clinicians and patients. Examples of some nursing practices that can be questioned are the automatic initiation of continuous fetal heart rate monitoring during labor for women without risk factors, use of physical restraints to manage delirium, keeping older hospitalized patients in bed or in a chair, and walking patients to routine care unless warranted by their conditions (ABIM Foundation, 2017).

OUTCOMES

The desired outcome for the nursing profession is that economic evaluations are incorporated into evaluations of nursing practice. This would provide additional information that informs decision making about services and best practices. The provision of nursing care requires resources. The environment for care is such that the judicious and equitable use of resources requires an economic evaluation. These evaluations provide support for the difficult decisions that must be made about which services and initiatives are funded in order to deliver high-quality care.

Summary

Economic evaluations of care along with outcome data at the micro and macro level are increasingly important in efforts to improve the quality of care while reducing costs. Initiatives are underway to increase the value of care by carefully examining alternative options, rewarding effective performance, and engaging patients to reduce the costs of care. Nurses are integral to the success of strategies to improve health care outcomes while reducing costs, and nurse leaders will be increasingly called on to demonstrate that with patient care and economic data.

ABIM Foundation. (2017). Choosing Wisely. Retrieved from http://www.choosingwisely.org

Centers for Medicare & Medicaid Services. (2016). National health expenditures 2015 highlights. Retrieved from https://www.cms.gov/Research-Statistics-Data-and-Systems/Statistics-Trends-and-Reports/National HealthExpend Data/Downloads/highlights.pdf

Josiah Macy Jr. Foundation. (2016). Registered nurses: Partners in transforming primary care: Recommendations from the Macy Foundation Conference on preparing registered nurses for enhanced roles in primary care. Retrieved from http://macyfoundation.org/publications/publication/conference-summary-registered-nurses-partners-in-transforming-primary-care

Rambur, B. (2015). *Healthcare finance, economics, and policy for nurses: A foundational guide.* New York, NY: Springer Publishing.

Saint, S., Greene, M. T., Kowalski, C. P., Watson, S. R., Hofer, T. P., & Krein, S. L. (2013). *JAMA Internal Medicine, 173*(10), 874–879. doi:10.1001/jamainternmed.2013.101

Silber, J. H., Rosenbaum, P. R., McHugh, M. D., Smith, H. L., Niknam, B. A., Even-Shoshan, O., ... Aiken, L. H. (2016). Comparison of the value of nursing work environments across different levels of patient risk. *JAMA Surgery, 151*(6), 527–536. doi:10.1001/jamasurg.2015.4908

Wang, L. Y., Vernon-Smiley, M., Gapinski, M. A., Desisto, M., Maughan, E. & Sheetz, A. (2014). Cost-benefit study of school nursing practices. *JAMA Pediatrics, 168*(7), 642–648. doi:10.1001/jamapediatrics.2013.5441

Wise, M. E., Scott, R. D., II, Baggs, J. M., Edwards, J. R., Ellingson, K. D., Fridkin, S. K., ... Jernigan, J. (2013).

National estimates of central-line associated infections in critical care patients. *Infection Control & Hospital Epidemiology, 34*(6), 547–554. doi:10.1086/670629

Uchida-Nakakoji, M., Stone, P. W., Schmitt, S., Phibbs, C., & Wang, Y. C. (2016). Economic evaluation of registered nurse tenure on nursing home resident outcomes. *Applied Nursing Research, 29,* 89–95. doi:10.1016/j.apnr.2015.05.001

■ HEALTH POLICY

Ruth Ludwick
Angela Contant

Overview

Every nurse has a role in policy. With more than 19 million nurses worldwide (World Health Organization [WHO], 2012), nurses share a distinctive lens for viewing patient care, health and illness, and the health care work environment. This lens provides acute sensitivity and understanding of broad global health care issues like access and quality, as well as clinical issues like infection control and staffing for patient care. As the professional who spends the most intimate time with patients, registered nurses practice at the crossroads of policy and the care patients receive. An often-seen example of this reality is the juncture between federal law and regulations related to advance directives and the personal decisions nurses help patients make regarding their end-of-life decisions, often at the hospital bedside. There may be further hospital-based policies related to advanced directives designed to minimize risk for the hospital and assure quality and efficiency (Bail, Cook, Gardner, & Grealish, 2009), perhaps creating more complexity to policy and the resulting practice. Thus, at its simplest, policy is a plan of action adopted, proposed, and/or implemented by a group or individual. However, as alluded to in the example about advance directives, the course of action may not be that simple.

Background

Policy can exist at many levels, including local, organizational, state, national, and global. Patton, Zalon, and Ludwick (2015) further categorize these levels as little "p" (local level) and big "P" (regional, state, national, or global). The organizational level can be a "p" or a "P" depending on the size of the organization.

The little "p" does not imply less importance, but is intended to convey scope. Examples of little "p" policies might mean making the business case for why children need recess time in inclement weather, or implementing a "no lift" policy in a clinical agency. Another example of an organizational "p" would be a particular organization's requirement for reassessment of patient's pain after opioid administration, including time frame and what type of monitoring equipment should be used such as the need for a pulse oximeter. Big "P" policies impact practice on a much larger scope. Examples of big "P" policies include state laws about registered nurse staffing ratios or laws protecting health workers like those protecting nurses against violence. Federal laws, for example, the highly debated Patient Protection and Affordable Care Act (PPACA) also impact patients and our work as nurses.

There are numerous forces shaping the need for nurses' active involvement in policy. The need for new policies may be a result of accreditation requirements, value-based purchasing initiatives, financial implications, public health concerns, or organizational goals. One example of forces that can impact hospital policy is the combined influence of the recommendations of the Institute of Medicine (IOM) and Magnet® designation requirements. The IOM set forth in *The Future of Nursing: Leading Change, Advancing Health* (2011), that the nursing profession should increase its percentage of nurses with a baccalaureate degree in nursing (BSN) to 80% by the year 2020. Following their lead, the American Nurses Credentialing Center (ANCC) Magnet Recognition Program (ANCC, 2013) made it a requirement that organizations wishing to be designated as a Magnet organization must set a yearly goal and demonstrate their progress toward the end target of having 80% of their nurses possess at least a BSN. This has resulted in many organizations setting forth a policy to either hire only BSN-prepared nurses or requiring those who are newly hired within their organization to commit to completing their BSN in a specific time frame.

Clinical Aspects

ASSESSMENT

Many sources of problems in nursing and health care would be best solved with input from the nurses. These problems frequently arise from the daily care we provide as we observe and reflect on everyday occurrences like common patient complaints or workflow interruptions.

Often the works of policy that nursing has a unique lens for are clinical patient care issues and/or issues about the work environment that health care occurs in. Assessment, therefore, is not just focused on the problem and data about the problem, but must also include knowing the best evidence and who the stakeholders are.

Many times, policy change comes about because numerous factors align to create what may be called a window of opportunity. A window of opportunity is said to exist when changes in the internal or external environment occur, creating an opening for a policy issue to be pushed forward, either locally or beyond. Some of the recent legislative initiatives concerning advanced practice registered nurses (APRNs) might be attributed to access and quality issues. Nurses have been able to leverage, in the media and during patient care, the important role APRNs can have in improving the quality. Thus, the dynamic around access and quality has made the timing right and created a window of opportunity so that legislation favorable to APRNs might move forward (Clabo et al., 2012.

Thus, it is vital in planning for policy to find out about the contextual and environmental issues that relate to the problem at hand. One approach is to use a SWOT analysis that involves the examination of the unit's internal strengths (S) and weaknesses (W), and also identifies external opportunities (O) and threats (T). Common problems nurses encounter that might be assessed using a SWOT analysis include:

■ Falls with injuries

■ Use of patient care-sitters/companions

■ Use of rotating shifts

■ Increasing employment of nurses with BSNs

■ Alarm fatigue

■ Bullying or incivility

■ Violence against nurses

Policies are routinely reviewed on a regularly scheduled cycle. However, particular policies may be identified for review outside of that cycle because of legislative changes or new research evidence. You may be the one to note an outdated policy through reading the literature, previous work experience, or new knowledge obtained by attending classes or conferences. These updates to policies involve a different, often simpler, assessment that is lead by a person or a committee to change the policy. The assessment of these policy changes often focuses on finding and evaluating the current best evidence. Loversidge (2016) and Stevens

(2013) suggest using an evidence-based practice (EBP) approach to informing health policy. Thus, a key assessment component is finding the best evidence through literature and practice guideline searches and applying known rubrics for evaluating the quality of the evidence. Nurses are often familiar with using evidence to establish clinical guidelines to guide practice. The Emergency Nurses Association (ENA), for example, has established clinical practice guidelines (CPGs) around a variety of nursing practice problems, for example, capnography during sedation and verification of g-tube placement (ENA, n.d.).

NURSING INTERVENTIONS, MANAGEMENT, AND IMPLICATIONS

There are general considerations for becoming involved with policy, whether you are looking to be involved in little "p" (local level) or big "P" level of policy. The first step is learning how the system works. Identify how policy is developed where you work. Consider whether you need to brush up on the basics of civics, whether at the local, state, or national level. Second, identify a mentor or mentors who can help guide you. Third, join shared governance committees at work, your professional association, and at least one specialty association.

Nurses' associations can serve as a key vehicle for influencing policy, both nationally and globally . . . the majority of initial improvement(s) in the profession can be traced to the organized commitment of individuals working under the auspices of nursing associations. (Benton, 2012)

Once you are involved, there are basic stages to policy making that align with the nursing process (Patton et al., 2015, para. 6):

■ Recognize and identify a problem

■ Formulate policy

■ Implement the policy change

■ Monitor and evaluate the result

Much like the care of patients, the process is often cyclic and involves continued monitoring as policy making is an ongoing process. Other strategies include-setting an agenda, building capital, and working with the media. These latter skills are used more often when policy extends beyond the local level to public policy. If you are involved with changing your state's nursing practice act, for example, then these additional steps are required.

OUTCOMES

The expected outcome for policy work is that all nurses are active at some level of policy making. To achieve this outcome, full participation in committee work within unit-based or system-shared workplace governance and professional and interprofessional associations (e.g., the American Nurses Association) are expected. A relatively new means for nurses to become involved in local policy that has impact beyond the hospital setting is through legislative and policy committees based within your work institution. These expected engagement activities provide nurses the vehicle for evidence-based policy analysis of issues related to both patient quality and safety and the work environment.

Summary

Registered nurses play a vital part in the development of health policy. Each nurse has a role and can encompass many fronts at the little "p" (local level) and big "P" levels. Forces influencing nursing practice and health care delivery (e.g., accreditation requirements, value-based purchasing initiatives) are shaping the need for nurses to become more active participants in policy. Thus, there are many sources of problems in nursing and health care that would be best served with the addition of a nurse to guide or to have input into policy solutions.

American Nurses Credentialing Center. (2013). *2014 Magnet application manual*. Silver Spring, MD: Author.

Bail, K., Cook, R., Gardner, A., & Grealish, L. (2009). Writing ourselves into a web of obedience: A nursing policy analysis. *International Journal of Nursing Studies*, 46(11), 1457–1466. doi:10.1016/j.ijnurstu.2009.04.005

Benton, D. (2012). Advocating globally to shape policy and strengthen nursing's influence. *Online Journal of Issues in Nursing*, 17(1), 5. doi:10.3912/OJIN .Vol17No01Man05

Clabo, L. L., Giddens, J., Jeffries, P., Mcquade-Jones, B., Morton, P., & Ryan, S. (2012). A perfect storm: A window of opportunity for revolution in nurse practitioner education. *Journal of Nursing Education*, 51(10), 539-541. doi:10.3928/01484834-20120920-01

Emergency Nurses Association. (n.d.). Safe practice, safe care. Retrieved from https://www.ena.org/practice -research/research/CPG/Pages/Default.aspx

Institute of Medicine. (2011). *The future of nursing: Leading change, advancing health*. Washington, DC: National Academies Press. Retrieved from http://books.nap.edu/ openbook.php?record_id=12956&page=R1

Loversidge, J. M. (2016). A call for extending the utility of evidence-based practice: Adapting EBP for health policy impact. *Worldviews on Evidence-Based Nursing*, 13(6), 399–401. doi:10.1111/wvn.12183

Patton, R., Zalon, M., & Ludwick, R. (2015). Leading the way in policy. In R. Patton, M. Zalon, & R. Ludwick (Eds.), *Nurses making policy: From bedside to boardroom* (pp. 3–40). New York, NY: Springer Publishing.

Stevens, K. (2013, May 31). The impact of evidence-based practice in nursing and the next big ideas. *Online Journal of Issues in Nursing*, 18(2), 4. doi:10.3912/OJIN .Vol18No02Man04

World Health Organization. (2013). Enhancing nursing and midwifery capacity to contribute to the prevention, treatment, and management of non-communicable diseases. *Human Resources for Health Observer*, 12. Geneva, Switzerland: Author.

■ HOSPITAL ACCREDITATION

Catherine S. Koppelman

Overview

Throughout the United States, the delivery of safe, quality care and services is defined in standards and regulated by laws and agencies (The Joint Commission [TJC], 2016a). Assurance that hospitals provide care and services by these standards is accomplished via mandatory accreditation requirements that are tied to payment (TJC, 2016b). Some health care organizations also voluntarily apply for reviews by professional bodies to demonstrate excellence that exceeds regulatory and professional standards. Standards, regulatory surveys, and voluntary recognition reviews that apply to nursing define expectations of nursing practice in acute, ambulatory, and postacute settings.

Background

The Centers for Medicare & Medicaid Services (CMS) is a federally funded and operated agency that, among many functions, delegates health care reviews and accreditation to other bodies, both nationally and state level. At the national level, this process is conducted by awarding "deemed status" to organizations that review on behalf of CMS (TJC, 2016a). The largest of these organizations is TJC, which accredits 5,400 of the 5,627 hospitals in the country (American Hospital Association [AHA], 2016). TJC standards incorporate the CMS standards known as the *Conditions of Participation* (TJC, 2016b). A hospital accreditation includes all inpatient and ambulatory service sites in a health care organization. Accreditation status lasts for 3 years and then requires renewal. Failure to earn accreditation can prevent a hospital from receiving CMS funding for services, which effectively closes the hospital (TJC, 2016a).

TJC surveys are unannounced 3- to 5-day on-site visits conducted by several surveyors. This approach requires hospitals to be in a continual state of readiness. Evaluation of compliance with the standards involves a review of the written documents and clinical outcomes; interviews with leaders, providers, and patients; as well as observations of the care provision. The care of patients is traced from admission to discharge. Overall survey findings include the outcomes and/or deficiencies concerning the standards. Deficiencies must be remediated with quantifiable outcomes and time frames. Sometimes a follow-up survey is required to secure full accreditation (TJC, 2016c).

At the state level, departments of health are required by law to survey specific programs for licensure or certification. They also conduct hospital surveys following TJC deficiency reports and complete surveys based on patient/family complaints or sentinel events leading to patient harm (Public Health Law Center, 2015).

Health care organizations also have numerous opportunities for voluntary application to a professional body to verify excellence in a particular aspect of the organization's services. In the nursing profession, the highest recognition for excellence is the American Nurses Association Magnet® designation (ANCC, 2013). The Magnet standards are organized into five model components: Transformational leadership, structured empowerment; exemplary professional practice; new knowledge, innovation, and improvements; and empirical quality results. The review process includes a written self-report documenting how the nursing department excels in the standards and outcomes followed by a 4- to 5-day on-site visit with nurse appraisers. Magnet appraisers visit all units and meet with nurses in groups on all shifts. The award extends for a 4-year period and redesignation follows a similar process. Only 6% of hospitals globally earn this designation (ANCC, 2013).

Many nursing organizations award recognition for exceeding nursing standards in a particular specialty. Examples include the American Association of Critical-Care Nurses (AACN) Beacon Awards and the Emergency Nurses Association (ENA) Lantern Award. Both require reviews with a demonstration of outcomes that exceed the standards (AACN, 2016; ENA, 2016).

Clinical Aspects

ASSESSMENT

Hospital TJC accreditation standards include reviews of nursing care and nursing practice. Reviews include a random selection of nurses' licenses, certifications, orientation competency validation, annual performance evaluations, continuing-education attendance, and nurses' involvement in quality/safety improvements.

Standards relate to all steps of the nursing process. The areas of nursing assessment include history and physical appraisal with specific attention to interventions in the plan of care (POC) based on assessment data, frequency of assessments by level of care, congruent reporting of abnormal findings to the POC, skin assessments, fall risk assessments, pain level assessments, and response to changes in the POC.

NURSING INTERVENTIONS, MANAGEMENT, AND IMPLICATIONS

Patient education plans and discharge plans need to involve the patient/family and confirm understanding. State departments of health reviews require demonstration of practice in these same standards for nursing care.

One section of TJC standards include the National Patient Safety Goals (NPSGs; TJC, 2017). These are based on the most current evidence and are endorsed by national bodies such as the Agency for Healthcare Research and Quality (AHRQ). The NPSGs have been incorporated into the curricula for the education of nursing students and are incorporated in the Quality and Safety Education for Nurses (QSEN) competencies. Examples of NPSGs include appropriate handwashing, patient identification, medication reconciliation, medication administration, and use of a universal protocol before an invasive procedure. The laws that govern the practice of nursing, scope, and standards of nursing documents and the American Nurses Association *Code of Ethics* require practice according to defined standards that include TJC and department of health standards for nurses. The settings in which nurses practice (hospitals, ambulatory, and post-acute) integrate these same standards into policies and procedures, orientation, competencies, and annual evaluations. Medical record forms and electronic charting templates are designed to follow these standards for assessments, plans-of-care components, and discharge plans. Health care organizations use self-review of these standards and outcomes during evaluation of their quality and patient safety programs.

Standards adopted by organizations for review of excellence in nursing include and extend beyond accreditation standards. For example, one section of the Magnet document relates to shared governance and nurses' involvement in decisions that affect nurses, and another section relates to professional development and education opportunities offered by the hospital.

OUTCOMES

The ultimate aim of programs such as regulatory surveys, accreditation, patient safety goals, and excellence initiatives is to ensure achievement of standards regarding safe, quality care. For example, the mission of TJC states: "To continuously improve health care for the public, in collaboration with other stakeholders, by evaluating health care organizations and inspiring them to excel in providing safe and effective care of the highest quality and value."

Many studies and systematic reviews have been conducted to assess the effects of accreditation and patient safety standards. Results are mixed (Alkhenizan & Shaw, 2011; Brubakk, Vist, Bukholm, Barach, & Tiomsland, 2015). However, accreditation does provide senior leaders of healthcare organizations with data which can be compared to benchmarks and standards and indices measured for programs implemented to improve outcomes. In addition, such data is publicized by organizations such as the CMS such that the public can compare healthcare organizations and providers.

For nurses, practicing in hospitals recognized for excellence in nursing have the opportunity to more fully participate in professional practice in care delivery and professional development. Nurses seeking career opportunities should evaluate health care organizations from the standpoint of publicly reported quality outcomes and recognition awards for nursing.

Summary

Health care organizations are regulated to ensure safe quality care provision. Accreditation and regulatory reviews are mandated to ensure this purpose. Some hospitals pursue voluntary recognition for exceeding these standards. Practicing nurses must be knowledgeable about and provide care according to professional and regulatory standards. They should evaluate regulatory status and recognitions for hospitals and nursing departments in evaluating employment in career decisions.

American Association of Critical-Care Nurses. (2016). Be a beacon of excellence for your community, hospital and patients. Retrieved from https://www.aacn.org/nursing/beacon-awards

American Hospital Association. (2016). Fast facts on U.S. hospitals. Retrieved from https://www.aha.org/research/rc/stat-studies/fast-facts.shtml

American Nurses Credentialing Center. (2013). *Magnet application manual. Review 3.* Silver Spring, MD: The Center.

Brubakk, K., Vist, G., Bukholm, G., Barach, P., & Tiomsland, O. (2015). A systematic review of hospital accreditation: the challenges of measuring complex intervention effects. *BMS Health Service Research, 15*(280), 1–10. doi:10.1186/s12913-015-0933-x

Emergency Nurses Association. (2016). ENA Lantern Awards. Retrieved from https://www.ena.org/practice-research/practice/2016/Lantern Award/Pages/Test.aspx

Pham, H., Coughlan, J., & O'Malley, A. (2006). The impact of quality-reporting programs on hospital operations. *Health Affairs, 25*(5), 1412–1422 doi:10.1377/hlthaff.25.5.1412

Public Health Law Center. (2015). State & local public health: An overview of regulatory authority. Retrieved from https:www.public.healthlawcenter.org/sites/defaults/files/resources/phlc-fs-state-local-req-authority-publichealth-2015.o.pdf

The Joint Commission. (2016a). Facts about federal deemed status and state recognition. Retrieved from https://www.jointcommission.org

The Joint Commission. (2016b). Facts about Joint Commission accreditation standards. Retrieved from https://www.jointcommission.org

The Joint Commission. (2016c). Facts about the on-site survey process. Retrieved from https://www.jointcommission.org

The Joint Commission. (2017). Patient safety/national patient safety goals. Retrieved from https://jointcommission

■ INFECTION PREVENTION AND CONTROL

Irena L. Kenneley

Overview

Infection prevention and control practices are required to prevent transmission of infectious diseases in all health care settings. Infection prevention and control require a basic understanding of the epidemiology of diseases, including mode of transmission and factors that increase patient susceptibility to infection. Health care–associated infections (HAIs), acquired by patients while they are receiving health care for another condition, are currently one of the top 10 leading causes of death in the United States. The risk of acquiring an HAI is related to the mode of transmission of the infectious agent (e.g., *Clostridium difficile*, ventilator-associated pneumonia, carbapenem-resistant Enterobacteriaceae, methicillin-resistant *Staphylococcus aureus* [MRSA], etc.), the environment of care, type of patient-care activity or procedure being performed, and the underlying host defenses of the patient.

Background

Health care professionals have an important role in the prevention of HAIs. Although significant progress has been made in preventing some types of infections, there is much more work to be done. The Centers for Disease Control and Prevention's (CDC; 2016b) annual report, the *National and State Healthcare-Associated Infections Progress Report* (*HAI Progress Report*) describes national and state progress in preventing HAIs. Among national acute care hospitals, the most recent report (2014 data, published 2016) revealed that the burden of HAIs was an estimated 722,000 in U.S. acute care hospitals. In addition, about 75,000 patients with HAIs died during their hospitalizations. More than half of all HAIs occurred outside of the intensive care unit.

Measures can be taken to control and prevent HAIs in all settings. Research shows that when health care facilities, care teams, and individual doctors and nurses are aware of the infection problems and take specific steps to prevent them, rates of some targeted HAIs (e.g., central line-associated blood stream infection known as CLABSI) can decrease by more than 70% (CDC, 2016b). Prevention of HAIs is possible, but everyone must be dedicated and must make a conscious effort. Thus, the ultimate responsibility to protect patients from an infection transmitted in a health care setting includes clinicians, health care facilities and systems, public health, quality-improvement groups, and the federal government. Everyone working together results in improving patient care, protecting patients, and ultimately saving lives.

Clinical Aspects

ASSESSMENT

HAIs can happen in any health care facility, including hospitals, ambulatory surgical centers, end-stage renal disease facilities, and long-term care facilities. HAIs are commonly caused by bacteria, fungi, and viruses.

HAIs are a significant cause of illness and death—and they can have devastating emotional, financial, and medical consequences. At any given time, about one in 25 inpatients has an infection related to hospital care (CDC, 2016b). These infections lead to the loss of tens of thousands of lives and cost the already overburdened U.S. health care system billions of dollars each year (CDC, 2016b). The following elements raise the patient risk of HAIs:

- Catheters (bloodstream, endotracheal, and urinary)
- Surgery
- Injections
- Health care settings that are not properly cleaned and disinfected
- Communicable diseases passing between patients and health care workers
- Overuse or improper use of antibiotics

Common HAIs patients acquire in hospitals include:

- CLABSI
- *Clostridium difficile* infections
- Pneumonia
- MRSA
- Surgical site infections
- Urinary tract infections

Catheter-associated urinary tract infections (CAUTI) are the most commonly reported hospital-acquired condition, and the rates continue to rise. More than 560,000 patients develop CAUTI each year, leading to extended hospital stays, increased health care costs, and patient morbidity and mortality. RNs can play a major role in reducing CAUTI rates to save lives and prevent harm. The American Nurses Association (ANA) offers an innovative, streamlined, evidence-based clinical tool for CAUTI prevention developed by leading experts (ANA, 2016).

Each facility should categorize patients per infection risk group in a specific patient population. The development of the "patient risk groups" criteria are dependent on the facility's mix of patients. Nursing homes and ambulatory care delivery sites have very different populations, and the infection control risk assessment must reflect this fact (Association for Professionals in Infection Control and Epidemiology [APIC], 2015). The key principles used for risk assessment categorization of patients include:

- Inherent susceptibility to infection—patients with immunosupression are at greatest risk.

- Invasiveness—a healthy patient undergoing surgery is at greatest risk when sterile tissues are exposed to the operation room (OR) environment (Association of Perioperative Registered Nurses [AORN], 2016).

- Exposure to construction—dust created during construction can cause release and spread of bacteria and molds. The American Institute of Architects (AIA) and The Joint Commission (TJC) require documentation of the facility's Infection Control Risk Assessment (ICRA).

NURSING INTERVENTIONS, MANAGEMENT, AND IMPLICATIONS

Nurses have significant and unique opportunities to reduce the potential for hospital-acquired infections. Using their skills and knowledge, nurses can facilitate patient recovery while minimizing complications related to infections. CDC guidelines provide basic strategies for preventing infection and promoting positive patient outcomes (CDC, 2007).

HAIs are significant. Nursing-sensitive indicators are actions and interventions performed by the nurse when providing patient care in the scope of nursing practice (ANA, 2016). These interventions are central to the processes of nursing care and are often performed in partnership with other members of a multidisciplinary health care team. Nursing-sensitive patient outcomes represent the consequences or effects of nursing interventions and result in changes in the patient symptom management, functional status, safety, psychological distress, or costs (APIC, 2015).

The nurse leads the rest of the health care team in practicing prevention strategies to protect the patient from infection. Some basic strategies include (APIC, 2015; CDC, 2016a):

- The practice and promotion of hand hygiene

- Consistent use of aseptic technique

- Cleaning and disinfection practices

- Use of standard precautions

- Patient assessment and additional transmission-based precautions

- Patient education

- Use of safety devices

- Removal of unnecessary invasive devices as soon as possible

- Use of bundle strategies for infection prevention

- All are fit for duty

Communicable diseases have been transmitted to patients by health care workers who report for work when they are ill. Nurses have the responsibility to avoid compromising patient safety. "Fit for duty" includes meeting basic physical requirements for safely performing necessary functions of the job without compromising the patient safety. This means nurses and staff members are free of active symptoms of possible infection such as fever, cough, sore throat, and gastrointestinal illness (APIC, 2015). Health care workers should be vaccinated against preventable diseases such as hepatitis B and seasonal influenza. Personnel at risk for exposure to tuberculosis should be screened per recommendations.

OUTCOMES

Nurses play instrumental roles in planning, implementing, and evaluating infection prevention and control programs in health care organizations, along with competency, standard-setting, and development of other related policies at the national and international levels. Outcomes of infection prevention and control programs implemented by health care organizations can be evaluated at the individual patient, population, and system levels. Process evaluation includes indices such as hand-hygiene compliance and outcome evaluation includes data such as HIAs.

System-level data is reviewed in terms of patient safety goals, state regulatory and TJC requirements, and other standards and benchmarks. There is clear evidence that infection prevention and control programs can decrease the incidence of HIAs. For example, the (Ontario, Canada) Provincial Infectious Diseases Advisory Committee (PIDAC) reported that "Infection prevention and control (IPAC) programs have been shown to be both clinically effective and cost-effective, providing important cost savings in terms of fewer health care–associated infections, reduced length of hospital stay, less antibiotic resistance, and decreased costs of treatment for infections" (2008, p. 6).

Summary

HAIs are associated with high morbidity and mortality. According to the CDC, HAIs account for an estimated 722,000 infections and 75,000 associated deaths each year in American hospitals. A recent study found HAIs to be the sixth leading cause of death in the United States, costing the health care industry $6 billion annually. Government laws linking patient outcomes to health care provider reimbursement have ignited discussion in boardrooms across the country. The current economic climate has health care providers more concerned than ever about promoting and supporting strategies to ensure patient safety. Patients and their families are more informed about health care services and have expectations for quality patient outcomes.

American Nurses Association. (2016). Streamlined evidence-based RN Tool: Catheter associated urinary tract infection (CAUTI) prevention. Retrieved from http://nursingworld.org/CAUTI-Tool

Association of Perioperative Registered Nurses. (2016). *AORN guideline implementation topics*. Denver, CO: Author. Retrieved from https://www.aorn.org/guidelines/guideline-implementation-topics

Association for Professionals in Infection Control and Epidemiology. (2015). *APIC text of infection control and epidemiology*. Washington, DC: Author.

Centers for Disease Control and Prevention. (2007). 2007 guideline for isolation precautions: Preventing transmission of infectious agents in healthcare settings. Retrieved from https://www.cdc.gov/hicpac/pdf/isolation/Isolation2007.pdf

Centers for Disease Control and Prevention. (2016a). Guideline for hand hygiene in health-care settings. Retrieved from https://www.cdc.gov/handhygiene/providers/index.html

Centers for Disease Control and Prevention. (2016b). National and state healthcare-associated infections progress report. Retrieved from https://www.cdc.gov/HAI/pdfs/progress-report/hai-progress-report.pdf

Provincial Infectious Diseases Advisory Committee. (2008). *Best practices for infection prevention and control programs in Ontario*. Ontario, Canada: Ministry of Health and Long-Term Care.

■ NURSING LEADERSHIP

Catherine S. Koppelman

Overview

Many definitions of leadership have been written over the years. Components common to most definitions include influence of others and the effect on organizational outcome (McCleskey, 2014). Responsibility and potential for leadership in clinical practice rest with every RN. However, because nurses are predominantly employed by hospitals or health care systems, regulations and organizational structures are relevant to leadership. In this context, regulatory bodies require the presence of a nurse leader for nursing practice in health care organizations and that leader needs to hold particular credentials and qualifications (Centers for Medicare & Medicaid Services [CMS], 2008). It is important that nurses be knowledgeable about their ability to lead in clinical practice, as well as the structure of leadership authority over practice in employment organizations.

Background

Organizational structures are commonly designed to group like functions and related people to promote the purpose and goals of the organization (Daft, 2008). In hospitals, nursing services are organized according to the care and services provided by nurses who practice in diverse areas of specialization (e.g., inpatient units, operative services, emergency departments, and ambulatory clinics). Regulatory and accrediting bodies require that nursing services in hospitals function "under the direction of a registered nurse" and "a plan of administrative authority and delegation of responsibilities for patient care and nursing responsibilities, resources, etc. be defined" (CMS, 2008). The Joint Commission (TJC; 2009, p. 7) leadership standards further require that the nurse leader "has an active role in senior leadership, the governing body, and the medical staff." Although these nursing leadership positions have various titles, the most common is "chief nursing officer" (CNO).

The CNO is typically required to have 5 years of leadership experience and a master's degree in nursing or a related field (American Organization of Nurse Executives [AONE], 2009). Over the past few years, based on the Institute of Medicine (IOM)'s report on the future of nursing, the CNO is more commonly preferred/required to have earned a doctoral degree (IOM, 2011). Depending on the size of the organization, middle managers are responsible for the safety and quality across various subgroupings, functions, or specialties (e.g., critical care services, women's health services, pediatric services). In such a structure or entity, each patient care unit may have a nurse manager who is sometimes called a head nurse.

The scope of responsibility for CNOs has evolved and often expanded over time as health care systems have expanded across multiple hospitals, ambulatory settings, and communities or geographic areas. In complex networks, corresponding structures span a complex system for which one CNO may have a global responsibility, and, in that system, additional CNOs may be responsible for each hospital in the system. Regardless, the CNO role usually reports to the chief executive officer or the president of the system and each hospital.

Because of the complexity of organizations, CNOs may have line, staff, or matrix responsibility. When a CNO has line responsibility, authority extends to decisions about the distribution of resources, operations, employment status, and nursing practice. When a CNO has predominantly staff responsibility, authority extends to nursing practice and regulatory issues for nursing. In a matrix, responsibility includes some combination of line and staff authority (Daft, 2008). However, in keeping with the leadership standards of the accrediting bodies, all structures need to ensure that the CNO role represents nursing as a member of senior leadership, governing body, and medical leadership. The National Council of State Boards of Nursing (NCSBN) also requires the CNO or nurse leader designee to report misconduct relative to the nursing practice act by a nurse employed by the hospital or system (NCSBN, 2016).

The CNO leads the nursing organization based on a philosophy of nursing, vision for nursing, strategic plan, and standards of professional nursing practice. This requires specialized knowledge and competencies (AONE, 2015). Leadership styles are influential in the effectiveness of the leader. The transformational leadership style is characterized by influencing others through a vision of the future that motivates and engages the followers. Transformational leadership has demonstrated the most effective outcomes in nursing literature (Clavelle et al., 2012; Giltiaone, 2013). The American Nurses Credentialing Center (ANCC) manual for Magnet designation of a hospital for overall nursing excellence describes an entire chapter of transformational leadership standards for the CNO role (ANCC, 2014).

Clinical Aspects

ASSESSMENT

Leadership in clinical practice is the responsibility of every RN and advanced practice registered nurse (APRN). Characteristics of a professional nurse include accountability for self and others to known standards of care and the laws that govern nursing practice. These standards are also integrated into regulatory requirements. Nurses can influence others by consistently providing safe quality care in their practice and engendering respect for the role using best practice and strong patient advocacy. Professional self-identity

is central to one's leadership in nursing practice. For this reason, nurses should have mentors and serve as mentors in all areas of clinical practice.

The clinical environment in which the nurse practices can benefit or hinder professional development and professional practice. When considering potential employing organizations, the nurses need to assess the professional culture in the organization, evaluate the formal nurse leaders, and consider the leadership structure in the hospital. These variables directly influence nurse satisfaction and leadership in professional practice.

The nurse leader who is the most influential for an applicant is the one to whom that nurse reports. For staff nurses, that is most commonly the unit manager. Alignment of one's philosophy of nursing and values with the culture is also an important consideration. This can be assessed on an interview with questions to the head nurse about the scope of the nursing role, nursing department philosophy, position description for the RN, orientation program, and the performance evaluation process. All give the applicant a good sense of the "value for nursing" in the organization. Taking a tour or shadowing a nurse for a few hours can also provide deep insights into nursing satisfaction and perceived value. The applicant should ask direct questions about the model of nursing care and the nurse-to-patient ratio. Opportunities to learn through orientation, continuing education, or a clinical career ladder are also important questions in the applicant interview. Other aspects of the assessment include physician–nurse relationships and the potential for input in decision making through shared governance structures.

NURSING INTERVENTIONS, MANAGEMENT, AND IMPLICATIONS

The design of the nursing leadership structure is intended to represent and support nurses and nursing functions in the organization. Regulatory requirements also stipulate that the nurse leader must have authority and accountability for professional standards that are integrated into the hospital policy and procedure. The structure of nursing services leadership and regulations have the potential to facilitate the professional practices of the nurses within that organization. Have these discussions with the head nurse in the interview as part of your decision-making process about joining the organization.

Once employed, a nurse should participate in education focused on standards and policies during orientation and beyond. As a professional, seek ongoing feedback on your practice from your nurse manager and through the annual evaluation process. If practice improvement needs are identified in these processes, expect to collaborate in setting defined plans and goals for your development. As professionals, nurses are obligated to hold themselves accountable to standards and lifelong learning.

OUTCOMES

If serious practice deficiencies or misconduct are identified, including violations of professional standards that result in patient harm or place the patient at risk of serious harm, the CNO will be involved directly. The other areas of misconduct related to licensure requirements, ethics violations, and impairment because of chemical dependency or mental/emotional disturbances may also be of concern. All require taking the nurse involved off duty and mandate a report to the state board of nursing. The CNO consults with the hospital legal counsel as these steps are taken and provides support to the nurse throughout the process. The state board of nursing will investigate, determine a plan of action, and monitor the status of the nurse concerning continuing practice or revoke his or her license to practice (NCSBN, 2016).

The CNO is responsible for leading and sustaining a culture of professional practice, as well as a consistent value for nursing and patient safety (AONE, 2007). Practicing nurses need and want a leader who respects and motivates them professionally. The ways in which leaders do that include inspiring through vision, planning through strategy, executing that strategy to yield positive outcomes, maintaining excellence in patient care, and achieving the satisfaction of the nurses that provide that care. Visibility and access to the nursing leader are critical to the effectiveness of the role of representing the needs of patients/families and professional nurses.

Summary

Nursing leadership in clinical practice is the responsibility of every RN in providing care according to professional standards for practice. In the practice arena, regulatory bodies also require a nurse leader or CNO for overall nursing practice in hospitals and health care organizations. Nurses need to be knowledgeable about their ability to lead as well as the leadership structure and authority over the nursing practice in employing organizations that will affect nursing practice and professional development.

American Nurses Credentialing Center. (2014). *2014 Magnet application manual: Review 3*. Silver Spring, MD: Author.

American Organization of Nurse Executives. (2007). Guiding principles for the role of the nurse executive in patient safety. Retrieved from https://www.aone.org/resources/role_nurse_executive_patientsafety.pdf

American Organization of Nurse Executives. (2009). Position statement on educational preparations of nurse leaders. Retrieved from https://aone.org/resources/educational-preparation-nurseleaders.pdf

American Organization of Nurse Executives. (2015). Nurse executive competencies. Retrieved from https://www.aone.org/resources/nec.pdf

Centers for Medicare & Medicaid Services. (2008). CMS conditions of participation: Nursing service. Retrieved from https://www.cms.gov/transmittals/downloads/R37SOMA.pdf

Clavelle, J., Drenkard, K., Tullai-McGuiness, S., & Fitzpatrick, J. (2012). Transformational leadership practices of chief nursing officers in Magnet® organizations. *Journal of Nursing Administration, 42*(4), 195–201. doi:10.1097/01.NNA.0000420389.87789.b1

Daft, R. L. (2008). *Fundamentals of organizational structure. Organizational theory and design* (10th ed., pp. 88–136). Mason, OH: South-Western/Cengage.

Giltiaone, C. L. (2014). Leadership styles and theories. *Nursing Standard, 27*(41), 35–39. doi:10.7748/ns2013.06.27.41.35.e7565

Institute of Medicine. (2011). *The future of nursing: Leading change, advancing health*. Washington, DC: National Academies Press. Retrieved from https://www.nap.edu/read/12956/chapter/1

McCleskey, J. A. (2014). Situational, transformational and transactional leadership and leadership development. *Journal of Business Studies Quarterly, 5*(4), 117–130. Retrieved from https://jbsq.org/wp-content/uploads/2014/06June_2014_9.pdf

National Council of State Boards of Nursing. (2016). NCSBN discipline. Retrieved from https://www.ncsbn.org/discipline

The Joint Commission. (2009). Joint Commission leadership in healthcare organizations. Retrieved from https:www.jointcommission.org/assests/1/18/WP-Leadership-Standard

■ NURSING MANAGEMENT

Cynthia L. Danko

Overview

Management is defined as "leading and directing all or part of an organization through the deployment and manipulation of resources" (Marquis & Huston, 2015, p. 33). Management in health care today is a process that involves patients, personnel (caregivers), and resources. Those who manage are responsible for decision making, patient safety, quality outcomes, and staff development. Competent management requires leadership skills to organize the environment and support the professional caregivers to meet the goals of the facility or organization (Pihlainen, Kivinen, & Lammintakanen, 2016). Nursing management encompasses accountability and responsibility for patient outcomes and professional growth and is the link between administration and bedside care (American Organization of Nurse Executives, 2015). The management process, similar to the nursing process, involves assessment, problem identification, planning, interventions, and evaluation. Management in nursing practice is the foundation of safe patient care.

Background

Nursing management has taken many of its constructs from social, behavioral, and systems theories. The classic management style (developed in the early 20th century) used a structured approach to meet organizational goals and increase productivity. It was deemed effective as it addressed production, structure, and technology. However, by the 1930s, workers were frustrated with the "job" being the only focus of attention and the neoclassical management style emerged, which emphasized the human side of the workplace (Sarker & Khan, 2013). Interpersonal relationships with coworkers and supervisors became a priority. Highlighting the human side of the workplace and having employees feel valued was now the goal (Sarker & Khan, 2013). As the complexity of health care systems increased, it has become necessary for nursing management to evolve with the changes to maintain employee satisfaction, pursue quality care, and improve outcomes. A transformation to a systems approach management model was recently embraced by health care that integrates the relationships of the professional caregivers, links the clinical and support services, and sustains the work of the organization to achieve safety and quality outcomes (O'Grady & Malloch, 2016).

The role of management using a systems approach means matching the mission of the organization with the resources available (O'Grady & Malloch, 2016). Important concepts to understand in a systems management model include:

- Just culture—eliminating individual blame for errors (Institute of Medicine, 2000)
- Emotional intelligence—recognize, understand, and manage emotions (Marquis & Huston, 2015)
- Empowerment—control over work activities, competence (Boaman & Laschinger, 2014)
- Advocacy—supporting others to make informed decisions (Marquis & Huston, 2015)

Management in any system is a complex process. The manager must possess skills to protect patients, empower staff, and recognize personnel and clinical challenges that could lead to conflict. Leadership skills are necessary for a manager to be successful. At this point, it is important to point out that the terms "leadership" and "management" are many times used interchangeably. However, the concepts are very different in the realm of contemporary health care systems. Management is viewed as maintaining the status quo, planning, budgeting, problem solving, and organizing the unit. Management of care is directed by someone in an assigned position. Managers who possess effective leadership skills become successful in meeting the expectations of the patients, personnel, and their unit.

Leadership is viewed as defining a vision, encouraging and instigating change, and creating long-term goals for the organization (O'Grady & Malloch, 2016). Leaders can emerge in an informal or formal position. Formal leaders who have management skills are better able to assimilate the complex details and numerous projects that are in the scope of their role. Health care values both roles. As the care delivery processes continue to change and advance, managers and leaders need to have a wide variety of skills to meet all of the challenges facing health care in the future.

Clinical Aspects

ASSESSMENT

Managing a clinical unit usually involves 24-hour accountability for the care of the patients and the management of the staff. Factors considered by mangers during the decision-making process include: (a) patient care, (b) personnel, and (c) resources (finances and people).

NURSING INTERVENTIONS, MANAGEMENT, AND IMPLICATIONS

Each decision made by the manager has the potential to impact patient care so managers must be knowledgeable, informed, and flexible. In making decisions, nurse managers consider the factors of patient care, personnel, and resources.

The patient is the central focus of health care, and management can have a significant influence on patient outcomes and practice issues (Fleiszer, Semenic, Ritchie, Richer, & Denis, 2016). Patient safety and satisfaction are key components of the health care process. Managing patient care using the Quality and Safety Education for Nurses (QSEN) competencies allows for an organized and individualized process to avoid errors and improve outcomes (Sherwood & Zomorodi, 2014). The six QSEN competencies include patient-centered care, safety, teamwork and collaboration, evidence-based practice, quality improvement, and informatics. Used as a clinical framework, the QSEN competencies provide management with a structure to offer care that aligns with a systems approach to health care delivery.

In regard to the management factor of personnel, staff caring for patients need guidance and support in completing their clinical duties. Management has the responsibility and authority to provide a safe work environment and to encourage the growth and development of the clinical teams. Communication, conflict management, delegation, and decision making are skills that management should model and participate in. As the professional staff and support team engage with each other and the patients nurse managers should model and participate in communication, conflict management, delegation, and decision making. Effectively managing personnel issues and providing opportunities for staff to work to their potential has been shown to have a positive effect on staff outcomes and job satisfaction (Asamani, Naab, & Ofei, 2016).

Resource management can be the most challenging responsibility for the nurse manager. It includes finances (budgets), people (staffing), and the physical plant (work environment). Management continually prepares, monitors, and adjusts these resources based on patient census and acuity. Equipment and supplies are assessed for needs and they are kept in appropriate working order.

OUTCOMES

The three factors (patient care, personnel, and resources) provide a framework for evaluating the effectiveness of nursing management. Patient care can be evaluated through assessment of internal and external standards and benchmarks for quality and safety, such as patient experience indicators, patient health outcomes, and cost–benefit analyses. Outcomes of effective resource management can include efficient workflow, a positive work environment for staff, and creation of a culture of caring and quality. The nurse manager leads participation in organizational initiatives to improve processes and outcomes based on results of evaluation.

Summary

Providing quality health care today is a challenge. Management is a process that involves providing safe patient care, supporting health care professional teams, and maximizing resources to create a healthy work environment. Done well, management has a direct impact on job satisfaction, staff retention, and improved patient outcomes (Asamani et al., 2016).

American Organization of Nurse Executives. (2015). *AONE nurse manager competencies*. Chicago, IL: Author.

Asamani, J. A., Naab, F., & Ofei, A. M. A. (2016). Leadership styles in nursing management: Implications for staff outcomes. *Journal of Health Sciences*, 6(1), 23–36.

Boaman, S., & Laschinger, H. (2014). Engaging new nurses: The role of psychological capital and workplace empowerment. *Journal of Research in Nursing*, 20(4), 265–277.

Fleiszer, A. R., Semenic, S. E., Ritchie , J. A., Richer, M., & Denis, J. (2016). Nursing unit leaders' influence on the long-term sustainability of evidence-based practice improvements. *Journal of Nursing Management*, 24, 309–318. doi:10.1111/jonm.12320

Institute of Medicine. (2000). *To err is human: Building a safer health system*. Washington, DC: National Academies Press.

Marquis, B. L., & Huston, C. J. (2015). *Leadership roles and management functions in nursing: Theory and application* (8th ed.). Philadelphia, PA: Wolters Kluwer/Lippincott Williams and Wilkins.

O'Grady, T. P., & Malloch, K. (2016). *Person of the leader: The capacity to lead Leadership in nursing practice: Changing the landscape of health care* (2nd ed., pp. 87–126). Massachusetts, MA: Jones & Bartlett Learning.

Pihlainen, V., Kivinen, T., & Lammintakanen, J. (2016). Management and leadership competence in hospitals: A systematic literature review. *Leadership in Health Services*, 29(1), 95–110.

Sarker, S. I., & Khan, M. R. A. (2013). Classical and neoclassical approaches to management: An overview. *IOSR Journal of Business and Management*, 14(6), 1–5.

Sherwood, G., & Zomorodi, M. (2014). A new mindset for quality and safety: The QSEN competencies redefine nurses' roles in practice. *Nephrology Nursing Journal*, 41(1), 15–23.

■ NURSING PROCESS: SYSTEMS APPROACH

Shanina C. Knighton
Aniko Kukla
Mary A. Dolansky

Overview

Moving the nursing process to a systems approach is the key to competency in the delivery of high-quality and safe nursing care. The Institute of Medicine (IOM) has consistently advised that nurses be prepared to lead in all aspects of health care (IOM, 2003, 2011). In 2005, nurse leaders from academia, research, and clinical practice responded to the 2003 IOM report, *Health Professions Education: A Bridge to Quality*, through the Quality and Safety Education for Nurses (QSEN) project funded by the Robert Wood Johnson Foundation. Six QSEN competencies were created and disseminated: patient-centered care, teamwork and collaboration, evidence-based practice, quality improvement, informatics, and safety (Cronenwett et al., 2007). The competencies include knowledge, skills, and attitude (KSAs) dimensions that guide their implementation in both academia and practice through routes such as residency programs, nursing practice models, textbooks, clinical ladder programs, and performance appraisals. Today, the QSEN project has evolved into The Quality and Safety Education for Nurses Institute, an international forum that addresses health care improvement by providing quality and safety competencies for nurses at both the undergraduate, graduate, and practice levels (QSEN, 2016). Implementation of the KSAs of the QSEN competencies requires that nurses incorporate a systems approach into the nursing process.

Background

Nurses are comfortable using the nursing process to provide care tailored to the individual patient. However, they less often practice care that is congruent with the health care system. Specifically, they lack awareness about how the care of the individual patient influences patient population outcomes. The paradigm shift in nurses' thinking from individual patient-focused care to systems-focused care requires integration of critical thinking and systems thinking of frontline nurses (Dolansky & Moore, 2013). Systems thinking includes the examination of the cause and effect of complex problems to find solutions that improve the components of the greater whole (Stalter et al., 2016). Evidence supporting strategies on how to better engage nurses in systems thinking related to the quality of care is emerging (Phillips & Stalter, 2016; Phillips, Statler, Mckee, & Dolansky, 2016). In the following section, the QSEN competencies are described in the phases of the nursing process to illustrate the moving from the care of the individual to care about the system.

Clinical Aspects

ASSESSMENT

During the assessment phase of the nursing process, nurses collect and analyze data that includes information about the psychological, physiological, socioeconomical, spiritual, and cultural well-being of the patient. The patient-centered care QSEN competency provides frontline nurses with the KSAs to see the patient and/or caregiver as a full partner in the delivery of high-quality and safe care. Concerns are documented from the patient's perspective and expanded to consider how the patient and family concerns affect the system. The frontline nurse assesses the concerns of one patient and the system for areas of improvement such as processes and policies. Individual care assessments expand to care delivery models by assessing the ethical implications, quality, safety, cost, communication needs, and barriers from a patient's standpoint.

NURSING INTERVENTIONS, MANAGEMENT, AND IMPLICATIONS

During the *diagnosis phase* of the nursing process, the nurse's clinical judgment about the patient's response to actual or potential health conditions or needs is stated as a nursing diagnosis. For example, the nursing diagnosis of *fear and anxiety* can be related to the unfamiliar environment, lack of understanding of illness or disease process, financial concerns, or feelings of confinement. The evidence-based practice QSEN competency provides the KSAs to help nurses differentiate between evidence-based knowledge and clinical opinion, and helps determine whether the nurse's clinical judgment/rationale (nursing diagnoses) is appropriate. Systems thinking during the time of nursing diagnoses requires the use of evidence-based practice for accurate judgment about individual care and the system as a whole. For example, the nurse would assess what system changes are necessary to ensure that nurses deliver evidence-based care so that high-quality and safe care is given at all times.

During the *planning phase*, the nurse is expected to set measurable and achievable short- and long-range goals for the patient. The *quality-improvement* QSEN competency ensures that the nurse set short- and long-range goals to improve outcomes of care processes and test change. The nurse sets goals or aim statements that are specific, measurable, achievable, realistic, and timely (SMART) such as *the patient (individual care) and patients on the unit experience a reduction in fear/anxiety as evidenced by a 40% reduction of fear anxiety assessments from baseline to the last day of hospitalization.* Moving to the systems approach, measurement of fear/anxiety can be collected daily on all patients on the unit and recorded in the electronic medical record. This quality-improvement data strategy moves nurses to examine fear and anxiety using data-analytic strategies, such as control charts, to impact system improvements.

In the *treatment phase* of the nursing process, action steps are taken to meet the main objective of continuity of care. The *quality-improvement* QSEN competency facilitates the use of data for monitoring the outcomes of care processes and uses improvement methods to design and test change. Moving the nursing process to a systems approach includes the quality-improvement action steps of plan, do, study, and act (PDSA). PDSA cycles comprise the interventions and align with the nursing diagnoses/planning (SMART statement). Nurses can measure the effectiveness of the interventions over time using measurement tools such as run chart and control chart. For example, for patients with fear and anxiety, nurses can keep track of the implemented environmental changes and use process measures to determine whether any change has occurred. The QSEN competency of safety includes K, S, and A, which help minimize risk to patients and providers by monitoring individual performance and system effectiveness. Examples of strategies to promote safety include root cause analyses, personal accountability, the value of the nurses' role in preventing errors, check lists, error reporting, and memory reliance reduction.

The teamwork and collaboration inherent in QSEN competency are essential for the treatment phase. Nursing care is moved from intraprofessional teams to interprofessional teams to foster open communication, establish and maintain mutual respect, and share decision making with the main objective of achieving quality patient care. Nurses learn to communicate with members of the health care team openly; gain knowledge about roles, accountability, and scope of practice; and coordinate care with appropriate care team members resulting in fewer medical errors and enhanced patient care. They also acknowledge key interprofessional partners necessary to implement system change.

During the implementation/treatment phase, the care documented in the patient's record is used to evaluate the effectiveness of interventions, however, the QSEN competency *safety* advises the nurses on how to measure safety at the system level. KSAs emphasize timely documentation of nursing care and use of checklists, co-signatures, and communication handoff tools before and during the implementation of the interventions. For example, clinical competencies are based on checklists and guidelines. Nurses gain an understanding of why individual documentation is important to the systems and how the actions impact quality, safety, and costs.

OUTCOMES

During the *evaluation phase* of the nursing process, the patient's status and effectiveness of nursing care are continuously evaluated. QSEN competencies help nurses to see how their interventions affect the patient and to understand the interconnectedness of the patient-delivered intervention to unit outcomes. The QSEN competency of *informatics* serves as an important tool in the evaluation of outcomes, especially at the system level. Furthermore, it facilitates nurses' utility of information and technology in communication, error mitigation, and decision-making support. For example, nurses can use the nursing process and competencies to create, evaluate, and influence the use of documentation templates in electronic health records on workflow. A nurse, armed with the QSEN competencies when caring for patients, might recognize that some key parts of the pain documentation are missing from the pain reevaluation template. The nurse gathers similar experiences from colleagues and approaches the documentation workflow committee to process change that impacts the system and not just the individual patient. Frontline nurses, with the use of QSEN competencies, view the system as a tool to improve patient care instead of an institution that provides care.

Summary

The QSEN competencies provide nurses with a toolbox for expanding the nursing process from the care of the individual to care of the system. Over the past 12 years, the QSEN.org website has been used by more than 80,000 nurses to learn about quality and safety, as students and frontline nurses taught to "treat the underlying cause." To improve health care, "treating the underlying cause" must expand beyond examining the primary cause of illness in a specific patient, to addressing the fundamental causes of system failures that have led or can lead to errors and poor quality care.

Although it is difficult to predict exactly what the future of health care entails, it is important to prepare all health care professionals to participate in health care improvement efforts at the systems level. In alignment with health care improvement efforts, systems science has uncovered what it means for the 21st century health care provider to function as an authentic, patient-centered navigator in interdependent health systems that require the expanded and integrated thinking of all health care professionals (Gonzalo et al., 2015). Therefore, there is a compelling need to expand the contributions of nurses and optimize the scope of practice of nurses in acute-care practice settings to function as leaders of health care quality and safety. Altering the nursing process, supported by the QSEN competencies, to address both individual care and the systems of care leads to the provision of high-quality and safe care for all.

Cronenwett, L., Sherwood, G., Barnsteiner, J., Disch, J., Johnson, J., Mitchell, P., . . . Warren, J. (2007). Quality and safety education for nurses. *Nursing Outlook*, 55(3), 122–131.

Dolansky, M. A., & Moore, S. M. (2013). Quality and safety in nursing education: The key is systems thinking. *Online Journal of Issues in Nursing*, 18(3). doi:10.3912/OJIN .Vol18No03Man01

Gonzalo, J. D., Haidet, P., Papp, K. K., Wolpaw, D. R., Moser, E., Wittenstein, R. D., & Wolpaw, T. (2015). Educating for the 21st-century health care system: An interdependent framework of basic, clinical, and systems sciences. *Academic Medicine*, 92(1), 35–39. doi:10.1097/ ACM.0000000000000951

Institute of Medicine. (2003). Health professions education: A bridge to quality. Retrieved from https://www .nap.edu/catalog/10681/health-professions-education -a-bridge-to-quality

Institute of Medicine. (2011). *The future of nursing: Leading change, advancing health*. Washington, DC: National Academies Press.

Phillips, J. M., & Stalter, A. M. (2016). Integrating systems thinking into nursing education. *Journal of Continuing Education in Nursing*, 47(9), 395–397.

Phillips, J. M., Statler, A., Mckee, G., & Dolansky, M. A. (2016). Fostering future leadership in quality and safety in healthcare through systems thinking. *Journal of Professional Nursing*, 32(1), 15–24.

Quality and Safety Education for Nurses Institute. (2016). Project overview: The evolution of the Quality and Safety Education for Nurses (QSEN). Retrieved from http://qsen.org/about-qsen/project-overview

Stalter, A. M., Phillips, J. M., Ruggiero, J. S., Scardaville, D. L., Merriam, D., Dolansky, M. A., . . . Winegardner, S. (2016). A concept analysis of systems thinking. *Nursing Forum*. Advance online publication. doi:10.1111/ nuf.12196

■ PATIENT EXPERIENCE

Catherine S. Koppelman

Overview

Patient experience of care is important to the mission of health care organizations and providers of care. Studies show a positive relationship among patient experience, patient safety, and clinical effectiveness (Doyle, Lennon, & Bell, 2013). Patient experience outcomes are now publically reported by the federal government and tied to provider payment. In hospitals, patient satisfaction survey questions include nursing care-related measures that speak about what patients want and need from the nurses.

Background

Historically, hospitals voluntarily contracted with survey vendors to internally measure patient satisfaction outcomes dating back to 1985 (Siegrist, 2013). Subsequently, as an outgrowth of the Quality and Patient Safety movement across the United States, the Centers for Medicare & Medicaid Services (CMS) began to include patient satisfaction in its transparency and payment reforms. CMS collaborated with the Agency for Healthcare Research and Quality (AHRQ) to develop the first CMS patient satisfaction survey for hospitals known as the *Hospital Consumer Assessment of Healthcare Providers and Systems (HCAHPS)* in 2002 (CMS, 2014a). This instrument was approved by the National Quality Forum, deployed to organizations, and the results were reported by CMS for the first time in 2008. Then, the Affordable Care Act of 2010 tied quality and patient satisfaction outcomes to reimbursement. This led to a practice known as *value-based purchasing* that changed payment based on services provided to payment based on performance and improvement in outcomes (CMS, 2014a).

Comprehensive payment reforms at CMS began in 2013 with the intent to focus on the quality of care and the experience of the patient, as well as the services provided. Patient satisfaction was a component of the outcomes measured (CMS, 2014a). This measure accounts for 30% of the payment at risk. Payment at risk is based on a percentage of the inpatient prospective payment that is held in reserve until the outcomes are determined. Hospitals can earn a higher, lower, or full payment based on performance on these measures and improved performance over time (CMS, 2017).

In the current version of the survey, 18 items address patient satisfaction, and 10 items are publically reported (CMS, 2014b). All measures included in the HCAHPS survey are tracked over a rolling four quarters for patients who chose the highest ratings on the survey questions (CMS, 2014a). Typically, hospitals survey all adult patients after discharge from the hospital to home. The HCAHPS survey is one of many surveys from AHRQ collectively called *Consumer Assessment of Healthcare Providers and Systems* (*CAHPS*; CMS, 2014a). These CAHPS surveys now include the entire continuum of care sites, including doctor's offices, ambulatory surgery centers, dialysis, home care, and postacute facilities. The goal is to ensure quality care and patient satisfaction across the continuum of care and to link payment to performance. The practice of increasing the percentage of all Medicare payments based on pay for performance methodologies is expected to continue (CMS, 2014a).

Clinical Aspects

ASSESSMENT

Unlike patient safety and quality-improvement efforts, there is strong limited evidence to drive meaningful patient satisfaction interventions. This science is in the infancy stage. Many health care organizations learn "best practice" by participating in collaboratives with high-performing hospitals and rely on publications in the literature that as yet lack rigor and methodologic control. HCAHPS survey questions relative to nursing care provide insights into what patients consider to be important in a hospital experience. The majority of the 10 publicly reported items relate to nursing responsibilities.

NURSING INTERVENTIONS, MANAGEMENT, AND IMPLICATIONS

"Nursing communication" is the most influential measure concerning overall patient experience in the hospital. This measure has three subquestions, which include how often the nurses "treated me with courtesy and respect," "listened carefully," and "explained things in a way I could understand." The rating scale is (never, sometimes, usually, and always; CMS, 2014b). All three of these items address the nature of the nurse–patient relationship. Communication and empathy are the basis of a therapeutic relationship (Koloroutis, 2004). Strong interpersonal skills as well as an understanding of patient engagement processes in partnering with patients and families in the plan of care are fundamental to a patient feeling respected, understood, and knowledgeable in making decisions. According to the Institute of Patient Family Centered Care (IPFCC) the "sit down" round is emerging in the literature as a powerful way to convey a message of intent and connection to the person in the bed (IPFCC, 2015, p. 1). To be effective patient advocates, nurses need to attend to the patient's story and preferences. Teaching and mentoring, as well as the primacy of the therapeutic connection among nurses, patients, and families are critical to the profession and to those we serve. They must be introduced in nursing education and reinforced in practice.

OUTCOMES

Some of the best practices developed to promote patient safety may apply to efforts to improve patient satisfaction as well. For example, hourly rounds, which have been demonstrated to improve safety, have the added benefit of improving patient satisfaction as measured by several HCAHPS questions. These include "When using the call button, did you get help as soon as you needed it?" "Did you get help to the bathroom or the bedpan as soon as you needed it?" and "How often was your pain controlled?" Studies show a decrease in falls as well as call-light usage because of the proactive and regular visits of the nurses on hourly rounds (Meade, 2006). Timely interventions are based on reliably completing hourly rounds. This includes nursing supervision and accountability of completed delegated tasks to unlicensed personnel. Interdisciplinary collaboration on pain management effectiveness is needed to develop individualized plans for pain based on current standards and regular assessments of pain control.

HCAHPS questions on discharge preparation are drawn from care transition evidence-based interventions (Dreyer, 2014). Patients need to understand why they are taking specific medication as well as the side effects of medications. These are also direct questions on the HCAHPS survey. Teach-back methods have been found to be more effective in a patient's level of knowledge and self-care capability to perform functions properly (AHRQ, 2015). Discharge planning should include questions about the need for "help at home" and "what to do and look for in symptoms" after hospitalization. Teaching needs to be reinforced with written materials. These are all questions on the survey, but more important, they are fundamental standards for effective patient education (Dreyer, 2014).

Sustainability of effective nursing interventions and positive patient experience outcomes also relies on the clinical environment in which the nurses practice, as well as a patient-centered culture in the organization. Nurses need the equipment and resources to provide the care and the time with the patients. Leadership rounds are emerging as a best practice to reinforce a culture of patient centeredness. Nursing leadership rounds involving the chief nursing officer (CNO) to the firstline unit nurse managers on a normative basis have been shown to improve patient satisfaction outcomes (Morton, Brekhus, Reynolds, & Dykes, 2014). Such rounds are a powerful means of reinforcing the importance of the patient experience of care and nurses' experiences in providing that care.

Summary

There is a positive relationship between the patient experience of care and safe quality care delivery. This importance has been elevated across the health care industry by public reporting and payment reform for performance and improvement in patient satisfaction outcomes. Patient surveys include perceptions of nursing care. Nurses can learn so much from patient feedback so as to improve the outcomes of care and overall patient experience of care.

Agency for Healthcare Research and Quality. (2015). Use the teach-back method: Tool 5. Retrieved from: https://www.ahrq.gov/professionals/quality-patient-safety/quality-resources/tools/literacy-toolkit/healthlittoolkit2-tool5.html

Centers for Medicare & Medicaid Services. (2014a). HCAHPS: patients' perspective of care survey. Retrieved from https://www.cms.gov/Medicare/Quality-Initiatives-Patient-Assessment-instruments/HospitalQualityInits/HospitalHCAHPS.html

Centers for Medicare & Medicaid Services. (2014b). HCAHPS FAQ. Retrieved from https://www.cms.gov/Medicare/Quality-Initiatives-Patient-Assessment-Instruments/HospitalQualityInits/Downloads/HospitalHCAHPS FAQFactSheet201007.pdf

Centers for Medicare & Medicaid Services. (2017). Hospital value based purchasing. Retrieved from https://cms.gov/Medicare/Quality-Initiatives-Patient-Instruments/hospital-value- based-purchasing/ondes.html

Doyle, C., Lennon, L., & Bell, D. (2013). A systematic review of evidence on the link between patient experience and clinical safety and effectiveness. *BMJ OPEN, 2013*(1), e001570.

Dreyer, T. (2014). Care transitions: best practices and evidence based programs. Retrieved from http://www.chrt.org/publication/care-transition-best-practice-evidencebased-programs

Institute for Patient and Family Centered Care. (2015). Applying patient- and family-centered concepts to bedside rounds. Retrieved from https://www.ipfcc.org/resources/PH_RD- Applying_PFCC_Rounds_012009.pdf

Koloroutis, M. (Ed.). (2004). *Relationship-based care: A model for transforming practice*. Minneapolis, MN: Creative Healthcare Management.

Meade, C. (2006). Effects of nursing rounds on patients' call light use, satisfaction, and safety. *American Journal of Nursing, 106*(9), 60.

Morton, J. C., Brekhus, J., Reynolds, M., & Dykes, A. K. (2014). Improving the patient experience through nurse leader rounds. *Patient Experience Journal, 1*(2), 10.

Siegrist, R. B. (2013). Illuminating the art of medicine, patient satisfaction: History, myths and misperceptions. *AMA Journal of Ethics, 15*(11), 982–987.

■ POPULATION HEALTH

Deborah F. Lindell

Overview

Population health is defined as "the health outcomes of a group of individuals, including the distribution of such outcomes within the group" (Kindig & Stoddardt, 2003, p. 381). "Methods of population health allow health care professionals and systems of health care to assess the health status of, manage, and evaluate the effect of targeted programs on the health of populations at particular risk of poor health outcomes" (Kindig & Stoddardt, 2003, p. 381).

The concept of population health as a type of health that can be measured was first explored in 1994 (Evans, Barer, & Marmor, 1994). Citing several large-scale longitudinal studies, the authors expressed concern regarding the increasing focus on the health care system determinant (or biomedical paradigm) and less attention to the key influence of the other determinants of health, particularly social factors. In the following years, the concept of population health and need to consider all determinants of health received increasing attention. In 2003, Kindig and Stoddardt addressed the lack of clarity as to the meaning of population health by proposing the definition noted earlier, and the model of population health used widely today.

Background

Each year, nearly 900,000 (or 63%) of Americans die prematurely from the five leading causes of death—heart disease, cancer, chronic lower respiratory diseases, stroke, and unintentional injuries. Yet 20% to 40% of the deaths from each cause could be prevented. (Centers for Disease Control and Prevention [CDC], 2014, para. 1)

The burden of these health issues impacts not only mortality and morbidity but the quality of life and the rapidly rising, and unsustainable, financial costs of health care. Since the mid-20th century, tremendous strides in the treatment of disease have contributed to increasing the average life span of Americans.

However, it has become clear that attention must shift from acute, rescue-focused treatment of illness to health promotion and prevention and control of the disease. Health systems are directly impacted by health policies, standards, and regulations aimed at controlling costs and improving access to quality and outcomes of health care. In response, health systems are directing efforts toward improving the health of high-risk populations in addition to the traditional focus on episodic care of individuals. This entry discusses the evolution of the concept of population health, its role in today's health care systems, and its relevance for nursing.

In population health, health and illness are viewed as influenced by not just biologic factors but multiple, interacting determinants "the range of personal, social, economic, and environmental factors that influence health status" (Office of Disease Prevention and Health Promotion, 2016a, para 2). In *Healthy People 2020* objectives (Office of Disease Prevention and Health Promotion, 2016a), the determinants are grouped into five categories of policy making, social factors, health services, individual behavior, and biology and genetics.

In the United States, the goals of *Healthy People 2020* (Office of Disease Prevention and Health Promotion, 2016b) reflect the increasing attention to population health: "Attain high-quality, longer lives free of preventable disease, disability, injury, and premature death; achieve health equity, eliminate disparities, and improve the health of all groups; and create social and physical environments that promote good health for all" (para. 2). The CDC established a population health division and directs particular attention to the influence of the social determinants of health on disparities in access to health care and health outcomes.

In recent years, the term "population health" has been linked to the cost of health care. In 2007, the Institute for Healthcare Improvement (IHI) reported on the extremely high costs of health care with poorer outcomes in the United States than in many other countries and that the unacceptable concerns with safety and quality could only be addressed through attention to population health. The Triple Aim framework, an approach to optimizing health system performance, was introduced, which includes three dimensions: population health, experience of care (the Institute of Medicine's six elements of quality health care), and per capita cost (IHI, 2017). The Affordable Care Act incorporates the IHI's view of population health in that it incorporates programs aimed at improving access to care, reducing inequity of health outcomes, and promoting affordable, cost-effective care.

Clinical Aspects

Health care systems have responded to the initiatives stimulated by Kindig and Stoddardt, the IHI, ACA, and others such as The Joint Commission, Medicare, Medicaid, and other payers. Specialists in the emerging field of population health assessment and management are using information systems to identify and describe populations who use proportionally high amounts of services with poorer outcomes; they also plan, implement, and evaluate programs aimed at addressing determinants (especially social) impacting their health and use of resources, reducing use of costly services, and improving health outcomes.

Nursing can play key roles in these initiatives. According to the National Advisory Council on Nurse Education and Practice (NACNEP; 2016), nurses practicing in all health care settings should have a basic understanding of population health, roles, and expectations of health care systems regarding population health and of emerging opportunities for nurses in population health management.

ASSESSMENT

The scientific methods of epidemiology and bio-statistics are used to measure population health. Information health systems provide rapidly expanding interhealth system data to facilitate assessment of population health. Assessment includes the determinants of health, particularly the social determinant, as well as outcomes of population health. For example, in the IHI Triple Aim framework measures include life expectancy; mortality rates; health and functional status; disease burden (the incidence and/or prevalence of chronic disease); and behavioral and physiological factors such as smoking, physical activity, diet, blood pressure, body mass index (BMI), and cholesterol (as measured via a health risk appraisal; IHI, 2017).

An example of population health assessment is a "study of food insecurity in patients with high rates of inpatient hospitalization ('super-utilizers')," which found that 55% of the participants were either food insecure (30%) or marginally food secure (25%), 75% were unable to shop for food, and 58% were unable to prepare their food (Phipps, Singletary, Cooblall, Hares, & Braitman, 2016, p. 414).

Nursing's core practice includes a holistic perspective of health and a focus on health promotion and disease prevention. Direct care nurses should assess for social, emotional, and spiritual factors as well as biologic factors influencing health. For example, smoking is the leading cause of preventable death. Direct care nurses are the front line in meeting requirements, tied to reimbursement of health care organizations to ensure each inpatient is screened for smoking and tobacco use and cessation intervention provided as indicated.

NURSING INTERVENTIONS, MANAGEMENT, AND IMPLICATIONS

Nurses in direct care roles in inpatient and ambulatory settings have a responsibility to address all determinants assessed as influencing a patient's health. Interventions include strategies, such as motivational interviewing, to facilitate health promotion, disease prevention, and self-management of chronic illness; and referrals to appropriate resources such as social workers and programs such as smoking cessation in the organization or community.

There are also exciting opportunities for nurses in emerging system-level, population-focused roles such as population health management, transitional care coordination, and quality improvement. Doctor of nursing practice programs are evolving as well to prepare nurses for these roles. In population-health management, six strategies have been identified by which health care systems can build infrastructure to support population health: "(a) value-based reimbursement, (b) seamless care across all settings, (c) proactive and systematic patient education, (d) workplace competencies and education on population health, (e) integrated, comprehensive HIT that supports risk stratification of patients with real-time accessibility, and (f) mature community partnerships to collaborate on community-based solutions" (Health Research & Education Trust, 2014, p. 3). Nurses can play instrumental roles in these initiatives. For example, the Commonwealth Fund reported that "supportive housing programs that offer shelter to the homeless and a variety of medical and social services have had a dramatic impact on health outcomes and costs in communities that have implemented them" (Hostetter & Klein, 2014, para. 1).

OUTCOMES

Epidemiological and biostatistical approaches are foundational to understanding of population health and measuring the outcomes of population health management programs. Examples of possible metrics include (a) summary measures, (b) inequality measures, (c) health status, (d) psychological state, (e) ability to function, (f) access to health care, (g) clinical preventive services, and (h) cost of care (HRET, 2014, p. 3).

Summary

In "Reaching the End Game: Total Population Health," Pamela Cipriano noted,

Nurses are in a prime position to carry out the reconstruction of a new care delivery model that becomes a new business model. We only have to know when to help tip the seesaw in the direction of promoting and maintaining health. It will require us to change, too. (Cipriano, 2014, para. 8)

Centers for Disease Control and Prevention. (2014). Up to 40 percent of annual deaths from each of five leading US causes are preventable. Retrieved from https://www.cdc.gov/media/releases/2014/p0501-preventable-deaths.html

Cipriano, P. (2014). Reaching the end game: Total population health. *American Nurse Today*, 9(6). Retrieved from https://www.americannursetoday.com/reaching-the -end-game-total-population-health. Copyright © 2017. HealthCom Media. All rights reserved. AmericanNurse Today.com

Evans, R., Barer, M., & Marmor, T. (1994) *Why Are some people healthy and others not?-The determinants of health of populations.* New York, NY: Aldine de Gruyter.

Health Research & Educational Trust. (2014). *The second curve of population health.* Chicago, IL: Author. Retrieved from http://www.hpoe.org/pophealthsecondcurve

Hostetter, M., & Klein, S. (2014). In focus: Using housing to improve health and reduce the costs of caring for the homeless. Retrieved from http://www.commonwealth fund.org/publications/newsletters/quality-matters/2014/ october-november/in-focus

Institute for Healthcare Improvement. (2017). The IHI Triple Aim Initiative. Retrieved from http://www.ihi.org/ Engage/Initiatives/TripleAim/Pages/default.aspx

Kindig D., & Stoddart, G. (2003) What is population health? *American Journal of Public Health, 93*(3), 300–383.

National Advisory Council on Nurse Education and Practice. (2016). *Preparing nurses for new roles in population health Management.* Washington, DC: Health Resources and Services Administration.

Office of Disease Prevention and Health Promotion. (2016a). Determinants of health. In *Healthy People 2020.* Retrieved from https://www.healthypeople.gov/2020/about/ foundation-health-measures/Determinants-of-Health

Office of Disease Prevention and Health Promotion. (2016b). Framework. In *Healthy People 2020.* Retrieved from https://www.healthypeople.gov/sites/default/files/ HP2020Framework.pdf

Phipps, E., Singletary S., Cooblall, C., Hares, H., & Braitman, L. (2016). Food insecurity in patients with high hospital utilization. *Population Health Management, 19*(6), 414– 420. doi:10.1089/pop.2015.0127

■ QUALITY IMPROVEMENT

Aniko Kukla
Mary A. Dolansky
Shanina C. Knighton

Overview

The quality-improvement (QI) movement began in the United States in the early 1990s contemporaneous with the total quality management movement in business. QI gained momentum after repeated reports of inadequate quality and safety (Kelly, Vottero, & Christie-McAuliffe, 2014). QI is defined as, "the combined and unceasing efforts of everyone—healthcare professionals, patients, and their families, researchers, payers, planners and educators—to make the changes that will lead to better patient outcomes (health), better system performance (care) and better professional development (learning)" (Batalden & Davidoff, 2007, p. 2). As a response to the quality movement in health care, the Quality and Safety Education for Nurses (QSEN) initiative set out to transform nursing education by implementing quality and safety competencies to ensure that nurses had the knowledge, skills, and attitudes to improve their work. The QI competency is "Using data to monitor the outcomes of care processes and using improvement methods to design and test changes to continuously improve the quality and safety of health care systems" (Cronenwett et al., 2007, p. 127).

Background

The concern with quality in health care dates back to the late 19th to early 20th centuries, when Dr. Ernest Codman tracked his patients' posthospitalization outcomes and Florence Nightingale used Polar diagrams to record patient outcomes. These early efforts focused on quality but not on continuous quality improvement. In the 1960s, attention moved to identifying underperforming physicians. QI efforts during that time focused on performance below minimal standards and methods, such as mentoring, to correct consequential practice habits (Kelly et al., 2014).

Governing agencies began to promote uniformity of standards of physicians across the country. The Joint Commission (TJC; 2017) was founded in 1951 as a collaborative effort among several hospital and medical associations. Today, the overall number of health care organizations accredited and certified by the TJC is more than 21,000.

In the 1970s and 1980s, the focus of hospital quality switched from peer review of individual physicians to review of the performance of a group of physicians and hospitals by implementing standard practice guidelines. In the early 2000s, TJC's emphasis shifted from measuring and improving the outcomes of evidence-based care to hospitals seeking accreditation and a requirement to report core patient quality performance measures. The Centers for Medicare & Medicaid Services (CMS) and various insurance companies also started to require proof of accreditation before reimbursement occurred. In 2003, CMS implemented the Hospital Quality Initiative (HQI), which involved health care agencies voluntarily reporting their performance on the set of core quality measures onto a public website (CMS, 2013). In addition, in 2007, the CMS instituted a program in which 2% of reimbursement to hospitals was withheld and paid out based on health care agencies meeting predefined benchmarks, and care provided as a result of medication errors was not reimbursed any longer. In 2013, the Hospital Value-Based Purchasing Program was implemented, and incentives are now paid by CMS to hospitals if certain benchmarks and desired outcomes are met.

The most commonly used QI models and methods in health care are the Donabedian model, Deming's framework, and the Six Sigma and Six Sigma Lean models. Avedis Donabedian created a model more than 40 years ago that is still widely used and addresses structure "the condition under which care is provided," process "the activities that constitute health care," and outcome "changes (desirable or undesirable) in individuals and populations that can be attributed to health care" (Donabedian, 2003, p. 46). The structure can be anything that supports the delivery of care: staffing, skill mix, educational level of staff, resources, supplies, budget, and so forth. *Process* refers to how the care is delivered: through evidence-based practice guidelines, nursing process, standards of care, pathways, policies, staff satisfaction, and core measures. Outcomes are any measures that the hospital, staff, or outside agencies determine: hospital-acquired infections, hospital-acquired pressure injuries, fall rates, patient satisfaction, and so forth. Donabedian developed seven pillars of quality that were used in the Institute of Medicine's report, *Crossing the Quality Chasm*, which highlighted six aims for the health care system to deliver care that is safe, effective, patient-centered, timely, efficient, and equitable (Institute of Medicine, 2001; Kelly et al., 2014).

W. Edward Deming's PDSA model is frequently used in health care QI. Deming used concepts from industry, engineering, and management to create the System of Profound Knowledge, which includes an appreciation for a system, knowledge of variation, theory of knowledge, and psychology. The theory of knowledge uses PDSA cycles to rapidly test changes on a smaller scale, tweak the process if changes are necessary, and test again before the changes are implemented across a system.

The Six Sigma and Lean Six Sigma methodologies were adopted from management and applied to health care. The main goal of these models is to reduce variations in existing processes. Six Sigma is based on restricting variation to 3 standard deviations above or below the mean. The common-cause variations are observed when the data points fall in these 6 standard deviations. The steps used in Six Sigma are define, measure, analyze, improve, and control. The principles of lean methodology emphasize waste reduction in the process to increase efficiency. When the waste processes occur, nurses and other health care professionals create workarounds, and potentially, an error. Small improvements result in improved performance. Lean methods are easier to learn than the Six Sigma methods, which require statistical skills, but both models are very useful in practice (Kelly et al., 2014).

The Institute for Healthcare Improvement (IHI) uses the Model for Improvement to guide both the teaching and practice of QI. The Model for Improvement is based on three fundamental questions: What are we trying to accomplish? (creating an aim), How will we know the change is an improvement? (determining the measures), What change can we make that will result in improvement? (testing change). After the answers to these questions are determined, a continuous set of PDSA cycles is used to test the change (Ogrinc et al., 2012).

Clinical Aspects

ASSESSMENT

There is mounting pressure to produce sustainable improvement in patient outcomes, resulting in mandates for health care professionals to integrate QI methods into their daily work. QI begins with identifying a focus area. Topics studied include those mandated in national standards (such as central line-associated blood stream infections (CLABSI) as well as concerns identified at the organization, department, or nursing unit levels. If the organization is committed to continuous quality improvement, data is gathered and monitored on an ongoing basis so deviations from standards as well as improvement can be quickly identified.

NURSING INTERVENTIONS, MANAGEMENT, AND IMPLICATIONS

Best practices of QI include strategies such as using a systematic approach, forming a team of interprofessional stakeholders, gathering and analyzing data to understand the issue from diverse perspectives, and then establishing measurable aims. Based on the aims, a plan to address the issue is developed, implemented, and evaluated. As the demands to improve the safety and quality of health care intensify, nurses assume new roles in QI initiatives, and these roles require competencies related to leadership, project management, data analytics, design thinking, and innovation. As the founder of the QSEN initiative, Cronenwett stated that nurses not only need to perform patient care but also improve care (Cronenwett et al., 2007). In medicine, Batalden stated that QI is a shared responsibility among everyone from a new student nurse to physicians, nurses, and attending leaders and support staff (Ogrinc et al., 2012).

The QI movement and the QSEN initiative have raised awareness of the importance of academic–clinical partnerships to align the goals to both provide care and improve care. An example of this is the integration of graduate entry prelicensure nursing students in QI in their last semester of the program at the Frances Payne Bolton School of Nursing, Case Western Reserve University. During a leadership practicum, student nurses in teams of three to four work 1 day a week on an assigned unit with the nursing staff. The nursing students assess systems factors and implement an evidence-based QI process to measure the nursing process of care using Kamishibai cards (K-cards; Bercaw, 2013). K-cards are a tool used in daily rounding to provide real-time data and improve adherence to evidence-based protocols. This example demonstrates the power of students and staff working together to implement QI. The partnership addresses the lack of time nurses have to fully engage in QI as students contribute to the improvement efforts.

OUTCOMES

The ultimate aim of QI in health care is safe, effective, patient-centered care. Related aims include those of the particular improvement project, patient and staff satisfaction, compliance with internal and external standards, and sustainability of the organization. The extent to which the aims have been met is evaluated by ongoing monitoring and analysis of multistakeholder qualitative and quantitative data. In continuous QI, the interprofessional improvement team uses a cyclical process to plan, implement, and evaluate additional actions in response to the evaluation findings. Successful strategies may be spread throughout the organization.

Summary

The quality of care is now highly monitored by regulatory agencies and reimbursement is tied to quality outcomes. QI methods, such as the Model for Improvement, provide a structure for assessing, diagnosing, and treating the health system of care outcomes.

By incorporating the QSEN competencies into undergraduate and graduate nursing curricula and professional development initiatives, nurses can lead and sustain QI projects. A culture that incorporates continuous learning and leadership is the key to producing and sustaining high quality and safety outcomes (Frankel, Haraden, Federico, & Lenoci-Edwards, 2017).

Let the words of Donabedian (2003) guide us in our future work:

Systems awareness and systems design are important for health professionals, but they are not enough. They are enabling mechanisms only. It is the ethical dimensions of individuals that are essential to a system's success. Ultimately, the secret of quality is love. You have to love your patient; you have to love your profession, you have to love your God. If you have love, you can then work backward to monitor and improve the system. (p. 46)

Batalden P. B., & Davidoff, F. (2007). What is "quality improvement" and how can it transform healthcare? *Quality & Safety in Healthcare, 16*, 2–3.

Bercaw, R. G. (2013). *Lean, leadership for healthcare: Approaches to lean transformation.* Boca Raton, FL: CRC Press: Taylor & Francis.

Centers for Medicare & Medicaid Services. (2013). Hospital quality initiative. Retrieved from https://www.cms.gov/Medicare/Quality-Initiatives-Patient-Assessment-Instruments/HospitalQualityInits/index.html

Cronenwett, L., Sherwood, G., Barnsteiner, J., Disch, J., Johnson, J., Mitchell, P., . . . Warren, J. (2007). Quality and safety education for nurses. *Nursing Outlook, 55*(3), 122–131.

Donabedian, A. (2003). *An introduction to quality and assurance in health care* (p. 46). New York, NY: Oxford University Press.

Frankel, A., Haraden, C., Federico, F., & Lenoci-Edwards, J. A. (2017). *Framework for safe, reliable, and effective care. White paper.* Cambridge, MA: Institute for Healthcare Improvement and Safe & Reliable Healthcare.

Institute of Medicine. (2001). *Crossing the quality chasm: A new health system for the 21st century.* Washington, DC: National Academies Press.

Kelly, P., Vottero, B. A., & Christie-McAuliffe, C. A. (2014). *Introduction to quality and safety education for nurses: Core competencies.* New York, NY: Springer Publishing.

Ogrinc, G. S., Headrick, L. A., Moore, S. M., Barton, A. J., Dolansky, M. A., & Madigosky, W. S. (2012). *Fundamentals of health care improvement: A guide to improving your patient's care* (2nd ed.). Oakbrook Terrace, IL: Joint Commission Resources.

The Joint Commission. (2017). About the Joint Commission. Retrieved from https://www.jointcommission.org/about_us/about_the_joint_commission_main.aspx

What is Hospital Compare? (2017). Hospital compare. Retrieved from https://www.medicare.gov/hospitalcompare/about/what-is-HOS.html

▪ QUALITY AND SAFETY EDUCATION

Nadine M. Marchi

Overview

Prevention of errors and improvement of safety and quality are the key areas of focus in health care today. In 1999 and again in 2003, it was reported that between 44,000 and 98,000 patients in medical facilities die annually because of preventable errors (Institute of Medicine [IOM], 1999, 2003). Recent reports indicate that the incidence of preventable errors is even higher and may be the third leading cause of death in the United States (James, 2014; Makary & Daniel, 2016). One nursing response is Quality and Safety Education for Nurses (QSEN), a virtual community of nurses working to improve the safety and quality of patient care through activities in nursing education and practice.

Background

Over the past 10 years, patient advocacy groups, accreditation organizations, educational programs across professions, and the health care industry have implemented a variety of efforts aiming to reduce errors and improve quality and safety of patient care. Two examples include (a) changes in reimbursement for health care services so that they are based on the implementation of safety measures and (b) changing the culture so that when an error is made, the response is focused on learning and prevention of future errors rather than blame. A small improvement in safety was reported when after an error the emphasis was placed on eliminating the blame and encouraging patient and leadership engagement in the analysis of the error process (Wachter, 2010).

A third example is a response in nursing. From 2005 to 2012, the Robert Wood Johnson Foundation (RWJF) funded the QSEN project. The primary goal of QSEN is "to address the challenge of preparing future nurses with the knowledge, skills, and attitudes (KSAs) necessary to continuously improve the quality and safety of the health care systems in which they work" (QSEN Project Overview, 2012, para. 1). The initial principal investigator of the QSEN project was Linda Cronenwett, PhD, RN, FAAN, Dean of the University of North Carolina at Chapel Hill School of Nursing. RWJF funded four phases of QSEN from 2005 to 2012. During phases I to III, (a) the QSEN competencies (see later) with associated prelicensure and graduate-level knowledge, skills, and attitude statements were developed and published; (b) pilot schools integrated the competencies in their nursing programs; (c) the website QSEN.org was initiated; (d) an annual QSEN forum was held; (e) faculty development institutes were convened across the United States; and (f) nurses were included in the Veterans Affairs National Quality Scholars Fellowship Program. Phase IV was coordinated by the American Association of Colleges of Nursing (AACN) and offered enhancement of the graduate quality and safety competencies, free online learning modules, and graduate-level faculty development workshops.

In 2012, the QSEN initiative transitioned to the QSEN Institute and was housed at the Frances Payne Bolton School of Nursing, Case Western Reserve University. The QSEN website is an ongoing central electronic hub for the QSEN competencies, teaching strategies, and resources for faculty and nursing practice. The website is being further developed to include a variety of activities with the focus on quality and safety. In addition, the QSEN Institute continues to host an annual national forum to disseminate advances and research related to the QSEN competencies.

The IOM (2003) competencies along with broad input from nurses across the United States, were used to develop the six QSEN competencies and their definitions:

- *Patient-centered care*: Recognize the patient or designee as the source of control and a full partner in providing compassionate and coordinated care based on respect for patient's preferences, values, and needs.

- *Teamwork and collaboration*: Function effectively in nursing and interprofessional teams, fostering open communication, mutual respect, and shared decision making to achieve quality patient care.

- *Evidence-based practice (EBP)*: Integrate best current evidence with clinical expertise and patient/family preferences and values for the delivery of optimal health care.

- *Quality improvement (QI)*: Use data to monitor the outcomes of care processes and use improvement methods to design and test changes to continuously improve the quality and safety of health care systems.

■ *Safety*: Minimize the risk of harm to patients and providers through both system effectiveness and individual performance.

■ *Informatics*: Use information and technology to communicate, manage knowledge, mitigate error, and support decision making (Cronenwett et al., 2007).

Clinical Aspects

ASSESSMENT

An assessment of the quality and safety strategies to use to increase the knowledge, skills, and attitudes of students toward patient safety is a topic of many research studies. Although there are an increasing number of educational tools available to assist student learning, there is no clear indication of how involved students need to be to achieve the level of changes in knowledge, skills, and attitudes that might be expected to equate with an increased likelihood of application on graduation. The goal is to emphasize patient quality and safety in prelicensure nursing programs so that these concepts can then readily be transferred into nursing practice. The impact on clinical care of nurses who have been educated with a patient quality and safety focus has not been measured. The QSEN Institute continues to promote further nursing research and practice endeavors to improve patient quality and safety in the health care environment.

Patient quality and safety in the clinical environment can be accomplished by nurses in many aspects of patient care. The QSEN Institute can be a source of information for the nurse who is employing a quality and safety focus with patients. On the first encounter with a patient, the nurse should include quality and safety measures as part of the initial assessment. Then, using clinical reasoning, the nurse should analyze the patient situation and implement appropriate quality and safety measures. This is a crucial function of professional nursing practice and involves the entire health care team. The nurse can also become involved in the workplace with analysis and review of patient quality and safety measures to enhance overall patient care.

NURSING INTERVENTIONS, MANAGEMENT, AND IMPLICATIONS

Three main QSEN activities can assist the nurse to use quality and safety measures in clinical practice. These are the QSEN Institute National Forum, QSEN website resources for patient quality and safety, and QSEN teaching strategies. To practice nursing with a quality and safety focus, resources provided by the QSEN Institute have recommended some nursing interventions:

■ Use and verification of deep vein thrombosis prophylaxis for patients at risk

■ Prevention of pressure-injuries by performing skin assessments and initiating appropriate therapy

■ Patient teaching regarding medications so self-management of medication regimen is effective

■ Use of medication reconciliation to prevent adverse drug events

■ Use the situation, background, assessment, recommendation communication technique

■ Use Institute for Healthcare Improvement (Resar, Griffin, Haraden, & Nolan, 2012) bundles such as prevention of central line-associated bloodstream infection, prevention of obstetrical adverse events, prevention of ventilator associated pneumonia, sepsis prevention

■ Screen patients for risk for falls

■ Decrease catheter-associated urinary tract infections by monitoring patients with catheters closely

OUTCOMES

At the student level, achievement of the knowledge, skills, and attitudes (KSAs) specified in the QSEN competencies may be assessed through quantitative tests, case studies, simulation, and clinical practice. This data may be aggregated for program evaluation and, increasingly, the QSEN KSAs are being incorporated in standardized tests such as the NCLEX-RN® exam and curricula for new graduate RN residency programs.

The long-term aim is that nursing competence in the QSEN KSAs will contribute to the urgent need for improved safety and quality of patient care. Rigorous, longitudinal studies are needed to evaluate the extent to which these competencies are implemented in clinical practice and contribute to needed improvement in the six domains of healthcare quality: safe, effective, patient-centered, timely, efficient, and equitable (Agency for Healthcare Research & Quality, 2016).

Summary

Nurses are at the forefront of patient care and have a responsibility and potential to improve patient quality and safety. Many initiatives are focused on improving the quality and safety of health care. However, the QSEN Institute is a unique resource specific to nursing that is dedicated to moving patient quality and safety to the forefront of nursing practice.

Agency for Healthcare Research and Quality. (2016). The six domains of health care quality. Retrieved from https://www.ahrq.gov/professionals/quality-patient-safety/talkingquality/create/sixdomains.html

Cronenwett, L., Sherwood, G., Barnsteiner, J., Disch, J., Johnson, J., Mitchell, P., . . . Warren, J. (2007). Quality and safety education for nurses. *Nursing Outlook, 55*(3), 122–131.

Institute of Medicine. (1999). *To err is human: Building a safer healthcare system.* Washington, DC: National Academies Press.

Institute of Medicine. (2003). *Health professions education: A bridge to quality.* Washington, DC: National Academies Press.

James, J. (2014). A new, evidence-based estimate of patient harms associated with hospital care. *Journal of Patient Safety, 9*(3), 122–128. doi:10.1097/PTS.0b013e3182948a69

Makary, M. A., & Daniel, M. (2016). Medical error—The third leading cause of death in the U.S. *British Medical Journal, 353*, i2139.

Quality and Safety Education for Nurses. (2012). Project Overview: Evolution of the Quality and Safety Education for Nurses (QSEN) Initiative. Retrieved from http://qsen.org/about-qsen/project-overview

Resar, R., Griffin, F. A., Haraden, C., & Nolan, T. W. (2012). *Using care bundles to improve health care quality. IHI innovation series white paper.* Cambridge, MA: Institute for Healthcare Improvement.

Wachter, R. M. (2010). Patient safety at ten-unmistakable progress, troubling gaps. *Health Affairs, 29*(1), 165–173. doi:10.1377/hlthaff.2009.0785

■ SOCIAL DETERMINANTS OF HEALTH

Rita M. Sfiligoj

Overview

The World Health Organization (WHO) Commission on the Social Determinants of Health emphasizes that "Much of the global burden of disease and premature death is avoidable, and therefore unacceptable. It is inequitable" (WHO, 2008, p. 29). To mitigate social injustice, it is necessary to connect health care with social supports and services that address the broad range of social determinants of health (SDH) that impact the population's health and well-being (Heiman & Artiga, 2015).

SDH are conditions of the environment in which people are born, live, work, grow, play, and age that can affect and shape every aspect of their lives. The services and systems in this environment include policies, infrastructure, and other resources (WHO, 2008). An impoverished environment may lead to a compromised quality of life, including poor health, poor development, and restricted opportunities to flourish in society. The impoverishments are commonly identified as SDH and nurses see their impact every day. They care for individuals who are more susceptible to illness and those who experience complications or injury because of the influence of social determinants of health. With a complete assessment, the nurse can often associate these complications to low income, high stress, poor housing, lack of food, and/or unemployment—all social determinants of health. It is important that nurses, practicing in all settings, consider the SDH in planning and providing care.

Background

Social determinants of health include factors such as socioeconomic status, education, access to health care, transportation options, availability of community resources, social support, natural and physical environment (i.e., green space, work sites, recreational sites, and schools), housing, exposure to toxins, access to healthy food sources, and physical barriers in the community (Office of Disease Prevention and Health Promotion, 2016). Many of these factors affect the health of communities and individuals, particularly for individuals with disabilities and behavioral–mental health concerns. There is growing concern that SDH functions as both opportunities and barriers for individuals' efforts to engage in healthy behaviors (Heiman & Artiga, 2015).

Clinical Aspects

ASSESSMENT

Although physical findings, laboratory results, imaging, and history are important components of the patient assessment, the SDH is commonly overlooked. To enhance health outcomes, the nurse needs to assess each patient's SDH and determine whether they act as barriers or opportunities. The nurse, as a part of the health care team, needs to make informed and appropriate decisions about care based on this evaluation and understanding.

When obtaining a history from a patient, social details should be documented. Who does the patient live with? Does this individual have support from a caregiver in the household or the community? Can this individual afford medications? Can this individual afford food? Does this individual have to choose between eating and taking medications? Is this individual employed? What type of work does this individual do (does it require heavy lifting, standing for long periods of time, sitting at a desk)? What means of transportation are available (is transportation easily accessible)? Is this individual exposed to environmental hazards (smoke, paint fumes, lead)? In every case, the individual should be viewed holistically. There is strong, suggestive evidence that viewing an individual as more than just a system of organs, and taking into account the social context in the delivery of health care services, can have an important impact in improving health (Williams, Costa, Odunlami, & Mohammed, 2008).

NURSING INTERVENTIONS, MANAGEMENT, AND IMPLICATIONS

The nurse considers situations in which SDH impact health and other outcomes. For example, there is no known single cause for breast cancer. However, it is certain that genetics and environmental and social risk factors predispose to cancer. Furthermore, individuals in impoverished environments lack access to nutritious food, quality health care, and social support systems. As a result, their diagnoses are commonly assigned later in any illness and outcomes of cancer are likely to be more adverse (Fortune, 2016).

Child health outcomes follow a social gradient. Children who are born into families that are poor, less educated, or in poor health are more likely to develop serious chronic illness (Moore, McDonald, Carlon, & O'Rourke, 2015). Parents make choices about the quality of the environment for their children before and after birth. These choices are conditioned by SDH, such as material resources (i.e., finances and transportation), knowledge of health practice, and their health behaviors (i.e., diet, exercise, and tobacco use), as well as the behaviors of the communities they live in.

OUTCOMES

With a change in the landscape of health care, attention is being directed at the social needs of the patients.

Evidence has shown that interventions that target social needs improve health and reduce health care costs (Bachrach, Pfister, Wallis, & Lipson, 2014). When planning care, nurses, and the entire health care team, need to consider whether patients have transportation to follow-up appointments, funds to purchase medications, environmental factors that influence illnesses such as asthma, and knowledge and resources necessary for nutritious meals.

Summary

Social factors play a key role in influencing access to health care and health outcomes for individuals, families, and communities. Nurses and the entire health care team need to assess patients, including the SDH, holistically. Then the plan of care should include strategies to address social factors (individual, family, and community) identified as barriers to health promotion, prevention of disease, self-management of chronic illness, and overall optimal quality of life.

Bachrach, D., Pfister, H., Wallis, K., & Lipson, M. (2014). *Addressing patients' social needs: An emerging business case for provider investment.* New York, NY: Commonwealth Fund.

Fortune, M. L. (2016). The influence of social determinants on late stage breast cancer for women in Mississippi. *Journal of Racial and Ethnic Health Disparities, 4*(1), 1–8.

Heiman, H. J., & Artiga, S. (2015). Beyond health care: The role of social determinants in promoting health and health equity. *Health, 20,* 10.

Moore, T. G., McDonald, M., Carlon, L., & O'Rourke, K. (2015). Early childhood development and the social determinants of health inequities. *Health Promotion International, 30*(2), 102–115. doi:10.1093/heapro/dav031

Office of Disease Prevention and Health Promotion. (2017). Social determinants of health. In *Healthy People 2020.* Retrieved from https://www.healthypeople.gov/2020/topics-objectives/topic/social-determinants-of health

Williams, D. R., Costa, M. V., Odunlami, A. O., & Mohammed, S. A. (2008) Moving upstream: How interventions that address the social determinants of health can improve health and reduce disparities. *Journal of Public Health Management Practice, 11*(14), 8–17. doi:10.1097/01.PHH.0000338382.36695.42

World Health Organization Commission on Social Determinants of Health. (2008). *Closing the gap in a generation: Health equity through action on the social determinants of health: CSDH final report.* Geneva, Switzerland: Author.

■ TRANSITIONAL CARE COORDINATION

Nadine M. Marchi

Overview

The health care system of the United States has the highest costs in the world. It accounts for 17% of the gross domestic product of the United States and is expected to grow to 20% by 2020 because of the aging population, increased longevity, and increased chronic health problems (Centers for Medicare & Medicaid Services, Office of the Actuary, n.d.).

To provide efficient health care in the context of such expense, the Institute for Healthcare Improvement (IHI) formulated the "Triple Aim" of health care (Berwick, Nolan, & Whittington, 2008). The Triple Aim has a three-pronged goal: improve patient experience in quality and satisfaction, improve the health of populations, and reduce cost. One area of attention related to accomplishing the goals of the Triple Aim is discharge from the hospital. Medicare patients who have been discharged from the hospital are too commonly readmitted within 30 days (19.6%), and more are readmitted in 90 days (34%) (Jencks, Williams, & Coleman, 2009). The Medicare Payment Advisory Commission reports the readmission of patients in 30 days accounted for $15 billion of Medicare spending (National Transitions of Care Coalition, 2010). The period when patients move from the hospital to another facility or home is a time at which the risk for readmission is particularly high (Jing, Young & Williams, 2014). To address this concern, many institutions have developed transitional care coordination teams.

Background

Transitional care is defined as services focused on ensuring health care continuity, providing safe transfer to different levels of care, and reducing costs related to readmission (Naylor, Aiken, Kurtzman, Olds, & Hirschman, 2011). In response to requirements of the 2010 Affordable Care Act, and efforts of hospitals and payers to meet the Triple Aim, evidence-based transitional care programs have been expanded in acute care settings. The accountable care organization (ACO) is one component of the Affordable Care Act related to care transitions and Medicare reimbursement. An ACO is a group of doctors, hospitals, and other health care providers who have voluntarily joined to provide high-quality care and reduce cost. It is anticipated that if an ACO reduces cost and provides high-quality care, then patients and communities can achieve greater health quality and satisfaction as acute care institutions share in the savings produced for Medicare.

In most institutions, the transitional care team consists of a network of bedside nurses, nurse practitioners, nurse case managers, social workers, physical and occupation therapists, pharmacists, physicians, utility review nurses, and other relevant health care professionals who coordinate across the continuum of health care. The key to success in the process of care coordination is communication among all members of the team. The transition point between one level of care and another is the crucial link in the system. When a failed transition in care occurs, the collapse may be related to poor communication, inadequate education of patients and family caregivers, limited access to services, and absence of a follow-up person who ensures the continuity of care. In addition, health literacy issues and cultural differences can exacerbate the problem (Naylor & Keating, 2008).

Clinical Aspects

Best practices for care transition are still in the identification phase. Early research suggests that preparation for discharge should start on admission. Often this is led by a transitional care coordinator (TCC). Specific aspects of such planning are discussed in the following sections.

ASSESSMENT

A crucial component of the transitional care coordination process is the initial assessment, which must be completed in 24 hours of arrival at the acute care facility. The physician lists the patient as observation or admitted. An observation patient is one who could be admitted, but whose needs could likely be fulfilled on an outpatient basis. If the observation patient is not admitted or discharged in 24 hours, the cost of reimbursement for the acute care facility and patient is significant. The TCC conducts the initial assessment using explicit criteria to screen the patient and caregiver to identify postdischarge risks and needs. Then the physician is notified as to the future status of the patient regarding admission or discharge, preparation for discharge begins, and the patient does not get lost in the system.

NURSING INTERVENTIONS, MANAGEMENT, AND IMPLICATIONS

The role of the professional nurse includes ensuring patient-centered high-quality care and conserving the cost of care provided at a variety of levels and settings of health care. Nurses have a major role in the effective implementation of the transitional care process. The priority nursing problems for care coordination are (a) lack of patient resources for changes in level of care; (b) difficulty in obtaining approval from insurance providers for patients who need precertification; (c) health literacy issues with patients, plus patient and family agreement in plan of care; (d) physician timely discharge of patient; and (e) barriers to transition and potentially unsafe home environment.

After the initial assessment, the TCC continues to follow the patient and coordinate planning for discharge. A holistic approach is used that includes patient and caregiver, self-determination when possible, measures to ensure safety, cultural considerations, and assistance with navigation through the health care system (Bobay, Bahr, Weiss, Hughes, & Costa, 2015). The TCC coordinates planning to promote optimal health and avoid readmission. Examples of TCC activities include medication reconciliation, identifying barriers to transition, evaluating home safety, appraising the patient's abilities based on therapists' recommendations, communicating with providers, identifying an appropriate subsequent level of care, arranging follow-up appointments before leaving the hospital, identifying social service needs, making referrals, sending discharge summaries to primary care providers, following up on test results that return after discharge, conducting a nurse–to-nurse report at transition, and phone follow-up with the patient after discharge (Kripalani, Jackson, Schnipper, & Coleman, 2007; Mays, 2016). Specialty care coordinators perform the same functions but for a specific population.

Care coordination is a team effort. The patient's bedside registered nurse works with the TCC and social workers to assist in the transition process by providing high-quality nursing care, notifying the TCC of unanticipated discharge needs, and providing pre-discharge education for patient and caregiver that includes teach-back. The TCC, pharmacist, bedside nurse, nurse practitioner, therapists, and other health care providers participate in interprofessional rounds to discuss and coordinate the patient's transitional needs. This is usually conducted at the bedside with the patient and family caregiver involved in the process. The goal of interprofessional rounds is to improve team communication and provide safe, high-quality, coordinated care. The whole team assesses the patient situation, reviews goals, and makes a plan for transition.

OUTCOMES

The expected outcomes of transitional care coordination are to support optimal health of the patient and the organization in attaining the goals of the Triple Aim. By implementing a team approach to care coordination and assigning a care coordinator to be actively involved in each patient's transitional care, the hope is that patient satisfaction, improved health, and safety can be enhanced and cost of health care be reduced. The role of nursing in this process is of utmost importance through all transitions of care.

A particular concern during the transition process is the need to place more emphasis on addressing the social determinants of health, including consideration of transportation, caregiver support, emotional needs, and environmental requirements. As patients move from one care setting to another their social needs follow them. To ignore social needs places the transitional care coordination process at risk as these needs can impact readmission and discharge as much as physical needs (Shier, Ginsburg, Howell, Volland, & Golden, 2013).

Summary

Health care in the United States is fragmented and costly. Many hospitalized patients are discharged without the necessary resources and return for readmission. Transitional care coordination by an interprofessional team can identify and address these issues in the acute care setting before discharge and follow the patient while in the community. The model and interventions discussed in this section can promote improvement in the safety and quality of care, patient satisfaction with care, and the costs of care (Mays, 2016).

Berwick, D., Nolan, T., & Whittington, J. (2008). The triple aim: Care, health, and cost. *Health Affairs, 27*(3), 759–769. doi:10.1377/hlthaff.27.3.759

Bobay, K., Bahr, S. J., Weiss, M. E., Hughes, R., & Costa, L. (2015). Models of discharge care in Magnet hospitals. *Journal of Nursing Administration, 45*(10), 485–491.

Centers for Medicare & Medicaid Services, Office of the Actuary. (n.d.). National Healthcare Expenditure Projections, 2010–2020. Retrieved from http://www.sellers dorsey.com/news/FileManager/national_health_spending__2010_to_2020.pdf

Jencks, S. F., Williams, M. V., & Coleman, E. A. (2009). Re-hospitalizations among patients in the Medicare fee for service program. *New England Journal of Medicine, 360,* 1418–1428.

Jing, L., Young, R., & Williams, M. (2014). Optimizing transitions of care to reduce re-hospitalizations. *Cleveland Clinic Journal of Medicine, 81*(5), 312–320. Retrieved from http://www.ccjm.org/content/81/5/312.full

Kripalani, S., Jackson, A.T., Schnipper, J. L., & Coleman, E. A. (2007). Promoting effective transitions of care at hospital discharge: A review of key issues for hospitalists. *Journal of Hospital Medicine, 2,* 314–323.

Mays, G. P. (2016). Aligning systems and sectors to improve population health: Emerging findings and remaining uncertainties. Systems for Action. Retrieved from http://systemsforaction.org/projects/accreditation-and-multi-sector-contributions-population-health-activities/meetings/aligning-systems-and-sectors-improve-popula tion-health-emerging-findings-and-remaining-uncertainties

National Transitions of Care Coalition. (2010). Improving transitions of care findings and considerations of the "Vision of the National Transitions of Care Coalition." Retrieved from http://www.ntocc.org/WhoWeServe/PolicyMakers/tabid/90/ItemId/0/Default.aspx

Naylor, M. D., Aiken, L. H., Kurtzman, E. T., Olds, D. M., & Hirschman, K. B. (2011). Importance of transitional care in achieving health reform. *Health Affairs, 30*(4), 746–754. doi:10.1377/hlthaff.2011.0041

Naylor, M. D., & Keating, S. A. (2008). Transitional Care-moving patients from one care setting to another. *American Journal of Nursing, 108*(9), 58–62.

Shier, G., Ginsburg, M., Howell, J., Volland, P., & Golden, R. (2013). Strong social support services, such as transportation and help for caregivers, can lead to lower health care use and costs. *Health Affairs, 32*(3), 544–551. doi: 10.1377/hlthaff.2012.0170

HEALTH PROMOTION

■ HEALTH BEHAVIOR

Deborah F. Lindell

Overview

Individual behavior is one of the five broad, interacting, determinants of health: the range of personal, social, economic, and environmental factors that determine the health status of individuals or populations. The other determinants include policy making, social and physical health services, and biology and genetics (Office of Disease Prevention and Health Promotion, 2017; World Health Organization [WHO], 1998). Today, in the United States, preventable illness accounts for 80% of the burden of illness and 90% all health care costs as well as eight of the top nine leading categories of death. Human behavior, as a determinant of health, accounts for almost 40% of the risk associated with preventable premature deaths in the United States (National Institutes of Health, 2017). Promoting healthy behavior at the individual, family, population, and community levels is a critical element of national efforts to improve health outcomes by preventing and managing chronic illness. This entry concerns promoting healthy behavior in individuals.

Background

The WHO defines health behavior as, "any activity undertaken by an individual, regardless of actual or perceived health status, for the purpose of promoting, protecting or maintaining health, whether or not such behavior is objectively effective towards that end" (WHO, 1998, p. 8). The study of health behavior is interdisciplinary, with contributions from sciences such as sociology, psychology, anthropology, nursing, demography, epidemiology, and public health. Many theories aim to explain health behavior and/or behavior change, each with a unique perspective but with elements in common as well.

Examples of theories that aim to explain health behavior and their unique perspectives include the health belief model (beliefs about prevention of disease), social cognitive theory (self-efficacy), ecologic model (health behavior is influenced by factors at multiple levels, individual to societal and environmental), health promotion model (HPM; healthy lifestyle), and individual and family self-management theory (nursing view of self-management of chronic illness; National Institutes of Health, 2005; Pender, 2011; Ryan & Sawin, 2009).

The HPM, nurse-authored and tested and applied in research for more than 27 years, exemplifies the complex factors influencing health behavior (Pender,

2011). The HPM has three over-arching constructs: (a) personal factors, (b) behavior-specific factors, and (c) behavioral outcome. Personal factors include biological, psychological, and sociocultural characteristics as well as previous experiences with behavior change. Behavior-specific factors include perceived benefits and barriers, perceived self-efficacy, activity-related affect, interpersonal influences, and situational influences. Personal and behavior-specific factors directly influence a commitment to a plan of action which leads to the behavioral outcome or health promoting behavior. The personal and behavior-specific factors also influence immediate competing demands and preferences which, in turn, influence the behavioral outcome (Pender, 2011).

Examples of theories that consider the process of behavior change and their unique contributions include the HPM (commitment to a plan of action), theory of planned behavior (intention to engage in action), and the transtheoretical model (TTM; stages of change and decisional balance). Each model reflects the idea that behavior change is typically a multistep process with the TTM viewing behavior change as having five stages likely to be iterative rather than sequential (National Cancer Institute, 1998).

Clinical Aspects

Nurses contribute to promoting healthy behavior through theory development, research, and clinical practice. In all encounters, nurses have the opportunities and responsibilities to collaborate with the patient and family, and other health care providers (HCPs), to assist patients in making choices about their health behavior.

Tobacco use, the single most important risk factor in preventing and managing the top preventable causes of death in the United States, provides an example of counseling for behavior change. The U.S. Public Health Service recommends tobacco use status be assessed and recorded at every visit and smoking-cessation counseling is one of the options by which hospitals can meet The Joint Commission's performance measures accreditation requirement (The Joint Commission, n.d.).

ASSESSMENT

The first step in promoting healthy behavior is to assess factors influencing the patient's health and health behavior. The nurse appreciates that the factors influencing

health behavior are multiple, complex, and that they dynamically interact. Assessment can be guided by a specific theory or nurses can assess elements shared by most models of health behavior such as (a) self-efficacy is a core, modifiable factor; (b) knowledge is one factor among many and knowledge alone does not ensure behavior change; (c) the experience of previous efforts to modify one's health behavior influences the future efforts; (d) readiness to change; and (e) individual options and choices are impacted by multiple spheres of influence at the family, community, and societal levels such as cultural norms and practices, social support, and availability of resources.

Regarding the example of smoking cessation and given that nurses' time for health counseling may be limited, a few questions assess key factors: Have you tried to stop smoking in the past? What went well? What were the challenges? What did you do to deal with the challenges? Was it helpful? Do you have family or friends who support your efforts? How confident are you that you can stop smoking, on a scale of 1 to 5 or 1 to 7 (1 = not confident at all; 7 = highly confident). If you are interested in stopping smoking, what do you already know about the effects of tobacco on your body and second-hand smoke and tobacco cessation and treatment?

NURSING INTERVENTIONS, MANAGEMENT, AND IMPLICATIONS

Problems encountered in promoting healthy behavior are largely on the nursing side and are process related. Examples include appreciation of the complexity of health behavior and challenges of behavior change; knowledge and skill in evidence-based strategies to promote behavior change; recognition of the right of self-determination; and limitations in time, organizational structure, and reimbursement needed for promoting healthy behaviors.

With regard to smoking cessation, the nurse (a) recognizes that tobacco use is often an addiction, (b) accepts patients whose behavior is or has the potential to negatively influence their health, (c) avoids blaming patients whose efforts to stop using tobacco are not successful, and (d) offers positive feedback for patients who make progress in smoking cessation.

Nurses recognize that successful behavior change may require several attempts, is typically a multistep process that includes developing a plan for changing the behavior, and collaborate with the patient to set goals (wellness, disease prevention, or self-management) and plan, implement, and evaluate strategies to support healthy behaviors. Depending on the situation, interventions may focus on primary, secondary, or tertiary prevention. In tertiary prevention, self-management is a key factor in improving health outcomes of chronic illness. As part of an interprofessional team, nurses play key roles in supporting individuals and their families to engage in self-management behaviors (Ryan & Sawin, 2009).

When promoting patient-centered, health behavior change, nurses implement roles such as counselor, coach, and educator. Patients are assisted in examining the pros and cons, readiness and options for change, and make their decisions about behavior change. The techniques of motivational interviewing (open-ended questions, affirmation, reflective listening, and summarizing) are used with the goal of evoking change talk (a continuum of desire, ability, reasons, need, commitment/intention, activation, and taking steps; Miller & Rollnick, 2013).

Regarding counseling for tobacco use, *Helping Smokers Quit: A Guide for Clinicians* (Public Health Service, 2008) provides clear, practical, strategies that incorporate elements of the TTM and notes "Even brief tobacco dependence treatment is effective and should be offered to every patient who uses tobacco" (p. 1). Strategies include (a) ask about tobacco use at every visit (current, former, never), (b) advise all tobacco users to quit (use clear, strong, personalized language), (c) assess readiness to quit (if willing, provide resources and assistance; if unwilling, see step two; and, if willing to talk about quitting, help motivate the patient to identify reasons to quit in a supportive manner and build patients' confidence about quitting, (d) assist tobacco users with a quit plan, and (e) arrange follow-up visits. Additional points from the TTM include tailoring messages to the stage of change; behavior change is a circular rather than linear process; accept patients who relapse, and for former smokers, provide positive feedback and discuss challenges (National Cancer Institute, 2005). These strategies, and those of motivational interviewing can easily be adapted in counseling for other health concerns, as well.

OUTCOMES

The evaluation of interventions include assessing the process used and patient outcomes: Was the encounter patient centered, was the patient's autonomy in decision making acknowledged, and were the patient's preferences, values, and needs considered? (Quality and Safety Education for Nurses, 2007). Were techniques of counseling, coaching, motivational interviewing, and health education implemented according to the patient's interest in change? If the patient was interested in change, did he or she advance on the continuum of change talk?

Summary

Health behavior, a complex phenomenon, is a determinant of health and an important factor in prevention and self-management of illness. Health behavior change is a multistep, iterative process characterized by a degree of readiness to change. Nurses play important roles in assessing health behavior and readiness to change and supporting patients to set goals and change their behavior. The strategies to promote behavior change should be patient centered and use techniques of motivational interviewing in the roles of counselor, coach, and educator.

Miller, W. R., & Rollnick, S. (2013). *Motivational interviewing: Help people change* (3rd ed.). New York, NY: Guilford.

National Cancer Institute. (2005). *Theory at a glance: A guide for health promotion practice* (2nd ed.). Rockville, MD: National Institutes of Health, U.S. Department of Health & Human Services.

National Institutes of Health. (2017). Science of behavior change's health relevance. Office of Strategic Coordination—The Common Fund. Retrieved from https://commonfund.nih.gov/behaviorchange/public

Office of Disease Prevention and Health Promotion. (2017). Determinants of health. In *Healthy People 2020*. Retrieved from https://www.healthypeople.gov/2020/about/foundation-health-measures/Determinants-oHealth

Pender, N. (2011). Health promotion model manual. Retrieved from https://deepblue.lib.umich.edu/handle/2027.42/85350

Public Health Service. (2008). *Helping smokers quit: A Guide for clinicians*. Rockville, MD: U.S. Department of Health and Human Services.

Quality and Safety Education for Nurses. (2007). Prelicensure competencies. Retrieved from http://qsen.org/competencies/pre-licensure-ksas

Resnicow, K., Gobat, N., & Naar, S. (2015) Intensifying and igniting change talk in motivational interviewing: A theoretical and practical framework. *European Health Psychologist, 17*(3), 102–110.

Ryan, P., & Sawin, K. (2009) The individual and family self-management theory: Background and perspectives on context, process, and outcomes. *Nursing Outlook, 57*(4), 217–225. doi:10.1016/j.outlook.2008.10.004

The Joint Commission. (n.d.). Six core measure accreditation requirement. Retrieved from https://www.jointcommission.org/core_measure_sets.aspx

World Health Organization. (1998). Health promotion glossary. Retrieved from http://www.who.int/healthpromotion/about/HPR%20Glossary%201998.pdf

■ HEALTH EDUCATION

Rita M. Sfiligoj

Overview

Health education is "any combination of learning experiences designed to help individuals and communities improve their health, by increasing their knowledge or influencing their attitudes" (WHO, 2017, para. 1). Health education is an intervention strategy identified as an integral part of the nursing process. The nurse's aim is to collaborate with and empower the client-learner to avoid disease, make healthy lifestyle choices, and improve his or her health and the health of his or her family and community. Health education can be implemented at the individual, family, group, or community level.

Background

Today, the major health issues of concern in a society are heavily influenced by the lifestyle choices of its members. Nursing interventions around health education and support of lifestyle changes can help prevent or limit the impact of the prevalent chronic illnesses such as chronic obstructive pulmonary disease (COPD), hypertension, and diabetes mellitus type 2. For example, COPD readmissions and length of hospital stay decreased following a COPD health education program (Ko et al., 2014). In this case, education helped to improve health outcomes. As another example, a health education plan for transplant patients and their families in the intensive care unit decreased morbidity and mortality, and at the same time reduced costs and health resource consumption (Pueyo-Garrigues, San Martín Loyola, Caparrós Leal, & Jiménez Muñoz, 2016). Education can also help improve health outcomes in a community. For example, prevention of progression from prediabetes to diabetes is possible with the development of a lifestyle changing health education program (Tuso, 2014).

Whether the aim is disease prevention, health promotion, or self-management of chronic illness, nurses should consider that health behavior is a complex process influenced by multiple factors of which knowledge is one. Examples of the other factors influencing health behavior include perceived barriers and self-efficacy, interpersonal influences, previous related behavior, competing demands, and commitment to a plan (Pender, 2011).

Clinical Aspects

The steps in health education or teaching–learning parallel the nursing process: (a) assess the learner and include assessment of need and readiness to learn, (b) state a learning need(s) that is comparable to developing a diagnosis, (c) develop a teaching–learning plan designed to meet the learning needs and desired outcomes, and (d) evaluate the process and outcomes.

ASSESSMENT

This section focuses on assessment of the learner and can be applied to a family, group, or community. However, the education should also consider the two other dimensions of health education: the teaching–learning situation (such as the site and audiovisual aids) and the educator's perspective, knowledge of the topic, and experience in client education. Assessment of the learner involves engaging him or her to understand the characteristics, factors influencing learning, and learning interests and needs. Factors considered include:

- *Perception.* The perspectives of both the nurse and client regarding the learning situation.

- *Readiness to learn.* The client's willingness and ability to participate in a teaching–learning activity is influenced by other dimensions such as the level of health or wellness.

- *Motivation to learn.* Motivation is an internal state that drives human behavior. Maslow's hierarchy of needs is an example of a theory that can be applied to assessing a client's priority needs for teaching–learning.

- *The level of health or wellness.* Health education should be tailored to the client's level of physical–psychological–emotional health or wellness.

- *Socioeconomic factors.* These social determinants, which should be considered when planning health education, include the client's living situation, social support, financial resources, and priorities including health insurance, transportation, and employment.

- *Cultural factors.* Cultural considerations, also social determinants, include factors such as values, beliefs, language, practices, food preferences, dress, dietary patterns, mores, and ethnicity.

■ *Health literacy*. This key consideration refers to the capacity an individual has to communicate, process, and understand basic health information needed to make appropriate health-related decisions (Centers for Disease Control and Prevention [CDC], 2016).

■ *Generational differences*. Generational differences may reveal factors, such as use of the internet and social media that can influence learning.

■ *Communication challenges*. Hearing, visual, or speech impairments should be addressed to facilitate the maximal opportunity for learning (Miller & Stoeckel, 2011).

NURSING INTERVENTIONS, MANAGEMENT, AND IMPLICATIONS

Following assessment, the next step in health education is to develop a teaching–learning plan that includes outcome learning objectives, content for each objective, when/how/who will teach, and how each objective is evaluated. Behavioral outcome objectives are learner-centered, specific short-term outcomes that set the stage for the attainment of long-term goals. They are classified into three domains of learning: cognitive (intellectual), psychomotor (motor skills), and affective (attitudes and emotions; Bloom, 1984). Behavioral objectives indicate how the learner will *cognitively* apply information, perform *skills,* and *value* the learning. For example, behavioral objectives for education of transplant patients in the intensive care unit include knowledge: self-care information and anxiety reduction for the patient and family, skills: the ability to properly follow the skills as directed, and attitudes: indecisive attitudes that are experienced by transplant patients and families (Pueyo-Garrigues et al., 2016). Behavioral objectives are written in the SMART format: specific, measurable, achievable, relevant, and time phased (Evaluation Research Team, 2009).

Any educational plan needs to be tailored to meet the need of the learners and applied appropriately. The characteristics of the learner identified during the assessment, including age, social status, culture, and health literacy, guide the approach to health education. Useful strategies include storytelling, game playing, group activities, use of audiovisual materials and instructional technology, and role playing, which can complement more traditional education.

Desired health outcomes, specified in the SMART objectives, can be achieved through well-planned interventions. The teaching–learning design of the intervention is determined according to the data accumulated during the assessment phase. Motivation and readiness of the learner

are key aspects to be considered when developing the intervention. When developing interventions, resources, such as space, equipment, and partnerships, need to be determined. Interventions are developed to meet the needs of the learner and avoid barriers. Theory- and evidence-based interventions are the most effective health education interventions (Rimer, Glanz, & Rasband, 2001).

OUTCOMES

The evaluation process is a way to determine outcomes of the health education program and should include continuous reassessments. *Process* evaluation confirms that the education that was proposed is being implemented. Several questions can be used to evaluate whether the process is meeting the health education objectives: Is the selected individual, family, or population being reached? Is the format appropriate or does the location and/or meeting time need to be changed? Is the level of instruction proper for the selected population? *Impact* evaluation or immediate outcome of health education is completed at the conclusion of the teaching lesson. The impact can be measured with an evaluation tool to determine the knowledge, attitude, behavior, or skill level after a health education session. *Outcome* evaluation is the long-term effect, measuring the quality and quantity of the learner's long-term knowledge (Anderson & McFarlane, 2015).

Summary

The learning process in health education follows steps similar to the nursing process. An accurate assessment of the learner, the readiness to learn, and the barriers to avoid comprise the initial step. Determination of a learning need is followed by the development of behavioral objectives, intervention, and implementation of a plan for evaluation. A well-developed health education program can assist individuals, families, and communities with making lifestyle changes and improving their overall health.

Anderson, E. T., & McFarlane, J. (2015). *Community as partner: Theory and practice in nursing* (7th ed.). Philadelphia, PA: J. B. Lippincott.

Bloom, B. (1984). *Taxonomy of educational objectives: The Classification of educational goals.* New York, NY: David McKay.

Centers for Disease Control and Prevention. (2016, July). Learn about health literacy. Retrieved from https://www.cdc.gov/healthliteracy/learn/index.html

Evaluation Research Team. (2009). Writing SMART objectives. Evaluation Briefs, 3b. *Centers for Disease Control and Prevention.* Retrieved from https://www.cdc.gov/healthyyouth/evaluation/pdf/brief3b.pdf

Ko, F. W., Ngai, J. C., Ng, S. S., Chan, K.-P., Cheung, R., Leung, M.-Y., . . . Hui, D. S. (2014). COPD care programme can reduce readmissions and in-patient bed days. *Respiratory Medicine, 108*(12), 1771–1778.

Miller, M., & Stoeckel, P. (2011) *Client education: Theory and practice.* Sudbury, MA: Jones & Bartlett.

Pender, N., Murdaugh, C., & Parsons, M. A. (2011). *Health promotion in nursing practice* (6th ed.). Boston, MA: Pearson.

Pueyo-Garrigues, M., San Martín Loyola, Á., Caparrós Leal, M. C., & Jiménez Muñoz, C. (2016). Health education in transplant patients and their families in an intensive care unit. *Enferm Intensiva, 27*(1), 31–39. doi:10.1016/j.enfi.2015.11.002

Rimer, B., Glanz, K., & Rasband, G. (2001). Searching for evidence about health education and health behavior interventions. *Health Education and Behavior, 28*(2), 231–248.

Tuso, P. (2014). Prediabetes and lifestyle modification: Time to prevent a preventable disease. *Permanente Journal Summer, 18*(3), 88–93.

World Health Organization. (2017). Health education topics: Health education. Retrieved from http://www.who.int/topics/health_education/en

■ HEALTH LITERACY

Joseph D. Perazzo

Overview

Health literacy refers to the capacity an individual has to communicate, process, and understand basic health information needed to make appropriate health-related decisions (Centers for Disease Control and Prevention [CDC], 2016). An individual's health literacy can impact his or her ability to make informed decisions about his or her health and to navigate an increasingly complicated health care system. People with low health literacy tend to have more difficulty in adhering to prescribed treatments, are less likely to use preventative health, have increased emergency room visits and hospitalizations, are more hesitant to report symptoms and poor health, and are less likely to receive and understand warnings related to environmental health and safety (Advisory Committee on Training in Primary Care Medicine and Dentistry, 2015). Nurses are often charged with patient education in the clinical environment, the workplace, and the community. Nursing assessment of health literacy is crucial to tailor

the successful delivery of information to promote the health of populations in these settings.

Background

More than 90 million adults in the United States have low health literacy, a problem costing Americans more than $200 billion annually (U.S. Department of Health and Human Services [DHHS], 2010). Determinants of health literacy include a person's ability to locate, read, listen to, analyze, comprehend, process, and apply information in the context of health. Even people with average (or even above-average) literacy skills (e.g., reading, speaking, and numeracy skills) can be at risk of low health literacy (CDC, 2016). Low or limited health literacy has been linked to demographic factors (e.g., older age, racial/ethnic minority status), limited or no exposure to health-related terminology and information, confusion and misunderstanding regarding the health care system (e.g., health care coverage, system navigation), language barriers, varying cultural norms regarding health beliefs and decision making, miscommunication between health care workers and patients, learning disabilities and cognitive deficits, and lack of public health infrastructure to cater to varying literacy levels (CDC, 2016).

Health care professionals in clinical and community settings are constantly engaged in the exchange of health information, and should always consider the health literacy of their intended audience at both the individual and group levels. Crucial interactions in which health literacy is of particular concern include patient–provider discussions of diagnoses and treatment plans, informed-consent discussions and documents for procedures and research studies, development and distribution of patient educational materials (e.g., discharge instructions), education on medication adherence, discussions about vaccination and other preventative health behaviors, trainings on work safety, and public health warnings and advisories (CDC, 2016; DHHS, 2010). Health care workers can prevent injury and illness by diligently ensuring that information is presented in a way that is comprehensible to individuals with different levels of health literacy.

Clinical Aspects

ASSESSMENT

People with low health literacy may be embarrassed or ashamed of an inability to read, calculate, or comprehend health information, resulting in avoidance of health care interactions (CDC, 2016; DHHS, 2010). Health care professionals should approach patients in a private, sensitive manner to assess health literacy and determine the most effective communication techniques (e.g., language preference, print versus imagery). Health literacy assessments enable health care workers to tailor their approach based on an individual's specific needs. Clinicians can collect both quantitative (measurable) information using validated tests/questionnaires, as well as qualitative (observable) information while interacting with the patients. Common health literacy measurements include:

- The Rapid Estimate of Adult Literacy in Medicine-Revised (REALM-R; Bass, Wilson, & Griffith, 2003): A list of eight health-related words (e.g., "allergic," "directed") that individuals read out loud to the clinician. Inability to complete this measure may indicate limited literacy skills.

- The Test of Functional Health Literacy in Adults (TOFHLA; Parker, Baker, Williams, & Nurss, 1995): A 67-item measure that tests reading ability/comprehension and numeracy skills; scored from 0 to 100, with scores below 75 indicating potential literacy concerns.

- The Newest Vital Sign (Weiss et al., 2005): A six-item measure that includes reading ability and comprehension of a nutrition label; scored between 0 and 6, with less than five correct answers indicating potential literacy concerns.

In addition to these global measures of health literacy, scientists in a variety of clinical specialties (e.g., diabetes, HIV, heart disease) have created disease-specific health literacy measures that can provide clinicians with an idea of how well a patient understands a specific condition and its treatment. Clinicians can also gather important information about health literacy through observation and discussion with the patients. Common signs that may indicate an individual with low health literacy and/or limited basic literacy include:

- Failure or refusal to complete paperwork at appointments

- Avoidance of reading or calculation tasks (e.g., "I don't have my glasses, can you read it for me?")

- Inaccurate interpretation of written instructions (e.g., discharge paperwork)

- Contradiction between reported behaviors and objective measurements (e.g., laboratory values; CDC, 2016; DHHS, 2010)

Health care professionals who assess an individual's health literacy can take a patient-centered approach that enables the patient to better understand information exchanged and made informed decisions regarding care. Online health literacy tools are available from national health agencies (e.g., Agency for Healthcare Research and Quality [AHRQ]) to help health care professionals tailor their approach with individuals of varying levels of literacy.

NURSING INTERVENTIONS, MANAGEMENT, AND IMPLICATIONS

Across practice settings, nurses are responsible for health education. Types of health education encounters include discharge teaching in the hospital setting, work safety in the industrial setting, health screening, and health promotion in the community. Nurses not only assess health literacy but apply strategic interventions to help people with low health literacy to better understand and apply health information. The following interventions may be used as a framework to (a) determine whether the individual is at risk for poor outcomes because of low health literacy and (b) to tailor their approach to best serve the individual in a patient-centered manner. If appropriate, these interventions are also desirable when interacting with family members and/or loved ones caring for patients:

- Determine cultural norms/beliefs/preferences (e.g., social etiquette, decision-making authority, family involvement, language, health beliefs, and religious/spiritual beliefs)

- Use global and disease-specific (where available) health literacy measures to assess health literacy before teaching and determine whether standard-of-care education is sufficient to meet an individual/family's learning needs

- Assess current knowledge to identify areas in need of further teaching (e.g., clarifying misinformation, easing fear and uncertainty, filling in knowledge gaps)

- Use large and legible fonts, visual aids, videos, and plain language in learning materials to promote simple, effective, dynamic learning

- Focus on action-based skill building as opposed to memorization and/or calculation tasks

Create a follow-up schedule to reinforce learning after or between the encounters.

OUTCOMES

Nurses can use demonstration and the teach-back method as frameworks to confirm whether the outcome learning objectives have been met.

Summary

Health literacy is a factor that can determine an individual's ability to seek out, obtain, process, and apply health information. Low health literacy has been associated with increased mortality, increased emergency room visits and hospitalizations, delayed health care-seeking behavior, and an inability to adhere to care and treatment recommendations. Health care professionals across settings must consider the complexities associated with health literacy to successfully design health interventions. Nurses, often trusted with the education of patients in these settings, are particularly well positioned to assess health literacy and play a crucial role in tailoring interventions to best meet the needs of patients and communities. Assessment of health literacy and application of health literacy interventions lead to an increased understanding of health information and improve health outcomes across populations.

Advisory Committee on Training in Primary Care Medicine and Dentistry. (2015). Health literacy and patient engagement. Twelfth annual report to the Secretary of the United States Department of Health and Human Services and the Congress of the United States. Retrieved from http://www.hrsa.gov/advisorycommittees/bhpradvisory/actpcmd/Reports/twelfthreport.pdf-sthash.ilhls27E.dpuf

Bass, P. F., Wilson, J. F., & Griffith, C. H. (2003). A shortened instrument for literacy screening. *Journal of General Internal Medicine*, 18(12), 1036–1038.

Centers for Disease Control and Prevention. (2016). Learn about health literacy. Retrieved from https://www.cdc.gov/healthliteracy/learn/index.html

Parker, R. M., Baker, D. W., Williams, M. V., & Nurss, J. R. (1995). The test of functional health literacy in adults. *Journal of General Internal Medicine*, 10(10), 537–541.

U.S. Department of Health and Human Services. (2010). *National action plan to improve health literacy.* Washington, DC: Author.

Weiss, B. D., Mays, M. Z., Martz, W., Castro, K. M., DeWalt, D. A., Pignone, M. P., . . . Hale, F. A. (2005). Quick assessment of literacy in primary care: The newest vital sign. *Annals of Family Medicine*, 3(6), 514–522.

■ SELF-MANAGEMENT

Marym M. Alaamri

Overview

The growing number of individuals living with chronic illnesses represents a significant public health concern and warrants strategies to prevent, treat, and manage chronic illnesses. Self-management has been identified as a central element of effective chronic disease management. In self-management, individuals collaborate with health care providers to make appropriate health care decisions. This involves addressing multiple behavioral risk factors such as smoking, poor diet, lack of physical activity, and many other factors that predispose individuals to poor outcomes. Self-management is a promising approach to achieve positive health outcomes, reduce health care utility, and improve quality of life associated with chronic conditions.

Background

According to the U.S. Centers for Disease Control and Prevention (CDC), chronic diseases are responsible for seven in 10 deaths and nearly 90% of health care costs. Nearly half of all adults in America have at least one chronic condition and one quarter of all adults have two or more conditions (CDC, 2016; Ward, Schiller, & Goodman, 2014). Although the damaging effects of chronic illness are so prevalent and costly, they are also the most preventable of all health problems (Ward et al., 2014).

Living with chronic illness requires individuals to make decisions on a daily basis to manage the health conditions that impact multiple aspects of their lives. For those individuals, this is a lifelong responsibility. Self-management of chronic illness has been defined as a dynamic, interactive, and complex daily process that individuals use to manage their illnesses or maintain their health (Lorig & Holman, 2003). The concept of self-management has appeared in the health literature for nearly half a century and has been widely used when referring to patients living with chronic illness. Corbin and Strauss (1988) identify three self-management tasks that an individual must learn to manage his or her chronic illness successfully. The first self-management task includes adhering to pharmacological and nonpharmacological interventions. The second task relates to adapting to the new condition by maintaining, changing, and creating new meaningful behaviors. The last self-management task involves dealing with emotions associated with living with a chronic illness. To achieve these tasks, there are several skills essential for successful chronic disease management such as problem solving, decision making, resource utility, the formation of a patient–provider partnership, action planning, and self-tailoring (Lorig & Holman, 2003).

Several conceptual models have provided broader understanding to the management of chronic conditions. The Chronic Care Model and the Individual and Family Self-Management theory are among the most influential and widely used models to elucidate the complexity of self-management and the elements required to improve chronic illness care across various health conditions. Self-management is often used interchangeably with other related concepts such as self-care, self-efficacy, or patient activation. However, self-management is an overarching concept that involves aspects of other related concepts. Self-management of chronic illness incorporates both personal elements, such as self-efficacy and patient activation, as well as interpersonal elements, such as patient–provider communication. Although self-management is tailored to specific conditions, it spans the prevention spectrum by establishing healthy patterns of lifestyle (primary prevention), as well as providing strategies for the management of conditions (secondary and tertiary prevention; Grady & Gough, 2015).

Clinical Aspects

ASSESSMENT

Nursing assessment, in both inpatient discharge planning and community settings, requires a distinctively different approach from a model of patient self-management. The patient and caregivers are the primary managers of patient care. In accordance, the care is planned around the assessed definition of illness from the patient's subjective understanding and perspective. The nurse assesses the patient/caregiver understanding of how past self-management efforts might have influenced the current condition and need for hospitalization. From the beginning of the therapeutic relationship, the nurse must seek to understand the patient's interpretation of the disease and symptoms, as well as feelings and emotions related to the condition. In addition, nursing assessment from a self-management model includes the patient/caregiver motivation and readiness to implement recommendations and change health behavior. The nurse must also assess the patient/caregiver's self-efficacy, that is, the confidence in his or her ability to implement healthy behaviors and manage chronic illness. Finally, nursing assessment recognizes that the primary management of the illness takes place outside of health care settings such as hospitals or clinics; care planning must incorporate an understanding of the family, social, cultural, and environmental

context in which the patient lives his or her daily life (Bodenheimer, Lorig, Holman, & Grumbach, 2002).

NURSING INTERVENTIONS, MANAGEMENT, AND IMPLICATIONS

Nursing interventions directed toward prevention, symptom management, and treatment are also distinctive in a self-management model. A traditional model of patient education focuses on disease-related information, as well as selected technical skills to comply with prescribed tasks. Research has demonstrated that knowledge alone is inadequate for changing the patient behavior. In a self-management model, education focuses on teaching symptom assessment, problem-solving skills, and adjusting action plans. Self-management-based patient education also includes self-monitoring methods such as the use of diaries and logs. In a traditional model of patient–provider interaction, the patient is passive; the patient's goal is to comply with the recommended treatment plan. In the model of disease self-management, patient outcomes are achieved through patient–provider collaboration, shared goal setting, and patient activation. In the traditional hospital discharge, a nurse provides a care plan often based on treatment protocols, guidelines, and checklists. In a self-management model, the plan is tailored to the individual patient/caregiver motivation, self-efficacy, and social as well as physical environment. The patient/caregiver works with the nurse to develop a short-term plan and is provided strategies to monitor and adjust the plan based on long-term goals. In a self-management model, the patient is often referred to community-based self-management programs that target skills improvement, behavior modification, problem solving, and knowledge development in a context of social support. Skills training initiated by providers in the clinical setting can be expanded in program-based education and coaching that fosters the behavioral skills necessary to enhance patients' abilities to manage their illness effectively. These skills include:

- *Problem solving*: Defining problem, identifying possible solutions, implementing solutions, and evaluating outcomes
- *Decision making*: Seeking information, assessing symptoms, making lifestyle choices, and choosing individualized methods to manage chronic illnesses
- *Resource utility*: Developing skills to be able to seek out and use informational, social, and financial resources

■ *Patient–provider relationships*: Patient self-efficacy, communication strategies (shared goals and agenda, tailored information, and patient summary of key information)

■ *Take action*: Set realistic and measurable goals, develop short-term action plan, and identify alternatives

OUTCOMES

In the self-management model, the nurse and patient collaborate to assess whether the elements of the plan were implemented and the desired outcomes achieved. Preliminary research supports the effectiveness of self-management programs in improving clinical outcomes, quality of life, and use of health care resources (Bodenheimer et al., 2002; Lorig et al., 2010).

Summary

Self-management has emerged as a promising approach to the increasing public health challenge of chronic illness. Unlike traditional patterns of provider role and patient education, a model of self-management encourages patients to take a more proactive role in their health decisions and personalized action plans. Effective self-management requires that patients and providers work collaboratively in problem definition, goal setting, planning, education, counseling, support, and skill development. In an effective model of self-management, nurses and other health care providers in all settings need to develop planning and coaching skills required to support patients and caregivers as they assume responsibility to successfully manage their chronic illnesses, efficiently use health care resources, and achieve desired health outcomes.

Bodenheimer, T., Lorig, K., Holman, M., & Grumbach, M. (2002). Patient self-management of chronic disease in primary care. *Innovations in Primary Care*, 288(19), 2469–2475.

Centers for Disease Control and Prevention. (2016). Chronic diseases: The leading causes of death and disability in the United States. Retrieved from https://www.cdc.gov/chronicdisease/overview/#ref1

Corbin, J. M., & Strauss, A. (1988). *Unending work and care: Managing chronic illness at home*. San Francisco, CA: Jossey-Bass.

Grady, P. A., & Gough, L. L. (2015). Self-management: A comprehensive approach to management of chronic conditions. *Revista Panamericana de Salud Pública*, 37(3), 187–194.

Lorig, K. R., & Holman, H. R. (2003). Self-management education : History, definition, outcomes, and mechanisms. *Annals of Behavioral Medicine*, 26(1), 1–7.

Lorig, K. R., Ritter, P. L., Laurent, D. D., Plant, K., Green, M., Jernigan, V. B. B., & Case, S. (2010). Online diabetes self-management program: A randomized study. *Diabetes Care*, 33(6), 1275–1281.

Ward, B. W., Schiller, J. S., & Goodman, R. A. (2014). Multiple chronic conditions among US adults: A 2012 update. *Preventing Chronic Disease*, 11, 1–4. doi:10.5888/pcd11.130389

■ WELLNESS

Elizabeth R. Click

Overview

Emphasizing the importance of wellness is a key patient care delivery strategy for nurses. The Institute of Medicine's report on the future of nursing (2011) advocated for well care delivery by nurses as health care moves away from a primary focus on treatment of illness. The American Nurses Association (ANA) has communicated the importance of wellness care in nursing and challenges nurses to become healthier themselves so that patient well-being may be better addressed (ANA, 2017). Nurses can foster wellness in their patients through their activities as educators, advocates, and role models. They have the opportunity to focus on the importance of healthy eating, regular physical activity, stress management, avoidance of tobacco, supportive relationships, and a solid spiritual base as key components of a wellness-oriented lifestyle. This holistic perspective, seeking any opportunity to encourage wellness and healthy behaviors, is important in patient care and self-care.

Nurses are well positioned to provide wellness care in and outside of the health systems. Although nurses focus on acute health needs during inpatient care delivery, the power of nurses to emphasize disease prevention and wellness care delivery, as more care is delivered in the community rather than in the hospital, is significant. Leveraging educational opportunities to prepare future nurses for this work is necessary (Sickora & Chase, 2014).

Background

The foundation of wellness efforts in nursing began with the work of Florence Nightingale. Her focus on clean air, nutritious food, and healthy environments paved the way for better health. During the period of 1970 to 1990, in an environment of illness care, several authors described nurses as promoters of health, namely, Rozella Schlotfeldt (health-seeking behaviors, 1975), Nancy Milio (framework for prevention, 1976), and Nola Pender (health promotion model, 1982, revised 1996). Pender, Murdaugh, and Parsons (2011) described wellness as the absence of disease, as well as the actualization of human potential through goal-directed behavior, self-care, and healthy relationships with others and the environment.

These visionary nurses set the stage for wellness-oriented care delivery by today's nurses. The National Wellness Institute (NWI; 2017) identifies wellness as a conscious and positive process encompassing multidimensional and interconnected aspects of wellness (e.g., physical, social, intellectual, spiritual, emotional, and occupational). The U.S. Healthy People 2020 objectives highlight the need for nurse involvement in wellness focused advocacy, education, and care (Office of Disease Prevention and Health Promotion, 2016). Being familiar with these national wellness priorities is critical for nurses as they seek to enhance health and well-being of the patients and themselves.

Recently, the focus has been placed on the concept of "culture of health." The Robert Wood Johnson Foundation (2015) published a vision of this collective effort in which they proposed a population health model to achieve long-lasting change in health and well-being for individuals, communities, populations and in the U.S. health care systems. The important influence of social determinants of health on overall wellness and well-being was highlighted. The 10 principles incorporated in the Foundation's culture of health vision describe the multidimensional aspects of care efforts and the critical nature of building communities with health as a shared value (Plough, 2014). Nurses have the education and perspective necessary to lead this work, foster wellness in the patients' lives as well as their own, and build cultures of health in the health care systems (Martsolf et al., 2016).

Clinical Aspects

ASSESSMENT

When nurses raise awareness of lifestyle opportunities and other wellness growth areas, patients may identify healthy behaviors to adopt for positive change. Tools exist to conduct these wellness assessments. For example, Brown, Applegate, and Yildiz (2015) developed the Holistic Wellness Assessment (HWA), which has shown some effectiveness in identifying personal health needs in young adults. Guidance on patient-centered health risk assessments from the Centers for Disease Control and Prevention (Goetzel et al., 2011) provides additional assessment suggestions. Encouraging the nurses to participate in wellness assessment in the workplace increases awareness of personal needs and assists in implementing lifestyle behavior changes to maximize health. Not only is nurse well-being strengthened, but patient well-being is also positively affected when wellness assessment is implemented.

NURSING INTERVENTIONS, MANAGEMENT, AND IMPLICATIONS

Over the past few decades, the incidence of chronic disease has increased in the United States. Although the traditional illness-focused health care system is needed to assist people with health conditions, such as diabetes, hypertension, and cardiovascular disease, there is a growing awareness of the need for new care delivery strategies both in and outside of the hospital setting. Maintaining or improving health and well-being and helping individuals with health risks to improve their health condition(s) are important goals. Encouraging lifestyle practices to maintain or increase health and delay or avoid disease onset is achievable.

Academic programs focus on preparing the nurses to provide comprehensive care for patients. However, additional emphasis on the multiple determinants of health that impact populations is indicated (Mason, 2014). In nursing education, encouraging students to develop skills in behavior change helps them more positively impact health during their practice (Willis & Kelly, 2016). Strengthening nurses' knowledge base in nutrition, physical activity, stress management, sleep hygiene, smoking cessation, behavior change management, goal setting, and preventive services allows them to enhance their patients' lives.

Focusing on wellness and lifestyle behavior change practices in patient care strengthens health and addresses critical needs of patients with chronic conditions. Educating patients about the importance of nutritious, balanced meals in maintaining health is important. Encouraging 30 minutes of moderate-intensity physical activity at least 5 days a week enhances physical well-being. Guiding patients in deep breathing, guided imagery, and daily meditation practice strengthens individuals' ability to manage stress. Discussing the need for 7.5 to 8 hours of sleep each night promotes overall well-being. For current tobacco users, encouraging tobacco cessation is critical. When nurses educate patients about the impact of lifestyle on current health status and provide opportunities for daily skills practice, they positively impact current and future health behaviors.

As health care costs rise, more hospitals and health care systems are realizing the benefits associated with worksite wellness. Increasing the number of nurses who participate in these programs is critical. Nurses can promote well-being by encouraging self-care with their colleagues and by suggesting involvement in worksite programs available to their patients (Soldano, 2016). In addition, nurses may choose to foster greater health through a worksite wellness provider role.

OUTCOMES

Improved health and/or quality of life for nurses and patients is expected following incorporation of wellness education and practice in daily life. As nurses take better care of themselves and emphasize the critical wellness needs of their patients, increased levels of physical activity, improved nutrition, increased utility of stress management practices, and decreased tobacco use should occur. For example, Bailey and Dougherty (2014) found that a wellness program led by nurses improved access to care and health of migrant workers. Falsafi and Leopard (2015) explored the impact of an 8-week long mindfulness training intervention and found positive effects on depression and anxiety symptoms in low-income and uninsured patients. Encouraging physical activity led to more care-seeking behaviors in the employee populations (Katz & Pronk, 2014). Better health for all will occur as a result of wellness promotion and practice by nurses.

Summary

Nurses' educational backgrounds provide a comprehensive foundation on which wellness advocacy may be based. Participation in worksite wellness programs increase individual health and wellness for nurses and enhance patient well-being too. Emphasizing the value of daily healthy lifestyle behavior practice improve health and wellness.

American Nurses Association. (2017). Healthy nurse, healthy nation. Retrieved from http://www.nursing world.org/MainMenuCategories/WorkplaceSafety/Healthy-Nurse

Bailey, E. N., & Dougherty, A. (2014). A nurse-led wellness program for migrant backstretch workers. *Nursing Forum, 49*(1), 30–38.

Brown, C., Applegate, E. B., & Yildiz, M. (2015). Structural validation of the holistic wellness assessment. *Journal of Psychoeducational Assessment, 33*(5), 483–494.

Falsafi, N., & Leopard, L. (2015). Use of mindfulness, self-compassion, and yoga practices with low-income and/or uninsured patients with depression and/or anxiety. *Journal of Holistic Nursing, 33*(4), 289–297.

Goetzel, R. Z., Staley, P., Ogden, L., Stange, P., Fox, J., Spangler, J., … Richards, C. (2011). *A framework for patient-centered health risk assessments—Providing health promotion and disease prevention services to Medicare beneficiaries.* Atlanta, GA: U.S. Department of Health and Human Services, Centers for Disease Control and Prevention. Retrieved from http://www.cdc.gov/policy/opth/hra

Institute of Medicine. (2011). *The future of nursing: Leading change, advancing health.* Washington, DC: National Academies Press. Retrieved from http://books.nap.edu/openbook.php?record_id=12956&page=R1

Katz, A. l. S., & Pronk, N. P. (2014). The relationship between physical activity and care seeking heavier among employed adults. *Journal of Physical Activity & Health, 11*, 313–319.

Martsolf, G. R., Gordon, T., May, L. W., Mason, D., Sullivan, C., & Villarruel, A. (2016). Innovative nursing care models and culture of health: Early evidence. *Nursing Outlook, 64*, 367–376.

Mason, D. J. (2014). Where and how is health created? *Nursing Outlook, 62*, 162–163.

Milio, N. (1976) A Framework for prevention: Changing health-damaging to health-generating life patterns. *American Journal of Public Health, 66*, 435–439.

National Wellness Institute. (2017). The six dimensions of wellness. Retrieved from http://www.nationalwellness.org/?page=six_dimensions

Office of Disease Prevention and Health Promotion. (2016). *Healthy People 2020.* Washington, DC: U.S. Department of Health and Human Services. Retrieved from https://www.healthypeople.gov

Pender, N., Murdaugh, C., & Parsons, M. A. (2011). *Health promotion in nursing practice.* Boston, MA: Pearson.

Plough, A. L. (2014). Building a culture of health. *American Journal of Preventive Medicine, 47*(5), S388–S390.

Robert Wood Johnson Foundation. (2015). *From vision to action: Measures to mobilize a culture of health.* Princeton, NJ: Author.

Schlotfeldt, R. (1975). The need for a conceptual framework. In P. Verhonic (Ed.), *Nursing research* (pp. 3–25). Boston, MA: Little, Brown.

Sickora, C., & Chase, S. M. (2014). The transformational role of nursing in health care reform. *Journal of Nursing Education, 53*(5), 277–280.

Soldano, S. K. (2016). Workplace wellness programs to promote cancer prevention. *Seminars in Oncology Nursing, 32*(3), 281–290.

Willis, J., & Kelly, M. (2017). What works to encourage student nurses to adopt healthier lifestyles? Findings from an intervention study. *Nurse Education Today, 48,* 180–184.

Medical–Surgical Nursing

Section Editor: Jane F. Marek

An estimated 650,000 of the 3.1 million practicing registered nurses in the United States today are medical–surgical nurses (Academy of Medical–Surgical Nurses [AMSN], 2017; Kaiser Family Foundation [KKF], 2017). Medical–surgical nursing or "med–surg" is one of the first clinical courses taken as a nursing student and practicing nurses continue to draw and build upon that body of knowledge throughout their careers, regardless of their area of expertise. Medical–surgical nursing is truly the foundation for patient care and is considered a specialty, yet the scope of practice is much broader than other specialty areas. Practice settings are just as diverse; although medical–surgical nurses are typically employed in acute-care settings, they also practice in the community, ambulatory care, skilled nursing, primary care, and home care.

Medical–surgical nurses care for acutely ill patients with complex problems involving multiple body systems. To deliver safe and effective care to a diverse patient population, the med–surg nurse needs a broad base of knowledge. This section covers a wide range of common health problems typically encountered in acute-care settings. Content includes respiratory, cardiovascular, gastrointestinal, renal, neurologic, and endocrine disorders, and is a valuable reference for novice and experienced nurses in any health care specialty or practice setting.

Academy of Medical–Surgical Nurses. (2017). What is medical–surgical nursing? Retrieved from https://www.amsn.org/practice-resources/what-medical-surgical-nursing

Kaiser Family Foundation. (2017). Total number of professionally active nurses. Retrieved from http://www.kff.org/other/state-indicator/total-registered-nurses/?currentTimeframe=0&selectedDistributions=registered-nurse- rn&sortModel=%7B%22colId%22:%22Location%22,%22sort%22:%22asc%22%7D

- Addison's Disease *Yolanda Flenoury*
- Amyotrophic Lateral Sclerosis *Mary Jo Elmo*
- Anemia in Adults *Kerry Mastrangelo and Mary T. Quinn Griffin*
- Atelectasis *Ashley L. Foreman*
- Atherosclerosis *Kari Gali*
- Benign Prostatic Hyperplasia *Kelly Ann Lynn*
- Bladder Cancer *Dianna Jo Copley*
- Bowel Obstruction *Kelly Ann Lynn and Jane F. Marek*
- Brain Tumors *Peter J. Cebull*
- Cardiomyopathy *Elsie A. Jolade*
- Chronic Kidney Disease *Mary de Haan*
- Chronic Obstructive Pulmonary Disease *Christina M. Canfield*
- Colorectal Cancer *Visnja Maria Masina and Crina V. Floruta*
- Coronary Artery Disease in Adults *Kate Cook and Mary T. Quinn Griffin*
- Cushing Syndrome *Yolanda Flenoury and Jane F. Marek*
- Deep Vein Thrombosis *Kelly K. McConnell*
- Diabetes Insipidus *Danielle M. Diemer*
- Diabetes Mellitus *Mary Beth Modic*
- Diverticular Disease *Rhoda Redulla*
- Endocarditis *Courtney G. Donahue and Celeste M. Alfes*
- Fractures *Joseph D. Perazzo*
- Gallbladder and Biliary Tract Disease *Andrea Marie Herr*
- Gastric Cancer *Una Hopkins and Jane F. Marek*
- Gastritis *Maria G. Smisek*
- Gastroesophageal Reflux Disease *Kelly Ann Lynn*
- Gout *Maria A. Mendoza*
- Guillain–Barré Syndrome *Kathleen Marsala-Cervasio*
- Heart Failure *Arlene Travis*
- Hemolytic Anemia *Rebecca M. Lutz and Charrita Ernewein*
- Heparin-Induced Thrombocytopenia *Bette K. Idemoto and Jane F. Marek*
- Hiatal Hernia *Maricar P. Gomez*
- Human Immunodeficiency Virus *Scott Emory Moore*
- Hypertension *Marian Soat*

- Hyperthyroidism *Colleen Kurzawa*
- Hypothyroidism *Karen L. Terry*
- Inflammatory Bowel Disease in Adults *Ronald Rock*
- Leukemia *Marisa A. Cortese*
- Liver Cancer *Shannon A. Rives*
- Lung Cancer *Helen Foley*
- Lymphoma *Marisa A. Cortese and Jane F. Marek*
- Multiple Sclerosis *Alaa Mahsoon*
- Myasthenia Gravis *Jennifer Gonzalez*
- Obesity *Kelly Ann Lynn*
- Osteoarthritis *Mary Variath*
- Osteomyelitis *Mary Variath and Jane F. Marek*
- Osteoporosis *Maria A. Mendoza*
- Paget's Disease *Jacqueline Robinson*
- Pancreatic Cancer *Jennifer E. Millman*
- Parkinson's Disease *Peter J. Cebull*
- Peptic Ulcer Disease *Lisa D. Ericson and Deborah R. Gillum*
- Pericarditis *Heidi Youngbauer*
- Peripheral Artery Disease *Gayle M. Petty*
- Pernicious Anemia *Edwidge Cuvilly*
- Polycythemia Vera *Sarine Beukian*
- Prostate Cancer *Erin H. Discenza*
- Rheumatoid Arthritis *Susan V. Brindisi*
- Sepsis *Sharon Stahl Wexler and Catherine O'Neill D'Amico*
- Sickle Cell Disease *Consuela A. Albright*
- Sleep Apnea *Deborah H. Cantero, Leslie J. Lockett, and Rebecca M. Lutz*
- Spinal Stenosis and Disc Herniation *Steven R. Collier*
- Syndrome of Inappropriate Antidiuretic Hormone Secretion *Carrie Foster*
- Systemic Lupus Erythematosus *Merlyn A. Dorsainvil*
- Thrombocytopenia *Maria A. Mendoza*
- Tuberculosis *Christina M. Canfield*
- Valvular Heart Disease *Rebecca Witten Grizzle*

■ ADDISON'S DISEASE

Yolanda Flenoury

Overview

The adrenal glands are an important part of the endocrine system. They secrete vital hormones (glucocorticoids, mineralcorticoids, and androgens) that play a part in response to stress, blood pressure, sodium, potassium, and water balance (Michels & Michels, 2014). Addison's disease is an illness characterized by destruction of the adrenal glands. Adrenal gland destruction may occur because of an autoimmune process, infectious or fungal disease, medications, or malignancy. The goal in caring for these patients is the ability to recognize the disease, treat the symptoms, maintain their health status, and avoid a crisis state. Nurses play a vital role in providing education so that the patients can manage and treat their disease appropriately (Bornstein et al., 2016).

Background

In 1855, Thomas Addison published a book describing his patient case studies and subsequent autopsy findings. He described a disease in his patients that had an insidious onset and was characterized by patterns of progressive, distinctive skin discoloration, nausea, weakness, delirium, and weak pulse with the ultimate demise of the patient. On autopsy, he found that all of his patients had diseased adrenal glands (Addison, 1855).

Addison's disease can manifest as the result of autoimmune processes. This form of Addison's disease accounts for 70% to 90% of cases. The second most common cause of Addison's disease is caused by tuberculosis. A less common cause of Addison's disease includes pathological disorders that include fungal infections, malignancies, and medications (National Endocrine and Metabolic Disease Information Service, 2014). A good history, including geographic location and travel, is vital when making the diagnosis. Patients who live or have been in areas with a high prevalence of tuberculosis or other infectious diseases will have a higher proportion of Addison's disease caused by these conditions (Bornstein et al., 2016). In Western countries, the prevalence of Addison's disease had been estimated at 35 to 60 million people. In the first two decades of life, Addison's disease is diagnosed more often in males, more evenly divided in the third decade and then mostly female in the subsequent decades of life. The gender differential, however, shifts to female, if patients have polyglandular autoimmune syndrome, a condition in which more than one endocrine gland is destroyed (Nieman, 2016).

The adrenal glands have two layers, the cortex and the medulla. The adrenal cortex is responsible for the synthesis of cortisol, aldosterone, and androgens. Most notable in Addison's disease, the lack of cortisol leads to diminished hepatic and muscle glycogen stores, hepatic glucose output and hypoglycemia, muscle weakness, anemia, hyponatremia, and postural hypotension (Brandão Neto & Carvalho, 2014). Cortisol is a glucocorticoid hormone that is secreted in response to pituitary secretion of ACTH. Cortisol is also secreted in response to circadian rhythms, eating, activity, and in response to stress. Cortisol is secreted rapidly after the onset of a physical stressor. This lack of response and release of cortisol results in an addisonian crisis during times of physical stress, such as illness or surgery, and is characterized by shock, hypotension, and volume depletion (Michels & Michels, 2014). In Addison's disease, the distinctive darkening of the skin that can be seen around the neck, axilla, groin, and between digits is related to the ACTH- mediation stimulation of melanocytes (Michels & Michels, 2014). Patients with Addison's disease often have decreased levels of the mineralocorticoid aldosterone due to adrenal cortex destruction. Aldosterone deficiency can lead to hyponatermia, hyperkalemia, and hypotension (Quinkler, Oelkers, Remde, & Allolio, 2014).

Clinical Aspects

It is recommended that acutely ill patients with unexplained symptoms suggestive of Addison's disease (volume depletion, hypotension, hyperkalemia, hyponatremia, fever, abdominal pain, hyperpigmentation, or hypoglycemia) are tested to exclude Addison's disease as a diagnosis (Bornstein et al., 2016). Confirmatory testing with corticotropin-stimulation testing is recommended for patients who have suggestive symptoms. Patients who have severe adrenal insufficiency or are in an adrenal crisis should be treated with intravenous (IV) hydrocortisone to prevent life-threatening consequences, even in the absence of definitive test results (Bornstein et al., 2016).

Diagnosis of Addison's disease can be made using the short synacthen test, also known as the ACTH stimulation test. Peak cortisol levels less than 500 nmol/L indicate adrenal insufficiency. Measurement of plasma ACTH is recommended to establish diagnosis of Addison's disease (primary adrenal insufficiency) versus secondary adrenal insufficiency related to decreased ACTH levels. Plasma renin and aldosterone can also be measured to determine whether the patient has a mineralocorticoid deficiency (Bornstein et al., 2016).

Patients who have Addison's disease need to have glucocorticoid replacement therapy. Glucocorticoids can be replaced with hydrocortisone, cortisone acetate, or prednisolone. Generally, the doses of hydrocortisone and cortisone acetate are given in divided doses, with the largest in the morning to mimic the circadian cycle of cortisol release (Bornstein et al., 2016). If the patient has an aldosterone deficiency, he or she should also have mineralocorticoid replacement with fludrocortisone (Quinkler et al., 2014).

Patients who are having an adrenal crisis should be treated emergently with IV glucocorticoids and fluid resuscitation. The preferred drug is hydrocortisone, followed by prednisolone. Dexamethasone should be used if no other glucocorticoid is available (Bornstein et al., 2016).

ASSESSMENT

It is imperative that patients who have Addison's disease have a thorough medication reconciliation. The nurse needs to be aware that these patients cannot be without their glucocorticoid replacement and that the other routes of medication administration must be provided if the patient is unable to take oral doses. The nurse should collaborate with the other members of the medical team to facilitate medication adjustments in the face of worsening illness, surgical procedures, or labor to prevent an Addisonian crisis. Nursing assessment should include monitoring for worsening symptoms of adrenal insufficiency; hypotension, elevated potassium, decreased sodium, and hypoglycemia could indicate an impending crisis (Craven, 2016).

NURSING INTERVENTIONS, MANAGEMENT, AND IMPLICATIONS

Addison's disease is a chronic condition with the vast majority of the disease being managed at home by the patient. Nurses play a vital role in educating and advocating for patients with Addison's disease. Patients should be educated about the types of physical stressors (illness, surgery, severe injury, and pregnancy) that

can precipitate a crisis (Bornstein et al., 2016; Craven, 2016). Education should also include symptoms, such as fever, nausea and vomiting, anorexia, weakness, lethargy, and decreased urinary output, that may indicate an impending crisis state (Craven, 2016). Patient education should include the importance of medication timing to mimic normal cortisol release, as well as emergency medication dosing if they are having crisis symptoms in a nonhospital settings (Bornstein et al., 2016; Craven, 2016).

OUTCOMES

Nursing evaluation of treatment response to glucocorticoid replacement includes assessment of weight stability, postural hypotension, reported energy levels, and signs of glucocorticoid excess (cushighoid symptoms). Treatment response to mineralocorticoid replacement should be assessed by presence of postural hypotension, peripheral edema, and reported salt craving (Bornstein et al., 2016).

Summary

Addison's disease or primary adrenal insufficiency is a disease characterized by destruction of the adrenal glands. Cortisol produced by the adrenal gland plays a vital role in the body's response to stress, and helps to maintain blood pressure, sodium, potassium, and water balance. Without lifelong cortisol replacement, patients with Addison's disease are at risk for life-threatening hypovolemia, hypoglycemia, and hypotension. The goal in caring for these patients is the ability to recognize the disease, treat the symptoms, maintain their health status, and avoid a crisis state. The nurse is responsible for providing close observation and careful nursing assessments to monitor for signs of adrenal insufficiency. As most of the management of Addison's disease is done outside of a health care setting, medication and disease management education is crucial to help people with Addison's disease maintain their health.

Addison, T. (1855). In the constitutional and local effects of disease of the supra-renal capsules. Retrieved from https://archive.org/details/b21298786

Bornstein, S. R., Allolio, B., Arlt, W., Barthel, A., Don-Wauchope, A., Hammer, G. D., . . . Torpy, D. J. (2016). Diagnosis and treatment of primary adrenal insufficiency: An Endocrine Society clinical practice guideline. *Journal of Clinical Endocrinology and Metabolism*, 101(2), 364–389. doi:10.1210/jc.2015-1710

Brandão Neto, R. A., & de Carvalho, J. F. (2014). Diagnosis and classification of Addison's disease (autoimmune adrenalitis). *Autoimmunity Reviews*, 13(4–5), 408–411. doi:10.1016/j.autrev.2014.01.025

Craven, H. (2016). Physiological alterations of the endocrine system. In H. Craven (Ed.), *Core curriculum for medical-surgical nursing*. Sewell, NJ: Academy of Medical Surgical Nursing.

Michels, A., & Michels, N. (2014). Addison disease: Early detection and treatment principles. *American Family Physician*, 89(7), 563–568.

National Endocrine and Metabolic Disease Information Service. (2014). *Adrenal insufficiency and Addison's disease*. Washington, DC: U.S. DHHS.

Quinkler, M., Oelkers, W., Remde, H., & Allolio, B. (2015). Mineralocorticoid substitution and monitoring in primary adrenal insufficiency. *Best Practice & Research. Clinical Endocrinology & Metabolism*, 29(1), 17–24. doi:10.1016/j.beem.2014.08.008

■ AMYOTROPHIC LATERAL SCLEROSIS

Mary Jo Elmo

Overview

Amyotrophic lateral sclerosis (ALS) is a progressive neurodegenerative disease affecting both upper and lower motor neurons resulting in paralysis. It was first described in 1869 and became well known in the United States when famous New York Yankee baseball player Lou Gehrig was diagnosed with ALS in 1939 (Zarei et al., 2015). There is no cure for ALS and the disease is fatal with death occurring in most patients within 2 to 5 years of diagnosis. An estimated 20,000 to 30,000 people in the United States are living with ALS with an additional 5,000 newly diagnosed cases annually. Patient presentation varies, but ultimately all patients will have respiratory insufficiency, which is the most common cause of death. Because there is no cure, a primary goal in ALS is symptom management.

Background

ALS is frequently called an insidious disease with progression leading to diffuse muscle weakness, muscle wasting, dysarthria, dysphagia, and paralysis, including paralysis of the respiratory muscles. Men have a lifetime risk of ALS of 1:350 and women 1:500 (Salameh, Brown, & Berry, 2015). Only 10% of patients live more than 10 years (Paganoni, Karam, Joyce, Bedlack, & Carter, 2015). ALS is sporadic in 90% to 95% of cases and 5% to 10% of cases have familial ALS. The superoxide dismutase-1 (SOD1) gene mutation was the first identified and is the most common. An additional 18 gene mutations that cause familial ALS (FALS) have been discovered. Whether sporadic or familial, the presentations are similar with age of onset as the distinguishing feature. In ALS, the age of onset varies from 50 to 65 years old; in familial ALS the onset is generally 10 years earlier. Although the etiology of sporadic ALS is unknown, there are several risk factors. Smoking increases the probability of ALS because of inflammation, oxidative stress, and neurotoxicity associated with cigarettes. There is an association with lead and formaldehyde exposure and ALS, but a relationship between other heavy metals and chemicals has not yet been identified (Zarei et al., 2015). There is an increase in the rate of ALS in U.S. military personnel and ALS is now considered a 100% service connected disability (Weisskopf, Cudkowicz, & Johnson, 2015).

ALS is a diagnosis of exclusion and it takes an average of 11 months to confirm the diagnosis. In many patients, symptoms need to progress before a definitive diagnosis can be made (Nzwalo, de Abreu, Swash, Pinto, & de Carvalho, 2014). Common presenting symptoms include foot drop, weak hand grasp, or slurred speech. Regardless of where the weakness first presents, with disease progression weakness ultimately spreads, finally affecting the respiratory muscles (Paganoni et al., 2015).

Individual patients vary in presentation and severity of symptoms. It was once thought patients with ALS do not experience cognitive impairment, but up to 50% of persons will develop frontotemporal dementia (FTD). Pseudobulbar palsy, characterized by uncontrollable laughing or crying, is also seen in up to 50% of patients (Pattee et al., 2014). Bulbar symptoms, such as dysphagia and dysarthria, are the presenting symptoms in 30% of patients. The presence of bulbar symptoms puts patients at risk for sialorrhea, weight loss, dehydration, aspiration pneumonia, and inability to communicate. Muscle weakness or complete paralysis can affect the neck, limbs, and trunk, which may lead to complete dependence on caregivers. Paralysis of the respiratory muscle leads to respiratory failure. Central apnea and nighttime hypoventilation can occur independently from daytime respiratory function (Ahmed et al., 2016). ALS affects bowel and bladder function and 43% of persons with ALS have urinary incontinence and 46% have problems with constipation (Nübling et al., 2014). Depression can affect the patient and family members. Although there is no cure, there are management strategies to treat symptoms.

Clinical Aspects

The only U.S. Food and Drug Administration–approved medication to treat ALS is riluzole (Rilutek, Tegultik), which decreases the neurotoxic effects of glutamate. The use of riluzole prolongs survival by approximately 3 months and may delay the need for tracheostomy or dependence on a ventilator. Caring for the patient with ALS is highly complex and requires ongoing assessments. Because of the progressive nature of the disease, an intervention employed just a week ago may be obsolete the following week. Patients with ALS who attend a multidisciplinary clinic specializing in treatment of ALS have slightly improved life expectancy. Both the American Academy of Neurology and the European Federation of Neurological Services recommend ALS patients and their caregivers be referred to a multidisciplinary clinic (Zarei et al., 2015).

Respiratory failure is the leading cause of death in persons with ALS, making assessing and monitoring patients' respiratory function a priority of care. Serial pulmonary function testing and monitoring the forced vital capacity (FVC) results are recommended; there is a strong correlation between mortality and FVC less than 50%. The nurse should carefully assess the patient for signs of declining respiratory functioning. Data should be gathered regarding the patient's quality and amount of sleep. Does the patient wake up with headaches? Is the patient fatigued during the day? Is the patient sleeping with more than two pillows? The use of noninvasive ventilation (NIV) is recommended when the FVC falls to approximately 50% or sooner if the patient is symptomatic, hypercarbic, or has apnea confirmed by a sleep study (Ahmed et al., 2016). The use of NIV can prolong survival in ALS, but approximately 25% of patients are unable to tolerate the therapy (Ahmed et al., 2016). Patients should be assessed for tolerance and compliance with therapy at each visit. Diaphragmatic (phrenic nerve) pacing has been used as a means to prolong survival and improve sleep in persons with ALS, but the results are controversial (Robinson, 2016).

Effective airway clearance is crucial in ALS. Sialorrhea, or excessive drooling, is caused by muscle weakness leading to the inability to manage normal saliva production (Banfi et al., 2015). Anticholinergic medications, such as glycopyrolate, scopolamine, and hyoscyamine sulfate, can decrease saliva production but can also contribute to thickening of mucus. Weakness of the muscles that control cough contributes to the inability to manage saliva production and the inability to clear secretions from airways. Methods to assist in cough and airway clearance include using a mechanical insufflator/exsufflator device, air stacking followed by cough, or a cough-aid device. To ensure patients are receiving the correct therapy, it is crucial for nurses to recognize whether the patient is having a problem with managing saliva or clearing mucus.

ASSESSMENT

Assessing the patient's nutritional status, fluid volume balance, and weight is another important nursing consideration. Malnutrition and dehydration contribute to fatigue and may compound muscle weakness (Zarei et al. 2015). Patients should undergo a formal swallow study and be frequently assessed for the ability to chew/swallow food. Patients are at risk for aspiration and may benefit from a nutritional consult to determine the type and consistency of food or need for supplements. It is not uncommon for patients with upper extremity paralysis, even in the absence of bulbar symptoms, to forgo food and fluid so as not to be "too much of a bother" to their caregivers. A percutaneous endoscopic gastrostomy is recommended when a patient loses 10% of body weight or 10 pounds in a month. In addition, fluid intake needs to be monitored, especially as it may contribute to constipation.

Many patients identify the loss of speech or ability to communicate as the worst symptom of ALS (Paganoni et al., 2015). Nurses should assess and identify strategies to allow the patient to communicate. There are a myriad of augmentative alternative speech devices (AAC) that patients can use when they lose the ability to speak. Patients should be continually assessed for referral and evaluation for an AAC device. These devices can be controlled by eye gaze or head movements. Nurses should also be aware of voice banking, in which the patient's own voice is be stored for eventual transfer to the AAC when the need arises.

Depression and pseudobulbar affect (PBA) are frequently seen in persons with ALS. Anxiety and caregiver burden are also common. Medications can be used to treat depression and PBA. Nurses should be aware that depression is different from hopelessness and a wish to die. Quality of life does not always correlate with physical function in persons with ALS. In fact, quality of life is generally maintained in people with ALS and health care professionals frequently underestimate how ALS patients perceive their quality of life.

End-of-life care issues need to be addressed while the patient is able to communicate and make decisions.

Palliative care and hospice are options for the patient and family to discuss. Many multidisciplinary clinics have palliative caregivers as part of their team.

OUTCOMES

The focus of care for patients with ALS is managing dyspnea and pain. Before the disease progresses to respiratory insufficiency, the patient should be made aware of the various treatment options, including tracheostomy and invasive ventilation. In the United States, between 1.4% and 15% of patients with ALS choose to go onto invasive ventilation. The number is much higher in Japan, with as many as 45% of patients opting for mechanical ventilation. Patients who choose tracheostomy ventilation are typically younger, have young children, and are less likely to be depressed (Rabkin et al., 2006).

Summary

ALS is a progressive degenerative motor neuron disease with an average survival rate of 2 to 5 years from onset of symptoms. There is no cure but there are treatment strategies to manage symptoms and prolong life. Ensuring patients are optimizing respiratory therapies is key to prolonging survival in ALS. This includes non-invasive ventilation, airway clearance therapies, and sialorrhea management. Malnutrition and dehydration are associated with other complications. Discussions regarding end-of-life care, including palliative care, hospice, and tracheostomy, are crucial in ensuring patients are given treatment options when disease progression affects respiratory functioning.

Ahmed, R., Newcombe, R., Piper, A., Lewis, S., Yee, B., Kernan, M., & Grunstein, R. (2016). Sleep disorders and respiratory function in amyotrophic lateral sclerosis. *Sleep Medicine Reviews*, 26, 33–42. doi:10.1016/j.smrv.2015.05.007

Banfi, P., Ticozzi, N., Lax, A., Guidugli, G. A., Nicolini, A., & Silani, V. (2015). A review of options for treating sialorrhea in amyotrophic lateral sclerosis. *Respiratory Care*, 60(3), 446–454. doi:10.4187/respcare.02856

Nübling, G. S., Mie, E., Bauer, R. M., Hensler, M., Lorenzl, S., Hapfelmeier, A., . . . Winkler, A. S. (2014). Increased prevalence of bladder and intestinal dysfunction in amyotrophic lateral sclerosis. *Amyotrophic Lateral Sclerosis & Frontotemporal Degeneration*, 15(3–4), 174–179. doi:10.3109/21678421.2013.868001

Nzwalo, H., de Abreu, D., Swash, M., Pinto, S., & de Carvalho, M. (2014). Delayed diagnosis in ALS: The problem continues. *Journal of the Neurological Sciences*, 343(1–2), 173–175. doi:10.1016/j.jns.2014.06.003

Paganoni, S., Karam, C., Joyce, N., Bedlack, R., & Carter, G. T. (2015). Comprehensive rehabilitative care across the spectrum of amyotrophic lateral sclerosis. *NeuroRehabilitation*, 37(1), 53–68. doi:10.3233/NRE-151240

Pattee, G. L., Wymer, J. P., Lomen-Hoerth, C., Appel, S. H., Formella, A. E., & Pope, L. E. (2014). An open-label multicenter study to assess the safety of dextromethorphan/quinidine in patients with pseudobulbar affect associated with a range of underlying neurological conditions. *Current Medical Research and Opinion*, 30(11), 2255–2265. doi:10.1185/03007995.2014.940040

Rabkin, J. G., Albert, S. M., Tider, T., Del Bene, M. L., O'Sullivan, I., Rowland, L. P., & Mitsumoto, H. (2006). Predictors and course of elective long-term mechanical ventilation: A prospective study of ALS patients. *Amyotrophic Lateral Sclerosis*, 7(2), 86–95. doi:10.1080/14660820500515021

Robinson, R. (2016). Diaphragm pacing for ALS at crossroads following conflicting trial results. *Neurology Today*, 16(2), 18–21. doi:10.1097/01.NT.0000480659.79684.39

Salameh, J. S., Brown, R. H., & Berry, J. D. (2015). Amyotrophic lateral sclerosis: Review. *Seminars in Neurology*, 35(4), 469–476. doi:10.1055/s-0035-1558984

Weisskopf, M. G., Cudkowicz, M. E., & Johnson, N. (2015). Military service and amyotrophic lateral sclerosis in a population-based cohort. *Epidemiology*, 26(6), 831–838. doi:10.1097/EDE.0000000000000376

Zarei, S., Carr, K., Reiley, L., Diaz, K., Guerra, O., Altamirano, P. F., . . . Chinea, A. (2015). A comprehensive review of amyotrophic lateral sclerosis. *Surgical Neurology International*, 6, 171. doi:10.4103/2152-7806.169561

■ ANEMIA IN ADULTS

Kerry Mastrangelo
Mary T. Quinn Griffin

Overview

Anemia is one of the most common hematologic problems. The term "anemia" refers to a condition in which there is a decrease in the number of circulating red blood cells (RBCs), hemoglobin concentration, or the volume of packed cells (hematocrit) as compared with normal values. The most commonly accepted definition of anemia is the World Health Organization's (WHO) definition of a hemoglobin concentration less than 13 g/dL in men and less than 12 g/dL in women (Le, 2016). Older adults with anemia have increased hospitalizations and higher mortality rates making anemia a relevant public health concern in light of the predicted increase in the population aged 65 years and older. Anemia is associated with higher utilization of health care resources and an overall increase in morbidity and mortality (Le, 2016).

Background

The prevalence of anemia in the United States is estimated at 5.6% of adults with 1.5% of anemias diagnosed as moderate to severe. The prevalence of anemia in adults has increased from 4.0% to 7.1% over the years 2003 to 2012 (Le, 2016). Anemia is a common problem and is found in 20% to 30% of all hospitalized patients, making it a significant concern for nurses. Most anemias in adults result from blood loss, inadequate RBC production, or destruction of RBCs. Anemias are generally categorized according to cause or morphology.

Clinical manifestations of anemia are dependent on the degree of anemia and whether the anemia is acute or chronic. Common manifestations, regardless of the etiology, are fatigue, dyspnea with exertion, weakness, lightheadedness, palpitations, and pallor of the skin, mucous membranes, and conjunctiva. Tachycardia and hypotension occur as anemia becomes more severe. Severe anemia leads to increased cardiac output to compensate for tissue hypoxia, resulting in a systolic ejection murmur. Sustained tachycardia to compensate for the decreased hemoglobin concentration eventually leads to left ventricular failure. The most common types of anemia in adults are iron-deficiency anemia, hemolytic anemia, pernicious anemia, and anemia related to chronic diseases (Goodnough & Schrier, 2014).

Iron-deficiency anemia, classified as a microcytic anemia, is the most common cause of anemia worldwide and is due to inadequate absorption of iron or excessive blood loss. Predisposing factors for the development of this anemia are diets poor in iron-rich foods, history of gastric surgery, chronic aspirin or nonsteroidal anti-inflammatory drug (NSAID) use, chronic blood loss, and menorrhagia. An unusual symptom of iron-deficiency anemia is pica, the compulsive eating of nonfood substances such as clay, dirt, and ice.

In hemolytic anemias, the life span of the RBC, usually 120 days, is shortened resulting in an increase in circulating reticulocytes related to bone marrow compensation. This anemia is classified as a microcytic anemia seen in persons with hemoglobinopathies, thalassemias,

hereditary spherocytosis, glucose-6-phosphate dehydrogenase (G6PD), and blood transfusion reactions.

Pernicious anemia, also called *megoblastic anemia*, is classified as a macrocytic anemia and is characterized by large, immature, poorly functioning RBCs. The two most common causes are vitamin B_{12} deficiency and folate deficiency. This anemia is more prevalent in the fifth and sixth decade of life and in persons of Northern European descent. There is a progressive decrease in parietal cell function in the stomach, resulting in decreased production of intrinsic factor necessary for the absorption of vitamin B_{12}. Predisposing factors for pernicious anemia are a history of gastric surgery, chronic gastritis, chronic alcoholism, malnutrition, and use of certain drugs such as hydroxyurea, trimethoprim, zidovidine, and methotrexate. In addition to the common clinical manifestations seen in anemia, persons with pernicious anemia may present with a sore, beefy red tongue; angular cheilosis; parethesias in the extremities; and edema of the lower extremities.

Anemia of chronic disease (ACD), also referred to as *anemia of inflammation*, can be classified as normocytic or microcytic and is a result of decreased proliferation and shortened life span of RBCs. The reduction in RBCs is thought to be due to decreased erythropoietin and the release of proinflammatory cytokines. ACD is most commonly seen in the elderly and is associated with chronic kidney disease, autoimmune disease, malignancies, and inflammatory disorders such as rheumatoid arthritis and systemic lupus erythematosus.

Clinical Aspects

ASSESSMENT

History, physical exam, and laboratory testing are essential in evaluating the patient with anemia. Anemia is indicative of an underlying pathology and is never a normal finding. A thorough patient health history should include a comprehensive dietary history, current and past medical and surgical history, and a review of prescribed and over-the-counter medications. Specific questions should be directed toward a history of kidney or liver disease, malignancy, autoimmune disease, blood transfusions, weight loss, a decrease in appetite, color of stools, alcohol and NSAID use, and menstrual pattern. The aim of physical examination is to ascertain the severity and etiology of the anemia. The assessment should include the evaluation of the patient's general appearance, nutritional status, and observing the patient's skin, mucous membranes and conjunctiva for pallor or jaundice. Vital signs should be assessed for hypotension, tachycardia, dyspnea, and fever. In addition, a complete cardiac and abdominal exam noting the presence of murmurs or an enlarged liver or spleen should be performed.

The initial diagnostic workup for anemia should include a complete blood count (CBC) with differential, red cell indices, a peripheral smear, reticulocyte count, serum folic acid, serum vitamin B_{12}, serum iron, total iron-binding capacity (TIBC), ferritin level, and stool for occult blood (Cash & Glass, 2017). The reticulocyte count is of primary importance in diagnosis, as it reflects the early release of immature erythrocytes. The red cell indices and the peripheral smear include the mean corpuscular volume (MCV) measuring the average size of the RBC classifying the anemia as microcytic, macrocytic, or normocytic and the mean corpuscular hemoglobin (MCH) measuring the hemoglobin content per erythrocyte, classifying the color of the cell as hypochromic or normochromic. Serum iron studies, vitamin B_{12} and folate levels provide information to differentiate among the types of anemia. Stool for occult blood identifies blood loss contributing to anemia.

The treatment of anemia is tailored to the underlying cause. If anemia is the result of blood loss, the source must be identified. Iron-deficiency anemia and pernicious anemia require supplementation of iron, folate, or vitamin B_{12}. ACD will improve with recovery from the underlying disorder, although if recovery is not possible, transfusions and erythropoiesis-stimulating agents may be warranted (Goodnough & Schrier, 2014).

NURSING INTERVENTIONS, MANAGEMENT, AND IMPLICATIONS

Nursing-related problems include inadequate tissue perfusion related to decreased hemoglobin and activity intolerance related to fatigue. Nursing care should include monitoring of vital signs, monitoring of hemoglobin level, administering oxygen to maintain O_2 saturation greater than 90%, assessing skin color and capillary refill, providing frequent rest periods, administering prescribed medications, and patient teaching.

OUTCOMES

The major goal of medical management and nursing care is to identify and correct the underlying cause of the anemia and prevent tissue hypoxia leading to heart failure. The expected outcomes of nursing care are tolerance of normal daily activity, heart rate and blood pressure within normal

parameters, maintaining adequate tissue perfusion, adherence to prescribed therapy, and the absence of complications.

Summary

The prognosis of anemia depends on its underlying cause. The severity, etiology, onset, and patient comorbidities play a significant role in the prognosis. Nursing care should focus on the prevention of the most serious complications due to tissue hypoxia, hypotension, and cardiac insufficiency.

Cash, J., & Glass, C. (2017). *Family practice guidelines* (4th ed.). New York, NY: Springer Publishing.

Goodnough, L. T., & Schrier, S. L. (2014). Evaluation and management of anemia in the elderly. *American Journal of Hematology*, 89(1), 88–96. doi:10.1002/ajh.23598

Le, C. H. (2016). The prevalence of anemia and moderate-severe anemia in the U.S. Population (NHANES 2003–2012). *PLOS ONE*, *11*(11), e0166635. doi:10.1371/journal.pone.0166635

■ ATELECTASIS

Ashley L. Foreman

Overview

Atelectasis is a pulmonary complication that is the result of an injury, chronic disease process, or surgical intervention (Cabrera & Pravikoff, 2016). Atelectasis is defined as a reversible alveolar collapse typically resulting from obstruction of the airway serving the affected alveoli (Restrepo & Braverman, 2015; Schub, Uribe, & Pravikoff, 2016). More specific, it describes a decrease in the ability of alveolar spaces to inflate with oxygen, resulting in volume loss. The extent of involvement ranges from microatelectases that are undetectable on chest radiograph to complete lung collapse. Atelectasis can be acute or chronic. Chronic atelectasis is associated with chronic airway diseases, neuromuscular impairment, chest wall deformity, or lung cancer. Acute atelectasis is the most common complication of surgery. Postoperative atelectasis occurs in 90% of adults and children receiving anesthesia (Cabrera & Pravikoff, 2016). Prompt initiation of treatment is necessary to open the areas of obstruction and relieve symptoms. Techniques to mobilize secretions, improve ventilation, and reduce morbidity and mortality are priorities in the nursing management of patients with atelectasis.

Background

Atelectasis is defined as the collapse or incomplete expansion of the lung, and is classified into two broad categories, obstructive and nonobstructive (Ray, Bodenham, & Paramasivam, 2014). Although it is usually a benign finding, there is an inability of the alveoli to expand completely, leading to volume loss and progressive airway collapse. This affects systemic oxygenation by the loss of adequate ventilation to lung zones and inadequate gas exchange. Atelectasis caused by large airway obstruction is often linked to bronchial or metastatic tumors, inflammatory diseases (e.g., tuberculosis or sarcoidosis), or other foreign bodies. Atelectasis caused by small airway obstruction is associated with mucus plugging caused by inflammatory or infectious disease processes, including pneumonia, bronchitis, and bronchiectasis (Ray et al., 2014). Mechanisms associated with non-obstructive etiology or compressive atelectasis include large bullae (extensive air trapping), loss of contact between the visceral and parietal pleura (due to pleural effusion), or lack of surfactant production as seen in acute lung injury (ALI) or acute respiratory distress syndrome (ARDS).

Atelectasis affects up to 90% of patients undergoing major surgical procedures and can lead to postoperative pulmonary complications (PPCs). A PPC is any pulmonary abnormality that produces an "identifiable disease or dysfunction that negatively affects the clinical course after surgery" (Restrepo & Braverman, 2015, p. 97). Examples include aspiration pneumonias, interstitial/alveolar edema, gas exchange abnormalities, respiratory failure, weaning failure, pleural effusion, or pneumothorax. Atelectasis has been recognized as a contributor to prolonged hospitalizations, admissions to the intensive care unit (ICU), and increased health expenditures (Restrepo & Braverman, 2015). Respiratory complications are the leading cause of morbidity and mortality in patients with impaired cough or neuromuscular disease (American Association for Respiratory Care [AARC], 2015).

Three important physiologic mechanisms found to cause or contribute to the development of atelectasis include "external compression (limitation of alveolar expansion), alveolar gas resorption and surfactant impairment" (Restrepo & Braverman, 2015, p. 97).

- ■ *External compression.* During general anesthesia (GA), mechanical ventilation forces the alveoli to collapse by disrupting the existing negative pressure that maintains them in the open state (Restrepo & Braverman, 2015). Dependent regions of the lung are then more prone to atelectasis secondary to decreased ventilation and insufficient spontaneous drainage of secretions with gravity (Ferri, 2014). In anesthetized patients, muscle relaxation displaces the diaphragm, which results in compression of adjacent lung tissue. Other factors influencing the development of compression atelectasis include chest anatomy and respiratory muscle changes (e.g., restrictive lung disease; Restrepo & Braverman, 2015).

- ■ *Alveolar resorption.* In alveolar resorption atelectasis, lower areas of ventilation (relative to perfusion) are susceptible to collapse due to mucus plugging in the bronchioles. In a normal state, "lung regions that have low ventilation compared with perfusion have low alveolar oxygen tension when the fraction of inspired oxygen is low" (Restrepo & Braverman, 2015, p. 99). Nitrogen helps to provide surface tension to prevent alveolar collapse. With GA, the fraction of inspired oxygen is increased with the addition of supplemental oxygen. Alveolar oxygen tension (partial pressure of arterial oxygen) then rises. Ultimately, the loss of nitrogen and increases in oxygen through GA result in diminished alveolar volume (Restrepo & Braverman, 2015).

- ■ *Surfactant impairment.* Pulmonary surfactant is a phospholipid that reduces alveolar surface tension, improves alveolar stability, and prevents collapse of the alveoli at end expiration. Anesthesia has been shown to diminish stabilizing properties of surfactant. Cyclical opening and closing of the alveoli during GA with mechanical ventilation leads to reduced availability of surfactant. Excessive alveolar surface tension reduces functional residual capacity (FRC) and pulmonary compliance.

In adults, atelectasis is commonly identified as a postoperative complication. Surgery greatly increases the risk for atelectasis due to supine positioning, chest wall splinting, abdominal distention, poor clearance of secretions, airway obstruction, and impaired cough reflex (Schub et al., 2016). Other major risk factors in the adult population include mucus plugs from obstructive lung disease, obesity, smoking, neuromuscular disease or chest wall injury (pneumothorax). Right middle lobe (RML) syndrome, a type of chronic atelectasis, usually results from bronchial compression and obstruction by surrounding lymph nodes or scarring (Sharma, 2015). The likelihood of PPCs increases in patients with pre-existing conditions.

Clinical Aspects

A thorough history and physical assessment should be performed to guide the nursing care of patients at risk for atelectasis. Evidence-based nursing interventions to prevent and treat atelectasis should be used to improve quality and safety outcomes.

ASSESSMENT

Physical assessment findings and clinical presentation may include decreased or absent breath sounds, cough, shortness of breath, tachycardia and diminished chest expansion, low-grade fever or hypoxia (Ferri, 2014). Patients may also present with concurrent history of recent surgery (anesthesia), chronic bronchitis, endobronchial neoplasm, chest infection, or injury. Imaging studies, including chest radiograph or CT scans, are commonly performed to investigate symptoms and narrow differential diagnoses. On chest radiograph, areas of atelectasis would be seen as volume loss, a linear or wedge-shaped density or loss of contour of the hemidiaphragm (Watters, 2014). Intravenous contrast may be required for appropriate differentiation of the types of atelectasis (Sharma, 2015). In selected patients, fiberoptic bronchoscopy may be helpful in removing foreign bodies, or mucus plugs unresponsive to conservative measures. Bronchoscopy is used to evaluate endobronchial or peribronchial lesions (Ferri, 2014). Arterial blood gases may be used to identify hypoxemia and bacterial cultures of sputum and blood are helpful in identifying sources of infection.

NURSING INTERVENTIONS, MANAGEMENT, AND IMPLICATIONS

Various nonpharmacologic therapies promote adequate pulmonary ventilation and airway clearance. Deep breathing/coughing, repositioning, and early ambulation after surgery are effective methods. Other mechanisms, such as incentive spirometry (ICS), tracheal suctioning (as appropriate), chest physiotherapy, and postural drainage, are also effective in mobilizing secretions. These techniques can be used in both acute and chronic atelectasis (Ferri, 2014). Nursing care should be focused on reducing the work of breathing and promoting optimal oxygenation. In more select cases, continuous positive airway pressure devices have also been used to promote positive end expiratory pressure (PEEP). Patients on mechanical ventilation may be given recruitment maneuvers to improve gas exchange, along with utilizing aggressive ventilator-weaning protocols as appropriate. These interventions help to reduce pulmonary complications, length of stay, and minimize readmissions to the hospital.

Aerosolized medications, including bronchodilators, expectorants, and mucolytic agents, have been used to improve airway clearance, but there is limited research to support the efficacy of these medications. AARC (2015) recommends nonpharmacological approaches to airway clearance, in combination with an individualized plan that may include pharmacological intervention as appropriate.

OUTCOMES

The use of bronchodilators and corticosteroids in symptomatic patients with chronic obstructive pulmonary disease (COPD) is highly recommended to reduce inflammation and mucus production (AARC, 2015). Inhaled dornase alfa (Pulmozyme), a mucolytic agent, in combination with hypertonic saline is an approved treatment for patients with cystic fibrosis for sputum clearance (Bilton & Stanford, 2014). This medication can also be used for mechanically ventilated patients with atelectasis.

Summary

Although atelectasis is usually a benign finding, it is important that practicing nurses understand the background, clinical presentation, and nursing implications of atelectasis. Early identification of symptoms is key in the management of atelectasis. To improve patient safety and quality, approaches to care should be tailored to meet individual patient needs based on clinical presentation and risk factors. Continued research in this area is needed to determine efficacy of treatment options and to improve health outcomes for patients.

American Association for Respiratory Care. (2015). AARC clinical practice guideline: Effectiveness of pharmacologic airway clearance therapies in hospitalized patients. *Respiratory Care*, 60(7), 1073–1077.

Bilton, D., & Stanford, G. (2014). The expanding armamentarium of drugs to aid sputum clearance: How should they be used to optimize care? *Current Opinion in Pulmonary Medicine*, 20(6), 601–606. doi:10.1097/ MCP.0000000000000104

Cabrera, G., & Pravikoff, D. (2016). Quick lesson: Atelectasis, postoperative. *CINAHL Nursing Guide*. Ipswich, MA: EBSCO Publishing.

Ferri, F. F. (2014). *Ferri's clinical advisor 2014*. Philadelphia, PA: Elsevier/Mosby.

Ray, K., Bodenham, A., & Paramasivam, E. (2014). Pulmonary atelectasis in anaesthesia and critical care. *Critical Care & Pain, 4*, 236–244.

Restrepo, R. D., & Braverman, J. (2015). Current challenges in the recognition, prevention and treatment of perioperative pulmonary atelectasis. *Expert Review of Respiratory Medicine, 9*(1), 97–107. doi:10.1586/17476348.2015.996134

Schub, T., Uribe, L. M., & Pravikoff, D. (2016). Quick lesson: Atelectasis, in children. *CINAHL Nursing Guide.* Ipswich, MA: EBSCO Publishing.

Sharma, S. (2015). Lobar atelectasis imaging. *Medscape.* Retrieved from http://emedicine.medscape.com/article/353833-overview

Watters, J. R. (2014). A systematic approach to basic chest radiograph interpretation: A cardiovascular focus. *Canadian Journal of Cardiovascular Nursing, 24*(2), 4–10.

■ ATHEROSCLEROSIS

Kari Gali

Overview

Atherosclerosis is a progressive, inflammatory disease characterized by the formation of a fatty plaque in the intimal layer of medium- and large-size arteries. Derived from the Greek terms, "athero," which means gruel or wax, describing the fatty luminal plaque and "sclerosis," which means hardening corresponding to the fibrous cap on the plaque's edge. Atherosclerosis is considered one of the most lethal diseases in the world today (Ladich & Burke, 2016). Starting from childhood, fatty streaks develop and over time grow into atheromas (plaques) narrowing arteries and impairing blood flow. Clinical manifestations generally do not occur until at least 75% of the arterial lumen is blocked. Presenting in three general ways, atherosclerosis progresses into cardiovascular diseases, peripheral artery disease (PAD), and chronic kidney disease associated with renal stenosis.

According to the 2017 Heart Disease and Stroke Statistic Update, cardiovascular disease accounts for 33% of the deaths in the United States, killing over 800,000 Americans annually (American Heart Association [AHA], 2017). With more than 92 million Americans affected by cardiovascular heart disease or stroke, estimated care costs currently exceed $316 billion annually. Peripheral vascular disease affects 8 to 12 million Americans and renal artery disease affects 6.8% of the population older than 60 years, or approximately 2 million people. The disease burden of atherosclerosis as reflected by the associated diseases (cardiovascular disease including stroke, renal artery disease and PAD) is not sustainable in today's health care environment. Health care reform and the move toward value-based health care are requiring more cost-effective and quality outcomes. This entry presents evidence to direct the nursing care of individuals with atherosclerosis.

Background

Atherosclerosis is a preventable disease; however, the associated disease burden that is measured by cost, morbidity, and mortality has exceeded epidemic proportions. Atherosclerosis prevalence and incidence rates are generally reported according to the disease with which they are associated and not reported solely under atherosclerosis. The AHA reports that heart disease (coronary heart disease, hypertension, and stroke) is currently the number one killer in the United States (AHA, 2017). Although there has been a gradual decline in cardiovascular-related mortality in higher income countries between 1990 and 2010, cardiovascular disease still accounts for one in three deaths in U.S. citizens who are older than 35 years of age. Prevalence increases with age, male gender, and ethnicity. Fifty percent of Black American adults have some form of cardiovascular disease. The lifetime risk of developing cardiovascular disease for people 40 years old is 49% in men and 32% in females compared to people reaching 70 years, when the lifetime risk is 35% and 24%, respectively (Centers for Disease Control and Prevention [CDC] & National Center for Health Statistics [NCHS], 2015; Sanchis-Gomar, Perez-Quillis, Leischik, & Lucia, 2016). Stroke is the fifth leading cause of death in the United States, killing more than 130,000 Americans annually, or one death every 4 minutes (CDC & NCHS, 2015).

Stroke, the fifth leading cause of death in the United States, accounts for 5% of all deaths and is the second cause of death globally. Annually 795,000 Americans suffer from a stroke, with 76% of those being a first-time attack. Poststroke disability occurs in 90% of stroke victims, which can impact both physical and cognitive ability.

PAD is another high-burden disease with a predominant association to atherosclerosis. Atherosclerotic plaque impairs blood flow to the arms, legs, or pelvic region and affects nearly 8.5 million Americans, 12%

to 20% of whom are 60 years or older. A major challenge for PAD is that only 25% of individuals have a general awareness of the disease, prolonging diagnosis and treatment (CDC, 2016; Davies et al., 2017).

The pathogenesis of atherosclerosis begins with chronic endothelial injury, damage, and adaptive thickening. Atherogenic triggers include one or more of these insults: (a) physical injury, direct trauma, or turbulent blood flow (hypertension); (b) free radical and toxins in circulation (smoking, infection, inflammation); (c) hypercholesteremia (elevated low-density lipoprotein [LDL] or very low density lipoprotein [VLDL]); (d) chronically elevated blood glucose (insulin resistance or poor diet); or (e) high levels of homocysteine, which is toxic to the endothelium.

Once the endothelium is damaged, cytokines attract leukocytes (monocytes and t-lymphocytes) that adhere to the endothelium, squeezing underneath the endothelial cells. The endothelial cells change shape, the tight junctions relax and leaking fluid, lipoproteins, macrophages, and enzymes accumulate in the intima. The accumulation of lipids on the endothelium identified as the fatty streak development begins the atherosclerotic process, yet is considered reversible. As the plaque continues to increase in size an atheroma forms, followed by the addition of a fibrous cap resulting in a fibroma. Lipids, fibrous tissue, calcium, cellular debris, and capillaries form these complex lesions, which can hemorrhage, calcify, or ulcerate stimulating thrombotic lesion development. Plaques can either form in an asymmetric pattern or cover the entire vessel circumference and often develop where arteries bifurcate. Some arteries have a high propensity for atherosclerosis development, including the left ascending coronary artery, renal arteries, and branching areas of carotid arteries. Atherosclerotic plaque also weakens artery walls, increasing the risk of aneurysms. Clinical manifestations result from restricted flow of oxygen-rich blood and vary depending on the location, severity, and speed of occlusion from these plaques.

Clinical Aspects

ASSESSMENT

In coronary artery disease, also called coronary heart disease, atherosclerosis interrupts normal blood flow through the coronary arteries. Plaque can lead to the development of blood clots that can break off and partially or completely block blood supply to an area of the heart muscle. Angina pectoris is characterized by transient chest pain, which occurs from an imbalance in oxygen demand and supply to the coronary artery. Myocardial infarction (MI) occurs when blood flow is interrupted and the heart muscle is deprived of oxygen for a period of time, resulting in a cardiac muscle ischemia and necrosis. Symptoms characterizing an MI include chest pain, which may or may not radiate, shortness of breath, dizziness, nausea, diaphoresis, and anxiety. Nursing implications center on hemodynamic evaluation, including cardiac output monitoring and tissue perfusion assessment and pain management, including evaluating, documenting, and administering measures to reduce pain. Nursing care should focus on reducing knowledge deficits, promoting self-care, and self-efficacy to engage in self-care behaviors as evidenced by the maintenance of a therapeutic regimen.

A comprehensive approach to atherosclerosis is key to reducing death, disability, and the associated global economic burden. Prevention strategies aimed at minimizing risk have been identified and refined by large prospective observational studies such as the Framingham study. Targeting risk factors for both symptomatic and asymptomatic patients is the first step and a shift from traditional management, which focused on preventing recurrence. Enhanced understanding of nonmodifiable and modifiable risk factors provides an opportunity to modify disease progression. Nonmodifiable factors include age, gender, and family history, whereas modifiable factors can be both pathologic and lifestyle oriented. Population health focuses on addressing lifestyle factors and behavior modification in regard to smoking, diet, activity, obesity, and medication use in women (oral contraceptive pills and hormone replacement therapy). Pathologic modifiable factors are associated with specific diseases, including hyperlipidemia, diabetes mellitus, and hypertension and improving clinical outcomes.

Nursing care for atherosclerosis entails primary, secondary, and tertiary prevention strategies. Atherosclerosis may be asymptomatic, based on the percentage of blockage in an artery and the development of collateral circulation, or symptomatic, as seen in a specific disease such as occurs after myocardial infarction (MI). Applicable to populations, promotion of healthy lifestyle behaviors, including not smoking, consumption of a healthy diet, adequate physical exercise, and weight management play a role in each stage. Learning readiness, learning support, decision-making support, and self-management are all aspects of nursing care. Addressing knowledge deficits with evidence-based education can help minimize the negative consequence associated with negative lifestyle behaviors.

Improving cholesterol levels with lifestyle modifications is the first step in management of atherosclerosis in patients with known disease, targeting the levels of both LDLs and high-density lipoproteins (HDLs). New atherosclerotic cardiovascular disease (ASCVD) American College of Cardiology and American Heart Association (ACC/AHA) guidelines in 2013 recommend (a) secondary prevention by targeting patients with any known form of ASCVD, (b) secondary prevention by targeting patients with LDL levels greater than 190, (c) primary prevention in patients with diabetes mellitus (40–75 years of age) with LDL levels 70–189, and (d) primary prevention in a patient without diabetes but with a slightly elevated hemoglobin A1c (less than 7.5%; Stone et al, 2013). Diabetes and poor glucose control, hyperinsulinemia, and altered functioning of platelets affecting arterial endothelium contribute to the inflammatory process and the development of atherosclerosis. Diabetes is also associated with high lipid levels, obesity, and hypertension, which also impact the progression of atherosclerosis. Nursing care includes addressing knowledge deficits through education, facilitating adherence to a therapeutic regime, and minimizing the effects of hyperglycemia.

Summary

Atherosclerosis is a progressive disease at the root of many lethal diseases that cause significant disease burden across the globe. Nevertheless, atherosclerosis is preventable. Incorporating primary prevention strategies or modifiable in secondary and tertiary prevention strategies when providing nursing care can shift the paradigm toward reducing disease-related illness and suffering. Through the use of evidence-based guidelines to inform practice, nursing collaboratively can improve clinical outcomes associated with the management of atherosclerosis, facilitating lifestyle changes at both the individual and population level.

American Heart Association. (2017). Heart disease and stroke 2017 statistic updates. Retrieved from https://www.heart.org/idc/groups/ahamah-public/@wcm/@sop/@smd/documents/downloadable/ucm_491265.pdf

CDC. (2016). Peripheral Artery Disease (PAD) Fact Sheet. Retrieved from https://www.cdc.gov/dhdsp/data_statistics/fact_sheets/fs_pad.htm

CDC, NCHS. (2015). Underlying cause of death 1999–2013. Retrieved from https://wonder.cdc.gov

Davies, J. H., Richards, J., Conway, K., Kenkre, J. E., Lewis, J. E., & Mark Williams, E. (2017). Primary care screening for peripheral arterial disease: A cross-sectional observational study. *British Journal of General Practice, 67*(655), e103–e110. doi:10.3399/bjgp17X689137

Ladich, E., & Burke, A. (2016). Atherosclerosis pathology: The heart. *Medscape.* Retrieved from http://reference.medscape.com/article/1612610-overview

Sanchis-Gomar, F., Perez-Quillis, C., Leischik, R., & Lucia, A. (2016). Epidemiology of coronary heart disease and acute coronary syndrome. *Annals of Translational Medicine, 4*(13), 256.

Stone, N., Robinson, J., Lichtenstein, A., Merz, C. N., Blum, C., Eckel, R., . . . Wilson, P. (2013). 2013 ACC/AHA guidelines on the treatment of blood cholesterol to reduce atherosclerotic cardiovascular risk in adults. *Circulation,* 1–85. doi:10.1161/01.cir.0000437738.63853.7a

■ BENIGN PROSTATIC HYPERPLASIA

Kelly Ann Lynn

Overview

Benign prostatic hyperplasia (BPH) is a medical condition characterized by noncancerous overgrowth of prostatic tissue. Men with BPH often present with complaints of significant lower urinary tract symptoms (LUTS), which include a weak urinary stream, frequency and urgency of urination, and nocturia (Vuichoud & Loughlin, 2015). Patients suffering from BPH may be at risk for significant morbidity, including urinary retention, the formation of bladder stones, sepsis, and renal insufficiency. Nursing care for patients with BPH focuses on early diagnosis, education, psychosocial support, and management of symptoms and the medications prescribed to treat the symptoms.

Background

BPH is one of the most common conditions affecting older men. The incidence of BPH increases as men age. Moreover, it is associated with considerable morbidity that can adversely affect quality of life. According to the National Institute of Health, BPH can start as early as 40 years of age and is estimated to affect about 50% of men between the ages of 51 and 60 years. Approximately 90% of men will develop histologic evidence of BPH by age 80 years (Lepor, 2005). Symptomatic BPH and LUTS affects 50% to 75% of men aged 50 years and older, and 80% of men older than 70 years (Egan, 2016).

BPH treatment in the United States costs approximately $4 billion per year (Vuichoud & Loughlin, 2015). Given the progressive nature of BPH and the increase in average life expectancy, it is presumed that the cost of managing the symptoms of BPH will only rise.

The exact cause of BPH remains unclear. However, there are some indications that aging and the long-time exposure to male hormones play a significant role. According to the National Institute of Diabetes and Digestive and Kidney Diseases (NIDDK), part of the National Institutes of Health (NIH; 2014), men whose testicles are removed before they reach puberty do not develop BPH. This indicates that aging and hormone levels (testosterone, estrogen, dihydrotestosterone) may have a causative role in the development of BPH. Black and Hispanic men are at increased risk for developing BPH compared to White men (Kristal et al., 2007). Other factors that appear to increase the incidence of BPH include a history of prostatitis and obesity, indicating that inflammation may also play a role. Moreover, increased levels of physical activity appears to be associated with a decreased risk for clinical BPH.

Various terms are used to describe BPH and the resulting symptoms. BPH is often interchanged with "benign prostatic enlargement" (BPE). However, it is important to note that BPH is a histologic diagnosis that refers to a progressive increase in the number of stromal and epithelial cells in the prostate. This proliferative process is most prevalent in the prostate region adjacent to the urethra, known as the *transitional zone* (T-zone; Egan, 2016). Given its proximity to the urethra, BPH in the T-zone may be associated with significant urinary obstruction to the flow of urine. BPE, by contrast, describes increased volume of the gland. It is important to note that the size of the prostate does not always determine the severity of the symptoms.

BPH-associated symptoms are categorized into (a) voiding or obstructive symptoms and (b) storage or irritative symptoms. Voiding symptoms include hesitancy, a delay in the start of urine flow; weak urinary stream; straining to urinate; postvoid dribbling; urinary retention and overflow incontinence. Storage symptoms include those clinical indications related to instability of the detrusor muscle. That is, that the detrusor contracts without our consent, manifesting in bladder instability with complaints of frequency, urgency, and nocturia.

As the prostate increases in size, it can obstruct the flow of urine as it exits the bladder and passes through the prostatic urethra. If the patient is not treated for this progressive bladder outlet obstruction, he may develop acute or chronic urinary retention. Chronic urinary retention can quietly lead to the development of renal insufficiency, ultimately resulting in renal failure. Another adverse effect of chronic urinary retention is the deterioration of bladder muscle function. When the bladder is unable to empty adequately, impaired detrusor contractility will occur. Moreover, in time, functional deterioration of the detrusor muscle can contribute to chronic bladder outlet obstruction. Long-term impairment of the detrusor muscle may be irreversible. Untreated, chronic obstruction can also lead to the development of bladder diverticula as a result of the high pressure in the bladder. Additionally, hydronephrosis, hydroureter, and vesicoureteral reflux can result from prolonged, untreated prostatic obstruction.

The clinical significance of BPH and LUTS cannot be understated. BPH and LUTS symptoms (i.e., urgency and nocturia) are associated with increased incidence of falls in the elderly (Schimke & Schimke, 2014). Elderly patients with decreased mobility are particularly susceptible to falling while rushing to use the bathroom. Moreover, skin integrity can be compromised by urinary incontinence. Electrolyte imbalances may result from chronic obstruction. There is also considerable emotional distress associated with the BPH and LUTS symptom complex.

Clinical Aspects

ASSESSMENT

A thorough nursing assessment is essential to identify and characterize a patient's symptoms associated with BPH. This includes a comprehensive patient history with targeted questions related to voiding patterns (urinary stream, frequency, straining to void), history of urinary tract infections, bladder stones, and the incidence of incontinence and nocturia. The International Prostate Symptom Score (IPSS) is a quick, inexpensive, and effective screening tool that can help diagnose and track progress of BPH. Physical assessment should be thorough and address vital signs, particularly blood pressure. It is also essential to examine the patients' ankles and feet for signs of fluid retention. Percussion and palpation of the suprapubic area allow for the detection of significant bladder overdistention. Obtaining a postvoid residual to assess bladder emptying will further clarify the efficacy of bladder emptying for a given patient. Uroflowmetry can be used to measure the urine flow rate. Moreover, a review of essential laboratory values relating to the health of the urinary system is of great value. The urinalysis will help detect the presence of WBCs and RBCs in the urine; serum chemistry will assess for electrolyte imbalances and serum blood urea nitrogen (BUN) and creatinine levels, thus helping to evaluate renal function; prostate-specific antigen (PSA). PSA is often used to detect prostate cancer, an elevated PSA level may also be indicative of BPH or acute bacterial prostatitis.

The review of medications is an essential part of the nursing assessment. Some medications (i.e., diuretics) can cause urinary frequency and increase distress for patients with BPH. Medications can contribute to acute urinary retention. Oral decongestants and antihistamines can cause constriction in the bladder neck and should be avoided in men with BPH. Other medications can affect detrusor muscle contractility and should be used cautiously in patients with BPH. These medications include anticholinergic agents (e.g., tricyclic antidepressants, selective serotonin reuptake inhibitors (SSRIs), antispasmodics), calcium channel blockers, nonsteroidal anti-inflammatory drugs (NSAIDs), opioids, and anti-Parkinsonian agents.

Nursing assessment of BPH must include all three components: comprehensive, in-depth history; a physical examination with evaluation and interpretation of laboratory and diagnostic tests; and medication review. Any encounter with a male patient older than the age of 50 years (regardless of whether he reports a history of BPH) should address all of these issues.

NURSING INTERVENTIONS, MANAGEMENT, AND IMPLICATIONS

Nursing care of patients with BPH should be tailored to the patients' symptoms and clinical status. The focus of care should be the prevention of the serious consequences related to BPH, such as renal failure, urinary retention, and urinary sepsis. Optimizing urinary elimination will reduce incidence of stasis, urinary tract infections (UTIs), bladder stones, detrusor instability, and electrolyte imbalances. Nursing care must include comprehensive education and emotional support for patients and their families.

Nursing interventions will vary, based on the clinical presentation, the treatment course, and the long-term objectives for a given patient.

Patients with BPH need considerable education about their disease process, treatment options, and the side effects of medications that may be offered. Newly diagnosed patients will need considerable education surrounding the disease process, the treatment options, and symptom management. Many patients are diagnosed with BPH only after they present in acute urinary retention. Patients in acute urinary retention will need to be catheterized to drain the urine out of the bladder. Some patients will be discharged home with an indwelling Foley catheter and leg bag for several days to allow the bladder to recover and to give medications a chance to work. Other patients may be taught to self-catheterize. Both groups will rely on comprehensive nursing education to manage their catheters and urine output.

Patients who are unresponsive to medical management, or those who have frequent UTIs, develop bladder stones, and/or renal insufficiency may be referred for consideration for surgical intervention. These patients will need education about the planned surgery and specific issues related to the various surgical options (TURP, laser ablation). The details of the management of the indwelling catheter, and the signs and symptoms of infection need to be reviewed in detail. Moreover, patients should be advised that they will, most likely, experience retrograde ejaculation as a consequence of the surgery. This is not dangerous, but it can be alarming for patients who may not be aware of it before they experience it.

Patients opting for medical management of their symptomatic BPH will need education focusing on the various medications and their possible interactions. Caffeine, spicy foods, alcohol, and chronic constipation are all associated with an increase in the severity of LUTS that may be experienced. Nurses should counsel patients to avoid these items. Warm sitz baths may temporarily relieve symptoms of LUTS. Also, avoiding constipation tends to decrease lower urinary tract discomfort, in general.

Patients with BPH or LUTS are encouraged to empty their bladders every 2 to 4 hours. They are advised to restrict fluids after 6 p.m. to reduce the incidence of nocturia. Also, patients with dependent edema are encouraged to wear compression stockings and to elevate their lower extremities well before they go to bed. These maneuvers will help sleep quality.

BPH affects not only patients, but also their partners and families. Chronic illness can be a significant stressor. Nurses must offer patients and families an opportunity to process the complex emotions surrounding this disease.

OUTCOMES

The expected outcomes of evidence-based nursing care for patients with BPH are the prevention of serious consequences associated with the progression of this disease (renal failure, urinary retention, urinary sepsis) so as to increase the patient's quality of life, and decrease the incidence of adverse events, like falls related to nocturia.

Summary

BPH is recognized as a chronic health issue for many men aged 50 years and older. Early intervention and initiation of appropriate nursing care can prevent significant morbidity and result in better quality of life. As the population ages, the incidence of BPH will continue to rise. The symptoms associated with BPH are considerable and contribute to unnecessary suffering. Nursing support and education can help patients to better manage their symptoms to ease their distress and promote compliance with their care plans.

The clinical ramifications of BPH extend far beyond the prostate. In fact, prostate health is essential to men's overall health. Nursing plays a significant role in the successful management of BPH.

Egan, K. B. (2016). The epidemiology of benign prostatic hyperplasia associated with lower urinary tract symptoms: Prevalence and incident rates. *Urologic Clinics of North America*, 43(3), 289–297. doi:10.1016/j.ucl.2016.04.001

Kristal, A. R., Arnold, K. B., Schenk, J. M., Neuhouser, M. L., Weiss, N., Goodman, P., . . . Thompson, I. M. (2007). Race/ethnicity, obesity, health related behaviors and the risk of symptomatic benign prostatic hyperplasia: Results from the prostate cancer prevention trial. *Journal of Urology*, 177(4), 1395–400; quiz 1591. doi:10.1016/j.juro.2006.11.065

Lepor, H. (2005). Pathophysiology of lower urinary tract symptoms in the aging male population. *Reviews in Urology*, 7(Suppl. 7), S3–S11.

Schimke, L., & Schinike, J. (2014). Urological implications of falls in the elderly: Lower urinary tract symptoms and alpha-blocker medications. *Urologic Nursing, 34*(5), 223–229.

Vuichoud, C., & Loughlin, K. R. (2015). Benign prostatic hyperplasia: Epidemiology, economics and evaluation. *Canadian Journal of Urology, 22*(Suppl. 1), 1–6.

■ BLADDER CANCER

Dianna Jo Copley

Overview

Bladder cancer is classified by histological type. The most common type is urothelial carcinoma (previously known as *transitional cell carcinoma*), which is further divided into papillary and flat carcinomas based on the pattern of growth. Other less common types of bladder cancer include adenocarcinoma and squamous cell carcinoma. Bladder cancer is the sixth most common cancer in the United States with men three to four times more likely to develop it in their lifetime than women (American Cancer Society, 2017). Like many other types of cancers, both modifiable and nonmodifiable risk factors can increase a person's likelihood of developing bladder cancer. Nursing care can vary depending on the stage of the cancer and planned interventions. An individual's emotional and psychological well-being, in addition to physiological symptoms related to the bladder cancer and treatments, should be considered.

Background

According to the American Cancer Society, there will be approximately 79,030 new cases and 16,870 deaths related to bladder cancer in 2017. Incidence rates have been declining for both men and women, although bladder cancer deaths decline in women and remain stable in men (American Cancer Society, 2017). Women have a higher mortality rate and are more likely to experience recurrence after treatment (Pozzar & Berry, 2017). Caucasians are diagnosed at a rate twice as often compared to African Americans or Hispanic Americans (American Cancer Society, 2017). Age is another nonmodifiable risk factor, with approximately nine in 10 individuals with bladder cancer older than 55 years (American Cancer Society, 2017).

Smoking tobacco is the most significant modifiable risk factor contributing to an estimated 50% of bladder disease, especially urothelial carcinoma (Chang et al., 2017). Chang et al. (2017) note that current smoking impacts the risk of bladder cancer by a factor of 4.1 and former smokers by a factor of 2.2 compared to individuals who have never smoked. Risk factors, such as second-hand smoke and occupational exposure to carcinogens, contribute to bladder cancer risk (Chang et al., 2017). A history of bladder or other urothelial cancers, family history, and previous exposure to chemotherapy and/or radiation, especially pelvic, can also increase one's risk for bladder cancer (American Cancer Society, 2017). Prevention is aimed at reducing modifiable risk factors. The American Cancer Society (2017) notes that increasing fluids and a diet high in fruits and vegetables may reduce the risk of bladder cancer. Exposure to *Schistosoma haematobium* infection can increase an individual's risk for squamous cell carcinoma of the bladder, but is not common in the United States (Chang et al., 2017).

Staging is separated into clinical and pathological stage and the tumor-node-metastases (TNM) classification that is outlined by the American Joint Committee on Cancer (AJCC) is used (Chang et al., 2016). The clinical stage is based on the physical exam, histologic findings at the time of the transurethral resection of the bladder tumor (TURBT), and radiologic imaging (Chang et al., 2016). Pathological staging is also known as surgical staging and is based on the extent of the disease after surgical removal of the bladder and surrounding lymph nodes (Chang et al., 2016). Stage 0 is noninvasive carcinoma with no lymph node involvement; stage I means that the cancer has grown to the connective tissue, but not the muscle with no lymph node involvement; stage II indicates cancer has penetrated the muscle of the bladder wall with no lymph node involvement; and stage III means the cancer has penetrated the fatty tissue around the bladder and may have spread into the surrounding genitourinary structures, including the prostate, uterus, and vagina but not the pelvic or abdominal wall (American Cancer Society, 2017). Stage IV includes cancer that has penetrated into the pelvic and abdominal wall with or without lymph node involvement and cancer that has metastasized to distant lymph nodes or other organs (American Cancer Society, 2017). Of newly diagnosed bladder cancers, approximately 30% are muscle-invasive (Chou et al., 2016).

Bladder cancer, depending on stage and treatment, can greatly impact an individual's quality of life. Interventions and treatment can impact urinary and bowel function, sexual function, body image, and emotional/mental well-being. Bladder cancer treatment can impact fertility, which should be considered when an individual is making treatment decisions. Individuals with bladder cancer may experience anxiety, fear, and hopelessness related to the diagnosis and prognosis. Survival rate for all stages of bladder cancer at 5 years is approximately 77%; 5-year survival rate for stage 0 is 98%; I is 88%; II is 63%; III is 46%; and IV, which indicates metastasis has occurred, is 15% (American Cancer Society, 2017).

Treatment for bladder cancer varies depending on the stage. Nonmuscle invasive bladder cancer (NMIBC) may be treated with TURBT and/or intravesical therapy (Dunn, 2015). Frequently used medications for intravesical therapy include bacillus Calmette-Guerin (BCG), mitomycin C, and epirubicin (Chang et al., 2016). Muscle-invasive bladder cancer (MIBC) may be treated with a variety of treatment modalities, including surgery, radiation, chemotherapy, or a combination of modalities (Dunn, 2015). Surgical interventions include partial cystectomy, radical cystectomy (removal of bladder, prostate, seminal vesicles in males; bladder, uterus, fallopian tubes, ovaries, and anterior vaginal walls in females), and lymphadenectomy (Chang et al., 2017).

Patients who undergo a radical cystectomy will require a urinary diversion. Urinary diversions include incontinent conduit, continent cutaneous, or orthotopic neobladder. An ileal conduit, the most commonly performed incontinent conduit, consists of a stoma constructed of small intestine with the ureters transplanted into the ileal segment. The urine drains through the stoma created on the abdominal wall and is collected in an external drainage bag. A continent cutaneous diversion requires intermittent catheterization of a stoma on the abdominal wall. The orthotopic neobladder consists of forming a new reservoir for urine with a segment of small intestine; the urethra and ureters are anastomosed to the neobladder allowing normal urination after healing (Merandy, Morgan, Lee, & Scherr et al., 2017).

Individual decision making should be supported when treatments are discussed. Pozzar and Berry (2017) highlight that women are less likely to receive a continent urinary diversion and less likely to undergo lymph node dissection than men with bladder cancer. Including the patient's family and support network as appropriate is an important consideration during the patient's decision-making process (Pozzar & Berry, 2017).

Clinical Aspects

ASSESSMENT

Nursing assessment should begin with a thorough patient history. Signs and symptoms of bladder cancer include microscopic or macroscopic hematuria, frequency, urgency, dysuria, inability to empty the bladder, and pain in more advanced stages. Bladder cancer signs and symptoms can mimic other genitourinary diseases.

Diagnostic tests include urine cytology, urine culture, urine tumor markers, and imaging of the urinary tract (American Cancer Society, 2017). Imaging may include MRI, ultrasound, radiographs, CT, and an intravenous or retrograde pyelogram. A cystoscopy will be performed examining the patient's urethra and bladder (Chang et al., 2016). Nurses should ask patients about their baseline sexual function before treatment is started (Dunn, 2015).

Focused nursing assessment is dependent on the patient's treatment plan. For patients receiving chemotherapy, assessment should include monitoring for infection, including reduced white blood cell (WBC) counts and any adverse reactions to the chemotherapy. Patients who have undergone surgical interventions should be monitored for infection, delays in wound healing, and stoma viability.

NURSING INTERVENTIONS, MANAGEMENT, AND IMPLICATIONS

Nursing-related problems may include acute and/or chronic pain, anxiety, deficient patient knowledge, nausea, risk for bleeding and/or infection, impaired skin integrity, risk for sexual dysfunction, risk for disturbed body image, and risk for dysfunctional gastrointestinal motility. Considerations should always be made for enhanced coping and psychosocial support of the patient and family.

Nursing interventions always include providing support and encouraging verbalization of feelings related to the diagnosis of bladder cancer and treatments. Nurses should support the patient's preference regarding discussing sexual function and sexuality with his or her partner (Dunn, 2015).

OUTCOMES

Patient and family education should focus on the individual's treatment and adapted to accommodate any barriers in learning. For patients undergoing surgical intervention, the nurse should assess the patient's ability for self-care and discharge needs at the preoperative visit. Education should begin immediately as demonstration of self-care is essential to promote independence and reduce risk for readmission.

Summary

Bladder cancer is a diagnosis that individuals need to monitor for the rest of their lives, regardless of the treatment method. Nurses have long been trusted to educate and advocate for patients and are critical for individuals being evaluated for bladder cancer, during treatment, and into survivorship.

American Cancer Society. (2017). Bladder cancer. Retrieved from https://www.cancer.org/cancer/bladder-cancer.html

Chang, S. S., Bochner, B. H., Chou, R., Dreicer, R., Kamat, A. M., Lerner, S. P., . . . Holzbeierlein, J. M. (2017). Treatment of non-metastatic muscle-invasive bladder cancer: AUA/ASCO/ASTRO/SUO guideline. *Journal of Urology, 198*(3), 552–559. doi:10.1016/j.juro.2017.04.086

Chang, S. S., Boorjian, S. A., Chou, R., Clark, P. E., Daneshmand, S., Konety, B. R., . . . McKiernan, J. M. (2016). Diagnosis and treatment of non-metastatic muscle-invasive bladder cancer: AUA/SUO guideline. *Journal of Urology, 196*(4), 1021–1029. doi:10.1016/j.juro.2016.06.049

Chou, R., Selph, S. S., Buckley, D. I., Gustafson, K. S., Griffin, J. C., Grusing, S. E., & Gore, J. L. (2016). Treatment of muscle-invasive bladder cancer: A systematic review. *Cancer, 122*(6), 842–851. doi:10.1002/cncr.29843

Dunn, M. W. (2015). Bladder cancer: A focus on sexuality. *Clinical Journal of Oncology Nursing, 29*(1), 68–73.

Merandy, K., Morgan, M. A., Lee, R., & Scherr, D. S. (2017). Improving self-efficacy and self-care in adult patients with a urinary diversion: A pilot study. *Oncology Nursing Forum, 44*(3), E90–E100. doi:10.1188/17.ONF.E90-E100

Pozzar, R. A., & Berry, D. L. (2017). Gender differences in bladder cancer treatment decision making. *Oncology Nursing Forum, 44*(2), 204–209. doi:10.1188/17.ONF.204-209

■ BOWEL OBSTRUCTION

Kelly Ann Lynn
Jane F. Marek

Overview

Bowel obstruction is a complete or partial blockage in either the small or large intestine that prevents the passage of intestinal contents. Patients with bowel obstruction usually have other underlying comorbidities and may present with acute, constant, or intermittent abdominal pain; vomiting; and decrease or absence of bowel activity (flatus and bowel movement). Small bowel obstruction (SBO) accounts for 12% to 16% of U.S. hospital admissions for acute abdominal pain (Paulson & Thompson, 2015). Most patients with SBO are treated conservatively by inserting a nasogastric tube to decompress the bowel. Patients with adhesive SBO who are managed conservatively have a shorter length of stay, but also have a higher recurrence of SBO and higher readmission rates than patients treated surgically (Di Saverio et al., 2013). Failure to promptly diagnose and treat bowel obstruction may result in serious complications, including ischemic bowel, short-gut syndrome, perforation, intra-abdominal abscess, peritonitis, sepsis, and death. Mortality rates associated with SBO are dependent on early recognition and treatment and may be as high as 25% with ischemic bowel or if surgical intervention is delayed (Paulson & Thompson, 2015).

Background

Bowel obstruction can be classified as either nonmechanical/functional or mechanical/physical. Mechanical obstructions occur either inside (intraluminal) or outside of the bowel (extraluminal). Extraluminal obstructions can be due to scar tissue or an intra-abdominal mass compressing the bowel and obstructing the lumen. Functional obstructions result from disruption of the neurovascular supply to the bowel, preventing peristalsis or causing ischemia. Examples of functional bowel obstruction include ileus (most commonly postoperative), use of opioid analgesics, electrolyte imbalances, and mesenteric infarct. Physiologic ileus following abdominal surgery is a normal finding and typically resolves within 48 to 72 hours. Delayed return of gastrointestinal function (over 72 hours) following abdominal surgery is referred to as *postoperative adynamic* or *paralytic ileus* and is due to a variety of factors, including bowel manipulation, surgical trauma, stress response, opioid use, and perioperative interventions (Ge, Chen, & Ding, 2015). Chronic functional bowel obstruction can be caused by a neuromuscular disorder such as Parkinson's disease, diabetes, or Hirschbrung's disease (aganglionic megacolon).

The most common cause of SBO is postoperative intra-abdominal adhesions, accounting for 60% and 70% of all SBO (Di Saverio et al., 2013). Adhesion formation is more common in open than in laparoscopic procedures; other risk factors for abdominal adhesions include colorectal and gynecologic procedures, age older than 60 years, laparotomy within 5 years, and history of abdominal trauma, previous adhesions, or emergency surgery (Loftus et al., 2015). Abdominal adhesions can begin to form within a few hours following surgery. Other causes include hernia, inflammatory bowel disease, volvulus, intussusception, tumor, and adhesions resulting from pelvic inflammatory disease. Large bowel obstruction (LBO) is most frequently related to a neoplastic process, usually colon or ovarian cancer; other causes include strictures, diverticulitis, volvulus, or fecal impaction.

Patients typically present with cramping, intermittent abdominal pain, abdominal distention, nausea, vomiting, and inability to pass stool or flatus. Fever, tachycardia, and peritoneal signs (abdominal rigidity, rebound tenderness) are usually indicative of strangulation and ischemic bowel. Percussion may reveal tympany due to trapped air; bowel sounds are typically hyperactive in the early stages of obstruction as peristalsis attempts to overcome the obstruction; hypoactive or absent bowel sounds occur in the later stages of obstruction. Patients presenting with these symptoms, particularly in combination with history of abdominal or pelvic surgery, malignancy, or treatment with abdominal radiation, need immediate workup to determine the cause and location of the obstruction.

Prompt treatment is essential to prevent complications, particularly ischemic bowel, perforation, peritonitis, and dehydration. Patients without strangulation or ischemia can be managed conservatively with intravenous fluid resuscitation, nasogastric tube decompression, and bowel rest (Loftus et al., 2015). If the obstruction is not relieved within 48 to 72 hours, surgical intervention is recommended. Surgical intervention is indicated for strangulation, ischemia, or tumor; laparoscopic approach is preferred over open technique (Paulson & Thompson, 2015). Conservative management is not indicated for patients with signs of strangulation or peritonitis; these patients should be treated promptly with surgical intervention.

Clinical Aspects

ASSESSMENT

Nursing assessment of patients with a bowel obstruction begins with a comprehensive assessment of the history of present illness and presenting symptoms, surgical history, bowel function, and medication and dietary history. Physical assessment includes assessing vital signs, specifically temperature, blood pressure, and heart rate, to identify early signs of infection and volume depletion and a thorough abdominal assessment, including palpation and percussion of the abdomen. Measuring abdominal girth may be useful to monitor the degree of abdominal distention. It is important to note that flatus or bowel movement may occur before the obstruction is relieved if the stool or gas is below the level of obstruction. Therefore, one must not take bowel movement or flatus as sign of resolution of obstruction; the complete clinical picture must be considered.

Nurses should be alert for signs and symptoms of acute abdomen, including pain upon palpation, tension, rigidity, and increasing distension. Laboratory studies include assessment of the complete blood cell count; the white blood cell count may be elevated with strangulation and the hematocrit may be elevated due to dehydration. Serum lactate levels may be elevated due to dehydration or ischemia; serum chemistry panels should be assessed for electrolyte imbalances and metabolic acidosis. Abdominal x-rays are performed to evaluate for air/fluid levels, free air, distended bowel loops, and gas patterns; CT scan with water-soluble contrast can identify the location of the obstruction and characterize the degree of obstruction.

NURSING INTERVENTIONS, MANAGEMENT, AND IMPLICATIONS

Delayed return of gastrointestinal function following abdominal surgery is a major cause of increased length of stay and morbidity. Nurses can play a key role in preventing postoperative ileus by implementing interventions to promote return of bowel function and identifying patients at risk for developing postoperative ileus. Early ambulation; cautious use of opioid analgesics; frequent abdominal assessment, including auscultating for bowel sounds; and gradual resumption of diet are effective interventions to enhance recovery of GI function. Chewing gum after surgery is thought to enhance return of GI function by cephalic–vagal stimulation, but there is insufficient evidence to support this intervention.

Nursing care of patients with bowel obstruction should focus on resolution of the issue and prevention of serious consequences related to obstruction, specifically dehydration, perforation, peritonitis, and sepsis. Patients should receive information on the available treatment options, including conservative management with nasogastric (NG) tube and bowel rest, endoscopic management, including stenting for LBO, and surgery to relieve the cause of the obstruction. Patients are at risk for developing another bowel obstruction and should receive education to monitor their bowel habits and recognize early signs of recurrence. Education regarding signs of bowel obstruction should be included in the discharge teaching for patients following abdominal and pelvic surgery due to the risk of developing postoperative adhesions.

Nursing interventions will vary, based on the clinical presentation, location, and extent of the obstruction, treatment course, and the long-term objectives for a given patient. All patients will need education about the underlying conditions and various treatment options. It is essential that nurses partner with patients and their families to allow patients to make decisions regarding their treatment options. This is particularly important when caring for patients with bowel obstruction caused by malignancies. Nurses should allow patients and their families the opportunity to express their treatment goals and facilitate the decision-making process to maximize quality of life.

Initial treatment of patients with bowel obstruction begins with conservative symptom management while the diagnostic workup is completed. Patients are not permitted anything by mouth and an NG tube is usually passed and placed to intermittent suction to relieve distention and decompress the bowel. NG tubes should be assessed for placement and patency and oral care is imperative due to nothing per os (NPO) status. Patients are at risk for developing respiratory complications due to increased intra-abdominal pressure, and reluctance to cough and deep breathe often related to abdominal pain. Assessing and monitoring respiratory status and interventions to promote optimal respiratory function is a nursing priority.

Patients with bowel obstruction are at risk for fluid volume and electrolyte imbalance due to dehydration. Dehydration and electrolyte imbalances occur as a result of fluid loss from emesis, bowel edema, and loss of absorptive capacity. Careful assessment and documentation of intake and output (I&O) are essential as patients will require intravenous fluid resuscitation and electrolyte replacement.

Monitoring for infection and peritonitis is another important nursing intervention. Stasis of intestinal contents can result in overgrowth of intestinal flora and may lead to peritonitis. Other nursing interventions include pain management. A comprehensive assessment of symptoms and response to medications and interventions is essential.

OUTCOMES

The expected outcomes of evidence-based nursing care for patients with bowel obstruction are the return of bowel function and prevention of complications.

Summary

Bowel obstruction is a serious health issue that requires prompt intervention and comprehensive nursing care to prevent significant morbidity and adverse outcomes.

Nurses must partner with their patients to develop customized care plans to improve health and to prevent complications and recurrence.

Di Saverio, S., Coccolini, F., Galati, M., Smerieri, N., Biffl, W. L., Ansaloni, L., . . . Catena, F. (2013). Bologna guidelines for diagnosis and management of adhesive small bowel obstruction (ASBO): 2013 update of the evidence-based guidelines from the world society of emergency surgery ASBO working group. *World Journal of Emergency Surgery*, 8(1), 42. doi:10.1186/1749-7922-8-42

Ge, W., Chen, G., & Ding, Y.-T. (2015). Effect of chewing gum on the postoperative recovery of gastrointestinal function. *International Journal of Clinical and Experimental Medicine*, 8(8), 11936–11942.

Loftus, T., Moore, F., VanZant, E., Bala, T., Brakenridge, S., Croft, C., . . . Jordan, J. (2015). A protocol for the management of adhesive small bowel obstruction. *Journal of Trauma and Acute Care Surgery*, 78(1), 13–19; discussion 19. doi:10.1097/TA.0000000000000491

Paulson, E. K., & Thompson, W. M. (2015). Review of small bowel obstruction: The diagnosis and when to worry. *Radiologic Society of North America: Radiology*, 2(275), 332–342, doi:10.1148/radiol.15131519

■ BRAIN TUMORS

Peter J. Cebull

Overview

The tissue found in the central nervous system (CNS) is complex and at times is the site of abnormal cellular growth. For many patients, brain tumors represent a feared and often unexpected diagnosis. In 2012, there were 688,000 people living with a primary brain or CNS tumor in the United States. Although the diagnosis of tumor often incites fear of malignancy, the majority of tumors were benign, with only 37% of primary brain tumors in the United States diagnosed as malignant (Ostrom et al., 2015). Providing nursing care for a patient with a brain tumor can be a challenging endeavor that requires an understanding of the prevalence and background behind the diagnosis, as well as a familiarity with the key clinical aspects of this condition.

Background

A brain tumor is tissue in the brain or central spine that has undergone abnormal growth and has the potential to disrupt normal brain function. In 2016, the World Health Organization (WHO) revised the 2007 classification system for CNS tumors. Before this reclassification, tumors were generally defined based on histology. The most recent classification system recommends considering the genetic composition of the tissue through the identification of molecular markers in addition to the histological features. This current system identifies over 120 different types and subtypes of brain and spinal tumors (Louis et al., 2016).

Another important aspect of defining a brain tumor is relative malignancy. Brain tumors that originate from cells found in or near the brain and do not contain cancerous cells are considered benign. Well-defined borders with a lack of involvement of surrounding tissue also characterize benign tumors. The most common nonmalignant brain tumor is meningioma, representing 53.4% of all benign brain tumors diagnosed between 2008 and 2012 (Ostrom et al., 2015). Malignant brain tumors grow more quickly than benign tumors due to the rapid division of cancer cells. The borders of malignant tumors are typically less defined and often spread into surrounding tissue as the tumor grows, rapidly becoming life-threatening (National Brain Tumor Society [NBTS], 2017). The most common malignant brain tumor is glioblastoma (GBM) representing 46.1% of all malignant brain tumors diagnosed between 2008 and 2012 (Ostrom et al., 2015).

Finally, when classifying a brain tumor, it is essential to identify the origin of the cells. Primary brain tumors begin from abnormal cellular growth in brain cells. When malignant, these often spread to other parts of the brain though rarely metastasize to areas outside of the CNS. Secondary brain tumors, also called *metastatic tumors* are the most common type of brain tumor. They begin in cells outside of the CNS and are referred to by their location of origin (National Brain Tumor Society [NBTS], 2017).

In 2016, The Central Brain Tumor Registry of the United States reported a primary CNS tumor incidence rate of 22.36 cases per 100,000 persons in the United States. Of those cases, 7.18 represented malignant tumors. When isolated by gender, females have a higher incidence at 24.46/100,000. In 2017, an estimated 26,070 cases of primary malignant CNS tumors will be diagnosed and an estimated 16,947 deaths will occur (Ostrom et al., 2015).

Five-year survival rates are impacted by several factors. For men with a primary malignant CNS tumor diagnosed between 1995 and 2013, 33.5% survived 5 years following diagnosis, whereas 36.1% of women survived 5 years following the same diagnosis. For nonmalignant CNS tumors diagnosed during this time frame, there was a 90.4% 5-year survival rate (Ostrom et al., 2015). The age of a patient at the time of diagnosis also factors heavily into the likelihood of 4-year survival. There is an inverse correlation between 5-year survival and age of diagnosis of primary malignant CNS tumor. Of patients with primary CNS malignancies, approximately 73.8% of patients aged 0 to 19 years survived to 5 years, whereas 33.5% of patients aged 45 to 54 years survived 5 years following diagnosis. The prevalence of any primary CNS tumor is considerably lower in the 0 to 19 age group, at 35.4 per 100,000 compared to an overall prevalence of 221.8 per 100,000 (Ostrom et al., 2015).

Clinical Aspects

ASSESSMENT

One of the most valuable portions of any assessment is the patient's history. When providing nursing care for a patient diagnosed with a brain tumor, it is beneficial to obtain a history from both the patient and his or her primary caregiver, who is familiar with the patient's most recent signs and symptoms. After the history, the most essential portion of the nurse's assessment is a complete neurologic examination. This establishes critical baseline information on the patient's deficits and aids in identifying the evolution or addition of neurologic deficits.

Neurologic deficits will vary based on the size and location of the brain tumor in relation to the physiologic functions of the affected brain tissue. For example, destruction or distortion of cerebral tissue in the supratentorial (cerebral) region can cause deficits such as memory loss, aphasia, and cognitive impairment. Tumors affecting tissue in the infratentorial (cerebellar) region can cause ataxia and autonomic dysfunction. As a tumor grows and occupies space in the cranial vault, the increase in intracranial pressure (ICP) worsens the deficits. In addition to these specific assessments, appropriate nursing assessment also includes screening for common findings associated with the presence of a brain tumor: visual disturbances such as blurriness, double vision and cuts in the visual fields; alteration of mental status or personality not otherwise explained; nausea and vomiting not explained by other illness or gastrointestinal irritants; onset of seizures; and headaches rated as most severe in the morning with improvement or resolution as the day progresses.

The diagnosis of a brain tumor relies heavily on high-quality neuroimaging. MRI following injection of IV contrast is typically the initial diagnostic choice, to identify the presence or absence of vasculature in a questionable lesion. After diagnosis, CT is often used to evaluate progression of disease and response to interventions. Surgical biopsy is often indicated to gain the necessary histological information needed to make an exact diagnosis and classification based on the WHO grading criteria.

NURSING INTERVENTIONS, MANAGEMENT, AND IMPLICATIONS

Medical interventions for brain tumors can include nonsurgical options, such as chemotherapy and radiation for malignancies, as well as more invasive surgical approaches, for example, craniotomy, tumor excision, or stereotactic radiosurgery. Similarly, nursing-related problems can vary based on the elected medical interventions.

Examples of nursing-related problems associated with the disease process can include communication barriers resulting from aphasia, risk for falls and injuries related to gait ataxia, and maladaptation complicated by changes in cognitive function and personality. Examples of nursing-related problems associated with nonsurgical treatment can include managing the adverse effects of chemotherapy. Surgical treatment can present nursing problems, including risk of infection, postoperative intracranial bleeding, and complications due to swelling of brain tissue.

When addressing the potential problems facing a patient with a brain tumor, there are multiple interventions for nurses to implement. The following are several examples of common problems and appropriate interventions. Aphasia resulting from a tumor affecting the speech centers of the brain can become a barrier to communication. Depending on the expressive or receptive nature, a written-communication board and other nonverbal forms of expression can be offered by a nurse.

High risk for falls is a common complication of gait disturbance with infratentorial tumors. Assistive devices and gait belts reduce this risk, improving safety for both the patient and nurse.

Nausea and vomiting related to chemotherapy are a common, uncomfortable, and even dangerous side effect when uncontrolled. There are many medications used to manage nausea and vomiting associated with chemotherapy, including serotonin receptor (5-HT3) antagonists, steroids, and neurokinin-1 receptor antagonists. Dietary modifications can also be beneficial.

Risk of infection is associated with any surgical procedure, including craniotomy. Postoperatively, the nurse needs to attentively monitor for signs of local and systemic infection in addition to administering prophylactic parenteral antibiotics such as cefazolin (Ancef).

OUTCOMES

Cerebral edema is a common complication of both brain tumors and treatment modalities such as tumor excision or debulking. A nurse must be vigilant in assessing the patient to identify early signs of increased ICP and administering parenteral or oral corticosteroids such as dexamethasone (Decadron) to decrease inflammation.

Summary

The diagnosis of brain tumor can present many challenges to patients and their caregivers. It is important to understand the key features that differentiate benign, malignant, primary, and secondary CNS tumors. Recognizing the relative incidence of this diagnosis as well as the significant mortality associated with primary malignant tumors can inform the nursing process. As a nurse, performing a high-quality assessment is essential to both identify and anticipate the nursing problems associated with this diagnosis.

Louis, D. N., Perry, A., Reifenberger, G., von Deimling, A., Figarella-Branger, D., Cavenee, W. K., . . . Ellison, D. W. (2016). The 2016 World Health Organization classification of tumors of the central nervous system: A summary. *Acta Neuropathologica, 131*(6), 803–820. doi:10.1007/s00401-016-1545-1

National Brain Tumor Society. (2013). Understanding brain tumors. Retrieved from http://braintumor.org/brain-tumor-information/understanding-brain-tumors

Ostrom, Q. T., Gittleman, H., Fulop, J., Liu, M., Blanda, R., Kromer, C., . . . Barnholtz-Sloan, J. S. (2015). CBTRUS statistical report: Primary brain and central nervous system tumors diagnosed in the United States in 2008–2012. *Neuro-oncology, 17*(Suppl. 4), iv1–iv62. doi:10.1093/neuonc/nov189

■ CARDIOMYOPATHY

Elsie A. Jolade

Overview

Cardiomyopathies are a diverse group of diseases affecting the myocardium in which the heart muscle becomes abnormally enlarged, thick or rigid, thereby losing the ability to contract effectively with each heartbeat. In rare cases, the myocardium is replaced with scar tissue. As the disease progresses, the heart weakens, leading to heart failure, arrhythmias, and valvular problems (American Heart Association [AHA], 2017). Many cases of cardiomyopathies are idiopathic. The disease can also be secondary to genetic predisposition, infectious diseases, exposure to toxins, systemic connective tissue disease, infiltrative and proliferative disorders, or nutritional deficiencies (McCance & Huether, 2014).

Background

A more thorough understanding and classification system for cardiomyopathy has evolved in the past 50 years. The term was first proposed by Bridges in 1957 as an uncommon, noncoronary heart muscle disease. In 2006, the American Heart Association (AHA) categorized the disease as primary and secondary cardiomyopathies. Primary cardiomyopathies predominantly involve the heart, whereas secondary cardiomyopathies are accompanied by other organ system involvement. Most recent in 2016, the National Heart, Liver, and Blood Institute (NHLBI) placed cardiomyopathy in five categories: as hypertrophic, dilated, restrictive, arrhythmogenic right ventricular, and unclassified cardiomyopathy (NHLBI, 2016).

Hypertrophic cardiomyopathy (HCM) is characterized by enlargement of the myocardial cells and thickening of the walls of the ventricles. Usually the ventricles and septum thicken, creating narrowing or blockages in the ventricles, making it harder for the heart to effectively pump blood. HCM can also cause stiffness of the ventricles, changes in the mitral valve, and cellular changes in the heart tissue (NHLBI, 2016).

HCM is a very common condition and can occur without an obvious cause. It is usually inherited and affects men and women of any age equally (AHA, 2016). Clinical manifestations of HCM include dyspnea and chest pain in the absence of coronary artery disease. Postexertional syncope due to diminished diastolic filling and increased outflow obstruction is also common. Ventricular arrhythmias are common and sudden death may occur, often in athletes after extensive exertion (Porth, 2015).

Dilated cardiomyopathy (DCM) is characterized by progressive cardiac dilation and contractile (systolic) dysfunction (Porth, 2015). DCM occurs in adults 20 to 60 years old; it is more common in men than in women.

The disease frequently starts in the left ventricle, where the heart muscle begins to stretch, dilate, and thin, leading to enlargement of the chamber (AHA, 2016). DCM is a common cause of heart failure and the leading indication for heart transplantation. Clinical manifestations include dyspnea, orthopnea, and reduced exercise capacity. As the disease progresses, people in late-stage DCM often have ejection fractions (EF) of less than 25% (normal EF 50–66%). Thrombosis can form within the chambers of the heart and systemic emboli can occur in late stages of the disease (Porth, 2015).

Restrictive cardiomyopathy (RCM) is a rare form of myocardial disease in which ventricular filling is restricted due to excessive rigidity, but without thickening of the ventricular wall (Porth, 2015). The ventricles are nondilated, though there is impaired ventricular filling. RCM is less common than DCM and HCM and is idiopathic or associated with other disorders such as scleroderma, endomyocardial fibrosis, amyloidosis, and sarcoidosis. The most common clinical manifestation of RCM is right heart failure with systemic venous congestion, cardiomegaly, and dysrhythmias (McCance & Huether, 2014).

Arrythmogenic right ventricular cardiomyopathy (ARVC), also called *arrhythmogenic right ventricular dysplasia (ARVD)*, is a rare type of cardiomyopathy that occurs when the muscle tissue in the right ventricle is replaced with fatty or fibrous tissue leading to various rhythm disturbances, particularly ventricular tachycardia and, potentially, heart failure. More than 50% of ARVD cases are inherited as an autosomal dominant trait. ARVD ranks second to HCM as the leading cause of sudden cardiac death in young athletes. Clinical manifestations include palpitations, syncope, or cardiac arrest, usually in young- or middle-aged men (McCance & Huether, 2014; NHLBI, 2016).

Other types of cardiomyopathy include peripartum cardiomyopathy (PPCM) and Takotsubo cardiomyopathy. PPCM is a DCM that occurs in an otherwise healthy woman without a previously diagnosed cardiac disorder in the last month of pregnancy and up to 5 months postpartum. PPCM is manifested by signs of systolic dysfunction and heart failure for which there is no identifiable cause or evidence before the last month of pregnancy. It is the fifth leading cause of mortality during pregnancy. Diagnosis of PCCM is often delayed due to overlapping signs and symptoms of other pregnancy-related problems. Incidence is greater in Black, multiparous, or older women with twin fetuses or pre-eclampsia (McCance & Huether, 2014; Troiano, 2015).

Takotsubo cardiomyopathy, also called *broken heart syndrome*, is a transient reversible left ventricular dysfunction in response to profound psychological or emotional stress characterized by ventricular apical ballooning (McCance & Huether, 2014).

The mean age for onset is older than 60 years, with about 90% of cases occurring in postmenopausal women. Patients present with chest pain, electrocardiographic evidence of ST segment elevation myocardial infarct (STEMI), and impaired myocardial contractility without evidence of coronary disease.

Clinical Aspects

ASSESSMENT

An in-depth history and physical assessment are imperative to recognize, diagnose, and implement appropriate medical interventions early in the disease process. Clinical presentation of cardiomyopathies varies depending on the etiology and severity of the disease. Clinical manifestation, such as dyspnea, ventricular arrhythmias, orthopnea, reduced exercise capacity, syncope, and signs of right heart failure such as elevated jugular venous distension (JVD) and lower extremity edema, tend to occur in most types of the disease. Patients with ARVD typically present with palpitations, syncope, or cardiac arrest in young athletes. A systematic approach to family screening has contributed to better assessment of familial cardiomyopathies and allowed the identification of family members predisposed to disease based on the inheritance of cardiomyopathy-associated genes (Arbustini et al., 2014).

Diagnostic tests for cardiomyopathy include EKG to assess for heart rhythm abnormalities, 2D echocardiography to assess left ventricular EF, and Holter or event monitors to allow continuous monitoring of the heart's electrical activity for a full 24 to 48 hours. Other diagnostics include cardiac MRI to assess the shape and size of the heart, cardiac catheterization, and genetic testing through bidirectional DNA sequence analysis to identify specific gene mutations. Stress testing, chest radiography, and serum blood analysis for cardiac biomarkers are also performed (Porth, 2015).

OUTCOMES

Treatment goals for cardiomyopathy include managing any contributing factors, controlling signs and symptoms, slowing the progression of the disease, and reducing complications and the risk of sudden cardiac death. Methodologies include lifestyle changes, medications, surgical interventions, and implanted devices to prevent or treat arrhythmias.

Patient education focusing on lifestyle changes, such as smoking cessation, weight loss, avoidance of alcohol, stress management strategies, and compliance with the prescribed medication regimen for underlying diseases such as hypertension and diabetes mellitus, are also essential. Nurses traditionally take the lead in patient education; nurse-led interventions can result in a significant improvement in self-management and cardiac knowledge scores (Mackie et al., 2014).

Classes of medications used to treat cardiomyopathy include diuretics to remove excess fluid and reduce preload as well as beta-blockers, calcium channel blockers, and angiotensin-converting enzyme (ACE) inhibitors to control heart rate, reduce blood pressure, and slow the progression of the disease. Patients may be prescribed antiarrhythmics and anticoagulants (AHA, 2016). Some patients may need an automatic implantable cardioverter-defibrillator (AICD), which delivers an electrical impulse or shock to the heart when it senses a life-threatening change in the heart rhythm.

Summary

In conclusion, cardiomyopathy is a very complex disease with various etiologies that affect all ages. Advances in early recognition, diagnosis, and management of cardiomyopathy have resulted in better patient outcomes. An evidence-based approach to care is continually evolving and has improved the quality of life of patients with cardiomyopathy. Because cardiomyopathy often manifests with symptoms similar to heart failure, nurses have and will continue to play a leading role in patient education and other interventions for optimal heart failure management, which are known to contribute to better patient outcomes.

American Heart Association. (2016). What is cardiomyopathy in adults? Retrieved from http://www.heart.org/ HEARTORG/Conditions/More/Cardiomyopathy/What -Is-Cardiomyopathy-in-Adults_UCM_444168_Article .jsp#.WIVgVxsrLIU

Arbustini, E., Narula, N., Tavazzi, L., Serio, A., Grasso, M., Favalli, V., . . . Narula, J. (2014). The MOGE(S) classification of cardiomyopathy for clinicians. *Journal of the American College of Cardiology*, 3(64), 304–318.

Mackie, A. S., Islam, S., Magill-Evans, J., Rankin, K. N., Robert, C., Schuh, M., . . . Rempel, G. R. (2014). Healthcare transition for youth with heart disease: A

clinical trial. *Heart, 100*(14), 1113–1118. doi:10.1136/ heartjnl-2014-305748

McCance, K., & Huether, S. (2014). *Pathophysiology: The biologic basis for disease in adults and children* (7th ed.). New York, NY: Mosby.

National Heart, Lung, and Blood Institute. (2016). Types of cardiomyopathy. Retrieved from https://www.nhlbi.nih .gov/health/health-topics/topics/cm/types#

Porth, C. (2015). *Essentials of pathophysiology* (4th ed.). Philadelphia, PA: Lippincott Williams & Wilkins.

Troiano, N. H. (2015). Cardiomyopathy during pregnancy. *Journal of Perinatal & Neonatal Nursing, 29*(3), 222–228. doi:10.1097/JPN.0000000000000113

■ CHRONIC KIDNEY DISEASE

Mary de Haan

Overview

Chronic kidney disease (CKD) is defined as an abnormality in kidney function or structure lasting longer than 3 months that negatively impacts a person's health (Garcin, 2015; Smith, 2016). Most adults with CKD experience a progressive decrease in kidney function along with kidney damage, ultimately resulting in life-threatening kidney failure. Interdisciplinary management focuses on preventing kidney dysfunction in high-risk populations and delaying disease progression, while preventing or managing complications, in adults diagnosed with CKD (Vassalotti et al., 2016). Nursing care involves timely assessment, evidence-based interventions, health-promoting activities, and self-management education designed to support adults with CKD and members of their support system over the course of their disease.

Background

It is estimated that 26 million adults in the United States have CKD, with over 660,000 requiring life-sustaining renal replacement therapy (RRT), which involves hemodialysis (HD) or peritoneal dialysis (PD) or renal transplantation due to kidney failure (National Kidney Foundation [NKF], 2016; U.S. Renal Data System [USRDS], 2016). Each year in the United States, more deaths are attributed to kidney disease than either breast or prostate cancer (USRDS, 2016). In addition to morbidity and mortality, CKD disease creates a financial burden as well. In 2014, Medicare spending for persons aged 65 years or older with CKD exceeded $50 billion, or 20% of all Medicare spending in that age group (USRDS, 2016). The two principal causes of CKD in adults are diabetes mellitus and hypertension, with nearly half of all adults with CKD experiencing one or both disorders (NKF, 2016). The Centers for Disease Control and Prevention (CDC) estimate that more than 70% of all new cases of kidney failure can be attributed to diabetes and/or hypertension (CDC, 2015). Other disorders that can lead to CKD include chronic glomerulonephritis, polycystic kidney disease, systemic lupus erythematosus, congenital kidney malformations, and repeated acute kidney injury (CDC, 2015; NKF, 2016). Populations at increased risk for developing CKD include older adults (older than 60 years), persons with a family history of kidney disease, and select racial/ethnic groups (African Americans, Hispanics, Native Americans, and Pacific Islanders; CDC, 2015; NKF, 2016).

The diagnosis of CKD is made based on the presence of one or more markers of kidney damage and/or a decrease in estimated glomerular filtration rate (eGFR less than 60 mL/min/1.73 m^2; National Kidney Disease Education Program [NKDEP], 2014; Vassalotti et al., 2016). Markers of kidney damage include albuminuria (defined as greater than 30 mg or urine albumin/gram of urine creatinine for more than 3 months), abnormal urine sediment, disruption of electrolyte and fluid balance, and kidney abnormalities discovered by histology or imaging (NKDEP, 2014; Vassalotti et al., 2016). Although approximately one in 10 adults have some degree of CKD, not all progress to kidney failure (eGFR less than 15 mL/min/1.73 m^2). Adults with high-grade albuminuria, steady decline in eGFR, and poorly controlled blood pressure are more likely to experience disease progression (NKDEP, 2014).

Medical management of adults with CKD focuses on implementing appropriate treatment, monitoring the patient's progress and disease progression, screening for CKD complications, and providing self-management education (NKDEP, 2014). Specific interventions aimed at reducing CKD progression include blood pressure control (lesser than 140/90 mmHg), use of angiotensin-converting enzyme inhibitors (ACEIs) or angiotensin receptor blockers (ARBs) to control hypertension and reduce albuminuria, glycemic control (HbA$_1$C ~7%), and avoidance of nephrotoxic substances, such as nonsteroidal anti-inflammatory drugs (NSAIDs) and iodinated contrast dye (Smith, 2016; Vassalotti et al., 2016). Because cardiovascular disease is the leading cause of

death for adults with CKD, cardiac risk factors also need to be addressed and health-promoting interventions initiated (CDC, 2015). These interventions include weight management, diet therapy, implementation of an exercise routine, and, in select cases, the administration of statins (Smith, 2016; Vassalotti et al., 2016).

Adults with severely decreased kidney function (eGFR 15–29 mL/min/1.73 m^2) should receive education regarding approaching kidney failure and treatment options such as RRT, renal transplantation, or conservative treatment, including palliative care (NKF, 2015; Smith, 2016). The decision to initiate RRT (HD or PD) is based on the presence of signs and symptoms of uremia, evidence of protein-energy wasting, and the ability to safely manage complications with medical therapy alone (NKF, 2015).

Patient preference and lifestyle, along with risks and benefits of each form of therapy, should also be considered. HD is the most common form of RRT. It involves the use of a machine to filter a patient's blood through an artificial semipermeable membrane for the purpose of removing waste products and excess fluid and restoring electrolyte balance (National Institute of Diabetes and Digestive and Kidney Diseases [NIDDK], 2016; Winkelman, 2016). HD can be administered at a dialysis center (three times per week for 3 to 5 hours per session) or in the patient's home (five to seven times per week for 2 to 3 hours per session).

Although HD is the most efficient mode of RRT, it does require specially trained personnel to maintain and operate the dialysis machine; patients also need vascular access via a temporary dialysis catheter or arteriovenous (AV) fistula (NIDDK, 2016; NKF, 2015). Potential HD complications include hypotension, blood-borne infections, thrombosis of the AV fistula, and peripheral ischemia (Winkelman, 2016).

PD is used to filter fluids, electrolytes, and waste products from the peritoneum (similar to a semipermeable membrane) into dialysis fluid. This fluid (dialysate) is infused into the peritoneal space via a surgically implanted intra-abdominal silicone catheter.

The fluid is allowed to "dwell" for a prescribed period of time before being drained from the peritoneal space (NIDDK, 2016; Winkelman, 2016). This process is repeated several times within a 24-hour period. Exchanges can be done using continuous ambulatory PD (four to six exchanges with dwell times of 4 to 8 hours occurring 7 days/week) or continuous cycling PD (exchanges occur overnight while the patient is sleeping via an automated cycling machine; NIDDK, 2016). PD allows for greater flexibility of lifestyle and diet, as compared to HD, yet fewer than 10% of adults with kidney failure use this form of RRT.

Potential PD complications include abdominal discomfort, exit site and tunnel infections, and peritonitis (Winkelman, 2016; NIDDK, 2016).

Clinical Aspects

ASSESSMENT

Nursing plays an important role in screening high-risk populations for CKD, especially since kidney disease in its early stages is often asymptomatic (USRDS, 2016). A thorough history from adults at risk for or diagnosed with CKD is critical. It should include personal and family history of kidney injury or disease, cardiovascular disease, diabetes, and/or hypertension. The history should also address medication use (both prescribed and over-the-counter products), dietary habits, tobacco and alcohol usage, and exercise. Physical assessment should focus on cardiopulmonary status (presence of extra heart sounds and/or adventitious breath sounds, presence of dependent edema, reports of dyspnea and/or activity intolerance) and renal function.

Additional symptoms that may be reported in adults with CKD include fatigue, lethargy, difficulty concentrating, anorexia, muscle cramping, and pruritus (NKF, 2016; Smith, 2016). Laboratory testing includes an eGFR, urine albumin-to-creatinine ratio (UACR), serum blood urea nitrogen (BUN) and creatinine, and serum electrolytes (Smith, 2016). Because CKD impacts all body systems, screening for complications such as anemia (complaints of fatigue and dyspnea, decreased red blood cells [RBCs], hemoglobin, hematocrit, and iron stores), malnutrition (unintentional weight loss, muscle wasting, decreased serum albumin), mineral and bone disorders (calcium and phosphorus imbalance), depression, and decreased functional status is also warranted (NKDEP, 2014; Vassalotti et al., 2016).

NURSING INTERVENTIONS, MANAGEMENT, AND IMPLICATIONS

The focus of nursing care for adults with CKD is to manage problems and reduce the effects of complications (Garcin, 2015). Nursing-related problems that need to be addressed include excess fluid volume due to decreased kidney function; decreased cardiac function related to fluid overload and increased peripheral resistance; risk for infection and injury related to skin break-down, falls, vascular access occlusion, or PD catheter site contamination; fatigue related to uremia, anemia, and malnutrition; and impaired psychosocial integrity related to anxiety, depression, and hopelessness associated with the diagnosis of a progressive chronic illness (Winkelman, 2016).

Fluid balance, respiratory status, and cardiac function need to be assessed due to the potential for fluid volume overload, pulmonary edema, and/or heart failure. Interventions should include monitoring intake, output, and patient weight; assessing cardiopulmonary status; maintaining a position of comfort to facilitate adequate ventilation; and administering prescribed medications (diuretics, ACEIs, ARBs) to control blood pressure. Electrolyte imbalances, such as hypo/hypernatremia and hyperkalemia, are common and require diligent monitoring of laboratory values, heart rate and rhythm, and neurological status (Smith, 2016; Winkelman, 2016).

Infection is a potentially life-threatening occurrence for adults with CKD. Uremic pruritus can lead to excoriation and skin breakdown, whereas dialysis access devices offer routes of entry to pathogens. Patients need to be monitored for fever, malaise, and evidence of skin breakdown, redness, or edema—particularly at the dialysis access insertion sites. Sterile technique should be used whenever an HD vascular access device or PD catheter is in use.

Nutritional needs, including fluid balance, glycemic control, protein and phosphorus intake, and sodium/potassium balance, should be discussed in collaboration with a registered dietician (Garcin, 2015; Winkelman, 2016).

Psychosocial support and self-management education should be offered to all adults with CKD and members of their immediate support system. Support should include providing information regarding the CKD diagnosis, anticipated disease progression, and treatment options, as well as referral to counseling services and support groups (Winkelman, 2016; NKDEP, 2014).

OUTCOMES

Adults with CKD should maintain adequate cardiac function and optimal fluid and electrolyte balance. Nutritional needs should be met in order to maintain an adequate protein–calorie intake, regardless of the dietary restrictions that may be recommended based on their degree of kidney function. Adults with CKD should avoid injury and infection and should be involved in health-promoting activities designed to prevent or delay the progress of CKD and its complications.

Psychosocial and educational needs should be evaluated and effective coping mechanisms supported by all members of the interdisciplinary care team. Effective nursing care applies principles of patient-centered care, teamwork, collaboration, and communication to address each of these evidence-based expected outcomes (NKDEP, 2014; Winkelman, 2016).

Summary

Adults diagnosed with CKD must cope with a number of uncertainties in terms of physical, psychosocial, and lifestyle changes they will face. Nurses, as members of the interdisciplinary team focused on preventing or delaying the progression of CKD and its associated complications, play a vital role in providing evidence-based care, health-promoting activities, and education to provide support throughout the course of the disease.

Centers for Disease Control and Prevention. (2015). Chronic kidney disease issue brief. Retrieved from http://www.cdc.gov/diabetes/pdfs/progress/CKDBrief.pdf

Garcin, A. (2015). Care of the patient with chronic kidney disease. *MedSurg Matters, 24*(5), 4–7.

National Institute of Diabetes and Digestive and Kidney Diseases. (2016). Kidney disease education lesson builder: Choices for treatment of kidney failure. Retrieved from https://www.niddk.nih.gov/health-information/health-communication-programs/nkdep/a-z/Documents/ckd-primary-care-guide-508.pdf

National Kidney Disease Education Program. (2014). *Making sense of chronic kidney disease: A concise guide for managing CKD in the primary care setting* (NIH pub No. 14-7989).

National Kidney Foundation. (2015). KDOQI clinical practice guideline for hemodialysis adequacy: 2015 update. *American Journal of Kidney Disease, 66*(5), 884–930.

National Kidney Foundation. (2016). About chronic kidney disease. Retrieved from http://kidney.org/kidneydisease/aboutckd

Smith, C. A. (2016). Evidence-based treatment of chronic kidney disease. *Nurse Practitioner, 41*(11), 42–48. doi:10.1097/01.NPR.0000502790.65984.61

U.S. Renal Data System. (2016). *2016 USRDS annual data report: Epidemiology of kidney disease in the United States.* Bethesda, MD: National Institutes of Health, National Institute of Diabetes and Digestive and Kidney Diseases.

Vassalotti, J., Centor, R., Turner, B., Greer, R., Choi, M., Sequist, T.; National Kidney Foundation Kidney Disease Outcomes Quality Initiative. (2016). Practical approach to detection and management of CKD for the primary care clinician. *American Journal of Medicine, 129*(2), 153–162.

Winkelman, C. (2016). Care of patients with acute kidney injury and chronic kidney disease. In D. Ignatavicius & M. Workman (Eds.) *Medical surgical nursing: Patient-centered collaborative care* (8th ed., pp. 1411–1447). Philadelphia, PA: Elsevier.

■ CHRONIC OBSTRUCTIVE PULMONARY DISEASE

Christina M. Canfield

Overview

The Global Initiative for Chronic Obstructive Lung Disease (GOLD) defines chronic obstructive pulmonary disease (COPD) as a "common, preventable and treatable disease that is characterized by persistent respiratory symptoms and airflow limitation that is due to airway and/or alveolar abnormalities usually caused by significant exposure to noxious particles or gases" (GOLD, 2017, p. x). Disease severity is influenced by exacerbations and comorbidities. COPD causes significant morbidity and mortality worldwide. Cigarette smoking is a well-known risk factor for development of COPD.

Background

It is estimated that more than 380 million people are living with COPD worldwide. COPD was responsible for 3 million deaths in 2012 and is projected to be the third leading cause of death by 2020 (GOLD, 2017). An estimated $52 billion is spent on care of the individual with COPD annually in the United States. In developing countries, the economic burden shifts from direct and indirect medical costs to lost workplace and home productivity. In addition, COPD contributes to significant disability worldwide.

Exposure to cigarette smoke is the most widely known cause of COPD. However, genetic factors, such as hereditary alpha-1 antitrypsin deficiency, predispose individuals to development of COPD. Additional risk factors include occupational exposure to chemicals, dust, fumes, and air pollution. Previously, men were more likely to be diagnosed with COPD than women. However, women are just as likely to develop COPD as males (GOLD, 2017). Individuals who experienced conditions that affected lung growth during gestation and childhood may be more likely to develop COPD than those who did not.

Inflammation of the lung and airways is a normal response when exposed to cigarette smoke or other noxious agents. Chronic inflammation may cause destruction of the lung tissue and disrupt the physiologic mechanisms that normally repair the lungs. These changes lead to reduced airway diameter and lung fibrosis. Airway changes lead to trapping of gas during expiration. Reduced expiratory volume is noted during spirometry. Patients with COPD have a reduction in forced expiratory volume (FEV) when expiration is measured over 1 second. This measurement is called FEV_1. In addition to airway changes, increased effort to breathe may lead to retention of carbon dioxide (GOLD, 2017).

COPD is a chronic, progressive disease that is characterized by periods of worsening symptoms, or exacerbations. Exacerbations may be triggered by infection, pollutants, or exposure to respiratory irritants. Patients experience more severe symptoms during an exacerbation and may require hospitalization.

All patients who complain of shortness of breath, chronic cough, or sputum production should be evaluated for COPD, regardless of risk factor exposure. A cough productive of sputum is seen in up to one third of patients (GOLD, 2017). The patient will undergo testing via spirometry to determine the extent of airflow limitation. Criteria for severity of airflow limitation in COPD may be classified as mild, moderate, severe, or very severe according to spirometry criteria defined by the GOLD (2017).

COPD often presents as one part of a complex patient health picture. Up to 40% of patients diagnosed with COPD may also be affected by heart disease (Grindrod, 2015). Other associated conditions include diabetes, hypertension, osteoporosis, and depression.

Medical management of COPD often involves the use of inhaled medications. A combination of long- and short-acting inhalers may be used to optimize therapy. Patients require significant instruction to ensure proper use of inhaled medications and individual administration technique should be assessed before changing medication or assuming a therapy is not effective (GOLD, 2017).

Clinical Aspects

ASSESSMENT

The nurse should suspect COPD in patients who present with complaints of progressive dyspnea, cough, and mucus production. Dyspnea is thought to be a better predictor of mortality than FEV and should be assessed during each encounter. It is recommended that facilities adopt a dyspnea or breathlessness rating scale to ensure consistency among assessments (Miller, Owens, & Silverman, 2015). Assess for risk factors, including cigarette smoking, exposure to secondhand cigarette smoke, or occupational exposure. Other diseases that mimic the symptoms of COPD include tuberculosis, asthma, congestive heart failure, and interstitial lung disease.

Physical assessment findings may include the following:

- Use of accessory muscles
- Changes in chest shape
- Cyanosis due to impaired arterial oxygenation
- Clubbing of the fingers
- Crackles or wheezes upon auscultation
- Cough productive of sputum
- Weight loss or signs of malnutrition

NURSING INTERVENTIONS, MANAGEMENT, AND IMPLICATIONS

Nursing management of the patient with COPD includes frequent observations of physiologic and mental status. Changes in respiratory function may be reflected via pulse oximetry, laboratory results (i.e., arterial blood gas), and mental status assessment. The nurse must recognize changes in status and consider indications of impending or actual respiratory failure or worsening disease.

Patients with COPD are likely to experience imbalanced nutrition due to high calorie expenditure caused by systemic inflammation and increased work of breathing (Hodson, 2016).

Nursing-related problems and the patient-specific plan of care should include consideration of oxygen imbalance, inadequate respiration, altered nutrition, activity intolerance, and risk for infection.

Nursing interventions include vital sign monitoring with frequent monitoring of oxygenation, administration of oxygen as ordered, assessment of dyspnea and signs of respiratory distress, medication management with oral or inhaled medications and oral or intravenous antibiotics, and education of the patient and significant other(s). Initiate appropriate nutritional screening and obtain consultation as indicated. Discharge planning includes anticipation of use of oxygen at home, need for assistive devices, and identification of challenges in obtaining or paying for medications.

OUTCOMES

Expected outcomes for any patient with COPD include activity tolerance, maintenance of adequate oxygenation, adequate nutrition, and adherence to prescribed medication regimen.

Following an exacerbation, expected outcomes include increased tolerance of activity, stable vital signs, absence of signs and symptoms of active infection, decreased sputum production, and a return to baseline oxygen requirements. Research has demonstrated that patients who receive the influenza vaccine experience a significant reduction in the number of COPD exacerbations when compared to those who do not receive the vaccine (GOLD, 2017). Evidence of the effectiveness of the pneumococcal vaccine is limited but it remains recommended for all patients aged 65 years and older (GOLD, 2017).

Summary

COPD is a preventable and treatable disease that often exists as a comorbidity with other diseases. Effective management of COPD includes medication, nutrition, preservation of physical function, and infection prevention. Assess for smoking during every patient encounter and encourage smoking cessation in those who actively smoke. Cessation of smoking is beneficial and may slow progression of the disease.

Global Initiative for Chronic Obstructive Lung Disease. (2017). Global initiative for chronic obstructive lung disease—Global strategy for the diagnosis, management and prevention of COPD. Retrieved from http://gold copd.org/gold-2017-global-strategy-diagnosis-management-prevention-copd

Hodson, M. (2016). Integrating nutrition into pathways for patients with COPD. *British Journal of Community Nursing, 21*(11), 548–552. doi:10.12968/bjcn.2016.21.11.548

Miller, S., Owens, L., & Silverman, E. (2015). Physical examination of the adult patient with chronic respiratory disease. *MedSurg Nursing, 24*(3), 195–198.

■ COLORECTAL CANCER

Visnja Maria Masina
Crina V. Floruta

Overview

Colorectal cancer is the most common type of gastrointestinal cancer. Colorectal cancer is defined as the presence of a malignant mass of cells affecting the tissue of the large bowel (colon) or rectum. The etiology of colorectal cancer is multifactorial, involving genetic, environmental, and inflammatory factors that incite a sporadic genetic mutation in the gland cells of the epithelial lining of the affected tissue. These sporadic mutations of the colorectal tissue may result in dysregulated growth that can produce a malignant growth or tumor. Nurses play a key in role in helping patients understand their risk for colorectal cancer, strategies to minimize their risk and to detect early stages of the colorectal cancer, which is curable.

Background

Colorectal cancer is considered a disease of Western society; the incidence is relatively high in industrialized countries and low in less developed countries, such as those in Africa and Asia. In the United States, colorectal cancer is the third most common cause of cancer deaths following lung, prostate, and breast cancer in both men and women. The epidemiologic pattern of colorectal cancer suggests that diet and environmental factors play a major role in the pathogenesis of colorectal cancer (American Cancer Society [ACS], 2017).

Mortality rates have declined steadily in the past three decades, likely due to more effective screening programs and improvements in available treatment modalities. Trends in the declining incidence differ by age; however, for unknown reasons since 1992 there has been a 1.8% increase in the incidence of colorectal cancer in adults younger than age 50 years (ACS, 2017). In the United States, an estimated 95,520 new cases of colon cancer and 39,910 new cases of rectal cancer are expected to be diagnosed in 2017 (ACS, 2017).

The risk of colorectal cancer increases with age. Colorectal cancer occurs less frequently before age 40 years; 90% of cases occur after 50 years of age. The lifetime risk of developing colorectal cancer in the United States is approximately 5%. In addition to living in a Western society, risk factors for colorectal cancer include hereditary conditions such as familial adenomatous polyposis (FAP), inherited genetic conditions such as Lynch syndrome also known as *hereditary nonpolyposis colorectal cancer syndrome (HNPCC)*, ulcerative colitis or Crohn's colitis (more than 10 years), personal or family history of colon polyps or cancer, and type 2 diabetes mellitus. Modifiable factors that increase risk for colorectal cancer include obesity, physical inactivity, long-term smoking, high consumption of red or processed meat, low calcium intake, moderate to heavy alcohol consumption, and very low intake of fruits and vegetables (ACS, 2017).

With early detection, colorectal cancer is a preventable and highly curable disease. Early-stage colorectal cancer is typically asymptomatic, making screening necessary to detect disease early. Whatever the causative factors, most colorectal cancers and adenocarcinomas in particular, thought to develop from adenomatous or serrated polyps. Although not all polyps progress to cancer, the evidence supports that most colorectal cancers arise from polyps. It is widely accepted that colorectal cancer-related morbidity and mortality can be reduced through early detection, removal of small polyps, and treatment of early-stage disease. National organizations, including the American Cancer Society (ACS), American Society for Gastrointestinal Endoscopy (ASGE), the National Comprehensive Cancer Network (NCCN), and American College of Gastroenterology (ACG) have established screening guidelines for average and increased-risk individuals. Routine screening for colorectal cancer and adenomatous polyps is recommended for asymptomatic adults aged 50 years and older. However, the individual's age and history should inform the frequency and mode of screening for colorectal cancer. Of all the screening methods for colorectal cancer, colonoscopy is considered the gold-standard screening modality.

Clinical Aspects

ASSESSMENT

Colon and rectal cancers are frequently conjoined but each tissue has distinct patterns of presentation, staging, and management of affected malignant tissue. Colon cancer can be categorized as right-sided or left-sided lesions. Abdominal pain, palpation of a mass on the right side, change in bowel habits, anemia, and weight loss are symptoms of ascending (right-sided) colon cancer. Pain, change in bowel habits, hematochezia, and bowel obstruction are symptoms characteristic to descending or left-sided colon cancer.

The evaluation of colon cancer includes complete history and physical examination; colonoscopy; laboratory studies, including complete blood count (CBC) to evaluate for anemia, basic metabolic panel (BMP) and liver function testing; and carcinoembryonic

antigen (CEA), which has been found to provide some prognostic information and is used during surveillance. The tumor, node, and metastasis framework is used for staging colorectal cancer. Initial staging is done through radiographic imaging such as CT scans of chest, abdomen, and pelvis. MRI of the liver or PET scans are reserved for when metastatic lesions are suspected. Treatment options for colorectal cancer are dependent on the stage at diagnosis. Early-stage colorectal cancer is treated surgically; the majority of stage I and II cancers are curable by surgical resection. A combination of surgery, chemotherapy, and radiation are used to manage stage III and IV diseases. Patients are followed at regular intervals up to 5 years from the diagnosis to monitor recuperation and detect any evidence of recurrent disease.

Symptoms of rectal cancer include bright red blood mixed in stool, rectal bleeding, and change in bowel habits and or shape of stool, tenesmus, fatigue, anemia, and unintentional weight loss. Timely evaluation of symptoms is essential. In addition to the evaluation for colon cancer, patients with suspected rectal cancer undergo MRI of the pelvis for locoregional staging and a flexible or rigid proctoscopy to verify the location of the tumor in relation to the anal verge. Locally advanced rectal cancers (stage II and III) are treated through a multidisciplinary treatment approach consisting of neoadjuvant chemoradiation therapy, followed by surgical resection, and adjuvant chemotherapy.

OUTCOMES

Nurses play an important role in educating the public in recognizing early signs of colorectal cancer and following recommended screening guidelines. Nurses play an integral role in supporting and educating patients with colorectal cancer by being knowledgeable regarding risk factors, signs and symptoms, disease course, and current and emerging therapies. Timely patient–family education may minimize anxiety and promote compliance and self-management.

For patients undergoing surgical resection in whom formation of a stoma is possible, consultation with a wound ostomy and continence (WOC) nurse is beneficial. Choosing an appropriate stoma site, teaching stoma care, and counseling about living with a stoma makes the postoperative course smoother with less complications. Topics discussed at this initial visit include anatomy; stoma function and appearance; emptying and changing of the pouch system; obtaining supplies; and activities of daily living, including bathing/showering, diet, clothing, and sexuality (Mahoney, 2016).

Summary

Prevention and early detection are key to curing colorectal cancers. Nurses play a fundamental role in educating and supporting patients about a sensitive topic and helping individuals understand the importance of screening. If a diagnosis of cancer is made, the nurse plays a pivotal role in the patient's cancer treatment journey.

American Cancer Society. (2017). *Cancer facts and figures*. Atlanta, GA: Author.

Mahoney, M. (2016). Preoperative preparation of patients undergoing a fecal or urinary diversion. In J. Carmel, J. Colwell, & M. Goldberg (Eds.), *Wound, ostomy and continence nurses society core curriculum: Ostomy management* (pp. 99–112). Philadelphia, PA: Wolters Kluwer.

■ CORONARY ARTERY DISEASE IN ADULTS

Kate Cook
Mary T. Quinn Griffin

Overview

Coronary artery disease (CAD), defined clinically as a blockage or narrowing of the coronary vessels that impedes blood flow, is a common form of cardiovascular disease in adults. The disease continues to be a leading cause of death in the United States, claiming 385,000 lives annually (Ramos, 2014). CAD is the number one cause of death across ethnic groups in both developed and developing countries worldwide; thus it is considered a global crisis (Assimes & Roberts, 2016). There are a number of modifiable and nonmodifiable risk factors that identify patients at greatest risk for developing CAD. Initial nursing efforts must focus on accurate assessment of risk stratification and alteration of all modifiable risk factors identified. Patient management varies as a patient's disease progresses, and is depending on related clinical manifestations.

Background

The obstruction in blood flow associated with CAD is due to atherosclerosis, which occurs when fatty substances build up over time, forming a plaque that hardens the walls of the arterial blood vessels. Atherosclerosis begins when the innermost layer of the arterial vessels, the endothelium, is repeatedly subjected to injury. In response to this damage within the vessels, inflammatory processes occur, which, in turn, change the structure and biochemistry of the arterial walls. Macrophages are produced and transport lipids inside the walls of the arteries. Smooth muscle migrates into the areas of fatty accumulation, forming a plaque that may protrude into the vessel opening. Depending on the thickness of the plaque, this protrusion may be enough to restrict blood flow, causing ischemia. Plaques on the vessel walls are vulnerable to rupture, which can result in the sudden formation of a thrombus. A thrombus in a coronary vessel leads to obstruction of blood flow, and the potential for complications such as acute coronary syndrome or a myocardial infarction.

A variety of risk factors may, in combination, inflict the initial injury to the walls of the coronary vessels. Modifiable risk factors include elevated serum lipid levels, tobacco use, hypertension, diabetes mellitus, obesity, sedentary lifestyle, and stress. Nonmodifiable risks associated with CAD include age, family history of CAD, ethnicity, and gender. African Americans have a higher incidence of CAD than other racial groups. In terms of gender, males tend to have a higher likelihood of developing CAD at an earlier age when compared to females. Recent evidence suggests that the presence of high blood pressure, obesity, and high cholesterol have a similar effect on CAD-related outcomes in men and women. Prolonged tobacco use, however, is more hazardous to women. Women who have a history of specific pregnancy complications (such as preeclampsia or gestational diabetes), polycystic ovary disease, or early-onset menopause are at higher risk for morbidity and mortality related to CAD.

Patient teaching focuses on educating patients regarding prevention and management of modifiable risk factors. Collaborative management of patients with CAD varies greatly depending on physical manifestations and disease severity. Common interventions include pain management, pharmacological therapy, percutaneous coronary intervention (stenting), and coronary artery bypass graft.

Clinical Aspects

ASSESSMENT

In the absence of physical symptoms, such as angina pectoris, clinicians must rely on an accurate health history, risk assessment tools, and the observance of unexpected findings in the physical assessment to detect CAD. A three-generation family history and information related to age of onset of any known cases of CAD is useful in determining a patient's heritable risk (Assimes & Roberts, 2016). For patients who have not been diagnosed, risk factor assessment is a critical component of identifying patients at greatest risk. The American College of Cardiology and the American Heart Association recommend use of the Pooled Cohort Equations risk assessment scale to estimate the 10-year risk of atherosclerotic cardiovascular disease in patients (Goff et al., 2014). This scale uses an algorithm based on an individual's gender, age, race, total cholesterol laboratory values, along with history of hypertension, smoking, and diabetes to determine an individual's risk classification. The scale has been validated for use in both White and African American men and women.

A thorough physical assessment should be performed. Cardiovascular assessment related to decreased coronary perfusion, such as accurate blood pressure measurement in both arms, ankle–brachial index, heart rate, respiratory rate, pulse oximetry, capillary refill, and the quality and rhythm of bilateral pulses should be performed. Neck veins should be examined for distention, and the heart and lungs should be auscultated for adventitious sounds, indicative of fluid volume excess. The skin and mucous membranes should be assessed for color, temperature, and the presence of moisture.

Various laboratory tests are useful in determining a patient's risk for development of CAD. A fasting lipid profile (total cholesterol, low- and high-density lipoproteins, and triglycerides) is often performed to establish a baseline for patients. The information gained from this profile can be used to preventatively treat patients without CAD who are known to be at risk or to proactively treat patients diagnosed with CAD and reduce the chances of progression. C-reactive protein (CRP) is a measure of the level of inflammation in the body, and is considered a marker for cardiovascular risk. Elevated brain natriuretic peptide (BNP) and homocysteine levels are biomarkers associated with an increased risk for CAD and may be used as part of the diagnostic evaluation. Patients diagnosed with metabolic syndrome for diabetes are inherently at higher risk for cardiac disease. Therefore, fasting plasma glucose and hemoglobin A1c are also common diagnostic screenings.

There are several noninvasive imaging studies commonly associated with the detection of CAD. Exercise (for patients physically able to exercise) or pharmacological (if exercise is contraindicated) stress tests are often performed to determine the presence of ischemia (Ramos, 2014). If patients are asymptomatic but have a significant family history of CAD or a diagnosis of diabetes mellitus, a nuclear stress test may be useful in detecting disease. CT angiograms (CTAs) have the ability to visualize the coronary arteries and are a noninvasive method to detect the presence and severity of plaque in the vessel walls (Ramos, 2014).

NURSING INTERVENTIONS, MANAGEMENT, AND IMPLICATIONS

Nursing interventions, such as education, support, and behavioral counseling, have been proven effective in assisting patients diagnosed with or at risk for developing CAD. These interventions, however, can involve a costly and time-consuming process, and there is some debate regarding the proper methods for going about these interventions (Saffi, Polanczyk, & Rabelo-Silva, 2014). Behavioral counseling and education should be focused on modifiable risk factors that are placing patients at greater risk. Nurses can connect patients with community resources, such as weight management, exercise, and smoking cessation programs, which provide individuals with education, support, and accountability (Lachman et al., 2015).

Advances in treatment and cardioprotective medications have led to a recent decline in hospitalizations and mortality for patients with ischemic disease. Adherence to these medication regimens is critical for control of CAD-related symptoms; therefore, medication nonadherence could be considered a modifiable risk factor for complications (Lourenço et al., 2014). Nurse-conducted interventions for outpatients aimed at reinforcing the importance of prescribed treatments and identifying individual barriers to adherence to protocols appear to promote positive health behavior changes in clients.

OUTCOMES

Expected outcomes related to CAD vary depending on the clinical manifestations of the disease, as well as each patient's genetic risk and adherence to treatment protocols. Recent studies have shown that for patients at high genetic risk, management of modifiable risk factors is associated with a 50% lower risk of CAD (Khera et al., 2016). Therefore, nursing goals should focus on adherence to prescribed treatment and modification of risk factors in order to prevent disease progression and limit complications.

Summary

CAD is a broad term used to describe conditions that lead to blocked blood flow within the vessels that supply blood, oxygen, and nutrition to the heart. Patients diagnosed and treated for CAD are at high risk for reoccurrence and mortality. Genetic and modifiable lifestyle factors have long since been associated with susceptibility to this disease. Most recent, human genome studies based on an individual's genetic makeup have the potential ability to determine persons at highest risk for developing CAD as well as individuals who will best respond to therapy (Assimes & Roberts, 2016). Early identification and treatment of patients with CAD will lead to an increased quality of life for these patients coupled with decreased morbidity and mortality in this patient population.

Assimes, T. L., & Roberts, R. (2016). Genetics: Implications for prevention and management of coronary artery disease. *Journal of the American College of Cardiology*, *68*(25), 2797–2818. doi:10.1016/j.jacc.2016.10.039

Goff, D. C., Jr., Lloyd-Jones, D. M., Bennett, G., Coady, S., D'Agostino, R. B., Gibbons, R., . . . Tomaselli, G. F. (2014). 2013 ACC/AHA guideline on the assessment of cardiovascular risk: A report of the American College of Cardiology/American Heart Association Task Force on Practice Guidelines [published correction appears in *Circulation*, *129*(Suppl. 2), S74–S75]. *Circulation*, *129*(Suppl. 2), S49–S73. doi:10.1161/01.cir.0000437741.48606.98

Khera, A. V., Emdin, C. A., Drake, I., Natarajan, P., Bick, A. G., Cook, N. R., . . . Kathiresan, S. (2016). Genetic risk, adherence to a healthy lifestyle, and coronary disease. *New England Journal of Medicine*, *375*(24), 2349–2358. doi:10.1056/NEJMoa1605086

Lachman, S., Minneboo, M., Snaterse, M., Jorstad, H. T., Ter Reit, G., Scholte Op Reimer, W. J.; Response 2 Study Group. (2015). Community-based comprehensive lifestyle programs in patients with coronary artery disease: Objectives, design and expected results of Randomized Evaluation of Secondary Prevention by Outpatient Nurse Specialists 2 trial (RESPONSE 2). *American Heart Journal*, *170*(2), 216–222. doi:10.1016/j.ahj.2015.05.010

Lourenço, L. B., Rodrigues, R. C., Ciol, M. A., São-João, T. M., Cornélio, M. E., Dantas, R. A., & Gallani, M. C. (2014). A randomized controlled trial of the effectiveness of planning strategies in the adherence to medication for coronary artery disease. *Journal of Advanced Nursing*, *70*(7), 1616–1628. doi:10.1111/jan.12323

Ramos, L. M. (2014). Cardiac diagnostic testing: What bedside nurses need to know. *Critical Care Nurse*, *34*(3), 16–27; quiz 28. doi:10.4037/ccn2014361

Saffi, M. A., Polanczyk, C. A., & Rabelo-Silva, E. R. (2014). Lifestyle interventions reduce cardiovascular risk in patients with coronary artery disease: A randomized clinical trial. *European Journal of Cardiovascular Nursing*, *13*(5), 436–443. doi:10.1177/1474515113505396

■ CUSHING SYNDROME

Yolanda Flenoury
Jane F. Marek

Overview

The adrenal glands are an important part of the endocrine system and produce and secrete glucocorticoids, mineralocorticoids, and androgens. Cortisol, sometimes referred to as the stress hormone, is an adrenal glucocorticoid hormone regulated by the hypothalamus–pituitary–adrenal (HPA) axis. Cortisol is essential to homeostasis and regulates the body's physiologic response to stress, including maintaining blood glucose levels, immune response, blood pressure, and protein, carbohydrate, and fat metabolism. In 1912, Harvey W. Cushing identified the relationship between certain physical characteristics and a tumor in the pituitary gland, which became known as Cushing disease. Cushing syndrome, characterized by excess cortisol levels, refers to patients with the classic signs and symptoms described by Cushing, but the cause of the excess cortisol is not restricted to adrenocorticotropic hormone (ACTH)-secreting pituitary tumors.

Background

Cushing syndrome is estimated to affect 10 to 15 million people annually in the United States. The disease is more common in women than men and the median age at diagnosis is approximately 41 years (Lacroix, Feelders, Stratakis, & Nieman, 2015). Patients with active untreated Cushing syndrome have a mortality rate 1.7 to 4.8 times higher than the general population (Neiman et al., 2015). Most of the cases of Cushing syndrome are caused by the use of exogenous glucocorticoids, such as prednisone, used to treat other medical conditions. The majority of cases unrelated to steroid use are a result of ACTH-secreting pituitary adenomas. Less common causes of Cushing syndrome are adrenal tumors responsible for the excess release of cortisol, ectopic ACTH-secreting tumors associated with certain malignancies, and family history (Neiman et al., 2015).

Clinical manifestations of Cushing syndrome vary depending on the cause and duration of the excess cortisol levels. The typical manifestations of Cushing syndrome include central obesity with thin arms and legs, rounded or "moon" face, excess fat behind the neck and upper back, and weight gain (Quinn, 2016). Other manifestations include fatigue, mood swings, depression, increased thirst and urine output, amenorrhea, acanthosis on the neck, ruddy complexion, acne, thin skin that is easily bruised, hirsutism, and prominent purple striae on the abdomen, breasts, hips, and axilla (Urrets-Zavalía et al., 2016). On physical examination, patients with Cushing syndrome often have elevated blood pressure, muscle atrophy, and muscle weakness.

Diagnosis is based on the patient's history, presenting symptoms, laboratory tests, and imaging. No single laboratory test is specific for Cushing syndrome. The three laboratory tests recommended by the Endocrine Society are the 24-hour urine-free cortisol, late-night salivary cortisol, and the low-dose dexamethasone suppression test (Lacroix et al., 2016). The late-night salivary cortisol level is commonly used for initial screening and can be done at home by the patient at bedtime. Other tests to aid in diagnosis include midnight plasma cortisol levels, corticotropin-releasing hormone stimulation test, and a high-dose dexamethasone suppression test. Once the diagnosis of Cushing syndrome has been established, serum testing of morning ACTH levels is performed to differentiate between Cushing disease and ectopic ACTH syndrome. CT scans and/or MRI may be used to identify the location of the tumor causing the increased cortisol levels (Raff & Carroll, 2015).

Treatment for patients with Cushing syndrome depends on the etiology. Patients with Cushing syndrome related to steroid use who cannot be treated with other medications will generally have the dose reduced to diminish Cushing symptoms, but still treat their primary disease. There are several treatments for patients with ACTH-secreting pituitary tumors. The goal of surgical intervention for Cushing syndrome is removal of the tumor on the pituitary or adrenal gland. Endoscopic transsphenoidal surgery (microadenectomy or hypophysectomy) allows removal of the pituitary tumor without disrupting overall pituitary functioning (Neiman et al., 2015; Raff & Carroll, 2014). Many patients will eventually have normal HPA function, but pituitary function may be affected following extensive surgical resection. Patients who have had unsuccessful

surgeries or who are not surgical candidates may be treated with radiation (Neiman et al., 2015). Pituitary radiation is effective for only approximately 40% to 50% of patients; unfortunately it may take months to years for patients to report an improvement in their symptoms. Medications can be used alone or in conjunction with surgery and/or radiation to treat Cushing syndrome. Adrenal enzyme inhibitors used to control excess cortisol production include ketoconazole (Nizoral), mitotane (Lysodren), amnioglutethimide (Cytadren), and metyrapone (Metopirone; Neiman et al., 2015).

Clinical Aspects

ASSESSMENT

Excess cortisol levels can cause a wide variety of psychosocial and physiologic alterations. Patients with Cushing syndrome may have body-image issues related to skin changes, hirsutism, and weight gain. The nurse should assess patients for body-image disturbances and be able to provide resources and support and help patients develop effective coping mechanisms. It is important for the nurse to monitor for other cortisol-related adverse effects, such as depression, mood swings, diabetes, hypertension, hypokalemia, deep vein thrombosis, infection, and osteoporosis. Patients with adverse effects should be provided with education regarding management and treatment options, as well as referred to appropriate providers (Neiman et al., 2015). Extremely elevated cortisol levels impair immunity and increase the risk for opportunistic infections and sepsis. The nurse should provide education related to age-appropriate vaccines (influenza, pneumococcal, and herpes zoster) and administer as appropriate (Neiman et al., 2015).

OUTCOMES

The primary treatment for Cushing syndrome is surgical intervention. Major surgical complications following pituitary surgery include diabetes insipidus, venous thromboembolic events (VTEs), and infection. Postoperatively, the nurse must monitor the patient for signs of diabetes insipidus, including polyuria, polydipsia, dehydration, tachycardia, hypotension, hypernatremia, elevated serum osmolality, and decreased urine osmolality. As patients with Cushing syndrome are at an increased risk of infection, postoperative care should include a thorough surgical site assessment and careful monitoring of temperature and laboratory values for changes related to infection. There is a normal and expected decrease in ACTH levels following adrenalectomy, which will result in cortisol levels dropping below normal. It is important to monitor patients for signs of adrenal insufficiency such as hypoglycemia, hyponatremia, hyperkalemia, and hypotension. Patients who have had an adrenalectomy will need to take cortisol replacement therapy for a period after surgery to allow for recovery of the HPA axis. The nurse should ensure that the patient has a proper understanding of why and when to take the cortisol replacement to mimic normal physiological secretion (Neiman et al., 2015; Raff & Carroll, 2104).

Cushing syndrome can cause alterations in coagulation factors, putting patients at risk for VTE. Nurses should carefully monitor and assess patients for signs of deep vein thrombosis (DVT) and pulmonary embolism (PE). The nurse should also collaborate with other members of the health care team to ensure that the patient has appropriate perioperative mechanical and/or pharmacological DVT prophylaxis. Patients who have had surgery to treat Cushing syndrome are still at risk for thrombosis up to a year postoperatively. Patients should have education regarding the symptoms of DVT and PE and the importance of seeking emergency care if they occur.

Summary

Most cases of Cushing syndrome are caused by the use of exogenous steroids. Whatever the cause, treatment goals include maintaining normal serum cortisol levels, minimizing adverse effects of steroid use, and avoiding signs of adrenal insufficiency. Steroid replacement therapy may be indicated following surgical treatment of Cushing syndrome or following long-term glucocorticoid treatment until the HPA axis returns to normal. If exogenous steroid treatment is necessary, the dose should be tapered to the lowest effective dose for the shortest duration to achieve desired outcomes. If possible, systemic therapy should be avoided. If the patient's medical condition makes treatment with corticosteroids unavoidable, the use of steroid-sparing immunosuppressive agents may be helpful in minimizing adverse effects. Patients at risk for osteoporosis being treated with long-term glucocorticoid therapy should be evaluated for treatment with bisphosphonates. Patients should be taught how to recognize signs of adverse effects associated with glucocorticoid therapy,

including infection, VTE, osteoporosis, hyperglycemia, ulcers and gastrointestinal bleeding, and delayed wound healing.

Lacroix, A., Feelders, S., Stratakis, C. A., & Nieman, L. K. (2015). Cushing's syndrome. *Lancet*, *386*(9996), 913–927. doi:10.1016/50140-6736(14)61375-1

Neiman, L. S., Biller, B. M. K., Findling, J. W., Hassan Murad, M., Newell-Price, J., Savage, M. O., & Tabarin, A. (2015). Treatment of Cushing's syndrome: An Endocrine Society clinical practice guideline. *Journal of Clinical Endocrinology and Metabolism*, *100*(8), 2807–2831. doi:10.1210/jc.2015-1818

Quinn, L. (2016). The endocrine system. In H. Craven (Ed.), *Core curriculum for medical-surgical nursing* (5th ed., pp. 311–328). Pitman, NJ: Academy of Medical–Surgical Nurses.

Raff, H., & Carroll, T. (2015). Cushing's syndrome: From physiological principles to diagnosis and clinical care. *Journal of Physiology*, *593*(3), 493–506. doi:10.1113/jphysiol.2014.282871

Urrets-Zavalía, J. A., Espósito, E., Garay, I., Monti, R., Ruiz-Lascano, A., Correa, L., . . . Grzybowski, A. (2016). The eye and the skin in nonendocrine metabolic disorders. *Clinics in Dermatology*, *34*(2), 166–182. doi:10.1016/j.clindermatol.2015.12.002

■ DEEP VEIN THROMBOSIS

Kelly K. McConnell

Overview

Deep vein thrombosis (DVT) or venous thrombosis in the leg, pelvis, or upper extremity may result in a venous thromboembolic event (VTE). A DVT occurs when a thrombus or clot is formed and there is dysregulation of the fibrinolytic system that prevents the breakdown or reabsorbtion of a thrombosis within the lumen of a venous blood vessel. Consequently, DVTs can cause an obstruction of blood flow preventing the delivery of oxygen and vital nutrients to tissues, and results in ischemic tissue injury or necrosis. Nursing care of the adult with a DVT is focused on early detection and the implementation of appropriate nursing interventions to optimize outcomes and decrease further morbidity or life-threatening complications.

Background

According to the Centers for Disease Control and Prevention (CDC), the exact number of people affected by VTE disease, including DVT, is unknown. As many as 900,000 Americans annually are likely to be affected by VTE disease; it is estimated that nearly two thirds of these adults have a detectable DVT (CDC, 2015). For adults who develop DVTs, the risk of recurrence is approximately 7% despite pharmacotherapy (McNamara, 2017). Venous thromboses are highly morbid, the 1-month mortality rate is as high as 6% for DVTs although postmortem studies suggest that this rate is likely to be significantly underestimated (Behravesh et al., 2017). In addition to the risk for acute mortality and, despite timely initiation of pharmacotherapy, DVT complications can lead to persistent chronic disease caused by impaired venous return, known as *postthrombotic syndrome (PTS)*. Among those who have had a DVT, one half will have long-term complications, such as swelling, pain, discoloration, and scaling, in the affected limb after an acute DVT (CDC, 2015).

The Agency for Healthcare Research and Quality (AHRQ) suggests that DVT is one of the most common preventable causes of hospital deaths (AHRQ, 2016). The total estimated costs in the United States associated with VTE is between $13.5 and $69.5 billion, including an estimated cost of $10,000 to treat DVT plus any additional nonmedical expenses (AHRQ, 2016).

A DVT can occur when a vein's inner lining is damaged by physical, chemical, or biological factors. DVTs are primary located in the deep veins of the lower extremities but can also appear in the pelvis and upper extremities. Risk factors for DVT include a history of endothelial damage/dysfunction, venous stasis, and hypercoagulable states also known as *Virchow's triad*. Venous stasis can be caused by immobilization, including individuals on bedrest or who have recently been traveling for a long period of time or individuals with polycythemia, which can lead to endothelial injury. Endothelial damage/dysfunction causes include a history of smoking, hypertension, serious injuries or major trauma or surgery within the past 4 weeks, inflammation, and immune responses. Hypercoagulable causes of DVT include active malignancy (treatment within previous 6 months or palliative therapy), splenectomy, sickle cell disease, previous proven venous thromboembolism, reduced cardiac output (congestive heart failure), obesity, advanced age (older than 60 years old although DVTs can occur in any age), pregnancy and 6 weeks after childbirth, hormone replacement therapy and oral contraceptives, chronic obstructive pulmonary disease (COPD), chronic inflammatory disease of the digestive tract, varicose veins, and indwelling catheters and electrodes in great veins and right heart (CDC, 2015; National Institutes of Health [NIH], 2011). Approximately 5% to 8% of the U.S. population has one of several genetic risk factors, known as *inherited thrombophilias*, which increase the risk for thrombosis (CDC, 2015). Inherited diseases include factor V Leiden-acquired thrombotic disorder, antiphospholipid antibodies, heparin-induced thrombocytopenia, and thrombocytosis (NIH, 2011). There is also supporting evidence confirming that individuals with HIV have a higher incidence of clinically detected thromboembolic disease (NIH, 2011).

Clinical Aspects

ASSESSMENT

Nursing care of the patient with suspected DVT includes a review of the individual's history, physical assessment findings, laboratory and diagnostic findings. When obtaining a health history, risk factors leading to abnormal clotting should be identified and documented. When assessing an individual for DVT, it is important to understand that approximately only half of people show signs and symptoms. The signs and symptoms for DVT include unilateral pain or tenderness in the leg, which may be felt only when standing or walking, swelling to the extremity, warmth in the area that is swollen or painful, and redness or discoloration of the extremity (CDC, 2015). When symptoms develop slowly and without "classic" clinical symptoms for DVT, conducting a thorough physical assessment should be done in conjunction with laboratory and diagnostic tests to diagnose DVT in an effort to prescribe interventions that reduce the risk for VTE-associated morbidity and mortality.

In addition to physical assessment findings, there are several diagnostic and laboratory tests that can be used to confirm the diagnosis of DVT. The most common test for diagnosing DVT is ultrasound. If an ultrasound does not provide a clear diagnosis, a venography may be ordered. Other tests used to diagnose DVT include MRI and CT scanning. Laboratory tests may be recommended to help diagnose DVT. The D-dimer test measures a substance in the blood that is released when a blood clot dissolves. If there are high levels of the substance, a blot clot may be present but if the results are normal and there are few risk factors, DVT is unlikely (CDC, 2015). Additional blood tests may also be ordered for individuals at risk for an inherited blood clotting disorder, including those with reoccurring blood clots with unknown etiology or when blood clots are found in unusual locations (such as the liver, kidney, or brain) suggesting an inherited clotting disorder (NIH, 2011).

NURSING INTERVENTIONS, MANAGEMENT, AND IMPLICATIONS

DVT can be treated with systemic and endovascular approaches in an effort to improve the 5% all-cause mortality within 1 year attributed to VTE (Behravesh et al., 2017). Anticoagulants, including unfractionated heparin, low-molecular-weight heparin, and factor X_a inhibitors can be used to treat DVT. The duration of anticoagulant therapy is generally 6 months, but can vary depending on the individual patient.

Thrombin inhibitors may be used for patients unable to tolerate treatment with heparin. The use of thrombolytics is restricted to life-threatening or emergent situations due to their high risk for bleeding.

In addition to medications there are other treatments to prevent further complications from DVT, including a vena cava filter, thrombolysis, and compression stockings or intermittent pneumatic compression devices (IPCDs). A vena cava filter is inserted inside the vena cava and catches blood clots before they travel to the lungs, preventing a pulmonary embolism, but does not stop new blood clots from forming. Thrombolysis may be performed in severe cases of DVT when there is a risk for loss of limb. Compression stockings and IPCDs are used to reduce venous stasis and improve venous return from the lower extremities. Contraindications should be considered when implementing mechanical DVT interventions, including conditions that affect the lower extremities, conditions that compromise lower extremity blood flow, severe congestive heart failure, thigh circumference that exceeds the limit of the instructions, and sensitivity to latex (McNamara, 2017).

Nursing care of the patient with DVT should primarily focus on the prevention of worsening the condition and education related to controllable risk factors and prescribed pharmacotherapy management, including safe practices and the risk for bleeding.

Nursing interventions for individuals with DVT include minimizing positions that compromise blood flow; immobilizing limb and initiating bed rest to reduce risk of clot mobilization, elevating limb maintaining slight flexion while in bed; applying graduated compression stockings or IPCDs per protocol; assisting with progressive ambulation when allowed; applying a warm, moist compress as scheduled; assessing and reporting worsening signs or symptoms of DVT; administering analgesics as prescribed for pain and evaluating effectiveness; administering oxygen as ordered to maintain tissue perfusion; administering anticoagulants and thrombin inhibitors as ordered to reduce the risk of additional clotting; and monitoring laboratory values, including prothrombin time (PT)/international normalized ratio (INR) to assess warfarin (Coumadin) and activated partial thromboplastin time (aPTT) to assess heparin effectiveness and dosage.

Care of an individual with DVT includes checking for signs of complications, including pulmonary embolism, decreased tissue perfusion, and excessive bleeding, which can be life-threatening. Signs and symptoms of bleeding include obvious signs of bleeding (bruising, petechiae, petechial hemorrhaging in the sclera, hematuria, epitasis, blood in stool or oral cavity). Nurses should ensure good hydration to prevent increased blood viscosity; provide education pertinent to anticoagulation therapy, including dietary restrictions such as vitamin K-rich foods when taking warfarin (Coumadin) and there is risk for bleeding. For individuals of childbearing age, the nurse should discuss contraception choices as oral contraceptive therapy can increase the risk for DVT.

OUTCOMES

Individual outcomes are dependent on the management of DVT. The goals for DVT therapy include stopping blood clots from enlarging, preventing blood clots from becoming an embolism to the lung, and reducing the recurrence of future blood clots. In addition to goals of therapy, individuals should be monitored for common side effects, such as bleeding, from pharmacotherapy to treat DVT. Individuals undergoing DVT treatment are usually initially hospitalized and then monitored closely at home by having regular blood tests measuring coagulability and effectiveness of pharmacotherapy.

Summary

DVT can lead to worsening morbidity and mortality rates in individuals who go untreated. Early detection and management are vital to the outcomes for individuals with DVT. Nurses play a pivotal role in assessing, monitoring, and providing care for patients with DVT. Implementing appropriate nursing interventions can reduce the additional risks associated with DVT. Utilizing evidence-based nursing practice standards and recommended pharmacologic and nonpharmacologic measures when caring for individuals with DVT can promote better outcomes and decrease worsening morbidity and mortality rates.

Agency for Healthcare Research and Quality. (2016). *Executive summary: Preventing hospital acquired venous thromboembolism: A guide for effective quality improvement.* Rockville, MD: Author. Retrieved from https://www.ahrq.gov/professionals/quality-patient-safety/patient-safety-resources/resources/vtguide/vtguidesum.html

Behravesh, S., Hoang, P., Nanda, A., Wallace, A., Sheth, R. A., Deipolyi, A. R., . . . Oklu, R. (2017). Pathogenesis of thromboembolism and endovascular management. *Thrombosis, 3039713*, 1–13. doi:10.1155/2017/3039713

Centers for Disease Control and Prevention. (2015). Venous thromboembolism (blood clots). Retrieved from https://www.cdc.gov/ncbddd/dvt/data.html

McNamara, S. A. (2014). Patient safety first: Prevention of venous thromboembolism. *AORN Journal, 99*(5), 642–647. doi:10.1016/j.aorn.2014.02.001

National Institutes of Health. (2011). What is deep vein thrombosis? Retrieved from https://www.nhlbi.nih.gov/health/health-topics/topics/dvt

■ DIABETES INSIPIDUS

Danielle M. Diemer

Overview

Diabetes insipidus (DI), not to be mistaken with diabetes mellitus, is a rare disorder that can be debilitating. A hormone called *antidiuretic hormone (ADH)*, also referred to as *vasopressin*, helps regulate the kidneys' fluid balance of water and sodium. In DI, there is a deficiency, or lack of ADH. Large amounts of diluted and odorless urine are excreted and patients experience increased thirst (National Institute of Diabetes and Digestive and Kidney Disease [NIDDK], 2015). Nursing care for individuals with DI focuses on early recognition of intake and output to deliver appropriate nursing care and education to both the patients and their families.

Background

In the United States, three in 100,000 individuals are affected by DI. Most of the cases of DI develop in childhood or early adulthood (Cumulative Index to Nursing and Allied Health Literature [CINAHL], 2016).

There are four different types of DI. Neurogenic and nephrogenic are the most common types. Neurogenic DI (also known as *central DI*) is caused by a lack of ADH. This occurs when there is damage to the hypothalamus or pituitary gland or in some cases an inherited defected gene. Nephrogenic DI is caused by the kidneys' inability to respond to ADH. Certain medications, chronic kidney disease, or inherited gene changes can cause this type of DI (National Institute of Health [NIH], 2016). The other two less common forms of DI are dipsogenic and gestational. In dipsogenic DI (also known as *primary polydipsia*), individuals experience excess thirst resulting in increased fluid intake from a problem with the thirst mechanism. This form of DI is often associated with psychiatric disorders (Sanjay et al., 2016). Gestational DI can occur during pregnancy, usually in the third trimester. The abnormality is that the placenta prohibits the mother's ADH from working properly (Tritos, 2013).

There are several factors that contribute to an individual's risk for developing DI. Medications that interfere with the kidneys' reabsorption of water can place an individual at risk. Also adrenal insufficiency, sickle cell anemia, Langerhans cell histiocytosis, genetic problems, polycystic kidney disease, and increased levels of calcium in the blood place individuals at risk for DI (CINAHL Information Systems, 2016).

The most significant complication of DI is dehydration. If the DI is not treated and becomes severe, seizures, permanent brain damage, or death can occur (NIDDK, 2015). Other complications include mental status changes, fatigue, lethargy, tachycardia, hypotension, fever, headaches, decreased body temperature, hypernatremia, and hypokalemia (CINAHL Information Systems, 2016). Immediate medical attention is needed in individuals experiencing dizziness, confusion, or sluggishness (NIDDK, 2015).

Treatment is aimed at determining the underlying cause or the type of DI. This initial treatment and management may require hospitalization. Once treated, there are usually no severe problems or issues with early death (NIH, 2016).

Clinical Aspects

ASSESSMENT

It is important for nurses to obtain a thorough medical and family history. The documentation of the individual's physical assessment and laboratory data are also important. During the history, it is important for the nurse to ask what home medications the patient is taking. Lithium is an example of a medication to be aware of that can cause DI. Other questions to ask the individuals are whether they are experiencing symptoms of polydipsia, polyuria, or nocturia. Inquiring about a family history of DI is also an important question for the nurse to ask (NIH, 2016).

During the physical assessment, the nurse should focus on looking for signs of dehydration (NIDDK, 2015). Other assessment findings of DI include increased urine output (regardless of intake), water cravings, and possibly fevers (CINAHL Information Systems, 2016). Laboratory tests that can be ordered include urinalysis; 24-hour urine, serum and urine osmolality/osmolality; and fluid deprivation test. A CT scan or MRI could also be ordered (CINAHL Information Systems, 2016).

NURSING INTERVENTIONS, MANAGEMENT, AND IMPLICATIONS

Nursing care of an individual with DI should focus on preventing severe hydration. Some nursing-related problems include fluid volume deficit, sleep disturbances, activity intolerance/fatigue, anxiety, and patient/family knowledge deficit (Vera, 2012).

OUTCOMES

The expected outcomes of evidence-based nursing care focus on keeping the symptoms under control and preventing dehydration from progressing to severe dehydration. Nursing monitoring of intake/output is a key element to determine the reduction of progression of the disorder during treatment.

Summary

Individuals diagnosed with DI may initially need to be hospitalized. A thorough medical/family history and assessment can help with the early diagnosis of DI. Once the type of DI is determined, then treatment will help with preventing any long-term complications.

CINAHL Information Systems. (2016). *Quick lessons: Diabetes insipidus*. Glendale, CA: Author.

National Institute of Diabetes and Digestive and Kidney Disease. (2015). *Diabetes insipidus*. Washington DC: U.S. Department of Health and Human Services. Retrieved from http://www.niddk.nih.gov/health-information/health -topics/kidney-disease/diabetes-insipidus/pages/facts.aspx

National Institutes of Health. (2016). Diabetes insipidus. Retrieved from https://medlineplus.gov/ency/article/ 000377.htm

Sanjay, K., Abdual Hamid, Z., Sunil, M. J., Bipid, S., Subhanker, C., Awadhesh Kumar, S., . . . Harshad, M. (2016). Diabetes insipidus. *Indian Journal of Endocrinology and Metabolism, 20*(1), 9–21. doi:10.4103/2230-8210.172273

Tritos, N. (2013, July). Diabetes insipidus. In A. Klibanski & J. Schlechte (Eds.), *Fact sheet: Diabetes insipidus* (pp. 1–2). Retrieved from http://www.hormone.org/ questions-and-answers/2013/diabetes-insipidus

Vera, M. (2012). 3 Diabetes insipidus nursing care plans. Retrieved from http://nurselabs.com/diabetes-insipidus -nursing-care-plans

■ DIABETES MELLITUS

Mary Beth Modic

Overview

Diabetes mellitus (DM) is a serious, complex, and progressive disease. DM refers to a group of metabolic diseases in which the pancreas does not produce insulin or the body cannot effectively use the insulin that is made. This results in high blood glucose levels that are strongly associated with macrovascular complications (e.g., coronary heart disease, peripheral vascular disease, cerebrovascular) and microvascular complications (e.g., retinopathy, nephropathy, and neuropathy).

There are several different types of DM, most notably type 1, type 2, and gestational (American Diabetes Association, 2016a). Type 1 DM (T1DM) occurs when the beta cells of the pancreas are compromised by autoimmune insults. Individuals with T1DM do not have functional beta cells that produce insulin, resulting in their need for exogenous replacement of insulin. Type 2 DM (T2DM) occurs when the body becomes resistant to insulin due to the metabolic alterations that occur with obesity. Similar to individuals with T1DM, the beta cells of individuals with T2DM or heightened states of insulin, resistance eventually lose their secretory function, and exogenous insulin supplementation is required. By the time a person is diagnosed with T2DM, it is estimated that there is a 50% decline in beta cell function (Petznick, 2011). There are other types of DM that occur as a result of pregnancy, malnutrition, genetic disorders, surgery, and medications. However, these other subtypes of DM occur in 1% to 5% of the population.

Therefore, this entry focuses on the nursing care for individuals with T1DM and T2DM. Although all

DM care should be customized to the individual and context, nursing care for patients with DM is typically directed at normalizing blood glucose, promoting effective self-management practices, and assisting them to live a normal life (Schreiner, 2016).

Background

DM affects 23.6 million Americans and 422 million people worldwide, with 5% of those diagnosed with T1DM and 90% with T2DM (Centers for Disease Control and Prevention [CDC], 2014). The cost of diabetes in the United States is estimated at $245 billion—$176 billion attributed to medical expenditures and $69 billion to lost work and wages (CDC, 2014). African Americans, Hispanics, and Native Americans are at greater risk of developing T2DM than Caucasians. Complications of diabetes include heart disease, dyslipidemia, stroke, renal failure, blindness, and amputations. Diabetes is the seventh leading cause of death but is often underreported on death certificates (CDC, 2014). Diabetes is a significant public health concern as Americans grow older, consume more calorically dense foods, become more sedentary, and obese.

There are three laboratory studies that are used to diagnose diabetes. A fasting blood glucose of 126 mg/dL (7 mmol/L) or greater on two separate occasions constitutes a diagnosis of diabetes, blood glucose values between 100 and 125 mg/dL identify a person with prediabetes, and a test result less than 100 mg/dL is normal. A second diagnostic test is an oral glucose tolerance test (OGTT) that requires the individual to fast for 8 hours and drink 75 g of glucose. The individual's blood is drawn at 1 hour and 2 hours postingestion of the glucose. A glucose value of 200 mg/dL or greater at the 2-hour interval results in a diagnosis of diabetes. A glycated hemoglobin test also known as *A1c* measures the average glucose value in the blood for the previous 2 to 3 months. A test result of greater than 6.5%, which is equivalent to a glucose value of 140 mg/dL, also provides a diagnosis of diabetes (American Diabetes Association, 2016b).

Clinical Aspects

ASSESSMENT

A diagnosis of DM may be acute, in the case of T1DM, when a child is brought to the health care provider because of polyuria (excessive urination), polydipsia (excessive thirst), polyphagia (excessive hunger), and weight loss. Parents or caregivers have noted very wet diapers, excessive trips to the bathroom as well as extreme thirst, hunger and weight loss in their child. In the case of T2DM, many of the complications associated with diabetes are already present when a diagnosis of diabetes is rendered.

In addition to gathering an accurate past medical history of the person's type and duration of DM and performing a physical assessment, it is essential that the individual's perception of success in performing daily diabetes self-care activities be explored. Physical activity, dietary practices, frequency of blood glucose monitoring, medication adherence, presence and degree of stress, and sleep patterns should be examined (Meece, 2015). Frequency and severity of hypoglycemic events, if the individual is prescribed insulin, should be reviewed as persons with T1DM typically experience two symptomatic hypoglycemic events a week and one severe episode per year (Hanefield, Duetting, & Bramlage, 2013).

NURSING INTERVENTIONS, MANAGEMENT, AND IMPLICATIONS

Nursing care of the adult with DM is directed at normalizing blood glucose levels, preventing hypoglycemia and hyperglycemia crises, and assessing the individual's ability to safely manage his or her diabetes.

Individuals with DM may present to the emergency department in hyperglycemic crisis. There are two conditions that warrant hospitalization: Diabetic ketoacidosis (DKA) and hyperglycemic hyperosmolar syndrome (HHS). DKA is most common in individuals with T1DM and is a state of absolute insulin deficiency. Dehydration, accumulation of ketone bodies, and metabolic abnormalities are also present in DKA. When the body does not have enough insulin to get glucose into the cells, the cells use fat to provide fuel. The breakdown of fat produces fatty acids and ketones that build up in the bloodstream. The individual will present with complaints of nausea, polyuria, polydipsia, weakness, and fatigue. The kidneys work to get rid of the ketones and the glucose, which leads to ketonuria (ketone bodies in the urine) and glycosuria (glucose in the urine). Laboratory results that indicate severe DKA include glucose (greater than 250 mg/dL), pH (greater than 7.00), bicarbonate (greater than 18 mEq/L), anion gap (greater than 12), and presence of serum and urine ketones. The anion gap is a calculated laboratory value that identifies the cause of metabolic acidosis. Treatment for DKA includes fluid resuscitation, insulin therapy, correction of other metabolic derangements, and investigation of the precipitating cause.

HHS is a condition in which a person, often elderly with T2DM, presents with significant hyperglycemia, hyperosmolality, and dehydration. (Pasquel & Umpierrez, 2014). Laboratory results that indicate HHS include glucose (greater than 600 mg/dL), serum osmolality (320 mOsm/kg), pH (greater than 7.30), bicarbonate (greater than 15 mEq/L), anion gap (variable), and small amounts of serum and urine ketones. Treatment is focused on fluid replacement, and normalizing glucose, osmolality, and electrolytes. Underlying infections are the primary precipitators of HHS with 40% to 60% being caused by pneumonia and 5% to 16% produced by urinary tract infections (Pasquel & Umpierrez, 2014).

Hypoglycemia can be a life-threatening event. It results from too little food, too much exercise, alcohol consumption, an unusual eating pattern, or too much insulin. The glucose threshold alert value for hypoglycemia is 70 mg/dL and a clinically significant hypoglycemic event is defined at 54 mg/dL (American Diabetes Association, 2016b). The severity of the event is not determined by the glucose value, but rather by the severity of the symptoms. As the glucose begins to drop, individuals begin to feel anxious, irritable, and tachycardiac. In response to hypoglycemia, glucagon, a counter-regulatory hormone is released. If the hypoglycemic event is not attended too quickly, the glucose will continue to drop and the individual can lose consciousness, seize, become comatose, and die as a result of glucose deprivation to the brain.

Depression is a common comorbid condition in individuals with diabetes, affecting 15% to 20% of people with diabetes overall (Friis, Consedine & Johnson, 2015). Individuals who suffer with depression have greater difficulty in following their prescribed medical regimen. Feelings of fatigue, lack of appetite, and feelings of hopelessness can impede a person's ability to perform the requisite self-management practices that must be performed daily to achieve metabolic control.

Priority nursing interventions for the patient with diabetes include monitoring of blood glucose, preventing glucose excursions (hyper and hypoglycemia), coordinating insulin administration with blood glucose monitoring and meal consumption, trending and interpreting glucose results, and supporting the individual in successful diabetes self-care practices.

OUTCOMES

The expected outcomes of evidence-based nursing care are directed at optimizing glucose control. Effective diabetes management requires that the individual living with diabetes is recognized as the expert on his or her life. Nurses and other health care team members need to be vigilant to the daily obstacles that can impede a person's ability to eat healthfully, be physically active, take diabetes medication as prescribed, monitor blood glucose correctly, interpret glucose results accurately, and seek out medical attention appropriately. Referrals to outpatient diabetes self-management education (DSME) programs, medical nutrition therapy, social work, and case management are warranted when a person with diabetes is noted to be struggling to follow the self-care practices that have been recommended and prescribed.

Summary

A diagnosis of DM is life-altering. The self-management of DM requires vigilance and significant behavioral self-regulation to follow the prescribed regimen. Nurses have an integral role in educating, supporting, and affirming these individuals to prevent complications and assist them to flourish in living with diabetes.

American Diabetes Association. (2016a). Classification and diagnosis of diabetes: Section 2. *Diabetes Care, 40*(Suppl. 1), S11–S24. doi:10.2337/dc17-S005

American Diabetes Association. (2016b). Classification and diagnosis of diabetes: Section 6. *Diabetes Care, 40*(Suppl. 1), S48–S56. doi:10.2337/dc17-S009

Centers for Disease Control and Prevention. (2014). *National diabetes statistics report: Estimates of diabetes and its burden in the United States*. Atlanta, GA: U.S. Department of Health and Human Services. Retrieved from https://stacks.cdc.gov/view/cdc/23442

Friis, A., Consedine, N., & Johnson, M. (2015). Does kindness matter? Diabetes, depression, and self-compassion: A selective review and research agenda. *Diabetes Spectrum, 29*(4), 252–257. doi:10:1111/codi.12781

Hanefield, M., Duetting, E., & Bramlage, P. (2013). Cardiac implications of hypoglycemia in patients with diabetes—A systematic review. *Cardiovascular Diabetology, 135*(12), 1–11. doi:10.1186/1475-2480-12-135

Meece, J. (2015). Improving adherence through better conversation. *AADE in Practice, 3*(4), 52–57. doi:10.1177/2325160316639021

Pasquel, F., & Umpierrez, G. (2014). Hyperosmolar hyperglycemic state: A historic review of the clinical presentation, diagnosis and treatment. *Diabetes Care, 37*(11), 3124–3131. doi:10.2337/dc14-0984

Petznick, A. (2011). Insulin management of type 2 diabetes mellitus. *American Family Physician, 84*(2), 183–190.

Schreiner, B. (2016). Teaching across the life span. *AADE in Practice*, 2(4), 28–31. doi.10.1177/2325160315624888

■ DIVERTICULAR DISEASE

Rhoda Redulla

Overview

Diverticular disease is a very common gastrointestinal (GI) disorder that can lead to hospitalization; diverticular bleeding is the most common cause of GI bleeding (Mosadeghi, Bhuket, & Stollman, 2016). Diverticular disease is also the most common finding during colonoscopy (Mosadeghi et al., 2016). Diverticular disease includes diverticulosis and diverticulitis. Diverticula are outpouchings or herniations of the mucosa in the wall of the large intestine. Diverticulitis is inflammation of diverticula and diverticulosis is the presence of noninflamed diverticula. The clinical course of diverticular disease is varied. Many patients have asymptomatic diverticular disease, others may experience acute complications, such as GI bleeding, fistulae formation, or perforation, whereas others may have chronic diverticular disease.

Background

Diverticular disease is a common and increasing problem in developed countries such as the United States, Australia, United Kingdom, and France. Age is a strong risk factor; the prevalence increases with age. Over 50% of adults older than 70 years have diverticula and 80% remain asymptomatic; an estimated 20% of patients with diverticulosis will eventually develop diverticulitis (Strate, 2014). Men and women are equally affected. Diverticular disease accounts for approximately 814,000 hospitalizations per year in the United States and an estimated 2.7 million outpatient visits (Feuerstein & Falchuk, 2016).

Lifestyle factors have long been associated with diverticular disease. Diets low in fiber and lack of fecal bulk were thought to be major contributing factors to the disease, especially in Western countries. However, there is conflicting evidence that a high-fiber diet and frequent bowel movements result in a higher incidence of diverticular disease (Mosadeghi et al., 2016). Low dietary fiber is thought to increase colonic transit time and decrease the volume of stool, which in turn increases intraluminal pressure in the colon. Other theories attribute the formation of diverticula to changes in collagen synthesis in the bowel wall, abnormal colonic motility, and dysfunction of colonic neurotransmitters (Mosadeghi et al., 2015). Alterations in connective tissue, known as *collaginosis* or *herniosos*, are thought to be responsible for Saint's triad, which includes hiatal hernia, diverticulosis, and cholelithiasis. Chronic, low-grade inflammation is thought to play a role in patients with mild symptoms (symptomatic uncomplicated diverticular disease [SUDD]; Mosadeghi et al., 2016). Other factors contributing to diverticular disease include lack or decrease in physical activity, genetics, poor bowel habits (ignoring or suppressing the urge to have a bowel movement), obesity, aspirin, use nonsteroidal anti-inflammatory drug (NSAID) use, steroid use, alcohol consumption, diets high in red meat, and the effects of aging (Feuerstein & Falchuk, 2016; Mosadeghi et al., 2016).

Diverticula form when increased pressure within the lumen of the large intestine causes bowel mucosa to form pouches through defects in the colon wall. Meckel's diverticulum or true diverticula penetrate through all layers of the bowel wall, in contrast, pseudodiverticula only involve the mucosa and submucosal layers. The circular and longitudinal muscles often thicken or hypertrophy in the area affected by diverticula. This narrows the bowel lumen, increasing intraluminal pressure. Contraction of the muscles in response to normal stimuli, such as meals, may occlude the narrowed lumen, further increasing intraluminal pressure. Although diverticula can occur anywhere in the GI tract, they are commonly found in the sigmoid colon, which has the highest intraluminal pressure in the bowel (Morris, Regenbogen, Hardiman, & Hendren, 2014). The high pressure causes mucosa to herniate through the muscle wall, forming a diverticulum. Areas where nutrient blood vessels penetrate the circular muscle layer are the most common sites for diverticula formation. Bleeding can occur from a rupture in any of the vessels lining a diverticulum. The severity of bleeding ranges from mild rectal bleeding to hemorrhage, hypotension, and impending shock. Most episodes of bleeding are self-limiting but endoscopic evaluation may be warranted for evaluation and treatment (Strate, 2016).

The etiology of diverticulitis is not completely understood. Feces or undigested food may collect in the outpouchings causing obstruction, distention, and decreased blood supply. An overgrowth of colonic bacteria may result in inflammation, localized necrosis of the bowel wall, and microperforation. Diverticulitis can range from mild to severe; larger perforations may lead to abscess or fistula formation and peritonitis.

Clinical Aspects

ASSESSMENT

More than two thirds of patients with diverticular disease are asymptomatic. Symptoms depend on the location, severity of disease, and presence of inflammation and complications. The most common clinical finding is cramping left lower quadrant abdominal pain; other symptoms include constipation, diarrhea, bloating, and painless rectal bleeding (Thompson, 2016). Weakness and fatigue may also develop as the disease progresses. The clinical presentation of diverticulitis ranges from no signs of infection to acute peritonitis. Depending on the location and severity of the inflammation, other symptoms, such as nausea, vomiting, and a low-grade fever, may occur. The abdomen should be inspected for masses, distention, and tenderness. The older adult may only report vague abdominal pain. Diagnosis is made by history and physical examination. Diagnostic testing includes hemoglobin and hematocrit, white blood cell count, stool for occult blood, and abdominal x-rays to identify perforation. Upper GI series or barium enema can be used to locate diverticula, but should not be performed during periods of acute inflammation.

During assessment, the nurse obtains a health history focusing on the onset and duration of pain, dietary habits, bowel patterns, presence of rectal bleeding, usual activity level, and presence of other risk factors. For recurrent episodes, the diagnosis is usually determined with a focused history and physical examination by the health care provider (Strate, Peery, & Neumann, 2015).

NURSING INTERVENTIONS, MANAGEMENT, AND IMPLICATIONS

Applicable nursing diagnoses for the patient with diverticulitis include acute pain, altered bowel elimination pattern, and deficient knowledge. Nursing interventions are specific to presenting symptoms and decrease the risk of the potential complications of perforation, bleeding, and peritonitis. Interventions for pain management include administration of opioid analgesics to manage severe pain. The nurse should monitor the patient for signs of infection, including assessing the temperature every 4 hours; fever more than 38.3°C (101°F) may indicate increased inflammation or spread

of inflammation. The older adult may present with only a slight temperature elevation or change in mental status. The nurse also monitors the patient's vital signs, observing for signs of bleeding and fluid volume deficit. Monitoring the patient's fluid volume status is particularly important for patients presenting with diarrhea. Bowel rest is usually indicated, especially for the patient with acute diverticulitis. The patient should be monitored for fluid and electrolyte imbalances; IV fluid and electrolyte replacement may be indicated. Other nursing interventions include performing a complete abdominal assessment, monitoring for distention and tenderness every 4 to 8 hours or more often as indicated. Significant changes, based on an ongoing assessment, should be promptly reported to the provider.

Evidence on dietary modification, particularly a high-fiber diet to reduce the risk of complications, remains undefined (Stollman, Smalley, & Hirano, 2015). Known benefits have been inconsistent. A stool softener may be prescribed but laxatives are not indicated for the patient with diverticular disease. During acute exacerbations, laxatives and enemas are contraindicated due to their effects on intestinal motility.

OUTCOMES

A priority nursing intervention is to provide patient education on the disease process, prevention of complications, dietary modifications, and treatment regimen. The expected outcome for the patient with acute diverticulitis is to remain free from complications, including abscess formation, fistula, bowel perforation, peritonitis, and hemorrhage. The patient should also be able to verbalize knowledge of strategies to prevent further episodes of acute disease and complications.

Individuals who are overweight or obese are at increased risk for developing diverticular disease. Smoking may also increase the risk of developing the condition. Patient education therefore includes the importance of maintaining a normal weight and avoidance or cessation of smoking (Strate et al., 2015).

No evidence exists to support avoiding intake of nuts and seeds to reduce the risk for diverticulitis in patients with known diverticulosis. Intake of nuts, corn, popcorn, and berries is not associated with increased risk for diverticular disease. Risk reduction strategies include limiting intake of red meat, maintaining a regular exercise pattern, avoiding the use of NSAIDs, and avoiding activities that increase intra-abdominal pressure (Strate et al., 2015).

Patients with mild symptoms are usually managed on an ambulatory basis. Medical treatment for acute diverticulitis includes oral (metronidazole and ciprofloxacin or trimethoprim-sulfamethoxazole) or intravenous antibiotics and diet modification. Indications for hospitalization include the presence of complications (bleeding, fistula formation, peritonitis, dehydration), the inability to tolerate oral fluids, fever, persistent abdominal pain, the presence of significant comorbidities, or lack of adequate support at home. Management strategies include pain management and bowel rest. Intravenous antibiotics have routinely been administered to patients admitted with acute uncomplicated diverticulitis. The most recent guidelines recommend the selective, rather than routine use of IV antibiotics (Peery & Stollman, 2015; Stollman et al., 2015). This recommended change in practice is based on results indicating no significant difference in the time to resolution of symptoms, complications, duration of hospital stay, and risk of recurrence between patients treated with intravenous (IV) antibiotics versus those treated with IV fluids alone (Peery & Stollman, 2015). There is growing inclination to withhold antibiotics when there is no risk for complicated disease (Johnson, 2016; Peery & Stollman, 2015; Stollman et al., 2015).

Surgical resection of the diseased segment of colon is often indicated if there is no clinical improvement within 48 hours despite supportive therapy. Emergency surgery may be indicated for patients with bowel obstruction, perforation, fistula, abscess, or peritonitis. A colon resection is the most commonly performed procedure; a temporary or permanent colostomy may be necessary (Peery & Neumann, 2015). An evolving discussion related to surgical approach in recurrent diverticulitis is elective surgery. However, there is insufficient evidence to support the benefits of elective surgery as a treatment for diverticular disease (Stollman et al., 2015). If creation of an ostomy is a possibility, a consult with a wound, ostomy, and continence (WOCN) nurse should be initiated.

Summary

Diverticular disease has become increasingly common in recent years. Etiologic theories and the approach to treatment has also significantly evolved (Regenbogen, Hardiman, Hendren, & Morris, 2014).

Emerging evidence does not support the theory of a low-fiber diet as a major causative factor in the etiology of diverticular disease. A high-fiber diet has recently been linked to an increased risk of diverticulitis. More research is indicated before a change in practice occurs. Because of the evidence supporting the role of chronic low-grade inflammation in the etiology of diverticular disease, more research is needed to evaluate the effectiveness of mesalamine for symptom relief and prevention of diverticulitis (Mosadeghi et al., 2015). The benefit of probiotics has not been demonstrated, but they may be prescribed (Feuerstein & Falchuk, 2016). Nursing management includes supportive measures based on presenting symptoms and patient education to prevent recurrent episodes. Some cases of uncomplicated diverticulitis may not require antibiotics. However, in severe diverticulitis, hospitalization is required. Recurrent disease may also prompt the need for surgery.

Feuerstein, J. D., & Falchuk, K. R. (2016). Diverticulosis and diverticulitis. *Mayo Clinic Proceedings, 91*(8), 1094–1104. doi:10.1016/j.mayocp.2016.03.012

Johnson, D. (2016). New guidelines on acute diverticulitis: How will they change clinical practice? *Medscape.* Retrieved from http://www.medscape.com/viewarticle/857275

Morris, A. M., Regenbogen, S. E., Hardiman, K. M., & Hendren, S. (2014). Sigmoid diverticulitis: A systematic review. *Journal of the American Medical Association, 311*(3), 287–297. doi:10.1001/jama.2013.282025

Mosadeghi, S., Bhuket, T., & Stollman, N. (2015). Diverticular disease: Evolving concepts in classification, presentation, and management. *Current Opinion in Gastroenterology, 31*(1), 50–55. doi:10.1097/MOG.0000000000000145

Peery, A. F., & Stollman, N. (2015). Antibiotics for acute uncomplicated diverticulitis: Time for a paradigm change? *Gastroenterology, 149*(7), 1650–1651. doi:10.1053/j.gastro.2015.10.022

Regenbogen, S. E., Hardiman, K. M., Hendren, S., & Morris, A. M. (2014). Surgery for diverticulitis in the 21st century: A systematic review. *JAMA Surgery, 149*(3), 292–303. doi:10.1001/jamasurg.2013.5477

Stollman, N., Smalley, W., & Hirano, I. (2015). American gastroenterological association institute guideline on the management of acute diverticulitis. *Gastroenterology, 149*(7), 1944–1949. doi:10.1053/j.gastro.2015.10.003

Strate, L. L. (2014). Diverticular disease. National Institute of Diabetes and Digestive and Kidney Diseases. Retrieved from https://www.niddk.nih.gov/health-information/digestive-diseases/diverticulosis-diverticulitis

Strate, L. L., Peery, A. F., & Neumann, I. (2015). American Gastroenterological Association Institute technical review on the management of acute diverticulitis. *Gastroenterology, 149*(7), 1950–1976. doi:10.1053/j.gastro.2015.10.001

Thompson, A. E. (2016). Diverticulosis and diverticulitis. *Journal of the American Medical Association, 316*(10), 1124. doi:10.1001/jama.2016.3592

■ ENDOCARDITIS

Courtney G. Donahue
Celeste M. Alfes

Overview

Infective endocarditis (IE) is an inflammation of the endocardium, the endothelial membrane that lines the heart chambers and valves. IE is a potentially lethal disease that occurs when bacteria or fungi invade the bloodstream and the endocardial tissue. The epidemiology of IE has become more complex with the multitude of health care-associated factors that predispose the patient to infection (Baddour et al., 2015).

Background

IE is an uncommon infectious disease seen in approximately three to seven cases per 100,000 persons per year and deaths related to endocarditis are estimated to be one per 100,000 cases per year (Baddour et al., 2015). Although this disease is relatively rare, IE continues to have increased morbidity and mortality. IE is now the third or fourth most common life-threatening infection syndrome. Although the major risk factor for IE, rheumatic fever, has decreased significantly, the incidence of IE remains high. IE has changed from a disease primarily of the young, to one of the elderly, related to the fact that individuals are living longer with chronic heart disease and are having more invasive medical procedures (Josephson, 2014).

Patients most susceptible to acquiring IE include people who have congenital heart defects, damaged or artificial heart valves, or implanted medical devices in the heart or blood vessels. Other risk factors include poor dental hygiene and intravenous drug users. Furthermore, those undergoing invasive procedures and surgeries are at higher risk for bloodstream infections that can result in endocarditis (Josephson, 2014). The most common bacteria associated with IE are *Staphylococcus aureus, Enterococci, and Streptococci* organisms. The incidence of IE caused by *S. aureus* has increased and is now the most common causative organism in the industrialized world (Baddour et al., 2015).

Nosocomial infections acquired during a hospital stay contribute to the incidence of endocarditis. Nosocomial infections are acquired secondary to procedures, such as a pacemaker implantation, or various catheter insertions. These infections are more prevalent in men than in women with a ratio of 2:1 (Baddour et al., 2015). Signs and symptoms of IE include but are not limited to fever, malaise, and fatigue. A heart murmur, weight loss, and coughing are present in 35% of cases and small, painful petechiae (Osler's nodes) under the fingernails or toenails can also be present as well as small dark painless flat spots on the palms of the hands or soles of the feet (Janeway lesions).

Clinical Aspects

ASSESSMENT

IE is a relatively uncommon condition that presents with a multitude of noncardiac symptoms, making diagnosis of IE challenging (Josephson, 2014). The single most definitive test result is a positive blood culture. Current practice guidelines recommend at least three blood cultures from three different venipuncture sites to confirm diagnosis (Nishimura et al., 2014). The cultures enable the health care professional to determine which bacteria is the infective agent in the bloodstream. Treatment with antibiotics can then be determined regarding resistance and sensitivity.

Echocardiography is another common diagnostic marker used to diagnose IE using sound waves to create pictures of the heart, which may show damage. A transthoracic echo (TTE), which allows the health care professional to look at images of the patient's heart and determine whether there is vegetation on its structures may be ordered. If suspicion remains likely for diagnosis of IE, then a transesophageal echocardiogram (TEE) will also be ordered to provide additional information to support the diagnosis. An EKG may also be ordered as a supplement to determine whether there are any arrhythmias present (Nishimura et al., 2014).

NURSING INTERVENTIONS, MANAGEMENT, AND IMPLICATIONS

Nurses play a vital role in the care and detection of endocarditis. A thorough physical assessment can help detect the signs and symptoms of endocarditis. It is important to note that a complete and thorough medical and surgical history is crucial to knowing whether the patient has had a valve replacement, intravenous drug abuse, or cardiac history that would preclude the patient to IE.

Nurses also have a very important role in preventing IE. Sterile dressing changes of peripherally inserted central catheter (PICC) lines, intravenous lines, and arterial–venous fistulas are vital to preventing IE associated with central line bloodstream infections. Furthermore, providing comprehensive education on dental hygiene to both the patient and family can help prevent IE. Oftentimes, patients are not aware of how important their dental hygiene and dental prophylaxis are to their overall health and that poor dental hygiene is a precursor to acquiring IE. Daily adherence to a strict oral hygiene regimen along with routine visits to one's dentist who is aware of the patient's IE history is vital.

The two approaches to treating IE are the use of intravenous antibiotics for 2 to 6 weeks and cardiac surgery (Josephson, 2014). Infectious disease physicians collaborate with the primary care physician in determining the best choice of antibiotic. In some cases, the damage from the infection requires surgery to remove or repair a heart valve. Surgery is implicated in patients who have a vegetation of more than 10 mm in diameter. This is often seen in IE caused by fungi as this can become harder to treat. The proportion of patients undergoing surgery has increased to approximately 50% of those affected. Mortality from endocarditis usually occurs from congestive heart failure.

Endocarditis can continue to affect the patient after antibiotic therapy is initiated. The risk of embolization occurs in 22% to 50% of IE cases (Nishimura et al., 2014). Recent research has shown that the rate of embolic events dramatically decreases during and after the first 3 weeks of antibiotic therapy. Up to 65% of embolic events involve the central nervous system with more than 90% of these emboli lodged in the middle cerebral artery with the potential to cause a cerebrovascular accident, one of the many possible neurologic complications (Thuny et al., 2005). Despite the risk of emboli, anticoagulation therapy is controversial in patients post-IE. Some authorities recommend continuing anticoagulation therapy in patients with mechanical valve IE (Nishimura et al., 2014). However, most research concludes that it should be discontinued in all forms for at least 2 weeks in patients who have had an embolic event (Thuny et al., 2005).

OUTCOMES

Although IE is rare, it is a very serious disease. After antibiotic therapy, thorough follow-up is important to prevent a recurrence of endocarditis. Teaching the patient signs and symptoms to look for in endocarditis, including fever, malaise, and fatigue, is beneficial to preventing recurrence. A repeat echocardiogram is recommended to obtain a new baseline after treatment of the infection. A thorough dental evaluation is recommended to rule out all active sources of oral infection. All indwelling intravenous catheters used to infuse antibiotics should be removed immediately upon cessation of antibiotics. Developing heart failure is commonly seen in patients who experience IE. Follow-up for patients includes a thorough workup to determine whether any heart failure is present.

Summary

IE is a complex disease generally requiring management by a team of physicians and allied health care providers. Nurses are key members of the health care team and can greatly influence the outcome of the patient with endocarditis. It is important for nurses to closely assess their patients and identify those at increased risk for developing IE. Monitoring vital signs closely, drawing blood cultures regularly, and assessing the skin for peripheral embolization are key to patient outcomes. Nurses can also convey their knowledge of endocarditis to the patients and their families to assist them in understanding the disease process, management, and long-term care for this disease. With proper nursing and medical care, patients can return to their lives after IE, rejoining the community stronger than before.

Baddour, L. M., Wilson, W. R., Bayer, A. S., Fowler, V. G., Tleyjeh, I. M., Rybak, M. J., . . . Taubert, K. A. (2015). Infective endocarditis in adults: Diagnosis, antimicrobial therapy, and management of complications: A scientific statement for healthcare professionals from the American Heart Association. *Circulation, 132*(15), 1435–1486. doi:10.1161/CIR.0000000000000296

Josephson, L. (2014). Infective endocarditis: A review for nurses. *Dimensions of Critical Care Nursing, 33*(6), 327–340. doi:10.1097/DCC.0000000000000081

Nishimura, R. A., Otto, C. M., Bonow, R. O., Carabello, B. A., Erwin, J. P., Guyton, R. A., . . . Thomas, J. D. (2014). 2014 AHA/ACC guideline for the management of patients with valvular heart disease. *Journal of the American College of Cardiology*, 1–185. doi:10.1016/j.jacc.2014.02.536

Thuny, F., Di Salvo, G., Disalvo, G., Belliard, O., Avierinos, J. F., Pergola, V., . . . Habib, G. (2005). Risk of embolism and death in infective endocarditis: Prognostic value of echocardiography: A prospective multicenter study. *Circulation, 112*(1), 69–75. doi:10.1161/CIRCULATIONAHA.104.493155

■ FRACTURES

Joseph D. Perazzo

Overview

Fractures are a form of skeletal trauma in which the continuity of bone tissue is lost, often referred to as a "break." Fractures occur when the force exerted on a bone exceeds the pressure the bone can withstand, and can be the result of force as seen in traumatic injuries or the result of a weakened bone matrix as seen in osteoporosis. Fractures can occur in any bone and, depending on location and severity, can lead to chronic pain, deformity, and even permanent disability (American Academy of Orthopedic Surgeons [AAOS], 2017). Nursing care for people who experience fractures is focused on safety, preventing further injury, alleviating pain, assisting with self-care, education, and promoting rehabilitative efforts to regain mobility and function (Hinkle & Cheever, 2014).

Background

Fractures can affect individuals across the life span, but are most commonly seen in young males between 15 and 24 years of age and in adults aged 65 years and older (Huether & McCance, 2016). The causes and specific sites of fractures differ across the life span, with traumatic fractures (e.g., tibial, clavical, humeral) affecting younger persons, and fragility fractures (e.g., wrist, hip, ribs, and spine) having a higher incidence in older adults as the result of pathological bone loss (e.g., age, osteoporosis; Huether & McCance, 2016). Other fractures, such as those to the skull, hands, and feet, are also related to traumatic injury, including workplace accidents (AAOS, 2017). According to the Global Alliance of Musculoskeletal Health (Watkins-Castillo, Yelin, & Weinstein, 2017), health care providers treat more than 18 million fractures annually, a figure expected to increase substantially as the population of older Americans increases. Perhaps the most damaging aspect of fractures is the

potential for long-term physical and psychosocial complications, including chronic pain and disability (Watkins-Castillo et al., 2017). Fractures, along with other musculoskeletal injuries, cost Americans more than $200 billion annually in direct health care costs, and more than $70 billion in indirect costs due to disability and lost productivity (Watkins-Castillo et al., 2017).

There are many different categorizations and classifications of fractures, many outside the scope of this entry. Common fractures include:

- *Oblique*: Angular fracture (diagonal) caused by direct or indirect injury to bone

- *Transverse*: Horizontal fracture across the bone, direct or indirect injury to bone

- *Comminuted*: Multiple-segment fracture "shatter," caused by direct injury to bone

- *Linear*: Fracture along the vertical axis of the bone, caused by overuse

- *Depressed*: Fracture driven inward, seen in skull and facial fractures

- *Spiral*: Fracture twists around bone shaft, caused by rotating force (e.g., athletics)

- *Stress*: Bone matrix breaks in response to repeated loading and unloading (e.g., running)

- *Closed*: Fracture does not break the skin, caused by direct or indirect injury to bone

- *Open*: Fracture breaks through skin, caused by moderate to severe trauma

- *Pathologic*: Fracture at site of weakened bone matrix, caused by low bone mineral density (Hinkle & Cheever, 2014; Huether & McCance, 2016)

Although fractures can affect people of any age, certain groups have an elevated risk for fractures, including young people at high risk for trauma and overuse (e.g., athletes), as well as postmenopausal women and individuals with chronic diseases that decrease bone mineral density (e.g., cancer, HIV). Other risk factors for fractures include malnutrition, decreased physical function (fall risk), low body mass index (BMI), alcohol use, smoking, and taking medications known to weaken bone (e.g., glucocorticoids; Huether & McCance, 2016). A key difference between traumatic and nontraumatic fractures is the level of force, energy, or activity that resulted in fracture; stress fractures occur through repetitive force, traumatic fractures are caused by significant (moderate to severe) force, and fragility fractures can occur regardless of force because of weak bone, sometimes during normal daily activities (Hinkle & Cheever, 2014; Huether & McCance, 2016).

The pathophysiology of fractures is defined by the specific causes of the fracture, as well as the ability of the bone to regain integrity during the healing process. Fracture healing occurs in three phases: (a) the inflammatory phase (immediate: 4 weeks), (b) the repair phase (1–2 months), and (c) the remodeling phase (up to 6 months; Huether & McCance, 2016; Kalfas, 2001). In the inflammatory phase, a hematoma forms at the site of the injured bone, leading to infiltration of inflammatory cells and fibroblasts, leading to formation of granulation and vascular tissue that allows the process of repairing to begin. Mesenchymal cells that differentiate into bone-forming cells (osteoblasts) migrate to the area and new blood vessels are formed to deliver oxygen and nutrients (Huether & McCance, 2016; Kalfas, 2001). Soft new bone tissue (osteoid) and cartilage are woven to create a bridge between the fracture fragments, creating a soft, fragile "callus" that is mineralized and hardened in a process known as *ossification*. Immobilization is particularly important during this phase. In the remodeling phase, osteoblasts and bone resorption cells (osteoclasts) work together to repair the physical structure of the bone and provide tissue to strengthen the new bone (Hinkle & Cheever, 2014; Huether & McCance, 2016; Kalfas, 2001). Remodeling is promoted by mechanical forces (e.g., weight bearing), and continues over time to continually strengthen the new bone and remove bone tissue where necessary, resulting in healed bone with appropriate anatomical structure. From first response to postdischarge rehabilitation, clinical interventions drive this process through efforts to stabilize, align, immobilize, and eventually stimulate bones to promote optimal healing (Hinkle & Cheever, 2014; Huether & McCance, 2016; Kalfas, 2001).

Clinical Aspects

ASSESSMENT

Fractures are diagnosed and monitored using x-ray imaging that allows clinicians to determine the site and severity of a fracture and to determine a course of action that will promote optimal healing. Clinical fracture interventions vary depending on the type of fracture, but share the goal of accomplishing reduction, immobilization, and restoration of function (Hinkle & Cheever, 2014).

NURSING INTERVENTIONS, MANAGEMENT, AND IMPLICATIONS

Reduction refers to the process of placing bones in their appropriate anatomical alignment. In a closed reduction, bones are manually manipulated into alignment and held in place using casts, splints, or percutaneous pinning. In an open reduction, a surgical approach is used in which fracture fragments are aligned and held in place with the use of internal fixation devices (e.g., pins, screws, plates, nails; Hinkle & Cheever, 2014).

Immobilization refers to interventions designed to keep bones in appropriate anatomical position that will lead to proper healing. Specific immobilization interventions are chosen based on the site and severity of a fracture, and include casts, bandages, and splints, which are used for simpler fractures often for long bones. *Fixation* refers to external and internal fixators used to maintain alignment, often used with more severe or more complex fractures. Traction involves the use of pulling force to promote bone alignment and is especially important in maintaining overall anatomical alignment of the injured body part; this includes skin traction (e.g., Buck's extension traction) and skeletal traction (Brunner et al., 2014). Finally, functional restoration includes all efforts to help individuals regain use of the injured body part and includes all matter of physical rehabilitative efforts, ranging from gradual range of motion to vigorous physical activity (Hinkle & Cheever, 2014).

Immediately following injury, particularly in the case of open fractures, individuals can have significant bleeding caused by injuries directly and indirectly associated with the broken bones. One of the most serious complications occurs with open femoral fractures in which the femoral artery can be torn causing acute hemorrhage, and is treated by fracture stabilization and blood volume restoration. Another potential (though rarely fatal) complication associated with fractures are fat emboli that can gain access to the vascular compartment, leading to occlusion of blood vessels that supply vital organs. Compartment syndrome is a complication that occurs when one of the body's 46 anatomic compartments, such as those in the extremities, loses blood flow, potentially leading to necrotic tissue loss. Finally, during healing, the complication of nonunion can occur when bones are not properly aligned and can lead to loss of function, chronic pain, deformity, and crepitus (AAOS, 2017; Hinkle & Cheever, 2014; Huether & McCance, 2016).

Nursing care of adults who experience fractures is focused on promoting patient safety, preventing further complication to fractures, and promoting optimal healing. Priority nursing diagnoses include careful assessment of fracture sites and sites of fixation for swelling and signs of infection, assessing and managing pain, careful asepsis and proper positioning of fixation and traction devices, ensuring immobilization, promoting early mobility when appropriate, and providing emotional support and patient education regarding expectations related to prognosis, hospitalization, surgical interventions, and future limitations (Hinkle & Cheever, 2014; Huether & McCance, 2016).

OUTCOMES

The outcomes of priority nursing interventions are directly associated with promoting optimal fracture healing. Swelling and drainage at the fracture site can alert nurses to malalignment, further complication of injuries, or infections at fixation or surgical sites (Hinkle & Cheever, 2014; Huether & McCance, 2016). Pain, often quite significant, is common in the early stages of fracture healing, but should improve with time. Sudden onset of increased pain (not associated with movement) can be a sign of complicated healing or compartment syndrome. Patients should maintain immobilization until clinical assessments indicate that movement would not jeopardize healing or patient safety (Hinkle & Cheever, 2014). Nurses should ensure that the patient completes required range of motion and mobilization to prevent bone loss and promote bone remodeling. Finally, patients should understand timelines related to healing, mobility restrictions, and be educated about healing following clinical encounters, potential physical limitations they may encounter, and ways to promote bone remodeling, particularly those related to diet and physical activity (AAOS, 2017; Hinkle & Cheever, 2014; Huether & McCance, 2016).

Summary

Fractures are a significant injury that can affect people of all ages and affect many different parts of the body. Optimal healing of fractures requires timely intervention and careful assessment of injuries. Nurses play a vital role in helping patients to tolerate, maintain, and understand the phases of fracture healing, both in and out of the clinical environment, which help patients to regain as much function as possible following injury.

American Academy of Orthopedic Surgeons. (2017). Fractures (broken bones). Retrieved from http://orthoinfo.aaos.org/topic.cfm?topic=a00139

Hinkle, J., & Cheever, K. H. (2014). *Brunner & Suddarth's textbook of medical–surgical nursing*. Philadelphia, PA: Wolters Kluwer Health.

Huether, S. E., & McCance, K. L. (2016). *Understanding pathophysiology* (5th ed.). St. Louis, MO: Elsevier Health Sciences.

Kalfas, I. H. (2001). Principles of bone healing. *Neurosurgical Focus, 10*(4), E1. doi:10.3171/foc.2001.10.4.2

Watkins-Castillo, S. I., Yelin, E., & Weinstein, S. (2017). The burden of musculoskeletal diseases in the United States: Facts in brief. Retrieved from http://www.boneandjoint burden.org/facts-brief

■ GALLBLADDER AND BILIARY TRACT DISEASE

Andrea Marie Herr

Overview

The main function of the gallbladder is storage and release of bile. Most gallbladder disease is a result of inflammation of the gallbladder or obstruction of the biliary tree, usually by stones, causing biliary stasis. Common gallbladder problems are cholecystitis and cholelithiasis. Cholelithiasis, or gallstones, are crystallized deposits containing cholesterol and/or bilirubin (Tiderington, Lee, & Ko, 2016). Surgical management of gallstones is considered to be the gold standard and is safe and effective; more than 750,000 cholecystectomies are performed annually (Pak & Lindseth, 2016). Other less common conditions include gallbladder polyps and benign or malignant tumors. Disorders of the biliary tract include choledocholithiasis, primary sclerosing cholangitis, and cholangiocarcinoma.

Background

GALLBLADDER DISEASE

Gallbladder disease is the second most common gastrointestinal discharge diagnosis in U.S. hospitalizations (Pak & Lindseth, 2016). Gallstones affect 10% and 20% of the adult population; gallbladder disease is more prevalent in women (Pak & Lindseth, 2016). There are two main types of gallstones; the majority of stones are made up of cholesterol and are yellow-green-colored and pigment stones, which are brown or black and contain bilirubin. Inflammation of the gallbladder, or cholecystitis, can be acute or chronic and commonly occurs as a result of gallstones, but can occur without stones (acalculous cholecystitis). Acalculous cholecystitis is associated with a higher morbidity and mortality rate than calculous cholecystitis. Acalculous cholecystitis is associated with critically ill patients with sepsis, burns, or who are on mechanical ventilation.

Most patients with cholethiliasis are asymptomatic. When gallstones are acutely symptomatic, they commonly cause biliary colic, a result of transient blockage of a bile duct, which is characterized by right-upper-quadrant pain, often radiating to the back or right shoulder and lasting longer than 30 minutes and nausea and vomiting (Pak & Lindseth, 2016). Other more chronic symptoms include a dull ache, intolerance of fatty foods, dyspepsia, and increase in flatulence. The treatment and management of acute and chronic cholecystitis is laparoscopic cholecystectomy. Medical treatment includes shock-wave lithotripsy and medical dissolution therapy. Dissolution therapy, primarily with bile acids, has largely been replaced with cholecystectomy, but may be indicated for some patients. There is a high rate of stone recurrence following treatment (Tiderington et al., 2016).

Both malignant and benign tumors can be found in the gallbladder. Benign tumors that are found in the gallbladder are papillomas, adenomyomas, or cholesterol polyps. Malignant tumors of the gallbladder, primarily adenocarcinomas, are relatively rare, but are the most common and aggressive cancer of the biliary tract (Kanthan, Senger, Ahmed, & Kanthan, 2015). Risk factors for gallbladder cancer include chronic inflammation, gallstones, gallbladder polyps, age, female gender, obesity, genetics, and ethnicity (Kanthan et al., 2015). Abdominal ultrasound, CT, or MRI can identify the tumor location. An endoscopic ultrasound (EUS) with biopsy or endoscopic retrograde cholangiopancreatography (ERCP) with tissue sampling can be used for diagnosis. Treatment modalities include surgery, radiation, and chemotherapy, alone or in combination, depending on tumor staging and grading.

Surgery is the only curative approach to gallbladder cancer. However, only about 20% of tumors are diagnosed early enough for a surgical cure. Most patients with gallbladder cancer are asymptomatic, making early diagnosis difficult. Most gallbladder cancers are discovered incidentally or diagnosed at an advanced stage (Kanthan et al., 2015).

BILIARY TRACT DISEASE

Choledocholithiasis is a gallstone in the common bile duct and can cause biliary obstruction, biliary colic pain, elevated liver function tests, cholangitis, and gallstone pancreatitis. About 11% to 21% of patients with gallstones also have common bile duct stones (Costi, Gnocchi, Di Mario, & Sarli, 2014). Intraoperative cholangiography can identify stones in the biliary tree; ERCP can be performed for stone removal. Lithotripsy may be used to break up a very large stone for easier removal (Costi et al., 2014).

Primary sclerolsing cholangitis (PSC) is a chronic, idiopathic inflammatory disease of the bile ducts. The disease is characterized by fibrosis of the bile duct and ultimately leads to end-stage liver disease (Hirschfield, Karlsen, Lindor, & Adams, 2013). PSC is linked to inflammatory bowel disease (IBD); approximately 60% to 80% of patients with PSC also have IBD. PSC results in biliary strictures, recurrent cholangitis, and biliary cirrhosis; approximately 50% of patients eventually need a liver transplant (Hirschfield et al., 2013).

Cholangiocarcinoma is a rare cancer of the bile duct, and is classified as intra- or extrahepatic based on the location of the tumor. Risk factors include PSC and ulcerative colitis. Symptoms include signs of biliary obstruction, weight loss, and abdominal pain. Five-year survival rates vary from 15% to 30% for localized cancers to 2% for stage 4 malignancies (American Cancer Society [ACS], 2017). Most tumors are unable to be surgically removed. Treatment options include surgical resection, radiation/chemotherapy, and palliative therapy with biliary stenting to maintain biliary drainage.

Clinical Aspects

ASSESSMENT

An understanding of the risk factors associated with gallbladder disease is useful in helping nurses identify patients at risk, provide information regarding preventive strategies, and to provide education and resources for disease management (Pak & Lindseth, 2016). Patients at risk for cholelithiasis include females older than 40 years, Native American or Mexican American ethnicity, and obesity (Pak & Lindseth, 2016). Other risk factors include sedentary lifestyle, dyslipidemia, rapid weight loss, treatment with estrogen therapy, type 2 diabetes, and family history. Nursing interventions and management include healthy dietary and lifestyle changes, weight loss, nutrition guidance, education on signs/symptoms of gallstone disease, and strategies to reduce modifiable risk factors.

Choledocholithiasis is usually discovered at either the time of gallbladder surgery or when a patient presents with symptoms of biliary duct obstruction.

Diagnostic studies include complete blood count, liver function tests, and serum amylase and lipase to differentiate among types of gallbladder disorders and complications of gallbladder disease. Abdominal ultrasound and cholescintigraphy (hepatobiliary iminodiacetic acid [HIDA] scan) are commonly used to diagnose cholelithiasis and cholecystitis. Magnetic resonance cholangiopancreatography (MRCP) and ERCP are indicated if choledocholithiasis is suspected; ERCP can be used diagnostically or therapeutically to remove stones or place stents.

OUTCOMES

Patients may be hospitalized for acute cholecsytitis. Treatment consists of bowel rest, intravenous (IV) fluids, and IV antibiotics. Complications of cholecystitis include gangrenous gallbladder, perforation, and peritonitis. Surgical options include laparoscopic, percutaneous, and open cholecystectomy. Perioperative nursing care consists of pain management, prevention of postoperative complications, and discharge education. The nursing care for patients with gallbladder cancer is focused on perioperative care if the tumor is resectable and oncology care for a patient who may undergo chemotherapy and/or radiation as treatment.

Summary

Gallbladder disease is found in 10% to 20% of the adult population and is a frequent cause for hospitalization (Shabanzadeh, Sørensen, & Jørgensen, 2016). Gallstones are common in the population, but only a small percentage of patients with gallstones are symptomatic (Tiderington et al., 2016). A better understanding of the risk factors for gallbladder and biliary tract disease is beneficial for nurses to better provide education about reducing the risk of disease and preventing complications for those already diagnosed (Pak & Lindseth, 2016).

American Cancer Society. (2017). Survival statistics for bile duct cancers. Retrieved from https://www.cancer.org/cancer/bile-duct-cancer/detection-diagnosis-staging/survival-by-stage.html

Costi, R., Gnocchi, A., Di Mario, F., & Sarli, L. (2014). Diagnosis and management of choledocholithiasis in the golden age of imaging, endoscopy and laparoscopy. *World Journal of Gastroenterology*, 20(37), 13382–13401. doi:10.3748/wjg.v20.i37.13382

Hirschfield, G. M., Karlsen, T. H., Lindor, K. D., & Adams, D. H. (2013). Primary sclerosing cholangitis. *Lancet*, 382(9904), 1587–1599. doi:10.1016/S0140-6736(13)60096-3

Kanthan, R., Senger, J.-L., Ahmed, S., & Kanthan, S. C. (2015). Gallbladder cancer in the 21st century. *Journal of Oncology*, 2015, 967472. doi:10.1155/2015/967472

Pak, M., & Lindseth, G. (2016). Risk factors for cholelithiasis. *Gastroenterology Nursing*, 39(4), 297–309. doi:10.1097/SGA.0000000000000235

Shabanzadeh, D. M., Sørensen, T. L., & Jørgensen, T. (2016). Abdominal symptoms and incident gallstones in a population unaware of gallstone status. *Canadian Journal of Gastroenterology and Hepatology*, 2016, 9730687. doi:10.1155/2016/9730687

Tiderington, E., Lee, S. P., & Ko, C. W. (2016). Gallstones: New insights into an old story. *F1000Research*, 5, 1817. doi:10.12688/f1000research.8874.1

■ GASTRIC CANCER

Una Hopkins
Jane F. Marek

Overview

Cancer of the stomach is the third leading cause of cancer deaths globally, with an estimated 700,000 deaths occurring annually. Once the leading cause of cancer-related deaths in the United States, gastric cancer is now the 15th most common cancer. The decline in the incidence of stomach cancer in the United States is thought to be a result of recognition of risk factors, including *Helicobacter pylori* infection, poor refrigeration, and an increase in consumption of fresh foods and vegetables. Despite the declining incidence in the United States, the prognosis remains poor, because most patients are diagnosed with advanced stage disease and few, if any, curative options. This is clearly reflected when comparing the 5-year survival rates for stage 1 cancer (57%–71%) compared with stage 3 (9%–20%) and stage 4 (4%; American Cancer Society [ACS], 2017). The disease is more prevalent in Central and Eastern Europe, Central and South America, and Asia; more than 70% of gastric cancer is found in developing countries. The highest rate of gastric cancer is in Korea, followed by Mongolia and Japan (World Cancer Research Fund International [WCRFI], 2015). The ACS estimates 28,000 new cases of gastric cancer and 10,960 deaths for 2017 (ACS, 2017). In the United States, the incidence of gastric cancer is higher among Asian Americans, Pacific Islanders, Hispanics, Native

Americans, and African Americans, and least common among Whites.

Background

There are two types of gastric cancer: intestinal and diffuse. Most cases of gastric cancer are adenocarcinomas and histologically resemble cancers arising from the intestinal tract. Other types of gastric cancer include lymphomas, gastrointestinal stromal tumors, carcinoids, and squamous cell. Adenocarcinomas originate in the mucosal layer of the stomach and then spread outward. The liver is the most common site of metastasis (48%), followed by the peritoneum (32%), lung (15%), and bone (12%); the site of metastasis varies on location of the gastric lesion (Riihimäki et al., 2016).

Dietary and lifestyle factors impact the risk of gastric cancer. A diet high in salt; processed meat; fish, fried, pickled, and smoked foods; and low in fiber and fresh fruits and vegetables increase an individual's risk for gastric cancer. Obesity, smoking, and a family history of gastric cancer are also risk factors. Other contributing factors include *H. pylori* and Epstein–Barr infection, chronic atrophic gastritis, gastric ulcers, pernicious anemia, intestinal metaplasia, familial adenomatous polyposis, and hereditary nonpolyposis colorectal cancer (Lynch syndrome; Ajani et al., 2016).

Gastric cancer is generally asymptomatic until late stages when it has progressed through the muscularis and serosa layers of the stomach. Clinical manifestations include indigestion, dysphagia, loss of appetite, bloating, nausea, weight loss, melena, hematemesis, and pain in the upper abdomen. Gastric outlet obstruction, small bowel obstruction, pleural effusion, and jaundice may occur with advanced metastatic disease.

There are no routine screening guidelines for gastric cancer. Diagnostic tests include esophagogastroduodenscopy (EGD), endoscopic ultrasound, and upper gastrointestinal series and barium swallow. Chest x-ray, CT, and positron emission tomography may be indicated to evaluate for metastases. Tumor markers, such as carcinoembryonic antigen (CEA) and carbohydrate antigen (CA19-9), may be used to evaluate the effectiveness of treatment.

Once a diagnosis of gastric cancer has been made through biopsy, the tissue should be tested for human epidermal growth factor receptor 2 (HER-2/neu or HER-2) levels. This molecular marker was originally discovered in breast cancer and is associated with other malignancies, including gastric and gastroesophageal cancer. HER-2 overexpression in gastric cancer varies from 4.4% to 53.4% (Abrahao-Machado & Scapulatempo-Neto, 2016). Trastuzumab (Herceptin), a monoclonal antibody that targets HER-2, is approved for gastric cancer. Testing for HER-2 must be done to identify patients who might benefit from this treatment and other molecular HER-2 agents being evaluated for treatment of gastric cancer (Abrahao-Machado & Scapulatempo-Neto, 2016). Treatment for gastric cancer depends on the location, size, and staging of the tumor.

A multidisciplinary team consisting of surgeons, radiation oncologists, gastroenterologists, dieticians, and nurses offers the best approach to care. According to National Comprehensive Cancer Network guidelines, early-stage cancers are treated with endoscopic mucosal resection or partial or total gastrectomy (Ajani et al., 2016). Chemotherapy can be used preoperatively or postoperatively in addition to radiation depending on the tumor stage. Chemotherapy and radiation may be indicated for unresectable tumors and palliation.

Clinical Aspects

ASSESSMENT

Nurses play a significant role in teaching and supporting the patients and their families throughout the cancer continuum. From providing support as patients cope with a new diagnosis of gastric cancer, teaching about the expected outcomes following surgery, chemotherapy, or radiation, to advocating for patients and their families at the end of life, nurses are the primary caregivers.

When caring for patients who have undergone surgical treatment of gastric cancer, nurses can implement evidence-based interventions to improve patient outcomes. These interventions include an interactive education program about gastric cancer, treatment, and symptom management; the Modified Hospital Elder Life Program (HELP) consists of early mobilization, nutritional assistance, and therapeutic cognitive activities, and perioperative interventions, including self-management of pain, management of enteral and abdominal drains, and dietary education. These interventions resulted in a decrease in delirium and improvement in functional and nutritional status, improvement in patients' knowledge about the disease process and treatments, improvement in coping skills and quality of life, and reduced postoperative complications and improvement in quality of life (Gomes et al., 2016).

OUTCOMES

The goal of surgical treatment is to improve survival, reduce symptoms, and maintain quality of life with the minimal amount of adverse effects. Five-year survival rates following surgical treatment of gastric cancer have improved and have been reported to be as high as 33% to 50% (Shan, Shan, Morris, Golani, & Saxena, 2015). A systematic review of patients' health-related quality of life (HRQOL) scores following partial and total gastrectomy demonstrated that HQOL was negatively impacted 1-month postsurgery but returned to preoperative levels or better 1 year after surgery. Patients continued to have gastrointestinal symptoms 6 months after surgery. Patients who underwent partial gastrectomy had better HQOL scores in the physical, emotional, and functional status domains and returned to preoperative levels faster than patients who underwent total gastrectomy (Shan et al., 2015). Nurses can apply these findings by ensuring that the patients undergoing partial and total gastrectomy are prepared to experience a decline in overall health and functional status in the first few months following surgery and understand this will most likely improve with time.

Monitoring the patient's nutritional status following gastric resection or gastrectomy is a priority. If patients are unable to tolerate oral feedings, parenteral nutrition may be indicated until the patient is able to tolerate enteral feeding. Most patients experience dumping syndrome following gastric resection. The nurse can reassure the patient that these symptoms usually lessen or resolve after several months and teach the patient dietary modifications to reduce their occurrence. A nutritional consult should be initiated to plan strategies to best meet the patient's nutritional needs while in the hospital and after discharge. Most patients experience a 20% weight loss over the first 3 to 6 months after surgery. Following gastrectomy, the patients require lifelong injections of vitamin B_{12} due to the loss of parietal cells and intrinsic factor necessary for absorption of vitamin B_{12} in the ileum.

Summary

Gastric cancer continues to be a leading cause of cancer deaths worldwide and a global health concern, despite declining rates in the United States. Gastric cancer is difficult to diagnose early due to its nonspecific symptoms in early stages, which contribute to the poor prognosis associated with this disease. Screening for gastric cancer is controversial and varies by geographic region. Screening programs have been implemented in Korea, Japan, and other countries with a high incidence of gastric cancer, but there are no evidence-based recommendations for the United States. Infection with H. pylori is a known risk factor for gastric cancer, and testing and treating H. pylori is relatively easy and inexpensive. More research is needed to examine the effectiveness of screening for H. pylori infection as a method of reducing the incidence of gastric cancer, especially in countries where the disease is prevalent (Herrero, Parsonnet, & Greenberg, 2014). The World Health Organization identified evaluating the effectiveness of screening and treating H. pylori infection as a method to reduce the incidence of gastric cancer as a global priority (Wald, 2014). Clinical trials are underway in several countries. Nurses can play a role in prevention by health-promotion teaching and risk reduction strategies.

Management of the patient with gastric cancer depends on the health of the individual, stage of disease, and treatment modality. Maintaining quality of life, managing symptoms, and promoting optimal nutrition are priorities of care for patients with any stage of gastric cancer. Nurses can provide information regarding resources and psychosocial support for patients with unresectable disease as they face end-of-life decisions. A multidisciplinary approach and supportive care are essential components of care for the patients and their families throughout the disease process.

Abrahao-Machado, L. F., & Scapulatempo-Neto, C. (2016). HER2 testing in gastric cancer: An update. *World Journal of Gastroenterology, 22*(19), 4619–4625. doi:10.3748/wjg.v22.i19.4619

Ajani, J. A., D'Amico, T. A., Almhanna, K., Bentrem, D. J., Chao, J., Das, P., . . . Sundar, H. (2016). Gastric cancer, version 3.2016, NCCN clinical practice guidelines in oncology. *Journal of the National Comprehensive Cancer Network, 14*(10), 1286–1312.

American Cancer Society. (2017). What are the key statistics about stomach cancer? Retrieved from https://www.cancer.org/cancer/stomach-cancer/about/key-statistics.html

Gomes, N. C. R. P., Vilaca de Brito Santos, C. S., Rodrigues Bettencourt de Jesus, M. M. G., & da Silva Henriques, M. A. (2016). Effectiveness of nursing interventions in the postoperative recover of gastric cancer patients: A systematic literature review. *Journal of Nursing Referencia, 4*(11), 111–119. doi:10.12707/RIV16050

Herrero, R., Parsonnet, J., & Greenberg, E. R. (2014). Prevention of gastric cancer. *Journal of the American Medical Association, 312*(12), 1197–1198. doi:10.1001/jama.2014.10498

Riihimäki, M., Hemminki, A., Sundquist, K., Sundquist, J., & Hemminki, K. (2016). Metastatic spread in patients with gastric cancer. *Oncotarget*, 7(32), 52307–52316. doi:10.18632/oncotarget.10740

Shan, B., Shan, L., Morris, D., Golani, S., & Saxena, A. (2015). Systematic review on quality of life outcomes after gastrectomy for gastric carcinoma. *Journal of Gastrointestinal Oncology*, 6(5), 544–560. doi:10.3978/j.issn.2078-6891.2015.046

Wald, N. J. (2014). The treatment of *Helicobacter pylori* infection of the stomach in relation to the possible prevention of gastric cancer. In IARC *Helicobacter pylori* Working Group (Ed.), *Helicobacter pylori eradication as a strategy for preventing gastric cancer* (pp. 174–180). Lyon, France: International Agency for Research on Cancer. Retrieved from http://www.iarc.fr/en/publications/pdfs-online/wrk/wrk8/index.php

World Cancer Research Fund International. (2015). Stomach cancer statistics. Retrieved from http://www.wcrf.org/int/cancer-facts-figures/data-specific-cancers/stomach-cancer-statistics

■ GASTRITIS

Maria G. Smisek

Overview

Gastritis is inflammation or swelling of the mucosal lining in the stomach (Cohen & Hull, 2015; Porth, 2015). Gastritis can be acute or chronic in nature and is considered one of the most common problems affecting the stomach. The National Institute of Diabetes and Digestive and Kidney Disease (NIDDK) estimates 60 to 70 million people in the United States have some form of a digestive disease resulting in 36.6 million office visits, 21.7 million hospitalizations, 245,921 deaths, and a total cost of $141.8 billion in direct and indirect care (NIDDK, 2014b).

Background

Gastritis is a disorder affecting the mucosa of the stomach. The epithelial lining of the stomach is usually impermeable to the gastric secretions produced, creating a mucosal barrier. In gastritis, the mucosa undergoes inflammatory changes that can lead to ulceration or bleeding. Common threats affecting the integrity of the mucosal lining are irritation, infections (predominately *Helicobacter pylori*), injury to the stomach lining due to trauma or surgery or an autoimmune response (NIDDK, 2014c). Contributing factors include excessive alcohol intake, ingesting food contaminated with bacteria, gastroesophageal reflux, chemicals, infection, and surgical procedures or trauma. Severe gastritis can erode the mucosa, forming a peptic ulcer in the membrane of the esophagus, stomach, or duodenum (Cohen & Hull, 2015, NIDDK, 2014a).

Gastritis may be acute or chronic and presents as erosive or nonerosive. Erosive gastritis occurs when the stomach lining begins to wear down, exhibiting ulcerations and erosions. Nonerosive gastritis causes inflammation to the stomach lining without subsequent ulceration or erosion. Approximately 30% to 40% of the population of the United States develops an *H. pylori* infection, lying dormant for years before exhibiting signs and symptoms (Kulnigg-Dabsch, 2016; NIDDK, 2014b).

Acute gastritis is an acute episode of inflammation of the stomach mucosa, which is typically a self-limiting condition that resolves in several days postremoval of the aggravating agent. Damage to the stomach lining from inflammation can be a result of exposure to nonsteroidal anti-inflammatory drugs (NSAIDs); foods or liquids that have low acidity or high alkalinity, such as alcohol, coffee, and spicy foods, chemical agents, or radiation. A reduction in mucus production and/or an increase in acidity lead to tissue damage. Progression from acute to chronic disease depends on the affected location in the stomach. Extreme physiologic stress related to serious medical or surgical intervention weakens the mucosa making it susceptible to an acute hemorrhage gastritis (Porth, 2015).

Chronic gastritis is an absence of grossly visible erosion and chronic inflammatory changes to the epithelium that persists for more than 3 months (Cohen & Hull, 2015, NIDDK, 2014c). Without treatment, chronic gastritis may persist for years leading to atrophy of the glandular epithelium and serious complications. Chronic gastritis has three major types: *H. pylori* gastritis, chronic autoimmune gastritis, and chemical gastropathy (Porth, 2015). *H. pylori* gastritis is the result of *H. pylori* bacteria causing a chronic inflammation of the antrum and body of the stomach. Possible modes of transmission are fecal–oral, oral–oral, and environmental (Porth, 2015). The *H. pylori* bacteria interferes with the mucosal barrier of the stomach and damages its lining. Prevent infection by following good hygiene: eat only food washed and cooked properly, wash with soap and water after using the restroom and before eating. Damage to the stomach lining related to NSAIDs use, alcohol consumption, exposure to chemicals or trauma can progress from an acute phase to chronic if untreated.

Autoimmune gastritis is chronic inflammation that eventually results in mucosal atrophy. The immune system attacks healthy parietal cells in the lining of the stomach affecting iron and B_{12} absorption and consequently causing pernicious anemia (Kulnigg-Dabsch, 2016). Pernicious anemia is a decrease in red blood cells due to inability to absorb B_{12}. Chemical gastritis is the result of exposure to bilious, pancreatic, or duodenal secretions. This form is seen typically in clients with abdominal surgery such as gastroduodenostomy or gastrojejunostomy (Porth, 2015).

Clinical Aspects

ASSESSMENT

A detailed history, including prescription and over-the-counter medications used, past illnesses along with the onset, duration, relieving, and aggravating factors related to signs and symptoms of acute or chronic exposure, should be taken. Findings may include long-term use of known irritants: aspirin, other NSAIDs, or chemotherapy. Dietary history may identify poor nutritional habits, allergies, alcohol, coffee, and tobacco use. Travel history, especially to developing countries, can indicate exposure to *H. pylori* or other bacteria. Complaints of dizziness, fatigue, pallor, shortness of breath may indicate anemia secondary to gastrointestinal (GI) bleeding (NIDDK, 2014c; Porth, 2015; Sipponen, 2015). Epigastric pain, anorexia, nausea, and vomiting may reveal abdominal distension, bloating and tenderness on physical exam. It is important to recognize any episode of dark stools, blood in emesis or coffee grounds indicates bleeding (Cohen & Hull, 2015; NIDDK, 2014c; Porth, 2015).

Diagnostic studies can be invasive or noninvasive based on history and physical findings. A blood test identifies anemia and stool for occult blood indicates GI bleeding. A noninvasive urea breath test can identify *H. pylori*, whereas an upper endoscopy visualizes the anatomy of the stomach and duodenum. Signs of irritation or ulceration indicate active gastritis. A small biopsy taken during the procedure rules out *H. pylori* and direct treatment.

Following diagnosis, a plan of care is developed between the physician and the client. Successful treatment is indicated when the symptoms are resolved and, in the case of *H. pylori*, the bacteria is eliminated (Porth, 2015).

Nursing-related problems include pain (acute or chronic) related to disruption of mucosal lining of the stomach as evidenced by use of irritants (NSAIDs, smoking, extreme stress), infection (*H. pylori*), trauma or surgery and infection related to ulceration of duodenum as evidenced by *H. pylori* bacteria (via biopsy), burning pain in abdomen, anorexia, and weight loss.

NURSING INTERVENTIONS, MANAGEMENT, AND IMPLICATIONS

Nursing interventions include assessing the client's past and present pain level (using a 1 to 10 scale), assessing for signs of infection, administering pain medication and antibiotics as ordered, and educating the client on the effect irritants, such as NSAIDs, alcohol, coffee, and smoking, have on stomach mucosa. Teaching should include alternative treatment for discomfort, setting treatment goals, implications for revision of intervention depending on client response, and identifying patient understanding through verbalization and return demonstration. The nurse should also supply the patients and their families with a list of community resources to assist compliance.

OUTCOMES

Although some people with gastritis have no pain or discomfort, others have been living with pain and discomfort. Inflammation and swelling can cause destruction of the epithelial lining of the stomach. Left untreated, gastritis can lead to peptic ulcers, anemia, erosion, and hemorrhage. Complaints of epigastric pain or other GI symptoms and a history of exposure to GI irritants suggests gastritis. Management of gastritis is done by treating the underlying cause and reducing the amount of acid in the stomach. Repeated use of irritants and medications can exacerbate the condition leading to hospitalization and long-term treatment.

Summary

Patient education is a key element in the treatment of patients with gastritis. Education regarding *H. pylori* and the suspected mode of transmission can assist in preventing exposure (NIDDK, 2014c; Porth, 2015). Early diagnosis of gastritis and its causitive agent can facilitate a speedy recovery. Identifying client concerns regarding treatment plan, cost, and access to that treatment are an essential nursing responsibility.

Cohen, B. J., & Hull, K. L. (2015). *Memmlers's the human body in health and disease* (13th ed., pp. 432–458). Philadelphia, PA: Wolters Kluwer.

Kulnigg-Dabsch, S. (2016). Autoimmune gastritis. *Wiener Medizinische Wochenschrift, 166*(13), 424–430. doi: 10.1007/s10354-016-0515-55

National Institute of Diabetes and Digestive and Kidney Disease. (2014a). Definition & facts for peptic ulcers (stomach ulcers). Retrieved from https://www.niddk.nih.gov/health-information/digestive-diseases/peptic-ulcers-stomach-ulcers/definition-facts

National Institute of Diabetes and Digestive and Kidney Disease. (2014b). Digestive diseases statistics for the United States. Retrieved from https://www.niddk.nih.gov/health-information/health-statistics/Pages/digestive-diseases-statistics-for-the-united-states.aspx

National Institute of Diabetes and Digestive and Kidney Disease. (2014c). Gastritis. Retrieved from https://www.niddk.nih.gov/health-information/digestive-diseases/gastritis

Porth, C. M. (2015). Disorders of gastrointestinal function. In C. M. Porth (Ed.), *Essentials of pathophysiology* (4th ed., pp. 696–723). Philadelphia, PA: Wolters Kluwer.

Sipponen, P. M. H.-I. (2015, June 3). Chronic gastritis. *Scandinavian Journal of Gastroenterology, 50*(6), 657–667. doi:10.3109/00365521.2015.1019918

■ GASTROESOPHAGEAL REFLUX DISEASE

Kelly Ann Lynn

Overview

Gastroesophageal reflux is a normal process that occurs in healthy adults and children when stomach contents briefly back up or "reflux" into the esophagus. Gastroesophageal reflux disease (GERD) is a consensus diagnosis that refers to the bothersome symptoms or complications that occur as a result of gastroesophageal reflux (Vakil, van Zanten, Kahrilas, Dent, Jones, & Global Consensus Group, 2006). Patients with GERD may be at increased risk of developing esophageal stricture, Barrett's esophagus, and esophageal cancer (Francis et al., 2013; Katz, Gerson, & Vela, 2013). GERD has been indicated in increased morbidity related to aspiration, particularly with intubated patients and exacerbation of symptoms for patients with asthma. Nursing care of patients with GERD focuses on prevention of complications, education, and management of symptoms and medications.

Background

Incidence of GERD is fairly common and is reported to affect 20% to 30% of the U.S. population (Katz et al., 2013; Kleiman et al., 2013). GERD may affect up to 40% of the U.S. population (Francis et al., 2013; Vaezi et al., 2016). Although there is no significant demographic predisposition to GERD, incidence is lower in Eastern Asia as compared to Western Europe and North America (Lightdale & Gremse, 2013). GERD is present in both adult and pediatric populations.

The costs associated with GERD are astounding. Kleiman et al. (2013) reported 5.5 million U.S. outpatient visits in 2002 and 76,000 inpatient admissions in 2005 for GERD-related care, and over $10 billion spent on acid-reducing medications in 2004. Likewise, Francis et al. (2013) note national expenditures ranging from $9.3 billion to $12.1 billion for GERD-related care.

GERD is associated with weakness or malfunction of the lower esophageal sphincter (LES), which connects the esophagus to the stomach. GERD affects the LES, a muscle connecting the esophagus and stomach. Gastric contents back up, or reflux, into the esophagus due to changes in LES muscle tone or increased pressure below the sphincter. Other factors contributing to the pathophysiology of GERD include decreased esophageal motility, which may be related to underlying diseases like achalasia or possibly the result of allergies or other inflammatory reactions. Pregnancy, obesity, and hiatal hernias also increase the incidence of GERD.

Patients with GERD typically present with complaints of heartburn, regurgitation, and sour taste in the mouth. These are also called *esophageal symptoms*. Atypical presentation (extraesophageal symptoms) include chronic cough, hoarseness, sore throat, worsening oral health, recurrent earache and ear infections, and nocturnal asthma (Katz et al., 2013; Lightdale & Gremse, 2013). More bothersome symptoms include vomiting, pain, and difficulty swallowing.

Clinical Aspects

ASSESSMENT

A thorough nursing assessment is essential for patients with GERD. This includes a comprehensive patient history with targeted questions related to eating habits and symptom triggers and remedies. Physical assessment should include accurate measurement of the patient's height and weight. Swallowing ability and gag reflex must be assessed to determine risk for aspiration. Patients presenting with pain (chest pain radiating to neck, jaw, and arm) need immediate evaluation to rule out myocardial infarction (MI) and angina as GERD symptoms can mimic these life-threatening conditions.

Review of essential laboratory values includes cardiac enzymes to rule out MI for patients presenting with chest pain, complete blood count (CBC) to assess for anemia, serum chemistry to assess for electrolyte imbalances and malnutrition, and serum iron studies (transferrin, total iron binding capacity, transferring saturation, or ferritin) are collected to help differentiate if an anemia is related to an iron-deficiency or chronic inflammation.

Review of medications is an essential part of the nursing assessment. Anticholinergic medications may delay gastric emptying and should be used cautiously in patients with GERD. Some pain medications (i.e., nonsteroidal anti-inflammatory drugs [NSAIDs] and aspirin) may cause gastritis and GI bleeding and should therefore be avoided.

Older children and adult patients may be prescribed an 8-week course of a proton pump inhibitor (PPI) to alleviate symptoms of GERD as a first-line therapy. PPIs should be taken 30 to 60 minutes before the first meal of the day for maximum efficacy. It is essential to review the prescribed schedule for PPI administration as studies have shown up to 70% of primary care practitioners in the United States advised patients to take the PPI at bedtime (Katz et al., 2013). Nurses should counsel patients on the appropriate dose and timing of PPIs.

NURSING INTERVENTIONS, MANAGEMENT, AND IMPLICATIONS

Nursing care of patients with GERD should be tailored to the patients' symptoms and clinical status. The focus of care should be prevention of the serious consequences related to GERD. Optimizing compliance with medication, diet, and lifestyle modifications will reduce symptoms of GERD and promote quality of life.

It is important that the nurses involved in the care of patients with GERD educate patients on all aspects of treatment and management. All medications should be reviewed for potential adverse interactions and side effects. Patients should be educated on proper administration of medications to maximize the effective relief of symptoms.

Knowledge of simple lifestyle modifications and medication therapy may be the only measures needed to reach treatment goals. Patients who are unresponsive to medical management and who are experiencing considerable distress from symptoms may be referred for esophageal testing (endoscopy, esophageal pH study, manometry) and/or surgical intervention. These patients need education about the planned interventions and specific issues related to various surgical options (fundoplication, myotomy). Symptoms can be alleviated by educating patients and their families about dietary recommendations and lifestyle modifications. Some eating habits can help manage symptoms of heartburn and reflux. Patients should be advised to practice mindful eating in a calm and relaxed environment, chew thoroughly, and avoid eating while standing. Remind patients to eat small meals and snacks to avoid overeating and abdominal distention. Dinner should be a lighter meal and patients should wait 2 to 3 hours after eating before they lie down.

Some foods and beverages cause the LES to relax and thus increase gastric secretions and acid level in the stomach subsequently causing "heartburn" and reflux symptoms. Patients should be educated to stay away from foods that are known to exacerbate symptoms. These include fruits and vegetables like bell peppers, tomatoes, and tomato sauce; citrus fruits and juices; beans; and cabbages. Heavy, high-fat, and fried foods should be avoided as well as spicy food, mints, and chocolate. Caffeine, carbonated beverages, and alcohol, especially red wine, should be avoided.

Patients should be encouraged to consume a healthy diet of lean protein, low-fat dairy products, heart-healthy fats, and whole grains. Some dietary additions that may alleviate symptoms include ginger, Chamomile tea, and fermented foods (i.e., kimchee, sauerkraut, kefir, tempeh, miso, plain yogurt, or kombucha). Keeping a food journal may help patients identify foods that trigger symptoms. Once a patient has achieved thorough and complete remission of symptoms through medication and lifestyle modifications, he or she may slowly reintroduce foods one at a time to ensure that they do not exacerbate symptoms.

Patients with GERD are encouraged to adopt healthy lifestyle habits. Weight loss, avoiding alcohol and smoking, and incorporating stress-reducing behaviors (exercise, yoga, meditation) all correlate with symptom relief. Patients should avoid tight clothing as this can increase pressure on the LES and exacerbate symptoms. Likewise, lying flat can promote reflux so patients are encouraged to sleep on several pillows.

Management of GERD symptoms centers around lifestyle and diet modification. Adherence to these modifications may cause stress for patients and their families. Parents of children and babies with GERD may become hypervigilant about the child's appetite, nutrition intake, and eating behaviors. This may lead to increased anxiety and tension around meals. Nurses must offer patients and their families support and encouragement as they manage their symptoms.

OUTCOMES

The expected outcomes of evidence-based nursing care for patients with GERD are effective management of symptoms and medications prescribed to treat them, increased quality of life, decreased incidence of serious consequences of GERD like aspiration pneumonia and exacerbation of asthma, and reduced sequelae of disease (i.e., Barrett's esophagus, esophageal adenocarcinoma).

Summary

GERD is a complicated health issue that can affect people of all demographics. The symptoms of GERD can adversely affect quality of life. Diagnosis can be elusive and effective management may rely on trial and error. Nursing care is essential to supporting patients through this process while promoting compliance with care plans and minimizing unnecessary distress and morbidity.

Francis, D. O., Rymer, J. A., Slaughter, J. C., Choksi, Y., Jiramongkolchai, P., Ogbeide, E., . . . Vaezi, M. F. (2013). High economic burden of caring for patients with suspected extraesophageal reflux. *American Journal of Gastroenterology*, *108*(6), 905–911. doi:10.1038/ajg.2013.69

Katz, P. O., Gerson, L. B., & Vela, M. F. (2013). Guidelines for the diagnosis and management of gastroesophageal reflux disease. *American Journal of Gastroenterology*, *108*(3), 308–328; quiz 329. doi:10.1038/ajg.2012.444

Kleiman, D. A., Sporn, M. J., Beninato, T., Metz, Y., Crawford, C., Fahey, T. J., & Zarnegar, R. (2013). Early referral for 24-hour esophageal pH monitoring may prevent unnecessary treatment with acid-reducing medications. *Surgical Endoscopy*, *27*(4), 1302–1309. doi:10.1007/s00464-012-2602-z

Lightdale, J. R., & Gremse, D. A.; Section on Gastroenterology, Hepatology, and Nutrition. (2013). Gastroesophageal reflux: Management guidance for the pediatrician. *Pediatrics*, *131*(5), e1684–e1695. doi:10.1542/peds.2013-0421

Vaezi, M. F., Brill, J. V., Mills, M. R., Bernstein, B. B., Ness, R. M., Richards, W. O., . . . Patel, K. (2016). An episode payment framework for gastroesophageal reflux disease. *Gastroenterology*, *150*(4), 1019–1025. doi:10.1053/j.gastro.2016.02.037

Vakil, N., van Zanten, S. V., Kahrilas, P., Dent, J., & Jones, R.; Global Consensus Group. (2006). The Montreal definition and classification of gastroesophageal reflux disease: A global evidence-based consensus. *American Journal of Gastroenterology*, *101*(8), 1900–1920; quiz 1943. doi:10.1111/j.1572-0241.2006.00630.x

■ GOUT

Maria A. Mendoza

Overview

Gout is a hereditary disease caused by deposits of uric acid crystals (monosodium urate) in the peripheral joints leading to inflammation. The most common site of inflammation is usually in the metatarsophalangeal joint of the great toe. Gout is also known as *gouty arthritis* and is the most common form of inflammatory arthritis. From 2007 to 2008, the National Health and Nutrition Survey (NHANES) found that 3.9% (8.3 million) of adults (20 years and more) self-reported a diagnosis of gout, a 1.2% increase over the past decade (Centers for Disease Control and Prevention [CDC], 2016). Men are afflicted more often (5.9%) than women (2.0%) with Black men affected about twice as often as White men (10.9% vs. 5.8%) (CDC, 2016). Data from the Health Professionals Follow-up Study showed an increased risk of all-cause mortality and cardiovascular disease mortality in men with gout (CDC, 2016). A diagnosis of gout has been associated with a poor quality of life (CDC, 2016). The major challenge to nurses caring for patients with gout is managing pain during acute episodes as well as preventing recurrent attacks.

Background

Gout can become a chronic disease with long remissions followed by acute exacerbations. Acute attacks are caused by excessive intake of rich food and alcohol, particularly beer. Gout is a complex disorder with both genetic and environmental risk factors, including increased age, hyperuricemia, dietary habits (intake of alcohol, sweetened beverages, fructose, seafood, meat, dairy product, coffee, and vitamin C), diuretic use, obesity, insulin resistance and metabolic syndrome, and impaired kidney function (Fuerst, 2015; Hainer, Matheson, & Wilkes, 2014; Harding, 2016).

Urates, a form of uric acid, are by-products of purine metabolism, a substance present in all body tissues and foods. Urates are excreted through the kidneys to maintain a serum uric acid level between 4 and 6.8 mg/dL. Increased production coupled with decreased excretion of urates results in hyperuricemia (serum level greater than 6.8 mg/dL). It is interesting to note that hyperuricemia does not always progress to gout unless there is crystallization of urates, resulting in inflammation.

The clinical presentation of gout includes extremely painful, inflamed, tender joints. It can involve any joint in the body but the metatarsophalangeal joint of the great toe is a common site because of the increased pressure on this joint during walking. Patients also report weakness, nausea, chills, and frequent urination. Untreated gout can lead to serious injury. Urate crystals can accumulate in the kidneys, leading to stone formation, and in the joints (tophi). Tophi are found in the fingers and in cartilage, such as the ears, and can lead to inflammation, scarring, and deformity. Appearance of tophi is commonly referred as *tophaceous gout*. A definitive diagnosis of gout is made through synovial fluid analysis for urate crystals in the affected joint. However, in primary care, a diagnosis of gout may be made through the patient's history and clinical presentation, including a rapid acute onset of symptoms, unilateral metatarsophalangeal joint involvement, and prior episodes (Harding, 2016). The uric acid level is not diagnostic as half of the patients with acute gout have normal levels; obtaining a baseline value is recommended to monitor the effectiveness of therapy (Harding, 2016; Qaseem, Harris, & Forciea, 2016).

Clinical Aspects

ASSESSMENT

The nurse should perform a comprehensive history to determine the presence of the aforementioned risk factors. Physical assessment includes vital signs, height and weight, body mass index (BMI), examination of the involved joint, signs of insulin resistance markers such as acanthosis nigricans, and assessment for tophi in joints and ears. Laboratory screening for uric acid may be ordered as well as examination of the synovial fluid from joint aspirate to look for urate crystals.

NURSING INTERVENTIONS, MANAGEMENT, AND IMPLICATIONS

Applicable nursing diagnoses for the patient with gout include pain, acute or chronic; deficient knowledge; and impaired physical mobility.

The following interventions are primarily based on the American College of Physician's guidelines for managing the patient with gout (Qaseem et al., 2017).

Medication and dietary adherence is of primary importance during prophylactic treatment. The nurse is responsible for teaching the patient about the actions, side/adverse effects, and proper administration of prescribed medications. Acute attacks of gout are managed with pharmacologic treatment. Numerous randomized controlled trials (RCTs) show that colchicine and non-steroidal anti-inflammatory drugs (NSAIDs), such as naproxen, indomethacin, and sulindac, are effective in controlling pain in acute gout. Gastrointestinal adverse effects are common and these medications should be taken with food. Corticosteroids are used in acute exacerbations and their inflammatory effect is equivalent to NSAIDs. Patients should be taught signs of adverse effects of NSAIDs and steroids. Patients should be taught to avoid aspirin and niacin, which can precipitate acute episodes by raising uric acid levels.

To prevent flares, patients should observe some dietary restrictions. Foods high in purine, such as organ meats, beef, lamb, pork, and seafood, are to be avoided. Other food restrictions include sugar-sweetened drinks and fruit juices containing high-fructose corn syrup, vegetables and fruits high in vitamin C, nuts, whole grains, and legumes. The patient should be encouraged to drink at least eight glasses of fluids daily to prevent uric-related urolithiasis. Excessive emotional and physical stress, surgery, and acute illness can also cause a flare. The evidence on dietary counseling showed mixed results. A randomized controlled study by Holland and McGill (2014) demonstrated that diet education resulted in significant improvement in knowledge of the intervention group but had no effect on serum urate level at 6 months.

Urate-lowering therapy is considered in patients with tophi, a history of two or more acute episodes of inflammation per year, stage 2 or higher chronic kidney disease (CKD), or a history of urolithiasis. RCTs show that the use of low-dose colchicine and NSAID or NSAID alone is effective in reducing the risk of acute attacks in patients initiating urate-lowering therapy. Allopurinol is the first line of treatment, gradually titrated every 2 to 5 weeks to reach desired serum uric acid level. Lower doses are used in patients with significant CKD. A more expensive medication, febuxostat, does not require dose adjustment in CKD. Probenecid is prescribed for patients with contraindications to either allopurinol or febuxostat with no history of urolithiasis and creatinine clearance above 50 mL/min. The nurse should inform the patient not to take aspirin, which would cancel the effects of the drug. Prophylaxis may continue for 3 months in persons without tophi and up to 6 months if tophi are present.

Nonpharmacological pain management, such as topical ice application on the affected joints 30 minutes four times a day, nonweight bearing on affected joints, and bedrest, are recommended during severe attacks.

The nurse plays a supportive role during acute episodes that affect the functional and mobility status of the patient. The environment has to be assessed to ensure patient safety. Provisions of safety and mobility aids may be necessary. Emotional support should be provided as needed.

Summary

Gout is an inflammatory disease of the peripheral joints caused by accumulation of urate crystals with both genetic and environmental risk factors. Typical presentation is an acute onset of unilateral joint redness, swelling, and pain. Analysis of synovial fluid from the involved joint for presence of urate crystals is the gold standard for diagnosing gout, but diagnosis is usually made from history and clinical presentation in primary care. Gout is managed by pharmacologic treatment during acute episode and as prophylaxis. The nurse's responsibility is supporting the patient in managing symptoms, reducing flares, and monitoring effects of therapy. Patient education related to diet counseling, medication teaching, and lifestyle modification is an important part of nursing care.

Centers for Disease Control and Prevention. (2016). Arthritis. Retrieved from https://www.cdc.gov/arthritis/basics/gout.html

Fuerst, M. L. (2015). How common is gout in the United States, really? *Rheumatology Network, 11*(11), 649–662.

Hainer, B. L., Matheson, E., & Wilkes, R. T. (2014). Diagnosis, treatment, and prevention of gout. *American Family Physician, 90*(12), 831–836.

Harding, M. (2016). An update on gout for primary care providers. *Nurse Practitioner, 41*(4), 14–21; quiz 21. doi:10.1097/01.NPR.0000481510.32360.fa

Holland, R., & McGill, N. W. (2015). Comprehensive dietary education in treated gout patients does not further improve serum urate. *Internal Medicine Journal, 45*(2), 189–194. doi:10.1111/imj.12661

Qaseem, A., Harris, R. P., & Forciea, M. A.; Clinical Guidelines Committee of the American College of Physicians. (2017). Management of acute and recurrent gout: A clinical practice guideline from the American College of Physicians. *Annals of Internal Medicine, 166*(1), 58–68. doi:10.7326/M16-0570

■ GUILLAIN–BARRÉ SYNDROME

Kathleen Marsala-Cervasio

Overview

Guillain–Barré syndrome (GBS) is the most common acute inflammatory polyneuropathy characterized by rapid, progressive, and symmetrical neuromuscular paralysis (Willison, Jacobs, & van Doorn, 2016). The annual incidence in the United States is 0.6 to 1.9 per 100,000 persons per year with 0.6 per 100,000 cases in children, and 2 to 7 per 100,000 persons per year in the elderly (Willison et al., 2016). It is believed that this disease is an autoimmune disorder triggered by infections, surgery, or vaccinations (Walling & Dickson, 2013). A severe manifestation of the disease triggers respiratory failure in approximately 25% of all cases and is fatal in 5% to 10% of cases worldwide (Walling & Dickson, 2013). GBS requires intensive nursing care to identify rapid progression and intervention as well as specific teaching and rehabilitation. Early detection of GBS is crucial to management of the syndrome.

Background

GBS is a fulminant polyradiculoneuropathy, characterized by progressive weakness and diminished to absent myotatic reflexes (Willison et al., 2016). First reported in the literature in 1834, this syndrome is believed to be triggered by infection stimulating an antiganglioside antibody production (Rajabally & Uncini, 2012). In approximately 70% of cases of GBS, symptoms occurs 1 to 3 weeks after an acute infectious process (Rajabally & Uncini, 2012). The organisms most commonly involved are *Campylobacter jejuni*, *Mycoplasma pneumonia*, *Haemophilus influenza*, cytomegalovirus, Epstein–Barr virus, and influenza (Willison et al., 2016). According to Rajabally and Uncini (2016), the administration of antirabies, influenza, and swine flu vaccines were all associated with an increase in the incidence of GBS.

Clinical Aspects

Clinical features of GBS include areflexia, progressive limb weakness initially in the legs, and uncommon sensory loss to the bulbar, facial, and respiratory function within 2 to 4 weeks after onset, the time of maximum severity of symptoms (Willison et al., 2016). Typically, after a month of symptom onset, remyelination occurs and the recovery process begins, lasting from weeks to years, often with residual effects.

Additional GBS symptoms include autonomic dysfunction and pain. Pain is the first reported symptom accompanied with numbness and tingling in the hands and feet bilaterally (Willison et al., 2016). Progressive symmetrical weakness occurs from the distal to proximal extremities with diminished reflexes, proprioception, and vibratory sensation (Moore & Shepard, 2014). Autonomic dysfunction may be characterized by arrhythmias, blood pressure instability, respiratory dysfunction, dysphagia, dysarthria, and facial paralysis. Children initially present with the inability to walk in over 50% of GBS cases; rarely is the syndrome seen in infants (Willison et al., 2016). Recently, Zika virus and dengue fever have been responsible for reported cases of GBS outside the United States (van den Berg et al., 2014).

ASSESSMENT

Assessment for GBS begins with a history, specifically asking about either viral gastrointestinal or respiratory infections in the 2 weeks prior to symptom onset. Physical findings may include difficulty in walking, numbness in the hands and feet, body weakness, and functional decline in the prior few days. As GBS progresses, there is fever and bladder and bowel dysfunction (van den Berg et al., 2014). Laboratory tests may include a cytological examination of cerebral spinal fluid, which usually reveals an increased level of protein. Immunoglobulins and serum protein electrophoresis may have decreased levels of immunoglobulin (IgA). Blood tests may reveal cytomegalovirus or Epstein–Barr virus, and stool cultures may identify *C. jejuni*. Other diagnostic studies may include nerve conduction velocity studies, electromyography, electrocardiogram, and pulmonary function tests. Plasma exchange therapy and intravenous immune globulin therapy have been shown to haste recovery (Rosen, 2012).

NURSING INTERVENTIONS, MANAGEMENT, AND IMPLICATIONS

Initial nursing assessment consists of a history, complete physical, and psychosocial evaluation of potential signs or symptoms of GBS. Documentation must include recent travel as well as recent viral illnesses, vaccinations, and surgeries. Recent and current

medications should be reviewed with the medical team. A neurological assessment should include the Glasgow Coma Scale, particular evaluation of muscle strength in all extremities, and questions for the presence of numbness and tingling of extremities, particularly the lower extremities. Filaments may be used for extremity sensory assessment. A complete set of vital signs should include oxygen saturation and a pain assessment. The respiratory system is thoroughly evaluated. If the patient is in a monitored environment, all vital signs should be continuously monitored with alarm settings on to identify any deviations quickly. As the nurse proceeds to continue assessing the patient, specific questions about bladder and bowel incontinence will be evaluated.

Safety is a priority and nurses should include a fall-prevention protocol that includes three rails up, call bell in reach, and frequent checks for activities of daily living. Weakness can also lead to other injuries like burns from hot drinks. Skin breakdown may occur and therefore prevention is key and implementation of skin care protocols a priority. Constant observation for incontinence is necessary to prevent skin breakdown. Patients with GBS should be on aspiration precautions with oxygen and suction at the bedside and the head of the bed up. Venous thrombosis prevention by passive or active range of motion, intermittent pneumatic compression devices, or anticoagulant prophylaxis may be indicated. Referral to physical therapy, plus occupational and speech therapy for swallowing assessment may be indicated. The nurse should ensure communication, assess coping mechanisms, screen for depression, and plan for rehabilitation with the patients and their families.

OUTCOMES

The administration of corticosteroids has not demonstrated any benefit to prognosis. Supportive therapy includes pain management, monitoring vital signs, frequent respiratory assessments, and a focus on preventing complications while hospitalized. Neurological problems will persist in up to 20% of patients with GBS, and one half of these patients will be severely disabled (van den Berg et al., 2014).

Summary

GBS is potentially life-threatening; no cure is known. A history and physical findings with specific questions by the registered nurse (RN) can identify early symptoms and intervention. GBS requires an interdisciplinary approach to care, recovery, and long-term rehabilitation. Increased awareness of GBS screening is vital in a time of identification of new organisms, that is, Zika, increased use of vaccinations, and increased surgical interventions.

Moore, A. S., & Shepard, L. H. (2014). Myasthenia gravis vs. Guillain–Barré syndrome—What's the difference? *Nursing Made Incredibly Easy, 12*(4), 20–30.

Rajabally, Y. A., & Uncini, A. (2012). Outcome and its predictors in Guillain–Barre syndrome. *Journal of Neurology, Neurosurgery, and Psychiatry, 83*(7), 711–718. doi:10.1136/jnnp-2011-301882

Rosen, B. A. (2012). Guillain–Barré syndrome. *Pediatrics in Review, 33*(4), 164–70; quiz 170. doi:10.1542/pir.33-4-164

van den Berg, V., Walgaard, C., Drenthen, J., Fokke, C., Jacobs, B., & van Doorn, P. (2014). Guillain–Barré syndrome: Pathogenesis, diagnosis, treatment, and prognosis. *Neurology*, (10), 469–482.

Walling, A. D., & Dickson, G. (2013). Guillain–Barré syndrome. *American Family Physician, 87*(3), 191–197.

Willison, H. J., Jacobs, B. C., & van Doorn, P. A. (2016). Guillain–Barré syndrome. *Lancet, 388*(10045), 717–727. doi:10.1016/S0140-6736(16) 00339-1

■ HEART FAILURE

Arlene Travis

Overview

Heart failure (HF) is a common condition associated with significant mortality, morbidity, reduction in quality of life, and health care costs. Nurses play an important role in the care of patients with HF. Well-informed nurses, skilled in the care of patients with HF, make significant contributions to the health and well-being of these patients.

HF is a syndrome characterized by the inability of the heart to supply the body with sufficient blood and oxygen to meet its metabolic needs. HF is a chronic condition, with no cure, characterized by flares in disease severity, requiring lifelong management to control symptoms and maintain optimal cardiac function. Patients with HF are subject to episodes of rapid worsening of symptoms, at which point chronic HF becomes acute HF (also known as *acute decompensated HF*), which usually requires hospitalization.

HF is a major public health problem and a global epidemic, affecting approximately 25 million people worldwide and 5.8 million in the United States (Ambrosy et al., 2014; Roger, 2013). The incidence of HF increases sharply with age (Go et al., 2012) and the number of people with HF is expected to rise dramatically due to the aging of the world's population. The number of Americans with HF is projected to increase from 5.8 million in 2012 to 8.5 million by 2030. One of five Americans will develop HF in their lifetime, and about 50% of patients with HF die within 5 years of diagnosis (Centers for Disease Control and Prevention [CDC], 2015). HF is one of the leading causes of hospitalizations in the United States and is responsible for 1 million hospitalizations every year (Pfuntner, Wier, & Stocks, 2013). Costs associated with HF place a significant economic burden on the health care system. In 2012, the cost of HF care in the United States was about $32 billion, and is anticipated to soar to $70 billion by 2030 (Heidenreich et al., 2013.) Hospitalizations account for the majority of the costs of caring for HF patients.

Background

HF begins when an event or insult to the heart impairs its ability to function, causing a reduction in cardiac output (CO). HF can be classified as ischemic or nonischemic depending on the underlying cause. The majority of patients (65%) have ischemic HF. In ischemic HF, decreased oxygenation of the myocardium, usually caused by coronary artery disease, results in decreased CO. In nonischemic HF, factors, such as hypertension or valve disease, cause the decrease in CO.

HF is categorized as systolic or diastolic. This distinction is based on the ejection fraction (EF), a measure of left ventricular (LV) function. EF is measured as the percentage of blood (which has filled the LV in diastole) that is pumped out during systole. In systolic HF (also known as *HF with reduced EF*), the EF is below normal. In diastolic HF (also known as *HF with preserved EF*), the EF remains normal or even high. Diastolic HF is caused by impaired ventricular filling during diastole, resulting in insufficient volume available to be pumped from the LV, whereas systolic HF is caused by impaired pumping action of the LV during systole.

CO (the volume of blood pumped by the heart in 1 minute) is determined by heart rate (HR) and stroke volume (SV), the volume of blood that is pumped from the LV in one myocardial contraction (systole). SV is determined by the interaction of three factors: *preload, afterload,* and *contractility. Preload* refers to volume of blood that fills the heart, *contractility* refers to the force with which the ventricle contracts, and *afterload* refers to the resistance the heart must overcome for blood to exit the ventricle (Butler, 2012).

When CO is reduced, the body attempts to compensate by activating mechanisms that affect both SV and HR (Rogers & Bush, 2015). HR is controlled by the sinoatrial node (SA), which is influenced by the sympathetic nervous system (SNS). Sympathetic activation is one of the key pathophysiologic mechanisms underlying HF; when the CO drops, the SNS is stimulated and HR increases.

Another underlying pathophysiologic process of HF is activation of the renin–angiotensin–aldosterone system (RAAS). As a result of decreased CO, renal perfusion is decreased. As a compensatory mechanism, the RAAS is activated causing the release of angiotensin II and aldosterone. Angiotensin II raises blood pressure (BP), increases afterload, and stimulates aldosterone production, which then leads to sodium and fluid retention and increased preload.

Initially, compensatory mechanisms are successful in restoring CO; however, this is short lived. In fact, these compensatory mechanisms have unintended consequences that actually cause the syndrome of HF. Activation of the SNS increases HR, temporarily restoring CO, but also places additional stress on an already struggling heart, which tires, and CO falls. Activation of the RAAS increases preload and afterload, which initially raise CO; however, additional strain is placed on the heart, and CO decreases even more. Compensatory mechanisms are reactivated over and over in response to successive reductions in CO, and a self-perpetuating cycle of unintended consequences (reduced CO and fluid and sodium retention) is established, which causes HF.

Clinical Aspects

The clinical presentation of HF is directly related to unintended effects of compensatory mechanisms. Reduced CO causes reduced oxygen delivery to the body tissues, causing symptoms of fatigue, activity intolerance, and alterations in mental status. Sodium and fluid retention cause edema, orthopnea, weight gain, pulmonary congestion, dyspnea, and pulmonary edema.

ASSESSMENT

Understanding the pathophysiology of HF is crucial in guiding patient assessment. Patients with HF should be assessed for orientation, cognition, mood, energy level, and activity tolerance, as these reflect CO and tissue oxygenation. Lungs should be auscultated for crackles, which result from volume overload and impaired cardiac function. The heart should be auscultated for rate and rhythm, and for the S3 heart sound, which indicates increased intravascular volume. Cardiac murmurs may reflect valve disease and a displaced apical impulse suggests cardiac enlargement.

Patients should be assessed for indications of fluid retention, such as peripheral edema, anasarca, jugular venous distention, and abdominal distention. Patients with chronic HF may have reduced appetite and nutritional deficiencies. Body weight and changes in weight are critical assessments for HF patients. Increasing weight is a sign of worsening HF, and a weight gain of more than 2 pounds in 1 day or 5 pounds in a week is a red flag and should be reported to the provider.

Vital signs are critical assessments for HF patients. An elevated BP increases afterload, reducing CO. Low blood pressure may reflect insufficient CO, which can compromise tissue oxygenation. Increased HR, especially at rest, is an indicator of cardiac dysfunction. Arrhythmias interfere with cardiac function and should be addressed. Respiratory rate and shortness of breath increase with worsening HF.

Laboratory tests include a metabolic panel and brain natriuretic peptide (BNP). Hyponatremia is associated with poor outcomes in HF patients, as is renal dysfunction. BNP is a hormone produced by the ventricles in response to volume overload and is elevated in persons with HF. BNP levels less than 100 pg/mL indicate no HF, if greater than 400 pg/mL HF is likely; clinical judgment should be used for findings within those ranges. As HF severity increases, BNP levels also increase; with effective treatment of HF, BNP levels should decrease. Patients hospitalized for acute HF should have BNP measured upon admission and in preparation for discharge. Chest x-rays shows size and position of the heart as well as pulmonary congestion. Echocardiography is done to evaluate LV function and determine the EF.

In addition to physical assessment, nurses should assess patients' knowledge and understanding of HF and their role in disease management. HF requires a significant amount of self-management and patients who understand the disease process and management strategies have better outcomes (Yancy et al., 2013).

These assessments allow the nurse to plan appropriate patient education. Health literacy should also be assessed and patient teaching should be tailored to the patient's health literacy level.

NURSING INTERVENTIONS, MANAGEMENT, AND IMPLICATIONS

Pharmacologic therapy and lifestyle modification are the cornerstones of HF management. Medications used to treat HF block or reduce the effects of compensatory mechanisms. Beta-adrenergic antagonists (beta blockers) and angiotensin-converting-enzyme-inhibitors (ACEI) and angiotensin II receptor blockers (ARB) are mainstays of pharmacologic therapy for HF. Beta blockers act by reducing the negative effects of catecholamine stimulation on the myocardium by inhibiting SNS activity. ACEI, ARB, and aldosterone antagonists all block the effects of RAAS activation.

Diuretics, especially the loop diuretics furosemide and bumetanide, are almost always used in the treatment of HF, as they mobilize and eliminate fluid, reduce shortness of breath, and reduce the demand on the heart due to fluid overload. Devices, such as implantable cardiac defibrillators (ICD), may be used to decrease risk of sudden cardiac death. Biventricular pacemakers for "cardiac resynchronization therapy" may be used to optimize synchronous operation of all four chambers of the heart. Newer medications for HF include ivabradine, which directly reduces HR and valsartan-sacubitril, a potent inhibitor of the RAAS (Yancy et al., 2013.) Nursing interventions include patient education on therapeutic effects and side effects and on the importance of adherence to a medication regimen.

Lifestyle modifications for HF patients usually include some fluid and sodium restriction; however, these should be individualized for each patient. Patients with HF should be taught the benefits of smoking cessation and advised to remain physically active and exercise as tolerated to prevent deconditioning. Essential self-management activities include taking medications as directed, adhering to dietary recommendations, attending follow-up appointments, remaining active, understanding the signs and symptoms of worsening failure, and monitoring daily weight (Yancy et al., 2013). Nursing interventions to support lifestyle modification include counseling and teaching patients about risk factor reduction, disease and symptom management, diet, activity, and self-management strategies. Nurses play a key role in patient education and motivation and are often the primary educators for the patients and their families.

OUTCOMES

The desired outcomes of treatment for patients with HF are preventing mortality due to HF, preventing progression of disease, optimizing quality of life, and preventing hospitalizations. Adherence to medical and lifestyle recommendations supports these goals. Patients with HF have the highest rates of unplanned (within 30 days) readmission of all discharge diagnoses. In 2015, 22% of Medicare HF patients had unplanned readmissions (Medicare.gov, 2016). The Centers for Medicare & Medicaid Services (CMS) can impose financial penalties on hospitals with excessive readmissions. In 2016, an estimated 75% of U.S. hospitals were subject to financial penalties for readmissions (Rice, 2015), representing millions of dollars of lost revenue.

Nurses can play a key role in reducing avoidable readmissions as they have primary responsibility for patient education and discharge preparation. Nurses are ideally positioned to evaluate patient readiness for discharge in areas such as (a) knowledge of disease process, (b) physical and functional status, and (c) anticipated support at home, and can intervene if necessary. Patients evaluated by nurses as having low readiness for discharge have higher risk for readmission. Lack of social support is related to poor outcomes in patients with HF (Weiss, Costa, Yakusheva, & Bobay, 2013), and nurses may intervene by involving social services or case management to obtain needed assistance. HF may also cause cognitive impairment and depression, which increase readmission risk. Nurses can assess patients for these problems and mobilize the health care team for management strategies if indicated. Managing HF can be challenging and demoralizing to patients, and nurses can provide much-needed counseling, emotional support, and encouragement.

Summary

HF is a complex problem with significant mortality and impact on patient quality of life that is influenced by medical, individual, social, and health care delivery system factors. Incidence and prevalence increase dramatically with an aging population. Management by multidisciplinary teams that include nurses is associated with better patient outcomes. Nurses will be called on to practice to the full extent of their scope to meet the health care needs of millions of HF patients, and are ideally positioned to use their knowledge and skills to improve outcomes and prevent readmissions in this growing patient population.

Ambrosy, A., Fonarow, G., Butler, J., Chioncel, O., Greene, S., Vaduganathan, M., . . . Gheorghiade, M. (2014). The global health and economic burden of hospitalizations for heart failure. *Journal of the American College of Cardiology*, *63*(12), 1123–1133. doi:10.1016/j.jacc.2013.11.053

Butler, J. (2012). An overview of chronic heart failure management. *Nursing Times*, *108*(14/15), 16–20. Retrieved from http://www.nursingtimes.net/clinical-archive/cardiology/an-overview-of-chronic-heart-failure-management/5043315.fullarticle

Centers for Disease Control and Prevention. (2015). Heart failure fact sheet. Retrieved from http://www.cdc.gov/dhdsp/data_statistics/fact_sheets/docs/fs_heart_failure.pdf

Go, A., Mozaffarian, D., Roger, V., Benjamin, E., Berry, J., Borden, W., . . . Turner, M. (2012). Heart disease and stroke statistic—2013 update: A report from the American Heart Association. *Circulation*, *127*(1), e6–e245. doi:10.1161/cir.0b013e31828124ad

Heidenreich, P., Albert, N., Allen, L., Bluemke, D., Butler, J., Fonarow, G., . . . Trogdon, J. G. (2013). Forecasting the impact of heart failure in the United States: A policy statement from the American Heart Association. *Circulation: Heart Failure*, *6*(3), 606–619. doi:10.1161/hhf.0b013e318291329a

Medicare.gov. (2016). Medicare hospital comparison of care. Retrieved from https://www.medicare.gov/hospitalcompare/search.html

Pfuntner, A., Wier, L., & Stocks, C. (2013). Statistical brief #162: Most frequent conditions in U.S. hospitals, 2011. Healthcare Cost and Utilization Project, Agency for Healthcare Quality and Research. Retrieved from http://www.hcup us.ahrq.gov/reports/statbr

Rice, S. (2015). Most hospitals face 30-day readmissions penalty in fiscal 2016. Modern Healthcare. Retrieved from http://www.modernhealthcare.com/article/20150803/NEWS/150809981

Roger, V. (2013). Epidemiology of heart failure. *Circulation Research*, *113*(6), 646–659. doi:10.1161/circresaha.113.300268

Rogers, C., & Bush, N. (2015). Heart failure. *Nursing Clinics of North America*, *50*(4), 787–799. doi:10.1016/j.cnur.2015.07.012

Weiss, M., Costa, L., Yakusheva, O., & Bobay, K. (2014). Validation of patient and nurse short forms of the readiness for hospital discharge scale and their relationship to return to the hospital. *Health Services Research*, *49*(1), 304–317. doi:10.1111/1475-6773.12092

Yancy, C. W., Jessup, M., Bozkurt, B., Butler, J., Casey, D., & Drazner, M., . . . Wilkoff, B. L. (2013). 2013 ACCF/AHA guideline for the management of heart failure: A report of the American College of Cardiology Foundation/American Heart Association task force on practice guidelines. *Circulation*, *128*(16), e240–327. doi:10.1161/cir.0b013e31829e8776

■ HEMOLYTIC ANEMIA

Rebecca M. Lutz
Charrita Ernewein

Overview

Hemolytic anemia (HA) is the expression of an underlying disease process. Hemolysis of the red blood cell (RBC) is a form of anemia resulting from the decrease in circulating RBCs (Barcellini & Fettizzo, 2015; Manchanda, 2015). HA may be acute or chronic, mild to severe, intravascular or extravascular, inherited or acquired (Bunn, 2017; Doig, 2015; Manchanda, 2015). An in-depth patient history, with the benefit of laboratory testing, aids diagnosis. Treatment is based on the differentiation of the underlying pathology (Cornett, 2017).

Background

Anemia is a general term indicating a decrease in circulating RBCs caused by a disease or deficiency and characterized by a decrease in the hemoglobin or hematocrit levels (Manchanda, 2015). Anemia results from a decrease in RBC production, an increase in RBC destruction, with an inability of the bone marrow to sufficiently compensate for the hemolysis, or a decrease in total blood volume (Barcellini & Fettizzo, 2015; Doig, 2015; Manchanda, 2015). The World Health Organization (WHO) estimated that 1.62 billion persons (24.8%) worldwide are affected by some form of anemia (WHO, 2008). The impact of HA on morbidity and mortality, quality of life, and levels of disability is linked to the severity of the underlying disorder and available treatment.

The RBC is produced by the bone marrow through the process of erythropoiesis. With a life span of 120 days, the primary function of the RBC is the exchange of gases within the body. Hemoglobin, a protein within the RBC, binds to oxygen in the lungs for transport to the tissues. In the event of hemolysis, decreasing levels of circulating oxygen stimulate the release of erythropoietin from the kidneys. Erythropoietin stimulates bone marrow to increase RBC production. Increased RBC production allows the body to compensate for hemolysis (Bunn, 2017; Doig, 2015; Manchanda, 2015).

Inherited hemolytic disorders result from intracellular (intrinsic) defects of the cell, enzyme deficiencies resulting in altered cell metabolism, or hemoglobin disorders (Bunn, 2017; Doig, 2015; Manchanda, 2015). Hereditary disorders include spherocytosis, elliptocytosis, xerocytosis, and stomatocytosis. The most common form, hereditary spherocytosis, is an autosomal dominant mutation. Glucose-6-phosphate dehydrogenase (G6PD) deficiency, an enzymatic disorder, is the most common X-linked chromosomal disorder. Inherited hemoglobin disorders, such as sickle cell (autosomal recessive) and thalassemia (autosomal dominant), result in acute, chronic, or episodic HA.

Acquired hemolytic disorders result from extracellular (extrinsic) factors such as infections, trauma, chemical exposures, or immunological disorders (Bunn, 2017; Doig, 2015; Manchanda, 2015). Acquired hemolytic disorders result from an array of causes: bacterial or protozoal infections, mechanical heart valves or dialysis, chemical exposure to toxins such as drugs or venoms, or autoimmune or alloimmune responses. Autoimmune hemolytic anemia (AIHA) results from the production of antibodies: immunoglobulin G (IgG; warm agglutinin syndrome) or immunoglobulin M (IgM; cold agglutinin syndrome).

Clinical Aspects

ASSESSMENT

Clinical manifestations of HAs are dependent on the type and severity of the anemia (Barcellini & Fettizzo, 2015; Cornett, 2017). The most direct indicators of the clinical severity of HAs are the hemoglobin level and the level of hemolysis. Hemoglobin values at diagnosis are also important predictors of patient outcomes, correlating with the risk of death and multiple therapy lines (Barcellini & Fettizzo, 2015). Clinical presentation of patients with HA is influenced by the onset of the anemia, focusing on whether the onset was abrupt or gradual. Close monitoring of hemoglobin levels is a critical component in disease management and treatment response evaluation (Barcellini & Fettizzo, 2015).

Signs and symptoms of HA vary based on the type and severity of the disease and directly arise from hemolysis. Mild cases of HA may present without signs and symptoms. The most common symptom of all types of anemia is fatigue (Cornett, 2017). Clinically, the main signs of HA include jaundice, splenomegaly, and dark urine. Patients may also present with fatigue, pallor, dizziness, hypotension, shortness of breath, and tachycardia (Cornett, 2017; Doig, 2015).

Laboratory features of HA specifically relate to the hemolysis and erythropoietic response of the bone marrow (Cornett, 2017). Diagnostic testing initially includes a complete blood count (CBC), peripheral smear, reticulocyte count, serum bilirubin, lactate dehydrogenase (LDH), haptoglobin alanine aminotransferase (ALT), and a Coombs test (Capriotti & Frizzell, 2016). If HA is suspected, specific testing would be required for a definitive diagnosis of a specific type of HA.

Nursing assessment and interventions for patients with potential anemia involve the collection of subjective and objective data. The nurse should collect a detailed review of patients' medical history, medications, and their family medical history. Frequent monitoring of vital signs and oxygen saturation is also indicated. The nurse should be proficient in understanding laboratory values. Appropriate nursing diagnoses applicable to patients with HA include hypoxemia, activity intolerance based on fatigue, risk for injury, and deficient knowledge. Specific nursing interventions are dependent on the etiology of the HA. Interventions should be directed at establishing balance in daily activities while safely integrating rest and exercise. Patient education, monitoring, and follow-up are significant in relation to promoting positive patient outcomes (Cornett, 2017).

Treatment of HA varies based on the type, cause, and severity of the disease. Age, family medical history, and overall health are other factors that affect treatment. Management also includes blood transfusions, medications, surgery, plasmapheresis, blood and bone marrow transplants, and lifestyle changes (Bass, Tuscano, & Tuscano, 2014). Blood transfusions are required to treat severe or life-threatening HA. Medicines, primarily glucocorticoids, are the mainstay in treating some types of HA, especially AIHA. Plasmapheresis, a process that removes antibodies from the blood, can be used to treat immune HA after other treatments have failed. Splenectomy can stop or reduce high rates of RBC destruction (Bass et al., 2014). The goals of treatment include reducing or stopping RBC destruction, increasing RBC count to therapeutic levels, and treatment of the underlying cause of the condition.

OUTCOMES

There are many causes of HA and positive outcomes depend on the cause and severity (Cornett, 2017). Mild HA may require no treatment; yet severe HA requires prompt treatment to avoid mortality. Some causes of acquired HA can be prevented. Avoidance of triggers is effective in certain types of HA. Acquired forms of HA may resolve if the cause is identified and treated (Bass et al., 2014). Ongoing treatment may be required for inherited HA (Cornett, 2017).

Summary

HAs are a group of heterogeneous diseases, inherited or acquired, causing challenges in diagnosis and treatment (Barcellini & Fettizzo, 2015). With over 1.62 billion persons affected by anemia, the impact of HA is based on the underlying disorder and available treatment options. Signs and symptoms of HA vary based on the type and severity of the disease, yet clinically, the main signs of HA include jaundice, splenomegaly, and dark urine (Cornett, 2017). Although diagnostic testing, medical management, and nursing interventions vary based on the type, cause, and severity of the disease, the goals of treatment remain consistent to improve long-term patient outcomes.

Barcellini, W., & Fettizzo, B. (2015). Clinical application of hemolytic markers in the differential diagnosis and management of hemolytic anemia. *Disease Markers, 2015*, 635670. doi:10.1155/2015/635670

Bass, G., Tuscano, E., & Tuscano, J. (2014). Diagnosis and classification of autoimmune hemolytic anemia. *Autoimmune Reviews, 13*, 560–564. doi:10.1016/j.autrev.2013.11.010

Bunn, H. F. (2017). Overview of the anemias. In J. C. Aster & H. F. Bunn (Eds.), *Pathophysiology of blood disorders* (2nd ed., pp. 32–46). New York, NY: McGraw-Hill. Retrieved from http://accessmedicine.mhmedical.com.ezproxy.hsc.usf.edu/book.aspx?bookid=1900

Cornett, P. (2017). Hemolytic anemia. In E. Bope & R. Kellerman (Eds.), *Conn's current therapy* (pp. 371–376). Philadelphia, PA: Elsevier.

Doig, K. (2015). Introduction to increased destruction of erythrocytes. In E. Keohane, L. Smith, & J. Walenga (Eds.), *Rodak's hematology: Clinical principles and applications* (5th ed., pp. 348–356). St. Louis, MO: Elsevier. Retrieved from http://site.ebrary.com/lib/univsouthfl/reader.action?docID=11073954

Manchanda, N. (2015). Anemias: Red blood cell morphology and approach to diagnosis. In E. Keohane, L. Smith, & J. Walenga (Eds.), *Rodak's hematology: Clinical principles and applications* (5th ed., pp. 284–296). St. Louis, MO: Elsevier. Retrieved from http://site.ebrary.com/lib/univsouthfl/reader.action?docID=11073954

World Health Organization. (2008). Worldwide prevalence of anemia 1993–2005. Retrieved from http://apps.who.int/iris/bitstream/10665/43894/1/9789241596657_eng .pdf

■ HEPARIN-INDUCED THROMBOCYTOPENIA

Bette K. Idemoto
Jane F. Marek

Overview

Heparin-induced thrombocytopenia (HIT) is an abnormal clotting response to heparin and a complication of heparin therapy in susceptible patients. Heparin is an anticoagulant that has been used for more than 90 years as prophylaxis and treatment of venous or arterial clots in a variety of conditions, including venous thromboembolic disease (deep vein thrombosis [DVT] and pulmonary embolus [PE]), acute coronary syndrome, atrial fibrillation, and cerebrovascular accident. Heparin is also used during transfusions, dialysis, and to maintain patency of some venous access devices. A normal platelet count ranges from 150,000 to 450,000 platelets per microliter of blood. Thrombocytopenia or low platelet count can range from mild to severe and places the patient at an increased risk for bleeding. Unfortunately, patients treated with heparin for anticoagulation may experience a paradoxical clotting response thought to be related to an antibody-mediated cascade. Diligent monitoring of the platelet count after exposure to heparin is important for early detection of this abnormal response, known as HIT.

Background

The clotting mechanism involves a complex reaction of cell activation, adhesion, and platelet aggregation. This reaction can be lifesaving by stopping bleeding; however, overactivation may result in the formation of blood clots or thrombi. Blood clots within vessels and organs can lead to skin necrosis, limb ischemia and possible amputation, end-organ damage, and death.

Over 30 years ago, clinicians began to report case studies with thrombocytopenia in patients who had been exposed to heparin. These patients presented with an abrupt decline in platelet count and paradoxical platelet aggregation. Central features of the HIT syndrome include thrombocytopenia and increased platelet aggregation. HIT may develop within hours or up to 14 days after initiation of heparin therapy. Type 1 HIT is a nonimmunologic response that occurs within hours of exposure to heparin and results in a mild transient thrombocytopenia. Type 1 HIT is usually self-limiting and heparin therapy may be continued with close monitoring to detect possible clotting. In contrast, type 2 HIT typically occurs 5 to 10 days after exposure to heparin and is a potentially life-threatening clotting response that activates an immune response resulting in clotting complications (Greinacher, 2015).

It is believed that HIT is caused by the development of antibodies that stimulate platelets after administration of heparin. Heparin and platelet factor 4 (PF4) bind to form an antigen (immunoglobulin [IgG]) in susceptible patients, depending on the particular type of heparin administered, unfractionated heparin (UFH), or low-molecular weight heparin (LMWH). An altered immune response leads to the formation of HIT antibodies (heparin-PF4 antibodies), which in turn, activate the prothrombotic microparticles leading to thrombocytopenia and thrombosis. This thrombosis has occasionally been called *white clot syndrome*.

Although all patients treated with heparin are at risk for developing HIT antibodies, most persons will not develop type 2 HIT. It is estimated that 1% to 8% of patients treated with heparin may develop antibodies, but only half of those develop arterial or venous thrombosis. Patients at increased risk include those with extended periods of prophylactic anticoagulation such as following orthopedic or cardiopulmonary bypass surgery. A higher incidence of type 2 HIT is seen in postoperative patients treated with UFH than patients treated with LMWH (Junqueira, Zorzela, & Perini, 2017). Type 2 HIT risk factors include Caucasian race, female, and age more than 66 years. Contributing factors include previous exposure to heparin, with or without HIT or heparin-induced thrombocytopenia and thrombosis (HITT).

Clinical Aspects

ASSESSMENT

The clinical signs of type 2 HIT include ecchymosis at the heparin injection site and pain, weakness, numbness, and redness or swelling of the extremity. Limb ischemia is seen with DVT; thrombus can cause pulmonary emboli, stroke, acute myocardial infarction, all of which would require anticoagulation. Systemic reactions include chills, fever, dyspnea, and chest pain. Unlike most heparin reactions that result in active bleeding, HIT usually does not cause bleeding, rather patients will develop venous thromboembolism or HITT.

Diagnosis of HIT can be challenging; failure to recognize HIT may result in thrombosis, amputation, or death. Inaccurate diagnosis may result in thrombosis or hemorrhage. Other causes of thrombocytopenia include sepsis with disseminated intravascular coagulation, liver disease, immune thrombocytopenia, and medications (Warkentin, 2016). Many clinicians use the 4-T score to differentiate HIT from other causes of thrombocytopenia (Crowther et al., 2014). Each criterion has a maximum point value of 2; a total score of 0–3 indicates low probability of HIT, 4–5 intermediate probability, and 6–8 high probability. The 4 scoring criteria (4-Ts) are *thrombocytopenia* severity (platelet count greater than 50% and platelet nadir greater than or equal to 20), *timing* of platelet count fall (clear onset between days 5 and 14 or less than or equal to 1 day prior heparin exposure within 30 days), *thrombosis* or other sequelae, and the likelihood of *other* causes of thrombocytopenia. Obesity is associated with increased rates of HIT in patients in critical care units and patient "thickness" could be considered the 5th T in the 4-T scoring system (Bloom et al., 2016). The 4-T score is used in conjunction with other patient assessment data to determine the diagnosis of HIT. The patient with HIT may present with multiple symptoms, including signs of DVT, PE, or stroke and other symptoms, including flushing, chills, fever, dyspnea, and chest pain. Laboratory assessment includes platelet count less than 50,000/mm^3 or sudden drop of 30% to 50% from baseline; heparin-induced platelet aggregation (HIPA) assay, serotonin release assay (SRA) to identify the HIT antigen, and enzyme-linked immunosorbent assay (ELISA) used to detect the HIT antigen, although false positives and lack of specificity limit the usefulness of the test (Nagler, Bachmann, ten Cate, & ten Cate-Hoek, 2016).

NURSING INTERVENTIONS, MANAGEMENT, AND IMPLICATIONS

Management includes recognition of patients at risk for HIT and assessing the patient for other possible causes of thrombocytopenia. Judicious use of heparin according to clinical practice guidelines can reduce unnecessary or prolonged treatment with heparin, thus reducing the risk of HIT. Early mobilization, exercise, and prevention of dehydration may all decrease the need for prophylactic subcutaneous heparin therapy, thus decreasing exposure to heparin and ultimately the risk of HIT. Discharge teaching should include education about HIT, risk factors, and signs and symptoms of HIT that may occur after discharge and before follow-up medical appointments. Patients should be taught to report unusual bruising and signs and symptoms of DVT and PE immediately to the provider.

Early recognition and diagnosis results in improved patient outcomes (Al-Eidan, 2015). All nurses should be aware of the potential for HIT. Strict guidelines and evidence-based interventions regarding maintenance of central venous access devices, implanted ports, and hemodialysis catheters should be followed to avoid unnecessary exposure to heparin. Ongoing physical assessment is important for early recognition and prevention of complications of HIT. Medication teaching should include a clear communication about exposure to heparin and delayed side effects of heparin after discharge.

OUTCOMES

The current standard for anticoagulation and heparin therapy is to obtain both baseline and ongoing laboratory values to monitor the platelet count, the major indicator of HIT. Evidence-based guidelines from the American College of Chest Physicians (ACCP; Garcia, Baglin, Weitz, & Samama, 2012) provide the standard of care for anticoagulation practices. The expertise of hematologists and vascular medicine specialists is an integral part of the interdisciplinary team's plan to manage patients with this complex phenomenon.

General principles of care of patients with HIT include immediate cessation of all heparin (including flushes, coated catheters, dialysate), laboratory testing to confirm the presence of the HIT antigen, alternative anticoagulation measures until the risk of thrombosis is satisfactorily eliminated, careful monitoring of the platelet count, and ongoing assessment for new thrombotic events (McGowan et al., 2016). Administering platelets is not recommended because they may exacerbate the hypercoagulable state.

The ACCP (Garcia et al., 2012) recommends limiting platelet transfusions to patients with severe thrombocytopenia and bleeding or those undergoing an invasive procedure with an increased risk of bleeding. Warfarin is not recommended as it can make the thrombosis worse in HIT; warfarin therapy should not be initiated until the platelet count has recovered to a minimum of 150×10^9/L. Patients should be treated with alternative anticoagulation; bivalirudin (Angiomax) and argatroban (Acova) are direct thrombin inhibitors currently approved for intravenous use in the United States (Garcia et al., 2012). Nursing care should follow the evidence-based guidelines, which have been specified for interdisciplinary teams (Vaughn et al., 2014).

Summary

Although the occurrence of HIT is infrequent, HIT can have devastating outcomes, such as DVT, PE, limb amputation, and death. It is imperative that nurses and all members of the health care team understand the devastating effects of unrecognized and untreated type 2 HIT. Efforts to limit unnecessary exposure to heparin are crucial. Patients receiving heparin must be carefully monitored with routine assessment of the platelet count. Discharge education regarding activity and recognizing the signs and symptoms of HIT is essential for prevention and early detection of HIT or HITT. Future trends include the development of selective anticoagulants with decreased side effects and sensitive diagnostic laboratory tests to adequately detect HIT and alternatives for anticoagulation.

Al-Eidan, F. A. (2015). Pharmacotherapy of heparin-induced thrombocytopenia: Therapeutic options and challenges in the clinical practices. *Journal of Vascular Nursing, 33*(1), 10–20. doi:10.1016/j.jvn.2014.07.001

Bloom, M. B., Zaw, A. A., Hoang, D. M., Mason, R., Alban, R. F., Chung, R., . . . Margulies, D. R. (2016). Body mass index strongly impacts the diagnosis and incidence of heparin-induced thrombocytopenia in the surgical intensive care unit. *Journal of Trauma and Acute Care Surgery, 80*(3), 398–403; discussion 403. doi:10.1097/TA.0000000000000952

Crowther, M., Cook, D., Guyatt, G., Zytaruk, N., McDonald, E., Williamson, D., . . . Warkentin, T. E. (2014). Heparin-induced thrombocytopenia in the critically ill: Interpreting the 4Ts test in a randomized trial. *Journal of Critical Care, 29*(3), 470.7–470.15. doi:10.1016/j.jcrc.2014.02.004

Garcia, D. A., Baglin, T. P., Weitz, J. I., & Samama, M. M. (2012). Parenteral anticoagulants: Antithrombotic therapy and prevention of thrombosis, 9th ed: American College of Chest Physicians evidence-based clinical practice guidelines. *Chest, 141*(2 Suppl.), e24S–e43S. doi:10.1378/chest.11-2291

Greinacher, A. (2015). Heparin-induced thrombocytopenia. *New England Journal of Medicine, 373*(19), 1883–1884. doi:10.1056/NEJMc1510993

Junqueira, D. R., Zorzela, L. M., & Perini, E. (2017). Unfractionated heparin versus low molecular weight heparins for avoiding heparin-induced thrombocytopenia in postoperative patients. *Cochrane Database of Systematic Reviews, 2017*(4), CD007557. doi:10.1002/14651858.CD007557.pub3

McGowan, K. E., Makari, J., Diamantouros, A., Bucci, C., Rempel, P., Selby, R., & Geerts, W. (2016). Reducing the hospital burden of heparin-induced thrombocytopenia:

Impact of an avoid-heparin program. *Blood, 127*(16), 1954–1959. doi:10.1182/blood-2015-07-660001

Nagler, M., Bachmann, L. M., ten Cate, H., & ten Cate-Hoek, A. (2016). Diagnostic value of immunoassays for heparin-induced thrombocytopenia: A systematic review and meta-analysis. *Blood, 127*(5), 546–557. doi:10.1182/blood-2015-07-661215

Vaughn, D. M., Mazur, J., Foster, J., Lazarchick, J., Boylan, A., & Greenberg, C. S. (2014). Implementation of a heparin-induced thrombocytopenia management program reduces the cost of diagnostic testing and pharmacologic treatment in an academic medical center. *Blood, 124*(21), 4848.

Warkentin, T. E. (2015). Heparin-induced thrombocytopenia in critically ill patients. *Seminars in Thrombosis and Hemostasis, 41*(1), 49–60. doi:10.1055/s-0034-1398381

■ HIATAL HERNIA

Maricar P. Gomez

Overview

Hiatal hernia is a condition in which abdominal contents, most commonly of the stomach, protrude through the esophageal hiatus in the diaphragm, and into the thoracic cavity. Hiatal hernias are common in Western countries, specifically in the adult population, affecting more women than men (Qureshi, 2016). Nursing care of patients with hiatal hernia is often directed at assessment of symptoms and education to minimize symptoms and severity of herniation.

Background

Hiatal hernias are classified as either sliding or paraesophageal. Sliding, or type I, hiatal hernias constitute about 90% of hiatal hernia cases and occur when the gastroesophageal junction (GEJ) slides freely in and out of the thorax during changes in position or intraabdominal pressure. Paraesophageal hernias (PEH) are further categorized by extent of herniation (types II, III, or IV). In type II hernias, the gastric fundus migrates above the diaphragm while the GEJ remains in the native subdiaphragmatic position. Type III is a combination of both types I and II, whereas the GEJ and gastric fundus protrude into the thorax through a pathologically widened esophageal hiatus. Finally, type IV refers to the presence of other abdominal visceral contents within the hernia sac such as omentum, spleen, pancreas, colon, or small bowel (Kohn et al., 2013).

Most adults with hiatal hernias are asymptomatic. Symptoms caused by hiatal hernias are a result of intermittent obstruction of the gastrointestinal tract and a lax or unsupported lower esophageal sphincter allowing reflux. Obstruction is a result of a herniated intrathoracic stomach compressing the adjacent esophagus along with angulation of the GEJ when stomach becomes progressively displaced into the chest. Rarely, patients develop acutely severe chest or epigastric pain and/or severe vomiting due to complications of volvulus or strangulation. Volvulus occurs when the intrathoracic stomach twists and subsequently obstructs the gastrointestinal tract. Strangulation of the stomach is a consequence of acute gastric volvulus. The blood supply to the stomach is interrupted and, if emergent surgery is not performed, gastric ischemia, necrosis, and even perforation of the stomach can ensue (Cohn & Soper, 2017).

The true incidence is difficult to approximate given that many people with hiatal hernias are asymptomatic and never diagnosed. Certain chronic conditions increase the propensity of developing hiatal hernia, including obesity, pregnancy, and abdominal ascites. These conditions promote herniation of organs from the positive pressure environment within the abdomen to a negative pressure environment within the thorax. The frequency of hiatal hernias increases with age, from 10% in patients younger than 40 years to 70% in patients older than 70 years (Qureshi, 2016). This is because as patients age, the diaphragmatic muscle and surrounding membranes around the hiatus weakens and loses elasticity (Roman & Kahrilas, 2014).

Hiatal hernias can be treated both medically and surgically. Conservative therapy should be initiated at first, particularly lifestyle changes and administration of pharmacologic agents. Surgery is usually reserved for symptomatic hernias that are refractory to pharmacologic therapy, or cases where there is bowel obstruction or ischemia.

Clinical Aspects

ASSESSMENT

Diagnosis is supported by an accurate history and diagnostic tests, whereas physical examination is nonspecific. While taking a patient's history, the registered nurse should assess for symptoms and related aggravating factors that indicate the presence of a hiatal hernia. Patients with sliding hiatal hernias typically endorse gastroesophageal reflux disease (GERD) symptoms like reflux, heartburn, or regurgitation, whereas patients with PEH indicate obstructive symptoms like postprandial fullness, epigastric pain, bloating, nausea, emesis, dysphagia, or retching. Atypical symptoms include cough, dyspnea, laryngitis, vocal hoarseness, dental erosions, or chest discomfort, which may also be related to different health processes. Any sign of acute chest pain and dysphagia in a patient with a known hiatal hernia can suggest incarceration. This is a medical emergency and providers should be notified immediately (Kohn et al., 2013). Auscultating the lungs for rhonchi can imply presence of pulmonary complications. Inquire about recurrent pneumonias, which can be due to silent aspiration. Question the patient regarding any history of anemia, hematochezia, melena, or hematemesis, which can be a result of Cameron's ulcers. A nutritional assessment with attention to unintentional weight loss or signs of dehydration may help identify the need for supplemental nutrition via parenteral nutrition or placement of a temporary feeding tube. In addition, since obesity is a significant risk factor for hiatal hernias, weight should be monitored. Explore the patient's social history, including smoking and alcohol use, as well as any stressors, which can exacerbate GERD symptoms. Medication reconciliation and checking for compliance also helps influence treatment planning.

NURSING INTERVENTIONS, MANAGEMENT, AND IMPLICATIONS

Nursing diagnoses include knowledge deficit about the disorder, diagnostic tests and treatments; acute pain related to dysphagia, reflux, gastric distention, impaired perfusion to herniated stomach; imbalanced nutrition due to inadequate consumption of body requirements related to dysphagia or reflux; and risk for aspiration due to dysphagia or regurgitation.

The most consequential role of a nurse caring for a patient with a hiatal hernia is health teaching. Because obesity is a significant risk factor, weight reduction is paramount. Refraining from wearing constricting clothing around the abdomen also helps decrease intra-abdominal pressure. Encourage patients to chew well, eat slowly, and to eat small amounts to prevent gastric distention. Remaining upright for 1 hour after eating, waiting at least 2 to 3 hours after last meal of the day, and sleeping with head of bed elevated at least 30° helps foster esophageal emptying, prevents aspiration of regurgitated contents, and prevents upward migration of hernia. Advise patients to avoid certain trigger foods (e.g., chocolate, fatty foods, fried foods), which can aggravate symptoms. Because alcohol, nicotine, and caffeine immediately decrease lower esophageal sphincter pressure, encourage patients to stop smoking and eliminate alcohol and caffeine. If psychological stress seems to cause symptoms, discuss coping mechanisms and stress management techniques.

If elective surgery is planned, discuss the benefits of weight loss with the patient before surgery. Obesity is also a risk factor for dehiscence and hernia recurrence postoperatively (Cohn & Soper, 2017). Tobacco abusers should refrain from smoking at least 4 weeks before surgery or as prescribed by the surgeon. Smoking increases the risk of postoperative deep vein thrombosis and, due to the effects of impaired oxygen uptake, cells in the surgical wound receive less oxygen. In turn, this delays wound healing and increases the chance of infection. Reinforce any preoperative instructions and ensure that any blood-thinning agents are documented and held for the appropriate length of time. To ease anxiety, it is helpful to prepare the patient for what to expect after surgery, for example, incisions, presence of tubes, diet, activity, length of stay, and/or postoperative restrictions.

OUTCOMES

As a result of thorough and reinforced health education, patients should increase compliance with therapy and instruction. Execution of nursing interventions postoperatively helps to identify complications early and prevent poor outcomes. Reassessment after nursing interventions are performed is important to determine treatment success or the need for alternative therapy.

Treatment of hiatal hernias is usually indicated for GERD. Proton pump inhibitors (PPIs) are more effective than histamine$_2$ receptor antagonists in healing esophagitis and decreasing the incidence of esophageal strictures, both complications of chronic GERD. Although generally safe, PPIs can cause adverse effects. Long-term PPI use has been associated with decreased bone density. Although the risk for osteoporosis is low, judicious use of PPIs in postmenopausal women who are at risk for hip fractures is recommended. Patients at risk for osteoporosis should have bone mineral density testing; treatment for osteoporosis may be indicated. In addition, PPIs have been linked to decreased intestinal magnesium absorption resulting in low serum magnesium levels. Before treatment with PPIs, patients should have baseline magnesium levels assessed and repeated at intervals. Intermittent studies and meta-analyses have also indicated that PPIs increase likelihood of development and recurrence of *Clostridium difficile* infection (Roman & Kahrilas, 2014). Patients should be instructed to report any persistent diarrhea to the provider. Finally, in 2011, the U.S. Food and Drug Administration (FDA) advised avoiding concurrent use of clopidogrel (Plavix) with omeprazole or esomeprazole because together they significantly reduce the antiplatelet activity of clopidogrel (FDA, 2011).

Summary

Most hiatal hernias are asymptomatic, but in some people hiatal hernia slowly worsen and may eventually require treatment. Rarely, a life-threatening complication may present acutely and require emergent surgery. Modifiable risk factors include maintaining a healthy weight, smoking cessation, and moderate alcohol consumption.

Cohn, T. D., & Soper, N. J. (2017). Paraesophageal hernia repair: Techniques for success. *Journal of Laparoendoscopic and Advanced Surgical Techniques. Part A*, 27(1), 19–23. doi:10.1089/lap.2016.0496

Kohn, G. P., Price, R. R., Demeester, S. R., Zehetner, J., Muensterer, O. J., Awad, Z. T., . . . Fanelli, R. D. (2013). Guidelines for the management of hiatal hernia—A SAGES guideline. Retrieved from https://www.sages.org/publications/guidelines/guidelines-for-the-management-of-hiatal-hernia

Qureshi, W. A. (2016). Hiatal hernia. *Medscape*. Retrieved from http://emedicine.medscape.com/article/178393-overview

Roman, S., & Kahrilas, P. J. (2014). The diagnosis and management of hiatus hernia. *British Journal of Medicine*, 349, g6154. doi:10.1136/bmj.g6154

U.S. Food and Drug Administration. (2011). Safety information—clopidogrel bisulfate tablet. Retrieved from https://www.accessdata.fda.gov/drugsatfda_docs/appletter/2011/020839s055ltr.pdf

■ HUMAN IMMUNODEFICIENCY VIRUS

Scott Emory Moore

Overview

HIV is a retrovirus, most often transmitted through sexual activity or the sharing of needles or syringes, that affects approximately 1.2 million people in the United States (AIDS.gov, 2015; Centers for Disease Control and Prevention [CDC], 2016). The retrovirus attacks its hosts' immune cells (CD4$^+$ T cells among others). There is no known cure for HIV, and, if undiagnosed and untreated, HIV can progress to AIDS. AIDS, the most advanced stage of HIV, results from the suppression of the immune system to the point of failure (Selik et al., 2014). However, with early diagnosis, connection to HIV care, combined antiretroviral therapy (cART), and viral suppression, HIV can be rendered a chronic illness. Nursing care for adults with HIV/AIDS should focus on limiting infections, symptom management, and the psychosocial implications of HIV/AIDS.

Background

In 1981, the illness that would come to be known as AIDS was first discussed as a probable association between a rare *Pneumocystis* pneumonia and homosexual activity among men in Los Angeles, California (CDC, 1981). Since then, AIDS has been shown to develop as a result of HIV infection. HIV is a retrovirus that incorporates its genetic code into the DNA of T-lymphocyte cells. HIV uses its host cell to replicate its genetic code and build new HIV viruses to infect other cells. In some cases, the HIV host cells become dormant making it difficult for the immune system to remove the virus or cART to affect the virus (Gallo & Montagnier, 2003).

There are two types of HIV: HIV-1 and HIV-2. HIV-1 is the most common type of infection in the United States, but there are cases of HIV-2 in the United States, although it is more common in western Africa than the United States. It is also possible to be infected with both HIV-1 and HIV-2. In addition to the two types of HIV, there are multiple groups within each type, and groups can have subtypes. These subtypes each have their own unique nature such as increased resistance to specific drugs, or increased successful transmission rates. In North America, HIV-1, group M, subtype B is the most common virus causing HIV infection (Hemelaar, 2012).

Initial diagnosis of HIV in an adult is usually based on laboratory data using multiple tests. The first type of testing used usually consists of an HIV antibody screening, which if found to be reactive (positive result), leads to confirmatory testing using another type of test that uses a differing mechanism for testing the presence of HIV or HIV antibodies (Selik et al., 2014). HIV-1 viral load testing, for example, would be an acceptable test to confirm a reactive antibody screen. Once diagnosed, staging is the next step of clinical classification of HIV. HIV is classified into one of five possible classifications, 0, 1, 2, 3, or unknown. Stage 0 is the earliest stage of HIV infection, considered to be the first 180 days since the last known negative test until the first positive HIV test. If the time since last negative test is greater than 180 days then HIV staging (stages 1, 2, 3, and unknown) is based on clinical criteria, CD4$^+$ T-lymphocyte count or percentage of total lymphocytes, and/or diagnosis of an opportunistic illness (Selik et al., 2014). When criteria for stage 0 are met, regardless of the presence of clinical criteria for the other stages, the patient is categorized as stage 0. If there is no information for the clinical criteria for staging then the initial stage is unknown, but, as with those with initial staging of 0, the progression of the disease will rely on the CD4$^+$ T-cells and/or the presence of an opportunistic illnesses. Stage 3 is also known as AIDS, and it is defined as having less than 200 CD4$^+$ T-cells, or less than 14% of all lymphocytes are CD4$^+$ and/or an opportunistic illness is present (Selik et al., 2014).

HIV affected approximately 1.2 million people in the United States, and approximately 36.7 million people worldwide at the end of 2015 (CDC, 2016; World Health Organization [WHO], 2016). In the United States in 2015, a total of 39,513 people were diagnosed with HIV and 18,303 people with AIDS (CDC, 2016).

Men who have sex with men continue to make up the majority of new diagnoses, 83% in 2014 (CDC, 2016). HIV disproportionately affects African Americans and Hispanic Americans, accounting for 44% and 24%, respectively of estimated new HIV diagnoses in the United States in 2014 (CDC, 2016). Older adults are a growing group of newly infected individuals, with 17% of new diagnoses in 2014 occurring in people aged 50 years and older. Of those newly diagnosed individuals who are 55 years old and older, 40% are diagnosed with AIDS because of delayed identification of the disease. Other groups at risk for HIV infection include people who are incarcerated, intravenous-drug users, of lower socioeconomic status, and people who trade sex for money or drugs (CDC, 2016).

The age-adjusted death rate for HIV was 2.0 per 100,000 people in 2014, down from 10.2 in 1990. Advanced stage HIV can leave a patient open to opportunistic illnesses ranging from cancers, such as Kaposi sarcoma, lymphoma, and cervical cancer, to microbial infections, including mycobacterium, toxoplasmosis, and candidiasis of the esophagus, bronchi, trachea, or lungs. In addition, the presence of HIV-associated encephalopathy and wasting syndromes can also be hallmarks of AIDS (Selik et al., 2014).

Clinical Aspects

ASSESSMENT

An HIV/AIDS-related assessment should include some disease-specific questions such as length of HIV diagnosis; which providers treat their HIV/AIDS; which cART regimen, if any, the patient is on; what time(s) of day he or she takes the cART; if the patient takes the medication as scheduled; if patient has any history of AIDS-defining illnesses. Other things of note in the assessment of these patients may be related to some of the risk factors for HIV such as substance use/abuse, trading sex for drugs or money, and screening for abuse, depression, malnutrition, and failure to thrive. Although the screening and diagnostic testing for the presence of HIV are important for diagnosis of HIV, CD4$^+$ T-cell count, viral load, hemoglobin, hematocrit, renal function, and white blood cell count results are more useful during the care of HIV$^+$ patients.

NURSING INTERVENTIONS, MANAGEMENT, AND IMPLICATIONS

It is less likely that HIV/AIDS is the principle reason for the patient needing nursing care; however, in addition to monitoring and treatment of the primary condition it is important to be aware of the compounding nature that HIV/AIDS may have on dealing with the presenting illness. The symptoms and features associated with HIV/AIDS can lead to certain complications, including delayed wound healing or inability to fend off infections (local or systemic) related to immune system deficiency, difficulty with participation in physical therapy secondary to fatigue, forgetfulness, and cognitive dysfunction related to the virus. Thus, nurses should be aware of the following: hydration, infection prevention, nutrition, polypharmacy, social support, stigma, and symptom management (e.g., cognitive dysfunction, depression, fatigue, pain, sleep disturbances, wasting). Each of these has specific associations with HIV/AIDS, but for most patients there are not any specific differences for nursing care of HIV/AIDS patients.

Polypharmacy and related complications are concerning for adults living with HIV/AIDS as they may take multiple medications for chronic illnesses or opportunistic infection prophylaxis in addition to their cART. Patients with HIV/AIDS may benefit greatly from a social work consult to ensure that they are aware of the various public services available to them. In addition to need for social support, HIV/AIDS-related stigma must be addressed. Not every HIV⁺ patient has disclosed his or her status, thus it is imperative for nurses to be informed about which people, if any, know about the patient's HIV status (Relf & Rollins, 2015).

OUTCOMES

The measure of optimal outcomes in patients living with HIV/AIDS are evaluated by whether and how consistently a patient is engaged in HIV care. The HIV care continuum spans levels of engagement ranging from unengaged, undiagnosed HIV through fully engaged, regular HIV-specific care (Gardner, McLees, Steiner, Del Rio, & Burman, 2011). When patients with HIV/AIDS need nursing care, it is important to assess the extent of their engagement in HIV-specific care.

Summary

With cART treatment, people with HIV/AIDS are living longer than they did in the 1980s. Although some patients are being diagnosed at stage 3 (AIDS), the patient's laboratory values may return to stage 1 or 2 levels as a result of treatment of the virus and AIDS-associated illness. Identification and evaluation of HIV/AIDS-related symptoms and patient advocacy are key parts of ensuring the best outcomes.

AIDS.gov. (2015). How do you get HIV or AIDS? Retrieved from http://www.aids.gov/hiv-aids-basics/hiv-aids-101/how-you-get-hiv-aids/index.html

Centers for Disease Control and Prevention. (1981). Pneumocystis pneumonia. *Morbidity and Mortality Weekly Report, 30*(21), 250–252.

Centers for Disease Control and Prevention. (2016). HIV in the United States: At a glance. Retrieved from https://www.cdc.gov/hiv/statistics/overview/ataglance.html

Gallo, R. C., & Montagnier, L. (2003). The discovery of HIV as the cause of AIDS. *New England Journal of Medicine, 349*(24), 2283–2285. doi:10.1056/NEJMp038194

Gardner, E. M., McLees, M. P., Steiner, J. F., Del Rio, C., & Burman, W. J. (2011). The spectrum of engagement in HIV care and its relevance to test-and-treat strategies for prevention of HIV infection. *Clinical Infectious Diseases, 52*(6), 793–800. doi:10.1093/cid/ciq243

Hemelaar, J. (2012). The origin and diversity of the HIV-1 pandemic. *Trends in Molecular Medicine, 18*(3), 182–192. doi:10.1016/j.molmed.2011.12.001

Relf, M. V., & Rollins, K. V. (2015). HIV-related stigma among an urban sample of persons living with HIV at risk for dropping out of HIV-oriented primary medical care. *Journal of the Association of Nurses in AIDS Care, 26*(1), 36–45. doi:10.1016/j.jana.2014.03.003

Selik, R., Mokotoff, E., Branson, B., Owen, S., Whitmore, S., & Hall, H. (2014). Revised surveillance case definition for HIV infection-United States, 2014. *Morbidity and Mortality Weekly Report, 63*(RR03), 1–10.

World Health Organization. (2016). Global summary of the AIDS epidemic 2015. Retrieved from http://www.who.int/hiv/data/epi_core_2016.png?ua=1

■ HYPERTENSION

Marian Soat

Overview

Hypertension (HTN) in adults, if not detected early and treated appropriately, can lead to myocardial infarction (MI), renal failure, stroke, and death (James et al., 2014). According to the Centers for Disease Control and Prevention (Yoon, Fryar, & Carroll, 2015), approximately 77.9 million American adults suffer from HTN, which is defined by the Eighth Joint National Committee (JNC8) as blood pressure (BP) that is equal to or greater than 140/90 mmHg. Because patients with HTN often present with no symptoms, the disease is difficult to diagnose, and controlling HTN is a challenge for health care providers (Wozniak, Khan, Gillespie, & Sifuentes, 2016). Nursing care for adults with HTN is focused on regular monitoring of signs and symptoms, a strict medication regimen, and compliance with lifestyle modifications.

Background

BP is the force exerted by the blood against the walls of the blood vessels. The extent of that force depends on both the cardiac output and the resistance of blood vessels. Optimal BP is generally defined as the level above which minimal vascular damage occurs. High BP is a condition in which the force of the blood against the artery walls is strong enough that, over an extended period of time, it may cause health problems such as heart disease (Hedegaard, Hallis, Rvn-Neilsen, & Kjeldsen, 2016).

Specifically, HTN is equated with BP higher than 140/90 mmHg if the patient is younger than 60 years, and higher than 150/90 mmHg for patients older than 60 years, according to the JNC 8 (2014). The overall occurrence is similar between men and women but differs with age: for those younger than 45 years, HTN is more common in men; for those older than 65 years, it is more common in women.

Worldwide, more than 1 billion adults are afflicted with HTN, causing more than 9 million deaths per year (Ettehad et al., 2016). Many patients are unaware of their elevated BP because they are asymptomatic. Symptoms experienced by patients are in the form of headaches, shortness of breath, or nosebleeds. Unfortunately, these signs and symptoms are not specific to HTN, and often do not occur until HTN has reached a severe or life-threatening stage.

There are two types of HTN. Primary, or essential HTN, tends to develop gradually over many years and for most adults, there is no identifiable cause. Secondary HTN appears suddenly, often caused by an underlying condition, resulting in a higher level BP than that attributed to primary HTN. Various conditions can lead to secondary HTN, including renal disease, obstructive sleep apnea, and thyroid disease. Certain medications, such as birth control pills, cold remedies, decongestants, over-the-counter pain relievers, and some prescription drugs, as well as illegal drugs such as cocaine and amphetamines, may cause an elevation in BP. Alcohol abuse or chronic alcohol use may cause an elevation in BP (Rapsomaniki et al., 2014).

A hypertensive "crisis" is a significant increase in BP that threatens to cause a stroke. Extremely high BP—a systolic pressure of 180 mmHg or higher or a diastolic pressure of 120 mmHg or higher—may damage blood vessels, which become inflamed and may leak fluid or blood and, as a result, the heart may not be able to pump blood effectively. Causes of a hypertensive emergency include noncompliance with antihypertensive medication or interaction between medications. In addition, an adult with HTN may experience a hypertensive crisis while having a stroke, an MI, an aortic rupture, or convulsions.

A hypertensive crisis is divided into two categories: urgent and emergent. In an urgent hypertensive crisis, the BP is extremely high but there is no evidence of end-organ damage. In an emergent hypertensive crisis, the BP is extremely high and resulting organ damage is indicated. An emergent hypertensive crisis can be associated with life-threatening complications. The adult may experience severe chest pain and/or a severe headache, accompanied by confusion and blurred vision, nausea, vomiting, severe anxiety, shortness of breath, seizures, and unresponsiveness. If an adult displays these symptoms along with highly elevated BP, that person will need immediate medical attention, including hospitalization for treatment with oral or intravenous medications (Ettehad et al., 2016).

Clinical Aspects

ASSESSMENT

A crucial component for effective nursing care for the patient with HTN is a comprehensive physical examination and medical history, as well as ongoing assessment, according to NANDA International (formerly the North American Nursing Diagnosis Association) (Herdman & Kamitsuru, 2014). Adults at risk for developing HTN should be noted and reported on regularly. Risk factors for HTN include excess weight, sedentary lifestyle, and noncompliance with medications.

As the patient's history is assessed, the nurse should evaluate reports of extreme fatigue, intolerance for activities, sudden weight gain, swelling of extremities, and progressive shortness of breath. These symptoms may indicate poor ventricular function or impending cardiac failure.

Proper equipment must be used in taking a BP, including a quality stethoscope and BP cuff. The patient should be relaxed, with his or her upper arm at the level of the heart. The nurse should remove any excess clothing that would interfere with the reading and the patient should remain still and quiet during the BP reading.

The nurse should check central and peripheral pulses. Bounding carotid, jugular, radial, or femoral pulses may be a sign of HTN. Pulses in the lower extremities may be diminished, indicating vasoconstriction. When auscultating heart and breath sounds, an S4 sound is common in a patient with HTN due to increased arterial pressure. Presence of crackles and/or wheezing may indicate pulmonary congestion secondary to developing heart failure. The nurse should observe skin color, moisture, temperature, and capillary refill time as pallor may be due to peripheral vasoconstriction. Dependent and general edema may indicate heart failure as well as renal or vascular impairment (Bauer, Briss, Goodman, & Bowman, 2014). The nurse should be sure to check laboratory data, including cardiac markers, complete blood count, electrolytes, arterial blood gases, blood urea nitrogen, and creatinine. Recording and reporting laboratory data can identify contributing factors to HTN, as well as indicate organ damage.

NURSING INTERVENTIONS, MANAGEMENT, AND IMPLICATIONS

Nursing management of the adult with HTN should focus on relieving stress by providing a calm environment while hospitalized. In order to decrease stimulation and promote relaxation, activities should be minimized. If needed, the adult should have scheduled uninterrupted rest times. The adult may need assistance with self-care activities, which will decrease the physical stress that can affect BP (Bauer et al., 2014).

Nursing care for the adult with HTN should emphasize compliance with a therapeutic regimen, lifestyle modifications, and prevention of complications. These restrictions can help manage fluid retention with a hypertensive response, which will decrease cardiac workload. Adults with HTN should be encouraged to quit smoking, reduce sodium intake to a maximum of 2,400 mg/day, and participate in moderate to vigorous activity 3 to 4 days per week, averaging 40 minutes a session per day (James et al., 2014).

Cigarette smoking can significantly increase the risk of cardiovascular disease, including HTN. A full assessment of the adult's smoking activity should be obtained, including identifying and documenting tobacco use. Nursing care involves encouraging the adult to quit smoking with the help of medication as well as a referral to a smoking-cessation counselor. If the adult is not willing to quit smoking immediately, he or she should be provided with smoking-cessation information for future use.

Adults with HTN should be placed on a healthy diet, such as the dietary approaches to stop hypertension (DASH) diet. The DASH diet is plant focused, rich in fruits, nuts, and vegetables. It is low fat, incorporating nonfat dairy, lean meats, fish, and poultry, and including whole grains and heart-healthy fats. The DASH diet emphasizes limiting portion sizes, eating a variety of foods, and ensuring an adequate amount of nutrients. There is also a lower sodium DASH diet, in which the adult can consume up to 1,500 mg of sodium a day. The DASH diet encourages limited alcohol consumption; the Dietary Guidelines for Americans recommend up to two drinks a day for men and one for women.

According to the American Heart Association (Brook et al., 2013), physical activity reduces not only HTN but also the risk of coronary artery disease, stroke, and type 2 diabetes. Adults with HTN should be encouraged to engage in regular physical activity, from moderate to vigorous, which can include brisk walking, swimming, and bicycle riding. Even while hospitalized, adults with HTN should be encouraged to engage in physical activity such as a walking regimen. Long term, the nurse should encourage the adult to maintain this activity, which may be supported by walking with a spouse, a friend, or in a group.

The adult with HTN should be encouraged to participate in activities that help alleviate stress, such as breathing exercises, muscle relaxation, and yoga. Nursing care should encourage long-term stress reduction, such as education in stress management, a plan for balancing work/life activities, and adequate rest (Oza & Garcellano, 2015).

The hypertensive patient may be prescribed one or more of the following initial drugs of choice for HTN, according to the JNC8 guidelines: angiotensin-converting-enzyme (ACE) inhibitor (ACE-I), angiotensin receptor blocker (ARB), calcium channel blocker (CCB), and a thiazide diuretic. Nursing care should emphasize and monitor the adult's strict compliance with his or her medication therapy, which is vital to the success of a program for reducing HTN.

OUTCOMES

Desired outcomes for the adult with HTN include maintaining BP within an individually accepted range as well as a stable cardiac rhythm and rate (James et al., 2014). If goal BP is not reached within a month of treatment, an increase of the dose of the initial drug, or a second drug, may be warranted. Nursing care then involves monitoring BP, ensuring compliance with medication, and noting and reporting any side effects such as increased fatigue or shortness of breath. This care regimen should be maintained until goal BP is reached.

Summary

Adults diagnosed with HTN should be monitored closely, as complications from the disease can escalate. Recommendations for BP control, including treatment levels, goals, and drug therapy, should be based on evidence as well as on considerations specific to the individual. For adults with HTN, the benefits of adopting lifestyle changes, including a healthy diet, weight control, and regular exercise, should be stressed to aid in BP control (James et al., 2014).

Bauer, U. E., Briss, P. A., Goodman, R. A., & Bowman, B. A. (2014). Prevention of chronic disease in the 21st century: Elimination of the leading preventable causes of premature death and disability in the USA. *Lancet*, *384*(9937), 45–52.

Brook, R. D., Appel, L. J., Rubenfire, M., Ogedegbe, G., Bisognano, J. D., Elliott, W. J., . . . Rajagopalan, S. (2013). Beyond medications and diet: Alternative approaches to lowering blood pressure: A scientific statement from the American Heart Association. *Hypertension, 61*(6), 1360–1383.

Ettehad, D., Emdin, C. A., Kiran, A., Anderson, S. G., Callender, T., Emberson, J., . . . Rahimi, K. (2016). Blood pressure lowering for prevention of cardiovascular disease and death: A systematic review and meta-analysis. *Lancet, 387*(10022), 957–967. doi:10.1016/S0140-6736(15)01225-8

Hedegaard, U., Hallas, J., Ravn-Nielsen, L. V., & Kjeldsen, L. J. (2016). Process- and patient-reported outcomes of a multifaceted medication adherence intervention for hypertensive patients in secondary care. *Research in Social and Administrative Pharmacy, 12*(2), 302–318. doi:10.1016/J.SAPHARM.2015.05.006

Herdman, T. H., & Kamitsuru, S. (Eds.). (2014). *Nursing diagnoses: Definitions & classification 2015–2017.* Chichester, UK: Wiley Blackwell.

James, P. A., Oparil, S., Carter, B. L., Cushman, W. C., Dennison-Himmelfarb, C., Handler, J., . . . Ortiz, E. (2014). Evidence-based guideline for the management of high blood pressure in adults report from the panel members appointed to the Eighth Joint National Committee (JNC 8). *Journal of the American Medical Association, 311*(5), 507–520. doi:10.1001/jama.2013.284427 Retrieved from http://jamanetwork.com/journals/jama/fullarticle/1791497

Oza, R., & Garcellano, M. (2015). Nonpharmacologic management of hypertension: What works? *American Family Physician, 91*(11), 772–776.

Rapsomaniki, E., Timmis, A., George, J., Pujades-Rodriguez, M., Shah, A. D., Denaxas, S., . . . Hemingway, H. (2014). Blood pressure and incidence of twelve cardiovascular diseases: Lifetime risks, healthy life-years lost, and age-specific associations in 1.25 million people. *Lancet, 383*(9932), 1899–1911.

Wozniak, G., Khan, T., Gillespie, C., & Sifuentes, L. (2016). Hypertension control cascade: A framework to improve hypertension awareness, treatment, and control. *Journal of Clinical Hypertension, 18*(3), 232–239. doi:10.1111/jch.12654. Epub 2015 Sept 4

Yoon, S. S., Fryar, C. D., & Carroll, M. D. (2015). *Hypertension prevalence and control among adults: United States, 2011–2014.* NCHS data brief, no 220. Hyattsville, MD: National Center for Health Statistics.

■ HYPERTHYROIDISM

Colleen Kurzawa

Overview

Hyperthyroidism (HT) occurs as a result of overfunction of the thyroid gland, which leads to an excess of thyroid hormone (TH) in the body (De Leo, Lee, & Braverman, 2016). According to De Leo et al. (2016), 1% to 3% of people in the United States will develop thyroid disease, HT increases with age, and the prevalence of HT is greater in females. TH increases metabolism and protein synthesis, which affects all major organs. Persons with HT may present with mild to severe manifestation depending on the amount and period of time of hypersecretion of TH. Nursing care of persons with HT focuses on prevention and treatment of complications.

Background

HT refers to an excess of TH that is synthesized and secreted by the thyroid gland, and *thyrotoxicosis* refers to excess circulating TH no matter what the source (De Leo et al., 2016). Patients with excessive TH will display an increased basal metabolic rate, increased cardiovascular function, increased gastrointestinal function, and increased neuromuscular function; weight loss; heat intolerance; and problems with fat, protein, and carbohydrate metabolism (Lemone, Burke, Bauldoff, & Gubrud, 2015; Melmed, Polonsk, Larsen, & Kronenberg, 2016). Several factors that cause HT are excessive thyroid-stimulating hormone (TSH) receptor stimulation (Graves' disease), autonomous TH secretion (toxic multinodular goiter), destruction of follicles in the thyroid with release of TH (infection, thyroiditis), and extrathyroidal sources of TH (overmedication; Lemone et al., 2015; Melmed et al., 2016). The most common causes of HT are Graves' disease and toxic multinodular goiter (Ross et al., 2016).

Worldwide, the prevalence of HT varies with the degree of iodine insufficiency in populations; especially at risk are pregnant women, children, and the elderly (De Leo, 2016; Devereaux & Tewelde, 2014). In the United States, the prevalence of HT is 1.2%, with 0.5% overt HT and 0.7% subclinical HT (Devereaux & Tewelde, 2014; Ross et al., 2016). Subclinical HT ranges from 1% to 10% in different populations and increases with age (Mitchell & Pearce, 2016). Grade I subclinical HT results when the TSH is low but detectable, and grade II subclinical HT results when TSH is suppressed (Mitchell & Pearce, 2016). About 76% of grade I subclinical HT goes back to euthyroid state (normal) and only 12.5% of grade II subclinical HT returns to the euthyroid state (Mitchell & Pearce, 2016). Patients with grade II subclinical HT have a 3.1% chance of progressing to a clinical HT in

7 years and patients with grade I subclinical HT have a 0.5% chance of progressing to a clinical HT in 7 years (Mitchell & Pearce, 2016). According to Ross et al. (2016), subclinical HT populations that are asymptomatic should be treated at 65 years and older when there is cardiac disease and osteoporosis. The percentages of females who develop HT are 1% to 2%, and it is 0.1% to 0.2% for males (Melmed et al., 2016). The prevalence of thyroiditis is 10% to 15% and toxic adenoma is 3% to 5% (Devereaux & Tewelde, 2014).

Graves' disease is caused by thyroid-stimulating autoantibodies (Melmed et al., 2016). Graves' disease typically includes a triad of symptoms: goiter (swelling of the thyroid gland), exophthalmos (protruding eyes), and skin problems. About 80% of all hyperthyroid cases are Graves' disease with an incidence of 1 per 1,000, and it is greater in females 30 to 60 years of age with a family history of thyroid problems (Melmed et al., 2016).

In pregnancy, the most common cause of HT is Graves' disease. The incidence of HT is five to nine per 1,000 pregnant women per year (De Leo et al., 2016). Postpartum thyroiditis in the mother is transient and may develop anywhere from 6 weeks to 6 months after childbirth (Devereaux & Tewelde, 2014). The fetus is also at risk before birth because thyroid antibodies are able to cross the placenta (De Leo et al., 2016).

HT in children is rare but if not treated it may lead to serious complications with growth and development (Srinivasan & Mirsra, 2015). The incidence of HT per 1,000 young children is 0.44 and in adolescents it is 0.26 (Endocrine Society, 2017). Graves' disease accounts for 95% of HT cases (Srinivasan & Mirsra, 2015). Subclinical HT prevalence in children is 0.7% (Endocrine Society, 2017).

Thyroid storm is an uncommon complication of HT but has an extremely high mortality rate (Devereaux & Tewelde, 2014). Thyroid storm is accelerated HT and accounts for 1% to 2% of admissions for HT (Devereaux & Tewelde, 2014; Mohananey et al., 2016). Thyroid storm occurs abruptly in patients being treated incompletely or may be precipitated by infection, trauma, surgical emergency, radiation thyroiditis, diabetic ketoacidosis, and toxemia during pregnancy (Melmed et al., 2016). Manifestations are the result of an extreme metabolic state and include irritability, tachycardia, vomiting, high temperature, profuse sweating, delirium, or psychosis, eventually leading to apathy, stupor, and coma (Lemone et al., 2015; Melmed et al., 2016). According to Mohananey et al. (2016), the mortality rate from thyroid storm has decreased over the past several years (60% in 2003, 21% in 2011).

Clinical Aspects

ASSESSMENT

TH in the body acts to increase metabolism and protein synthesis. Manifestations are similar to problems such as increased sympathetic nervous system stimulation (Lemone et al., 2015; Melmed et al., 2016). Physical manifestations are cardiovascular (hypertension, tachycardia, arrhythmias, and edema); protein, carbohydrate, and lipid metabolism (increased appetite, weight loss, and aggravation of diabetes mellitus); nervous system (nervousness, emotional liability, exaggerated movements, tremors of tongue, hands, eyelids, and fatigue); eyes (blurred vision, photophobia, lacrimation, and exophthalmos); respiratory (dyspnea); gastrointestinal (diarrhea, hepatomegaly, jaundice, nausea, vomiting); musculoskeletal (muscle weakness, pathologic fractures, increased excretion of calcium and phosphorus, osteoporosis, and osteomalacia); skin (warm and moist, fine hair, soft nails); reproductive (delayed sexual maturity, amenorrhea, reduced fertility, gynecomastia, and erectile dysfunction; Melmed et al., 2016).

Nursing assessments should include a thorough health history and physical examination. The health history should focus on family prevalence of thyroid disease, menstruation history, gastrointestinal problems, weight changes, and medication use (Lemone et al., 2015). Physical assessment should center on vital signs and an examination of skin, eyes, cardiovascular, gastrointestinal, reproductive, musculoskeletal system, and other systems (Lemone et al., 2015).

Laboratory results that demonstrate elevated TH, low TSH (elevated pituitary tumor), elevated triiodothyronine (T3)/thyroxine (T4), and erythrocyte sedimentation rate would indicate HT. Other tests may include a protein-binding inhibition assay and bioassay. The radioactive iodine uptake (RAIU) will be elevated. A thyroid ultrasound may indicate the presence of a nodular thyroid gland and a thyroid scan may confirm hyperfunctioning nodules.

Nursing diagnosis for the person with HT should be individualized and take into consideration all possible effects on major organs and metabolism. The most common health problems include cardiovascular, visual, nutrition, and body image (Lemone et al., 2015). Persons may have increased blood pressure, tachycardia, and dyspnea. Vital signs should be monitored, activity and rest need to be balanced, and stress should be decreased with relaxation interventions

(Lemone et al., 2015). Disturbed sensory perception due to diplopia, photophobia, and eye changes can put the patient at risk for falls. Patients should wear dark glasses, use artificial tears, and elevate the head of bed (Melmed et al., 2016). Imbalanced nutrition (less than body requirements) is due to the hypermetabolic state induced by HT. The patient should understand the need to check weight daily and keep a record. Collaboration with a dietician is important to help ensure patients consume adequate amounts of carbohydrates and proteins in relation to their metabolic demand (Lemone et al., 2015). Disturbed body image and anxiety are due to changes with eyes, hair loss, perspiration, sexual changes, and mood changes (Lemone et al., 2015). Good communication skills are necessary to build a trusting relationship that allows the person to verbalize her or his feelings and perceptions of the illness. Finally, the nurse needs to clarify any misconceptions and provide information.

Summary

There is no cure for HT, and so the primary focus is on maintenance of the disease process and alleviation of related symptoms. Nurses need to assist the patient in the identification of stress-relieving activities and emphasize the need for a trusting relationship with health care professionals. Nursing care is centered on education and health promotion. Patients need to be aware that medication regimens will be lifelong so they will need to be educated on ways to monitor their symptoms and what side effects to report. If radioactive iodine therapy or surgery is required, then postprocedure care is initiated. With treatment for HT, the person must understand signs and symptoms of hypothyroidism and thyroid storm.

De Leo, S., Lee, S. Y., & Braverman, L. E. (2016). Hyperthyroidism. *Lancet, 388*(10047), 906–918.

Devereaux, D., & Tewelde, S. Z. (2014). Hyperthyroidism and thyrotoxicosis. *Emergency Medicine Clinics of North America, 32*(2), 277–292.

Endocrine Society. (2017). Endocrine facts and figures. Retrieved from http://endocrinefacts.org/health-conditions/thyroid/4-hyperthyroidism

Lemone, P., Burke, K., Bauldoff, G., & Gubrud, P. (2015). *Medical–surgical nursing: Critical thinking in patient care* (6th ed.). Upper Saddle River, NJ: Pearson.

Melmed, S., Polonsk, K. S., Larsen, P. R., & Kronenberg, H. M. (2016). *Williams textbook of endocrinology* (13th ed.). Philadelphia, PA: Elsevier.

Mitchell, A. L., & Pearce, S. H. (2016). Subclinical hyperthyroidism: First do no harm. *Clinical Endocrinology, 85*(1), 15–16.

Mohananey, D., Villablanca, P., Bhatia, N., Agrawal, S., Murrieta, J. C., Ganesh, M., . . . Ramakrishna, H. (2016). Trends in incidence, management and outcomes of cardiogenic shock complicating thyroid storm in the United States. *Circulation, A18332,* 134. Retrieved from http://circ.ahajournals.org/content/134/Suppl_1/A18332.short

Ross, D. S., Burch, H. B., Cooper, D. S., Greenlee, M. C., Laurberg, P., Maia, A. L., . . . Walter, M. A. (2016). 2016 American Thyroid Association guidelines for diagnosis and management of hyperthyroidism and other causes of thyrotoxicosis. *Thyroid, 26*(10), 1343–1421.

Srinivasan, S., & Misra, M. (2015). Hyperthyroidism in children. *Pediatrics in Review, 36*(6), 239–248.

■ HYPOTHYROIDISM

Karen L. Terry

Overview

Hypothyroidism is an endocrine disorder characterized by insufficient circulating levels of the thyroid hormones thyroxine (T4) and triiodothyronine (T3). Primary hypothyroidism occurs when there is either reduced thyroid hormone or impaired thyroxine synthesis by follicle cells. Central hypothyroidism occurs when the hypothalamic–pituitary axis is damaged. Hypothyroidism consists of two subsets referred to as *secondary* and *tertiary*. Deficient pituitary thyroid-stimulating hormone (TSH) production is considered secondary hypothyroidism. Deficient hypothalamic thyroid-releasing hormone (TRH) production is considered tertiary hypothyroidism (March, 2016).

Hypothyroidism is more prevalent in less developed countries, but has decreased overall due to routine iodine supplementation in salt, flour, and other food staples. Worldwide, insufficient iodine intake is the most common cause of hypothyroidism, whereas autoimmune disease is the most common cause in the Unites States (Orlander et al., 2016). The focus of nursing care for adults with hypothyroidism is on symptom management and the delivery of nursing interventions that prevent or reduce complications during care and recovery as it relates to the severity of the disease at the time of diagnosis.

Background

Hypothyroidism is easily treatable and reversible. If left unchecked, severe hypothyroidism can lead to coma and death. Garber et al. (2012) noted in the American Association of Clinical Endocrinologists (AACE) guidelines that TSH, T3, and T4 levels need to be carefully interpreted to diagnose hypothyroidism. Not all patients with abnormal lab results will be diagnosed with hypothyroidism or be treated with hormones. Most patients need to be symptomatic, have TSH levels greater than 4.5 mIU/L and low levels of thyroid hormone to receive hormone replacements (Garber et al., 2012). In addition, diagnosis of primary or central hypothyroidism will also help determine how medical treatment ensues. Possible causes of primary hypothyroidism could include chronic lymphocytic (autoimmune) thyroiditis, postpartum thyroiditis, subacute (granulomatous) thyroiditis, drug-induced hypothyroidism, and iatrogenic hypothyroidism. Possible causes of central hypothyroidism could include pituitary and hypothalamus tumors, lymphocytic hypophysitis, Sheehan syndrome, history of brain irradiation, medications, congenital nongoiterous hypothyroidism type 4, and thyrotropin-releasing hormone resistance or deficiency (Orlander et al., 2016). Partial or complete surgical removal of the thyroid gland can also result in hypothyroidism.

Hypothyroidism is more prevalent in women with low body mass index during childhood (Orlander et al., 2016). In the landmark National Health and Nutrition Examination Survey (NHANES) 1999 to 2002, the frequency of hypothyroidism was noted to increase with age and the prevalence was higher in Whites and Mexican Americans than in African Americans, with 3.7% of the U.S. population reporting hypothyroidism or TSH levels exceeding 4.5 mIU/L (Aoki et al., 2007). In the United States, according to the National Institute of Diabetes and Digestive and Kidney Diseases (NIDDKD), 4.6% of the population reported hypothyroidism, and subclinical hypothyroidism affects 1% to 10% of the population (NIDDKD, 2016).

If untreated and allowed to progress, severe hypothyroidism worsens metabolic abnormalities and leads to coma and death in adults. Severe hypothyroidism in infants causes cretinism and irreversible mental retardation. Hypothyroidism and its treatment, if diagnosed before severe advancement and permanent damage, have a good prognosis, and abnormal signs and symptoms reverse fairly well with thyroid hormone replacement. Quality-of-life measures have also been noted to significantly improve in just 6 weeks of treatment (Orlander et al., 2016).

Clinical Aspects

ASSESSMENT

Key to the nursing process in caring for the patient with hypothyroidism is a thorough assessment, including history, physical, laboratory findings, and diagnostic or imaging studies (March, 2016). Early in the disease process, compensatory mechanisms maintain T3 hormone levels, but as time and stressors continue, these mechanisms fail and T3 production or release decreases. Patients present different clinical presentations depending on how long the hypothyroidism has occurred or how severe the suppression of thyroid hormone. Documentation of an accurate timeline is important as well as its onset, duration, and severity of signs and symptoms. Medical, surgical, and family history are obtained, with particular attention to risk factors for hypothyroidism. Common medications that have the potential to cause hypothyroidism include amiodarone, interferon alpha, rifampin, phenytoin, lithium, and carbamazepine (Orlander et al., 2016).

Common symptoms of hypothyroidism include fatigue, weight gain, puffy face, goiter, cold intolerance, joint or muscle pain, constipation, dry skin, dry or thinning hair, heavy or irregular menses, fertility problems, depression, bradycardia, and decreased sweating. Common risk factors for developing hypothyroidism include family history of hypothyroidism, goiter, radiation to neck, past thyroid surgery, Sjögren's syndrome, lupus, rheumatoid arthritis, type 1 diabetes mellitus, 6 months postpartum, and pernicious anemia (NIDDKD, 2016).

During physical examination particular attention to the presence of goiter or delayed relaxation of deep tendon reflexes can be significant indicators of hypothyroidism (March, 2016). Goiter may present as difficulty swallowing or hoarse voice and not necessarily an enlarged neck mass. Common lab abnormalities for hypothyroidism include elevated TSH, with low T3 and/or T4 levels. Imaging studies are used to evaluate lesions/tumors; chest radiography can show enlarged heart/pleural effusions; sinus bradycardia and other electrophysiological changes can be noted with EKG evaluation (March, 2016).

NURSING INTERVENTIONS, MANAGEMENT, AND IMPLICATIONS

Nursing care of the patient is dependent on the severity of hypothyroidism at the time of diagnosis. Patients with long-standing hypothyroidism can present with myxedema, which leads to coma and death. Nursing problems would include mental deterioration, decreased cardiac output, impaired spontaneous ventilation, activity intolerance, and loss of skin integrity (NANDA, n.d.). Assessment of mental and neurological status changes, adequate cardiopulmonary support to maintain tissue perfusion, pressure ulcer prophylaxis, and psychosocial support for the family are priorities. In addition to ventilation and fluid support, nursing would administer proper intravenous dosage of levothyroxine with stress glucocorticoids and perform cardiac assessments. Continued review of laboratory data would determine subsequent levothyroxine dose adjustments.

In less critically ill patients, symptoms are less life threatening and affect quality of life. Nursing-related problems include constipation, disturbed body image, imbalanced body temperature, and knowledge deficits. Focus is on maintaining normal bowel function, addressing altered self-concept due to possible weight gain and hair loss, maintaining temperature control, and addressing knowledge deficit related to lack of information about the disease process and self-care (Belleza, 2016).

Patients need to know to take their thyroid hormone with water 30 minutes prior to any other medication and food. Levothyroxine drug interactions can occur among many medications, including iron, aluminum, magnesium, calcium carbonate, cimetidine, sucralfate, and caffeine. Teach patients not to stop medication; replacement therapy is usually needed for life. Genetic studies are helping develop combination hormone therapies that promise improved efficacy.

OUTCOMES

Expected outcomes for the proper management of severe hypothyroidism are improved cardiac status and normal breathing patterns, activity participation and return to independence, and intact skin integrity. For patients with less severe hypothyroidism, outcomes would include normal bowel function, improved body image and thought process, maintenance of normal body temperature, and proper administration of medications and self-care (Belleza, 2016). Overall, patients should return to normal metabolic states.

Summary

Hypothyroidism is a common endocrine disorder that is easily treated. Nursing care and interventions are aimed at symptom relief and reduction of complications during recovery. Severity and advancement of the hypothyroidism will affect patient clinical presentation; therefore, nursing interventions and care plans must be individualized to meet the patient's needs at the time of diagnosis. Genetic studies may help in identifying patients who would benefit from pharmacogenomics. Thyroid hormone treatment reverses symptoms, helps return patients to normal metabolic states, and improves quality of life.

Aoki, Y., Belin, R. M., Clickner, R., Jeffries, R., Phillips, L., & Mahaffey, K. R. (2007). Serum TSH and total T4 in the United States population and their association with participant characteristics: National Health and Nutrition Examination Survey (NHANES 1999–2002). *Thyroid*, *17*(12), 1211–1223. doi:10.1089thy.2006.0235

Belleza, M. (2016). Hypothyroidism: Nursing care management and study guide. *Nurse Study Guides (medical-surgical nursing)*. Retrieved from http://nurseslabs.com/hypothyroidism

Garber, J. R., Cobin, R. H., Gharib, H., Hennessey, J. V., Klein, I., Mechanick, J. I., . . . Woeber, K. A. (2012). Clinical practice guidelines for hypothyroidism in adults: Cosponsored by the American Association of Clinical Endocrinologists and the American Thyroid Association. *Endocrine Practice*, *18*(6), 988–1028.

March, P. (2016). *Quick lesson: Hypothyroidism in adults*. Glendale, CA: CINAHL Information Systems.

NANDA. (n.d.). Nursing diagnosis list for 2015–2017. Retrieved from http://health-conditions.com/nanda-nursing-diagnosis-list-2015-2017

National Institute of Diabetes and Digestive Kidney Diseases. (2016). Hypothyroidism (underactive thyroid). Retrieved from http://www.niddk.nih.gov/health-information/health topics/endocrine/hypothyroidism

Orlander, P. R., Varghese, J. M., Freeman, L. M., Griffing, G. T., Davis, A. B., Bharaktiya, S., . . . Ziel, F. H. (2016). Hypothyroidism. *Medscape*. Retrieved from http://emdecine.medscape.com/article/122393-overview

■ INFLAMMATORY BOWEL DISEASE IN ADULTS

Ronald Rock

Overview

Inflammatory bowel disease (IBD) is a chronic autoimmune disease of unknown etiology characterized by periods of remission and exacerbation. Crohn's disease (CD) and ulcerative colitis (UC), the two chronic conditions of IBD, are characterized by chronic uncontrolled inflammation of the gastrointestinal (GI) tract causing edema, ulceration, bleeding, and profound fluid and electrolyte losses (Centers for Disease Control and Prevention [CDC], 2016). IBD has been associated with decreased quality of life and extensive morbidity, and often results in complications requiring hospitalization and surgical intervention (CDC, 2016). Overall, an estimated 3.1 million, or 1.3% of U.S. adults are diagnosed with IBD (CDC, 2016). Nursing care of the adult with IBD focuses on management of fluid and electrolyte imbalances, nutritional deficiencies, infections, chronic pain, and body-image disturbances (Burkhalter et al., 2015).

Background

Although the etiology of IBD is unknown, evidence suggests that normal intestinal flora trigger an abnormal immune reaction resulting in an overactive, inappropriate, and sustained inflammatory response. According to the CDC (2016), UC is slightly more common in males, ex-smokers, and nonsmokers, whereas CD is more frequent in women and smokers. Diagnosis of IBD is usually made before age 30 years, with peak incidences from 14 to 24 years and a second smaller peak in the sixth decade. Caucasians, individuals of white-collar occupations, and persons of Ashkenazi Jewish decent are more susceptible to IBD than other racial, occupational, and ethnic subgroups (CDC, 2016). Diet, oral contraceptive use, perinatal and childhood infections, and atypical mycobacterial infections are thought to play a role in developing IBD (CDC, 2016).

CD often presents in adolescence and is more prevalent in women than in men. Although the etiology of CD is unknown, it is associated with a mutation in the NOD2 gene (Wilkins, Jarvis, & Patel, 2011). UC is more common in North America and Europe than in other regions. Risk factors for UC include a history of recent infection with *Salmonella* or *Campylobacter*, and a family history of the disease (Adams & Bornemann, 2013).

Both disorders are characterized by extraintestinal manifestations, most commonly affecting the skin, eyes, mouth, and joints; the hepatobiliary, renal, and pulmonary systems can also be affected. In addition, persons with IBD are at increased risk for developing osteoporosis and colon cancer. CD is characterized by transmural inflammation of the bowel wall and can occur anywhere in the GI tract from the mouth to the anus, but most often involves the terminal ileum and colon. Typically, ulcerations are deep and longitudinal, penetrating between islands of inflamed edematous mucosa, characterized by the classic "skip lesions" and cobblestone appearance. Because the inflammation penetrates the entire bowel wall, microscopic leaks can allow bowel contents to enter the peritoneal cavity, resulting in abscess, fistulae, or peritonitis.

In contrast, UC typically starts in the rectum and moves proximally in a continuous pattern toward the cecum, different than the typical skip lesions of CD. Although there is sometimes mild inflammation in the terminal ileum, UC is primarily a disease of the colon and rectum. In UC, inflammation and ulcerations occur in the mucosal layer of the large intestine, hence fistulae and abscess formation are rare.

IBD is a chronic lifelong condition with significant health and economic costs. Based on data from 2004, IBD accounts for approximately 1,300,000 physician visits and 92,000 hospitalizations in the United States each year (CDC, 2016). In addition, 75% of patients diagnosed with CD and 25% of patients with a diagnosis of UC will require surgery (CDC, 2016). Mortality and morbidity of IBD are more closely linked to acquired coexisting conditions, such as infection, thrombus, or chronic disease, than the disease itself (Kassam et al., 2014). In 2008, direct treatment costs for patients with IBD were greater than $6.3 billion, whereas indirect costs were $5.5 billion, and these are anticipated to rise without a cure (CDC, 2016).

Clinical Aspects

ASSESSMENT

Patients with IBD may present with a variety of unspecific and overlapping features, making the differential diagnosis a challenge compounded by the lack of a single gold standard diagnostic test to distinguish between UC and CD (Tontini, Vecchi, Pastorelli, Neurath, &

Neumann, 2015). The first step of diagnosis is a complete patient history addressing the onset, severity, and pattern of symptoms, especially frequency and consistency of bowel movements. The history focused on risk factors and possible alternative diagnoses should include recent travel, exposure to antibiotics, food intolerance, medications, smoking, and family history of IBD. Common symptoms of IBD include abdominal pain, diarrhea, fatigue, fever, GI bleeding, and weight loss. Physical evaluation should include heart rate, blood pressure, temperature, and body weight; abdominal examination may reveal tenderness, distention, or masses. An anorectal examination should be performed as one third of patients have a perirectal abscess, fissure, or fistula at some time during the illness (Wilkins et al., 2011).

Laboratory tests are useful for diagnosing IBD, assessing disease activity, identifying complications, and monitoring response to therapy. Initial testing often includes white blood cell count; platelet count; measurement of hemoglobin, hematocrit, blood urea nitrogen, creatinine, liver enzymes, and C-reactive protein; and erythrocyte sedimentation rate. Stool culture and testing for *Clostridium difficile* toxin should also be considered to rule out an infectious cause of diarrhea. Endoscopic or colonoscopic biopsy is valuable in the diagnosis and differentiation of UC from CD.

Treatment goals for patients with IBD are achieving remission and preventing exacerbations and complications. Medical management focuses on relieving symptoms, controlling inflammation, and healing of intestinal mucosa. Pharmacologic treatment is initiated early in the disease and is based on a step-down or step-up approach; medications include biologics (tumor necrosis factor alpha inhibitors), corticosteroids, immunomodulators (azathioprine [AZA] and 6-mercaptopurine [6-MP]), antibiotics, and aminosalicylates. Surgery is indicated to treat complications or when medical management fails to control the disease. Surgical options vary depending on the type and severity of IBD and include drainage of abscesses, fistula repair, strictureplasty, bowel resection (with or without ostomy formation), and colectomy. Patients with CD who undergo multiple resections of the small intestine may develop short bowel syndrome. Short bowel syndrome is associated with several complications, including acid/base and fluid/electrolyte imbalances, malabsorption, vitamin and mineral deficiencies, and renal stones. Persons with CD often experience disease recurrence even with surgical intervention, whereas removal of the diseased colon in UC may be considered curative.

NURSING INTERVENTIONS, MANAGEMENT, AND IMPLICATIONS

An individual with IBD will journey through the health care system at different points, from initial investigation and diagnosis, through emergency care, admission, surgery (planned or emergent), postoperative care and discharge, education regarding management of associated medical conditions, and follow-up care with routine IBD management (Foskett, 2013). Because of systemic involvement, a multidisciplinary team approach is recommended. No single model of care is appropriate for all patients all the time; care may be delivered in hospital, shared between hospital and primary care, or through supported self-managed care (Foskett, 2013). Nursing care of patients with IBD focuses on managing fluid and electrolyte imbalances, malabsorption and nutritional deficiencies, infections, chronic pain, and body-image disturbances specific to the individual needs of patients (Burkhalter et al., 2015).

OUTCOMES

The main goal of treatment of IBD is to improve the patient's condition and health-related quality of life (HRQOL; Peyrin-Biroulet et al., 2016). Unfortunately, the physical well-being of the patient with IBD is not the only nursing concern. The uncertainty and chronicity of the disease and the lack of a definitive cure require nursing to be aware of other HRQOL indictors for this patient population. With the increasing incidence of IBD in the United States, identifying interventions to address the patient's psychosocial and physiologic needs and determining the impact of disease on the individual's activities of daily living (Iglesias-Rey et al., 2014) are essential.

Summary

Adults diagnosed with IBD may experience chronic or acute manifestations of CD or UC. The disease may result in long-term medical management and/or surgery. Evidence-based medical and surgical nursing care is critical in managing this patient population. In combination with physiologic, pharmacologic, and, if needed, psychological therapy, patients suffering with this potentially debilitating disease can be effectively managed.

Adams, S. M., & Bornemann, P. H. (2013). Ulcerative colitis. *American Family Physician, 87*(10), 699–705.

Burkhalter, H., Stucki-Thür, P., David, B., Lorenz, S., Biotti, B., Rogler, G., & Pittet, V. (2015). Assessment of inflammatory bowel disease patient's needs and problems from a nursing perspective. *Digestion, 91*(2), 128–141.

Centers for Disease Control and Prevention. (2016). Prevalence of inflammatory bowel disease among adults aged ≥18 years—United States, 2015. *Morbidity and Mortality Weekly Reports 28;65*(42), 1166–1169. doi:10.15585/mmwr.mm6542a3

Foskett, K. (2013). Inflammatory bowel disease—Patient engagement and experience. *Journal of Community Nursing, 27*(3), 29–32.

Iglesias-Rey, M., Barreiro-de Acosta, M., Caamaño-Isorna, F., Rodríguez, I. V., Ferreiro, R., Lindkvist, B., . . . Dominguez-Munoz, J. E. (2014). Psychological factors are associated with changes in the health-related quality of life in inflammatory bowel disease. *Inflammatory Bowel Diseases, 20*(1), 92–102.

Kassam, Z., Belga, S., Roifman, I., Hirota, S., Jijon, H., Kaplan, G. G., . . . Beck, P. L. (2014). Inflammatory bowel disease cause-specific mortality: A primer for clinicians. *Inflammatory Bowel Diseases, 20*(12), 2483–2492.

Peyrin-Biroulet, L., Panés, J., Sandborn, W. J., Vermeire, S., Danese, S., Feagan, B. G., . . . Rycroft, B. (2016). Defining disease severity in inflammatory bowel diseases: Current and future directions. *Clinical Gastroenterology and Hepatology, 14*(3), 348–354.c17.

Tontini, G. E., Vecchi, M., Pastorelli, L., Neurath, M. F., & Neumann, H. (2015). Differential diagnosis in inflammatory bowel disease colitis: State of the art and future perspectives. *World Journal of Gastroenterology, 21*(1), 21–46.

Wilkins, T., Jarvis, K., & Patel, J. (2011). Diagnosis and management of Crohn's disease. *American Family Physician, 84*(12), 1365–1375.

■ LEUKEMIA

Marisa A. Cortese

Overview

Leukemia is a malignancy of the blood. Cells of the blood develop in the bone marrow. The bone marrow is the site of production for erythrocytes (red blood cells [RBCs]) and leukocytes (white blood cells [WBCs]), as well as thrombocytes (platelets). There were approximately 60,140 new cases of leukemia diagnosed in the United States in 2016 (National Cancer Institute Surveillance, Epidemiology, and End Results Program [NCI SEER], 2017). Leukemia is often treated with chemotherapy, which may cause adverse effects for the patient (National Cancer Institute, 2017).

Background

Leukemia is a malignancy in which immature cells or ineffective WBCs (lymphoblasts) grow rapidly within the bone marrow. These lymphoblasts begin to accumulate in the bone marrow and eventually replace normal cells. This causes anemia, neutropenia, and thrombocytopenia. Leukemia can be classified as either an acute or chronic condition.

There are two types of acute leukemia found in the adult population: acute lymphoblastic leukemia (ALL) and acute myeloid leukemia (AML; National Cancer Institute, 2017). ALL and AML are both aggressive types of leukemia. ALL is caused by the rapid proliferation of lymphoblasts (immature lymphocytes), whereas AML is caused by the rapid growth of myeloblasts (immature myeloid cells; National Cancer Institute, 2017).

Acute leukemia can spread to other parts of the body such as the lymph nodes, spleen, liver, and central nervous system (CNS). Some of the common signs and symptoms found in acute leukemia are fatigue, fever, night sweats, bruising/bleeding easily, unexplained weight loss, swollen lymph nodes, and frequent infections (National Cancer Institute, 2017).

When patients present with symptoms of acute leukemia, a thorough history and physical examination with laboratory tests that include a complete blood count with differential, chemistry panel, and coagulation tests need to be performed. A bone marrow biopsy and aspiration is performed in order to determine the extent of the disease and to test for genetic mutations, which may show prognostic factors (National Cancer Institute, 2017).

A patient's prognosis and treatment plan depends on a number of factors that include age, comorbidities, CNS involvement, and chromosomal abnormalities in the bone marrow (Gaynor et al., 1988; Hoelzer et al., 1988). The standard treatment for patients with acute leukemia is chemotherapy and possible allogeneic hematopoietic stem cell transplantation (HSCT). Allogeneic HSCT is a process in which stem cells are collected from a donor and infused into a patient who has received a combination of chemotherapy and immunosuppressive therapy. This will promote bone marrow recovery (Ezzone, 2013).

There are two types of chronic leukemia found in the adult population: chronic lymphocytic leukemia (CLL) and chronic myelogenous leukemia (CML). CLL and CML are both slow-growing cancers. CLL is caused by bone marrow making too many lymphocytes, whereas CML is caused by a distinct genetic abnormality found on the Philadelphia chromosome (Dighiero & Hamblin, 2008; Goldman & Melo, 2003).

Patients diagnosed with CLL or CML may have symptoms of fatigue, fever, or night sweats. Patients with CLL may develop enlarged lymph nodes (Dighiero & Hamblin, 2008; Goldman & Melo, 2003).

Similar to those patients diagnosed with acute leukemia, a complete medical workup must be performed. The following examinations and testing should be performed: a thorough history and physical examination, laboratory tests, including complete blood count with differential and a chemistry panel. A bone marrow biopsy and aspiration is performed in order to determine the extent of the disease and to test for genetic mutations that may show prognostic factors (National Cancer Institute, 2017).

A patient's prognosis and plan of care are dependent on age, comorbidities, and the presence or absence of specific chromosomal abnormalities found in the blood and/or bone marrow (Dighiero & Hamblin, 2008; Goldman & Melo, 2003). The standard treatment for CLL is chemotherapy. Patients diagnosed with CML are treated with agents called *tyrosine kinase inhibitors*, which stop the enzyme that produces the malignant cells from forming (Dighiero & Hamblin, 2008; Goldman & Melo, 2003).

Clinical Aspects

ASSESSMENT

Patients diagnosed with an acute or chronic leukemia will need to be monitored closely for adverse events during their treatment. It is important to assess patients for potential fever, infection, and other complications that may be found during their initial workup as well as follow-up assessments during active treatment. Patients should be asked during their assessments whether they have had any recent fever, night sweats, chills, bleeding or bruising, abdominal pain, or frequent infections. On physical examination, a patient may appear pale and feverish; have swollen lymph nodes in the neck, armpit, or groin; have swelling of the abdomen; and/or have an enlarged spleen (National Cancer Institute, 2017).

A patient undergoing treatment for leukemia is at risk for infection. The risk factors associated are the lack of mature WBCs, immunosuppression, and bone marrow suppression due to chemotherapy. To prevent infection in patients with leukemia, it is important to educate patients as well as their families on protecting from sources of pathogens or infection. Patients and their families need education on good handwashing techniques to reduce the risk of the patient receiving an infection from others. A neutropenic diet that restricts eating fresh fruits and vegetables should be followed. These foods should be properly washed, peeled, and/or cooked. The patient's temperature should be monitored closely for temperature elevations (Shelton, 2013).

Inability to cope with their diagnosis and treatment can be an issue for many patients diagnosed with leukemia. The patient may express an intense fear or anxiety. Evaluating anxiety and supporting coping mechanisms can help manage a patient's fear and anxiety. Nurses should encourage patients to use stress management techniques such as deep breathing exercises and guided imagery. If needed, a nurse should refer the patient to social work for further assistance (Bush, 2013).

Patients may also develop malnutrition and volume depletion from chemotherapy. This loss may be due to nausea, vomiting, anorexia, and/or fever. Maintaining adequate fluid volume should be managed by monitoring urine input and output. Daily weights should be obtained. Patients should be encouraged to eat and drink to reduce anorexia. Monitor blood pressure (BP) and heart rate (HR) frequently; a change may reflect hypovolemia (Held-Warmkessel, 2013).

OUTCOMES

The expected outcomes for patients undergoing treatment for leukemia are to prevent/reduce the risk of infection and promote a safe environment. Patients need to be educated on preventing dehydration and maintaining adequate fluid volume. Patients should appear relaxed and be able to rest/sleep (Shelton, 2013).

Summary

Leukemia is a blood cancer that is treated by chemotherapy. Whether the leukemia is acute or chronic, nurses need to be aware of the risk factors and potential side effects of chemotherapeutic agents. Identifying infection and deficit volume in a timely manner is important. Proper education regarding treatment, side effects, and potential risks is needed for all patients and their families.

Bush, N. J. (2013). Psychosocial management. In B. H. Gobel, S. Triest-Robertson, & W. H. Vogel (Eds.), *Advanced oncology nursing certification* (pp. 637–631). Pittsburgh, PA: Oncology Nursing Society.

Dighiero, G., & Hamblin, T. J. (2008). Chronic lymphocytic leukaemia. *Lancet, 371*(9617), 1017–1029.

Ezzone, S. A. (2013). Blood and marrow stem cell transplantation. In B. H. Gobel, S. Triest-Robertson, & W. H. Vogel (Eds.), *Advanced oncology nursing certification* (pp. 261–262). Pittsburgh, PA: Oncology Nursing Society.

Gaynor, J., Chapman, D., Little, C., McKenzie, S., Miller, W., Andreeff, M., . . . Gee, T. (1988). A cause-specific hazard rate analysis of prognostic factors among 199 adults with acute lymphoblastic leukemia: The Memorial Hospital experience since 1969. *Journal of Clinical Oncology, 6*(6), 1014–1030.

Goldman, J. M., & Melo, J. V. (2003). Chronic myeloid leukemia—Advances in biology and new approaches to treatment. *New England Journal of Medicine, 349*(15), 1451–1464.

Held-Warmkessel, J. (2013). Cardiac, gastrointestinal, neurologic, and ocular toxicities. In B. H. Gobel, S. Triest-Robertson, & W. H. Vogel (Eds.), *Advanced oncology nursing certification* (pp. 261–262). Pittsburgh, PA: Oncology Nursing Society.

Hoelzer, D., Thiel, E., Löffler, H., Büchner, T., Ganser, A., Heil, G., . . . Rühl, H. (1988). Prognostic factors in a multicenter study for treatment of acute lymphoblastic leukemia in adults. *Blood, 71*(1), 123–131.

National Cancer Institute. (2017). Leukemia. Retrieved from http://www.cancer.gov/types/leukemia

National Cancer Institute Surveillance, Epidemiology, and End Results Program. (2017). Cancer stat facts: Leukemia. Retrieved from http://seer.cancer.gov/statfacts/html/leuks.html

Shelton, B. (2013). Myelosuppression. In B. H. Gobel, S. Triest-Robertson, & W. H. Vogel (Eds.), *Advanced oncology nursing certification* (pp. 261–262). Pittsburgh, PA: Oncology Nursing Society.

■ LIVER CANCER

Shannon A. Rives

Overview

Liver cancer is one of the leading cancers worldwide (Singal & El-Serag, 2015). Liver cancer can be primary or a result of metastasis. A primary tumor originates in the liver. Hepatocellular carcinoma (HCC) is the most common primary tumor and is often the consequence of underlying liver disease (Ryerson et al., 2016). Cholangiocarcinoma is cancer of the bile ducts and may occur in the intrahepatic biliary ducts. A secondary tumor is caused by metastasized tumor cells to the liver from other organs. The liver is a common site for metastases from breast, colon, bladder, kidney, ovarian, pancreatic, and lung cancer. Liver cancer is often found parenthetically because liver-specific symptoms may be absent or overlapping with chronic liver disease. Screening algorithms can be useful for early recognition; treatment options are selected by weighing risks and benefits. Nursing care is influenced by the treatment regimen, but overall education and support for patients and their families is needed throughout the process.

Background

Liver cancer is more common in sub-Saharan Africa and Southeast Asia than in the United States (American Cancer Society [ACS], 2016). Each year, liver cancer affects approximately 31,000 Americans (22,000 men and 9,000 women) and the incidence rate of liver cancer in the United States continues to rise (U.S. Cancer Statistics Working Group, 2017). Worldwide estimates of newly diagnosed events of hepatocellular carcinoma (HCC) exceeded 750,000 cases (Schütte, Balbisi, & Malfertheiner, 2016). Chronic liver disease has affected the incidence rates of HCC in the United States, which have continually increased in recent decades (Singal & El-Serag, 2015; Mittal et al., 2016). Chronic hepatitis B and C (HBV/HCV) infections are prominent risk factors for developing HCC; infection rates in the United States range from 850,000 to 2.2 million and 2.7 million to 3.5 million, respectively (Ryerson et al., 2016). Other risk factors include nonalcoholic steatohepatitis (NASH), type 2 diabetes mellitus, obesity, tobacco use, excessive alcohol use, exposure to aflatoxins (produced by fungi found on crops such as corn and peanuts), male gender, Asian descent, and genetic disorders (hemochromatosis; Ryerson et al., 2016; Schütte, Balbisi, & Malfertheiner, 2016; Schütte, Schulz, & Malfertheiner, 2016).

Five-year survival rates vary based on the stage and type of liver cancer. For persons with localized cancer, the 5-year survival rate is approximately 31%, compared to stage 4 cancer with metastases, for which the 5-year rate is approximately 3% (ACS, 2016). Currently, the average 5-year survival rate is around 15% (Mittal et al., 2016). Early detection is the cornerstone of an optimal treatment plan, but, unfortunately, HCC is not easily detected through objective and subjective data collection. For high-risk patients, screening usually includes an abdominal ultrasound and determination of an alpha-fetoprotein level (AFP; Singal & El-Serag, 2015). A diagnosis can be established based on a combination of factors, including the presence or absence of underlying liver disease, characteristics of the tumor, increased serum markers (AFP greater than 500 ng/mL), CT scan or MRI results, and/or histological findings from biopsy (Pagana & Pagana, 2014; Singal & El-Serag, 2015).

Treatments for liver cancer include surgical intervention (partial hepatectomy or liver transplant), tumor ablation, embolization, targeted therapies, chemotherapy, and radiation. Transarterial chemoembolization (TACE) involves placement of a catheter in the hepatic artery to deliver chemotherapy and embolization agents directly to the tumor. The procedure is performed in interventional radiology and utilizes fluoroscopy and contrast media. Tumor characteristics, such as size, location, grade, and staging and the individual patient condition, are dynamics that impact the course of treatment.

Most cases of HCC are seen in patients with cirrhotic livers (Schütte, Schulz, & Malfertheiner, 2016). In chronic liver disease, the hepatocytes are injured from exposure to harmful agents (excessive fat, alcohol, excessive iron, or viral infection). Hepatocyte destruction activates vitamin A-storing hepatic stellate cells, situated in the space between the capillaries and liver cells, which yield collagen proteins and other elements that assist in creating a fibrin mesh (Benyon & Iredale, 2000). The fibrin mesh is similar to scar tissue that develops in the wound-healing process and lies between the hepatocytes and capillaries that supply oxygenated blood from the hepatic artery and nutrient-rich blood from the portal vein. The liver is a regenerative organ and will attempt to repair itself; if the offending agent is removed, there is potential for the scar tissue to be broken down and the fibrosis may resolve to some degree.

In patients with cirrhosis, continuous injury and inflammation lead to the development of a thick and tough fibrin mesh. Over time, the fibrin mesh will disrupt the normal architecture of the liver, producing nodular structures (this gives the liver a bumpy surface). Even in this altered state, the liver will still attempt to repair itself by producing more hepatocytes, but these new cells may have mutations.

Clinical Aspects

ASSESSMENT

Although signs and symptoms of liver cancer may be ambiguous or absent, accurate collection of objective and subjective data is still an essential part of patient care. As the tumor increases in size, the patient may report a feeling of fullness after eating or pain in the right side of the abdomen. An increase in the symptoms associated with the patient's underlying liver disease may be the first sign of liver cancer. A thorough patient history is important to identify potential risk factors for liver disease such as exposure to viruses, alcohol consumption, intravenous drug use, components of the metabolic syndrome, and genetic disorders. If the patient has an established diagnosis of cirrhosis, it is important to determine the cause and stage, as well as the presence of symptoms. Transition from compensated cirrhosis to decompensated cirrhosis can be hastened by the presence of a tumor. The patient should be assessed for any personal or family history of cancer, nutritional status, changes in appetite, unintentional weight loss, presence of abdominal pain, changes in bowel activity, and any respiratory symptoms. Objectively, a focused physical assessment should include inspecting for signs of liver disease, abdominal distention and other physical abnormalities of the abdomen, auscultating bowel sounds, and palpating and percussing for hepatomegaly and masses.

In the tertiary setting, the patient's treatment regimen will impact the nurse's daily focus. For example, postprocedural assessment of lower extremity pulses is relevant for a patient following chemoembolization. Following surgical resection, patients should have pain levels and respiratory status monitored, while evaluating for organ rejection is pertinent for transplant recipients. In general, monitoring for signs and symptoms of respiratory problems, infection, hypoglycemia, bleeding, weight gain, fluid and electrolyte imbalances, and cognitive changes is ongoing. Laboratory results can also offer some clues into the patient's condition. Trending liver enzymes, bilirubin, prothrombin time, and albumin levels all assess liver function. A compromised liver can cause a decrease in renal function so blood urea nitrogen (BUN) and creatinine levels are followed.

NURSING INTERVENTIONS, MANAGEMENT, AND IMPLICATIONS

Nursing has the opportunity to utilize primary and secondary prevention strategies to decrease the risk of liver disease and liver cancer whether in the community, ambulatory office, or acute care setting. Health-promotion strategies should include teaching the patient how to avoid HBV, including sex safe practices, stressing the avoidance of needle sharing, promoting HBV vaccination for at-risk populations, and adhering to safety measures that prevent transmission in the hospital. Current recommendations suggest persons born between 1945 and 1965 should be tested for HCV (Ryerson et al., 2016). For the patient who tests positive, treatment with antivirals should be discussed. High-risk patients should also be encouraged to keep any follow-up appointments with the medical team.

OUTCOMES

Decreasing a patient's risk factors for developing HCC should be an expected outcome. The HBV vaccine can offer a defense from the virus and can reduce the rate of HCC cases (Schütte, Balbisi, & Malfertheiner, 2016). Currently, there is no vaccine for HCV; however, achieving sustained virological response using HCV antiviral medication therapy lessens the risk of HCC (Schütte, Balbisi, & Malfertheiner, 2016). An increase in testing for HCV will identify infected people and treatment can be offered.

Summary

Liver cancer is a cause of cancer deaths worldwide. A diagnosis of liver cancer drastically decreases life expectancy and can be devastating to a patient and the family. Nursing plays a vital role in caring for patients with liver cancer by providing education and psychosocial support. Identifying patients at risk, particularly persons with a history of chronic liver disease, is the first step in early recognition and treatment of liver cancer. Prevention and surveillance through education and testing are interventions that can be integrated across the continuum of care.

American Cancer Society. (2016). Liver cancer survival rates. Retrieved from https://www.cancer.org/cancer/liver-cancer/detection-diagnosis-staging/survival-rates.html

Benyon, R. C., & Iredale, J. P. (2000). Is liver fibrosis reversible? *Gut*, *46*(4), 443–446.

Mittal, S., Kanwal, F., Ying, J., Chung, R., Sada, Y. H., Temple, S., . . . El-Serag, H. B. (2016). Effectiveness of surveillance for hepatocellular carcinoma in clinical practice: A United States cohort. *Journal of Hepatology*, *65*(6), 1148–1154.

Pagana, K. D., & Pagana, T. J. (2014). *Mosby's manual of diagnostics and laboratory tests* (5th ed.). St. Louis, MO: Elsevier Mosby.

Ryerson, A. B., Eheman, C. R., Altekruse, S. F., Ward, J. W., Jemal, A., Sherman, R. L., . . . Kohler, B. A. (2016). Annual report to the nation on the status of cancer, 1975–2012, featuring the increasing incidence of liver cancer. *Cancer*, *122*(9), 1312–1337.

Schütte, K., Balbisi, F., & Malfertheiner, P. (2016). Prevention of hepatocellular carcinoma. *Gastrointestinal Tumors*, *3*(1), 37–43.

Schütte, K., Schulz, C., & Malfertheiner, P. (2016). Nutrition and hepatocellular cancer. *Gastrointestinal Tumors*, *4*(2), 188–194. doi:10.1159/000441822

Singal, A. G., & El-Serag, H. B. (2015). Hepatocellular carcinoma from epidemiology to prevention: Translating knowledge into practice. *Clinical Gastroenterology and Hepatology*, *13*(12), 2140–2151.

U.S. Cancer Statistics Working Group. (2017). *United States cancer statistics: 1999–2014 incidence and mortality web-based report*. Atlanta, GA: Department of Health and Human Services, Centers for Disease Control and Prevention, and National Cancer Institute. Retrieved from http://www.cdc.gov/uscs

■ LUNG CANCER

Helen Foley

Overview

Lung cancer is the leading cause of cancer death in the United States for both men and women (Seigel, Miller, & Jemal, 2016). If detected in its early stages, lung cancer can be cured surgically. Yet, lung cancer is commonly diagnosed only after it has spread to other sites within the lung or body. Lung cancer has been widely associated with cigarette smoking, although other risk factors, such as exposure to radon, various occupational chemical exposures, and secondhand smoke, play a role, which has resulted in stigma and the misconception that all lung cancer patients have a history of smoking. In fact, lung cancer is a disease of advanced age. The median age of a lung cancer patient at diagnosis has been estimated at 71 years, and two thirds of all patients diagnosed are between the ages of 65 and 84 years (National Cancer Institute Surveillance, Epidemiology, and End Result Program [NCI SEER], 2016).

Nursing care of the patient with lung cancer focuses on support of the patient through diagnosis and treatment. This includes symptom management for symptoms arising from the disease itself or the treatment. Nurses play important roles in primary and secondary prevention, treatment, and symptom management.

Nurses are also instrumental in addressing quality-of-life issues, coordinating the care delivery team, and preparing patients and families for end of life. Nurses are the primary caregivers at end of life and are an important part of every hospice care team.

Background

According to the American Cancer Society, lung cancer is the most prevalent cancer in men, after prostate cancer, and the second most prevalent cancer in women (ACS, 2016a). Histology or cell type is important for both prognosis and treatment. Lung cancers are divided into two main groups, non-small cell lung cancer (NSCLC) and small cell lung cancer (SCLC). Mesothelioma is often grouped with lung cancer, but it is actually a malignancy of the pleura, or lining of the lungs, associated with asbestos exposure, and will not be discussed here.

NSCLC, primarily adenocarcinoma cell type, accounts for more than 80% of all lung cancers, and almost 100% of lung cancer found in nonsmokers (Sherry, 2017). Staging matters for both survival and treatment. Early-stage lung cancers are amenable to surgery or surgery and radiation (stages 1 and 2) and carry a 5-year survival rate of 49% for stage 1 and 30% for stage 2. Stage 3 cancers may be treated with a combination of chemotherapy and radiation and have a 5-year survival rate of 14% or less. Stage 4 lung cancer, which has spread to other organs or the opposite lung at the time of diagnosis, also treated with chemotherapy and radiation, has a 5-year survival rate of 1% (ACS, 2016b).

New treatments, such as immune therapy and targeted therapies for NSCLC, are offering increasing survival for some patients. Immune therapies utilize immune checkpoint inhibitor antibodies to help harness the body's own immune system to fight the cancer (Knoop, 2016). Although less toxic overall, they have their own set of side effects resulting from the activation of the body's immune system, and currently are very expensive. Scientists are still determining which patients are most likely to benefit from these treatments. Like chemotherapy, they require intravenous infusion in a specialized treatment center. Targeted therapies are directed at particular biomarkers in the cancer and include agents such as epidermal growth factor receptor (EGFR) mutations and anaplastic lymphoma kinase (ALK) gene fusions. Targeted therapies are generally oral agents

reserved for the small percentage of patients who have a particular mutation in their cancer (Knoop, 2016) and require genetic testing of the tumor. These mutations are more often found in female nonsmokers (Sherry, 2017).

SCLC makes up less than 20% of all lung cancers, but is considered a rapidly growing cancer, and is almost always associated with a smoking history. Seventy-five percent of patients with SCLC are diagnosed with extensive, late-stage disease (Knoop, 2016). Treatment of limited-stage and extensive-stage SCLC is generally chemotherapy with and without radiation therapy. Prophylactic cranial radiation is almost always recommended due to the high frequency of metastasis to the brain. Median survival for limited-stage SCLC is 14 to 20 months; median survival for extensive-stage SCLC is 9 to 11 months, but can be as short as a few weeks (Knoop, 2016).

Clinical Aspects

ASSESSMENT

Nurses in every setting have a role in secondary prevention by identifying patients who are current smokers. Nurses should assess the patient's readiness to quit, provide motivation, and help the patient find appropriate resources for smoking-cessation strategies. The American Lung Association and National Comprehensive Cancer Network (NCCN) have excellent resources and guidelines to help patients stop smoking (American Lung Association, 2016; NCCN, 2017). Nurses also have a role in identifying patients who meet the current lung cancer screening criteria established by the U.S. Preventive Services Task Force and supported by the American Cancer Society and the NCCN network. Screening criteria are adults aged 55 to 80 years with a 30-pack-year smoking history, current smokers, or those who have quit in the last 15 years. The current recommendation is annual screening using low-dose CT scan of the chest (U.S. Preventive Services Task Force, 2016).

Nurses play a key role in educating patients about various aspects of treatment and assessing their tolerance of the treatment. Early identification and treatment of side effects will contribute to increased quality of life. Neutropenia, esophagitis, swallowing issues, taste alterations, hair loss, and skin erythema and breakdown are especially common in patients receiving concurrent chemotherapy and radiation.

OUTCOMES

Nurses also provide symptomatic treatment and palliative care for patients with lung cancer. These symptoms, including pain, cough, dyspnea, fatigue, and poor appetite, affect quality of life for the patient and cause distress for family members. Accurate assessment, appropriate referrals, and supportive counseling by the nurse can improve the quality of life for the patient and family. A lung cancer diagnosis is a crisis for both the patient and family members. Lung cancer patients are likely to experience physical, spiritual, psychological, and social distress. Appropriate identification of disturbance in one or more of these quality-of-life domains and timely intervention or referral by the nurse can lead to improved patient outcomes. The importance of palliative care in lung cancer patients should not be underestimated. A study of lung cancer patients showed that when lung cancer patients had palliative care service provided in conjunction with standard cancer care, they had higher satisfaction with their care and lived an average of almost 3 months longer than those who received standard care alone (Temel et al., 2010).

Nurses play a vital role in helping patients with advanced care planning and identifying their goals for care and end-of-life preferences. Nurses are often relied on to communicate these issues to the health care team, and serve as advocates for patients and families. This requires the nurse to have good communication skills and comfort in addressing sensitive issues. Oncology nurses benefit from end-of-life training through such programs as those offered by the American Association of Colleges of Nursing's End-of-Life Nursing Education Consortium (ELNEC).

Summary

Lung cancer is a devastating diagnosis for patients and their families. Eighty percent of patients diagnosed with lung cancer will die from their disease (NCI SEER, 2016). Lung cancer is associated with significant symptom and treatment burdens that have longstanding impact on the patient's quality of life. The development of new treatments in the last few years offers hope for patients for prolonged survival and some even have a better side-effect profile than chemotherapy and radiation.

Patients benefit from good nursing care along the disease continuum, from diagnosis to death. Nurses play a vital role in assessing and managing bothersome side effects, educating patients, monitoring treatment and treatment-related problems, and coordinating the care team. Lung cancer patients benefit when nurses are able to comfortably and openly discuss goals of care and end-of-life issues with patients and their families.

American Cancer Society. (2016a). Facts and figures. Retrieved from https://www.cancer.org/cancer/non-small-cell-lung-cancer/detection-diagnosis-staging/survival-rates.html

American Cancer Society. (2016b). Non-small cell lung cancer survival rates by stage. Retrieved from http://www.cancer.org/cancer/non-smallcelllungcancer/detectiondiagnosis-staging/survival-rates.html

American Lung Association. (2016). Stop smoking. Retrieved from http://www.lung.org/stop-smoking

Knoop, T. (2016). Lung cancer. In C. H. Yarbro, D. Wujcik, & B. H. Holmes (Eds.), *Cancer nursing: Principles and practice* (8th ed., pp. 1679–1720). Burlington, MA: Jones & Bartlett.

National Cancer Institute Surveillance, Epidemiology, and End Result Program. (2016). Cancer of the lung and bronchus cancer stat facts. Retrieved from http://seer.cancer.gov/statfacts/html/lungb.html

National Comprehensive Cancer Network. (2017). Clinical practice guidelines in oncology. Smoking cessation. Version 1.2017. Retrieved from http://www.nccn.org/professionals/physician_gls/pdf/smoking.pdf

Sherry, V. (2017). Lung cancer: Not just a smoker's disease. *American Nurse Today, 12*(2), 16–21.

Siegel, R. L., Miller, K. D., & Jemal, A. (2016). Cancer statistics, 2016. *CA: A Cancer Journal for Clinicians, 66*(1), 7–30.

Temel, J. S., Grier, J. A., Muzicansky, A., Gallagher, E. R., Admane, S., Jackson, V. A., . . . Lynch, T. J. (2010). Early palliative care for patients with metastatic non-small cell lung cancer. *New England Journal of Medicine, 363*(8), 733–742.

U.S. Preventive Services Task Force. (2016). Final update summary: Lung cancer screening. Retrieved from http://www/uspreventativeservicestaskforce.org/Page/Document/Update Summary Final/Lung-cancer-screening

■ LYMPHOMA

Marisa A. Cortese
Jane F. Marek

Overview

Lymphoma is a cancer of the lymphatic system and can appear anywhere in the body. The primary purpose of the lymphatic system is to fight infection. Both B- and T-lymphocytes play a key role in fighting infection by regulation of the immune system and production of cytokines and antibodies. B-lymphocytes are produced in the bone marrow and T-lymphocytes are produced by the thymus gland. Lymphomas are divided into two types: Hodgkin's lymphoma (HL) and non-Hodgkin's lymphoma (NHL), named after the British pathologist Thomas Hodgkin who described the disease in 1832. Both of these lymphomas can occur in children and adults.

There were approximately 81,080 new cases of lymphoma diagnosed in the United States in 2016 (National Cancer Institute [NCI], 2017a). The 5-year survivor rate for HL is approximately 85%, for NHL 69%; the 10-year survival rate decreases for both lymphomas (80% and 58%, respectively; Rummel, 2015). HL is generally considered a curable disease, but treatments may cause profound adverse effects for the patient.

Background

Genetic and environmental factors contribute to the development of lymphomas. Environmental influences include exposure to pesticides, benzenes, or radiation; occupations at increased risk include farmers, chemists, and persons employed in the rubber, petroleum, plastics, and synthetic industries (Rummel, 2015). Both lymphomas are more common in Caucasians than in any other racial group. Persons who have received an organ transplant or are being treated with immunosuppressive drugs are at increased risk for developing the disease.

HLs are caused by alterations in lymphocytes resulting in large, abnormal lymphocytes in the lymph nodes called *Reed–Sternberg cells*; most HLs are derived from B-lymphocytes. Most persons with HL are diagnosed between the ages of 15 and 35 years or over 65 years. Risk factors for developing HL include male gender, history of infection with Epstein–Barr or HIV, or having a first-degree relative with HL. The common signs and symptoms of HL are lymphadenopathy, hepatomegaly or splenomegaly, unexplained fever, night sweats, unintentional weight loss, pruritus, and fatigue (Rummel, 2015). Patients often experience pain in the enlarged lymph nodes after alcohol intake.

NHL refers to a group of lymphatic cancers derived from B-lymphocytes, T-lymphocytes, or natural killer cells; the majority of NHL originates from B-cells. NHL can be indolent or aggressive. Indolent lymphoma tends to spread slowly and has few signs and symptoms. Aggressive lymphoma spreads quickly, and the patient may have many signs and symptoms, some of which can be severe. Most lymphomas are diagnosed in persons aged 65 to 74 years. Additional risk factors include a history of any of the following: organ transplant; previous cancer treatment; inherited immune disorder; autoimmune disease; or infection with HIV/AIDS, human T-lymphotropic virus type I, Epstein–Barr virus, or *Helicobacter pylori*.

The most common sign of NHL is lymphadenopathy anywhere in the body. Other clinical manifestations include hepatomegaly or splenomegaly, unexplained fever, fatigue, unintentional weight loss, decreased appetite, and skin rash or pruritus (Shankland, Armitage, & Hancock, 2012). Patients with lymphomas may also present with symptoms specific to the tumor location, for example, a chest lesion may cause respiratory problems or chest pain.

Patients diagnosed with lymphoma require a complete medical workup. A thorough history and physical examination and laboratory tests, including complete blood count with differential and chemistry panel, should be performed. Other causes of lymphadenopathy and symptoms of lymphoma must be ruled out. A lymph node biopsy is necessary for diagnosis; bone marrow aspiration and biopsy may be performed to check for metastasis. Following biopsy, staging is done to determine the extent of the disease and to guide treatment. A PET or CT scan can be useful in determining the extent of disease.

A patient's prognosis is dependent on age, comorbidities, staging, and the presence or absence of specific chromosomal abnormalities found in the blood and/or bone marrow (Rummel, 2015). The prognosis is also dependent upon the presence of systemic symptoms, or B-symptoms. B-symptoms include fever more than 38°C for 3 consecutive days, unintentional weight loss of more than 10% body weight in 6 months, and drenching night sweats (Carbone, Kaplan, Musshoff, Smithers, & Tubiana, 1971).

The standard treatment is chemotherapy, immunotherapy, or radiation therapy, alone or in combination. Patients with indolent NHL may be followed and monitored closely, rather than undergo treatment. Patients with relapsed/refractory disease may undergo a hematopoietic stem cell transplant (NCI, 2017b).

Clinical Aspects

ASSESSMENT

The nurse should assess the patient for risk factors and specific symptoms associated with lymphoma, including a history of viral illness or cancer treatments; fever;

night sweats; chills; bleeding or bruising; and abdominal pain or frequent infections. A thorough medication history should be elicited, paying particular attention to immunosuppressant use, which may increase the risk of lymphoma. On physical examination, a patient may appear pale and feverish, and have enlarged lymph nodes in the neck, armpit, or groin or present with a rash (Rummel, 2015).

Patients with a large tumor burden and certain types of high-grade NHL are at increased risk for tumor lysis syndrome (TLS). TLS occurs as a result of cancer treatments, which cause rapid destruction of neoplastic cells resulting in hyperkalemia, hypocalcemia, hyperphosphatemia, and hyperuricemia. TLS can occur with the administration of chemotherapy, radiation therapy, biotherapy, glucocorticoids, or general anesthesia. This is a potentially life-threatening condition that can cause metabolic disturbances such as acute kidney injury, seizures, cardiac arrhythmias, metabolic acidosis, or death (Cope, 2013). An elevated lactate dehydrogenase, renal insufficiency, or dehydration before therapy can indicate an increased risk for developing TLS (Ikeda, Jaishankar, & Krishnan, 2016).

Prevention of infection is a nursing priority; patients with lymphoma are at increased risk for infection due to the disease process and also as an adverse effect of treatment. Interventions should focus on preventing infection, preventing injury, decreasing fatigue, and promoting optimal nutrition. The patient and family should be included in the teaching, so they can continue preventive strategies at home.

The nurse/patient navigator is an important resource to support and guide patients and their families across the cancer continuum (Rummel, 2015). The nurse navigator functions as part of a multidisciplinary team to assist patients in dealing with the financial, communication, treatment, psychosocial, and logistical barriers faced when dealing with cancer. They play a key role in patient education and support patients after treatment as they transition to survivorship (Rummel, 2015). The role of the nurse navigator is supported by the Academy of Oncology Nurse & Patient Navigators and the American College of Surgeons Commission on Cancer (Rummel, 2015).

The goal of treatment is to achieve a cure and maintain the patient's quality of life. The desired outcomes for patients undergoing treatment for lymphoma are to prevent/reduce the risk of infection and complications. Patients must be carefully monitored during and after care treatment for adverse effects and realize the importance of follow-up care.

Summary

The prognosis for patients with lymphoma varies depending on the individual patient, type of lymphoma, and stage of disease. Advances in treatment have led to increased survivorship for patients with both NHL and HL. Nurses working in any setting may encounter patients with lymphoma along any stage of the cancer continuum. Knowledge of the risk factors, disease process, and treatment modalities can enable nurses to provide quality and evidence-based care to these patients.

Carbone, P. P., Kaplan, H. S., Musshoff, K., Smithers, D. W., & Tubiana, M. (1971). Report of the Committee on Hodgkin's Disease Staging Classification. *Cancer Research*, 31(11), 1860–1861.

Cope, D. G. (2013). Metabolic emergencies. In B. H. Gobel, S. Triest-Robertson, & W. H. Vogel (Eds.), *Advanced oncology nursing certification* (pp. 568–574). Pittsburgh, PA: Oncology Nursing Society.

Ikeda, A. K., Jaishankar, D., & Krishnan, K. (2016). Tumor lysis syndrome. *Medscape*. Retrieved from http://emedicine.medscape.com/article/282171-overview#a5

National Cancer Institute. (2017a). Cancer stat facts: Lymphoma. Retrieved from http://seer.cancer.gov/statfacts/html/nhl.html

National Cancer Institute. (2017b). Lymphoma. Retrieved from http://www.cancer.gov/types/lymphoma

Rummel, M. (2015). Non-Hodgkin lymphoma and Hodgkin lymphoma: The role of the nurse navigator in improving patient outcomes. *Journal of Oncology Navigation & Survivorship*, 6(3), 3–10.

Shankland, K. R., Armitage, J. O., & Hancock, B. W. (2012). Non-Hodgkin lymphoma. *Lancet*, 380(9844), 848–857.

■ MULTIPLE SCLEROSIS

Alaa Mahsoon

Overview

According to the National Multiple Sclerosis Society (2016), multiple sclerosis (MS) is a chronic condition that damages the myelin sheath (demyelination) that surrounds nerve fibers in the brain, spinal cord, and optic nerves. Demyelination causes impaired nerve conduction that creates neurological problems. According to Alroughani, Akhtar, Ahmed, Behbehani, and Al-Hashel (2016), MS is an immune-mediated disease because the immune cells in the central nerves system (CNS) are attacked by an unknown antigen. Clinical pictures of patients with MS differ from person to person. However, early symptoms might involve numbness, tingling, or weakness in the extremities; visual changes; impaired balance; and urinary frequency and urgency. Besides physical deterioration of the disease, MS can be psychologically destructive for patients and their families. Therefore, nursing care is crucial for patients' physical and psychological stability and well-being.

Background

According to the National Multiple Sclerosis Society (2016), MS prevalence among the U.S. population is not well studied because health care providers are not required to report cases of MS; because of its invisible symptoms individuals have MS and do not know it. However, there are 2.3 million reported cases worldwide. MS is more prevalent in women and Whites. The rate of MS is also high among individuals between the ages of 40 and 59 years as well as non-Hispanics in the United States. The Centers for Disease Control and Prevention indicate that in the United States the rate varies from 58 to 95 cases per 100,000 population (Dobson et al., 2016). However, the prevalence rate varies among regions and ages worldwide. Variation in ultraviolet (UV) radiation exposure among regions accounts for the geographic difference between MS prevalence estimates. Disparately, adults between the ages of 40 and 59 years have higher chances of contracting the disease compared to children.

Social, environmental, and biological factors contribute to the development of MS. MS is regarded as a significant cause of disability in young people. The etiology of the disease is unknown. Genetic factors increase an individual's risk by 2% to 4% and are present in 30% of individuals without MS. Thus, relatives of patients with MS have an increased chance of getting the disease due to their genetic predisposition (Moccia et al., 2016). Environmental factors, such as radiation exposure, are also likely to influence disease susceptibility. Despite the lack of data demonstrating a link between exposure to bacteria and development of MS, an association is known to exist (Moccia et al., 2016).

Social determinants are also linked with race; MS is more prevalent in Whites with higher socioeconomic status than in Hispanics and other ethnic groups. Research further indicates that the prevalence and incidence of MS increases with age (Jelinek et al., 2016). The rise in the prevalence rate is influenced by prolonged survival of patients with MS, whereas the incidence rate is affected by the risk factors identified. MS is often regarded as a highly variable illness and poses a fundamental challenge to health care providers. More than 50% of people who have MS experience clinical symptoms such as brain lesions.

Clinical Aspects

The etiology of MS is not clear; however, clinical manifestations often link complex interactions between the immune system and environmental and genetic factors. The associated negative impact affects patients' disability over time, primarily when the onset of treatment is late or when clinicians are not familiar with the immunopathogenesis, natural course, and symptoms of the disease. MS also reduces the quality of life, causing premature disability and an increased mortality rate (Dilokthornsakul et al., 2016).

Nursing process or care, as well as quality-improvement processes, has a significant role in reducing the adverse effects of the clinical condition in context. MS creates the need for increased efficacy and safety of the treatment methods provided. Nurses have a critical role in facilitating the start and management of the treatment options in MS. However, the nurse's role has evolved over the years as they are now required to establish collaborative partnerships with patients and other health care providers. Nurses also have a vital role in helping the patients understand the available treatment options as well as understanding their diseases. They also help encourage the patient's adherence and management of treatment to promote positive outcomes (Riemann-Lorenz et al., 2016).

MS nurses have also expanded their role and training or set of skills due to increased changes in the treatment paradigm. MS also requires a broad range of clinical options, dosing schedules, and addressing the risk factors, which has created the need for nurses and other health care providers to enhance their professional training and development. Nursing care and process improvement should be based on a patient-centered approach that addresses the patient needs to improve positive outcomes. The process of care provided can include different steps such as assessment stage, problem identification, nursing intervention, and outcomes evaluation.

ASSESSMENT

The assessment phase includes a stage during which nurses will be involved in identifying the relevant history of the patients because genetic factors are key risk factors in MS. Patient history presents a chance to understand the association between risk of MS and genetics. This information helps to shape the intervention methods adopted. The patient's physical condition is evaluated so as to provide diagnostic data to the nursing care and process improvement teams to promote positive outcomes (Jelinek et al., 2016).

NURSING INTERVENTIONS, MANAGEMENT, AND IMPLICATIONS

The nursing-related problems that are responsive to nursing interventions or process change may include communication problems and teamwork issues. As such, the care model that should be adopted for MS patients includes a collaborative approach to care that involves both the patients and other care providers to promote positive outcomes. The approaches are also responsive to process change because they are influenced by patient needs and available interventions.

MS has no cure; however, care providers can use their positions to reduce the adverse effects or patient suffering by providing nursing interventions that address identified needs. The most appropriate nursing interventions and management options necessary to address MS include the provision of patient-centered care and a collaborative approach to care. The methods offer a chance to include both the care providers and the patients in their care. The methods serve as evidence-based interventions that promote the likelihood of shaping patient outcomes. Nurses can also support the implementation of early treatment of the disease. The evidence-based approaches used provide an opportunity to reduce the associated adverse effects and provide the health care institutions an opportunity to shape patient care (Jelinek et al., 2016).

OUTCOMES

In most cases, the use of a collaborative approach to patient-centered care among other evidence-based practices promotes positive outcomes. However, given the fact that MS is not curable, the available interventions provide a chance to manage the condition, especially when early intervention is provided. Hence, the expected outcomes of the proposed interventions for MS include a reduction in the overall mortality rate, improved quality and safety of care provided, and positive results for patients.

Summary

MS is a critical health condition that often leads to negative outcomes such as patient disability. Research has identified key risk factors of genetic and environmental issues. Although MS does not have a cure, care providers can utilize different interventions to manage the condition based on the disease pathogenesis. The evolution of treatment options has created the need to have an active collaboration between care providers and the patients. Nurses have a fundamental role in helping patients understand the available treatment options as well as their medical condition. They are expected to improve their professional skills to ensure expertise in the ever-changing therapies for MS. Future trends may influence the delivery of nursing care and improve patient outcomes and treatment options or therapies. Therefore, the role of MS nurses will continue to evolve over time; better management can be shaped by involving patients in their care and establishing a collaborative approach among care providers.

Alroughani, R., Akhtar, S., Ahmed, S., Behbehani, R., & Al-Hashel, J. (2016). Is time to reach EDSS 6.0 faster in patients with late-onset versus young-onset multiple sclerosis? *PLOS ONE, 11*(11), e0165846.

Dilokthornsakul, P., Valuck, R. J., Nair, K. V., Corboy, J. R., Allen, R. R., & Campbell, J. D. (2016). Multiple sclerosis prevalence in the United States commercially insured population. *Neurology, 86*(11), 1014–1021.

Dobson, R., Ramagopalan, S., Topping, J., Smith, P., Solanky, B., Schmierer, K., . . . Giovannoni, G. (2016). A risk score for predicting multiple sclerosis. *PLOS ONE, 11*(11), e0164992.

Jelinek, G. A., De Livera, A. M., Marck, C. H., Brown, C. R., Neate, S. L., Taylor, K. L., & Weiland, T. J. (2016). Lifestyle, medication and socio-demographic determinants of mental and physical health-related quality of life in people with multiple sclerosis. *BMC Neurology, 16*(1), 235.

Moccia, M., Palladino, R., Lanzillo, R., Carotenuto, A., Russo, C. V., Triassi, M., & Brescia Morra, V. (2017). Healthcare costs for treating relapsing multiple sclerosis and the risk of progression: A retrospective Italian cohort study from 2001 to 2015. *PloS One, 12*(1), e0169489.

The National Multiple Sclerosis Society. (2016). Multiple sclerosis. Retrieved from http://www.nationalmssociety .org/What-is-MS

Riemann-Lorenz, K., Eilers, M., von Geldern, G., Schulz, K.-H., Köpke, S., & Heesen, C. (2016). Dietary interventions in multiple sclerosis: Development and pilot-testing of an evidence based patient education program. *PLOS ONE*, *11*(10), e0165246. doi:10.1371/journal.pone.0165246

■ MYASTHENIA GRAVIS

Jennifer Gonzalez

Overview

Myasthenia gravis (MG) is an acquired autoimmune disease characterized by fluctuating skeletal muscle weakness and fatigability that increases with exercise and improves with rest (Drachman & Amato, 2014). MG can develop into a lifelong chronic neuromuscular disease resulting in periods of exacerbation, remission, and sometimes crises of bulbar, ocular, facial, and respiratory muscles requiring medication adjustment and immunotherapy treatments (Drachman & Amato, 2014). MG occurs in both genders and all ethnic groups, although it is more common in women under the age of 40 years and men older than 60 years (National Institute of Neurological Disorders and Stroke [NINDS], 2010). Nursing care of adults with MG should focus on symptom identification, psychosocial assessment, patient education on medication regimens, and airway management during MG crises.

Background

MG is the most common disorder involving the neuromuscular junction (NMJ). There are approximately 36,000 to 60,000 cases of MG in the United States with a prevalence of 14 to 20 cases per 100,000 people (Howard, 2015); MG affects more than 700,000 people worldwide (Sanders et al., 2016). Over time, the ability to understand functions of the NMJ, autoimmunity, and role of the thymus gland has been attributed to an increase in survival rates and overall life span of patients with MG (NINDS, 2010). An international task force convened by the Myasthenia Gravis Foundation of America created a consensus guide for treatment goals, minimal manifestations, remission, crises, and additional statements to guide clinicians in the management of MG (Sanders et al., 2016).

In many cases of MG, muscle weakness and fatigability occur from a decrease or lack of acetylcholine

receptors (ACh-Rs) available at the NMJ during normal muscle contraction (Drachman & Amato, 2014). ACh, released by neurons at the NMJs, produces action potentials that stimulate contraction of skeletal muscles by depolarizing the muscle membrane (Drachman & Amato, 2014). In some forms of MG, ACh-R antibodies are released as an immune response causing rapid turnover of ACh-Rs, blockage of ACh-R sites, and impairment to the postsynaptic muscle membrane where depolarization occurs (Drachman & Amato, 2014). Symptoms generally become apparent when the number of ACh-Rs is approximately 30% of normal.

The thymus gland is responsible for immune development in childhood and is believed to play a role in the immune response in certain subtypes of MG (NINDS, 2010). Conditions of the thymus, such as hyperplasia or thymomas, may be an indication for thymectomy, resulting in realignment of the immune system and the potential for symptom reduction or cure (NINDS, 2010). Early-onset MG is characterized by positive ACh-R antibodies, thymic hyperplasia, and onset of symptoms younger than 40 years (Livesay, 2012). Persons with late-onset MG are typically diagnosed after age 40 years; have a normal thymus gland; and have positive antibodies for ACh, titin, and ryanodine receptors (Livesay, 2012). Most persons with MG have anti-ACh-R antibodies. Patients without anti-ACh-R antibodies are classified as having seronegative myasthenia gravis (SNMG). Many patients with SNMG have antibodies against muscle-specific tyrosine kinase (MUSK). The MUSK receptors are another component in the NMJ needed for successful neurotransmission for muscle contraction. Patients with this subtype of MG are usually female, diagnosed before age 40, and have normal thymus glands (Livesay, 2012).

Clinical Aspects

ASSESSMENT

The Myasthenia Gravis Foundation classified MG into five main types and several subtypes based on severity of symptoms, ranging from Class I with ocular muscle weakness to Class V with respiratory muscle weakness requiring intubation. Clinical manifestations of MG include muscle weakness that fatigues with repetitive movement and improves with rest. Muscle weakness is usually symmetrical with normal sensory function and deep tendon reflexes. As previously discussed, there are different subtypes of MG with varying clinical presentation. There are two clinical forms, referred to as ocular myasthenia gravis (OMG) and generalized myasthenia gravis (GMG). Approximately 85% of patients have OMG and present with fluctuating ocular involvement that does not progress to other muscles (Drachman & Amato, 2014). Other ocular symptoms include ptosis, diplopia, ocular palsy, and nystagmus (Smith, 2016). Within 2 years of OMG diagnosis, 50% of patients will progress to the GMG form with involvement of bulbar, facial, and limb muscles (American Association of Neuroscience Nursing [AANN], 2013). An adult with bulbar dysfunction will have symptoms such as dysphagia, dysphonia, and dysarthria (Smith, 2016). Snarling or expressionless face and flattening of the nasolabial fold are characteristic of facial muscle involvement (AANN, 2013). Persons with extremity involvement display weakness in the neck and upper extremities (AANN, 2013). Respiratory muscle involvement can cause dyspnea, hypoventilation, and respiratory failure requiring intubation and mechanical ventilation.

Diagnosis of MG is based on the patient's history and physical examination and bedside and serologic testing. Bedside testing includes the ice test and edrophonium test, but these tests should not be used as the sole means of diagnosis. The ice test can be useful for patients with ptosis in differentiating MG from other disorders. In the ice test, an ice pack is placed over the patient's eyes for 2 to 5 minutes; the cold should limit anticholinesterase activity, allowing for more availability of ACh. The test is considered positive if the eyelid elevates 2 mm following application of ice (Nair, Patil-Chhablani, Vankatramani, & Gandhi, 2014). The administration of intravenous edrophonium will show a rapid relief of symptoms if the MG type is responsive to acetylcholinesterase (ACh-E; AANN, 2013).

Serum laboratory tests include anti-ACh-R antibodies; 80% of patients with GMG will test positive (Nair et al., 2014). Adults with OMG may have negative anti-ACh-R antibody results but it is thought to be related to low detectable levels and should not be used to confirm the diagnosis (Drachman & Amato, 2014). Other laboratory testing includes antistriated muscle antibody testing, present in the majority of patients younger than 40 years of age with thymoma, and anti-MUSK antibody testing.

Other diagnostics may be indicated based on the patient's symptoms. A new onset of ocular symptoms may require a head CT scan or MRI to rule out brain lesions (Drachman & Amato, 2014). CT and MRI may also be performed to evaluate the thymus gland. Vital capacity is used to measure lung function when respiratory muscles are involved. Muscle strength and EMG (electromyography) should be included in the clinical workup.

NURSING INTERVENTIONS, MANAGEMENT, AND IMPLICATIONS

Nursing care of the adult with MG should focus on symptom management, psychosocial support, and medication compliance and administration. ACh-E inhibitors, such as pyridostigmine (Mestinon), can slow the degradation of ACh, allowing more availability of the neurotransmitter at the NMJ, thereby improving muscle activity (AANN, 2013). Excess ACh can result in cholinergic crisis, so it is important for nurses to teach patients the importance of taking their medications as prescribed, and also the side effects and signs and symptoms of overdose. Immunosuppression through administration of azathioprine (Imuran) or cyclosporine can also be used for immune-mediated MG. Patient education regarding immunosuppressives is required to ensure safety. The side effects associated with immunosuppressive therapy, including infection, nephrotoxicity, hepatotoxicity, and bone marrow suppression, warrant the need for close physician monitoring when initiating these medications (AANN, 2013).

Priority nursing problems related to the care of patients with MG include the management and identification of myasthenia crisis. Myasthenia crisis is a life-threatening complication characterized by severe respiratory muscle weakness and frequent bulbar weakness that may necessitate intubation and mechanical ventilation. Patients are at increased risk for aspiration due to excessive drooling and muscle weakness. Symptoms of MG may be potentiated by stress, surgery, or medications such as certain antibiotics, beta blockers, and muscle relaxers (Drachman & Amato, 2014). During MG crisis, immune-modulating therapy and plasmapheresis to remove circulating antibodies can aid in symptom management. Administration of intravenous immunoglobulin G (IVIG) is used to bind antibodies, permitting an increased availability of ACh during crisis (AANN, 2013). In addition to understanding the therapies used during crises, nurses should also consider the psychosocial aspects of the patient experiencing the crisis and during other uncertain periods of the disease such as exacerbations. Education points should include energy conservation, identification of triggers, when to seek medical attention, and information about professional organizations that may provide additional support.

OUTCOMES

Patients in remission with minimal ocular symptoms, such as eyelid weakness, may have their medication dose decreased or discontinued (Sanders et al., 2016). Mortality rates in adults with MG are between 4% and 8% and have continued to improve; the highest mortality rates occur within the first 2 years of diagnosis (AANN, 2013; Livesay, 2012). Prognosis is better in those whose disease remains restricted to ocular involvement; less favorable prognoses are associated in persons with thymomas (AANN, 2013).

Summary

MG can be accurately identified by clinical assessment, serological testing, and clinical diagnostic testing, although adults with mild weakness may require an extensive workup due to the need for differential diagnosis to rule out other causes of muscle weakness (NINDS, 2010). Medications that increase availability of ACh are a key component of symptom management in persons with MG. Many adults with MG can have a normal life. Immune-modulating therapies have allowed for treatment of MG crisis and have been attributed to improved prognosis (Sanders et al., 2016). Nurses should provide holistic care that involves chronic disease management such as medication coaching, symptom relief and prevention, community support, and patient and family education.

American Association of Neuroscience Nursing. (2013). Care of the patient with myasthenia gravis. AANN Clinical Practice Guidelines Series. Retrieved from http://www.myasthenia.org/LinkClick.aspx?fileticket=I2Imja5gU4s%3D&tabid=101

Drachman, D. B., & Amato, A. A. (2014). Myasthenia gravis and other diseases of the neuromuscular junction. In D. Kasper, A. Fauci, & S. Hauser (Eds.), *Harrison's principles of internal medicine*. Retrieved from http://accessmedicine.mhmedical.com/content.aspx?bookid=1130&sectionid=79756727

Howard, J. F. (2015). Clinical overview of myasthenia gravis. Retrieved from http://www.myasthenia.org/HealthProfessionals/ClinicalOverviewofMG.aspx

Livesay, S. (2012). Neurologic problems. In J. G. W. Foster & S. S. Prevost (Eds.), *Advanced practice nursing of adults in acute care* (pp. 223–227). Philadelphia, PA: F. A. Davis.

Nair, A. G., Patil-Chhablani, P., Vankatramani, D. V., & Gandhi, R. A. (2014). Ocular myasthenia gravis: A review. *Indian Journal of Ophthalmology, 62*(10), 985–991. doi:10.4103/0301-4738.144987

National Institute of Neurological Disorders and Stroke. (2010). Myasthenia gravis fact sheet (Publication No. 10-768). Washington, DC: DHHS. Retrieved from https://www.ninds.nih.gov/Disorders/Patient-Caregiver-Education/Fact-Sheets/Myasthenia-Gravis-Fact-Sheet

Sanders, D. B., Wolfe, G. I., Benatar, M., Evoli, A., Gihus, N. E., Illa, I., . . . Narayanaswami, P. (2016). International consensus guidance for management of myasthenia gravis. *Neurology, 87*(4), 419–425. doi:10.1212/WNL.0000000000002790

Smith, D. (2016). The neurologic system. In H. Craven (Ed.), *Core curriculum for medical–surgical nursing* (5th ed., pp. 407–460). Pitman, NJ: Academy of Medical–Surgical Nurses.

■ OBESITY

Kelly Ann Lynn

Overview

Obesity is a chronic metabolic disease that is associated with considerable morbidity and mortality. Obesity has been identified as a contributing factor for the development of several significant diseases, including type 2 diabetes mellitus (DM), hypertension (HTN), coronary artery disease (CAD), peripheral vascular disease, nonalcoholic fatty liver disease (NAFLD), osteoarthritis (OA), obstructive sleep apnea (OSA), and many cancers (colon, breast, ovarian; Hahler, 2002; Lobstein et al., 2015; Ng et al., 2014). Obesity also contributes to fertility and reproductive issues, depression, and dementia. Rates of obesity are rising in virtually all populations: in adults and children, and in developed and developing countries. Underscoring the significant impact of obesity on population health, the incidence of obesity is rising and has been described as a *global pandemic* (Ng et al., 2014). Nursing care of patients with obesity must focus on prevention, early intervention, and effective interventions that reduce morbidity and mortality associated with obesity and resultant disease.

Background

Obesity is defined as having a body mass index (BMI) greater than 30; a BMI between 25 and 29.9 is considered overweight. According to the Centers for Disease Control and Prevention (CDC), approximately 69% of adults in the United States are overweight, with more than one third (78.6 million) of these considered obese (CDC, 2015). Worldwide, obesity has more than doubled since 1980. The World Health Organization (WHO) statistics for 2014 are shocking: nearly 39% of adults or 1.9 billion people were overweight or obese; 41 million children younger than the age of 5 were overweight or obese (WHO, 2016). These statistics are very alarming, particularly when considering the propensity for illnesses and morbidity, disability, and mortality attributed to obesity and high BMI.

BMI is a universally accepted scale for assessing healthy weight and it refers to weight in kilograms divided by height in meters squared (BMI = kg/m^2). It is important to note that BMI is not an exact measurement. Muscle weighs more than fat and thus someone with a high muscle mass may have a deceptively high BMI. Likewise, someone with low muscle mass may have a misleading BMI. Waist circumference is another metric that is essential to assessing for obesity. Men should have a waist circumference less than or equal to 40 inches and women should have a waist circumference less than or equal to 35 inches.

Obesity is a complex disease and often has several contributing factors; obesity may be the result of genetic, metabolic, hormonal, and/or emotional issues. Emerging research suggests obesity may result from sleep deprivation, infection, exposure to endocrine-disrupting chemicals (EDCs), certain medications, and changes to the gut microbiome, among others (McAllister et al., 2009). Obesity is a major health concern because it is a precursor to other serious health conditions. The burden of disease-related obesity is massive. Nurses must address BMI, diet, and lifestyle with patients to prevent the devastating sequelae related to obesity.

Clinical Aspects

ASSESSMENT

A thorough nursing assessment is essential for all patients with obesity. This includes a comprehensive patient history with targeted questions related to eating habits, activity level, and reproductive/menstrual history. Physical assessment should be thorough and address vital signs, particularly height, weight, waist circumference, heart rate, and blood pressure. To evaluate circulation and identify areas of skin breakdown or infection, a thorough skin assessment is essential. It is imperative that nurses perform a comprehensive psychosocial assessment to identify underlying or associated mental health conditions, specifically depression.

Moreover, a review of essential laboratory values is of utmost importance. The urinalysis will help detect for the presence of glucose in the urine; serum chemistry will assess for electrolyte imbalances, cholesterol and lipid panel, fasting blood sugar, hemoglobin A1c for blood sugar control, serum albumin and vitamin B_{12} levels for malnutrition, blood urea nitrogen (BUN) and creatinine levels to evaluate renal function, thyroid function tests, liver enzymes and liver panel, and erythrocyte sedimentation rate (ESR or sed rate) to detect inflammation.

The review of medications is an essential part of the nursing assessment as some medications can contribute to obesity. These include psychotropic medications, antidiabetic drugs, antihypertensives, steroid hormones and contraceptives, antihistamines, and protease inhibitors (McAllister et al., 2009).

Nursing assessment of obesity must include all three components: comprehensive, in-depth history; a physical examination with evaluation and interpretation of laboratory and diagnostic tests; and medication review. Any encounter with patients with an elevated BMI (greater than or equal to 25) should address all of these issues.

NURSING INTERVENTIONS, MANAGEMENT, AND IMPLICATIONS

Nursing care of obese and overweight patients should focus on lifestyle and weight management. Prevention of the serious consequences related to obesity, specifically diabetes, cancer, and cardiovascular events, is the goal of care. Partnering with patients and championing their efforts will contribute to their success. Patients should be counseled on all available treatment options, including medical management, bariatric surgery, and endoscopic procedures that will help them be successful in reversing obesity. Patients must be encouraged to approach their care as a series of lifestyle changes rather than a diet, exercise, and medication program. Lowering BMI will reduce the incidence of diabetes, cardiovascular disease, urinary retention, and urinary sepsis. Nursing care must include comprehensive education and emotional support for patients and their families.

Nursing interventions will vary based on the clinical presentation, the treatment course, and the long-term objectives for a given patient. All patients will need considerable education about healthy lifestyle, their disease process, treatment options, and the side effects of medications that may be offered.

Some patients will be offered medical management to facilitate weight loss. These patients will require in-depth education about the medications, side effects, and potential interactions with other medications taken. Patients who choose bariatric surgery will need to be educated about the planned surgery and specific issues related to the various surgical options (gastric bypass, sleeve gastrectomy, laparoscopic adjustable band, duodenal switch). The details of the postoperative diet, management of nausea, and the signs and symptoms of infection need to be reviewed in detail. Similarly, patients opting for endoscopic intervention (endoscopic gastroplasty, endoscopic balloon) will need to be educated specific to these procedures.

Obese patients need guidance to adopt healthier lifestyle behaviors. They need to make healthier food choices by reducing sugar and simple carbohydrates in favor of nonstarchy vegetables and high-quality lean protein. Nurses should help patients develop a healthy relationship with food by discouraging emotional eating and disordered eating patterns (i.e., binging and craving). Food should be seen as a source of life. It must be emphasized to obese patients that every meal offers an opportunity to nourish their physical being.

Patients are encouraged to increase their activity level, starting off slowly and gradually increasing in intensity. Also, patients should be encouraged to adopt effective stress management techniques to reduce emotional eating and promote wellness. Walking, yoga, and meditation are all excellent stress reducers.

In addition, patients must be encouraged to improve their sleep habits. Adults should get 7 hours of sleep per night; children and adolescents need more. Sleep is essential to weight loss and overall health. This may be particularly difficult for obese people because they often suffer from OSA as a comorbidity of their obesity. Patients with OSA will need more intervention to ensure that they get the recommended amount of sleep.

Obese patients are often marginalized. Nurses must advocate for this vulnerable patient group to ensure that they get the appropriate care needed. All treatment areas must have appropriate seating and equipment (blood pressure cuffs, gowns) to ensure the safety and dignity of these patients.

Obesity is a multifaceted disease that affects not only patients, but also their partners and families. Nurses must offer patients and families an opportunity to process the complex emotions surrounding this disease.

OUTCOMES

The expected outcomes of evidence-based nursing care for patients with obesity are the prevention of serious consequences associated with the progression of this disease (diabetes, cancer, cardiovascular disease) so as to increase the patient's quality of life, and decrease the incidence of developing comorbid conditions.

Summary

Obesity medicine is a new specialty that recognizes that the condition is a disease, and that treating obesity is the best way to prevent diabetes. Early intervention and initiation of appropriate nursing care can prevent significant morbidity and result in better quality of life. Nurses must partner with their patients to develop customized care plans to reduce weight, improve health, and prevent progression of disease. Nursing support and education can help patients to choose healthier lifestyle behaviors and ease their distress and to promote compliance with their care plans.

Centers for Disease Control and Prevention. (2015). Adult obesity facts. Retrieved from http://www.cdc.gov/obesity/data/adult.html

Hahler, B. (2002). Morbid obesity: A nursing care challenge. *Medsurg Nursing, 11*(2), 85–90.

Lobstein, T., Jackson-Leach, R., Moodie, M. L., Hall, K. D., Gortmaker, S. L., Swinburn, B. A., . . . McPherson, K. (2015). Child and adolescent obesity: Part of a bigger picture. *Lancet, 385*(9986), 2510–2520. doi:10.1016/S0140-6736(14)61746-3

McAllister, E. J., Dhurandhar, N. V., Keith, S. W., Aronne, L. J., Barger, J., Baskin, M., . . . Allison, D. B. (2009). Ten putative contributors to the obesity epidemic. *Critical Reviews in Food Science and Nutrition, 49*(10), 868–913.

Ng, M., Fleming, T., Robinson, M., Thomson, B., Graetz, N., Margono, C., . . . Abraham, J. P. (2014). Global, regional, and national prevalence of overweight and obesity in children and adults during 1980–2013: A systematic analysis for the Global Burden of Disease Study 2013. *Lancet, 384*(9945), 766–781. doi:10.1016/S0140-6736(14)60460-8

World Health Organization. (2016). Obesity and overweight fact sheet. Retrieved from http://www.who.int/mediacentre/factsheets/fs311/en

■ OSTEOARTHRITIS

Mary Variath

Overview

Osteoarthritis (OA) is characterized as a chronic, degenerative, inflammatory disease that can affect any joint or structural component of a joint (Gomes et al., 2016; Kang et al., 2016). OA is the most common form of arthritis, and a leading cause of pain and disability globally. Middle-aged adults and the elderly are likely to experience symptoms of OA, which is consistent with the increased prevalence of OA among persons aged 45 years and older (Kapoor, 2015). Although OA can affect any joint, the hip and knee joints are commonly affected and can contribute to significant reductions in quality of life among those affected by OA. Nursing care for persons living with OA should consider nonpharmacological therapies in combination with pharamaceuticals to minimize pain and maintain the physical functioning of the affected joint (Uthman et al., 2014).

Background

In the United States, OA is a prevalent and disabling chronic condition. According to the Organization for Economic Cooperation and Development, about 28.5% men and 27.9% women in the United States are affected with OA (Kang et al., 2016). Advanced age is a factor associated with OA. In fact, it is estimated that individuals who are aged 70 years and older have a higher likelihood of having OA than persons aged 50 to 60 years (Kang et al., 2016). The incidence of OA has also been linked to obesity. Obesity has shown to drastically increase the incidence of OA of the knee in men and women (Kapoor, 2015). Thus, advanced age and obesity have been established as major risk factors for the development and progression of OA. Other risk factors include gender, race and ethnicity, genetics, nutrition, smoking, traumatic injury, and type 2 diabetes mellitus (Frey, Hügle, Jick, Meier, & Spoendlin, 2016; Huebner et al., 2016; Kang et al., 2016; Kapoor, 2015).

The relative significance of certain risk factors may differ from joint to joint, for early versus end-stage OA, for development as opposed to progression of disease, and for radiographic versus symptomatic disease. Although it is well established that the risk of developing OA increases dramatically with age; age is not the sole determinant of developing the disease.

Genetic, environmental, metabolic, and biochemical factors or a combination of these may result in more severe outcomes. Furthermore, inactivity of the joint may result in accelerated cartilage degradation. Sometimes the progressive loss of articular cartilage can be accompanied by alterations of the underlying structures, such as subchondral bone alteration. Besides, synovial tissue inflammation may be observed leading to synovitis, resulting in the initiation and/or progression of OA. Together, these structural changes produce the symptoms of joint pain, restriction of motion, crepitus with motion, joint effusions, and deformity.

Clinical Aspects

ASSESSMENT

Symptoms of OA are localized and not systemic, and include pain, bony enlargement, crepitation, tenderness to palpation, reduced range of movement, deformities, and overall functional limitation. Distal interphalangeal nodes called *Heberden's nodes* are a bony enlargement that are classic signs of hand OA; Bouchard's nodes in proximal interphalangeal joints are common in women. In advanced hip OA, leg length discrepancy and muscular atrophy, secondary to joint splinting for pain relief, may be noticed.

With spine OA, weakness and/or numbness in the arms and legs may result from nerve root impingement due to osteophytes. Localized warmth, an indication of inflammation, such as synovitis, may be noted in knee or hand OA. Individuals may experience one or more of these symptoms leading to pain and disability.

Joint pain and joint disability are the dominant symptoms of OA and the primary reason individuals seek medical help. The pain generally is described as mechanical in nature with a gradual onset, that increases with increased joint use but is relieved by rest in early stages. Pain, even at rest, especially at night, indicates severity of the condition. Joint stiffness, especially early-morning stiffness due to prolonged periods of inactivity, is another typical sign of OA. However, stiffness associated with OA is relieved with increased activity unlike persistent stiffness in rheumatoid arthritis. Together, pain and stiffness result in functional impairment of the joint.

In addition to assessing for local symptoms, diagnostic investigations such as diagnostic imaging, including radiographic assessment and MRI, which play a pivotal role in ruling out OA, also help. These tests assist in early diagnosis, grading, and monitoring of OA. CT, ultrasound, and nuclear medicine are also used to assess OA, although the role these play is very limited (Salat, Salonen, & Veljkovic, 2015).

These methods are generally used to stage the severity of the disease condition. Although there are no specific blood tests to rule out OA, an elevated erythrocyte sedimentation rate (ESR) indicates synovitis. Synovial fluid assessment can be performed to differentiate between OA and other forms of arthritis.

NURSING INTERVENTIONS, MANAGEMENT, AND IMPLICATIONS

Because OA is a chronic progressive disease with localized symptoms, primary nursing care should focus on assessing for the severity of pain, extent of deformity, functional disability, and examination of diagnostic imaging and laboratory data to confirm OA. The next step is to choose the appropriate steps to help slow the disease progression, damage, and disability, while managing the symptoms at the same time. Although there is no cure for OA, there are myriad treatment options to manage the symptoms, which include pharmacological and nonpharmacological options (Sepriano et al., 2015).

The pharmacological management of OA is currently based on a wide spectrum of therapeutic options to relieve pain, improving the physical function and quality of life. The American College of Rheumatology guidelines recommend topical capsaicin; topical nonsteroidal anti-inflammatory drugs (NSAIDs); oral NSAIDs, including cyclooxygenase inhibitors; and tramadol (Roubille, Pelletier, & Pelletier, 2015). However, the rapid-acting symptomatic treatments for OA consist mainly of analgesics and NSAIDs. Among them, acetaminophen remains the first-line therapeutic agent because of its cost-effectiveness, efficacy, and safety. Opioids and duloxetine are two other often-used agents. If the symptoms are not severe, topical NSAIDs, such as capsaicin and lidocaine patches, are reported to be effective (Roubille et al., 2015). The non-NSAIDs, such as corticosteroids that are anti-inflammatory drugs, and hyaluronic acid, which is a glycosaminoglycan component for the maintenance of joint homeostasis, are administered as intra-articular treatments in severe conditions (Roubille et al., 2015).

Other OA drugs with disease-modifying properties are being developed, such as slow-acting drugs for OA that are believed to reduce joint pain and slow structural disease progression in the joint. In addition, cartilage changes, bone remodeling, and synovial inflammation control are the types of studies in progress. Furthermore, a few promising therapies might emerge, such as platelet-rich plasma, bone remodeling modulators, and inflammatory inhibitors (Roubille et al., 2015).

Nonpharmacological intervention is directed toward self-management programs. Examples include muscle strengthening, low-impact aerobic exercises on land and in water; weight loss; physical therapy; and neuromuscular education (Schachar & Ogilvie-Harris, 2015). Surgery may be considered for individuals whose function and mobility remain compromised and are refractory to pharmacological and nonpharmacological interventions. Surgical interventions for OA include arthroscopy, osteotomy, arthrodesis, and total joint arthroplasty.

OUTCOMES

The intended outcomes of any type of intervention include pain management, providing comfort, minimizing activity intolerance, and ineffective functional and role performance.

Affected individuals learn self-management therapies, including land and/or water aerobic exercises, to improve activities of daily living and provide coping mechanisms.

Summary

OA is a chronic degenerative disorder, causing pain and limitation of movements due to gradual deterioration and inflammation of articular cartilage and joints, resulting in major physical and functional limitations. OA can affect any joint; however, hip and knee joints have a higher prevalence, with higher incidence of OA of the knee due to its weight-bearing function, resulting in a declining quality of life of the individual. Individuals older than 45 years are most often affected. The incidence of OA has risen with the escalation of obesity in the population. Because there is no cure for OA, the primary focus is symptomatic management using pharmacological or nonpharmacological therapies. Pain management, disease-progression control, and deformity prevention are the expected outcomes.

Frey, N., Hügle, T., Jick, S. S., Meier, C. R., & Spoendlin, J. (2016). Type II diabetes mellitus and incident osteoarthritis of the hand: A population-based case-control analysis. *Osteoarthritis and Cartilage, 24*(9), 1535–1540.

Gomes, W. F., Lacerda, A. C., Brito-Melo, G. E., Fonseca, S. F., Rocha-Vieira, E., Leopoldino, A. A., . . . Mendonça, V. A. (2016). Aerobic training modulates T cell activation in elderly women with knee osteoarthritis. *Brazilian Journal of Medical and Biological Research, 49*(11), e5181.

Huebner, J. L., Landerman, L. R., Somers, T. J., Keefe, F. J., Guilak, F., Blumenthal, J. A., . . . Kraus, V. B. (2016). Exploratory secondary analyses of a cognitive-behavioral intervention for knee osteoarthritis demonstrate reduction in biomarkers of adipocyte inflammation. *Osteoarthritis and Cartilage, 24*(9), 1528–1534.

Kang, K., Shin, J. S., Lee, J., Lee, Y. J., Kim, M. R., Park, K. B., & Ha, I. H. (2016). Association between direct and indirect smoking and osteoarthritis prevalence in Koreans: A cross-sectional study. *BMJ Open, 6*(2), e010062.

Schachar, R., & Ogilvie-Harris, D. (2015). Osteoarthritis: Joint conservation strategies. In M. Kapoor & N. N. Mohammad (Eds.), *Osteoarthritis* (pp. 155–169). Cham, Switzerland: Springer International.

Sepriano, A., Roman-Blas, J. A., Little, R. D., Pimentel-Santos, F., Arribas, J. M., Largo, R., . . . Herrero-Beaumont, G. (2015). DXA in the assessment of subchondral bone mineral density in knee osteoarthritis—A semi-standardized protocol after systematic review. *Seminars in Arthritis and Rheumatism, 45*(3), 275–283.

Toupin April, K., Rader, T., Hawker, G. A., Stacey, D., O'Connor, A. M., Welch, V., . . . Tugwell, P. (2016). Development and alpha-testing of a stepped decision aid for patients considering nonsurgical options for knee and hip osteoarthritis management. *Journal of Rheumatology, 43*(10), 1891–1896.

■ OSTEOMYELITIS

Mary Variath
Jane F. Marek

Overview

Osteomyelitis (OM) is inflammation of the bone caused by a variety of infectious organisms (i.e., bacteria, fungi, or viruses) that results in tissue destruction of the affected bone. OM is a complex disease in its pathophysiology, clinical presentation, and management, making accurate diagnosis and treatment a challenging process. The symptoms of OM include history of local inflammation, erythema, and/or swelling. In addition, patients with OM may present with low-grade fever, malaise, and fatigue, along with nonspecific chronic pain at the site of infection (Malhotra, Schulz, & Kallail, 2015). OM may affect any bone, resulting in progressive bone destruction and the formation of sequestra. OM can be acquired through contiguous spread from adjacent soft tissue, joint, and blood infections or direct inoculation of microorganisms into the bone as a result of trauma or surgery (Malhotra et al., 2015). Other risk factors include diabetes, vascular insufficiency, dialysis treatment, intravenous drug use, and immunosuppression. If untreated, OM can become a life-threatening illness due to bacteremia and sepsis. Therefore, early diagnosis, identification of the causative organism, and prompt treatment can prevent recurrent infection, chronic disease, and complications.

Background

OM is an ancient disease and is one of the most difficult infectious diseases to diagnose and treat (Malhotra et al., 2015). OM can affect people of all ages. Major causative bacterial organisms include *Pseudomonas aeruginosa, Staphylococcus aureus, Streptococcus pyogenes,* and *Streptococcus pneumoniae.* Infection with drug-resistant organisms is of particular concern. For unknown reasons, *Haemophilus influenzae* type B is shown to affect joints rather than bones alone. In addition, fungal or mixed bacteria are associated with skull, vertebral, and/or long bone OM. In fact, about 75% to 95% of skull OM is reported to be of fungal origin (Johnson & Batra, 2014; Peltola & Pääkkönen, 2014).

Bacteria can reach the bone through direct inoculation from traumatic wounds, open fractures, or implanted hardware; by spreading from adjacent tissue affected by various infections, such as cellulitis and septic arthritis; or by hematogenous spread following bacteremia. OM resulting from hematogenous spread is more common in children; boys are more commonly affected than girls. In developed countries, approximately eight in 100,000 children are affected with OM annually; in developing countries, the incidence is higher, especially in resource-poor places where patients present with advanced disease and survivors experience serious and long-lasting complications (Peltola & Pääkkönen, 2014). Salmonella species are reported to be a common cause of OM in developing countries as well as in patients with sickle cell disease. OM usually results from adjacent tissue inflammation and infection, as in the case of OM of the skull as a result of contiguous spread from an infected sinus or penetrating trauma (Malhotra et al., 2015). Skull base OM, although rare, is associated with a 10% to 20% mortality rate and primarily affects patients with diabetes and/or immunocompromised men in their 60s (Conde-Diaz et al., 2017).

Pyogenic vertebral OM generally occurs as an acute OM infection in patients older than 55 years. The estimated incidence of vertebral OM has increased in recent years to four to 10 per 100,000 persons annually in high-income countries, increasing the economic burden of the disease (Bernard et al., 2015).

Treatment depends on the etiology of the infection. Debridement of the affected bone was once considered the primary method of treatment; however, long-term systemic antimicrobial therapy has since replaced debridement as the first-line therapy (Conde-Diaz et al., 2017; Johnson & Batra, 2014). In severe cases, antimicrobial therapy needs to be continued for several weeks to avoid recurrent or chronic infection.

Surgical intervention is indicated if the patient does not respond to antimicrobial treatment or has persistent soft tissue infection, joint infection, or bony abscess. Goals of surgical management are debridement of necrotic bone and tissue, management of dead space, restoration of vascular supply, and adequate wound closure. Surgical techniques include bone debridement and resection, stabilization using an external fixator (including the Ilizarov technique), revascularization procedures, and, as a last resort, amputation. Infection following fracture fixation and prosthetic joint infection may result in removal of the hardware, systemic antibiotic therapy, and fracture fixation or joint revision after resolution of infection. Local antibiotic therapy with antibiotic-impregnated beads (antibiotic bead pouch) and spacers may be considered with joint infections and open fractures complicated with OM. In persons with extensive soft tissue involvement, hyperbaric oxygen treatment, vacuum-assisted wound closure (VAC), and skin grafting may be indicated.

Clinical Aspects

ASSESSMENT

Long-bone OM is classified by the Cierny–Mader system that is used to guide treatment. Symptoms of OM may include pain, persistent sinus tract or wound drainage, poor wound healing, and presence of fever. Bony necrosis may not occur for 6 weeks after the onset of infection (Spencer, 2015). Further, if signs and symptoms are less severe, the individual may be slow to seek medical care, in which case bone deterioration may continue without treatment. Therefore, a thorough history and physical assessment are critical to determine the initial injury, infection, or precipitating event.

OM can be classified as acute if the duration of the illness has been less than 2 weeks, subacute for a duration of 2 weeks to 3 months, and chronic for duration longer than 3 months. Classic clinical manifestations in children include inability to walk, fever and focal tenderness, visible redness and swelling around the affected bone. Symptoms are dependent on the affected bone. For example, spinal OM in adults is characteristically manifested as back pain, whereas pain on a digital rectal examination suggests sacral OM.

Diagnosis is determined by the patient's history and clinical presentation and diagnostic testing. Laboratory testing is nonspecific to OM and includes complete blood count and differential, C-reactive protein, and erythrocyte sedimentation rate. Bone biopsy and wound and blood cultures are performed to identify the causative organism and to develop the antibiogram (Peltola & Pääkkönen, 2014). Selection of imaging techniques is based on clinical findings. In some cases, plain radiographs may be sufficient for diagnosis. If plain films are normal or inconclusive, MRI is most sensitive for OM; CT or scintigraphy can also be used, especially if a long bone is affected or if symptoms are not localized.

OUTCOMES

Nursing interventions include managing pain, monitoring neurovascular status of the affected extremity, administering antibiotic therapy, preventing further infection, supporting and immobilizing the affected area, preventing further injury, teaching the patient and family about medications, antibiotic therapy, treatments, prognosis, and rehabilitation therapy. Nurses can take an active role in infection-control education, which will help to control OM development and prevent complications (Spencer, 2015).

Summary

OM usually involves long-term treatment, and recurrence rates are high. Prompt identification of the offending organism and appropriate antibiotic therapy are key in optimizing patient outcomes. Because of the complexity of the illness, a multidisciplinary team approach is necessary. Physical and occupational therapy referrals are often indicated and the patient may require help with activities of daily living and the use of assistive devices until weight-bearing is permitted. Due to the length of treatment, psychosocial support of the patient and family is an important intervention. Treatment goals include limb preservation and prevention of complications, including pathologic fracture and further injury, flexion contractures and muscle atrophy, and systemic complications. Identification of persons at risk and prevention of infection are important nursing considerations.

Bernard, L., Dinh, A., Ghout, I., Simo, D., Zeller, V., Issartel, B., . . . Therby, A. (2015). Antibiotic treatment for 6 weeks versus 12 weeks in patients with pyogenic vertebral osteomyelitis: An open-label, non-inferiority, randomised, controlled trial. *Lancet, 385*(9971), 875–882.

Conde-Díaz, C., Llenas-García, J., Grande, M. P., Esclapez, G. T., Masiá, M., & Gutiérrez, F. (2017). Severe skull base osteomyelitis caused by *Pseudomonas aeruginosa* with successful outcome after prolonged outpatient therapy with continuous infusion of ceftazidime and oral ciprofloxacin: A case report. *Journal of Medical Case Reports, 11*(1), 48.

Johnson, A. K., & Batra, P. S. (2014). Central skull base osteomyelitis. *Laryngoscope, 124*(5), 1083–1087.

Malhotra, B., Schulz, T., & Kallail, K. J. (2015). When anemia, atypical plasma cells, and a lytic bone lesion are not myeloma: An unusual presentation of osteomyelitis. *Kansas Journal of Medicine,* 151–152.

Peltola, H., & Pääkkönen, M. (2014). Acute osteomyelitis in children. *New England Journal of Medicine, 370*(4), 352–360.

Spencer, D. (2015). Implications of underlying pathophysiology of osteomyelitis in diabetics for nursing care. MSN StudentScholarship. Paper 68. Retrieved from http://digitalcommons.otterbein.edu/stu_msn/68

■ OSTEOPOROSIS

Maria A. Mendoza

Overview

Osteoporosis is a chronic, progressive disease characterized by low bone mass density resulting in bone fragility and predisposition to fracture. Approximately 12 million people have osteoporosis in the United States, a number that is expected to rise to 14 million in 2020, of whom 80% are women (Cosman et al., 2015). One and a half million Americans have osteoporotic fractures (Jeremiah, Unwin, Greenawald, & Casiano, 2015), resulting in disability and decreased quality of life and the need for long-term nursing home care (Jeremiah et al., 2015).

Osteoporosis is considered a "silent" disease because it is asymptomatic, with many patients going undiagnosed and untreated until a fracture occurs (Cosman et al., 2015; Lorentzon & Cummings, 2015).

The major role of nursing in caring for patients with osteoporosis is in fracture prevention (Smeltzer & Qi, 2014). The impact of osteoporosis is significant, both in the effects on the patient and the economic burden. Assessing risk, assisting the patient to identify modifiable factors, and collaborating on a plan for lifestyle modification to help maintain bone health are important nursing interventions.

Background

Bone health is maintained by a dynamic process of formation and resorption. In osteoporosis there is imbalance in these processes caused by decreased bone formation, increased resorption, or both. Bone loss may be localized or generalized due to disuse or immobilization. Osteoporosis is divided into three types. Type I is related to aging and has two forms: postmenopausal (occurring in women after menopause) and senile (occurring in both genders age 65 and older). Type II usually occurs in younger individuals secondary to an underlying disease such as hyperthyroidism or multiple myeloma. Type III is found in women with amenorrhea associated with eating disorders. This section only discusses type I osteoporosis.

The most common sites for osteoporotic-related fractures (fragility fractures) are the hip, spine, and distal radius (Colles' fracture). Fractures are treated with surgical intervention, open reduction and internal fixation, or total or hemiarthroplasty for hip fractures; kyphoplasty or vertebroplasty for vertebral compression fractures; and closed or open reduction for Colles' fractures. Patients are at increased risk for another fracture following an osteoporotic fracture.

The nonmodifiable risk factors of osteoporosis include age (50 years and older), female gender, family history of osteoporosis, previous fracture (increase in risk by 86%), ethnicity (Caucasian and Asian), menopause/hysterectomy (due to decreased estrogen), inflammatory bowel disease, rheumatoid arthritis, systemic lupus erythematosus, hyperparathyroidism, hyperthyroidism, thin body frame, and primary/secondary hypogonadism (androgen deficiency) in men. Modifiable risk factors include long-term glucocorticoid therapy, excessive alcohol consumption, smoking, poor nutrition, vitamin D deficiency, gastric bypass surgery, eating disorders, insufficient weight-bearing exercise, low dietary calcium intake, certain medications (e.g., antiseizure, thyroid replacement, and selective serotonin reuptake inhibitors), and frequent falls (Cosman et al., 2015; Jeremiah et al., 2015).

Fracture risk assessment can be accomplished in a variety of ways. The fracture risk assessment tool (FRAX) is a valid online assessment tool that assesses the 10-year risk of osteoporotic fracture based on the individual's risk factors. There are limitations to this tool and it should be used in conjunction with clinical judgment. Other methods include bone mineral density (BMD) by dual-energy x-ray absorptiometry (DXA), quantitative computerized tomography (QCT), and hip structure analysis (HSA; Imai, 2014). BMD testing is the most common method used to identify fracture risk and evaluate the patient's response to treatment. The bone density in the hip and spine is measured and compared against established norms (peak BMD of a healthy 30-year-old adult) to give a T-score. The World Health Organization has established criteria for T-scores. A normal T-score is within +1 to –1 standard deviation (SD). Low bone density is between 1 and 2.5 (–1 to 12.5 SD). A level of 2.5 SD or lower is diagnostic of osteoporosis and more than 2.5 SD plus one or more osteoporotic fractures is considered severe osteoporosis (Cosman et al., 2015). BMD is recommended for women at age 65 years or may be done before 65 years on those who are at an increased risk for fractures (Cosman et al., 2015). There is no strong evidence to recommend biennial frequency of testing and no evidence to recommend DXA testing in men (Cosman et al., 2015).

The process of bone remodeling produces biochemical markers such as serum C-telopeptide, urinary telopeptide, serum bone-specific alkaline phosphatase, and aminoterminal propeptide (Jeremiah et al., 2015). These biochemical markers can predict fracture risk and rapidity of bone loss. They can also predict the magnitude of BMD and patient adherence to osteoporosis therapy.

Clinical Aspects

ASSESSMENT

In addition to assessing for the risk factors listed earlier, the nurse should also include an evaluation of the patient's nutritional status, dietary intake of calcium and vitamin D, alcohol consumption, smoking, and exercise habits (weight-bearing and resistive-type exercise and walking). Physical assessment includes height/weight; body mass index (BMI); vital signs, including orthostatic blood pressure and pulse; posture and balance; functional status (mobility, activities of daily living [ADL] abilities); and neurological and cardiovascular status. Physical findings include increased thoracic kyphosis; loss of height over time generally due to fractures of the vertebrae; and fractures in the wrist, hips, and other sites that may occur as disease progresses. Pain from a hip fracture is usually manifested by a report of groin pain, whereas vertebral compression fracture is characterized by acute localized pain after a fall/lifting episode. The area of the spine palpated will be tender to touch.

Diagnostic laboratory tests, such as alkaline phosphatase, calcium, liver and kidney function tests, complete blood count, thyroid-stimulating hormones, parathyroid hormone, total testosterone (men), estradiol (women), 25-hydroxyvitamin D, and urinary calcium, are usually done to diagnose primary and secondary causes of osteoporosis (Jeremiah et al., 2015).

NURSING INTERVENTIONS, MANAGEMENT, AND IMPLICATIONS

Applicable nursing diagnoses for the patient with osteoporosis include risk for injury/falls, acute pain, impaired mobility, and deficient knowledge.

The following interventions are based on the recommendations by the National Osteoporosis Foundation (Cosman et al., 2015) developed by an expert committee regarding prevention, risk assessment, diagnosis, and treatment of osteoporosis.

Risk assessment and counseling on risk of osteoporosis and fractures. The nurse should obtain a history of risk factors listed earlier. Patient engagement to understand the implications of the risk factors and to plan a lifestyle modification regimen to decrease risk is imperative for success. The nurse can play a major role in multidisciplinary teams or programs that increase awareness of osteoporosis screening and treatment in the community and long-term care facilities (Smeltzer & Qi, 2014).

Nutritional and lifestyle counseling to maintain healthy bone. The recommended calcium intake from food and supplements is 1,200 mg daily for women 51 years and older and 1,000 mg daily for all adults aged 19 to 50 and men 51 years and older. The best source for calcium is from food; calcium supplements may cause constipation and increase the risk for kidney stones. The data regarding the association between cardiovascular disease and calcium supplementation are controversial. There does not appear to be an association between calcium supplementation (up to 2,000–2,500 mg/day) and cardiovascular disease risk in healthy adults (Chung, Tang, Fu, Wang, & Newberry, 2016). Patients should be advised not to take calcium supplements in doses over 500 mg at one time to maximize absorption. Vitamin D recommendation is 800 to 1,000 IU per day for adults aged 50 years and older. The major dietary source of vitamin D is vitamin D-fortified milk (400 IU/quart). Fortification with vitamin D may also be found in other foods such as soy milk, juices, and cereals. The nurse should recommend reading food labels for nutritional information. The nurse should also provide information about the effects of smoking and alcohol on bone health and counsel the patient regarding smoking cessation and moderate alcohol intake.

OUTCOMES

The nurse should encourage patients to engage in a lifelong, regular, weight-bearing and muscle-strengthening exercise regimen to increase bone density and improve balance, posture, strength, and agility. Examples of beneficial exercises include walking, jogging, Tai Chi, stair climbing, dancing, and yoga. Patients should be cautioned not to begin a vigorous exercise program before being evaluated by their provider.

The goal of patient education is behavior change. To increase the effectiveness of education, the nurse can personalize the information to make it more relevant and to motivate the patient toward behavior change. For example, using the significance of the patient's BMD score in tailoring lifestyle changes or monitoring the progress of bone health would be more effective than merely providing information (Smeltzer & Qi, 2014).

Fall prevention. There are numerous risk factors for falls. They can be categorized into environmental (e.g., loose rugs, poor lighting, and lack of assistive devices), medical (e.g., age, anxiety, agitation, sensory impairment, cardiac dysfunction, medications, and malnutrition), and neurological/musculoskeletal (e.g., kyphosis and impaired balance, transfer, and mobility). The nurse should identify patients who are at risk for falls and implement safety measures for fall prevention.

Pharmacologic therapy. The role of the nurse in pharmacologic therapy is primarily providing medication education, monitoring for adverse effects and the effectiveness of treatment, and patient adherence. Bisphosphonates are the first-line therapy for postmenopausal women to reduce the risk for hip and vertebral fractures. There are many other medications to treat osteoporosis, including calcitonin, estrogens, selective estrogen receptor modifiers (SERM),

tissue-selective estrogen complex, and parathyroid hormone. The nurse is responsible for becoming familiar with the patient's medications, her or his pharmacokinetics, administration, adverse effects, and nursing implications.

Summary

Osteoporosis is the most common metabolic bone disease and is caused by low bone mass density, progressive deterioration of bone tissue, and microarchitecture resulting in bone fragility and predisposition to fracture. Osteoporosis is a common problem worldwide and its prevalence is increasing. There are an estimated 200 million women in the world with osteoporosis and a fragility fracture occurs every 3 seconds (Tabatabaei-Malazy, Salari, Khashayar, & Larijani, 2017). It is a silent disease that generally affects older women with increased incidence after menopause. The nurse plays a major role as a member of the interdisciplinary team who focuses on prevention, detection, and treatment of osteoporosis. Education regarding bone health is an important health-promotion topic for at-risk adults, as well as for younger individuals to develop healthy bones and prevent osteoporosis.

Chung, M., Tang, A. M., Fu, Z., Wang, D. D., & Newberry, S. J. (2016). Calcium intake and cardiovascular disease risk: An updated systematic review and meta-analysis. *Annals of Internal Medicine, 165,* 856–866. doi:10.7326/M16-1165

Cosman, F., de Beur, S. J., LeBoff, M. S., Lewiecki, E. M., Tanner, B., Randall, S., & Lindsay, R. (2015). Erratum to: Clinician's guide to prevention and treatment of osteoporosis. *Osteoporosis International, 26*(7), 2045–2047.

Imai, K. (2014). Recent methods for assessing osteoporosis and fracture risk. *Recent Patents on Endocrine, Metabolic, & Immune Drug Discovery, 10*(2), 48–59. doi:10.2174/1872214808666140118223801

Jeremiah, M. P., Unwin, B. K., Greenawald, M. H., & Casiano, V. E. (2015). Diagnosis and management of osteoporosis. *American Family Physician, 92*(4), 261–268.

Lorentzon, M., & Cummings, S. R. (2015). Osteoporosis: The evolution of a diagnosis. *Journal of Internal Medicine, 277*(6), 650–661.

Smeltzer, S. C., & Qi, B. B. (2014). Practical implications for nurses caring for patients being treated for osteoporosis. *Nursing: Research and Reviews, 4,* 19–33. doi:10.2147/NRR.S36648

Tabatabaei-Malazy, O., Salari, P., Khashayar, P., & Larijani, B. (2017). New horizons in treatment of osteoporosis. *Daru, 25*(1), 2.

■ PAGET'S DISEASE

Jacqueline Robinson

Overview

Paget's disease of the bone, or osteitis deformans, is a metabolic bone disease that is characterized by both excessive bone resorption and subsequent compensatory bone formation. However, because both processes occur at such an accelerated rate, the bone that forms is exaggerated, more vascular, and fragile. This bone growth leads to deformities and complications if left untreated and these complications are often the presenting symptoms that lead to the diagnosis of the disease itself. The risk for Paget's disease increases with age; in fact, the disease is very uncommon in patients younger than 40 years (National Institutes of Health [NIH], 2011). Nursing care of the patient with Paget's disease is focused on the prevention of complications, the importance of follow-up care once a diagnosis is made, and ongoing education of the patient and family members.

Background

The exact prevalence of Paget's disease is unknown due to the fact that it is often not diagnosed until complications occur or until visible signs manifest. Of those cases that are diagnosed, the disease is more common in men and individuals with increasing age (Nebot Valenzuela & Pietschmann, 2017). However, there are cases when patients who are in their teens and 20s have Paget's disease with a familial inheritance, which affects the bones of the skull, face, and hands, as well as increasing the person's risk for hearing loss (NIH, 2011). The disease is most common in those of Northwest European decent, particularly those from Britain (NIH, 2011).

Unlike other metabolic, noninflammatory diseases of the bone, Paget's disease does not affect the entire skeleton; rather, it affects one or several bones in an area. If a single bone is affected, it is monostotic; if multiple bones are affected, it is polystotic. The most common sites include the skull, femur, tibia, spine, and thorax. There is an increase in both osteoclast and osteoblast activity in the affected area. First, the osteoclasts cause accelerated bone resorption; to compensate for this loss, osteoblasts then accelerate formation. However, this rate is grossly accelerated and leads to highly vascular, disorganized, fibrotic bone that results in overgrowth and deformity (Nebot Valenzuela & Pietschmann, 2017).

Although the exact cause of Paget's disease is unknown, there are studies that suggest both a genetic and environmental component. The familial form of Paget's disease that accounts for one third of cases is linked to a gene mutation of sequestosome-1 (SOSTM-1) in 46% of patients with the disease within the same family (Audet et al., 2016). Other studies suggest a link to a virus, some even suggest the measles virus. Due to a decline in the virus in certain areas, environmental influences have also been suggested as an influence on development (Audet et al., 2016). Viral components have been obtained from the nuclei of osteoclasts from patients positively diagnosed with Paget's disease (Nebot Valenzuela & Pietschmann, 2017).

Although many patients with Paget's disease of the bone are asymptomatic, many suffer from complications that lead them to seek treatment and subsequent diagnosis. In addition, the potential deformity to the affected area(s) not only affects quality of life from an aesthetic point of view but also from a functional standpoint.

Clinical Aspects

ASSESSMENT

The signs and symptoms of Paget's disease of the bone range from a complete absence of symptoms to symptoms specific to a particular affected body area, all the way to systemic manifestations. The patient may simply complain of bone pain in the affected area or surrounding joint space. The systemic manifestations include the potential for high cardiac output heart failure. Due to the fact that the lesions that develop are highly vascular and that this constant cycle of osteoclast and osteoblast activity leads to an increase in metabolic demand, there is an increase in the workload of the heart (Nebot Valenzuela & Pietschmann, 2017).

If the skull is involved, the entire cranium will increase in size; therefore, the face will look smaller. Due to the potential for increased pressure on the cranial nerves, the patient may suffer from hearing loss. The patient may have other neurologic complications, including headaches, tinnitus, and, in rare cases, a buildup of cerebrospinal fluid (Muschitz, Feichtinger, Haschka, & Kocijan, 2016). The patient with lower extremity involvement will have an altered gait with a waddling appearance. The long bones may bow and the patient will appear bowlegged even at rest. If the area is extensive, the surrounding joints can be affected, causing stress on the cartilage leading to osteoarthritis (Muschitz et al., 2016). Rigidity of the thorax and spine is also possible if they are involved in the pathology. Paralysis has been reported as well as pinched spinal nerves (NIH, 2011). Osteosarcoma is a rare complication that can be diagnosed via bone biopsy (NIH, 2011). Fractures are the most common presenting symptom and complication of Paget's disease.

Diagnosis of Paget's disease is made by simple radiograph of the area. Early lesions are osteolytic, whereas older lesions that are more progressed are sclerotic and bone growth is as much as 8 mm/year (Muschitz et al., 2016). A bone scan may be ordered to determine the extent of the disorder and the activity of the cells. Finally, a bone biopsy will be done to confirm osteosarcoma.

The gold standard in terms of diagnosis as well as follow-up on the progression of the disease and treatment outcomes is serum levels of alkaline phosphatase (ALP). This enzyme is produced by bone cells and thus is in excess in patients with Paget's disease as osteoblasts continue to produce incompetent bone. A level twice the normal serum level is considered positive for Paget's disease (NIH, 2011). The serum ALP is sent after treatment is implemented and family members of persons with Paget's disease should also have serum ALP levels sent every 2 to 3 years after the age of 40 (NIH, 2011). The frequency of serum ALP levels after initiation of treatment is based upon the regimen chosen for the patient, with the most potent therapy requiring less frequent follow-up.

Bisphosphonates are the treatment of choice for Paget's disease. These medications prevent fractures and halt disease progression but do not reverse the damage that has already occurred (Kumar, Selviambigapathy, Kamalanathan, & Sahoo, 2016). They work by inhibiting osteoclasts and promoting apoptosis (Muschitz et al., 2016). The ideal bisphosphonate is intravenous zoledronate (Muschitz et al., 2016). This medication is highly nephrotoxic and has also been known to cause flu-like side effects. However, it holds the highest efficacy and therefore requires the least follow-up care. Other bisphosphonates are not as potent and will continue to need more frequent ALP levels.

NURSING INTERVENTIONS, MANAGEMENT, AND IMPLICATIONS

Pain management is a focus of nursing care for some patients, not only with the diagnosis of Paget's disease but also with the complication of osteoarthritis and the pinched nerves that are possible. Nursing must encourage weight-bearing activity to prevent disuse and promote full range of motion. Weight-bearing activity also inhibits bone resorption. Pain may also be relieved by altering hot and cold soaks and emersion therapy. Finally, administration of ordered nonsteroidal antiinflammatory medications and acetaminophen may be necessary. Nurses must also encourage their patients to maintain a healthy weight to reduce the burden on the joints and bones.

Safety is another top priority for nursing care of the patient with Paget's disease. The goal is to avoid fractures. A key is to prevent falls. Encourage the use of assistive devices when warranted such as walkers and canes, focusing education on their proper use. Grab bars, hand rails, nonskid mats, and proper lighting must be installed in the home for safety. A thorough evaluation of the home environment for anything that could place a patient at risk for tripping or loss of balance, such as throw rugs, power cords, and clutter, must be done with the patient, also including the patient's family and/or significant others.

Communication is a focus for the patient with hearing impairment. Although bisphosphonates have shown to halt disease progression and prevent fractures, not all hearing issues have reversed. Thus, nursing interventions aimed at improving communication is key for day-to-day functioning of the hearing-impaired patient with Paget's disease.

Finally, the nurse must stress the importance of follow-up care. Testing serum ALP levels for patients diagnosed with the disease is necessary to determine the progression of the disease as well as the efficacy of treatment efforts. It is also crucial that family members of the patient also be tested due to the clear familial link that has been identified.

OUTCOMES

The expected outcomes of nursing care focus on the prevention of complications and pain management. The need for follow-up care as well as an evaluation of the patient's home environment for safety and health promotion is also paramount. Maintaining safety and self-esteem in the home environment is the goal. If a patient does suffer a complication, the nursing care will be reprioritized based on the specific problem.

Summary

The diagnosis of Paget's disease of the bone is often made after a complication has occurred or a radiograph of an adjacent area has revealed the characteristic findings of the disease. It is confirmed with serum ALP levels being twice the normal range. Although there is no specific cause known and there is no cure, there are therapies aimed at halting progression and preventing complications, with bisphosphonates being the primary pharmacologic choice. Nurses play a key role in the prevention of complication and the maintenance of safety as well as encouraging patients to remain compliant with follow-up care.

Audet, M. C., Jean, S., Beaudoin, C., Guay-Bélanger, S., Dumont, J., Brown, J. P., & Michou, L. (2016). Environmental factors associated with familial or non-familial forms of Paget's disease of bone. *Joint Bone Spine, 84*(6), 719–723. doi:10.1016/j.jbspin.2016.11.010

Kumar, R., Sevianbigapathy, J., Kamalanathan, S., & Sahoo, J. (2016). Stress fractures healing with bisphosphonates in Paget's disease. *Joint Bone Spine, 84,* 91. doi:10.1016./j/jbspin.2016.01.010

Muschitz, C., Feichtinger, X., Haschka, J., & Kocijan, R. (2017). Diagnosis and treatment of Paget's disease of bone: A clinical practice guideline. *Wiener medizinische Wochenschrift, 167*(1–2), 18–24.

National Institute of Health. (2011). Questions and answers about Paget's disease of bone. Retrieved from http://www.bones.nih.gov

Nebot Valenzuela, E., & Pietschmann, P. (2017). Epidemiology and pathology of Paget's disease of bone—A review. *Wiener medizinische Wochenschrift, 167*(1–2), 2–8.

■ PANCREATIC CANCER

Jennifer E. Millman

Overview

Pancreatic cancer is one of the most aggressive malignancies. Although it accounts for just 3% of all cancers in the United States and 7% of all cancer-related deaths (American Cancer Society [ACS], 2016), it is particularly problematic because patients are usually diagnosed with advanced stage cancer that is refractory to aggressive medical care. The only curative treatment for pancreatic cancer is surgical resection. However, more than 80% of patients have nonresectable lesions at the time of diagnosis (De La Cruz, Young, & Mack, 2014). Nursing care of patients with pancreatic cancer should focus on the delivery of holistic care for the patients and their family system.

Background

The incidence of pancreatic cancer ranges between one and 10 cases per 100,000 people worldwide and is more common in men and in developed countries (Ryan, Hong, & Bardeesy, 2014). In the United States, it is the eighth leading cause of cancer death among men and ninth among women (Ryan et al., 2014). The risk of developing pancreatic cancer increases with age; the median age at diagnosis is 71 years (Ryan et al., 2014). Almost all patients are diagnosed after age 45 years, and two thirds of cases are diagnosed after age 65 years (ACS, 2016). The ACS (2016) estimates there were 53,070 new cases of pancreatic cancer and approximately 41,780 deaths due to the disease, annually (ACS, 2016). The lifetime risk of developing pancreatic cancer is about 1.49% or one in 67 persons (Becker, Hernandez, Frucht, & Lucas, 2014).

Pancreatic cancer is notable for its unique biological features. Characteristics include the presence of KRAS (Ki-ras2 Kirsten rat sarcoma viral oncogene homolog) oncogene mutation (greater than 90%), progression from a precursor lesion, and an affinity for local invasion and distant metastasis (Ryan et al., 2014). Most pancreatic cancers arise from microscopic precursor lesions called *pancreatic intraepithelial neoplasia* (PanIN), which is a noninvasive epithelial lesion arising in the pancreatic ducts (Jaloudi & Kluger, 2017). Many pancreatic cancers begin as precancerous growths in the pancreas. With more advanced imaging techniques, it is possible to identify more pancreatic cysts before they develop into cancer. Precancerous growths, such as mucinous neoplasms (MCNs) and intraductal papillary mucinous neoplasms (IMPN), warrant monitoring as they may progress to cancer over time (ACS, 2016). Rapidly growing lesions or lesions connecting to the main pancreatic duct are suggestive of malignancy and may lead to surgical resection.

The pancreas is made up of exocrine and endocrine cells. The islets of Langerhans are endocrine cells that produce insulin and glucagon and regulate blood glucose levels. Most of the pancreas consists of acinar cells that secrete the digestive enzymes lipase, amylase, and protease. The majority of pancreatic tumors are exocrine in origin; 95% of exocrine pancreatic cancers are pancreatic adenocarcinoma (ACS, 2016). Pancreatic endocrine tumors account for less than 5% of pancreatic cancers (ACS, 2016).

Smoking is strongly associated with pancreatic cancer; 20% to 30% of pancreatic cancers may be caused by smoking (ACS, 2016). Other modifiable risk factors include overweight or obesity and workplace exposure to chemicals used in dry cleaning and metal-working. Unmodifiable risk factors include increased age, male gender, African American race, family history of pancreatic cancer, and inherited genetic disorders (ACS, 2016). Up to 10% of pancreatic cancers have a hereditary component and 20% of those have a genetic mutation (Becker et al., 2014). Genetic risk factors include hereditary breast and ovarian cancer syndrome (BRCA1), Lynch syndrome, familial adenomatous polyposis, hereditary pancreatitis, cystic fibrosis, and familial atypical multiple mole melanoma syndrome (Becker et al., 2014).

Diabetes, chronic pancreatitis, cirrhosis of the liver, and *Helicobacter pylori* infection may increase the risk of pancreatic cancer (ACS, 2016). More research is needed regarding the role of alcohol, diet, and physical inactivity in the development of pancreatic cancer. Health-promotion teaching should focus on smoking cessation, maintaining a healthy weight, limiting alcohol intake, and limiting exposure to toxic chemicals (ACS, 2016).

Clinical Aspects

ASSESSMENT

More than two thirds of pancreatic cancer tumors originate in the head of the pancreas, resulting in biliary obstruction (De La Cruz et al., 2014). Presenting symptoms caused by biliary obstruction include abdominal pain, jaundice, pruritus, dark urine, and pale stools. Other more nonspecific symptoms caused by tumors of the tail or body include anorexia, weight loss, early satiety, nausea, and dyspepsia (De La Cruz et al., 2014).

Practitioners should keep in mind that physical findings of pancreatic cancer can vary based on the stage of cancer at diagnosis. Patients who present in the early stages of pancreatic cancer may have no abnormal physical findings on examination. In contrast, patients with advanced pancreatic cancer with liver involvement may present with a palpable gallbladder with mild, painless jaundice (Courvoisier's sign); migratory thrombophlebitis (Trousseau's sign of malignancy), or supraclavicular lymphadenopathy (Virchow node), which is indicative of metastatic abdominal malignancy (De La Cruz et al., 2014).

The pancreas CT protocol, a triphasic cross-sectional imaging, is the standard for diagnosis and staging when patients present with a high suspicion of pancreatic cancer. In cases for which a CT scan is contraindicated, MRI or magnetic resonance cholangiopancreatography (MRCP) can be useful. If a pancreatic mass is seen on imaging, an endoscopic ultrasound with fine-needle aspiration or biopsy is indicated for tissue diagnosis (National Comprehensive Cancer Network [NCCN], 2017). If no obvious mass is seen on cross-sectional imaging and there is no evidence of metastatic disease, then further workup should include endoscopic ultrasound, endoscopic retrograde cholangiopancreatography (ERCP), MRI, and MRCP (NCCN, 2017). Cancer antigen 19-9 (Ca 19-9), a tumor marker clinically significant in pancreatic ductal adenocarcinoma, can be used for diagnosis and prognosis and to monitor the patient's response to treatment. Ca 19-9 is not tumor specific and is not a sufficient screening tool (De La Cruz et al., 2014); it is elevated with several other conditions, including pancreatitis, cirrhosis, biliary tract disease, and other malignancies (De La Cruz et al., 2014).

Surgical resection is the primary treatment method for pancreatic adenocarcinoma. However, only 15% to 20% of patients are candidates for surgical resection when diagnosed (NCCN, 2017). Even with surgery, the prognosis is poor; the 5-year survival rate of patients who undergo surgical resection is only 20% (NCCN, 2017). The decision of whether or not a patient is a candidate for surgical resection should be determined by a multidisciplinary board at a large volume center (NCCN, 2017). Prognosis depends on the tumor grade and staging at the time of diagnosis. Contraindications to surgical resection include the presence of metastatic liver disease or direct involvement of the superior mesenteric artery, inferior vena cava, aorta, celiac axis, or hepatic artery (Jaloudi & Kluger, 2017).

The choice of surgical procedure depends on the location of the tumor. Surgical options include pancreaticoduodenectomy (with or without pylorus sparing), total pancreatectomy, and distal pancreatectomy. Pancreaticoduodenectomy, or Whipple procedure, is indicated for tumors of the head of the pancreas. Tumors of the body and tail are rarely resectable as they cause fewer presenting symptoms and at diagnosis are typically discovered at a more advanced stage. These types of tumors are better treated by distal pancreatectomy. Endoscopic procedures for nonresectable pancreatic cancer include radiofrequency ablation of the bile duct and celiac plexus neurolysis for pain management. Endoscopic retrograde pancreaticoduodenectomy for stent placement and biliary decompression may be indicated for patients with jaundice or cholangitis due to biliary tract obstruction.

Chemotherapy and radiation can be used as adjuvant or neoadjuvant therapy and to treat patients with nonresectable disease. The key chemotherapeutic agents used for patients with advanced pancreatic cancer are gemcitabine (Gemzar), FOLFIRINOX regimen (5-fluorouracil, leucovorin, irinotecan, and oxaliplatin), and nab-paclitaxel (Abraxane). In 2011, treatment with the FOLFIRINOX regimen was shown to prolong overall survival by more than 4 months than treatment with gemcitabine alone (Hronek & Reed, 2015).

Nurses are present during administration of chemotherapy and typically provide care and support when patients experience adverse events (Hronek & Reed, 2015). Thus, it is imperative that nurses know how to manage toxicities from chemotherapy. Toxicities include pancytopenia, peripheral neuropathy, fatigue, anorexia, stomatitis, nausea, and vomiting. Nurses should also monitor patients for depression.

OUTCOMES

Nurses must have a comprehensive understanding of surgical complications and adverse events from chemotherapy as well as an understanding of the psychosocial implications of the diagnosis of pancreatic cancer.

Perioperative nursing considerations for the patient undergoing Whipple procedure include interventions to prevent respiratory complications, hemorrhage, venous thromboembolic events, infection, hepatorenal failure, fluid volume deficit, and nutritional deficits (Jaloudi & Kluger, 2017). Patients who present with jaundice are at risk for coagulopathies, malabsorption, malnutrition, and pruritus (Jaloudi & Kluger, 2017). Pruritus will improve with biliary decompression and symptoms may be managed with an antihistamine. Blood glucose levels should be monitored and some patients may require insulin supplementation. Patients with pancreatic cancer may be at risk for developing pancreatic exocrine insufficiency, which can be managed with pancreatic enzyme supplements.

Summary

Treatment of pancreatic cancer remains challenging. Nurses play a crucial role in educating patients about the disease and supporting patients and families as they cope with the diagnosis of pancreatic cancer. It is essential that nurses are knowledgeable regarding presenting symptoms of pancreatic cancer, treatment modalities, supportive care, and symptom management. Health-promotion teaching should be geared toward risk reduction strategies, especially smoking cessation. Goals for future research include improving screening methods and early detection of pancreatic cancer, especially for high-risk populations.

American Cancer Society. (2016). Pancreatic cancer. Retrieved from https://old.cancer.org/acs/groups/cid/documents/webcontent/003131-pdf.pdf

Becker, A. E., Hernandez, Y. G., Frucht, H., & Lucas, A. L. (2014). Pancreatic ductal adenocarcinoma: Risk factors, screening, and early detection. *World Journal of Gastroenterology, 20*(32), 11182–11198.

De La Cruz, M. S., Young, A. P., & Ruffin, M. T. (2014). Diagnosis and management of pancreatic cancer. *American Family Physician, 89*(8), 626–632.

Hronek, J. W., & Reed, M. (2015). Nursing implications of chemotherapy agents and their associated side effects in patients with pancreatic cancer. *Clinical Journal of Oncology Nursing, 19*(6), 751–757.

Jaloudi, J., & Kluger, M. D. (2017). Pancreatic cancer. In G. Nandakumar (Ed.), *Evidence based practices in gastrointestinal & hepatobiliary surgery* (pp. 566–588). New Delhi, India: JP Medical.

National Comprehensive Cancer Network. (2017). NCCN clinical practice guidelines in oncology: Pancreatic adenocarcinoma. Retrieved from https://www.nccn.org/professionals/physician_gls/pdf/pancreatic.pdf

Ryan, D. P., Hong, T. S., & Bardeesy, N. (2014). Pancreatic adenocarcinoma. *New England Journal of Medicine, 371*(11), 1039–1049.

■ PARKINSON'S DISEASE

Peter J. Cebull

Overview

Parkinson's disease (PD) is a progressive neurodegenerative condition characterized by a lack of the neurotransmitter dopamine, which regulates movements and emotions. According to the Michael J. Fox Foundation for Parkinson's Research, more than 60,000 new cases are diagnosed each year with no definitive cure available. Though the exact cause of this disease remains unknown, genetics and environmental factors play a role in the development and progression of PD.

The definitive characteristic of PD is the progressive death of dopaminergic neurons in the brain. The resulting lack of sufficient dopamine in the basal ganglia leads to the classic Parkinsonian movements most commonly associated with the disease, although numerous nonmotor symptoms can manifest earlier in the disease course. Research indicates that other neurotransmitters outside the basal ganglia are also affected during disease progression (Kalia & Lang, 2015).

PD results from both a genetic predisposition and environmental influences on susceptible genes. The only definitive diagnostic tool used to confirm PD is postmortem histological analysis to identify the degraded dopaminergic neurons or the presence of abnormal groupings of proteins called *Lewy bodies*. The exact role Lewy bodies play in PD and some forms of dementia is being investigated. Because the treatments for PD are largely symptomatic rather than curative, symptoms are treated after onset and modified as they progress. A diagnosis of exclusion is usually made based on various criteria that contribute to an overall compelling clinical picture (Kalia & Lang, 2015).

Globally, PD is the most prevalent neurodegenerative disease following Alzheimer's disease. Gender is regarded as a major risk factor; three males are affected by the disease for every two females. The most significant factor in PD risk is age; there is an exponential increase of prevalence and incidence in persons younger than 80 years, with the peak age at onset occurring in a person's 70s. As the U.S. population ages, the number of Americans affected by this disease is projected to increase by as much as 50% by 2030. For this reason, a working understanding of this disease is of considerable importance to nurses who will be caring for older Americans.

Clinical Aspects

ASSESSMENT

When assessing a person with PD, it is important to understand the key signs associated with the disease: bradykinesia, rigidity, and resting tremor. Bradykinesia, or slow movements, characterize this disease. Often, the first motion in an action is the most challenging, such as taking the first step when walking or swallowing food later in the disease course. Speech can also be affected for the same reason, causing decreased volume of voice and dysarthria. Other manifestations of this sign occur when walking: a person's arms will often stop swinging as they normally would and facial muscles do not move as easily as they once did, creating a baseline mask-like expression.

Muscle rigidity occurs with decreased use; muscles stiffen, resulting in resistance to both passive and active range of motion throughout the body, especially in the knee and elbow joints. The classic tremor associated with PD is a resting tremor, which occurs while the person is not using a particular muscle group for a specific task. For example, asking a person with a Parkinsonian tremor to write his or her name will reduce the hand tremor once the person is holding the pen; however, the tremor will still interfere with the ability to conduct the smooth fine-motor movements needed for handwriting. In addition to assess for the motor symptoms of PD, it is important to also screen for depression, cognitive difficulties, and issues with the bladder, digestion, and circulation as these also manifest at various stages throughout the disease course (U.S. National Library of Medicine [NLM], 2015).

NURSING INTERVENTIONS, MANAGEMENT, AND IMPLICATIONS

Providing nursing care for a person with PD requires anticipating and understanding the various problems the disease can present. Because of the impaired, disordered movements, there is an increased risk for falling. The lack of control over fine motor and possible cognitive dysfunctions later in the disease course can impair a person's ability to complete activities of daily living (ADL). The treatments of the disease can be both surgical (deep-brain stimulation) and nonsurgical. Medications used to treat the motor symptoms of PD include levodopa (precursor to dopamine), dopamine agonists, catechol-O-methyltransferase (COMT) inhibitors, monoamine oxidase (MAO) B inhibitors, and anticholinergics. Other medications may be prescribed for sleep disorders, dementia, and depression, which are common in persons with PD. Hallucinations and psychosis may be treated by reducing or stopping the dose of one of the medications used to treat the motor symptoms of PD. Levodopa is the most effective medication used to treat bradykinesia, tremor, and rigidity. To improve efficacy of the levodopa, it is combined with carbidopa (Sinemet). The patient must be carefully monitored for the adverse effects associated with long-term therapy with levodopa–carbidopa and dopamine agonists.

The person with PD is at increased risk for falling and injury due to slowing of movements and even "freezing" of movement altogether. A common gait associated with PD is a propulsive, shuffling, small-stepped gait that makes tripping over small objects, such as rugs, or climbing stairs a major hazard and risk for serious injury related to falls. A nurse can conduct a thorough environmental review and work with a patient and his or her caregivers to reduce these hazards.

Lack of fine-motor control is characteristic of this disease because of bradykinesia, tremor, and stiffness. A person who experiences these symptoms, which are typically worse in the mornings and just before the next dose of medications, can have significant difficulty with ADL. Planning ADL and arranging for assistance as needed can be a key nursing intervention to improve the quality of life for a person with PD.

Speech and swallowing can be affected, creating a potential communication barrier and risk for aspiration. The nurse can offer more time and alternative methods of communication when necessary. Dysphagia can be identified by a simple swallowing test. If swallowing difficulty is detected, the nurse can refer the patient for more advanced testing and consult with a nutritionist to recommend dietary modifications to reduce the risk of aspiration. This is a simple but potentially life-saving intervention as one choking incident can result in serious lifelong deficits and even death.

Adverse effects of dopamine agonist therapy are a problem commonly experienced by almost all patients with this disease who take any one of a number of dopamine agonist medications. The most widely used medication to treat PD is levodopa–carbidopa (Sinemet). As therapy continues and the disease progresses, higher doses of the medication are necessary. The nurse needs to monitor the patient for adverse effects such as orthostatic hypotension, hallucinations, excessive daytime sleepiness, dyskinesia, and increased impulsivity or atypical behavior (NLM, 2015). These effects of dopamine-agonist treatment can significantly affect the life of the patient and his or her family. A nurse can intervene by recognizing and educating the patient and caregivers about adverse effects and to notify the prescribing health care provider if they occur.

Summary

PD is a progressive neurodegenerative disorder characterized by a lack of the neurotransmitter dopamine. PD primarily affects older adults, a rapidly increasing population in the United States. Nurses are in a unique position to assess, identify problems, and intervene to improve the quality of life for patients with PD. Although deaths from the disease itself are rare, the common causes of

PD-related death are complications related to symptoms such as impaired gait and dysphagia (NLM, 2015).

OUTCOMES

It is important for nurses to understand the stages of disease progression and that patients may go undiagnosed for a significant period of time before the classic motor signs of PD appear. In addition to neuromuscular symptoms, including tremors, bradykinesia/akinesia, and rigidity, the patient's mood and cognition may be affected. The pathophysiology of this disease has also been related to dementia (Lewy body), and depression is an even more common manifestation of patients who are faced with this progressive, life-altering diagnosis (NLM, 2015). All patients with PD should be screened for depression. Although the motor symptoms are often the first and most emphasized feature, these other problems can prove just as debilitating and dangerous, warranting an equal emphasis from health care providers. Through informed, evidence-based nursing care of persons with PD, patient outcomes and morbidity and mortality can be positively influenced.

Kalia, L. V., & Lang, A. E. (2015). Parkinson's disease. *Lancet, 386*(9996), 386, 896–912. doi:10.1016/S0140-6736(14)61393

The Michael J. Fox Foundation Parkinson's Disease. (n.d.). Understanding Parkinson's disease. Retrieved from https://www.michaeljfox.org/understanding-parkinsons/index.html?navid=understanding-pd

U.S. National Library of Medicine. (Ed.). (2015). Parkinson's: Overview. Retrieved from https://www.ncbi.nlm.nih.gov/pubmedhealth/PMH0076679

■ PEPTIC ULCER DISEASE

Lisa D. Ericson
Deborah R. Gillum

Overview

Peptic ulcer disease (PUD) is inflammation of the gastrointestinal mucosa of the stomach and/or duodenum, which can lead to gastric or duodenal ulcers. The major causes of PUD are *Helicobacter pylori* infections and the chronic use of nonsteroidal anti-inflammatory drugs (NSAIDs). Although the prevalence of PUD has declined significantly since 1992, it still affects 4.5 million people in the United States, with an additional half a million newly diagnosed cases each year (Anand, 2017; Lee, 2014). Treatment goals include eradication of *H. pylori*, discontinuation of NSAID use, promotion of ulcer healing, and control of other precipitating risk factors.

Background

PUD is a disruption of the mucosal and submucosal layers of the stomach and/or duodenum, which results in the body's inability to adequately protect the epithelium from the effects of gastric acid and pepsin. Under normal conditions, a physiologic balance exists between gastric acid secretion and mucosal defense, but PUD develops when there is an imbalance between the body's protective factors and aggressive factors that can damage the gastric mucosa (Anand, 2017; Ignatavicius & Workman, 2016; Konturek & Konturek, 2014). PUD includes three types of ulcers: (a) gastric ulcers that develop in the antrum of the stomach near the acid-secreting mucosa and which usually are the result of *H. pylori* infection, (b) duodenal ulcers that occur within 2 cm of the pylorus and are related to high gastric acid secretion, and (c) stress ulcers that typically occur secondarily to an acute medical crisis or trauma (Ignatavicius & Workman, 2016; Lee, 2014).

Contributing PUD risk factors can be endogenous, such as gastric acid and pepsin, or exogenous, such as *H. pylori* infection, NSAIDs, alcohol consumption, smoking, obesity, or stress (Anand, 2017; Chuah et al., 2014; Konturek & Konturek, 2014). *H. pylori* and NSAID use are the most common causes of PUD. *H. pylori* colonizes in the gastric mucosa and is typically transmitted via the fecal–oral route during early childhood. This bacterium can remain dormant for decades, and although it does not cause illness in most people, it can lead to mucosal inflammation and epithelial cell necrosis, resulting in PUD (Anand, 2017; Ignatavicius & Workman, 2016). Ulcers with an indeterminate cause are termed *idiopathic* and tend to occur with older age, multimorbidity, recent surgery, sepsis, and medications other than NSAIDs (Konturek & Konturek, 2014).

Approximately 4.5 million people in the United States are affected annually by PUD, accounting for more than 507,000 hospitalizations and costing $4.85 billion yearly (Anand, 2017; Laine, 2016). In the United States, the prevalence of *H. pylori* among patients older than 60 years ranges between 40% and 60%, whereas 20-year-olds have a prevalence of 20%. It is rarely diagnosed in children (Anand, 2017; Fashner & Gitu,

2015; Lee, 2014). An additional contributing factor that increases the risk of PUD in older adults includes the number of high-risk medications they are prescribed (e.g., antiplatelet drugs, warfarin, and selective serotonin reuptake inhibitors; Fashner & Gitu, 2015). Although in the past PUD occurred more frequently in males, recent trends show that the gap is narrowing; males have an 11% to 14% lifetime occurrence rate, whereas females have an 8% to 11% lifetime occurrence rate (Anand, 2017; Lee, 2014). People of lower socioeconomic status also have higher rates of PUD, possibly related to higher rates of *H. pylori* infection (Lee, 2014).

PUD prognosis is excellent once the cause of the ulcer is identified. With eradication of *H. pylori* infection, avoidance of NSAIDs, and the appropriate use of antisecretory therapy, most patients are successfully treated (Anand, 2017). First-line therapy of *H. pylori* eradicates more than 80% of infections (Fashner & Gitu, 2015). The mortality rate has decreased modestly in the past 20 years and is approximately 1 death per 100,000 cases. Including all patients with duodenal ulcers, the mortality rate due to ulcer hemorrhage is 5%. If the ulcer should perforate and surgery is required, the mortality risk is 6% to 30%. Several factors are associated with higher mortality rates, including location of the ulcer (perforated gastric ulcers have twice the mortality than perforated duodenal ulcers), shock at the time of admission, immunocompromised state, cirrhosis, renal insufficiency, age older than 70 years, delay of initiation of surgery for more than 12 hours after presentation, and comorbidities (e.g., cardiovascular disease or diabetes mellitus; Anand, 2017).

Clinical Aspects

ASSESSMENT

On history and physical examination, the most common symptoms include nausea and vomiting; hematemesis (vomiting of blood); melena (passage of dark, "tarry" stools that contain blood); pyrosis (heartburn); dyspepsia (indigestion) described as sharp, burning, or gnawing; pain or tenderness in the mid- or upper-epigastric region; pain in the epigastric region after eating; and hyperactive bowel sounds initially that become hypoactive as the disease progresses (Anand, 2017; Ignatavicius & Workman, 2016; Konturek & Konturek, 2014).

Common complications of PUD are perforation, hemorrhage, and pyloric obstruction. Perforation is a medical emergency and clinical manifestations may include sudden, sharp pain; tender, rigid, board-like abdomen (associated with peritonitis); fetal positioning; and absent bowel sounds (Ignatavicius & Workman, 2016).

The current standard for diagnosing PUD is an esophagogastroduodenoscopy (EGD). Endoscopy provides an opportunity to view the ulcer to determine active bleeding and to attempt hemostasis, if necessary. EGD also allows for biopsy of the gastric mucosa to detect the presence of *H. pylori* (using a rapid urease test) and cytologic studies to rule out cancerous cells (Anand, 2017; Ignatavicius & Workman, 2016; Konturek & Konturek, 2014). A nuclear medicine scan may be ordered if perforation or hemorrhage is suspected (Ignatavicius & Workman, 2016).

NURSING INTERVENTIONS, MANAGEMENT, AND IMPLICATIONS

Interventions for nursing include four goals: (a) eliminate *H. pylori* infections, (b) reduce pain, (c) heal ulcers, and (d) prevent reoccurrence. No single medication has been successful in treating *H. pylori*, thus a combination of agents is used. This combination, referred to as *PPI-triple therapy*, includes a proton pump inhibitor (PPI), such as pantoprazole, and two antibiotics (clarithromycin and tetracycline or metronidazole; Fashner & Gitu, 2015). These medications are prescribed for 10 to 14 days. Some providers add bismuth (Pepto-Bismol) to the PPI-triple therapy, which prevents *H. pylori* from binding to the mucosal lining to stimulate mucosal protection. Hyposecretory medications are used to reduce pain by reducing gastric acid secretions. These medications include PPIs (pantoprazole, omeprazole) and histamine blocking agents (H2 receptor antagonist), such as ranitidine and famotidine. Antacids, such as aluminum hydroxide and magnesium hydroxide, can also be used to buffer gastric acid and prevent the formation of pepsin. Mucosal barrier protectors, such as sucralfate, can be used to reduce pain, heal ulcers, and prevent reoccurrence (Ignatavicius & Workman, 2016).

Patient teaching should address peptic ulcer reoccurrence. Patients should avoid alcohol and tobacco as they stimulate gastric acid secretion. During the acute phase of the illness, patients ought to adhere to a bland diet and avoid foods that cause an increase in symptoms. The role of nutrition therapy in PUD management is controversial and no evidence exists to support dietary restrictions. Treatment other than medications is focused on stress reduction, which can be promoted through yoga, guided imagery, and hypnosis (Ignatavicius & Workman, 2016). Other nursing care will include measures to reduce anxiety, maintain nutritional requirements, and help the patient become knowledgeable about the management and prevention of ulcer recurrence (Belleza, 2016).

OUTCOMES

The prognosis for patients with PUD is excellent. Patients are treated successfully with *H. pylori* eradication, avoidance of NSAIDs (lifestyle triggers), and antisecretory therapy. Safety issues are addressed with patient education regarding medication adherence and lifestyle modifications (Ignatavicius & Workman, 2016).

Summary

H. pylori and chronic NSAID use remain the most common contributing factors associated with PUD (Lee, 2014). Quality of life and expected outcomes are excellent for those diagnosed with PUD with appropriate teaching regarding risk factors to prevent reoccurrence (Ignatavicius & Workman, 2016). Successful patient outcomes are promoted through thorough patient education, including the role of *H. pylori* and NSAIDs in PUD development, the importance of adhering to the medical treatment, and avoidance of lifestyle triggers (Lee, 2014).

Anand, B. S. (2017). Peptic ulcer disease. *Medscape*. Retrieved from http://emedicine.medscape.com/article/181753-overview#a5

Belleza, M. (2016). Peptic ulcer disease. Retrieved from https://nurseslabs.com/peptic-ulcer-disease

Chuah, S. K., Wu, D. C., Suzuki, H., Goh, K. L., Kao, J., & Ren, J. L. (2014). Peptic ulcer disease: Genetics, mechanism and therapies. *BioMed Research International, 2014*, 898349. doi:10.1155/2014/898349

Fashner, J., & Gitu, A. C. (2015). Diagnosis and treatment of peptic ulcer disease and *H. pylori* infection. *American Academy of Family Physicians, 91*(4), 236–242.

Ignatavicius, D. D., & Workman, M. L. (2016). *Medical-surgical nursing: Patient-centered collaborative care*. St. Louis, MO: Elsevier.

Konturek, P. C., & Konturek, S. J. (2014). Peptic ulcer disease. In E. Lammert & M. Zeeb (Eds.), *Metabolism of human diseases* (pp. 129–135). Vienna: Springer Publishing. doi:10.1007/978-3-7091-0715-7_21

Laine, L. (2016). Upper gastrointestinal bleeding due to a peptic ulcer. *New England Journal of Medicine, 374*(24), 2367–2376. doi:10.1056/NEJMcp1514257

Lee, L. (2014). First consult: Peptic ulcer disease. *ClinicalKey*. Retrieved from https://www.clinicalkey.com/#!/content/medical_topic/21-s2.0-1014794

■ PERICARDITIS

Heidi Youngbauer

Overview

Acute pericarditis is an inflammation of the pericardium with or without pericardial effusion (Adler & Charron, 2015), and is diagnosed in approximately 5% of patients with nonischemic chest pain in North America and Western Europe (Imazio, Gaita, & LeWinter, 2015). The true incidence and prevalence of acute pericarditis are difficult to measure, as low-risk patients are rarely admitted to hospitals (Doctor, Shah, Coplan, & Kronzon, 2016), and many cases may resolve without a diagnosis (Imazio et al., 2015). Acute pericarditis most commonly affects middle-aged individuals (Doctor et al., 2016; Imazio et al., 2015), with the mean age of patients ranging from 41 to 60 years, and is responsible for 0.1% (Adler & Charron, 2015) to 0.2% (Imazio et al., 2015) of hospital admissions.

Patients with acute pericarditis typically present with clinical symptoms of precordial chest pain, worse on inspiration and when the patient is placed supine. A physical assessment may reveal a pericardial friction rub and diffuse ST segment elevation on electrocardiogram (Cremer et al., 2016; Doctor et al., 2016). Depending on the underlying etiology of the disease process, orthopnea, palpitations, mild fever, weakness, and cough may also be reported by patients with acute pericarditis (Adler & Charron, 2015). Therefore, this entry provides information on evidence-based nursing care to optimize the outcomes of patients presenting with pericarditis.

Background

Pericarditis is an inflammation and irritation of the membrane surrounding the heart and may be defined as acute, incessant, recurrent, or chronic depending on recurrence and duration of symptoms (Adler & Charron, 2015; Cremer et al., 2016). According to Cremer et al. (2016), acute pericarditis is common and responsive to appropriate treatment; however, up to 30% of patients will develop complications or recurrent attacks.

The pericardium is a double-walled avascular sac that functions to protect the heart against infection and spread of malignancy (Doctor et al., 2016), provides lubrication, and secures the heart to the mediastinum (Adler & Charron, 2015). The pericardium is composed of a fibrous outer layer called the *parietal pericardium* and a mesothelial inner layer called the *visceral pericardium*, which adheres to the epicardium (Hoit, 2016). The pericardial space between the two layers normally contains 25 mL to 50 mL of fluid, which serves as a lubricant to reduce friction on the epicardium as the heart pumps (Doctor et al., 2016), as well as to equalize forces over the surface of the heart (Hoit, 2016).

The pericardium has a relatively simple structure, with the response to injury limited to the exudation of fluid, fibrin, and inflammatory cells (Hoit, 2016). This inflammatory response leads to the classic symptoms of sharp, pleuritic chest pain relieved with a forward-leaning position (Doctor et al., 2016). Complications of acute pericarditis result when fluid continues to accumulate, leading to a pericardial effusion or a life-threatening condition called *cardiac tamponade*, which compresses the heart, preventing it from normal function (Adler & Charron, 2015). Chronic recurrences and long-term inflammation can result in another complication called *constrictive pericarditis* in which the pericardium loses elasticity and constricts the heart, causing a form of heart failure secondary to a noncompliant pericardium (Miranda & Oh, 2016).

The typical classification of pericardial disease is according to etiology, which may be infectious or non-infectious (Cremer et al., 2016; Doctor et al., 2016), as the pericardium may be affected by infectious, autoimmune, neoplastic, iatrogenic, traumatic, and metabolic disease (Adler & Charron, 2015). Patients should be screened and considered for specific etiology according to their epidemiological background, as the etiology of pericarditis varies depending on geographic location (Doctor et al., 2016). The majority of pericarditis cases in developing countries have an infectious cause, whereas the majority of cases in Western Europe and North America are categorized as idiopathic and are presumed to be viral after unremarkable diagnostic workup (Imazio et al., 2015). Tuberculosis accounts for about 70% of pericarditis diagnoses in developing countries, with a 25% to 40% mortality rate at 6 months postdiagnosis, as many have a concomitant diagnosis of HIV (Imazio et al., 2015). In developed countries, when the specific etiology of pericarditis is identified, the underlying causes include neoplastic disease (5%–10%), systemic inflammatory diseases and pericardial injury syndromes (2%–7%), tuberculous pericarditis (4%), and purulent pericarditis (less than 1%; Imazio et al., 2015, p. 1499). The increasing use of cardiovascular interventions in developed countries, combined with the aging population, also increases the possible risk of pericardial complications, as even minor intracardiac bleeding can lead to pericarditis (Imazio et al., 2015).

Clinical Aspects

ASSESSMENT

Meticulous history and physical examination are necessary to differentiate pericarditis in the patient with acute chest pain (Doctor et al., 2016). The most common presentation of pericarditis is chest pain (Adler & Charron, 2015; Doctor et al., 2016; Imazio et al., 2015), typically sudden in onset and sharp in nature (Doctor et al., 2016). The clinical diagnosis of acute pericarditis may be made with two of the following criteria: precordial chest pain that is worse with inspiration and improved with upright position, pericardial friction rub, electrocardiogram changes that include widespread ST elevation, and pericardial effusion (Adler & Charron, 2015; Cremer et al., 2016). Additional supportive findings include elevated inflammatory markers, including C-reactive protein (CRP), erythrocyte sedimentation rate (ESR), and white blood cell (WBC) count, and evidence of inflammation by imaging (Adler & Charron, 2015; Cremer et al., 2016).

Echocardiography is an important imaging technique to detect pericardial fluid as well as the effects on the heart (Doctor et al., 2016), and is recommended in all patients with acute pericarditis (Adler & Charron, 2015). Patients with acute pericarditis and no additional signs and symptoms that predict higher risk of complications are often successfully treated as outpatients (Cremer et al., 2016). However, those patients with high-risk features, including fever, history of immunosuppression, history of trauma, or evidence of severe pericardial effusion, should be hospitalized for more intensive monitoring of possible complications (Doctor et al., 2016).

Pericarditis is categorized according to the duration of symptoms, with the first attack of pericardial inflammation considered acute pericarditis (Cremer et al., 2016; Doctor et al., 2016). Acute pericarditis has a good long-term prognosis, with risks of adverse events or the development of complicated pericarditis relatively rare (Adler & Charron, 2015). Hemodynamic compromise, such as cardiac tamponade, develops rarely and more often in patients with underlying etiology of malignancy or tuberculosis (Adler & Charron, 2015). Myocardial involvement occurs in about 15% of patients with acute pericarditis, although usually it has a benign course (Cremer et al., 2016). The risk of developing constrictive pericarditis is low (less than 1%) for idiopathic and viral pericarditis, intermediate (2%–5%) for autoimmune and malignant etiologies, and high for bacterial (20%–30%) etiologies (Adler & Charron, 2015; Hoit, 2016).

Recurrence of pericarditis, or pericarditis lasting longer than 4 to 6 weeks, is considered a complicated form of the disease (Cremer et al., 2016). Risk for developing complicated pericarditis is associated with early use of corticosteroids, a lack of response to nonsteroidal anti-inflammatory drugs (NSAIDs), and elevated CRP levels (Cremer et al., 2016). The absence of colchicine as treatment is also associated with an increased risk of developing a complicated or recurrent form of pericarditis (Cremer et al., 2016).

OUTCOMES

Patients diagnosed with acute pericarditis have acute pain, anxiety related to the diagnosis, and a risk for activity intolerance due to the disease process of pericarditis. Recommended treatment includes aspirin or NSAIDs, along with gastric protection with colchicine recommended as adjunct therapy to reduce recurrence rates (Adler & Charron, 2015; Imazio et al., 2015). In the presence of acute pain, patients should be assisted to a position of comfort. Education should include information regarding medications and side effects as well as instruction to avoid strenuous exercise until resolution of symptoms and normalization of CRP, electrocardiogram changes, and echocardiogram findings (Adler & Charron, 2015). Steroids are infrequently prescribed and not recommended as first-line therapy for acute pericarditis, although they may be used in cases of pericarditis refractory to NSAIDs or contraindications to the use of aspirin, NSAIDs, or colchicine (Adler & Charron, 2015). Patients should be assured that outcomes are generally positive when pericarditis is diagnosed promptly and the treatment regimen and recommendations are followed.

Summary

The most recent guidelines regarding diagnosis and treatment of pericarditis emphasize the importance of a thorough physical examination and history in diagnosing acute pericarditis, as the criteria for diagnosis may be obtained with an initial physical examination and electrocardiogram (Adler & Charron, 2015). Although the etiology of pericarditis is varied, the majority of cases in Western Europe and North America are presumed viral, with an unremarkable diagnostic workup (Imazio et al., 2015). The recommended treatment of acute pericarditis can typically be outpatient based and includes aspirin or NSAIDs with adjunct colchicine and exercise restriction (Adler & Charron, 2015). Nursing interventions include nonpharmacologic approaches to relieve pain, education, and support. Overall, the long-term prognosis for patients with acute pericarditis is good with rare complications when the recommended treatment regimen is followed (Doctor et al., 2016).

Adler, Y., & Charron, P. (2015). The 2015 ESC guidelines on the diagnosis and management of pericardial diseases. *European Heart Journal, 36*(42), 2873–2874.

Cremer, P. C., Kumar, A., Kontzias, A., Tan, C. D., Rodriguez, E. R., Imazio, M., & Klein, A. L. (2016). Complicated pericarditis: Understanding risk factors and pathophysiology to inform imaging and treatment. *Journal of the American College of Cardiology, 68*(21), 2311–2328.

Doctor, N. S., Shah, A. B., Coplan, N., & Kronzon, I. (2016). Acute pericarditis: Review. *Progress in Cardiovascular Diseases, 59*(2017), 349–359. doi:10.1016/j.pcad.2016.12.001

Hoit, B. D. (2016). Pathophysiology of the pericardium. *Progress in Cardiovascular Diseases, 59*(2017), 341–348. doi:10.1016/j.pdad.2016.11.001

Imazio, M., Gaita, F., & LeWinter, M. (2015). Evaluation and treatment of pericarditis: A systematic review. *Journal of the American Medical Association, 314*(14), 1498–1506.

Miranda, W. R., & Oh, J. K. (2016). Constrictive pericarditis: A practical clinical approach. *Progress in Cardiovascular Diseases, 59*(4), 369–379. doi:10.1016/j.pcad.2016.12.008

■ PERIPHERAL ARTERY DISEASE

Gayle M. Petty

Overview

Peripheral artery disease (PAD), previously referred to as *peripheral vascular disease, peripheral arterial occlusive disease*, or *arteriosclerosis obliterans*, is a varying vascular disease primarily caused by aneurysmal, atherosclerotic, and thromboembolic pathophysiologic processes. These pathophysiologic processes alter the normal structure and function of the arteries. PAD is a common, acute, and chronic condition that affects a large proportion of the adult population worldwide (Hirsch et al., 2006). Patients present with a range of signs and symptoms, and often require emergent revascularization, surgical interventions, or amputation.

Background

Commissioned by the American Heart Association in 2008, the Atherosclerotic Peripheral Vascular Disease Interdisciplinary Working Group came together with the goal to develop programs that will facilitate prevention and treatment of peripheral atherosclerotic diseases (Creager et al., 2008). As a result, definitions for vascular disease nomenclature were recommended. The term *vascular diseases* should refer to all diseases of arteries, veins, and lymphatic vessels. *Atherosclerotic vascular disease* refers to diseases of arteries caused by atherosclerosis (Creager et al., 2008). The 2011 American College of Cardiology (ACC)/American Heart Association (AHA) focused update of the guideline for the management of patients with PAD (updating the 2005 guideline) refers to PAD as peripheral "artery" disease and anatomically identifies lower extremity, renal and mesenteric arteries, and abdominal aortic as the arteries referenced when discussing PAD (Rooke et al., 2011).

The major cause of PAD is atherosclerosis (Hirsch et al., 2006). Risk factors are age related and include a history of cigarette smoking, diabetes, dyslipidemia, hypertension, and hyperlipidemia (Gerhard-Herman et al., 2016). The prognosis of patients with PAD is characterized by an increased risk for cardiovascular ischemic events, such as myocardial infarction or stroke, due to concomitant coronary artery disease and cerebrovascular disease (Gerhard-Herman et al., 2016). Etiologies for PAD beyond atherosclerosis and thromboembolic processes include familial, acquired, inflammatory, or aneurysmal. Establishment of an accurate etiology is necessary if individual patients are to receive ideal treatment (Hirsch et al., 2006).

Clinical Aspects

PAD can involve the aorta, renal and mesenteric arteries, and arteries of the lower extremities. Patients with PAD should receive a comprehensive program of guideline-directed medical therapy (GDMT), including structured exercise and lifestyle modification, to reduce cardiovascular ischemic events and improve functional status (Gerhard-Herman et al., 2016). Smoking cessation is a vital component of care for patients with PAD who continue to smoke (Gerhard-Herman et al., 2016). Patients with PAD should be prescribed a guideline-based program customized to each patient's risk profile that includes pharmacotherapy to reduce cardiovascular ischemic events and limb-related events (Gerhard-Herman et al., 2016). Prescribed pharmacotherapy classifications may include antiplatelets, statins, antihypertensives, oral anticoagulants, and cilostazol (Gerhard-Herman et al., 2016).

ASSESSMENT

Identification and prevention of disease progression before ischemic symptoms become severe are the health care goals for patients with PAD. Patient assessment should focus on any reports of ischemic rest pain, exertional limitation, or a history of walking impairment (Gerhard-Herman et al., 2016). Patients may describe walking limitation characteristics such as fatigue, aching, numbness, or pain in the buttock, thigh, calf, or foot (Hirsch et al., 2006).

Several key physical examination assessment components for PAD include the following: auscultation of both femoral arteries for the presence of bruits; palpation of the femoral, popliteal, dorsalis pedis, and posterior tibial pulse sites; and evaluation of lower extremity pulse intensity. The pulse intensity should be recoded numerically as follows: 0, when the pulse is absent; 1, when the pulse is diminished; 2, when the pulse is normal; and 3, when the pulse is bounding (Gerhard-Herman et al., 2016). As part of the physical examination, patients' shoes and socks should be removed and the feet should be inspected, noting the color, temperature, and integrity of the skin. An abnormal lower extremity pulse examination, a vascular bruit, a non-healing lower extremity wound, and lower extremity gangrene are all suggestive of PAD (Gerhard-Herman et al., 2016). Additional findings may include lower extremity color changes, including pallor, when elevated and dependent rubor (Gerhard-Herman et al., 2016).

The most cost-effective, low-risk tool for detecting PAD is the resting ankle–brachial index (ABI; Aboyans et al., 2012). The resting ABI is obtained by measuring systolic blood pressure (SBP) at the arms (brachial arteries) and ankles (dorsalis pedis and posterior tibial

arteries) in the supine position using a Doppler device (Gerhard-Herman et al., 2016). The ABI is the ratio of the ankle SBP—the numerator of the ratio—to either arm's highest brachial artery SBP—the denominator for the ratio. The numerator for the calculation of the ABI incorporates the SBP of the posterior tibial or the dorsalis pedis artery separately or is the average of both. It can be performed quickly for each lower extremity and has high validity and good reproducibility (Diehm et al., 2012; Gerhard-Herman et al., 2016). An ABI can be an indicator of atherosclerosis at other vascular sites and can serve as a prognostic marker for cardiovascular events and functional impairment, even in the absence of PAD symptoms.

Individuals performing the ABI should have basic knowledge of vascular anatomy, physiology, and the clinical presentation of PAD, as well as a basic understanding of how a Doppler device functions. The normal ABI ranges from 1.00 to 1.40; findings less than or equal to 0.90 are abnormal and values of 0.91 to 0.99 are considered borderline. Values greater than 1.40 indicate noncompressible arteries (Diehm et al., 2012; Gerhard-Herman et al., 2016).

NURSING INTERVENTIONS, MANAGEMENT, AND IMPLICATIONS

Patients with asymptomatic PAD can acutely progress to a situation requiring emergent interventions. Acute limb ischemia arises when a rapid or sudden decrease in limb perfusion threatens tissue viability (Gerhard-Herman et al., 2016). This may be the first manifestation of artery disease in a previously asymptomatic patient.

The hallmark clinical symptom and physical examination signs of acute limb ischemia include the six "Ps": pain, pallor, pulselessness, poikilothermia, paresthesias, and paralysis (Gerhard-Herman et al., 2016; Hirsch et al., 2006). Determining whether a patient with acute limb ischemia has a salvageable or nonviable extremity is crucial. An urgent evaluation is necessary to preserve the limb and prevent systemic illness or death as a result of the metabolic abnormalities associated with tissue necrosis. The ACC/AHA acute limb ischemia guidelines should be followed when performing the evaluation (Gerhard-Herman et al., 2016).

OUTCOMES

Patients with acute limb ischemia and a salvageable extremity should undergo an emergent evaluation leading to prompt endovascular or surgical revascularization. Patients with acute limb ischemia and a nonviable extremity will most likely require an amputation of the diseased limb (Gerhard-Herman et al., 2016).

Summary

Peripheral arterial diseases encompass diseases of the aorta, renal and mesenteric, and the lower extremity arteries. Etiologies may vary, but the majority of PAD is caused by atherosclerosis. Early identification using ABI and GDMT interventions can delay the disease progression and prevent life-threatening cardiovascular ischemic events.

Aboyans, V., Criqui, M. H., Abraham, P., Allison, M. A., Creager, M. A., Diehm, C., . . . Treat-Jacobson, D. (2012). Measurement and interpretation of the ankle-brachial index: A scientific statement from the American Heart Association. *Circulation, 126,* 2890–2909. doi:10.1161/ CIR.0b013e

Creager, M. A., White, C. J., Hiatt, W. R., Criqui, M. H., Josephs, S. C., Alberts, M. J., . . . Rocha-Singh, K. J. (2008). Atherosclerotic peripheral vascular disease symposium II: Executive summary. *Circulation, 118,* 2811–2825, doi:10.1161/CIRCULATIONAHA.108 .191170

Gerhard-Herman, M. D., Gornik, H. L., Barrett, C., Barshes, N. R., Corriere, M. A., Drachman, D. E., . . . Walsh, M. E. (2016). AHA/ACC guideline on the management of patients with lower extremity peripheral artery disease: Executive summary. *Circulation.* doi:10.1161/ CIR.0000000000000470

Hirsch, A. T., Haskal, J. Z., Hertzer, N. R., Bakal, C. W., Creager, M. A., Halperin, J. L., . . . Reigal, B. (2006). ACC/AHA 2005 guidelines for the management of patients with peripheral arterial disease (lower extremity, renal, mesenteric, and abdominal aortic). *Circulation, 113,* e463–e654. doi:10.1161/ CIRCULATIONAHA.106.174526

Rooke, T. W., Hirsch, A. T., Mirsa, S., Sidawy, A. N., Beckman, J. A., Findeiss, L. K., . . . Zierler, R. E. (2011). ACCF/AHA focused update of the guideline for the management of patients with peripheral artery disease (updating the 2005 guidelines). *Journal of the American College of Cardiology, 58*(19), 2020–2045. doi:10.1016/j.jacc.2011.08.023

■ PERNICIOUS ANEMIA

Edwidge Cuvilly

Overview

Pernicious anemia (PA), also known as *vitamin B$_{12}$ deficiency*, is the most common vitamin deficiency in the world, affecting at least 3% of those aged 20 to 39 years, 4% of those aged 40 to 59 years, and 6% of those 60 years and older (Shipton & Thachil, 2015). PA is an insidious complex disorder, provoking a sequelae of modifications in the immunological, hematological, gastrointestinal, and neurological system over a period of time that could be fatal if left untreated. Even though PA has been found in practically every ethnic group, the highest prevalence is among individuals from Northern European countries, mainly the United Kingdom and Scandinavia (Bizzaro & Antico, 2014). Nursing care is essential in detecting the early signs and preventing the clinical manifestations of PA across the life span.

Background

PA is a macrocytic anemia caused by the inability of gastric parietal cells to produce intrinsic factor (IF). IF is a gastric protein secreted by parietal cells to allow the absorption of an adequate amount of vitamin B$_{12}$ in the diet. Vitamin B$_{12}$ is found in animal food bound to a protein that is broken down after ingestion, then further broken down in the stomach by pepsin and hydrochloric acid to release free vitamin B$_{12}$. The free vitamin B$_{12}$ is bound to IF secreted by gastric parietal cells until they bind to mucosal cell receptors in the ileum, where they gets absorbed and can be used for intracellular processes. Vitamin B$_{12}$ is an important micronutrient that aids in the formation of erythrocytes in the bone marrow. When there is a deficiency of vitamin B$_{12}$, erythrocytes are prematurely released into the systemic circulation and have a shortened life span because the premature erythrocytes are prone to early destruction, thus resulting in a reduced erythrocyte count and a state of anemia.

PA occurs as a clinical manifestation of autoimmune gastritis. Autoimmune gastritis is a disease process in which parietal cells are destroyed and a subsequent reduction in the IF results in a vitamin B$_{12}$ deficiency, or PA. Vitamin B$_{12}$ is responsible for erythropoiesis and myelin synthesis; when symptoms are present, vitamin B$_{12}$ deficiency is detected, then swift action to initiate treatment is necessary to reverse or prevent further continuation of damage.

Due to a broad spectrum of symptoms associated with severe consequences of untreated vitamin B$_{12}$ deficiency, screening is essential for high-risk patients to guarantee a quick delivery of treatment. In the elderly, the prevalence of vitamin B$_{12}$ deficiency increases with age and 20% of those 60 years or older are more prone to acquiring a vitamin B_{12} deficiency (Shipton & Thachil, 2015).

There is no gold standard test to diagnose vitamin B_{12} deficiency, but the World Health Organization (WHO) defined PA as having a hemoglobin concentration less than 13 g/dL for men and less than 12 g/dL for women, mean corpuscular volume (MCV) more than 100 fL, and a serum vitamin B_{12} level less than 200 pg/mL (Sun, Wang, Lin, Chia, & Chia, 2013). A low serum vitamin B_{12} that is less than 200 pg/mL is an indicator for prompt initiation of vitamin B_{12} supplementation. However, the lack of accepted value creates a vague demarcation of what is consider deficiency (Wong, 2015). In order to make a distinction between PA and other causes of low vitamin B_{12}, serum autoantibodies are imperative. Anti-IF antibody assay is the preferred test due to high specificity (more than 95%; Shipton & Thachil, 2015).

The distinction between autoimmune gastritis and other causative factors (e.g., vegetarian/vegan diet, alcoholism, poor diet) becomes important when assessing vitamin B_{12} deficiency among the elderly. The main etiology of vitamin B_{12} in the elderly can be separated into two categories: first, inadequate dietary intake (vegetarian, alcohol consumption) and impaired absorption of vitamin B_{12} (PA, atrophic gastritis, postgastrectomy). In spite of the preconception that the most common cause of vitamin B_{12} deficiency in the elderly is inadequate dietary intake, studies have shown the opposite.

Clinical Aspects

ASSESSMENT

The basic clinical features of PA are commonly associated with hypersegmented neutrophils and megaloblastic maturation of erythrocytes, sores on the tongue associated with loss of papillae, and atrophic glossitis, achlorhydria, and neurologic symptoms (paresthesia and ataxia; Bunn, 2014). A complete blood count will often confirm a low hemoglobin, hematocrit, and red blood cell count. Morphological changes of the erythrocyte are likely to occur where there is a high MCV. The megaoblastic shape of the erythrocytes contributes to clinical manifestations of anemia accompanied by pallor, fatigue, weakness, palpitations, dyspnea upon exertion, chest pain, and angina.

OUTCOMES

Evidence-based nursing care should focus on the assessment of risk factors and early identification of clinical

manifestations related to PA or vitamin B_{12} deficiency. Devalia, Hamilton, and Molloy (2014) reported that the interpretation of the results should take into consideration these clinical manifestations. Clients with anemia, neuropathy, glossitis, and suspected PA should be tested for anti-IF antibodies. The specification of oral or intramuscular supplementation of vitamin B_{12} should be guided by the results of the laboratory testing, which can inform the etiology of the vitamin B_{12} deficiency.

Summary

PA or vitamin B_{12} deficiency is a treatable condition that has profound effects on the health of an individual. Nursing care for clients with PA or vitamin B_{12} deficiency should include a comprehensive physical assessment and review of pertinent laboratory tests to inform nursing management. The goal of nursing interventions for clients with PA or vitamin B_{12} deficiency is to prevent the sequelae of physiological derangements that can occur as the result of the cellular changes that occur with untreated PA or vitamin B_{12} deficiency.

Bizzaro, N., & Antico, A. (2014). Diagnosis and classification of pernicious anemia. *Autoimmunity Reviews, 13*(4–5), 565–568.

Bunn, H. F. (2014). Vitamin B_{12} and pernicious anemia—The dawn of molecular medicine. *New England Journal of Medicine, 370*(8), 773–776.

Devalia, V., Hamilton, M. S., & Molloy, A. M. (2014). Guidelines for the diagnosis and treatment of cobalamin and folate disorders. *British Journal of Haematology, 166*(4), 496–513.

Shipton, M. J., & Thachil, J. (2015). Vitamin B_{12} deficiency—A 21st century perspective. *Clinical Medicine, 15*(2), 145–150.

Sun, A., Wang, Y. P., Lin, H. P., Chia, J. S., & Chia, C. P. (2013). Do all the patients with gastric parietal cell antibodies have pernicious anemia? *Oral Diseases, 19*, 381–386.

Wong, C. W. (2015). Vitamin B_{12} deficiency in the elderly: Is it worth screening? *Hong Kong Medical Journal, 21*, 155–164.

■ POLYCYTHEMIA VERA

Sarine Beukian

Overview

Polycythemia vera (PV) is characterized by a mutation in a single amino acid that renders the Janus kinase 2

(JAK2) enzyme constitutively active. This induces cytokine-independent proliferation of cell lines that express erythropoietin (EPO) receptors and cause these cells to become hypersensitive to cytokines. Therefore, more proerythroblasts and erythrocytes are formed than are physiologically needed. PV is often discovered as an incidental finding in laboratory work or while seeking medical care in the midst of a thrombotic or hemorrhagic complication. It carries a pronounced symptom burden and can progress to myelofibrosis (9%–21% of individuals) or acute leukemia (3%–10%; Stein et al., 2015).

Background

PV is defined as elevated red blood cells (RBCs), hematocrit (Hct), and hemoglobin (Hgb) laboratory values; PV is also referred to as *erythrocytosis*. PV is further categorized as relative and absolute. Relative PV applies to patients suspected of polycythemia but are found to have a normal RBC mass and a smaller than normal plasma volume, which could be caused by dehydration. Absolute PV applies to true increase in RBC mass, which is further divided into primary and secondary PV based on etiology. The latter is more common and is caused by chronic hypoxia, EPO-producing tumors, or medications such as erythropoiesis-stimulating agents. Hypoxia stimulates EPO and increases RBC count due to bone marrow (BM) stimulation. Living in higher altitudes, smoking, carbon monoxide poisoning, chronic obstructive pulmonary disease, or heart failure can cause hypoxia. Primary polycythemia results from congenital or acquired mutations, and it includes PV and other rare familial conditions (Tefferi & Barbui, 2015). PV is one of the myeloproliferative neoplasms (MPN), alongside primary myelofibrosis and essential thrombocytopenia, among others (Tefferi & Barbui, 2017). Nearly all patients with PV hold a JAK2 mutation, involving exon 14 with JAK2V617F (96%) or exon 12 (3%; Tefferi & Barbui, 2017).

Prevalence (22 cases per 100,000 people) and yearly incidence rates are high (1.3 cases per 100,000 for women and 2.8 cases per 100,000 for men). Risk factors include old age, White race, or Ashkenazi Jewish ancestry. Male predominance with an average age of 61 years at the time of diagnosis has been reported (Scherber & Mesa, 2016; Stein et al., 2015; Tefferi & Barbui, 2015).

Patients often present with fatigue, night sweats, bone pain, fever, weight loss, splenomegaly associated with early satiety, atypical chest pain, paresthesias, and aquagenic pruritus (particularly when in contact with warm or hot water; Stein et al., 2015; Tefferi & Barbui, 2015). Patients are at risk for thrombosis at 2.5% to 4% per year. This includes cerebrovascular accidents, acute coronary syndrome, and thrombosis of the hepatic, portal, and mesenteric veins. Microvascular symptoms, such as headache, visual change, dizziness, erythromelalgia (erythema, warmth, and pain in distal extremities—most commonly palms and soles), also commonly occur and overwhelmingly perturb quality of life, with a mortality rate of 37% (Stein et al., 2015).

Persistent erythrocytosis without an obvious trigger requires workup. Presence of symptoms suggestive of a MPN should add to clinical suspicion. JAK2V617F mutation and EPO levels should be checked. Presence of the mutation makes PV a likely diagnosis. If the mutation is not present and EPO levels are normal or elevated, PV is unlikely, and other causes need to be considered. If the EPO levels are subnormal, then JAK2 (exon 12) should be checked; its presence makes the diagnosis of PV likely. However, its absence requires a BM biopsy. The World Health Organization revised its criteria for the diagnosis of PV in 2016, which includes a combination of the following: elevated Hgb/Hct levels, increased RBC mass, BM biopsy showing hypercellularity, presence of JAK2 mutation, and subnormal serum EPO level. BM biopsy is not always needed to establish the diagnosis of PV (Tefferi & Barbui, 2017).

Medical therapy has shown promising results in the prevention of thrombotic events and reducing symptom burden. However, it has failed to show a difference in disease progression or improvement in survival rates. Median survival in PV is 14 years with aggressive medical therapy, including phlebotomy. The median survival is significantly reduced to 2 years when aggressive medical therapy and the target Hct of less than 45% is not maintained (Tefferi & Barbui, 2015, 2017). Medical therapy for the prevention of thrombosis is based on risk stratification: age older than 60 years and history of thrombosis are markers of high risk. One exception is low-dose aspirin therapy: with no specific contraindication, it is prescribed to all patients regardless of risk-factor profile. It can help with managing symptoms related to microvascular complications. A twice-a-day regimen can be helpful in those who are resistant to a daily regimen or are at risk of arterial thrombus. High-risk patients who continue to be symptomatic, have extreme thrombocytosis, or are unable to tolerate phlebotomy (due to anemia) require treatment with cytoreductive therapy (Stein et al., 2015; Tefferi & Barbui, 2017).

The first line of therapy is hydroxyurea; other options are busulfan or interferon therapy, which lower the risk of thrombosis and leukemic transformation (Stein et al., 2015; Tefferi & Barbui, 2017). Busulfan shows a reduction in allele burden. Interferon therapy is prescribed to manage ongoing erythrocytosis, to reduce spleen size and control pruritus. JAK1/2 inhibitors, such as ruxolitinib, have gained a lot of interest with U.S. Food and Drug Administration approval in 2014. They have shown improvement in Hct control, splenic size reduction, and symptom burden. However, incidence of thrombosis, disease progression, and long-term safety remain questions that need to be addressed. Pipobroman is associated with a shorter survival, increased leukemic transformation, and a lower rate of fibrosis transformation. Radiophosphorus also increases the risk of leukemic transformation (Stein et al., 2015).

Clinical Aspects

ASSESSMENT

Nurses play a crucial role in identifying abnormal laboratory values and side effects of therapy, in educating and counseling patients about PV, and in appropriately intervening to reduce symptom burden and improve patients' quality of life. In the care of the patient with PV, nurses can start with assessment of the patient by reviewing the laboratory values, test results pertinent to PV, medication list, smoking history, medical and surgical history (conditions that cause chronic hypoxia), symptoms, and physical examination findings. Nursing diagnoses that apply to PV are fatigue, pain, (risk for) decreased cardiac tissue perfusion, risk for bleeding, risk for impaired skin integrity, imbalanced nutrition (patients consume less than body requirements because of early satiety), deficient knowledge regarding condition, impaired comfort related to itching, and (risk for) ineffective peripheral tissue perfusion. The following section serves as an example of a nursing care plan to discuss the last three symptoms mentioned.

Given the chronic nature of the disease, it is imperative to assess the patient's understanding of the disease process, symptoms, complications, medications, side effects, and signs and symptoms of complications such as thrombosis (Golden, 2003). Thereafter, the diagnosis of deficient knowledge can be utilized. The desired outcome would be for the patient to comprehend the disease process, medical therapy, and participate in decision making regarding therapy and interventions. Implementation can be through one-on-one discussions with the patient, providing or guiding him or her to the right resources and support groups. Evaluation should follow, in order to ensure comprehension and assessment for further needs.

All patients with PV are at risk of thrombosis. Assessment would include reviewing laboratory values, history of thrombosis, age, medications, medical history, cardiovascular risk factors, and physical examination. Nursing interventions include performing phlebotomy, medication administration, encouraging activity, and educating patients to avoid crossing legs or wearing tight-fitting clothes. Interventions specific to phlebotomy include the removal of 450 mL to 500 mL of blood every few days at first, and thereafter every 2 to 3 months in order to reach target Hct goal; encouraging hydration before and after phlebotomy; monitoring for orthostatic hypotension, headache, weakness, or chest pain postphlebotomy. Evaluation should be used as an opportunity to adjust care plans as necessary (Golden, 2003).

OUTCOMES

Aquagenic pruritus can be debilitating to PV patients. Assessment should include an observation of the patient's pattern of itching, asking the patient about the severity of the symptom, and a skin examination. Subsequently, the diagnosis can be made. One outcome is to relieve the patient or at least alleviate the symptom. Interventions include avoiding dry skin; hot temperature; encouraging tepid showers; drying the skin gently; administering antihistamines, antidepressants, or JAK inhibitors. Evaluation should follow with adjustments as necessary (Golden, 2003; Tefferi & Barbui, 2017).

Summary

PV affects about 148,000 people in the United States alone (Stein et al., 2015). JAK2 mutation remains the most important diagnostic test to identify PV. Phlebotomy and aspirin are the cornerstones of therapy. Patients' symptoms, life expectancy, and risk factors should be evaluated before selecting medical therapy for PV. One of the challenges is to identify and link elevated laboratory values to an underlying disease process; "more is not better" when it comes to RBC, Hgb, and Hct levels, as they may suggest PV.

Golden, C. (2003). Polycythemia vera: A review. *Clinical Journal of Oncology Nursing, 7*(5), 553–556.

Scherber, R. M., & Mesa, R. A. (2016). Elevated hemoglobin or hematocrit level. *Journal of the American Medical Association, 315*(20), 2225–2226.

Stein, B. L., Oh, S. T., Berenzon, D., Hobbs, G. S., Kremyanskaya, M., Rampal, R. K., . . . Hoffman, R. (2015). Polycythemia vera: An appraisal of the biology and management 10 years after the discovery of JAK2 V617F. *Journal of Clinical Oncology, 33*(33), 3953–3960.

Tefferi, A., & Barbui, T. (2015). Essential thrombocythemia and polycythemia vera: Focus on clinical practice. *Mayo Clinic Proceedings, 90*(9), 1283–1293.

Tefferi, A., & Barbui, T. (2017). Polycythemia vera and essential thrombocythemia: 2017 Update on diagnosis, risk-stratification, and management. *American Journal of Hematology, 92*(1), 94–108.

■ PROSTATE CANCER

Erin H. Discenza

Overview

Prostate cancer is the most common cancer in males following nonmelanoma skin cancer and is one of the leading causes of cancer death in males, exceeded only by lung cancer (Centers for Disease Control and Prevention [CDC], 2016). The manifestations, progressive course, and prognosis of the disease vary and are reliant on factors such as extent of the tumor, aggressiveness of the malignancy, comorbidities, and age of the patient (National Cancer Institute [NCI], 2017). The key focus of nursing care of the patient with prostate cancer should be good communication and patient education. There are numerous psychological aspects pertaining to the diagnosis and treatment of prostate cancer and these must be addressed to provide excellent patient-centered nursing care and to ensure desired outcomes.

Background

The prostate gland is located in the pelvis below the bladder and just in front of the rectum. The urethra travels through the center of the prostate. As men age, the prostate may grow benignly larger and cause urinary symptoms such as hesitancy. However, when the cells of the gland grow uncontrollably, cancer is suspected (American Cancer Society [ACS], 2017).

Although the incidence and mortality rates have decreased significantly among all races, prostate cancer remains the second most common cancer in males. According to the CDC (2016), 176,450 men were diagnosed with prostate cancer in 2013, and 27,681 men died from the disease. The NCI estimates those numbers will decrease in 2017 to 161,360 new cases and 26,730 deaths. The average age of diagnosis is 66 years (CDC, 2016).

The primary risk factors associated with prostate cancer are age, family history, and race. The older a man is, the greater his risk for developing prostate cancer. Men younger than 40 years rarely develop the disease, but the risk rises expeditiously after the age of 50 years. Approximately 60% of cases are found in men older than the age of 65 years (CDC, 2016; NCI, 2017). Family history may also affect a man's chance of developing prostate cancer. Having a first-degree relative diagnosed with prostate cancer increases an individual's risk, particularly if the relative was diagnosed at a young age; the risk increases with the number of affected relatives. African American males are at greater risk of developing the disease and are more than twice as likely to die as a result of the cancer. Geography may also play a role in the risk of developing prostate cancer. It is more common in North America and parts of Europe. The exact geographical impact is unknown, but it is posited that more extensive screening practices in developed countries or diets consisting of excessive amounts of red meat or high-fat dairy products may be a contributor to this phenomenon (ACS, 2017).

The early stages of prostate cancer rarely yield symptoms, but in advanced stages the symptoms can be detrimental to the patient's quality of life. The most common symptoms are lower urinary tract symptoms (LUTSs) and include urinary urgency, hesitancy, nocturia, dysuria, and incontinence. Other symptoms include blood in the urine or semen; intractable pain in the back, hips, or pelvis; painful ejaculation; and erectile dysfunction (ED). If the cancer spreads to the bone, there may also be spontaneous fractures (ACS, 2017; CDC, 2016).

Clinical Aspects

ASSESSMENT

Extensive history taking and a complete physical examination are the first steps in the assessment process. Because genetics may play a part in the risk of developing the disease, the nurse should be aware of any family history of prostate cancer. A digital rectal examination (DRE) is also useful in determining whether the prostate is enlarged. The clinician inserts a finger into the rectum to estimate the size of the gland and to feel for lumps or other anomalies (CDC, 2016). Prostate-specific antigen (PSA) is a protein secreted by the prostate. When higher PSA levels are found in the serum, the clinician may suspect cancer but other causes must be ruled out. PSA is specific to the prostate, but it is not specific to cancer (Paterson, Alashkham, Windsor, & Nabi, 2016). Certain medications, medical procedures, infections of the prostate, and enlargement of the prostate can all be possible origins of elevated serum PSA (CDC, 2016).

If cancer is suspected, a transrectal ultrasound guided-needle biopsy is the most common method for a definitive diagnosis (NCI, 2017). MRI produces a clearer picture and is sometimes used for biopsy and to determine whether the cancer has spread outside of the prostate gland. It is important to note that antibiotics may be prescribed prophylactically due to the increased risk of sepsis after needle biopsy (NCI, 2017).

NURSING INTERVENTIONS, MANAGEMENT, AND IMPLICATIONS

There are many factors to be considered when deciding on a treatment strategy for prostate cancer. They include the age of the patient and his life expectancy, comorbidities, stage and grade of the cancer, potential for cure, and possible side effects of the treatment modalities (Williams, Hemphill, & Knowles, 2017).

Active surveillance (AS), including a PSA test and DRE every 6 months, is rapidly becoming a preferred method of management due to the slow progression of the disease. This treatment requires active patient participation in the medical decision-making process (Jayadevappa et al., 2017). When the cancer is confined to the gland and the patient's life expectancy is at least 10 years, therapy with curative intent is most often selected. The most common procedure in this instance is radical prostatectomy (RP), in which the surgeon removes the entire gland (NCI, 2017). Urinary incontinence and ED are both major side effects of RP. If left untreated, the patient's quality of life is severely impacted, leading to depression, anxiety, and decreased feelings of well-being (Jayadevappa et al., 2017).

Radiation therapy (RT) is also a choice for low-grade cancer that is confined to the prostate gland, but may also be used in more advanced cases (ACS, 2017; Williams et al., 2017). RT is accomplished by either external beam radiation or brachytherapy, an implanted RT. Compared with RP, RT is associated with higher risk of hospitalization, need for open surgical procedures, and development of secondary malignancies (Williams et al., 2017).

A relatively new treatment method involves the development of new-generation genomic biomarkers and tissue-based gene expression tests. These biomarkers can indicate whether a prostate cancer is more aggressive than average and more likely to metastasize; however, there are no available recommendations regarding the routine use of these tests (Eapen & Meng, 2017).

Other treatment modalities include cryotherapy, hormone therapy, chemotherapy, and vaccine treatments (ACS, 2017). The choice of treatment method is an important one that should be based not only on the aforementioned factors, but also on the potential for negative impact on quality of life.

The nursing-related problems and the associated nursing interventions are directly related to the diagnosis and treatment of the disease. Many of the problems arise from the psychological impact of the side effects of treatment, such as anxiety and deficient knowledge related to the diagnosis and treatment plan, as well as sexual dysfunction related to effects of treatment. The interventions for these problems are based on open communication and patient education. A more patient-centered approach is needed to support patients and their caregivers to reduce anxiety and encourage self-management. Nurses must also better understand the role of culture, spirituality, and religion in their patients' treatment course (Allchorne & Green, 2016; Baker, Wellman, & Lavender, 2016; Paterson et al., 2016; Williams et al., 2017).

OUTCOMES

The goal of evidence-based nursing care is to ameliorate the effects of the devastating diagnosis of cancer, as well as the psychosocial ramifications of the therapies. Reduction of stress and increased ability to cope are paramount. Patient education must be a key focus as the patient moves from diagnosis to treatment to survivorship. Open lines of communication between the patient and the nurse are of utmost importance to the patient's well-being and quality of life. Along with the psychosocial needs of the patient, there are the problems of pain caused by the procedures, urinary problems such as retention, and infection risks that must be addressed by the nurse. The objective is symptom management. With good nursing care, the prospect of full recovery to prediagnosis functionality is excellent.

Summary

Although prostate cancer is one of the most common cancers in men and a leading cause of cancer death, it can be treated and cured successfully. The treatment modalities induce several undesirable side effects, but these can be mitigated with excellent nursing care. Evidence-based nursing interventions include patient education and open lines of communication, and are vital to the attainment of desired outcomes.

Allchorne, P., & Green, J. (2016). Identifying unmet care needs of patients with prostate cancer to assist with their success in coping. *Urologic Nursing, 36*(5), 224–232.

American Cancer Society. (2017). About prostate cancer. Retrieved from https://www.cancer.org/cancer/prostate -cancer/about.html

Baker, H., Wellman, S., & Lavender, V. (2016). Functional quality-of-life outcomes reported by men treated for localized prostate cancer: A systematic literature review. *Oncology Nursing Forum, 43*(2), 199–218.

Centers for Disease Control and Prevention and National Cancer Institute, U.S. Department of Health and Human Services. (2016). United States cancer statistics: 1999– 2013 incidence and mortality web-based report [Data file]. Retrieved from https://nccd.cdc.gov/uscs

Eapen, R. S., & Meng, M. V. (2017). Role of molecular bio-markers in localized prostate cancer. *Urology Times, 45*(4), 14–16.

Jayadevappa, R., Chhatre, S., Wong, Y. N., Wittink, M. N., Cook, R., Morales, K. H., . . . Gallo, J. J. (2017). Comparative effectiveness of prostate cancer treatments for patient-centered outcomes: A systematic review and meta-analysis (PRISMA Compliant). *Medicine, 96*(18), e6790.

National Cancer Institute. (2017). *PDQ Prostate cancer treatment.* Bethesda, MD: Author. Retrieved from https://www.cancer.gov/types/prostate/hp/prostate -treatment-pdq

Paterson, C., Alashkham, A., Windsor, P., & Nabi, G. (2016). Management and treatment of men affected by metastatic prostate cancer: Evidence-based recommendations for practice. *International Journal of Urological Nursing, 10*(1), 44–55.

Williams, S., Hemphill, J. C., & Knowles, A. (2017). Confidence of nursing personnel in their understanding of the psychosocial impact of prostate cancer. *Urologic Nursing, 37*(1), 23–30.

■ RHEUMATOID ARTHRITIS

Susan V. Brindisi

Overview

There are hundreds of different types of arthritis. Rheumatoid arthritis (RA) is one specific type that is considered an autoimmune disease that occurs when antibodies in the body attack the joints. Inflammation occurs in the synovium, the joint lining, which then causes cartilage inflammation. If cartilage inflammation goes unchecked irreversible damage can occur, narrowing the joint space, which can cause loose and unstable joints, joint deformity, and pain. Complications of RA include systemic damage of the heart, lungs, and gastrointestinal tract. RA is a chronic health condition that can be a comorbidity for nurses caring for patients in every setting. Pain management and a clear understanding of current medication treatments are a priority for the nurse taking care of the RA patient. Knowledge of disease progression and its stage will determine the nursing care. It is also important to know what the patient can or cannot do in terms of activities of daily living. Knowledge of assistive devices, including mobility aids, is also essential in the care of the RA patient.

Background

RA is commonly defined as a chronic inflammatory disease of unknown etiology that attacks the articular structures and lining of the joints or synovium (Pinto & Schub, 2016). The disease can cause joint deformity, pain, swelling, tenderness, and various extra-articular manifestations. There is no cure for RA; however, it can go into remission (Schub & Uribe, 2016). According to the Arthritis Foundation (2017), 1.5 million Americans have RA and it is more common in women between 30 and 60 years of age. In men, RA is more common later in life. RA is common in families, although it can manifest in individuals without a family history. RA is also more common in Native Americans. According to Schub and Holle (2016), approximately 50% of patients with RA become disabled after 10 years of disease onset. The overall mortality rate in patients with RA is 2.5 times that of the general population and globally, RA occurs in all people and in all countries.

Clinical Aspects

ASSESSMENT

A diagnosis of RA is made based on classification criteria developed by the American College of Rheumatology/European League Against Rheumatism, 2015 version. A diagnosis of RA includes the presence of synovitis in at least one joint that is not explained by another disease; a calculated score of the number and site of joints involved allows for zero to five possible points. The smaller joints (hand, wrist, feet) score a higher number in that RA tends to effect smaller joints first. After the smaller joints, the larger weight-bearing joints may be affected. Joint symptoms are usually bilateral and symmetrical. Also included are blood tests: a positive serum rheumatoid factor and symptom duration.

Early signs and symptoms of RA can include joint pain, stiffness, fatigue, lethargy, and anorexia. Patients may present to emergency rooms with flare-ups of RA later in the disease progression. Patients with RA may participate in rehabilitation multiple times throughout the course of their lives. Working closely with physical and occupational therapists can improve quality of life and independence for the RA patient. The certified rehabilitation registered nurse (CRRN) serves as a clinical expert and important part of the rehab team in the care of the RA patient.

Serious systemic problems can arise if RA is not treated. These problems can affect the skin, eyes, muscles, blood vessels, heart, and lungs (Pinto & Schub, 2016; Schub & Uribe, 2016). Cardiovascular disease is one serious systemic problem. This is likely due to chronic inflammation that is combined with the often sedentary lifestyle of the RA patient, who might also be overweight. Complications of RA can also include temporomandibular joint disease. This could impair the patient's chewing and ability to eat. In addition, the following can also occur: infection, osteoporosis, lymphadenopathy, and peripheral neuritis. Additional potential complications of RA include pericarditis, pleuritis, pleural effusion, cervical spine instability, anemia, gastrointestinal problems, Sjögren's syndrome, Felty syndrome, lymphoma, and other cancers. Mental health issues include anxiety and depression (Schub & Holle, 2016).

NURSING INTERVENTIONS, MANAGEMENT, AND IMPLICATIONS

Pharmacologic management has progressed in the past 10 years and has made RA a more manageable condition. Drug therapy can slow the progression of RA and treat symptoms. According to Schub and Uribe (2016), drug therapy is most effective when initiated in the early stages of the disease. Disease-modifying antirheumatic drugs (DMARDs) are often the first line of therapy. These include methotrexate, hydroxychloroquine, sulfasalazine, and leflunomide. A second type of drug therapy includes tumor necrosis factor-alpha (TNF-α) antagonists. These include drugs such as etanercept, infliximab, and adalimumab. There are other biologic agents not targeting TNF-α that can reduce inflammation. This includes abatacept, which is a fusion protein that inhibits T-cell activation. Combinations of these agents can often treat RA. Side effects include infection and increased risk of cancer.

Pain management is an important part of RA management. Nonsteroidal anti-inflammatory drugs (NSAIDs) can be used for swelling and pain. They relieve symptoms but do not stop the progression of RA as do the biologic agents. Steroids, especially corticosteroids like prednisone or hydrocortisone, can also be used to decrease inflammation. Other pain management includes acetaminophen, codeine, hydrocodone, morphine, and topical capsaicin (Schub & Uribe, 2016). Nonpharmacologic approaches to treating RA-associated pain include hot and cold therapy and guided imagery.

The nurse assessing the RA patient needs to know the current stage of the disease. In unidentified RA, the nurse can refer to laboratory assessment data and a rheumatologist to make the initial diagnosis. The nurse must assess vital signs and all systems to identify risk for or actual systemic complications. During a clinical assessment, the nurse can palpate the joint for pain, swelling, warmth, erythema, lack of function, or boggy tissue (Smeltzer & Bare, 2004). RA can also cause fever, weight loss, fatigue, anemia, lymph node enlargement, lymphedema, and Raynaud's phenomena (Smeltzer & Bare, 2004). The nurse should note any decreased range of motion and assess for mobility status. Because the RA patient can also experience anorexia, the nurse must also weigh the patient and include a thorough nutrition assessment. RA nursing care includes managing pain, sleep disturbance, altered mood, and limited mobility (Smeltzer & Bare, 2004).

Nursing interventions include application of heat and cold, massage, position change, using a firm mattress, use of splints and pillows, administering antiinflammatory medications as well as other disease-modifying medication. Patient teaching about managing pain and continually monitoring joints in order to maximize lifestyle needs are paramount. The nurse should encourage verbalization about the disease, assessing the need for physical and/or occupational therapy, promoting the use of assistive devices, and encouraging rest after periods of activity. Patient teaching on pain management and medication regimen is a priority to manage activity with RA. Patient teaching should include helping the patient to identify activities that interfere with self-care activities and devising a plan to manage the difficult activities of daily living. Additional nursing interventions include teaching use of appropriate assistive devices for self-care and making a referral to a community agency for help.

OUTCOMES

Expected outcomes as a result of the nursing care of the RA patient focus on the patient living fully and managing disability associated with RA. The patient and family should be comfortable with identifying and managing pain exacerbation, proficient with the use of mobility devices, and identifying community resources that support full living with RA.

Summary

Living with RA is manageable especially with early intervention. Nursing management of RA is crucial to the patient living a fulfilling lifestyle. Teaching must focus on management of disease progression, medication management, positioning, mobility, assistive devices, and working to maintain a healthy lifestyle so that the patient will achieve a positive state of living. Future trends may reflect a larger percentage of patients going into remission as biologic medications for RA become more prevalent.

Arthritis Foundation. (2017). Rheumatoid arthritis. Retrieved from http://www.arthritis.org/about-arthritis/types/rheumatoid-arthritis/what-is-rheumatoid-arthritis.php

Pinto, S., & Schub, T. (2016). *Arthritis, rheumatoid arthritis (evidence-based care sheet)*. Glendale: CA: CINAHL Information Systems, a division of EBSCO Information Services.

Schub, T., & Holle, M. N. (2016). *Arthritis, rheumatoid: Complications (quick lesson)*. Glendale, CA: CINAHL Information Systems, a division of EBSCO Information Services.

Schub, T., & Uribe, L. M. (2016). *Arthritis: Rheumatoid: Drug therapy (quick lesson)*. Glendale, CA: CINAHL Information Systems, a division of EBSCO Information Services.

Singh, J. A., Saag, K. G., Bridges, L. S., Akl, E. A., Bannuru, R. R., Sullivan, M. C., . . . McAlindon, T. (2016). Arthritis and rheumatology: 2015 American College of Rheumatology guideline for the treatment of rheumatoid arthritis. *Arthritis & Rheumatology*, 68(1), 1–26. doi:10.1002/art.39480

■ SEPSIS

Sharon Stahl Wexler
Catherine O'Neill D'Amico

Overview

Sepsis is defined as the presence of infection in conjunction with a systemic inflammatory response. The response of the body to infection leads to life-threatening organ dysfunction. Septic shock is defined as sepsis that results in tissue hypoperfusion, hypotension requiring vasopressors, and elevated lactate levels (Howell & Davis, 2017). It is difficult to provide incidence or prevalence data for sepsis as there is no confirmatory diagnostic test for sepsis; diagnosis is based on the evidence of infection and the clinical judgment of the provider (Epstein, Dante, Magill, & Fiore 2016). Sepsis is common and is a leading cause of death, contributing to one third to one half of deaths in hospitalized patients. Patients who develop sepsis have an increased risk of complications and death and face higher health care costs and longer treatment.

Background

Older adults have increased susceptibility to sepsis. This increased susceptibility is due to the many normal age-related changes as well as increased number of comorbid conditions present in many older adults (Umberger, Callen, & Brown, 2015). It is estimated that up to 65% of patients who develop severe sepsis in the United States are older than 65 years (Umberger et al., 2015). Recent years have seen the development of sepsis "bundles" to deal with this serious issue. Major recommendations in these bundles include a focus on identifying infection, managing infection, fluid resuscitation, the use of vasopressors in patients with septic shock, and mechanical ventilation as indicated (Howell & Davis, 2017).

Clinical Aspects

Sepsis is defined as the presence of infection together with systemic manifestations of infection. Sepsis is frequently associated with other conditions such as pneumonia, intestinal obstruction, gallbladder disease, pyelonephritis, or peritonitis. Sepsis is an important complication of major trauma, burns, cancer, and major surgical procedures. Urosepsis is common in older adults. General signs and symptoms of sepsis include fever (often with shaking chills), increased respiratory rate, impaired mental status, and either warm or cold skin.

ASSESSMENT

Diagnostic criteria for sepsis include a documented or suspected infection and some of the following general manifestations, which include alterations in body temperature (fever or hypothermia), increased heart rate, increased respiratory rate, altered mental status, a positive fluid balance, or significant edema and hyperglycemia in the absence of diabetes. Inflammatory manifestations may include leukocytosis, leukopenia, elevated plasma C-reactive protein, elevated plasma procalcitonin, or a normal white blood cell count with more than 10% immature forms. Hemodynamic manifestations include arterial hypotension. Organ dysfunction variables may include arterial hypoxemia, acute oliguria, increased creatinine, coagulation abnormalities, thrombocytopenia, hyperbilirubinemia, or absent bowel sounds.

Diagnostic testing for sepsis includes a variety of laboratory studies, including a complete blood count (CBC), blood cultures, and urine cultures. The specific laboratory study recommended depends on the suspected cause of sepsis, for example, a central line infection would include a culture of the catheter tip. A CBC may show an elevated or low white blood cell count, anemia, or thrombocytopenia. Imaging studies that may be helpful in the diagnosis of sepsis also depend on the suspected cause. A chest x-ray is indicated to rule out pneumonia and other pulmonary causes. An abdominal ultrasound is useful when there is a suspected biliary tract obstruction. An abdominal CT or MRI may be useful in assessing other intra-abdominal sources of infection.

Hospitalized patients and individuals presenting in a local emergency room may or may not have the "usual signs of infection," including elevated body temperature; skin lesions; inflammatory signs and symptoms affecting the gastrointestinal, respiratory, or urinary tract. Some individuals, particularly older adults, may present with nonspecific and nonlocalized symptoms, including complaints of not feeling well, no elevation of body temperature, or family members who indicate that the individual is experiencing changes in usual behavior or complaints of inability to do usual tasks (Englert & Ross, 2015; Quan et al., 2013; Umberger et al., 2015). A thorough history followed by head-to-toe assessment of these individuals and individuals who present with the usual signs of infections and inflammation should be initiated by the nurse (Agency for Healthcare Research and Quality [AHRQ], 2013; Umberger et al., 2015).

NURSING INTERVENTIONS, MANAGEMENT, AND IMPLICATIONS

Individuals with other identified comorbidities are at greater risk for having sepsis (Englert & Ross, 2015; Novosad et al., 2016; Quan et al., 2013; Umberger et al., 2015). These comorbidities, which increase the risk for sepsis, include age greater than 75 years, immunosuppression (cancer and cancer treatments, treatment with corticosteroids), recent invasive procedure or surgery, diabetes, cardiovascular diseases, chronic kidney disease, and chronic obstructive pulmonary disease, indwelling urinary catheters, or intravenous access (Novosad et al., 2016; Quan et al., 2013; Umberger et al., 2015).

Initial management of sepsis typically includes transfer to a hospital setting if the patient is not in an acute care setting. Within the acute care setting, transfer to an intensive care setting for close monitoring and treatment is usually indicated. Swan–Ganz catheterization is frequently used to help manage fluid status. Supportive therapy to maintain organ perfusion and respiration is initiated based on individual patient presentation. Empiric antibiotic therapy is initiated followed by antibiotic therapy that is specific to the infecting organism presumed to be the source of the sepsis. Appropriate antibiotics to treat sepsis are usually combinations of two or three antibiotics given at the same time. Surgery may be indicated to drain or remove the source of infection.

The interdisciplinary team initiates the following laboratory tests: blood gases, including glucose and lactate measurement, blood culture, CBC, C-reactive protein, blood urea nitrogen (BUN) and electrolytes, creatinine, and clotting screening. Central intravenous access is initiated in addition to any peripheral access that was initiated during the assessment. Based on the AHRQ (Quan et al., 2013) criteria, acute care facilities begin intravenous fluid bolus and broad spectrum antibiotics are initiated within 1 hour after the lactate and blood cultures are obtained. Intravenous fluids are given as a bolus of 500 mL within 15 minutes. The broad spectrum antibiotics recommended are typically those in the penicillin, sulfonamides, glycopeptide, and aminoglycoside classes. Antibiotics are to be initiated immediately after the blood cultures are obtained and within 1 hour of meeting the criteria that sepsis is likely. Usually two medications are prescribed in combination based on the assessment and the likely source of the initial infection.

The individual with sepsis or septic shock is moved to the intensive care unit (ICU) where additional measures to support hypovolemia, ventilation and oxygenation, and urinary output are initiated and level of consciousness is monitored closely. Life-support measures include the administration of fluids and vasopressors, anticoagulation, mechanical ventilation, and oxygen supplementation. Changes in the antibiotic regimen and monitoring the effectiveness of the treatment should be continuously evaluated. As the individual responds to the antibiotics and vasopressor use is diminished, the individual can be moved out of the critical care environment.

OUTCOMES

Sepsis in the adult and older adult is a medical emergency requiring quick and effective action by the interdisciplinary team. Early recognition of sepsis may be the best hope for a positive outcome (Howell & Davis, 2017). Multiple authors cite early recognition and initiation of treatment as the factor that decreases the odds that the patient will die from sepsis (DeBacker & Dorman, 2017; Howell & Davis, 2017; Stoller et al., 2016). It has been noted recently that sepsis accounts for more hospital readmissions than any of the four conditions currently tracked by the federal government for guiding reimbursement and quality care, and remains one of the leading causes of death for hospitalized patients (DeBacker & Dorman, 2017; Mayr et al., 2017). Studies identify that despite new treatments and early-recognition practices, 20% to 45% of those diagnosed do not survive (Novosad et al., 2016; Stoller et al., 2016). The recognition of this problem has led to the development of interdisciplinary best practices for

the early identification and treatment of sepsis of the hospitalized adult and older adult.

The prognosis of a patient with sepsis is related to the severity of the sepsis, the underlying condition of the patient, and the stage at which the sepsis is diagnosed. Patients with sepsis and no signs of organ failure at the time of diagnosis have about a 15% to 30% chance of death. Elderly patients have the highest death rates (DeBacker & Dorman, 2017).

Because the sepsis morbidity and mortality rate is high, nurses and the interdisciplinary staff must keep families informed about the potential outcomes for the individual. The nurse and the interdisciplinary team need to be aware of the advanced directives that are in place before and during aggressive resuscitation as well as the potential for progressive organ failure. Planning for the end of life or palliative care should be considered if the individual or the family want to limit resuscitation measures (Englert & Ross, 2015; Quan et al., 2013; Umberger et al., 2015). Discharge instructions by the nurse to the individual and family should include instructions about symptoms to monitor, how to seek medical attention if these symptoms occur, including how to get urgent medical attention (Quan et al., 2013). The nurse should provide the individual and the family time to ask questions and address concerns, including whether this will happen again, how to prevent it from happening again, and details of arrangements made for the care of any residual treatments (tracheostomy care, peripherally inserted central catheter [PICC] line care; Quan et al., 2013).

Summary

Sepsis is a medical emergency with significant morbidity and mortality. It is a leading cause of hospitalization and mortality for patients of all ages. Older adults are of particular risk due to the many normal age-related changes and possible multiple comorbidities, making diagnosis a challenge. The role of the nurse in caring for patients with sepsis begins with infection prevention and progresses to recognition of the signs and symptoms of sepsis and the early initiation of fluids, vasopressors, and antibiotics for the treatment of sepsis. Current treatment of sepsis includes the use of bundles to simplify the complex processes of care of the patient with sepsis.

DeBacker, D., & Dorman, T. (2017). Surviving sepsis guidelines: A continuous move toward better care of patients with sepsis. *Journal of the American Medical Association.* Advance online publication. doi:10.1001/

jama.2017.0059. Retrieved from http://jamanetwork.com/pdfaccess.ashx?url=/data/journals/jama/0

Englert, N. C., & Ross, C. (2015). The older adult experiencing sepsis. *Critical Care Nursing Quarterly, 38*(2), 175–181.

Epstein, L., Dantes, R., Magill, S., & Fiore, A. (2016). Varying estimates of sepsis mortality using death certificates and administrative codes—United States, 1999–2014. *Morbidity and Mortality Weekly Report, 65*(13), 342–345.

Howell, M. D., & Davis, A. M. (2017). Management of sepsis and septic shock. *Journal of the American Medical Association, 317*(8), 847–848.

Mayr, F. B., Talisa, V. B., Balakumar, V., Chang, C. H., Fine, M., & Yende, S. (2017). Proportion and cost of unplanned 30-day readmissions after sepsis compared with other medical conditions. *Journal of the American Medical Association, 317*(5), 530–531.

Novosad, S. A., Sapiano, M. R., Grigg, C., Lake, J., Robyn, M., Dumyati, G., . . . Epstein, L. (2016). Vital signs: Epidemiology of sepsis: Prevalence of health care factors and opportunities for prevention. *Morbidity and Mortality Weekly Report, 65*(33), 864–869.

Quan, H., Eastwood, C., Cunningham, C. T., Liu, M., Flemons, W., De Coster, C., & Ghali, W. A.; IMECCHI investigators. (2013). Validity of AHRQ patient safety indicators derived from ICD-10 hospital discharge abstract data (chart review study). *BMJ Open, 3*(10), e003716.

Stoller, J., Halpin, L., Weis, M., Aplin, B., Qu, W., Georgescu, C., & Nazzal, M. (2016). Epidemiology of severe sepsis: 2008-2012. *Journal of Critical Care, 31*, 58–62.

Umberger, R., Callen, B., & Brown, M. L. (2015). Severe sepsis in older adults. *Critical Care Nursing Quarterly, 38*(3), 259–270.

■ SICKLE CELL DISEASE

Consuela A. Albright

Overview

Sickle cell disease is a heritable, chronic disorder of the blood. Abnormalities in the composition of hemoglobin give red blood cells a sickle shape and affect the viscosity, life span, and oxygen-carrying capacity of the cell. Sickle cell disease affects multiple organs, including the brain, heart, eyes, lungs, kidneys, liver, and spleen. Acute symptoms may lead to organ damage, organ failure, and death. Care for persons with acute exacerbation of sickle cell disease should focus on reversal of symptoms through replacement of red blood cells, hydration, oxygenation, pain management, and early recognition and treatment of underlying causes to prevent secondary complications (Yawn et al., 2014).

Background

The National Heart, Lung, and Blood Institute (NHLBI) reports that sickle cell disease affects individuals of African, Hispanic, Southern European, Middle Eastern, and Asian Indian descent (NHLBI, 2016). The Centers for Disease Control and Prevention (CDC) estimate that approximately 100,000 Americans are currently affected by sickle cell disease (CDC, 2016). Sickle cell disease is caused by an autosomal recessive inheritance; a child born with sickle cell disease receives two copies of the recessive gene, one from each parent. One of every 365 African American children born in the United States has sickle cell disease, and one of every 16,300 Hispanic American children born in the United States has sickle cell disease (CDC, 2016).

All children born in the United States are tested for sickle cell disease and sickle cell trait with newborn screening. One in 13 African American babies is born with one copy of the sickle cell gene, known as sickle cell trait. Carriers of sickle cell trait do not exhibit any symptoms of sickle cell disease (CDC, 2016). Individuals with sickle cell trait have a 50% chance of passing the trait to their children, and two carriers of sickle cell trait have a 25% chance of conceiving a child with sickle cell disease (CDC, 2016).

Sickle cell disease is the result of a point mutation of the amino acids at the sixth position of the beta chain of the hemoglobin molecule. Normal adult hemoglobin (HbA) contains glutamic acid at the sixth position of the beta chain, whereas sickle hemoglobin (HbS) has valine at its sixth position. HbS makes red blood cells sickle shaped, rigid, and sticky (Yosmanovich, Rotter, Aprelev, & Ferrone, 2016). HbS is sensitive to dehydration, hypoxia, infectious processes, and temperature changes; these stressors trigger clumping of red blood cells in the vascular space, known as sickle cell crisis.

The long-term effects of sickle cell disease are the result of vaso-occlusion in sickle cell crises. Damage to the neurologic, cardiovascular, respiratory, renal, musculoskeletal, hepatic, and genitourinary systems causes complications secondary to sickle cell disease. Chronic pain is another secondary complication of sickle cell disease. The prognosis for an individual with sickle cell disease is dependent on the type and severity of sickle cell disease. Patients with HbSS and HbS/β^0 thalassemia experience marked severity of disease than do patients with HbSC, HbS, and HbS/β^+ thalassemia. Rarer forms of sickle cell disease are HbSD, HbSE, and HbSO, and each varies in severity (CDC, 2015). The mean age of mortality for sickle cell patients by disease type is HbSS

(35.19 years), HbSC (44.47 years), HbS/β⁰ thalassemia (41 years), and HbS/β⁺ thalassemia (30.5 years; Ngo et al., 2014).

Sickle cell disease presents once levels of fetal hemoglobin (HbF) fall and HbS levels rise between 6 and 12 months (Bender & Douthitt Seibel, 2014). HbF has a high affinity for oxygen and inhibits sickling of blood cells. The life span of a sickled blood cell is 10 to 20 days, compared to healthy red blood cells' life span of 100 to 120 days, causing a decrease in the number of circulating mature red blood cells, resulting in an anemic state (NHLBI, 2014). Adult and pediatric patients may present with yellowing of the sclera (icterus), a sign of jaundice. Jaundice is caused by rapid lysis of red blood cells, buildup of excess bilirubin in tissues, and inability of the liver to process bilirubin at the same rate of cell lysis (Bender & Douthitt Seibel, 2014).

Clinical Aspects

ASSESSMENT

History and physical assessment are key to treating a patient in sickle cell crisis. A detailed medical history, including the type of sickle cell disease, should be taken. The history must also include information about the onset, duration, and location of symptoms, and baseline vital signs, paying close attention to pulse oximetry. Ongoing, thorough physical assessment and vital sign monitoring will alert a nurse in the acute care setting to changes from baseline in the patient's condition.

Sickle cell crises vary in presentation, but pain is a hallmark finding. Pain may be localized to the head, face, bones, abdomen, back, or chest with a sudden, severe onset. Vaso-occlusion in the brain is a risk for stroke in children and adults with sickle cell. Strokes in children with sickle cell are responsible for long-term cognitive deficits. The initial presentation of sickle cell crisis in a young child could present as painful swelling of the hands and feet (dactylitis). Adults may report hand and foot pain, as well as pain in the long bones of the upper and lower extremities. Male patients may experience priapism, a penile erection caused by vaso-occlusion. Abdominal pain in a patient with sickle cell crisis should be evaluated to rule out splenic sequestration, a life-threatening complication in which sickled red blood cells become trapped in the spleen, causing a drop in the volume of circulating red blood cells, leading to hypovolemic shock. Splenic sequestration may require surgical removal of the spleen (Bender & Douthitt Seibel, 2014).

Acute chest syndrome is a complication of sickle cell disease affecting adults and children alike. A vaso-occlusive crisis decreases perfusion of the lungs and leads to respiratory failure and death. Acute chest syndrome is triggered by infection, pneumonia, respiratory disease, emboli, or any other stressor that initiates hypoxemia and sickling. Clinically, acute chest syndrome is defined as new pulmonary infiltrate on chest x-ray, accompanied by fever, hypoxemia, tachypnea, wheezing, or cough (Bender & Douthitt Seibel, 2014).

A nurse should anticipate diagnostic testing and laboratory workup for appropriate treatment of symptoms. Diagnostic testing will include chest x-ray, CT scan, complete blood count with differential, electrolytes, renal function panel (blood urea nitrogen [BUN]/creatinine), urinalysis, hepatic function (alanine transaminase [ALT], bilirubin), blood culture, and arterial blood gases.

OUTCOMES

The goal of treatment for sickle cell crisis is immediate reversal of symptoms and treatment of the underlying cause (Lentz & Kautz, 2017). The amount of sickled blood cells may require exchange transfusion, in which the recipient's blood is phlebotomized and replaced in equal volumes with donor blood to reduce the amount of sickled blood in circulation. Intravenous fluid resuscitation reverses dehydration. The nurse should be prepared to administer analgesics, supplemental oxygen, and pharmacologic treatment of the underlying cause to prevent deterioration of the patient's condition. Initiation of treatment with hydroxyurea may also occur in the acute care setting. Hydroxyurea increases the levels of HbF, which increases the amount of normal red blood cells in circulation (Yawn et al., 2014).

Summary

Sickle cell disease is a lifelong condition of varying severity. Patients with sickle cell disease may have frequent admissions to the acute care setting for exacerbation of symptoms. Pain in the patient with sickle cell anemia is poorly understood in the acute care setting, as it is chronic and patient responses to pain vary significantly among individuals. Nurses in the acute care setting should be reminded that pain is a very real symptom of sickle cell crisis that should be assessed frequently and treated as needed. Aggressive treatment of sickle cell crisis and underlying causes of symptoms is necessary to prevent life-threatening complications of the disease.

Bender, M. A., & Douthitt Seibel, G. (2014). Sickle cell disease. Retrieved from https://www.ncbi.nlm.nih.gov/books/NBK1377

Centers for Disease Control and Prevention. (2015). Sickle cell trait. Retrieved from https://www.cdc.gov/ncbddd/sicklecell/traits.html

Centers for Disease Control and Prevention. (2016). Data & statistics. Retrieved from https://www.cdc.gov/ncbddd/sicklecell/data.html

Lentz, M. B., & Kautz, D. D. (2017). Acute vaso-occlusive crisis in patients with sickle cell disease. *Nursing, 47*(1), 67–68.

National Heart, Lung and Blood Institute. (2014). Sickle cell anemia. Retrieved from https://www.ncbi.nlm.nih.gov/pubmedhealth/PM

National Heart, Lung, and Blood Institute. (2016). Who is at risk for sickle cell disease? Retrieved from https://www.nhlbi.nih.gov/health/health-topics/topics/sca/atrisk

Ngo, S., Bartolucci, P., Lobo, D., Mekontso-Dessap, A., Gellen-Dautremer, J., Noizat-Pirenne, F., . . . Habibi, A. (2014). Causes of death in sickle cell disease adult patients: Old and new trends. *Blood, 124*(21), 2715. Retrieved from http://www.bloodjournal.org/content/124/21/2715

Yawn, B. P., Buchanan, G. R., Afenyi-Annan, A. N., Ballas, S. K., Hassell, K. L., James, A. H., . . . Tanabe, P. J. (2014). Management of sickle cell disease: Summary of the 2014 evidence-based report by expert panel members. *Journal of the American Medical Association, 312*(10), 1033–1048.

Yosmanovich, D., Rotter, M., Aprelev, A., & Ferrone, F. A. (2016). Calibrating sickle cell disease. *Journal of Molecular Biology, 428*(8), 1506–1514. doi:10.1016/j.jmb.2016.03.001

■ SLEEP APNEA

Deborah H. Cantero
Leslie J. Lockett
Rebecca M. Lutz

Overview

Sleep apnea (SA) results in daily functional impairment and increases the patient's risk of multisystem health disorders. SA is characterized by repetitive apneic cycles that result in disrupted sleep. Categories of SA include obstructive sleep apnea (OSA) and central sleep apnea (CSA). Management of SA requires a long-term, multidisciplinary approach aimed at decreasing apneic episodes, thereby improving long-term health outcomes.

Background

SA is a chronic condition resulting in repeated cycles of apnea or intermittent episodes of decreased inspiratory effort (hypopnea). An apneic or hypopneic episode typically lasts a minimum of 10 seconds (Kasper et al., 2016). With each apneic or hypopneic episode, the oxygen saturation level decreases. With apneic episodes, increasing the partial pressure of carbon dioxide in the circulatory system, an individual is prone to recurrent cycles of arousal, and even awakenings, while sleeping (Semelka, Wilson, & Floyd, 2016; Zinchuk & Thomas, 2017).

The most common form of SA is OSA. In OSA, there is thoracic and diaphragmatic respiratory effort; however, the airway is partially or completely obstructed. Airway obstruction in the upper airway is due to pharyngeal muscle relaxation with collapse (Chesnutt & Prendergast, 2017). In contrast, CSA is associated with decreased or ineffective respiratory drive as a result of impaired stimulation from central nervous system injury or medications (Zinchuk & Thomas, 2017).

SA occurs across the life span. OSA is diagnosed in approximately 4% of the population, although research estimates that up to 24% of the population is undiagnosed (DiNapoli, 2014). Of all the sleep-related breathing disorders, approximately 10% are CSA in origin (Zinchuk & Thomas, 2017). Risk factors include obesity, family history of SA, age 40 to 70 years, male gender, being postmenopausal, endocrine-associated conditions, certain anatomical features, central nervous system disorders, and opioid use (Kasper et al., 2016; Semelka et al., 2016). Untreated SA increases the risk of cardiac complications due to effects on the sympathetic nervous system (Kasper et al., 2016). This impacts quality of life as patients often exhibit excessive daytime sleepiness, potential changes in mood or cognition, and increased risk for occupational injury (DiNapoli, 2014).

Clinical Aspects

ASSESSMENT

Nursing assessment begins with a thorough health history to identify key aspects to guide nursing interventions. History includes investigation of regular snoring, apneic gasps, and daytime drowsiness as well as apnea reported by a sleeping partner (Avidan & Kryger, 2017). Additional assessment would include use of opiates, morning headache, excessive sleepiness, sleep duration, decreased concentration, poor memory, and motor vehicle accidents related to sleepiness.

Safety considerations regarding anesthesia and post-operative recovery should also be evaluated (Avidan & Kryger, 2017). Modifiable contributing risk factors, such as obesity, smoking, and alcohol intake, should be noted. All findings should be recorded for other providers.

Objective assessment includes the observance of physical characteristics, including excessive weight, short thick neck, and any evidence of upper airway narrowing such as tonsillar hypertrophy. Secondary conditions to assess include associated hypertension (HTN), congestive heart failure (CHF), arrhythmias, myocardial infarction, and cor pulmonale (Obstructive Sleep Apnea Task Force of the American Academy of Sleep Medicine, 2009). A thorough head-to-toe assessment is necessary to inform the nurse in developing a care plan, promoting optimal health for the patient, and preventing complications.

The clinical characteristics of OSA and CSA may overlap, and definitive diagnosis is made with a poly-somnography (PSG) sleep study (Obstructive Sleep Apnea Task Force of the American Academy of Sleep Medicine, 2009; Zinchuk & Thomas, 2017). The PSG study and the apnea–hypopnea index (AHI) allow the provider to distinguish between OSA and CSA (Zinchuk & Thomas, 2017). Medicare guidelines for the initiation of therapy for continuous positive airway pressure (CPAP) parameters include: (a) AHI greater than 15, eligible for CPAP and (b) AHI of 5 to 14, eligible if excessive sleepiness, HTN, or cardiovascular disease is documented (Downey, 2017).

Once treatment is initiated, nurses should continually assess and monitor for evidence of hypoxia or hypoxemia. In addition, nurses should focus on interventions regarding assessment, education, and interdisciplinary referrals. This is particularly important because compliance is a documented issue within this population. Therefore, education is critical for the patient's understanding of the increased risk for complications associated with SA (DiNapoli, 2014). Adherence, comfort, knowledge of therapy, and readiness to learn should also be assessed.

Using principles of adult learning and patient-centered care, nurses should convey the pathophysiology, risk factors, natural history, and clinical consequences of SA to both the patient and the caregiver (DiNapoli, 2014). This encourages engagement in the treatment plan. Including the caregiver is also important due to the potential for neurocognitive and physiological consequences of hypoxia, which may limit the patient's full understanding of SA and therefore limit compliance with therapy (DiNapoli, 2014; Obstructive Sleep Apnea Task Force of the American Academy of Sleep Medicine, 2009). On initiation of therapy, and with all subsequent reevaluations, education on CPAP device usage and cleaning procedures, sleep position, and good sleep hygiene is essential (Downey, 2017; Obstructive Sleep Apnea Task Force of the American Academy of Sleep Medicine, 2009). Risk reduction education on the impact of weight loss, sleep positions, alcohol avoidance, and risks of driving while drowsy should be included to promote self-care with this chronic condition (Obstructive Sleep Apnea Task Force of the American Academy of Sleep Medicine, 2009).

OUTCOMES

Interdisciplinary referrals for care collaboration, including respiratory therapy, sleep specialists, and group behavioral therapy, have demonstrated increased compliance (DiNapoli, 2014). Prompt attention to adverse effects of CPAP (nasal stuffiness, dry eyes, skin irritation, and claustrophobia) and adjustments in the treatment plan promote compliance (DiNapoli, 2014; Downey, 2017). Finally, follow-up with the provider to evaluate effectiveness within 2 months is recommended (Downey, 2017). The major outcomes of the interventions include patient report of resolution of sleepiness, patient/spouse satisfaction, adherence to therapy, and improvement in quality of life (Freedman, 2017; Obstructive Sleep Apnea Task Force of the American Academy of Sleep Medicine, 2009).

Summary

SA, whether obstructive or central, disrupts sleep patterns and may result in increased morbidity and mortality. Causes of SA are variable, therefore medical and nursing interventions must also be customized for each patient. Nursing care begins with a thorough assessment of the physical, social, and psychological impact SA has on the patient's quality of life. Nursing interventions include an emphasis on patient and caregiver education aimed at improving understanding and compliance. The primary goal of care is to decrease the frequency of apneic episodes, improve quality of life, and ultimately decrease multiorgan impairment or death.

Avidan, E. Y., & Kryger, M. (2017). Physical examination in sleep medicine. In M. H. Kryger & T. Roth (Eds.), *Principles and practice of sleep medicine* (6th ed., pp. 587–606). Philadelphia, PA: Elsevier. Retrieved from http://www.sciencedirect.com.ezproxy.lib.usf.edu/science/article/pii/B9780323242882000593

Chesnutt, M. S., & Prendergast, T. J. (2017). Pulmonary disorders. In M. A. Papadakis, S. J. McPhee, & M. W. Rabow (Eds.), *Current medical diagnosis & treatment 2017* (56th ed). New York, NY: McGraw-Hill. Retrieved from http://accessmedicine.mhmedical.com.ezproxy.hsc.usf.edu/content.aspx?bookid=1843&sectionid=135704883

DiNapoli, C. M. (2014). Strategies to improve continuous positive airway pressure: A review. *Journal of Nursing Education and Practice, 5*(2), 110–116. doi:10.5430/jnep.v5n2p110

Downey, R. (2017). Obstructive sleep apnea. *Medscape.* Retrieved from http://emedicine.medscape.com/article/295807-overview

Freedman, N. (2017). Positive airway pressure treatment for obstructive sleep apnea. In M. H. Kryger & T. Roth (Eds.), *Principles and practice of sleep medicine* (6th ed., pp. 1125–1137). Philadelphia, PA: Elsevier. Retrieved from http://www.sciencedirect.com.ezproxy.lib.usf.edu/science/article/pii/B978032324288200115X

Kasper, D. L., Fauci, A. S., Hauser, S. L., Longo, D. L., Jameson, J., & Loscalzo, J. (2016). Sleep apnea. In D. L. Kasper, A. S. Fauci, S. L. Hauser, D. L. Longo, J. Jameson, & J. Loscalzo (Eds.), *Harrison's manual of medicine* (19th ed., pp. 745–746). New York, NY: McGraw-Hill. Retrieved from http://accessmedicine.mhmedical.com/Book.aspx?bookid=1820

Obstructive Sleep Apnea Task Force of the American Academy of Sleep Medicine. (2009). Clinical guideline for the evaluation, management and long-term care of obstructive sleep apnea in adults. *Journal of Clinical Sleep Medicine, 5*(3), 263–276. Retrieved https://www.ncbi.nlm.nih.gov/pmc/articles/PMC2699173

Semelka, M., Wilson, J., & Floyd, R. (2016). Diagnosis and treatment of obstructive sleep apnea in adults. *American Family Physician, 94*(5), 355–360. Retrieved from http://www.aafp.org/afp/2016/0901/p355.html

Zinchuk, A. V., & Thomas, R. J. (2017). Central sleep apnea: Diagnosis and management. In M. H. Kryger & T. Roth (Eds.), *Principles and practice of sleep medicine* (6th ed., pp. 1059–1074). Philadelphia, PA: Elsevier. Retrieved from http://www.sciencedirect.com.ezproxy.lib.usf.edu/science/article/pii/B9780323242882001100

■ SPINAL STENOSIS AND DISC HERNIATION

Steven R. Collier

Overview

Spinal stenosis and disc herniation are common findings in the general population. Spinal stenosis has been defined in many studies as having a spinal canal dimension of 10 mm or less in the anterior–posterior plane of measurement, and the symptoms of pain, paresthesias, and dysesthesias in the legs. Although these patients may have spinal stenosis diagnosed by imaging, they are not always symptomatic (Kalichman et al., 2009). Disc herniation is defined as a focal projection of disc material into the spinal canal or neural foramina greater than 3 mm and may be situated posteriorly, cephalad, caudally, or can form a free-floating disc fragment (Fardon et al., 2014). Nursing care for these patients focuses on rehabilitation, mobilization, identification of surgical emergencies, and perioperative care for patients treated with surgical intervention.

Background

Neck pain and low-back pain are common medical conditions in the United States and around the world. The global prevalence of neck pain is 4.9% and is 6.5% in the United States (March et al., 2014). Low-back pain has a global prevalence rate of 9.4% and 7.7% in the United States (March et al., 2014). Neck pain tends to occur at a younger age with a mean age of 45 years, and is more common in females, whereas back pain peaks later in life with a mean age of 80 years and is seen more frequently in males (March et al., 2014). Spinal stenosis and disc herniation are leading causes of neck pain and low-back pain.

Lumbar spinal stenosis occurs most often in patients who are 65 years or older and occurs slightly more often in men than in women (Weinstein et al., 2008). The findings for cervical stenosis are similar, with the incidence increasing with advancing age, and occurring slightly more often in men than in women (Nagata et al., 2012). Risk factors include being overweight, having elevated body mass index (BMI), occupations involving manual labor, and for men, diabetes (Abbas et al., 2013). Smoking was not linked to an increased risk of spinal stenosis (Abbas et al., 2013). Spinal stenosis can be caused by degenerative disc disease (DDD), spondylosis, spondylolisthesis, hypertrophy of the ligamentum flavum, tumors, cysts, infection, and congenital narrowing of the spinal canal. Lumbar stenosis can occur at any level in the lumbar spine, but occurs more frequently at L4–L5, then L3–L4 centrally; neural foraminal stenosis occurs most frequently at L5–S1, followed by L4–L5 (Ishimoto et al., 2013). Cervical stenosis is noted most frequently at C5–C6, followed by C4–C5, then C6–C7 (Nagata et al., 2012).

The diagnosis of cervical spinal stenosis is made by a combination of MRI/CT findings of decreased spinal canal diameter and physical exam findings of arm and possibly leg paresthesias and dysesthesias, hyperreflexia, Hoffman's sign, up-going Babinski reflex, discoordination, and possibly gait instability (Nagata et al., 2012). Diagnosis of lumbar spinal stenosis is made by a combination of MRI/CT findings of decreased spinal canal diameter and physical exam findings of leg paresthesias and dysesthesias that can occur at rest, but are exacerbated with ambulation or standing and spinal extension, and usually improve with rest or spinal flexion (Kreiner et al., 2013).

The incidence and prevalence of cervical disc herniation is difficult to define because approximately 10% of herniations found on imaging in persons younger than 40 years and 5% in persons more than 40 years are asymptomatic (Hammer, Heller, & Kepler, 2015). Cervical disc herniation may be caused by trauma or jobs that require heavy lifting or repeated stress to the spine (Hammer et al., 2015).

The mean age for diagnosis of lumbar disc herniation is 41 years and is slightly more prevalent in males than in females (Schroeder, Guyre, & Vaccaro, 2015). Risk factors include obesity, heavy lifting with twisting and bending, and family history of herniated disc (Schroeder et al., 2015). Patients with increased stress and time-sensitive jobs also appear to be at higher risk for lumbar disc herniation (Schroeder et al., 2015). The symptoms for cervical and lumbar disc herniation are largely the same as listed previously for stenosis, but can occur more acutely when the result of trauma.

Spinal disorders are a major source of health care spending. Patients with spine problems are more likely to limit their social interactions, have decreased physical functioning, and miss school or work than persons without spine disease.

Clinical Aspects

ASSESSMENT

Nursing management of patients with spinal stenosis and disc herniation is heavily reliant on an accurate physical assessment with a focus on the neurological exam. The history should focus on the temporal aspect of the onset of the pain or the decrease in neurological function. An accurate history of the patient's current and past medical problems, along with any interventional or surgical procedures should be recorded. Medication lists should be obtained and accurately verified for any history of spinal injections or use of immunosuppressants within the last several months.

The physical exam consists of a head-to-toe assessment focusing on the neurological exam. Special attention is paid to any areas of spinal tenderness with palpation, any deformities of the spine, or abnormal posture. Strength testing of all major extremity muscle groups along with reflex testing and sensation testing are crucial to accurate diagnosis. Special reflex testing should include testing for the Hoffman and Babinski reflexes and for clonus. The gait should be observed for any alterations, inability to heel or toe walk, and inability to walk heel to toe in a straight line. Rectal tone should be assessed if the patient reports any bowel or bladder incontinence, or saddle area anesthesia.

Imaging for patients with spine pain that is consistent with stenosis or disc herniation is often appropriate for MRI, or if contraindicated, CT imaging of the spine (Kreiner et al., 2014). Plain film x-rays can be helpful in the examination of posture, or initial rapid imaging for fracture, or checking of previous spinal hardware. There are no specific laboratory tests for spinal stenosis or disc herniation, but an elevated white blood cell count and C-reactive protein (CRP) may indicate spinal infection, although these findings are nonspecific.

NURSING INTERVENTIONS, MANAGEMENT, AND IMPLICATIONS

The nursing care of patients with spinal stenosis or disc herniation focuses on promoting mobility and managing pain. Many patients need assistance with mobility, and even assistance with passive and active range of motion (PROM and AROM). If bracing is used as treatment or postoperatively, assuring proper fit and application along with checking of the skin under the brace is required.

Patients with cervical stenosis with myelopathy or cervical disc herniation with Brown–Sequard syndrome can have special needs ranging from total care to assistance with toileting, feeding, and hydration. Patients with lumbar stenosis or disc herniation may require assistance with ambulation and range of motion, as well as assistance with bladder catheterization and bowel regimens for neurogenic bowel and bladder dysfunction. Cauda equina is characterized by an acute onset of severe radicular leg pain, bowel and bladder dysfunction, and saddle area anesthesia. Cauda equina is a surgical emergency and prompt recognition of symptoms is crucial; the degree of patient recovery depends on rapid diagnosis and treatment. The opioid epidemic must be taken into account when managing patients with spinal disorders. Acute spine pain can be appropriately managed with opiate pain medication; however, there is no sufficient evidence to support the use of opiates for the chronic management of spinal pain management (Simon, Conliffe, & Kitei, 2015).

OUTCOMES

Rapid identification of neurological changes based on serial neurological examinations is critical in preserving function and limiting loss of function in the patient with a spinal disorder. Evidence-based nursing interventions are similarly focused on preservation and maximization of neurological function. Promotion of rehabilitation and therapy with the use of AROM and PROM, along with medication management, supports the achievement of optimal patient recovery, and limits permanent disabilities from occurring.

Summary

Most patients diagnosed with spinal stenosis or disc herniation can usually be managed conservatively and return to their baseline functional status. Spinal stenosis and disc herniation are prevalent in the adult population and are a leading cause of disability and decreased productivity. Early intervention and recognition of neurological decline in these patients is essential and evidence-based rehabilitation leads to optimal recovery.

Abbas, J., Hamoud, K., May, H., Peled, N., Sarig, R., Stein, D., . . . Hershkovitz, I. (2013). Socioeconomic and physical characteristics of individuals with degenerative lumbar spinal stenosis. *Spine, 38*(9), E554–E561. doi:10.1097/BRS.0b013e31828a2846

Fardon, D. F., Williams, A. L., Dohring, E. J., Murtagh, F. R., Gabriel Rothman, S. L., & Sze, G. K. (2014). Lumbar disc nomenclature: Version 2.0: Recommendations of the combined task forces of the North American Spine Society, the American Society of Spine Radiology and the American Society of Neuroradiology. *Spine Journal, 14*(11), 2525–2545. doi:10.1016/j.spinee.2014.04.022

Hammer, C., Heller, J., & Kepler, C. (2015). Epidemiology and pathophysiology of cervical disc herniation. *Seminars in Spine Surgery, 28*(2), 64–67. doi:10.1053/j.semss.2015.11.009

Ishimoto, Y., Yoshimura, N., Muraki, S., Yamada, H., Nagata, K., Hashizume, H., . . . Yoshida, M. (2013). Associations between radiographic lumbar spinal stenosis and clinical symptoms in the general population: The Wakayama Spine Study. *Osteoarthritis and Cartilage, 21*(6), 783–788. doi:10.1016/j.joca.2013.02.656

Kalichman, L., Cole, R., Kim, D. H., Li, L., Suri, P., Guermazi, A., & Hunter, D. J. (2009). Spinal stenosis prevalence and association with symptoms: The Framingham Study. *Spine Journal, 9*(7), 545–550. doi:10.1016/j.spinee.2009.03.005

Kreiner, D. S., Hwang, S. W., Easa, J. E., Resnick, D. K., Baisden, J. L., Bess, S., . . . Toton, J. F. (2014). An evidence-based clinical guideline for the diagnosis and treatment of lumbar disc herniation with radiculopathy. *Spine Journal, 14*(1), 180–191. doi:10.1016/j.spinee.2013.08.003

Kreiner, D. S., Shaffer, W. O., Baisden, J. L., Gilbert, T. J., Summers, J. T., Toton, J. F., . . . Reitman, C. A. (2013). An evidence-based clinical guideline for the diagnosis and treatment of degenerative lumbar spinal stenosis (update). *Spine Journal, 13*(7), 734–743. doi:10.1016/j.spinee.2012.11.059

March, L., Smith, E. U., Hoy, D. G., Cross, M. J., Sanchez-Riera, L., Blyth, F., . . . Woolf, A. D. (2014). Burden of disability due to musculoskeletal (MSK) disorders. *Best Practice & Research: Clinical Rheumatology, 28*(3), 353–366. doi:10.1016/j.berh.2014.08.002

Nagata, K., Yoshimura, N., Muraki, S., Hashizume, H., Ishimoto, Y., Yamada, H., . . . Yoshida, M. (2012). Prevalence of cervical cord compression and its association with physical performance in a population-based cohort in Japan: The Wakayama Spine Study. *Spine, 37*(22), 1892–1898. doi:10.1097/BRS.0b013e31825a2619

Schroeder, G. D., Guyre, C. A., & Vaccaro, A. R. The epidemiology and pathophysiology of lumbar disc herniations. *Seminars in Spine Surgery, 28*(1), 2–7. doi:10.1053/j.semss.2015.08.003

Simon, J., Conliffe, T., & Kitei, P. Non-operative management: An evidence-based approach. *Seminars in Spine Surgery, 28*(1), 8–13. doi:10.1053/j.semss.2015.08.004

Weinstein, J. N., Lurie, J. D., Tosteson, T. D., Tosteson, A. N., Blood, E. A., Abdu, W. A., . . . Fischgrund, J. (2008). Surgical versus nonoperative treatment for lumbar disc herniation: Four-year results for the Spine Patient Outcomes Research Trial (SPORT). *Spine, 33*(25), 2789–2800. doi:10.1097/BRS.0b013e31818ed8f4

■ SYNDROME OF INAPPROPRIATE ANTIDIURETIC HORMONE SECRETION

Carrie Foster

Overview

Syndrome of inappropriate antidiuretic hormone secretion (SIADH) was first discussed in 1957 in relation to patients with bronchogenic lung carcinoma (Schwartz,

Bennett, Curelop, & Bartter, 1957). The classic description still holds true today. Characteristics of SIADH include hypotonic hyponatremia and inappropriate release of antidiuretic hormone (ADH) causing excessive renal water reabsorption, resulting in inadequately diluted urine (Grant et al., 2015). The causes of SIADH are multiple and varied, but generally fit into three categories: malignant disease; pulmonary, central nervous system (CNS) and genetic disorders; or medication induced (Spasovski et al., 2014).

Background

SIADH is a biochemical syndrome of euvolemic hyponatremia resulting from inappropriate secretion of ADH independent of plasma osmolality (Cuesta & Thompson, 2016). SIADH has been reported in association with many disease processes and as a complication from medications. Increased incidence is noted with conditions such as intracranial processes, lung carcinoma, and other pulmonary illness (Spasovski et al., 2014). An estimated 15% of patients with small cell lung cancer experience SIADH (Cuesta & Thompson, 2016). Generally, it is likely that about 5% to 10% of hospital admissions may have a component of SIADH, with highest rates in neurosurgical units (Cuesta & Thompson, 2016). SIADH is the most common cause of hyponatremia in specific patient populations, including nursing home residents and oncology patients (Shepshelovich et al., 2015). Recent data indicate the most frequent causes of SIADH include malignancy and as a result of administered medication (Shepshelovich et al., 2015). Morbidity and mortality are typically driven by the causative factor, with worse outcomes in malignancy-induced versus idiopathic or medication-induced SIADH, as the pathophysiology between the two processes is different.

The pathophysiology behind SIADH can vary by cause. In general, the sodium concentration in the plasma is the primary osmotic determinant of arginine vasopressin (AVP) secretion. AVP is the naturally occurring form of ADH found in humans, and is stored in the posterior pituitary gland. Baroreceptors and osmoreceptors detect changes in circulating volume depletion and hyperosmolality, and, as plasma osmolality rises, AVP secretion is stimulated. AVP is released from the posterior pituitary and binds to cell membranes of target tissues, causing an increase in water reabsorption and an increase in urine osmolality. Typically, AVP secretion stops when the plasma osmolality drops below 275 mOsm/kg. This

decrease in AVP causes increased water excretion, creating dilute urine. Malignancy-associated SIADH is usually the result of an ectopic secretion of AVP (Cuesta & Thompson, 2016). Tumors may cause SIADH by creating physical interference with the osmoregulatory pathways. The mechanism of action behind medication-induced SIADH is incredibly variable, but is commonly seen with cytotoxic agents (Cuesta & Thompson, 2016).

The most serious complications from SIADH primarily arise from too rapid correction of hyponatremia or rapid initial development. When osmolality changes faster than 10 mOsm/kg per hour, patients are at increased risk for cerebral herniation, central pontine myelinolysis, and severe neurological impairment (Grant et al., 2015). Risk factors for increased morbidity and mortality rates include being hospitalized, rapid onset of hyponatremia, and severity of hyponatremia (Mocan, Terhes, & Blaga, 2016). Hyponatremia can result in gait instability and neurological impairment, placing elderly patients at higher risk for falls (Mocan et al., 2016). Multifactorial SIADH is associated with increased mortality, with the etiology as the key prognostic indicator.

Clinical Aspects

ASSESSMENT

The primary presentation of a patient experiencing SIADH is usually related to hyponatremia, with two factors influencing presentation: degree of hyponatremia and rate of development (Mocan et al., 2016). Serum sodium less than 135 mmol/L is considered hyponatremia (Spasovski et al., 2014). Patients will have plasma serum osmolality less than 275 mOsm/kg as well as urine sodium concentration greater than 30 mmol/L with normal dietary salt and water intake (Grant et al., 2015). Depending on the rate of development and biochemical degree of hyponatremia, patients may be asymptomatic. Patients may have symptoms that correlate to increased ADH secretion, including increased thirst, chronic pain, symptoms associated with CNS or pulmonary tumors, head injury, or drug use. Rapid-onset hyponatremia can manifest with confusion, disorientation or change in mental status, muscle weakness, and decreased reaction times. Because the patient is often euvolemic, signs of fluid overload are typically absent (Mocan et al., 2016).

TREATMENT

SIADH is a diagnosis of exclusion, and can be made if a patient meets the established six essential criteria originally proposed by Schwartz, Bennett, Curelop, and Bartter in 1957 (Spasovski et al., 2014). The diagnostic criteria are effective serum osmolality less than 275 mOsm/kg; urine osmolality greater than 100 mOsm/kg at some level of decreased effective osmolality; clinical euvolemia; urine sodium concentration greater than 30 mmol/L with normal dietary salt and water intake; absence of adrenal, thyroid, pituitary, or renal insufficiency; and no recent use of diuretics. After a diagnosis has been made, the mainstay of treatment for SIADH is fluid restriction, the degree of which is driven by the patient's ability to excrete electrolyte-free urine (Grant et al., 2015). Fluid restriction allows for a more gradual correction of hyponatremia. Rapid correction of sodium imbalances can have catastrophic outcomes, including central pontine myelinolysis and permanent neurological deficits (Spasovski et al., 2014). Second-line treatments include increasing solute intake with 0.25 to 0.50 g/kg per day of urea or using a combination of low-dose loop diuretics and oral sodium chloride to correct electrolyte imbalance (Spasovski et al., 2014). If possible, it is important to treat and diagnose the underlying cause of SIADH, as this may correct symptoms.

NURSING INTERVENTIONS, MANAGEMENT, AND IMPLICATIONS

Patients with SIADH are typically euvolemic and normotensive, but clinical changes can be seen in severe or rapid-onset scenarios (Mocan et al., 2016). Nevertheless, nursing staff must be vigilant in monitoring fluid balance for patients with SIADH. Careful attention should be paid to fluid intake and urine output. Nurses should monitor skin turgor, condition of mucous membranes, and changes in weight, noting that rapid changes of 0.5 to 1 kg/day can be related to fluid status. Mental status assessments are critical in hyponatremic patients. Nurses must monitor level of consciousness, orientation, and presence of muscle weakness and alert providers to changes. Serious consequences of hyponatremia include seizure and coma, although this is unlikely in a patient with SIADH (Grant et al., 2015). Patients are at risk for neurological changes as sodium levels are being corrected and careful monitoring is critical during this period.

OUTCOMES

Best practice recommends correcting hyponatremia gradually, with the best patient outcomes occurring when correction occurs over 24 to 48 hours (Grant et al., 2015). Hyponatremia is the most clinically

significant problem with SIADH and is associated with multiple diseases. Hyponatremia may be a poor prognostic marker, but is not a disease state in itself. The prognosis for SIADH greatly correlates to the underlying cause. A complete recovery is commonly seen with drug or anesthesia-induced SIADH once the causative agent is removed. Effective treatment of a CNS or pulmonary infection also often results in correction of SIADH (Cuesta & Thompson 2016).

Summary

SIADH is a complex phenomenon with multiple etiologies. ADH is secreted independently of osmolality, placing the patient in a hyponatremic, hypoosmolar state. The excessive ADH secretion leads to renal water reabsorption and subsequent diuresis. The severity of symptoms is correlated to the degree of hyponatremia; patients most at risk are those with rapid onset of symptoms, or severe levels of hyponatremia. The current best practice for treatment is fluid restriction with gradual correction of sodium levels.

Nursing interventions revolve around careful monitoring of intake and output for patients with SIADH. Frequent and careful neurological assessment may be indicated for patients with severe hyponatremia, or during the process for corrections. Elderly patients are at an increased risk for falls due to gait instability and changes in mental status associated with hyponatremia, and should be assisted with ambulation. It is imperative that nursing staff notify providers to any acute changes in level of consciousness or orientation, as rapid correction of hyponatremia can have profoundly adverse side effects on neurological status. As the frontline caregivers, nursing staff should feel empowered to notice changes in their patient's assessment, intake and output, as well as abnormal lab values when caring for patients at risk or currently experiencing SIADH.

Cuesta, M., & Thompson, C. J. (2016). The syndrome of inappropriate antidiuresis (SIAD). *Best Practice & Research Clinical Endocrinology & Metabolism, 30*(2), 175–187.

Grant, P., Ayuk, J., Bouloux, P. M., Cohen, M., Cranston, I., Murray, R. D., . . . Grossman, A. (2015). The diagnosis and management of inpatient hyponatraemia and SIADH. *European Journal of Clinical Investigation, 45*(8), 888–894.

Mocan, M., Terhes, L. M., & Blaga, S. N. (2016). Difficulties in the diagnosis and management of hyponatremia. *Clujul Medical, 89*(4), 464–469.

Schwartz, W. B., Bennett, W., Curelop, S., & Bartter, F. C. (1957). A syndrome of renal sodium loss and hyponatremia probably resulting from inappropriate secretion of antidiuretic hormone. *American Journal of Medicine, 23*(4), 529–542.

Shepshelovich, D., Leibovitch, C., Klein, A., Zoldan, S., Milo, G., Shochat, T., . . . Lahav, M. (2015). The syndrome of inappropriate antidiuretic hormone secretion: Distribution and characterization according to etiologies. *European Journal of Internal Medicine, 26*(10), 819–824.

Spasovski, G., Vanholder, R., Allolio, B., Annane, D., Ball, S., Bichet, D., . . . Nagler, E.; Hyponatraemia Guideline Development Group. (2014). Clinical practice guideline on diagnosis and treatment of hyponatraemia. *Nephrology, Dialysis, Transplantation, 29*(Suppl. 2), i1–i39.

■ SYSTEMIC LUPUS ERYTHEMATOSUS

Merlyn A. Dorsainvil

Overview

The word *lupus* originates from the Latin word for wolf. Wolf, a legendary predator, is a fitting name for a disease that is referred to as *the cruel mystery* (Lupus Foundation of America, 2017). Lupus is a mystery because it has remained elusive for much of its long history. To date, its cause remains unknown and there is no known cure for it. Lupus is cruel for the various degrees of debilitation that it causes. Systemic lupus erythematosus (SLE) is an autoimmune disease that causes widespread inflammation throughout various body tissues, including the kidneys, heart, lungs, brain, and blood vessels. There are different types of lupus: (a) cutaneous lupus, (b) drug-induced lupus, and (c) neonatal lupus. However, SLE is the most common and serious type. SLE is a chronic disease marked by periods of flares and remissions. Symptoms can range from mild to life-threatening, but with effective management the prognosis can be good. It is estimated that 1.5 million Americans have SLE, with more than 16,000 new cases detected annually. Women of color and of childbearing age are two to three times more likely to develop SLE than Caucasians (Lupus Foundation of America, 2017).

Background

SLE is a chronic, autoimmune disease that causes widespread inflammation throughout the body. Individuals with SLE often present with generalized symptoms such as fatigue, fever, and weight loss. Diagnosis is made by a clinical assessment, ideally by an experienced rheumatologist. The American College of Rheumatology (ACR) has developed criteria for diagnosing SLE. Individuals are diagnosed with SLE if they report at least four of these symptoms, with no other cause:

- Rashes:
  - Butterfly-shaped rash over the cheeks—referred to as *malar rash*
  - Red rash with raised round or oval patches—known as *discoid rash*
  - Rash on skin exposed to the sun

- Mouth sores: sores in the mouth or nose lasting from a few days to more than a month

- Arthritis: tenderness and swelling lasting for a few weeks in two or more joints

- Lung or heart inflammation: swelling of the tissue lining the lungs (referred to as *pleurisy* or *pleuritis*) or the heart (pericarditis), which can cause chest pain when breathing deeply

- Kidney problem: blood or protein in the urine, or tests that suggest poor kidney function

- Neurologic problem: seizures, strokes, or psychosis

- Abnormal blood tests such as:
  - Low blood cell counts: anemia, low white blood cells, or low platelets
  - Positive antinuclear antibodies (ANA) test result
  - Certain antibodies that show an immune system problem (ACR, 2015).

Based on the ACR criteria for SLE, the estimated prevalence of SLE in the United States is 72.8 to 74.4 per 100,000 and the incidence is 5.5 to 5.6 per 100,000 of population. Prevalence of SLE is more than 2 times higher among African Americans than among Caucasians and the incidence is three times higher. The burden of the disease is on women, with nine to 10 times higher prevalence among women than men (Lim et al., 2014; Somers et al., 2014). The average age of diagnosis is 39 to 41 years (Lim et al., 2014; Somers et al., 2014).

The cause of SLE is unknown but, based on the disproportionate burden on women and people of color, it is believed to be linked to genetic and hormonal factors. Exogenous and endogenous environmental exposures, such as infections, ultraviolet light, and stress, are linked to SLE (Sakkas & Bogdanos, 2016). The most common clinical manifestations of SLE among new cases include (a) arthritis, (b) hematologic disorders, (c) and serologic disorders. African Americans have a higher proportion of renal disease and end-stage renal disease compared to Caucasians (Somers et al., 2014).

There is no cure for SLE and treatment is based on the severity of symptoms. Nonsteroidal anti-inflammatory drugs (NSAIDs) are commonly used to treat inflammation and pain. Antimalarial drugs are used to treat symptoms such as fatigue and rashes. The biologic belimumab was approved in 2011 by the U.S. Food and Drug Administration for the treatment of active, nonsevere SLE. And for severe symptoms of SLE, corticosteroids and immunosuppressants are prescribed (ACR, 2015).

SLE has among the highest 30-day hospital readmission rates among chronic conditions. Following hospitalization for SLE, about one in six patients return within 30 days. Patients who are more likely to be initially hospitalized and readmitted within 30 days with SLE are those who (a) are young, (b) are African American or Hispanic, and (c) have Medicare or Medicaid as the primary payer. Renal disease, thrombocytopenia, serositis, and seizures are the SLE manifestations that are associated with readmissions (Yazdany et al., 2014). Pregnant women with SLE are at increased risk for stillbirths and early-onset preeclampsia (Simard et al., 2017; Vinet et al., 2016). Hospital admissions can pose financial burdens to patients and result in high health care costs. The average cost of a hospitalized patient with SLE is $51,808.41 per year (Anandarajah, Luc, & Ritchlin, 2016). Further financial burden comes from loss of productivity and loss of work days. SLE also significantly impacts quality of life. Most of the symptoms of SLE are not visible to others; common symptoms, such as fatigue and joint pain, are experienced by the individual but are not apparent to others. Subsequently this limits the amount of social support, validation, and medical care that individuals suffering with SLE receive (Brennan & Creaven, 2016).

Clinical Aspects

ASSESSMENT

The invisibility of SLE (Brennan & Creaven, 2016) can lead to feelings of powerlessness among those suffering with the condition. A thorough nursing assessment can be the first step in putting a face to this invisible condition. The nursing assessment should begin qualitatively with a history, examining onset of symptoms as well as exacerbating and relieving factors. Psychosocial aspects should be examined also: How has the disease impacted the client's life? What types of support does the client currently have? The history should be followed with a comprehensive physical examination, with focused assessments to the following systems: dermatologic, cardiovascular, renal, musculoskeletal, neurological, and pain. Nurses should anticipate laboratory tests, including an ANA test, complete blood count, erythrocyte sedimentation rate, C-reactive protein, and urinalysis. Although no two people with SLE will present with identical symptoms, some symptoms are commonly seen. Rashes are a classical symptom and, at some stage in the disease process, individuals with SLE will present with a rash. Fatigue is often a common and initial complaint. Many clients will also have joint pain.

The goals of nursing care for the client with SLE are to control flare-ups, prevent damage to organs, and promote overall health. Nursing-related problems clients can experience include (a) fatigue related to SLE disease process, (b) disturbed body image related to rashes, and (c) social isolation due to overall lack of public awareness of SLE. Clients should be encouraged to see a rheumatologist for the medical management of SLE. In addition, clients should also have routine primary health care for overall health promotion. For women of childbearing age, primary care from a women's health provider is ideal. Clients with SLE should be encouraged to maintain healthy, balanced diets and exercise. Frequent rest periods and energy conservation techniques should be discussed with clients. Nurses can assist clients in identifying essential versus nonessential activities so that their energy can be put to the most productive use. Clients with rashes should avoid direct sunlight and use sunscreen whenever outdoors. Nurses can use advocacy skills to educate and raise awareness of SLE to family, friends, and the public.

OUTCOMES

The outcome of nursing care for the client with SLE should be the client's confidence in managing the disease and improved quality of life. This outcome is achieved when nurses utilize the Quality and Safety Education for Nurses (QSEN) competency of patient-centered care. Nurses assist clients in the process of self-discovery of how SLE impacts their body and lives and ways to mitigate any potential or actual damages.

Summary

SLE has been deemed a "cruel mystery" because little is known about this debilitating, chronic disease. There is no known cause, no known cure, and minimal epidemiological data. Therefore, it remains a mystery to the health care community and the public; those with SLE often suffer in silence. However, the Centers for Disease Control and Prevention has recently funded research throughout the United States to obtain more accurate estimates of the disease. With better estimates of SLE prevalence and incidence, more resources can be allocated for research. Organizations, such as the Lupus Foundation of America, promote advocacy, research, and support for the disease so that SLE will no longer be a mystery. Until a cause and cure are found, clients with SLE can live long, productive lives with effective medical management and self-management. Nurses can support clients with SLE in their self-management and help to increase public awareness of this chronic condition.

American College of Rheumatology. (2015). Lupus. Retrieved from http://www.rheumatology.org/i-am-a/patient-caregiver/diseases-conditions/lupus

Anandarajah, A., Luc, M., & Ritchlin, C. (2016). Hospitalization of patients with systemic lupus erythematosus is a major cause of direct and indirect healthcare costs. *Lupus, 26*(7), 1–6. doi:10.1177/0961203316676641

Brennan, K. A., & Creaven, A. M. (2016). Living with invisible illness: Social support experiences of individuals with systemic lupus erythematosus. *Quality of Life Research, 25*(5), 1227–1235.

Lim, S. S., Bayakly, A. R., Helmick, C. G., Gordon, C., Easley, K. A., & Drenkard, C. (2014). The incidence and prevalence of systemic lupus erythematosus, 2002–2004: The Georgia Lupus Registry. *Arthritis & Rheumatology, 66*(2), 357–368.

Lupus Foundation of America. (2017). What is lupus? Retrieved from http://www.lupus.org/answers/entry/what-is-lupus

Sakkas, L. I., & Bogdanos, D. P. (2016). Infections as a cause of autoimmune rheumatic diseases. *Auto-Immunity Highlights, 7*(1), 13.

Simard, J. F., Arkema, E. V., Nguyen, C., Svenungsson, E., Wikström, A. K., Palmsten, K., & Salmon, J. E. (2017). Early-onset preeclampsia in lupus pregnancy. *Paediatric and Perinatal Epidemiology, 31*(1), 29–36.

Somers, E. C., Marder, W., Cagnoli, P., Lewis, E. E., DeGuire, P., Gordon, C., . . . McCune, W. J. (2014). Population-based incidence and prevalence of systemic lupus erythematosus: The Michigan Lupus Epidemiology and Surveillance program. *Arthritis & Rheumatology, 66*(2), 369–378.

Vinet, É., Genest, G., Scott, S., Pineau, C. A., Clarke, A. E., Platt, R. W., & Bernatsky, S. (2016). Brief report: Causes of stillbirths in women with systemic lupus erythematosus. *Arthritis & Rheumatology, 68*(10), 2487–2491.

Yazdany, J., Marafino, B., Dean, M., Bardach, N., Duseja, R., Ward, M., & Dudley, R. (2014). Thirty-day hospital readmissions in systemic lupus erythematosus: Predictors and hospital and state-level variation. *Arthritis & Rheumatology, 66*(10), 2828–2836. doi:10.1002/art.38768

■ THROMBOCYTOPENIA

Maria A. Mendoza

Overview

Thrombocytopenia is a blood disorder characterized by low platelet (thrombocyte) count caused by deficient marrow production, increased destruction, and splenic sequestration. Normal platelet count is between 150,000 and 400,000/µL and thrombocytopenia in adults is defined as a platelet count below 150,000/µL (Krisnegowda & Rajashekaraiah, 2015).

Thrombocytopenia may be associated with many diseases and syndromes and in some cases is drug induced, making it the most common blood disorder (Izak & Bussel, 2014). It is common among hospitalized and critically ill adults. It is believed to be present in as much as 67.6% of adult patients on admission to the intensive care unit (ICU) and acquired by up to 44% of patients while in the ICU (Hui, Cook, Lim, Fraser, & Arnold, 2011). It may sometimes be the first sign of hematologic cancers. In many situations, the patient suffering from thrombocytopenia is clinically asymptomatic. Low platelet count is often found during a routine complete blood count (CBC) test. Patients with count less than 30,000/µL have potential for bleeding but it is generally a count below 10,000/µL that clinically presents with spontaneous bleeding from skin, wounds, or body cavities (Izak & Bussel, 2014).

Background

Platelets are tiny (1–3 µm) anucleated cells produced in the large bone marrow cells called *megakaryocytes*. The fragmentation of megakaryocytes in the presence of a hormone called *thrombopoietin* results in the release of platelets (1,000 platelets per megakaryocyte). The main functions of platelets are hemostasis and wound healing. Their sticky consistency plus ability to change shape make them efficient in sealing off the bleeding site.

Identifying the etiology of thrombocytopenia is part of the diagnostic process. The major laboratory tests are CBC, blood smear (to analyze blood cell morphology), and coagulation tests (prothrombin time and activated partial thromboplastin time). Other tests ordered to help with the differential diagnosis include direct Coombs, fibrinogen, D-Dimer, lactate dehydrogenase (LDH), alkaline phosphatase, liver and renal function tests, vitamin B_{12}, folic acid level, and serological tests. In some cases, a bone marrow biopsy may be performed.

Treatment of thrombocytopenia is directed at eliminating the etiology. However, in the majority of cases, the etiology is not very clear. First-line pharmacotherapy includes corticosteroids, intravenous immunoglobulin G (IV IgG), and intravenous anti-D (Krisnegowda & Rajashekaraiah, 2015). When first-line drugs have failed, immunosuppressants, such as azathioprine, cyclophosphamide, and cyclosporine, may be tried (Krisnegowda & Rajashekaraiah, 2015). The American Association of Blood Banks (AABB) recommends platelet transfusion in hospitalized adult patients with a platelet count of 10,000/μL or less to reduce spontaneous bleeding (Kaufman et al., 2015). Packed cell transfusion is administered to replace blood loss. In case of increased destruction of platelets by the spleen, a splenectomy (laparoscopic, if possible) may be done.

Clinical Aspects

ASSESSMENT

A comprehensive history helps to identify the etiology of the disease. The nurse is part of the health care team who may collect this information, which includes presence of family history of thrombocytopenia, recent infection (viral and bacterial), vaccinations, history of cancer, treatment with chemotherapy, pregnancy, recent travels (for possible exposure to malaria, dengue fever, rickettsiosis), recent transfusions, alcohol intake, dietary habits, risk factors for or history of HIV, and hepatitis C. A review of all medications with focus on medications started in the past 2 weeks should also be done. Verify symptoms such as muscle/joint pain, dizziness, persistent headache, blurred or double vision, and abdominal pain.

Physical assessment should include thorough examination of the skin to identify signs of bleeding such as ecchymosis (bruising), petechiae, purpura, and frank hemorrhage. Bleeding from body cavities is also checked, including the oral cavity (gums), eyes, nose (epistaxis), lungs (hemoptysis), gastrointestinal tract (hematemesis, melena, and occult bleeding), urinary tract (hematuria), and vaginal tract (vaginal bleeding or increased menstrual flow). A neurological assessment should be done, especially in patients at risk for and/or with suspicion of cerebral bleeding. Careful palpation for lymphadenopathy (enlarged lymph nodes) and for organomegaly of the liver and spleen should be performed. Skeletal malformations of the thumbs and forearm, and short stature present in certain forms of thrombocytopenia should be noted (Izak & Bussel, 2014).

NURSING INTERVENTIONS, MANAGEMENT, AND IMPLICATIONS

Patient education is needed to prevent bleeding and injury. The nurse reviews with the patient/family the disease condition, etiology (if known), complications, treatment, and how to prevent and manage bleeding. A review of all medications (prescribed and over-the-counter) should be done (Winkeljohn, 2013). General instructions should include medications to avoid such as aspirin and drugs containing aspirin. The patient is informed to check with health care provider before using over-the-counter medication. Promote activities to prevent bleeding such as using soft-bristle toothbrush, electric shaver when shaving, and emery board to trim nails. Patient should avoid using household tools, such as scissors, knives, and sharp objects, to prevent injuries. Counsel the patient not to drink alcohol. Patient has to check with his or her health care provider before undergoing dental work or other procedures that can cause bleeding. Patient should avoid heavy lifting, contact sports, and strenuous activities that can lead to a fall or injury. The patient/family should know what to report to the health care provider, such as observation of any kind of bleeding, as listed earlier. Teach the patient/family how to control bleeding such as applying pressure over a cut with a clean cloth or gauze until bleeding is controlled. Hemostatic agents, such as Gelfoam, may be used to cause vasoconstriction (Winkeljohn, 2013). The health care provider and emergency medical service phone numbers should be handy in case of emergency.

Teaching directed toward medication(s) prescribed to treat thrombocytopenia should be provided to patient/family. The nurse should teach proper administration and side/adverse effects of medications such as corticosteroids and other immunosuppressants.

For severe states of thrombocytopenia, a platelet transfusion may be included in the patient's plan of care. The nurse assists in the administration of a platelet transfusion and performs the following nursing interventions to ensure the patient's safety:

1. Obtain an informed consent after explaining the procedure, purpose, possible complications, and necessary monitoring during and after the procedure. Use the laboratory results to explain the need for transfusion and target levels posttransfusion (Winkeljohn, 2013). Proper identification of the patient before transfusion is imperative. The platelet bags and tubing should be checked for integrity. The procedure should be done under strict aseptic technique.

2. Establish baseline vital signs and lab values before transfusion. Allergic and hemolytic reactions, such as fever, isolated pruritus and urticaria, bronchoconstriction, hypotension, and shock, may occur. Febrile nonhemolytic transfusion reaction (FNHTR) with or without chills may occur within the first 4 hours of transfusion followed by normalization of the temperature within 48 hours. FNHTR is confirmed once bacterial infection and hemolytic causes are ruled out. Bacterial sepsis, caused by contaminated platelets, is manifested by high fever, chills, vomiting, tachycardia, hypotension, and shock.

3. Monitor patient's vital signs during and after transfusion. Check platelet count 15 minutes to 1-hour posttransfusion. As indicated, CBC, coagulation, and renal function tests are done. Continue to monitor for bleeding.

4. Maintain good oral hygiene using soft swabs, normal saline rinse, and mouthwash as appropriate to prevent dry mucous membranes and minimize bleeding.

OUTCOMES

The major role of the nurse in managing thrombocytopenia is to work and collaborate with the health care team to collect data and provide safe patient care. Nursing assessment includes a thorough history to identify etiology and a physical examination to check for bleeding. Patient education is very important to promote safety and prevent injuries that may lead to bleeding.

Summary

Thrombocytopenia is a common blood disorder defined as platelet count less than 150,000/μL. Etiology can be due to deficient marrow production, increased destruction, and splenic sequestration. Diagnosis is primarily established by laboratory studies. In few cases, bone marrow biopsy may be done to identify deficient marrow production. Treatment is focused on removing the causative factor. First-line drug therapy includes corticosteroids, IV IgG, and intravenous anti-D. Platelet transfusion may be necessary when platelet count falls below 10,000/μL and there is high risk of spontaneous bleeding.

Hui, P., Cook, D. J., Lim, W., Fraser, G. A., & Arnold, D. M. (2011). The frequency and clinical significance of thrombocytopenia complicating critical illness: A systematic review. *Chest, 139*(2), 271–278.

Izak, M., & Bussel, J. B. (2014). Management of thrombocytopenia. *F1000Prime Reports, 6*, 45.

Kaufman, R. M., Djulbegovic, B., Gernsheimer, T., Kleinman, S., Tinmouth, A. T., Capocelli, K. E., . . . Tobian, A. A. (2015). Platelet transfusion: A clinical practice guideline from the AABB. *Annals of Internal Medicine, 162*(3), 205–213.

Krisnegowda, M., & Rajashekaraiah, V. (2015). Platelet disorders: An overview. *Blood Coagulation and Fibrinolysis, 26*(5), 479–491. doi:10.1097/01.mbc .0000469521.23628.2d

Winkeljohn, D. (2013). Diagnosis, treatment and management of immune thrombocytopenia. *Clinical Journal of Oncology Nursing, 17*(6), 664–666. doi:10.1188/ 13.CJON.664-666

■ TUBERCULOSIS

Christina M. Canfield

Overview

A disease of historical significance, tuberculosis (TB) has caused more deaths worldwide than any other infectious disease, including plague, smallpox, and malaria (Heemskerk, Caws, Marais, & Farrar, 2015). One third of the world's population is infected with TB and there is one new case of TB diagnosed every 4 seconds (Centers for Disease Control and Prevention [CDC], 2016). Nurses must be aware of the risk factors associated with transmission, symptoms, and treatment of a TB infection.

Background

The global incidence of TB varies widely. In 2015 an estimated 10.4 million new cases of TB were identified worldwide. Incidence of TB is higher in underdeveloped countries. The World Health Organization

(Global Tuberculosis Report, 2016) reports that 60% of new cases were identified in just six countries: India, Indonesia, China, Nigeria, Pakistan, and South Africa. The CDC (2016) noted a rate of 3.0 cases per 100,000 persons in the United States in 2015. HIV-infected adults, persons born in foreign countries, and those of lower socioeconomic status make up the majority of active TB cases in the United States (Raviglione, 2015). TB is a treatable disease that may be cured; however, drug-resistant strains of *Mycobacterium tuberculosis* are becoming more prevalent. Untreated TB is often fatal and carries a 1-year mortality of 30%.

TB has been known by many names, including consumption, Pott's disease, shaky oncay, and the white plague (Heemskerk et al., 2015). It is a disease caused by the bacterium *M. tuberculosis*. Mycobacteria have a unique lipid-rich cell wall, which makes them resistant to many disinfectants and antibiotics. *M. tuberculosis* is an acid-fast bacilli (AFB) usually transmitted when an infectious person coughs, sneezes, or speaks. Droplets may remain suspended in the air for hours and then be inhaled into the airways. An infected individual may expel up to 3,000 infectious nuclei per cough. It is estimated that up to 20 contacts may be infected by each positive case. This is due to delays in pursuing care and in making a diagnosis (Raviglione, 2015).

TB transmission occurs in high population density locations such as hospitals, nursing facilities, prisons, and hostels (Heemskerk et al., 2015).

Clinical Aspects

Exposure to *M. tuberculosis* activates the immune system. In most cases, the body will contain the infection and form a granuloma around it. Cases in which the infection is controlled but not fully eliminated are referred to as *latent TB*. Latent TB may become an active infection if the infected individual suffers from an impaired immune system. In 5% to 10% of exposed individuals, the bacteria cannot be contained and TB occurs soon after the initial exposure. The lungs are affected in two thirds of TB cases and the middle and lower lungs are most commonly involved. Pulmonary TB may be asymptomatic or the infected individual may present with fever and pleuritic chest pain. In young children or immunocompromised individuals, TB may progress rapidly. All HIV-positive patients should be screened for TB (Heemskerk et al., 2015).

ASSESSMENT

Symptoms may mimic the flu and therefore patients may not immediately seek treatment. Diagnosis is commonly made based on finding evidence of AFB testing on a sputum sample.

Symptoms include:

- Fever
- Night sweats
- Weight loss
- Loss of appetite
- Malaise
- Weakness
- Cough
- Sputum (purulent or bloody)

NURSING INTERVENTIONS, MANAGEMENT, AND IMPLICATIONS

The nurse should suspect TB in the patient who presents with persistent cough and unexplained weight loss. A heightened suspicion should be given to patients who are infected with HIV, who are homeless, or who have emigrated from a county of high incidence of TB. Abnormal findings on a chest x-ray may lead to further testing. Follow the facility's procedure for use of personal protective equipment and establishing isolation. Anticipate placing the patient in a negative pressure airflow room.

The nurse should expect to collect or facilitate the collection of two to three samples gathered first thing in the morning on consecutive days (Raviglione, 2015).

There are four medications that are considered to be first-line agents for the treatment of active TB: isoniazid, rifampin, pyrazinamide, and ethambutol.

Patients will receive a 2-month initial course of all four medications followed by up to 4 months of rifampin and isoniazid. Up to 90% of patients will be cured following 6 months of active treatment (Raviglione, 2015). The long course of therapy and multiple medications required present a challenge for medication adherence. The multidisciplinary team may engage the assistance of a TB control program to help with medication management. Administration of medications using directly observed therapy (DOT) improves adherence to the medication regimen and is strongly recommended for individuals who require treatment for TB in the community setting. Medications provided during DOT are given directly to the patient by a health care provider or trained worker. The patient is monitored during administration to ensure that medications have been taken. Use of DOT is essential for patients with drug-resistant TB and those with HIV infection. The effectiveness of treatment is monitored by repeating sputum cultures.

Patients with known latent TB infections may also receive treatment with isoniazid. This treatment may last 9 months. Presence of HIV infection is the strongest risk factor associated with conversion of a latent TB infection to an active TB infection (Heemskerk et al., 2015).

There is only one vaccine available for prevention of TB. The bacillus Calmette-Guérin (BCG) vaccine has been administered around the world since 1921. The effectiveness of the vaccine varies from 0% to 80% and it has been found to be most effective in preventing meningitis associated with TB (Heemskerk et al., 2015).

The nurse should consider including the following problems and interventions when creating the patient-specific plan of care (Garvey, 2014): ineffective airway clearance, risk for impaired gas exchange, impaired nutrition, and knowledge deficit.

OUTCOMES

Expected nursing outcomes are focused on maintaining and improving oxygenation and nutrition while assuring adherence to prescribed therapies. The nurse should perform ongoing assessments of the patient's and significant other(s)' understanding of the medication regimen and actions necessary to prevent the spread of infection. Those who will be in close contact with the patient during the anticipated course of treatment must be able to verbalize an understanding of the signs and symptoms of TB and must know when to seek medical treatment.

Summary

The worldwide burden of TB remains significant. TB is a curable disease but commitment to completion of the long course of treatment requires significant personal effort, social support, and access to resources. Wide-scale elimination efforts hinge on the identification of an effective vaccine. The nurse must become familiar with the signs and symptoms of active TB infection to prevent the spread of disease and protect vulnerable individuals. Nursing care of the patient with active TB infection involves medication delivery, monitoring for adverse effects, and frequent education of the patient and his or her support systems.

Centers for Disease Control and Prevention. (2016). TB data and statistics. Retrieved from https://www.cdc.gov/tb/statistics/default.htm

Garvey, C. (2014). Respiratory disorders. In S. M. Nettina (Ed.), *Lippincott manual of nursing practice* (10th ed., 277–323). Philadelphia, PA: Lippincott Williams & Wilkins.

Global Tuberculosis Report. (2016). (1st ed., pp. 5–82). Retrieved from http://apps.who.int/iris/bitstream/10665/250441/1/9789241565394-eng.pdf?ua=1

Heemskerk, D., Caws, M., Marais, B., & Farrar, J. (2015). *Tuberculosis in adults and children* (1st ed., pp. 1–55). Springer International.

Raviglione, M. (2015). Tuberculosis. In D. Kasper, A. Fauci, S. Hauser, D. Longo, J. Jameson, & J. Loscalzo (Eds.), *Harrison's principles of internal medicine* (19th ed.). New York, NY: McGraw-Hill. Retrieved from http://accessmedicine.mhmedical.com/content.aspx?bookid=1130&Sectionid=79737003

■ VALVULAR HEART DISEASE

Rebecca Witten Grizzle

Overview

Valvular heart disease (VHD) encompasses health conditions affecting the four heart valves: aortic, pulmonic, mitral, and tricuspid. Common disorders include valvular stenosis and regurgitation; the aortic and mitral valves are most commonly affected. In the United States, the prevalence of VHD is 2.5% in the general population and 13% in persons over the age of 75 years (Iung & Vahanian, 2014). VHD results in significant morbidity and mortality and burden to the health care system (Moore, Chen, Mallow, & Rizzo, 2016). Therefore, patient management and quality of life are important concerns to nurses, especially those who care for special populations such as pediatric, athletic, obstetric, perioperative, and geriatric patients.

Background

The most common types of VHD among European populations are aortic stenosis (43%) and mitral regurgitation (32%), followed by aortic regurgitation (13%) and mitral stenosis (12%; Iung & Vahanian, 2014). In the United States, mitral valve disease is more prevalent than aortic valve disease and rates of both increase with age (Moore et al., 2016). The etiology of VHD is predominantly degenerative in nature, although rheumatic heart disease still accounts for many cases worldwide (Moore et al., 2016). The remaining causes are infective endocarditis, congenital heart disease, inflammatory processes, mediastinal radiation, or cardiotoxic drug exposure. Degeneration is the result of progressive calcification of the valve cusps in a process similar to atherosclerosis, although there are no known evidence-based strategies to slow its progression (Iung & Vahanian, 2014). The risk factors for progression of aortic valve calcification include age, hypertension, diabetes mellitus, hypercholesterolemia, hypercalcemia, and smoking (Carità et al., 2016). Rates of aortic valve calcification vary from person to person and may be influenced by genetic factors that result in higher plasma lipoprotein(a) levels (Rahimtoola, 2014).

Approximately one third of VHD patients are symptomatic, reporting significant chest pain, palpitations, shortness of breath, dizziness, and syncope (Moore et al., 2016). Medical management of symptomatic patients appears largely ineffective, and the only definitive treatment is repair or replacement of the affected valve. Thus, the risks and benefits of surgery must be considered given the patient's comorbidities, expected outcome, quality of life, and personal wishes. There were approximately 133,000 heart valve surgeries in 2013 in the United States partly due to the increasing incidence of transcatheter aortic valve implantation (TAVI) procedures (Miller & Flynn, 2015). The health care expenditure for all types of mitral and aortic valve diseases is estimated at $23.4 billion annually. Successful surgery decreases the patient's symptom burden and is seen as cost-effective compared to medical management in the long term (Moore et al., 2016).

Individuals with VHD are at higher risk of thromboembolic events due to changes in blood flow from valve pathology. However, the population also has higher bleeding risks such as age, hypertension, medication usage, liver dysfunction, alcohol use, and renal disease. Careful consideration must be given to patient selection for anticoagulation management. For example, the annual risk of thromboembolism among patients with mitral stenosis is 1% to 6% (Iung & Vahanian, 2014). However, patients with mitral valve disease were considerably undertreated with oral anticoagulants when compared to patients with aortic valve disease, even though their risk for stroke is much higher (Başaran et al., 2017).

Other comorbidities, such as atrial fibrillation, carry an elevated risk for stroke, based on the risk stratification score. In patients with nonvalvular atrial fibrillation, at least one third have significant valvular disease. Patients with significant valvular disease are at greater risk of stroke and simultaneously have higher risks for bleeding (Başaran et al., 2017). These caveats make patient management challenging and complex.

Living with VHD significantly impacts an individual's quality of life due to physical, psychological, and social factors (dos Anjos, Rodrigues, Padilha, Pedrose, & Gallani, 2016). Patients with VHD worry about exacerbations and decompensating, thus affecting their health self-perception. Fatigue, dyspnea, palpitations, chest pain, syncope, and edema affect their daily lives. Patients are prescribed an average of four medications. Diuretic use can have a significant impact on the individual's physical, social, and emotional well-being due to the drug's effects on activities of daily living. A high percentage of these patients are unemployed or on disability, and many have lower educational and income levels (dos Anjos et al., 2016). In addition, symptomatic aortic valve disease patients are more likely to have higher rates of depression and anxiety (Moore et al., 2016).

Clinical Aspects

ASSESSMENT

Special populations with different VHD management concerns include infants and children, adolescent and young adult athletes, pregnant women, and older adults. Nurses must continue to maintain physical assessment skills across the life span, particularly in auscultating cardiovascular sounds and documenting findings pertaining to rhythm, pitch, tone, timing, and radiation to carotid arteries and thorax. Nurses must also be able to anticipate patients' cardiac complaints and pose appropriate assessment questions to elicit signs and symptoms. In short, patients with VHD must be properly assessed in order to be efficiently diagnosed, evaluated, and treated. Diagnostic tests, such as electrocardiogram, chest radiography, and echocardiography, are used to evaluate cardiac function to determine the extent of valve pathology. Cardiac stress testing is discouraged in symptomatic VHD patients.

Symptomatic or undiagnosed heart murmur in surgical patients may present a dilemma to the perioperative team. Given the high prevalence of untreated aortic stenosis among older adults, the perioperative team may consider obtaining an echocardiogram to evaluate cardiac function and valvular anatomy. A higher degree of suspicion is supported by the presence of signs and symptoms of heart failure, history of heart failure and worsening dyspnea, or dyspnea of unknown origin (Fleisher et al., 2014). Research findings suggest that patients with severe aortic stenosis can undergo noncardiac surgery if consideration is given to enhanced anesthetic management. Careful monitoring with an arterial line to monitor and prevent hypotension on induction and during anesthesia will help prevent intraoperative events, by maintaining the pressure gradient to overcome the stenotic aortic valve (Rahimtoola, 2014).

The American Heart Association and American College of Cardiology updated management guidelines for patients with VHD, including recommendations regarding dental prophylaxis, diagnostic imaging, surgical intervention, prosthetic valve selection, and anticoagulation (Nishimura et al., 2017). These recommendations highlight the need for a comprehensive team approach for care of patients with VHD. Although nurses may not be central in the medical decision making, they are essential in supporting, teaching, and advocating for these patients. Nurses' integral involvement on a dedicated heart team provides clinical leadership for promoting excellent outcomes among VHD patients (Lauck, McGladrey, Lawlor, & Webb, 2016).

Perioperative nursing interventions include monitoring for hemodynamic instability, such as hypotension, bleeding, tamponade, and arrhythmias. Patients are at risk for paravalvular leak, ventricular dysfunction, atrioventricular conduction abnormalities, atrial fibrillation, and pulmonary hypertension. All are conditions that can lead to decompensation. In general, patients undergoing aortic and mitral procedures have higher risk than those undergoing pulmonic and tricuspid procedures. Postoperative patients need frequent neurological assessments to evaluate for stroke or transient ischemic attacks (Miller & Flynn, 2015). Anticoagulation therapy is often indicated, requiring careful lifelong follow-up care.

OUTCOMES

Nurses play an important role in teaching and supporting patients in the management of VHD. Patient education for this population focuses on smoking cessation, health-promotion strategies, medication therapies,

anticoagulation monitoring, thromboembolic risk reduction, and endocarditis prophylaxis. Nurses have a unique perspective in that they can promote lifestyle changes while addressing diverse social, cultural, emotional, and financial concerns (McLachlan, Sutton, Ding, & Kerr, 2015). By understanding the influence of socioeconomic factors on the clinical management of VHD patients, nurses can plan more effective interventions that are tailored to the individual patient's needs (dos Anjos et al., 2016).

Summary

VHD is a worldwide concern affecting newborns to older adults, although prevalence increases with age. Patients should be evaluated thoroughly if they exhibit signs and symptoms of VHD. Given the tremendous implications for morbidity and quality of life, a team approach is needed to determine the best plan of care. Often surgical valve repair or replacement is the only definitive treatment in symptomatic severe VHD. Patients will require lifelong monitoring and continuous support. Nurses play a key role in planning patient management strategies that are tailored to the individual's needs. Trends indicate more catheter-based procedures will increase the demand for highly trained nurses who can care for the growing population of VHD patients.

Başaran, Ö., Dogan, V., Beton, O., Tekinalp, M., Aykan, A. Ç., Kalaycioglu, E., . . . Biteker, M. (2017). Impact of valvular heart disease on oral anticoagulant therapy in nonvalvular atrial fibrillation: Results from the RAMSES study. *Journal of Thrombosis and Thrombolysis, 43*(2), 157–165.

Carità, P., Coppola, G., Novo, G., Caccamo, G., Guglielmo, M., Balasus, F., . . . Corrado, E. (2016). Aortic stenosis: Insights on pathogenesis and clinical implications. *Journal of Geriatric Cardiology, 13*(6), 489–498.

dos Anjos, D. B., Rodrigues, R. C., Padilha, K. M., Pedrosa, R. B., & Gallani, M. C. (2016). Influence of sociodemographic and clinical characteristics at the impact of valvular heart disease. *Revista Brasileira De Enfermagem, 69*(1), 33–39.

Fleisher, L. A., Fleischmann, K. E., Auerbach, A. D., Barnason, S. A., Beckman, J. A., Bozkurt, B., . . . Wijeysundera, D. N. (2014). 2014 ACC/AHA guideline on perioperative cardiovascular evaluation and management of patients undergoing noncardiac surgery: Executive summary: A report of the American College of Cardiology/ American Heart Association Task Force on Practice Guidelines. *Circulation, 130*(24), 2215–2245.

Iung, B., & Vahanian, A. (2014). Epidemiology of acquired valvular heart disease. *Canadian Journal of Cardiology, 30*(9), 962–970.

Lauck, S. B., McGladrey, J., Lawlor, C., & Webb, J. G. (2016). Nursing leadership of the transcatheter aortic valve implantation Heart Team: Supporting innovation, excellence, and sustainability. *Healthcare Management Forum, 29*(3), 126–130.

McLachlan, A., Sutton, T., Ding, P., & Kerr, A. (2015). A nurse practitioner clinic: A novel approach to supporting patients following heart valve surgery. *Heart, Lung & Circulation, 24*(11), 1126–1133.

Miller, S., & Flynn, B. C. (2015). Valvular heart disease and postoperative considerations. *Seminars in Cardiothoracic and Vascular Anesthesia, 19*(2), 130–142.

Moore, M., Chen, J., Mallow, P. J., & Rizzo, J. A. (2016). The direct health-care burden of valvular heart disease: Evidence from US national survey data. *ClinicoEconomics and Outcomes Research, 8*, 613–627.

Nishimura, R. A., Otto, C. M., Bonow, R. O., Carabello, B. A., Erwin, J. P., Fleisher, L. A., . . . Thompson, A. (2017). 2017 AHA/ACC focused update of the 2014 AHA/ACC guideline for the management of patients with valvular heart disease: A report of the American College of Cardiology/American Heart Association Task Force on Clinical Practice Guidelines. *Journal of the American College of Cardiology, 70*(2), 252–289.

Rahimtoola, S. H. (2014). The year in valvular heart disease. *Journal of the American College of Cardiology, 63*(19), 1948–1958.

Neonatal Nursing

This section consists of the more common pathologic processes encountered in neonatology, which is a subspecialty of pediatrics. Neonatal nurses work in newborn nurseries and in different levels of neonatal intensive care units (NICU) around the world.

Neonatal nurses are a unique group of individuals because not only do they care for a very fragile population, but often, they must do so in a high-tech and fast-paced NICU environment that requires advanced skills and knowledge. The neonatal bedside nurse provides education to mothers and families on every topic from bathing a newborn to changing a tracheostomy tube. From attending deliveries, to administering medications, to grieving with a family as their infant is dying, neonatal nurses are at the bedside.

The neonatal nurses must have a strong foundation in pathophysiology, pharmacology, psychology, and ethics. They must keep up to date with ever-changing technology; support families in crisis; and stay current with nursing, medical, and other scientific literature.

A multidisciplinary team approach is necessary in providing the best care to both healthy and ill neonates, but at the heart of this care is the neonatal nurse. They are the most integral component of this specialty area. Their greatest strength is their role as advocates to protect and support infants and their families during a stressful, vulnerable time of life. There are many challenges as a neonatal nurse, however, there are just as many rewards.

- ABO Incompatibility *Donna M. Schultz and Mary F. Terhaar*
- Acute Renal Failure *Christine Horvat Davey*
- Anemia of Prematurity *Barbara Greitzer Slone*
- Apnea of Prematurity *Amy Bieda*
- Bronchopulmonary Dysplasia *Amy Bieda*
- Decreased Pulmonary Blood Flow *Jennifer Johntony and Jodi Zalewski*
- Extremely Low-Birth-Weight Infant *Jenelle M. Zambrano*
- Gastroesophageal Reflux *Suzanne Rubin*
- Gastroschisis and Omphalocele *Beverly Capper*
- Hirschsprung's Disease *Anne M. Modic*
- Hydronephrosis *Charlene M. Deuber*
- Hyperbilirubinemia *Donna M. Schultz and Mary F. Terhaar*
- Hypertension *Mary F. Terhaar*
- Hypoglycemia *Tina Di Fiore*
- Hypoxic Ischemic Encephalopathy *Ke-Ni Niko Tien*
- Increased Pulmonary Blood Flow *Jennifer Johntony and Jodi Zalewski*
- Infant of a Diabetic Mother *Mary F. Terhaar*
- Intraventricular Hemorrhage *Helene M. Lannon*
- Late Preterm Infant *Donna A. Dowling*
- Meconium Aspiration Syndrome *Rae Jean Hemway*
- Necrotizing Enterocolitis *Charlene M. Deuber*
- Respiratory Distress Syndrome *Mary Ann Blatz*
- Retinopathy of Prematurity *Mary Ann Blatz*
- Sepsis *Karla Phipps*
- Substance Abuse/Opioid Withdrawal *Helene M. Lannon*
- Thermoregulation *Paula Forsythe*

■ ABO INCOMPATIBILITY

Donna M. Schultz
Mary F. Terhaar

Overview

ABO incompatibility is the single, most common form of isoimmune hemolytic anemia in the Western world, occurring in 12% to 15% of all pregnancies (Roberts, 2008). The condition occurs when maternal blood type differs from fetal blood type. Most often, the condition arises in a blood type O mother who carries a blood type A or B fetus; although it can be present in a blood type A or B mother who carries a fetus of a different blood type. In 3% to 4% of these pregnancies, maternal red blood cells (RBCs) cross the placenta and interact with fetal cells, triggering complications, including anemia and hyperbilirubinemia (Basu, Kaur, & Kaur, 2011).

ABO incompatibility is one of the hemolytic anemias. Due to the antenatal administration of Rhogam (anti-D gamma globulin), Rh isoimmunization has decreased, leaving ABO incompatibility as one of the most common causes of hemolytic disease (HD).

Background

Blood types are assigned to correspond to the surface antigen on the RBC. Type A blood carries A-antigens on the surface of the RBC along with anti-B antibodies. Type B blood carries B-antigens on the surface along with anti-A antibodies. Type AB blood carries both A and B antigens on the surface, but neither anti-A nor anti-B antibodies. Finally, type O blood carries neither A nor B antigens, but both anti-A and anti-B antibodies. Each blood type recognizes cells from the same type when it encounters corresponding antigens that matches its own. Conversely, antibodies mobilize, clump, and hemolyze blood cells, which carry antigens different from their own.

The reason type O blood is the universal donor is because it carries no antigen to trigger hemolysis and rejection. The mother with type O blood has no antigen on the surface of her RBCs and so the fetus with a dissimilar blood type will not hemolyze maternal cells. However, her blood does carry anti-A and anti-B antibodies. When O negative cells of the mother cross into fetal circulation, the anti-A and anti-B antibodies they carry attack and hemolyze fetal cells, which lowers the RBC count and elevates the levels of waste products, including bilirubin. This is the mechanism by which ABO incompatibility leads to anemia and hyperbilirubinemia.

Clinical Aspects

ASSESSMENT

Actual, symptomatic HD occurs in fewer than 1% of infants affected by ABO incompatibility. The primary symptom is hyperbilirubinemia and the presentation is generally mild, particularly if the Coombs-direct antibody test (DAT) is negative.

Bilirubin causes jaundice, which is easily visible to the eye. However, visualization is an unreliable indicator of the severity of disease or risk. For this reason, routine screening is important, especially for infants with deeply pigmented skin (American Academy of Pediatrics Subcommittee on Hyperbilirubinemia [AAP], 2004).

Infants with ABO incompatibility should be closely monitored and their bilirubin levels plotted to determine their level of risk for hyperbilirubinemia. Diagnosis of ABO incompatibility can be quickly established shortly after the birth. A blood type and DAT should be determined for all infants born to mothers with blood type O. Infants found to have a blood type of A or B, who also have a positive DAT, have a confirmed diagnosis of ABO incompatibility. However, a positive test does not indicate that severe hyperbilirubinemia will develop. It is important and necessary to evaluate the risk of HD. Serial bilirubin levels, a complete blood count (CBC), reticulocyte count, and history of a sibling who was treated for significant hyperbilirubinemia are all predictors for HD (Bhat & Kumar, 2014).

Bilirubin levels for term newborns are typically drawn at the time of the metabolic screening and repeated at 8-hour intervals through discharge or initiation of phototherapy. However, with ABO incompatibility, hyperbilirubinemia is often seen within the first 24 hours of life. Bilirubin levels are plotted over hours of life and correlated to the risk of hyperbilirubinemia. The result is a four-zone risk stratification for newborns in which zone 1 is low risk, zone 2 is low-intermediate risk, zone 3 is high-intermediate risk, and zone 4 is high risk (Bhutani, Johnson, & Sivieri, 1999). Use of this nomogram is best practice for monitoring newborns with hyperbilirubinemia (AAP Committee for Hyperbilirubinemia, 2004).

Phototherapy is used for infants whose bilirubin levels rise into the moderate to high-risk zone (Bhutani, Vilms, & Hamerman-Johnson, 2010). Bilirubin levels that are critical may require intravenous immunoglobulin (IVIG), or more rarely, an exchange transfusion (Smits-Wintjens et al., 2013).

Among newborns who receive phototherapy, roughly 50% will also have evidence of hemolysis on their CBC analysis (Bhat & Kumar, 2012). Hemolytic anemia occurs when the infant's RBCs break down faster than normal in relation to the mother's antibodies. Maternal antibodies may remain in the infant for a few weeks after birth. As a result, the infant may require a blood transfusion.

NURSING INTERVENTIONS, MANAGEMENT, AND IMPLICATIONS

Nurses are integral to identifying and closely monitoring risk factors for ABO incompatibility and hyperbilirubinemia. Mothers with blood type O need to be quickly identified so that their infant's blood can be typed and screened. The health care providers responsible for the infants care need to be notified with the results of the lab work so the infant can be closely monitored for hyperbilirubinemia and hemolysis (AAP Committee for Hyperbilirubinemia, 2004).

The infant with ABO incompatibility will benefit from breastfeeding early and at frequent intervals. For the infant whose mother who does not elect to breast-feed, small frequent feedings are beneficial. Both keep the infant well hydrated, which helps to clear the by-products of hemolysis and reduce the risk of kernicterus, which results from unmanaged hyperbilirubinemia.

Oral intake and urine output are monitored closely. The jaundiced infant may be fatigued, may have low muscle tone, and or lethargy. All of these findings may contribute to difficulty feeding and mild dehydration. Often, the baby may require intravenous (IV) fluid. The urine may be darker in color because the infant elimi-nates bilirubin in the urine as well as the stool.

Parents need to understand the importance of pro-viding adequate fluid intake and recording urine and stool output. Because exclusively breastfed infants and those born before 38 completed weeks of gestation face increased risk for clinically significant hyperbilirubine-mia, nurses need to teach families about the risks asso-ciated with hyperbilirubinemia. This understanding enables parents to advocate for their babies after they are discharged from the hospital (Centers for Disease Control and Prevention [CDC], n.d.).

Nurses must also be knowledgeable about the types of therapies used for treatment of ABO incompatibility: phototherapy, IVIG administration, and exchange trans-fusion. Each treatment modality has risks associated with it and nurses must be aware of these risk factors so that symptoms can be identified early, if they occur.

OUTCOMES

Rarely does ABO incompatibility cause major sequelae in infants. Severe anemia as a result of hemolysis is known to occur. Kernicterus, as a result of extremely high bilirubin levels, is decreased with early and aggres-sive phototherapy.

Summary

Although ABO incompatibility is easily detected and primary treatment is close monitoring and photother-apy, it is important to ensure screening for HD. It is the most common type of isoimmune hemolytic ane-mia in the United States; can be diagnosed easily and early; and primary treatment, including adequate fluid intake and phototherapy, presents low risk and low cost. More severe forms of neonatal ABO incompati-bility and HD are rare, but easily detected and treated. Nursing plays an integral role in the identification of at-risk newborns. Guidelines should be in place so that nurses may track bilirubin levels in hours of life on the nomogram.

Best practices include development and adher-ence to evidence-based protocols for hyperbilirubine-mia screening that include universal screening of all babies at 12 to 24 hours of life. Bilirubin levels (either transcutaneous or serum) should be plotted in hours of life on the nomogram to determine risk (Cabra & Whitfield, 2005).

Nurses must also be aware of treatment modalities and their risk factors. In addition, nurses must prepare their families well by educating them on risk factors of hyperbilirubinemia, treatment, and appropriate fol-low-up in the primary care setting until bilirubin levels start to decline.

American Academy of Pediatrics Subcommittee on Hyperbilirubinemia. (2004). Management of hyperbili-rubinemia in the newborn infant 35 or more weeks of gestation. *Pediatrics, 114*(1), 297–316. Retrieved from http://pediatrics.aappublications.org/content/114/1/297 .long

Basu, S., Kaur, R., & Kaur, G. (2011). Hemolytic disease of the fetus and newborn: Current trends and perspectives. *Asian Journal of Transfusion Science, 5*(1), 3–7.

Bhat, R. Y., & Kumar, P. C. (2012). Morbidity of ABO hae-molytic disease in the newborn. *Paediatric International Child Health, 32*(2), 93–96.

Bhat, R. Y., & Kumar, P. C. (2014). Sixth hour transcutane-ous bilirubin predicting significant hyperbilirubinemia in ABO incompatible neonates. *World Journal of Pediatrics, 10*(2), 182–185.

Bhutani, V. K., Johnson, L., & Sivieri, E. M. (1999). Predictive ability of a predischarge hour-specific serum bilirubin for subsequent significant hyperbilirubinemia in healthy term and near-term newborns. *Pediatrics, 103*(1), 6–14.

Bhutani, V. K., Vilms, R. J., & Hamerman-Johnson, L. (2010). Universal bilirubin screening for severe neonatal hyperbilirubinemia. *Journal of Perinatology, 30*(Suppl.), S6–S15.

Cabra, M. A., & Whitfield, J. M. (2005). The challenge of pre-venting neonatal bilirubin encephalopathy: A new nurs-ing protocol in the well newborn nursery. *Proceedings, 18*(3), 217–219.

Centers for Disease Control & Prevention. (n.d.). Jaundice & kernicterus: Guidelines and tools for health professionals. Retrieved from http://www.cdc.gov/ncbddd/jaundice/hcp.html

Roberts, I. A. (2008). The changing face of haemolytic disease of the newborn. *Early Human Development, 84*(8), 515–523. doi:10.1016/j.earlhumdev.2008.06.005

Smits-Wintjens, V. E., Rath, M. E., van Zwet, E. W., Oepkes, D., Brand, A., Walther, F. J., & Lopriore, E. (2013). Neonatal morbidity after exchange transfusion for red cell alloimmune hemolytic disease. *Neonatology, 103*(2), 141–147.

■ ACUTE RENAL FAILURE

Christine Horvat Davey

Overview

Acute renal failure (ARF), also known as *acute kidney injury*, is a reversible acute decline in renal function with rapid onset (Devarajan, 2017). ARF is marked by a decrease in glomerular filtration rate, an inability of the kidneys to regulate fluid and electrolyte homeostasis as well as an increase in serum creatinine and blood urea nitrogen levels (Andreoli, 2009). The exact incidence of infant ARF is unknown. Nursing care for infants with ARF focuses on determination and treatment of the underlying cause with early medical management to decrease long-term sequelae.

Background

After birth, the kidneys undergo a maturation process and continue to further adapt, which is a vital element in prevention and management of neonatal ARF (Nada, Bohachea, & Askenazi, 2017). The number of nephrons present at birth is attributed to genetic and fetal environmental factors and range from 300,000 to 1.8 million per kidney (Nada et al., 2017). Premature infants with ARF can be at an increased risk for long-term kidney issues depending on the status of their nephrons (Nada et al., 2017). The incidence of ARF is rising in relation to increased use of advanced medical technology for infants who are critically ill or experience chronic conditions (Devarajan, 2017).

ARF in infants is rarely caused by a primary renal issue, but rather caused by reversible prerenal failure due to poor perfusion of kidneys, acute tubular necrosis, or cortical necrosis (Coulthard, 2016). Hypotension is the primary cause of poor perfusion and can be caused by cardiac failure, hypovolemia, vasodilation associated with sepsis, multiple organ failure, or a combination of these (Coulthard, 2016). There are several additional factors associated with an increased risk for development of ARF in infants, including premature birth, birth weight, nephrotoxicity, genetics, hypoxia, ischemia, acute injury, or illness. Premature birth can lead to a low nephron count and incomplete nephrogenesis, contributing to an increased risk for the development of ARF. A low birth weight places infants at a higher risk for developing ARF (Arcinue, Kantak, & Elkhwad, 2015). Nephrotoxin-induced ARF is often related to hospitalization because hospitalization poses an increased risk for exposure to medications that are nephrotoxic (Sutherland et al., 2013). In addition to environmental factors, there may be genetic risk factors for ARF. Several candidate polymorphisms have shown an association with ARF (Andreoli, 2009).

The diagnosis of ARF is most often based on characteristic signs and symptoms: edema, decreased urine output, hematuria, and/or hypertension with abnormal laboratory results, especially an abnormal serum creatinine level. A normal serum creatinine level for an infant is 0.2 to 0.4 mg/dL (18–35 µmol/L; Devarajan, 2017). Diagnostic use of serum creatinine levels can present issues. Following ARF, serum creatinine is an insensitive and delayed measure of decreased kidney function (Andreoli, 2009). Serum creatinine may not increase until a 50% or higher reduction in glomerular filtration rate is present (Devarajan, 2017). In addition, if dialysis is initiated as a treatment, serum creatinine levels cannot be measured accurately. An abnormal urinalysis can also indicate ARF, though individuals with prerenal ARF may display a normal urinalysis. Urinalysis is most often utilized to determine the underlying cause of ARF. Regardless of the limitations posed by serum creatinine levels in this diagnosis, it is presently the best laboratory test for diagnosis of ARF in infants.

The ability to classify causes of ARF can lead to early and targeted medical interventions. ARF in infants is often multifactorial. Causes of ARF can be prerenal, renal (intrinsic), and postrenal. Prerenal ARF signifies a functional alteration without actual kidney damage (Nada et al., 2017). This can present as a rise in serum creatinine levels, nitrogen retention, and oliguria. Several factors can lead to prerenal ARF, including decreased renal perfusion, increased capillary permeability, decreased oncotic pressure, and medication exposure. Decreased renal perfusion can result from hypotension, decreased cardiac output, and decreased intravascular volume (Nada et al., 2017). Increased capillary permeability can be due to sepsis. Exposure to certain medications prenatally or postnatally, such as nonsteroidal anti-inflammatory drugs (NSAIDs) and angiotensin-converting enzyme (ACE) inhibitors, can also contribute to prerenal ARF.

Renal ARF is characterized by persistent functional alterations that are not appropriately corrected and lead to kidney damage and acute tubular necrosis (Nada et al., 2017). Renal ARF can be caused by vascular compromise, renal artery thrombosis, renal infarction, or medications. Vascular compromise can be induced by bilateral renal vein thrombosis, which is often seen in umbilical artery catheter malposition (Nada et al., 2017). Medications known to induce renal ARF include antimicrobial medications such as aminoglycosides, gentamicin, acyclovir, intravenous immunoglobulin (IVIG), and radiocontrast agents.

Postrenal ARF is the least common form and is often caused by intrinsic obstructions, such as tumors, fungal balls, or may be congenital (Nada et al., 2017). Urethral strictures due to traumatic bladder cauterization or malfunctioning indwelling urinary catheters can also cause postrenal ARF (Nada et al., 2017). Correction of the obstruction usually results in renal function improvement.

Clinical Aspects

ASSESSMENT

As soon as the diagnosis of known or suspected ARF is determined, further assessment is dedicated to identifying the underlying cause. This evaluation includes an accurate record of an individual's physical assessment, medical history, and laboratory data. The physical assessment should focus on signs and symptoms related to alterations in renal function. These assessment findings include oliguria or anuria, edema, hematuria, and or hypertension (Devarajan, 2017). Nursing responsibilities include accurate blood pressure measurement, assessment for edema, or volume depletion (indicated by dry mucous membranes, decreased skin turgor, tachycardia, orthostatic falls in blood pressure, and decreased peripheral perfusion), recent weight gain, signs of system disease (rash or joint disease), enlarged palpable kidneys (may indicate renal vein thrombosis), and or enlarged bladder (may indicate urethral obstruction; Devarajan, 2017).

An accurate history is essential because there is often a known etiologic factor that predisposes an infant to ARF. These factors include heart failure, shock, or a preceding streptococcal infection seen in patients with poststreptococcal glomerulonephritis (Devarajan, 2017). Laboratory data to monitor when there is a concern for alterations in renal function include elevation of serum creatinine and/or blood urea nitrogen levels, abnormal urinalysis, hyperkalemia, hyponatremia, or less often hypernatremia, metabolic acidosis, hypocalcemia, and/or hyperphosphatemia. Renal imaging can also be performed or on rare occasions a kidney biopsy may be conducted to determine underlying cause. Utilization of an accurate physical assessment, medical history, and laboratory data can facilitate initiation of proper and timely nursing care that can positively impact patient outcomes.

NURSING INTERVENTIONS, MANAGEMENT, AND IMPLICATIONS

Nursing care of infants with ARF should focus on treatment of ARF and prevention of long-term sequelae. Nursing care includes monitoring of vital signs, including maintenance of proper blood pressure, daily weights, strict accurate measurement of intake and output, maintenance of proper electrolyte balance and nutrition, determination of underlying cause and correction of the cause, initiation of treatment such as hemodialysis if necessary, peritoneal dialysis or continuous renal reperfusion therapy (CRRT), monitoring of laboratory data, and psychological support for the family unit.

OUTCOMES

The anticipated outcomes of nursing evidence-based practice focus on treatment of ARF and prevention of long-term sequelae. Early determination of ARF based on signs, symptoms, and laboratory data as well as prompt correction of the underlying cause facilitate positive outcomes. Urine output is a key indicator for management of ARF in infants due to the fact that low urine volumes limit fluid administration and, in turn, restrict nutrition (Coulthard, 2016). A primary focus in reversing ARF is correction of hypotension. Therefore, corrective measures include fluid resuscitation, cardiac inotropic support, correcting coagulopathies, and treating infections (Coulthard, 2016). It is vital to avoid fluid overload and inadequate nutrition. In addition to correction of underlying causes of ARF and management of signs and symptoms, treatment options can include hemodialysis, peritoneal dialysis, and CRRT.

Effective nursing care outcomes should result in correction of ARF without long-term sequelae.

Summary

It is of utmost importance to recognize the early signs and symptoms of ARF as well as to differentiate among prerenal, intrinsic, and postrenal failure. Morbidity and mortality are dependent on the etiology of the renal failure. Early recognition and medical management can facilitate positive outcomes and decrease incidence of long-term sequelae.

Andreoli, S. P. (2009). Acute kidney injury in children. *Pediatric Nephrology, 24*(2), 253–263.

Arcinue, R., Kantak, A., & Elkhwad, M. (2015). Acute kidney injury in ELBW infants (< 750 grams) and its associated risk factors. *Journal of Neonatal–Perinatal Medicine, 8*(4), 349–357.

Coulthard, M. G. (2016). The management of neonatal acute and chronic renal failure: A review. *Early Human Development, 102,* 25–29.

Devarajan, P. (2017). Acute kidney injury: Still misunderstood and misdiagnosed. *Nature Reviews Nephrology, 13*(3), 137–138.

Nada, A., Bonachea, E. M., & Askenazi, D. J. (2017). Acute kidney injury in the fetus and neonate. *Seminars in Fetal & Neonatal Medicine, 22*(2), 90–97.

Sutherland, S. M., Ji, J., Sheikhi, F. H., Widen, E., Tian, L., Alexander, S. R., & Ling, X. B. (2013). AKI in hospitalized children: Epidemiology and clinical associations in a national cohort. *Clinical Journal of the American Society of Nephrology, 8*(10), 1661–1669.

■ ANEMIA OF PREMATURITY

Barbara Greitzer Slone

Overview

Anemia of prematurity, anemia in preterm infants, or neonatal anemia are interchangeable terms used to refer to a low hemoglobin (Hb) or hematocrit (Hct) concentration of more than 2 standard deviations below the mean for postnatal age. It is a major problem encountered in neonatal intensive care units (NICUs) (Colombatti, Sainati, & Trevisanuto, 2016). Blood transfusions, administration of iron, and erythropoiesis-stimulating agent administration are common nursing care measures in NICUs to address this clinical issue. There is also a role for the nurse in the promotion of delayed cord clamping for the prevention of anemia in this cohort of patients (Katheria, Truong, Cousins, Oshiro, & Finer, 2015).

Background

All infants experience a drop in their Hb/Hct levels after birth in the first few weeks of life. This is called *physiologic anemia of the newborn* and it may go unnoticed. In preterm infants, the anemia is more pronounced and the drop is faster, often presenting with symptoms, including pallor, tachypnea, poor feeding, poor growth, lethargy, and tachycardia and frequently requiring treatment (Gardner, 2016). Anemia of prematurity is present in all preterm infants, but may not cause symptoms. Infants equal to or less than 32 weeks gestation often require blood transfusions, one citation estimating 80% of infants less than 32 weeks gestation require transfusion (Colombatti et al., 2016).

Anemia of prematurity presents with normocytic, normochromic, hyporegenerative anemia, and this can be determined when evaluating the results of the complete blood count (CBC). The reticulocyte count is the index that reveals the bone marrow's response to the anemia; a higher count indicates more new red blood cells are being manufactured.

Preterm infants, particularly those at 32 weeks or less, frequently require myriad medical interventions to assist the infant to breathe, digest nutrients, and maintain homeostasis. These medical interventions require frequent blood sampling to assess their adequacy. The preterm infant is ill equipped to respond to this demand for blood sampling. Preterm infants frequently are iron deficient, nutritionally deficient, and suffer from other chronic illnesses, which all contribute to their anemia.

Erythropoiesis, or the making of new red blood cells, is a complex phenomenon in a newborn infant and quite different from that of an adult. During human gestation, blood formation initially occurs in the yolk sac; during the second trimester, this moves to the liver, spleen, and lymph nodes. Finally, in the last half of gestation, the bone marrow takes over (Colombatti et al., 2016). Premature infants are still in the process of switching over to erythropoiesis in the bone marrow. Newborns are also born with a predominance of fetal Hb, which carries a higher affinity for oxygen and is necessary for intrauterine life. The fetal Hb has a shorter life span and in the first few weeks after birth, the newborn will switch over to adult Hb, resulting in a more rapid increase in destruction of red blood cells. As the newborn transitions from the hypoxic intrauterine environment to the oxygen-rich postnatal environment, erythropoietin production is decreased, resulting in less production of red blood cells. The preterm newborn in this physiologic milieu is predisposed to anemia.

Iron deficiency is an additional contributing factor to the severity of anemia of prematurity. Iron stores at birth are largely obtained in the last trimester of pregnancy. Children developing iron deficiency in the first year of life are more at risk for developing neurocognitive sequelae, with poorer school performance and memory tasks (Kling & Coe, 2016). Factors that contribute to decreased iron stores include prematurity; multiple gestation; male gender; small size for gestational age; large size for gestational age; and maternal factors of obesity, diabetes, placental dysfunction, stress, ethnicity, low socioeconomic status, and maternal iron deficiency anemia (Kling & Coe, 2016).

Erythropoiesis-stimulating agents (erythropoietin), once widely used to aid in the prevention of anemia of prematurity, have come into disfavor. There has been an association between use of these agents and cancers in adults (Hitti, 2017). In the newborn population, there is limited evidence for the efficacy of this therapy and in a Cochrane review published in 2014, the authors concluded that the administration of epoetin alfa did not significantly reduce or increase any clinically important adverse outcomes (Aher & Ohlsson, 2014). These agents are no longer being routinely used in most NICUs.

There is a growing body of evidence for delayed cord clamping in the delivery room and its positive effect on decreasing the incidence and severity of anemia in the preterm infant. This practice essentially provides the patient with additional cells from the blood supply of the placenta (World Health Organization, 2012). Here the nurse can educate the family and be supportive of her or his delivery-room colleagues.

Clinical Aspects

ASSESSMENT

The laboratory assessment of anemia of prematurity is largely done by obtaining a CBC of the infant. The evaluation of the Hb and Hct is dependent on the gestational age of the infant, chronological age of the infant, and the need for oxygen therapy. The severity of the infant's illness also needs to be considered. In general, the sicker the infant, the greater the need for a higher Hgb/Hct.

NURSING INTERVENTIONS, MANAGEMENT, AND IMPLICATIONS

Nursing is integral to evaluating infants for anemia. On physical examination, pallor, increased work of breathing, substernal and intercostal retractions, tachycardia, or tachypnea can all be indicators of anemia. Anemia also frequently presents with apnea, bradycardia, desaturations, lethargy, poor feeding, or tachypnea after feeds and poor growth.

An astute nurse can assess these symptoms and ensure that the patient is receiving appropriate treatment by describing the infant's vital signs, feeding tolerance, and changes in oxygen requirements to the care provider. In addition, the nurse should ensure that there is a regular, systematic surveillance of all the preterm infants to determine whether intervention is required. Typically, in clinical practice, surveillance includes a CBC differential and a reticulocyte count.

Prevention of anemia is by attentiveness to the necessity of all blood sampling for laboratory tests, careful attention to obtaining only the minimal amount of blood needed for each test, and vigilance during blood sampling to prevent extraneous loss. The mainstay of treatment is a blood transfusion. Packed red blood cells that are irradiated and leukocyte poor are used. They must be typed and cross-matched for each individual patient. Consent from the parent or guardian must be obtained. The usual dose is 15 mL/kg given over 3 hours intravenously. Exposure to multiple donors can be limited by the use of small aliquots of blood sourced from the same donor. In infants who are chronically ill with lung disease and who require ventilatory support, the transfusion can be followed by a dose of furosemide to minimize the effects of the additional fluid on the cardiovascular system of the patient. Transfusion-related gut injury concerns have led many practitioners to keep patients on nothing-per-os status (NPO) for 3 hours prior to, during, and 3 hours posttransfusions. This requires that the nurse evaluates the blood sugar levels of the patient before, during, and after the infusion.

Iron supplementation is routinely given to infants who are able to tolerate full feeds. The iron may be in a liquid multivitamin form or may be given separately. The role of the nurse is to ensure that all infants are given iron supplementation in the nursery and to provide parental education on the administration of the supplement and importance of continuing iron therapy at home.

OUTCOMES

Infants with anemia of prematurity may demonstrate apnea, poor growth patterns, and cardiovascular compromise if not treated. Anemia of prematurity is a transient, physiologic process that is exacerbated by multiple blood draws when the infant is ill and rapid growth during the recovery phase. Anemia of prematurity will resolve with good nutrition, careful monitoring of the hemoglobin and reticulocyte count, and iron supplementation.

Summary

Anemia of prematurity is a common problem in neonatal intensive care. Nurses can play a pivotal role in the prevention, recognition, and treatment of this problem. This can prevent both short-term and long-term consequences and neurodevelopmental sequelae in this patient population.

Aher, S. M., & Ohlsson, A. (2014). Early erythropoietin for preventing red blood cell transfusion in preterm and/or low birth weight infants. *Cochrane Database of Systematic Reviews, 2014*(4). doi:10.1002/14651858

Buonocore, G. (2014). Erythropoietin use in the newborn. *Italian Journal of Pediatrics, 40*(Suppl. 2), A41. Siena, Italy: Biomed Central.

Colombatti, R., Sainati, L., & Trevisanuto, D. (2016). Anemia and tranfusion in the neonate. *Seminars in Fetal and Neonatal Medicine, 21*, 2–9.

Gardner, S. L. (2016). *Merenstein & Gardner's handbook of neonatal intensive care* (8th ed.). St. Louis, MO: Elsevier.

Hitti, M. (2017). WebMD: Cancer home. Retrieved from http://www.webmd.com/cancer/news/20171108/anemia-drugs-change-black-box-warning#1

Katheria, A. C., Truong, G., Cousins, L., Oshiro, B., & Finer, N. N. (2015). Umbilical cord milking versus delayed cord clamping in preterm infants. *Pediatrics, 136*, 61–69.

Kling, P. J., & Coe, C. L. (2016). Iron hemostasis in pregnancy, the fetus, and the neonate. *NeoReviews, 12*(11), e657–e664.

World Health Organization. (2012). *Delayed clamping of the umbilical cord to reduce infant anemia.* Geneva, Switzerland: Author.

■ APNEA OF PREMATURITY

Amy Bieda

Overview

Apnea of prematurity (AOP) is a common clinical problem affecting premature infants that is related to developmental immaturity. By definition, it is the cessation of breathing for more than 15 to 20 seconds accompanied by bradycardia (heart rate less than 80 beats/min) and desaturations (SpO_2 less than 80%; Zhao, Gonzales, & Mu, 2011). AOP is inversely related to gestational age (Eichenwald & AAP Committee on Fetus and Newborn, 2016). The majority of infants with a birth weight less than 1,000 g and a gestational age less than 28 weeks at birth develop AOP (Morton & Smith, 2016). It is rarely experienced by infants born at greater than 37 weeks gestational age (Fairchild et al., 2016). Neonatal intensive care unit (NICU) nurses are at the forefront of managing infants with AOP.

Background

Apnea is classified as central, obstructive, or mixed. Central apnea is the complete termination of respirations, which occurs due to the immaturity of the brainstem and resultant poor control of the central respiratory drive. Obstructive apnea occurs when there is no airflow within the upper airway, particularly at the level of the pharynx, while the infant continues to have respiratory effort. Mixed apnea involves an event of central apnea that is directly followed by or preceded by an obstructive apnea event. The majority of premature infants experience mixed apnea, which occurs as an episode of apnea and bradycardia with desaturation. AOP needs to be distinguished from periodic breathing in which pauses in respiration last for as long as 20 seconds and alternate with breathing. Newborns of all gestational ages will have periodic breathing, which is a normal variant of respiration in the neonate. However, if the respiratory pause lasts more than 20 seconds, it is considered apnea and requires ongoing observation and may require treatment.

Due to the immaturity of the respiratory system, premature infants have an altered response to hypoxia and hypercapnia. In response to hypoxia, infants experience ventilatory depression, which is a transient increase in respiratory rate followed by a decrease in spontaneous respirations below the infant's baseline respiratory rate. This pattern may recur over several weeks. Various neurotransmitters are involved in hypoxic ventilatory depression. In response to hypercapnia, premature infants have a decreased respiratory rate and prolonged exhalation, unlike adults, who will increase their respiratory rate when hypercapnic (Darnall, 2010). Hypercapnic ventilatory response is primarily mediated by central chemoreceptors.

The laryngeal chemoreflex is involved in the control of breathing. This reflex protects the lungs from aspiration. However, in the premature infant, an exaggerated response to stimulation of the laryngeal mucosa can lead to apnea, bradycardia, and hypotension. The passage of a feeding tube or vigorous suctioning of an infant is an example of stimulation that can trigger a bradycardic episode, followed by apnea. As infants mature, the laryngeal chemoreflex matures to respond more often by coughing and less often by apnea and swallowing (Thach, 2007). This laryngeal chemoreflex is mediated through superior laryngeal nerve afferents.

Although AOP is primarily attributed to physiologic immaturity, other factors may contribute. Functional residual capacity, the air left in the lung after an exhalation, is decreased due to pulmonary immaturity and increased chest wall compliance. This results in increased work of breathing for the infant, the development of diaphragmatic fatigue, and apnea. Apnea occurs more often during rapid eye movement (REM) sleep when infants have more paradoxical breathing than during quiet sleep. The mechanism of sucking, swallowing, breathing, and esophageal function is complex and requires physiologic maturity lacking in premature infants (Lau, 2015). Premature infants have difficulty coordinating this process with resultant apneic episodes during feeds.

Infants are traditionally obligate nose breathers. Irritation of the mucous membranes from a nasogastric tube and frequent suctioning of the nares contributes to swelling of the mucous membranes of the nasal passages with resultant obstruction of the nares. This in turn, may cause apnea.

Clinical Aspects

ASSESSMENT

AOP may be idiopathic. However, it is also a symptom of multiple pathologic conditions in the infant, including infection, intraventricular hemorrhage, seizures, electrolyte imbalance, inborn errors of metabolism, congestive heart failure, patent ductus arteriosus, anemia, necrotizing enterocolitis, and temperature instability. The association between gastroesophageal reflux (GER) and AOP is controversial. Although there is a temporal relationship, cause and affect have not been established.

In premature infants, pathologic conditions may present concurrent with apnea, cyanosis or pallor, and hypotonia and this is called *secondary apnea*. It is critical that the evaluation of an infant occurs in a timely fashion if an infant develops apnea or has increased apneic events.

In addition to the physical evaluation, it is important to read both the mother's and the infant's birth history to determine whether there are any factors that predispose to apnea. A complete blood count (CBC) and C-reactive protein (CRP) will assess for infection and anemia. A lumbar puncture may be necessary if the infant's history and current condition clinically indicate it. Electrolytes should be evaluated to assess for possible metabolic causes. A head ultrasound (HUS) may be needed to rule out intraventricular hemorrhage (IVH). A chest x-ray is done to assess respiratory and cardiac status.

NURSING INTERVENTIONS, MANAGEMENT, AND IMPLICATIONS

The nurse at the bedside is instrumental in the care of the infants with AOP. Cardiorespiratory and pulse oximetry monitors assist the nurse in monitoring apneic events. Documentation of apnea, bradycardia, and desaturation episodes is paramount. The nurse needs to document any event that occurs prior to the apnea; the length of the apnea; if the apnea is associated with a bradycardia, including how low the heart rate falls; if a desaturation occurred, how low the desaturation fell, as well as how long the desaturation lasted; any change in color; what intervention the nurse performed; and the infant's response to that intervention. Infants usually respond to gentle stimulation if they become apneic. In the event that the infant does not respond to the stimulation, the nurse needs to initiate bag-and-mask ventilation.

Positioning of the infant is extremely important. The nurse must assess the infant's alignment and keep the head at midline without extension or flexion of the neck. Term and healthy preterm infants should be placed supine, but it is not known whether preterm infants may benefit from prone or side-lying positions to help decreased apneic events (Bredemeyer & Foster, 2012).

Keeping premature infants in a neutral thermal environment is a basic tenant of neonatal nursing. Rapid changes in temperature have resulted in apneic events in infants (Gardner, Hines, & Nyp, 2016). Keeping an infant at the lower end of the neutral thermal environment, rather than the upper end, may help decrease the number of apneic events.

Respiratory support is commonly required. A number of noninvasive support measures, including high-flow nasal cannula, synchronized nasal intermittent positive-pressure ventilation (SNIPPV), nasal bi-level positive airway pressure (N-BiPAP), nasal continuous positive airway pressure (CPAP), and bubble CPAP may be required for an infant who does not respond to gentle stimulation or bag-and-mask ventilation. Sicker infants may require mechanical ventilation.

Medications are commonly used. Methylxanthines, such as caffeine citrate, aminophylline, and theophylline, are pharmacologic treatment modalities for AOP. Caffeine citrate is preferred because it only requires daily dosing, has a longer half-life, and a wider therapeutic index. Nurses should give caffeine in the morning in order to prevent disruption of sleep–wake patterns. Nurses need to be cognizant of the side effects of caffeine citrate therapy such as jitteriness, tachycardia, and feeding intolerance. Doxapram is another medication that has been used for treatment of AOP for over four decades in Europe, but is not used in the premature infant population in the United States because it contains benzyl alcohol.

Anemia may play a role in AOP. Increase in apneic events may occur at the time the premature infant's hemoglobin has fallen to its physiologic nadir. Treatment for AOP with packed red blood cell transfusions is controversial. Blood transfusions are usually reserved for infants with severe anemia who are having multiple apneic events daily.

OUTCOMES

Nurses play a critical role in the prevention and treatment of AOP. The sophisticated monitoring equipment available today alerts nurses when an infants' status is changing, but medical device alarm safety is a major patient safety issue. The majority of the equipment used in the hospital has some type of alarm system. Due to the number of false alarms triggered, nurses, as well as all members of the health care team have become sensory overloaded and desensitized. This is known as *alarm fatigue* (Sendelbach & Funk, 2013). As a result, health care team members may ignore, override, or turn off alarms (Tanner, 2013). Alarm fatigue has resulted in avoidable deaths. Most NICUs have set parameters for cardiorespiratory and pulse oximetry monitors. However, education needs to be ongoing to ensure safe patient care.

Summary

AOP is a common clinical problem and reflects physiologic immaturity. Current treatment modalities include xanthine therapy and noninvasive ventilator support. As infants mature the number of apneic events and the interval between apneic events should decrease in order to discharge the infant home safely. Parents need

extensive education, including infant cardiopulmonary resuscitation. Close, accurate monitoring and documentation of all apneic events is an important component of infant care and the ultimate responsibility of the bedside nurse.

Bredemeyer, S., & Foster, J. (2012). Body positioning for spontaneously breathing preterm infants with apnoea. *Cochrane Database of Systematic Reviews, 2012*(6), CD004951. doi:10.1002/14651858.CD004951.pub2

Darnall, R. A. (2010). The role of CO_2 and central chemoreception in the control of breathing in the fetus and the neonate. *Respiratory Physiology and Neurobiology, 173*(3), 201–212.

Eichenwald, E. C., & AAP Committee on Fetus and Newborn. (2016). Apnea of prematurity. *Pediatrics, 137*(1), e20153757.

Fairchild, K., Mohr, M., Paget-Brown, A., Tabacaru, C., Lake, D., Delos, J., . . . Kattwinkel, J. (2016). Clinical associations of immature breathing in preterm infants. Part 1: Central apnea. *Pediatric Research, 80*(1), 21–27.

Gardner, S., Hines, M., & Nyp, M. (2016). Respiratory disease. In S. Gardner, B. Carter, M. Enzman Hines, & J. Hernandez (Eds.), *Merenstein & Gardner's handbook of neonatal intensive care* (pp. 647–673). St. Louis, MO: Elsevier.

Lau, C. (2015). Development of suck and swallow mechanisms in infants. *Annals of Nutrition and Metabolism, 66*(5), 7–14.

Morton, S., & Smith, V. (2016). Treatment option for apnoea of prematurity. *Archives of Disease in Children-Fetal and Neonatal Edition, 101*, 352–356.

Sendelbach, S., & Funk, M. (2013). Alarm fatigue: A patient safety concern. *AACN Advanced Critical Care, 24*(4), 378–386.

Tanner, T. (2013). The problem of alarm fatigue. *Nursing for Women's Health, 17*(2), 153–157.

Thach, B. (2007). Maturation of cough and other reflexes that protect the fetal and neonatal airway. *Pulmonary Pharmacology and Therapeutics, 20*(4), 365–370.

Zhao, J., Gonzalez, F., & Mu, D. (2011). Apnea of prematurity: From cause to treatment. *European Journal of Pediatrics, 170*(9), 1097.

■ BRONCHOPULMONARY DYSPLASIA

Amy Bieda

Overview

Bronchopulmonary dysplasia (BPD) is a multifactorial disorder that evolves in infants born prematurely. These infants require some degree of mechanical ventilation and have an oxygen requirement due to respiratory distress (Davidson & Berkelhamer, 2017). Extremely premature infants are at the highest risk of developing BPD because it usually occurs at a pivotal stage of lung development. With the advent of postnatal corticosteroids, surfactant therapy, and improved ventilator management, the survival rate has increased, resulting in infants with this long-term morbidity. Infants with BPD may have prolonged hospitalizations and multiple hospital readmissions, especially during the first year of life. Approximately 10,000 to 15,000 infants are diagnosed yearly in the United States, with a prevalence of males over females (Jensen & Schmidt, 2014).

Background

Northway, Rosan, and Porter (1967) first described BPD in a group of moderate to late premature infants who developed pulmonary changes on chest radiograph with respiratory failure related to long-term mechanical ventilation and prolonged exposure to high levels of oxygen. These changes included areas of atelectasis and marked scarring with hyperinflation, pulmonary fibrosis, and smooth muscle hypertrophy in the pulmonary vasculature. This description is referred to as "classic" BPD.

The introduction of surfactant therapy in the early 1990s, increased use of antenatal steroids, and improvements in ventilator technology changed the clinical presentation of BPD (Jensen & Schmidt, 2014) and a new pathophysiology emerged. In this group of infants, alveoli formation may stop or there may be a decrease in alveolar growth. Lung changes include less pulmonary fibrosis, inflammation, and smooth muscle hypertrophy with an increase in lung fluid and damage to vascular development. These changes are derived from an interruption in lung development rather than barotrauma and volutrauma from mechanical ventilation and was labeled the "new" BPD.

In 2001, the National Institute of Child Health and Human Development (NICHD) proposed a change in the definition of BPD in infants less than 32 weeks gestational age. This definition was based on the severity of lung disease and the need for supplemental oxygen at 28 days of life and/or method of ventilatory support at 36 weeks postmenstrual age. However, due to wide practice variations in neonatal intensive care units (NICUs) and the spectrum of the severity of this disease, the new definition has limitations (Davidson & Berkelhamer, 2017).

Antenatal risk factors, such as chorioramnionitis, lack of antenatal steroids, and fetal growth restriction, have been implicated as prenatal risks for the development of BPD. The risk factor of chorioramnionitis is controversial due to its complex nature. Empirical research suggests that inflammation increases surfactant production and promotes lung maturation (Davidson & Berkelhamer, 2017), whereas animal models suggest lung injury. There are multiple confounders making it difficult to determine a causal relationship.

Antenatal steroids are a primary prophylactic treatment of women who are in preterm labor (ACOG [American Congress of Obstetricians and Gynecologists] Committee on Obstetric Practice, 2011) and their use has contributed to decreased respiratory distress syndrome (RDS) and morbidities common in premature infants. Although antenatal steroids stimulate lung maturation in the fetus, it has not decreased the rate of BPD.

Low birth weight is a robust predictor of BPD, especially in infants less than 28 weeks gestational age. Increased rates of BPD and aberrant pulmonary outcomes have also been demonstrated in preterm infants who are small for gestation age (SGA) or have intrauterine growth restriction (IUGR) at delivery (Poindexter & Martin, 2015).

Clinical Aspects

ASSESSMENT

Infants born extremely premature are in the canalicular stage of lung growth and mechanical ventilation interferes with normal lung development. Mechanical ventilation can contribute to volutrauma (increased lung volume or lung stretching) and barotrauma (excessive ventilator pressures) resulting in lung overdistention. As a result, there is a cycle of continuous injury to the lung with healing and rehealing (Gardner, Hines, & Nyp, 2016).

In addition, very sick infants may be exposed to high levels of supplemental oxygen therapy for prolonged periods. Hyperoxia causes acute pulmonary injury to the developing lung, resulting in inflammation, pulmonary edema, and thickening of the alveolar membrane. In addition to hyperoxia, preterm infants lack antioxidant mediators contributing to cytotoxic oxygen free radical production resulting in oxidative stress and further lung injury (Gien & Kinsella, 2011).

Infants with a patent ductus arteriosus (PDA) and persistent left-to-right (systemic to pulmonary) shunting of blood may have increased pulmonary circulation resulting in increased interstitial fluid. Increased interstitial fluid results in impaired pulmonary function and prolongs the need for mechanical ventilation as well as increases the need for supplemental oxygen, which contribute to the pathology of BPD (Gien & Kinsella, 2011). Infants with severe BPD may also develop pulmonary hypertension and cor pulmonale (right-sided heart failure).

An increased incidence of BPD has also been associated in infants with RDS who receive large volumes of fluid in the first few days of life. In a Cochrane review (Bell & Acarregui, 2014), careful regulation of fluid intake in premature infants may reduce the risk of BPD.

BPD in premature infants has been associated with postnatal nosocomial infection. Gram-positive and negative bacteria, cytomegalovirus (CMV), and adenovirus have been shown to increase the systemic inflammatory response in the lungs, resulting in the production and release of pro-inflammatory cytokines. Prolonged antibiotic use especially during the first week of life has also been implicated (Novitsky et al., 2015).

NURSING INTERVENTIONS, MANAGEMENT, AND IMPLICATIONS

In addition to surfactant therapy, which decreases the duration of mechanical ventilation and reduces the incidence of BPD, multiple modes of noninvasive respiratory modalities that do not require intubation/mechanical ventilation are available. Often infants are given surfactant via the endotracheal tube and then extubated to continuous positive airway pressure (CPAP), high-flow nasal cannula (HFNC), bi-level positive airway pressure (BIPAP), or nasal intermittent positive pressure ventilation (NIPPV). Permissive hypercapnia is a strategy that may reduce the risk of lung injury by accepting higher values of $PaCO_2$ while using lower tidal volumes and inspiratory pressures. This is to evade pulmonary overdistention.

Corticosteroids, such as dexamethasone, which reduce lung inflammation and improve gas exchange, may judiciously be used in the treatment of infants. Corticosteroids facilitate weaning and extubation from mechanical ventilation, but the medication has side effects, including hyperglycemia, hypertension, infection, and gastrointestinal bleeding, especially if given in the immediate postnatal period. Longitudinal studies have established that corticosteroids contribute to smaller head growth and abnormal neurological outcomes, including cerebral palsy (CP; Khetan, Hurley,

Spencer, & Bott, 2016). The type of corticosteroid, dose, and timing of initiation of therapy have not been determined (Onland, De Jaeger, Offringa, & vanKaam, 2017).

Other pharmacologic agents can be used in the treatment of BPD. Intravenous (IV) caffeine, if started in the first 3 days of life, helps in decreasing the incidence of BPD. Diuretics, such as furosemide (IV and oral), are loop diuretics used to treat the interstitial alveolar edema that is commonly seen. Thiazides, such as chlorothiazide and spironolactone, are also used. There is less electrolyte imbalance with the use of thiazides, which may decrease the need for furosemide.

Bronchodilators, such as albuterol and ipratropium bromide, can also be used to reduce reactive airway disease and help increase lung compliance. Premature infants at birth have low body stores of vitamin A, an antioxidant that is important in surfactant synthesis and the repair of lung epithelial cells. The administration of vitamin A starting after delivery may be useful in reducing oxygen use at 36 weeks postmenstrual age.

A PDA is usually treated either by surgical ligation, coil occlusion performed in a cardiac catheterization laboratory, or medically with either IV indomethacin or IV ibuprofen. All treatment modalities have associated risks. Current controversy exists as to whether to treat a PDA because the majority of them close spontaneously. Many centers are using a more cautious approach that includes clinical assessment of the infant, fluid restriction, and diuretic therapy.

Nutrition is an integral component in the management of premature infants. Postnatal growth is slower in infants with BPD and many have failure to thrive. These infants have high energy expenditure coupled by poor caloric intake, feeding difficulties, including oral aversion; complications of respiratory disease and may be fluid restricted on diuretic therapy resulting in poor linear growth and inadequate weight gain. Early enteral nutrition and increased protein in calorie-dense formula or fortified maternal breast milk are of prime importance in improving lung growth, lung repair, decreasing the risk and severity of BPD, and improving neurologic outcomes (Poindexter & Martin, 2015).

Caring for the infant with BPD requires a strong interdisciplinary team of neonatologists, pulmonologists, nurses, nutritionists, physical therapists, occupational therapists, social workers, and child life specialists. Nurses must have in-depth knowledge of the pathophysiology of BPD, arterial and capillary blood gases, medications, oxygen therapy, ventilator management, nutrition, and growth and development.

This group of infants can be challenging to care for and should have a dedicated core of nurses who understand not only the infant's physiologic status and recognition of any changes from baseline, but must understand the infant's nuances in behavior and responses to treatment.

Parent education is an ongoing process because these infants can be in the hospital for an extended period. Nurses must not only promote parent infant bonding but also help parents engage in socialization, language development, and emotional support of their infant.

OUTCOMES

Depending on the severity of BPD, these infants will have varying degrees of pulmonary sequelae. They are at greater risk for ongoing lung problems, especially lower respiratory infections. As a result, these infants have a higher rate of readmission to the hospital during the first year of life. Infants with BPD also have a higher rate of asthma and reactive airway disease. Many of these infants have cardiovascular problems that require long-term monitoring. The long-term health outcomes of these infants as older adults is relatively unknown.

Summary

BPD is a chronic condition that primarily affects premature infants. Current treatment modalities, such as noninvasive respiratory support, gentle ventilation, pharmacologic agents, and optimal nutrition, are imperative. However, the prevention of BPD is challenging and at the core of this is preventing premature birth.

American Congress of Obstetricians and Gynecologists Committee on Obstetric Practice. (2011). Opinion No. 475: Antenatal corticosteroid therapy for fetal maturation. *Obstetrics and Gynecology, 117*(2, Pt. 1), 422–424. doi:10.1097/AOG.0b013e31820eee00

Bell, E., & Acarregui, M. (2014). Restricted versus liberal water intake for preventing morbidity and mortality in preterm infants. Cochrane Neonatal Group. *Cochrane Database of Systematic Reviews, 2014,* 1–26. doi:10.1002/14651858.CD000503.pub3

Davidson, L., & Berkelhamer, S. (2017). Bronchopulmonary dysplasia: Chronic lung disease of infancy and long-term pulmonary outcomes. *Journal of Clinical Medicine, 6*(4), 4. doi:10.3390/jcm6010004

Gardner, S., Hines, M., & Nyp, M. (2016). Respiratory diseases. In C. Gardner, H. Enzman, & J, Hernandez (Eds.), *Merenstein and Gardner's handbook of neonatal intensive care* (pp. 565–643). St. Louis, MO: Elsevier.

Gien, J., & Kinsella, J. P. (2011). Pathogenesis and treatment of bronchopulmonary dysplasia. *Current Opinion in Pediatrics, 23*(3), 305–313.

Jensen, E. A., & Schmidt, B. (2014). Epidemiology of bronchopulmonary dysplasia. *Birth Defects Research Part A, Clinical and Molecular Teratology, 100*(3), 145–157.

Khetan, R., Hurley, M., Spencer, S., & Bhatt, J. M. (2016). Bronchopulmonary dysplasia within and beyond the neonatal unit. *Advances in Neonatal Care, 16*(1), 17–25; quiz E1.

Northway, W. H., Rosan, R. C., & Porter, D. Y. (1967). Pulmonary disease following respirator therapy of hyaline-membrane disease. Bronchopulmonary dysplasia. *New England Journal of Medicine, 276*(7), 357–368.

Novitsky, A., Tuttle, D., Locke, R. G., Saiman, L., Mackley, A., & Paul, D. A. (2015). Prolonged early antibiotic use and bronchopulmonary dysplasia in very low birth weight infants. *American Journal of Perinatology, 32*(1), 43–48.

Onland, W., De Jaegere, A. P., Offringa, M., & van Kaam, A. (2017). Systemic corticosteroid regimens for prevention of bronchopulmonary dysplasia in preterm infants. *Cochrane Database of Systematic Reviews, 2017*(1), CD010941. doi:10.1002/14651858

Poindexter, B. B., & Martin, C. R. (2015). Impact of nutrition on bronchopulmonary dysplasia. *Clinics in Perinatology, 42*(4), 797–806. doi:10.1016/j.clp.2015.08.007

■ DECREASED PULMONARY BLOOD FLOW

Jennifer Johntony
Jodi Zalewski

Overview

Decreased pulmonary blood flow results from the shunting of deoxygenated blood from the right side of the heart to the oxygenated left side of the heart (Nelson, Hirsch-Romano, Ohye, & Bove, 2015). Infants born with heart defects that cause a decrease in pulmonary blood flow present with cyanosis and hypoxemia due to a lack of blood flow to the lungs. The systolic and diastolic pressures on the right side of the heart exceed those on the left due to some form of obstruction to pulmonary blood flow, leading to this right-to-left shunting. Congenital heart defects (CHD) that result in decreased pulmonary blood include tetralogy of Fallot (TOF), pulmonary atresia, tricuspid atresia, and pulmonary stenosis.

Background

TOF accounts for approximately 4% of CHDs (Nelson et al., 2015). The classic description of TOF includes (a) the presence of a ventricular septal defect, (b) some form of right ventricular outflow track obstruction, (c) overriding of the aorta, and (d) right ventricular hypertrophy (Schroeder, Delaney, & Baker, 2015). The degree of cyanosis is often determined by the severity of the right ventricular outflow tract obstruction. The obstruction to the right ventricular outflow tract in TOF patients can start below the pulmonary valve and extend all the way out to the branches of the pulmonary arteries. If the obstruction is severe and degree of cyanosis is significant in the neonatal period, a palliative or temporizing procedure is often performed to increase oxygen saturation thereby increasing pulmonary blood flow (Schroeder et al., 2015). Complete repairs are generally performed in the first year of life. The operative mortality for total correction of TOF is less than 3% (Schroeder et al., 2015).

Pulmonary atresia is a relatively rare defect and accounts for approximately 1% of all congenital heart lesions (Park, 2016). In this disorder, the pulmonary valve is absent or atretic and the intraventricular septum can be either intact, or accompanied by a ventricular septal defect. This particular anatomy, in which the intraventricular septum is intact, leads to an absence of blood exiting the right ventricle into the main pulmonary artery (Nelson et al., 2015). Patients born with this disorder must have an interatrial communication (either atrial septal defect or patent foramen ovale) or the presence of a patent ductus arteriosus (PDA) to allow for adequate pulmonary blood flow and cardiac output after birth. To maintain patency of the ductus arteriosus, intravenous prostaglandin E1 (PGE1) is administered (Park, 2016). The size of the right ventricle and pulmonary arteries determines the type and success of surgical repair. If the size of the right ventricle and pulmonary arteries is adequate, a two-ventricular repair can be performed. If the size or function of the right ventricle is inadequate, a single ventricle palliative approach may be necessary (Nelson et al., 2015). The survival rate of pulmonary atresia varies and is determined by a biventricular repair, single ventricle palliation, or cardiac transplantation.

Tricuspid atresia accounts for 1% to 3% of all CHDs (Park, 2016). Tricuspid atresia, a complete lack of a tricuspid valve, results in the absence of direct communication between the right atrium and right ventricle (Nelson et al., 2015). Pulmonary blood flow is achieved when deoxygenated blood flows or shunts across an atrial septal defect from the right atrium to the left atrium, then to the left ventricle, through a ventricular septal defect and out to the lungs (Schroeder et al., 2015). The complete mixing of oxygenated and unoxygenated blood in the left atrium results in systemic desaturations and hypoxemia (Schroeder et al., 2015). This particular lesion is treated in three stages. The first-stage palliation for the majority of patients occurs in the newborn period and is the placement of a systemic to pulmonary artery shunt (modified Blalock–Taussig shunt) to maintain adequate pulmonary blood flow. The second procedure, referred to as the *Glenn procedure*, connects the superior vena cava directly to the pulmonary artery. In the third procedure, the Fontan, a direct connection between the inferior vena cava and pulmonary artery is created, thus completing the full separation of oxygenated and deoxygenated blood. All blood flow to the lungs is now passive and the single ventricle is solely responsible for pumping oxygenated blood to the body. The overall survival for tricuspid atresia is approximately 83% at 1 year, 70% at 10 years, and 60% at 20 years (Nelson et al., 2015).

Isolated pulmonary stenosis accounts for 10% of all CHDs and is defined as a thickening of the pulmonary valve at the entrance of the main pulmonary artery (Darst, Collins, & Miyamoto, 2016). This thickened pulmonary valve leads to variable levels of obstruction to pulmonary blood flow resulting in an increase in the right ventricular pressure that can be potentially life threatening (Darst et al., 2016). Neonates with severe pulmonary valve obstruction and minimal pulmonary blood flow present with cyanosis at birth (Darst et al., 2016). To minimize the patient's degree of cyanosis, the patency of the ductus arteriosus must be established with prostaglandins. Then the decision to treat the patient with either a balloon angioplasty of the pulmonary valve or surgical treatment with the placement of a modified Blalock–Taussig shunt is made. Long-term outcomes after balloon valvuloplasty are favorable; however, restenosis or valve incompetence may occur later in life (Schroeder et al., 2015).

Clinical Aspects

ASSESSMENT

Patients born with TOF can either present with cyanosis at birth, or develop it over time as the subvalvular obstruction increases (Darst et al., 2016). The patient's physical examination is positive for a grade II to IV/VI systolic ejection murmur that is heard best at the left sternal border in the third intercostal space and radiates to the lungs. Extreme cyanosis or hypoxic episodes occur causing severe "blue spells" or "tet spells." Hypercyanotic spells are defined as a sudden onset of cyanosis or deepening of cyanosis. Infants have dyspnea, alterations in consciousness from irritability to syncope with a decrease or disappearance of the systolic murmur (Darst et al., 2016).

Infants with pulmonary atresia present with cyanosis at birth and as the ductus arteriosus closes, they become more cyanotic (Darst et al., 2016). These patients have a continuous murmur due to the PDA (Park, 2016). To maintain pulmonary blood flow, patency of the ductus must be achieved with infusion of prostaglandins until surgery can be performed (Darst et al., 2016).

Infants with tricuspid atresia usually present with cyanosis at birth as well as tachycardia, tachypnea, and increased work of breathing (Schroeder et al., 2015). If there is a significant increase in pulmonary blood flow, they may develop symptoms of congestive heart failure, such as sweating, tachypnea, poor oral intake and increased time to orally feed, resulting in poor weight gain (Darst et al., 2016). A grade III/VI systolic murmur from the ventricular septal defect (VSD) is often heard at the lower left sternal border (Park, 2016).

Patients with pulmonary stenosis have variable presentations. Those with mild pulmonary stenosis are usually asymptomatic. Infants with severe pulmonary stenosis present often with hypoxic spells, failure to thrive, and right-heart failure (Nelson et al., 2015). The murmur of valvular pulmonary stenosis is an ejection click heard best at the upper left sternal border. A low-pitched murmur indicates less severe pulmonary stenosis (Park, 2016). Those patients may be followed symptomatically with mild to moderate pulmonary stenosis. Catheter-based intervention or surgical intervention should be considered for a gradient higher than 50 mmHg, progressive ventricular hypertrophy, or new tricuspid regurgitation.

NURSING INTERVENTIONS, MANAGEMENT, AND IMPLICATIONS

Nursing-related issues for infants with decreased pulmonary blood flow can vary depending on the lesion. These infants can experience cyanosis, dyspnea, tachycardia, irritability, and feeding difficulties.

It is important to become informed about the infant's cardiac anatomy and baseline clinical presentation in order to intervene when changes occur. The nurse should assess and record heart rate, respiratory rate, breath sounds, blood pressure, and pulse oximetry readings. Oxygen administration and nasopharyngeal suctioning may be required to maintain appropriate pulse oximetry and reduce respiratory distress. Any prescribed cardiac medications need to be given at the scheduled time and monitor for any side effects or signs and symptoms of toxicity, which should be reported and documented (Schroeder et al., 2015).

The nurse can decrease cardiac demands by minimizing unnecessary stress and stimulation. Nursing interventions must focus on providing maximum rest and comfort care such as offering nonnutritive sucking and swaddling. In order to promote energy conservation, nursing must organize activities that allow for uninterrupted sleep (Schroeder et al., 2015). In order to provide adequate nutrition, infants should be fed in a semiupright position and be offered small, frequent feedings.

Cyanotic infants must be well hydrated to maintain good cardiac output and to minimize their risk for cerebral vascular accidents due to polycythemia (Schroeder et al., 2015). Infants with decreased pulmonary blood flow are at risk for hypercyanotic spells, which occur suddenly and are typically observed in the setting of extreme agitation or painful stimulation. The interventions to reverse hypercyanotic spells centers around promoting an increase in pulmonary blood flow and include the following: place infant in a knee–chest position, calm the infant with comfort measures, administer 100% oxygen, give intravenous morphine, begin fluid replacement and volume expansion (Schroeder et al., 2015).

In any patient born with a cardiac defect, alteration in parenting related to the perception of the infant as vulnerable may exist. These families experience periods of shock, followed by tremendous anxiety, and oftentimes fear that their child may die (Schroeder et al., 2015). Nurses are instrumental in dealing with parental stress, provide support and education, and participate as an interdisciplinary team member in order to care for both the infants and their families.

OUTCOMES

Patients with congenital heart disease have outcomes specific to evidence-based nursing practice that focus on assisting the patient to demonstrate an improvement in cardiac function, a decrease in cardiac demands, and optimal blood flow to the lungs (Schroeder et al., 2015). Improvement in cardiac function occurs when there is a decrease in the afterload of the heart, thereby increasing the overall cardiac output.

Summary

Infants born with TOF, pulmonary atresia, tricuspid atresia, and pulmonary stenosis are at increased risk for decreased pulmonary blood flow due to an interruption of blood flow leaving the right side of the heart and entering the lungs. They may experience cyanosis, feeding issues, and inadequate weight gain. Many of these infants undergo palliative or corrective surgery within the first few weeks of life. Understanding each specific patient's cardiac anatomy is imperative to caring for the infant effectively. Providing efficient and holistic nursing care to hospitalized infants with congenital heart disease results in increased survival and quality of life in this vulnerable patient population.

Darst, J. R., Collins, K. K., & Miyamoto, S. D. (2016). Cardiovascular diseases. In W. W. Hay Jr., M. J. Levin, R. R. Deterding, & M. J. Abzug (Eds.), *Current diagnosis & treatment pediatrics* (23rd ed., pp. 601–625). New York, NY: McGraw-Hill.

Nelson, J. S., Hirsch-Romano, J. C., Ohye, R. G., & Bove, E. L. (2015). Congenital heart disease. In G. M. Doherty (Ed.), *Current diagnosis & treatment: Surgery* (14th ed., pp. 423–454). New York, NY: McGraw-Hill.

Park, M. (2016). *The pediatric cardiology handbook.* Philadelphia, PA: Elsevier Saunders.

Schroeder, M., Delaney, A., & Baker, A. (2015). The child with cardiovascular dysfunction. In M. Hockenberry & D. Wilson (Eds.), *Wong's nursing care of infants and children* (10th ed., pp. 1251–1285). St. Louis, MO: Elsevier Mosby.

■ EXTREMELY LOW-BIRTH-WEIGHT INFANT

Jenelle M. Zambrano

Overview

Extremely low-birth-weight (ELBW) infants are defined as infants weighing less than 1,000 g at birth (Mandy, 2016; Sherman, 2014). In 2013, 8% of the approximate 550,000 preterm infants born in the United States were low-birth-weight infants (Mandy, 2016). Fewer than 1% of the low-birth-weight infant population consists of ELBW infants (Mandy, 2016; Morris, 2015). Although ELBW infants account for a small percentage of overall births, they are generally the most critically ill and at the highest risk for death and disability (Glass et al., 2015; Sherman, 2014). Care of the ELBW infant is complex and requires understanding the ELBW subgroups and the pathophysiologic processes associated with each subgroup (Papageorgiou & Pelausa, 2014). Care for these infants requires expert management beginning in the delivery room and continuing in the neonatal intensive care unit (NICU). Careful consideration is necessary when providing respiratory, thermoregulatory, and nutritional support, and neuroprotective care (Morris, 2015; Sherman, 2014).

Background

Prematurity, defined as birth before 37 weeks of gestation, is a significant contributor to infant and child morbidity and mortality and is associated with one third of all infant deaths in the United States (Glass et al., 2015). The rate of premature births in the United States had been on a steady rise during the 1990s and early 2000s, but had begun to decrease annually in the early 2010s. However, in 2015, the U.S. premature birth rate increased for the first time in 8 years from 9.57% to 9.63% (March of Dimes, 2016). Major risk factors for preterm births include multiple births (e.g., twins or triplets), history of preterm delivery, stress, infection, smoking and/or illicit drug use, and extremes in maternal age (e.g., mothers younger than 16 years, mothers older than 35 years; Mandy, 2016; Morris, 2015).

Of the 450,000 to 500,000 preterm births in the United States each year, fewer than 1% of these infants are ELBW (Mandy, 2016; Morris, 2015). ELBW infants can be classified into two subgroups: the first ELBW group consists of extremely premature infants who are appropriate for gestational age, and the second ELWB group consists of intrauterine growth-restricted infants who are small for gestational age, but not necessarily very premature (i.e., less than 27-week gestational age, Papageorgiou & Pelausa, 2014). Understanding the differences between these two subgroups is essential as the different pathophysiologic processes associated with each group may yield different responses and outcomes to the care provided.

Although perinatal care, technology, and understanding of the pathophysiology and needs of the ELBW infant have improved, ELBW infants remain at high risk for death, with 30% to 50% mortality and high risk for severe impairment with 20% to 50% long-term morbidity in survivors (Glass et al., 2015; Papageorgiou & Pelausa, 2014; Sherman, 2014). The risk of death increases with decreasing birth weight and gestational age, and both are associated with increasing immaturity. The infant mortality rates per 1,000 live births in the United States in 2013 were 124.6 for infants weighing 750 to 999 g, 394.3 for those weighing 500 to 749 g, and 853 for those weighing less than 500 g (Mandy, 2016). Risk factors for death and severe neurodevelopmental impairment in ELBW infants are bronchopulmonary dysplasia (BPD), brain injury, severe retinopathy of prematurity (ROP), infection, and cardiopulmonary resuscitation (CPR) in the delivery room. ELBW infants who received CPR in the delivery room were more critical with higher pneumothorax, grade III and IV intraventricular hemorrhage (IVH), and BPD rates, compared to those who did not receive CPR (Mandy, 2016). Therefore, successful management of the ELBW infant must begin in the delivery room.

Clinical Aspects

ASSESSMENT

A standardized, team approach, ideally consisting of an experienced neonatologist, nursing, respiratory, and social work in a level III facility, is essential for the proper management and care of the ELBW infant (Morris, 2015; Papageorgiou & Pelausa, 2014). This team approach should begin from the prenatal consultation and continue in the delivery room management of the ELBW infant and care in the NICU. Prenatal consultation should involve similar information, incorporating both national and hospital outcomes, open and honest dialogue, and understanding of family expectations in order to be supportive of the family's decisions, regardless of the members who comprise the team conducting the consultation (Morris, 2015; Sherman, 2014).

NURSING INTERVENTIONS, MANAGEMENT, AND IMPLICATIONS

In the management of the ELBW infant in the delivery room and in the NICU, it is important to be aware of the in utero environment from which the infant came and would have stayed in had the infant not been born prematurely. The infant's environment changes from a warm, fluid-filled, quiet, dark environment where movements are slow and supported to one that is bright, loud, invasive, exposed, full of stimulation, and movement is no longer supported (Morris, 2015).

The initial stages of care during the first few hours after birth determine the outcome of the ELBW infant. Umbilical cord clamping should be delayed 30 to 60 seconds after birth with the infant at a level below the placenta. Delayed cord clamping has been shown to improve transitional circulation, establish better red blood cell volume thereby reducing the need for blood transfusion as well as potentially reducing the risk of an IVH by 50% (Sherman, 2014).

A majority of ELBW infants require resuscitation. The goal of delivery resuscitation is to efficiently deliver the least amount of intervention needed to support normal gas exchange and decrease the potential for lung injury. Current practice recommendations for administering supplemental oxygen to the ELBW infant include basing administration on objective preductal oxygen saturation monitoring, using blended oxygen, and administering positive pressure for persistent cyanosis (Sherman, 2014). If positive pressure ventilation is necessary, low inspiratory pressure should be provided to avoid overinflation of the lungs and potential lung injury. Debate over the administration of surfactant in the first few minutes of an ELBW infant's life is still ongoing. In the NICU, most ELBW infants require respiratory assistance, ranging from nasal continuous positive airway pressure (CPAP) to intubation, to survive. Progressive weaning protocols that provide respiratory assistance on low peak inspiratory pressures and rates are thought to be more efficacious and help with nutrition advancement.

Thermoregulation is another important aspect in ELBW infant care. Due to their structurally and functionally immature skin and large body surface area, these infants lose heat quickly and are prone to cold stress, which can affect glucose, oxygenation, and acid–base balance. Neonatal Resuscitation Program recommendations include increasing delivery room temperature to 77°F to 80°F, preheating the radiant warmer, using a polyethylene bag without first drying the skin, and using a portable warming mattress (Morris, 2015). In the NICU, ambient humidity of 70% or higher for ELBW infants is recommended to decrease transepidermal water loss and heat loss. The fragility of the skin places the ELBW infants at risk for experiencing skin shearing and denuding and increases their risk of infection. Therefore, skin integrity preservation must be incorporated into their daily care and must include frequent skin condition assessments and repositioning of the infant a minimum of every 4 hours.

ELBW infants have limited nutritional reserves; immature nutrient absorption and metabolic pathways;

and have higher nutrient needs, which can cause them to rapidly enter into a catabolic state (Papageorgiou & Pelausa, 2014; Sherman, 2014). Introducing parenteral nutrition early as soon as these infants are stabilized prevents them from experiencing metabolic shock. In addition, early trophic feeds using colostrum, then breast milk, or donor milk and standardized feeding guidelines are recommended to improve feeding tolerance, stimulate gut motility and maturity, shorten the time to full feeds, and decrease length of stay (Morris, 2015).

OUTCOMES

Because ELBW infants are at increased risk for developing severe cognitive and motor impairments, modifications to the NICU environment are necessary to limit exposure to negative stimuli. Strategies to promote a neuroprotective environment include decreasing ambient light and noise, clustering care with minimal handling to allow for periods of uninterrupted sleep, and using positioning aids for containment (Sherman, 2014). These considerations, along with the respiratory, thermoregulatory, and nutritional considerations, comprise the care necessary to successfully manage the ELBW infant.

Summary

ELBW infants are generally the sickest infants; they have the highest rates of mortality of morbidity of infants. Care of the ELBW infant is complex and requires an expert team approach beginning at delivery. The goal of resuscitation is to efficiently deliver the least amount of intervention needed to support normal gas exchange and reduce the potential for lung injury. Strategies to promote respiratory, thermoregulatory, nutritional, and neuroprotective support must be consistently practiced to ensure comprehensive care of ELBW infants to improve their chances of survival.

Glass, H. C., Costarino, A. T., Stayer, S. A., Brett, C., Cladis, F., & Davis, P. J. (2015). Outcomes for extremely premature infants. *Anesthesia and Analgesia, 120*(6), 1337–1351.

Mandy, G. T. (2016). Incidence and mortality of the preterm infant. *UpToDate.* Retrieved from https://www.uptodate.com/contents/incidence-and-mortality-of-the-preterm-infant

March of Dimes. (2016). Preterm birth increases in the U.S. for the first time in eight years: 2016 March of Dimes premature birth report card reveals underlying geographic, racial/ethnic disparities. Retrieved from http://www.marchofdimes.org/news/preterm-birth-increases-in-the-us-for-the-first-time-in-eight-years.aspx

Morris, M. (2015). Care of the extremely low birth weight infant [PowerPoint slides]. Retrieved from https://www.anymeeting.com/WebConference/RecordingDefault.aspx?c_psrid=E950DF86884E31https://www.anymeeting.com/WebConference/RecordingDefault.aspx?c_psrid=E950DF86884E31

Papageorgiou, A., & Pelausa, E. (2014). Management and outcome of extremely low birth weight infants. *Journal of Pediatric and Neonatal Individualized Medicine, 3*(2), 1–6. doi:10.7363/030209

Sherman, J. (2014). Care of the extremely low birth weight (ELBW) infant. In M. T. Verklan & M. Walden (Eds.), *Core curriculum for neonatal intensive care nursing* (pp. 427–438). St. Louis, MO: Elsevier Saunders.

■ GASTROESOPHAGEAL REFLUX

Suzanne Rubin

Overview

Gastroesophageal reflux (GER) refers to uncomplicated, recurrent spitting and vomiting in healthy infants that resolves without intervention. It is considered physiologic and usually resolves before 12 months of life. GER occurs commonly in healthy infants and is a frequent topic of discussion with pediatricians, especially during the first several months of life. Symptoms include frequent nonbilious "spit up" after feedings that does not seem to cause problems. Weight gain, attainment of developmental milestones, and general contentment are noted. Clinical interventions for parents at this stage involve education and reassurance that resolution is likely by 12 months of life. Gastroesophageal reflux disease (GERD) is a more complicated, pathological form of reflux that causes alarming symptoms or leads to medical complications and may occur at any age. The esophageal manifestations of GERD can include heartburn, frequent regurgitation, and mucosal injury of the esophagus.

Background

A historical literature search shows a relative lack of reference to this disease process before the mid-19th century. Most likely this represents a lack of anatomical understanding of the disease process and identification. How and where the reflux condition initiated was not well understood before the invention of the rigid endoscopy and the first barium upper gastrointestinal radiologic studies in the 1960s (Modlin, Kidd, & Lye, 2003). At this time, major access to the esophageal lumen was developed and the understanding of anatomy and physiology began. Following use of this procedure, the development of pressure manometers and pH probes helped to document the relationship of acid secretion as well as the esophageal–gastric structure, physiology, and pathology. Understanding normal maturational changes in the infants' stomach and esophagus contributed to a better understanding of these processes. The association of infants with colic, feeding disorders, and regurgitation followed. Increasing awareness has permitted the development of additional diagnostic studies and treatment. GER is common in infants and usually is not pathological (Martin & Hibbs, 2016).

Clinical Aspects

GER is common in infants with regurgitation present in 50% to 70% of all infants, peaking at age 4 to 6 months, and typically resolving by 1 year. A small minority of infants with GER develop other symptoms suggestive of GERD, including irritability, feeding refusal, hematemesis, anemia, respiratory symptoms, and failure to thrive (Martin & Hibbs, 2016).

ASSESSMENT

Compared to full-term infants, premature infants are at increased risk for GER due to immaturity of feeding skills as well as immature or impaired anatomic and physiologic factors that limit reflux (such as transient relaxation of the lower esophageal sphincter). GER is more common in healthy preterm infants, in whom gastric fluids reflux into the esophagus as often as 30 or more times daily (Martin & Hibbs, 2016). Nursing assessment includes close monitoring of growth parameters, feeding and vomiting history, history of irritability, and other findings that may be related to pathologic reflux.

Older children may also experience GER, with symptoms similar to adults described. They may complain of heartburn, swallowing difficulty, or regurgitation into the oral cavity. Some syndromes have increased incidence of the disease due to anatomical differences, such as asthma, cystic fibrosis, hiatal hernia, developmental delays, or prior chest surgery. Weakened chest muscles or increased frequency of coughing can increase intra-abdominal pressure in the stomach, causing movement of stomach acids to the esophagus.

NURSING INTERVENTIONS, MANAGEMENT, AND IMPLICATIONS

Pediatric GER clinical guidelines for management of pediatric GER in clinical practice were published by the North American Society for Pediatric Gastroenterology, Hepatology, and Nutrition (NASPGHAN) and the European Society for Pediatric Gastroenterology, Hepatology, and Nutrition (ESPGHAN). These guidelines were adopted in 2009 by the American Academy of Pediatrics (AAP). Evidence-based progressive interventions start with a complete history and physical by the infant or child's primary pediatrician. If clinical findings include persistent vomiting/regurgitation and poor weight gain, further investigation may include calorie and diet counseling. When GER is accompanied by increasing symptoms, the consideration of thickened formula, an allergen-elimination diet (including most common offenders, such as milk and eggs, in mothers who breastfeed) may be an effective strategy to address GER in many patients. In particular, the AAP adopted guidelines emphasizing that milk protein allergy can cause a clinical presentation that mimics GERD in infants. Therefore, a 2- to 4-week trial of a maternal exclusion diet that restricts at least milk and egg is recommended in breastfeeding infants with GERD symptoms, whereas an extensively hydrolyzed protein or amino acid-based formula may be appropriate in formula-fed infants (Neu, Corwin, Lareau, & Marcheggiani-Howard, 2012).

Teaching families about the resolution of uncomplicated disease, possible etiology, and home interventions for GER can enhance adherence to recommended infant care. Because parents note different signs associated with reflux (fussiness, irritability, spitting up, arching of back), it may be difficult to know whether symptoms are caused by reflux or another discomfort such as gas or pain. Although many published reviews are available, there is lack of agreement in the scientific community as to the best intervention for infants. Symptoms most frequently monitored include irritability and regurgitation of feedings.

Specific interventions may vary from infant to infant. Combination interventions may be nonpharmacologic or pharmacologic. Activities aimed at soothing the infant include patting, touching, holding, massaging, or placing them in an infant swing.

Feeding modifications, such as thickened formulas, hydrolyzed formulas, elimination diet in breastfeeding mothers, upright positioning after feeding or small frequent feedings, may be initiated. Eliminating tobacco smoke in the home may be helpful. At this time, meta-analysis of all interventions does not show an advantage of one single intervention. It appears that the passage of time is the only consistent factor reducing irritability and spitting up, usually after 6 months of life (Neu et al., 2012). More research is needed in addition to anticipatory guidance for families of infants with GER and GERD.

When dietary management does not improve symptoms, consultation with a pediatric gastroenterologist may be required. Failure of caloric management should initiate complete blood count, urinalysis, and celiac disease screening (if infant older than 6 months). If any diagnostic findings are positive, management of these disease states is recommended.

Pharmacologic support, including buffering agents, oral acid suppression therapy or prokinetics, can be tried for effectiveness. Increasing severity may result in hospitalization for intensive feeding therapy or nasogastric (NG)/nasojejunal (NJ) feedings.

Pharmacological therapy involves two major classes of pharmacologic agents. These include acid suppressants and prokinetic agents. Acid suppressants include antacids, histamine-2 receptor antagonists (H2-blockers), and proton pump inhibitors (PPIs). The goal is to increase the pH of stomach secretions and reduce chemical trauma of the esophageal mucosa. Pro-kinetic agents strengthen the lower esophageal sphincter and aids in the stomach content emptying faster. These agents seems to be effective for longer episodes of reflux.

Antacids do not have a strong record of efficacy of relieving symptoms of GERD among infants and they may promote adverse events such as aluminum toxicity. Histamine-2 receptor antagonists can be effective against GERD, but decreasing response can develop within 6 weeks of initiation of treatment. These medications appear less effective than PPIs.

An alternative treatment for regurgitation of feedings severe GERD may be surgical intervention. The indications for surgical treatment are controversial. Generally, if all prior dietary and pharmacological treatments have been unsuccessful and chronic airway distress is persisting, a procedure called a *fundoplication* may benefit some infants. The most commonly performed procedure is the Nissen *fundoplication* in which the fundus of the stomach is wrapped around the lower esophagus. This procedure may be done laparoscopically.

OUTCOMES

Infants with severe reflux may be the most vulnerable population with GERD, due to risk of aspiration and subsequent poor airway protection (Wakeman, Wilson, & Warner, 2016). Although the outcome of a successful fundoplication may diminish future reflux episodes and aspiration, this population is generally more vulnerable as a surgical candidate and risk–benefit ratio should be calculated.

Summary

The establishment of standardized guidelines adopted by the AAP has emphasized evaluation and treatment using best practices for use by general pediatricians and pediatric subspecialists. The infant with uncomplicated recurrent regurgitation may require only conservative management. Parental education and anticipatory guidance may be all that is required. Weight gain and progression of developmental attainment of milestones is reassuring. Infants with recurrent regurgitation and symptoms, such as weight loss or apparent pain, may benefit from individual comfort or dietary interventions. When comfort or dietary adjustments are inadequate, there may be some efficacy in the use of pharmacological agents. Consultation with pediatric gastrointestinal specialty may be required, where additional diagnostic evaluation and pharmaceutical or surgical options may be further pursued. Current research is inconclusive as to a single most effective treatment.

Lightdale, J., Gremse, D., & Section on Gastroenterology, Hematology and Nutrition. (2013). Gastroesophageal reflux: Management guidelines for the pediatrician. *Pediatrics*, *131*(5), 1684–1685. doi:10.1542/peds.2013-0421

Martin, R., & Hibbs, A. M. (2016). Gastroesophageal reflux in premature infants. In A. G. Hoppin (Ed.), *UpToDate*. Retrieved from https://www.uptodate.com/contents/gastroesophageal-reflux-in-premature-infants

Modlin, I. M., Kidd, M., & Lye, K. (2003). Historical perspectives on the treatment of gastroesophageal reflux disease. *Gastrointestinal Endoscopy Clinics of North America*, *13*, 19–55.

Neu, M., Corwin, E., Lareau, S. C., & Marcheggiani-Howard, C. (2012). A review of nonsurgical treatment for the symptom of irritability in infants with GERD. *Journal for Specialists in Pediatric Nursing*, *17*, 177–192.

Wakeman, D. S., Wilson, N. A., & Warner, B. W. (2016). Current status of surgical management of gastroesophageal reflux in children. *Current Opinion in Pediatrics, 28*(3), 356–362.

■ GASTROSCHISIS AND OMPHALOCELE

Beverly Capper

Overview

Defects in the abdominal wall occur during the early stages of fetal development. Interruption in the normal development of the abdomen between 6 and 10 weeks of gestation prevents normal closure of the abdomen, and allows the abdominal organs to float freely in amniotic fluid (Lepigeon, Van Miegham, Maurer, Giannoni, & Baud, 2014). Abdominal wall defects increase neonatal mortality and morbidity, as well as the risk of preterm delivery, neonatal surgery, infection, digestive issues, and prolonged hospitalization. Gastroschisis and omphalocele are the two most common types of congenital abdominal wall defects in newborns (Corey et al., 2014). Gastroschisis occurs once in every 12,000 live births, and omphalocele occurs once in every 4,000 live births (Corey et al., 2014). The increase in incidence of gastroschisis over the past 10 years is concerning and unexplained (Bergholz, Boettcher, Reinshagen, & Wenke, 2014). Currently there is no fetal intervention for gastroschisis or omphalocele and a large number of these pregnancies result in preterm birth (Lepigeon et al., 2014). Surgical correction of gastroschisis and omphalocele is imminent after birth and best managed with a team of specialists (Insigna et al., 2014). Delivery ideally occurs in a center equipped to perform surgery and care for the newborn in a neonatal intensive care unit (NICU).

Background

The formation of the abdomen occurs during weeks 6 to 10 of fetal development. During this time, the abdomen lacks sufficient room to accommodate the growth of organs so the intestines naturally protrude into the umbilical cord and then at week 11 recede back into the abdomen (Rubarth & Van Woudenberg, 2016). Failure of the organs to recede prevents closure and allows organs to form outside the abdomen. Gastroschisis and omphalocele are both characterized by herniation of abdominal organs that may include the intestines, spleen, liver, or other organs (Corey et al., 2014). The presence of gastroschisis or omphalocele is generally detected prenatally on a routine ultrasound and an elevated maternal serum alpha fetoprotein (AFP; Lepigeon et al., 2014). Once a defect is identified, repeated ultrasounds are recommended throughout the remainder of the pregnancy to monitor the growth and well-being of the fetus (Lepigeon et al., 2014).

Although the etiology is unknown, there is evidence linking environmental factors and maternal smoking and alcohol ingestion, genitourinary infection during the first trimester, use of selective serotonin-reuptake inhibitors (SSRIs), and poor prenatal care (Insigna et al., 2014). The risk of gastroschisis is highest among women under 20 years of age, whereas the risk for omphalocele is noted in advanced maternal age.

A gastroschisis is herniation typically located to the right of the umbilicus and lacks a membrane or sac to cover the exposed organs. The defect is not associated with chromosomal defects and is classified as simple or complex. Simple gastroschisis has intestines or other organs outside the abdomen, whereas complex gastroschisis has additional pathologies of intestinal atresia, perforation, necrotic segments, or volvulus (Bergholz et al., 2014). Complex gastroschisis requires a longer hospitalization and is associated with more feeding complications.

The omphalocele is a midline abdominal wall defect located near the base of the umbilical cord with a thin membrane or sac covering the exposed organs. Omphalocele is frequently associated with Trisomy 13, 18, and 21 chromosomal defect; Beckwith–Wiedeman syndrome; and other congenital anomalies (Corey et al., 2014). Although the prevalence of omphalocele is lower than gastroschisis, it carries a higher mortality rate thought to be related to the associated congenital anomalies.

Perinatal treatment strategies for the timing and mode of the delivery remain controversial, but Lepigeon et al. (2014) reported evidence from a study that showed a decreased risk of sepsis and organ damage with induction of labor at 37 weeks. There is little evidence demonstrating a benefit of cesarean section over vaginal delivery. Surgical correction is needed shortly after birth to restore the integrity of the abdominal wall and to prevent damage to exposed organs (Insigna et al., 2014). Three surgical approaches described by Wu, Lee, and DeUgarte (2016) include a nonoperative strategy, primary closure, and a staged repair using a silo that contains eviscerated intestines.

The nonoperative procedure is a newer strategy, and is performed at the bedside by placing an umbilical flap to cover the opening in the abdomen. Primary closure is the preferred procedure and places the intestines and other organs back in the abdomen in one surgery. Staged repair may be necessary if swelling and inflammation of the intestines prevent a primary closure. The intestines remaining outside the abdomen are covered with a mesh silo and suspended over the abdomen. The intestines recede by gravity, and the silo is tightened daily to gently push the intestines into the abdomen.

Clinical Aspects

ASSESSMENT

Essential components for nursing care for the newborn include obtaining a thorough maternal history that includes the pregnancy and mode of delivery, as well as physical assessment of the newborn, laboratory data, and echocardiogram. These assessments help to properly identify risk factors and medications that may have had adverse effects on the newborn. The physical assessment of the newborn is focused on respiratory function and alterations that result from preterm delivery, low birth weight, and intrauterine growth retardation (IUGR). Of particular concern is the respiratory compromise attributable to increased intra-abdominal pressure, cold stress from heat loss through exposed organs, and changes in heart rate due to extreme fluid loss. The initial assessment confirms the differential diagnosis between gastroschisis and omphalocele based on the presence or absence of a sac surrounding the exposed organs. Caution is needed to protect the integrity of the organs themselves with both defects and specifically the sac in presence of an omphalocele. Laboratory data are monitored to evaluate electrolytes for the effectiveness of fluid resuscitation. After initial stabilization, physical assessment findings are evaluated for additional congenital anomalies and heart function is evaluated with a fetal echocardiogram.

NURSING INTERVENTIONS, MANAGEMENT, AND IMPLICATIONS

Nursing care of the newborn with gastroschisis or omphalocele is focused on prevention of complications during the immediate stabilization and throughout the neonatal recovery period. Nursing problems include maintaining thermoregulation, fluid resuscitation to maintain vascular perfusion and adequate ventilation, protection of herniated abdominal organs to maintain sac integrity and prevent organ damage, administration of broad spectrum antibiotics, decreased cardiac output from increased abdominal pressure following primary closure, optimization of gastric function to prevent ileus and long-term feeding problems, and provision of support for parents and family during a prolonged hospitalization.

Immediately after birth the exposed organs are covered with a nonadherent dressing and clear plastic bag to prevent heat and fluid loss, drying of organs, and to promote visualization. Use of a radiant warmer or the warm humidified environment of an isolette assists with thermoregulation. Fluid replacement may require volumes at twice the normal maintenance amounts and placement of an oral or nasogastric tube is needed for decompression and also to decrease the risk of aspiration. Enteral feedings may be delayed for several weeks requiring the insertion of a peripherally inserted central catheter (PICC) or central venous line to infuse total parental nutrition. Maternal or donor breast milk is the preferred nutrition and tolerance of human milk may help gain faster attainment of full enteral feeds. Postoperative care includes pain management, infection prevention, and feeding. Discharge preparation begins early, engaging the parent(s) in caring for their newborn and teaching normal newborn care and care specific to the comorbidities or congenital anomalies.

OUTCOMES

Prognosis is determined by the severity of the defect. Newborns with gastroschisis have an excellent recovery and the majority have no long-term health problems. Complex gastroschisis has greater feeding difficulties, and 4% to 10% of infants experience bowel obstruction requiring additional surgery and possibly resulting in short gut (Lepigeon et al., 2014). Omphalocele has a higher morbidity and mortality rate reflective of associated congenital anomalies. Parents may need counseling for future pregnancies and support for future hospitalizations.

Summary

Early prenatal diagnosis and delivery at a tertiary care center optimizes the stabilization and surgery for the newborn diagnosed with gastroschisis or omphalocele. Treatment is prolonged for complex gastroschisis and omphalocele averaging more than 1 month with costs exceeding $100,000 (Wu et al., 2016). Further research is needed to determine the etiology of gastroschisis and omphalocele.

Bergholz, R., Boettcher, M., Reinshagen, K., & Wenke, K. (2014). Complex gastroschisis is a different entity to simple gastroschisis affecting morbidity and mortality—A systematic review and meta-analysis. *Journal of Pediatric Surgery*, 49, 1527–1532. doi:10.1016/j.jpedsurg.2014.08.001

Corey, K. M., Hornik, C. P., Laughon, M. M., McHutchinson, K., Clark, R. H., & Smith, P. B. (2014). Frequency of anomalies and hospital outcomes in infants with gastroschisis and omphalocele. *Early Human Development, 90,* 421–424. doi:10.1016/j.earlhumdev.2014.05.006

Insigna, V., Lo Verso, C., Antona, V., Cimador, M., Ortolano, R., Carta, M., . . . Corsello, G. (2014). Perinatal management of gastroschisis. *Journal of Pediatric Neonatal Individual Medicine, 3*(1), e030113. doi:10.7363/03011

Lepigeon, K., Van Mieghem, T., Maurer, S. V., Giannoni, E., & Baud, D. (2014). Gastroschisis—What should be told to parents. *Prenatal Diagnosis, 34,* 316–326. doi:10.1002/pd.4305

Rubarth, L. B., & Van Woudenberg, C. D. (2016). Development of the gastrointestinal system: An embryonic and fetal review. *Neonatal Network, 35*(3), 156–158. doi:10.1891/0730-0832.35.3.156

Wu, X. J., Lee, S. L., & DeUgarte, D. A. (2016). Cost modeling for management strategies of uncomplicated gastroschisis. *Journal of Surgical Research, 205,* 136–141. doi:10.1016/j.jss.2016.06.039

■ HIRSCHSPRUNG'S DISEASE

Anne M. Modic

Overview

Hirschsprung's disease (HD) is also referred to as *congenital aganglionic megacolon* or *meconium plug syndrome.* Meconium plug syndrome is a broader diagnosis that correlates with a 13% incidence of Hirschsprung's (Keckler et al., 2008). HD is most found often in the sigmoid colon of the large intestine preventing normal contraction of the affected area and subsequently normal expulsion of stool.

Background

HD is a congenital disease in which ganglion nerve cells in the myenteric and submucosal plexi responsible for peristalsis and smooth muscle movement of the gut are absent from the intestine. This results from failure of the ganglion cells to migrate in a craniocaudal direction during the fifth through the twelfth week of gestation (Keckler et al., 2008). As a result, there is a continual state of contraction of the aganglionic segment of bowel and the internal anal sphincter preventing normal expulsion of stool.

Short-segment HD is defined by the absence of nerve cells in the sigmoid colon (Keckler et al., 2008). In long-segment disease, there is an absence of nerve cells throughout most or all of the large intestine, occasionally part of the small intestine, and rarely the entire intestinal tract. The proximal bowel subsequently becomes dilated due to normal function in an effort to pass stool. The incidence is approximately one in 5,000 live births. Occurrence of this disease is a 4:1 male-to-female ratio (Moore, 2016). HD accounts for 20% to 25% of intestinal obstruction in the neonatal period.

Historically, this was a fatal disease. In 1886, Hirschprung, a Danish pediatrician, presented two cases of infants at the Berlin Conference of German Society Pediatrics (Sergi, 2015). The infants' similar symptoms included absence of spontaneous bowel movements, abdominal distention, and episodes of diarrhea. Treatment consisted of laxatives and daily enemas. Both children died. The autopsies showed rectal narrowing, dilated loops of bowel, as well as some ulceration of the mucosa associated with thickening of the bowel wall (Sergi, 2015).

Significant HD research looking at the enteric nervous system (ENS) has been the focus of developmental neurobiologists and geneticists (Heanue & Pachnis, 2007; Moore, 2016). The ENS is the part of the parasympathetic nervous system that regulates smooth muscle movements and peristalsis of the gut. Developmental neurobiologists have been uncovering the molecular process of the migration, proliferation, and differentiation of neural crest cells responsible for the creation of the normal ENS. Geneticists have found a number of genetic expressions related to the development of HD. Biologic and genetic advances in HD have brought the focus to exploration for ENS stem cells.

Clinical Aspects

Clinical presentation of HD may occur from early in the neonatal period to 2 or 3 years of life and beyond. Older children often present with chronic constipation or enterocolitis. However, in 80% to 90% of cases, symptoms occur in the neonatal period (Parry, 2011).

ASSESSMENT

The neonate fails to pass meconium in the first 24 to 48 hours of life with varying symptoms of abdominal distention, poor feeding, vomiting, and occasionally enterocolitis. The physical examination varies from an abdomen that is soft and nondistended to tense with significant abdominal distention. A rectal examination may produce notable gas and explosive stool. Abdominal radiographs with contrast show dilated loops of bowel with lack of air in the rectum. A full-thickness or suction rectal biopsy is performed for histology to determine the presence or absence of ganglion cells. Bowel decompression is done followed by surgical intervention. The level of surgical repair is determined by ascending serial biopsies and frozen section biopsy to ascertain presence of ganglion cells.

The aganglionic portion of the bowel is resected; the normal bowel is attached to the anus in a primary pull-through procedure known as a *single-stage pull-through (SSPT)*. The Swenson, Soave, and Duhamel are the most common techniques used. Each of these procedures differs in how the connection between bowel and rectum is created. When there is long segment, higher level disease, enterocolitis or other bowel damage such as perforation, the aganglionic bowel is removed and an ostomy is created at the level of normal bowel in a multistage pull-through (MSPT). An ostomy takedown is done after the bowel is sufficiently healed and the healthy bowel is connected to the rectum. In general, SSPT is associated with improved outcomes (Sulkowski et al., 2014).

NURSING INTERVENTIONS, MANAGEMENT, AND IMPLICATIONS

Nurses are instrumental both in the diagnosis and care of infants with HD. Nurses must pay close attention to gastrointestinal (GI) status, including feeding tolerance and stooling patterns, particularly in the first 48 hours of life. Close monitoring by nurses is important due to the concern for perforation with intestinal distention proximal to the aganglionic area. Abdominal decompression with a nasogastric tube is critical. The inability of the neonate to orally feed and possible subsequent vomiting requires clinicians to follow electrolytes, hydration status, and nutritional needs closely. Total parenteral nutrition is standard nutritional support. Neonates should be closely monitored for sepsis or enterocolitis. Symptoms include temperature instability, abdominal distention, vomiting, explosive diarrhea that may be foul smelling or bloody, and, in advanced cases, septic shock. Treatment includes antibiotics, observation for signs of septic shock, nothing by mouth, and intravenous fluid support. Rectal saline washout is required before surgery when enterocolitis is present (Bucher, Pacetti, Lovvorn, & Carter, 2016).

In addition to normal postoperative care, the nurse must be diligent in monitoring electrolytes and maintaining hydration and nutrition as well as monitoring the abdominal status and/or ostomy site and preventing infection. Nurses are at the forefront of pain control for these infants. Opioids are generally used for immediate postop pain control with transition to acetaminophen. Parental nutrition and abdominal decompression are provided until GI function has been reestablished. Feeds can then be slowly initiated with close monitoring of feeding tolerance. At times, tolerance of elemental formula is better than standard formula. However, breast milk and breastfeeding are strongly recommended. Stooling patterns should be observed for normalcy. Significant constipation or diarrhea around areas of constipation may be indicative of strictures.

The presence of strictures requires rectal dilation. Hegar dilators are used with the size of the dilator increased over time. Symptoms include constipation or diarrhea around areas of significant constipation. Postoperative antibiotics are prescribed prophylactically for enterocolitis. Establishment and tolerance of enteral feeds as well as family education are necessary prerequisites before safe discharge. Family education for rectal dilation, symptoms of enterocolitis and, if needed, ostomy care should be provided (Malcolm, 2015).

OUTCOMES

Persistent constipation can occur with unresected areas of aganglionosis that may require further surgical intervention to remove the abnormal segment of bowel. HD patients generally are followed for at least 1 year postop. Ongoing issues require long-term follow-up and intervention. This may include enterocolitis and/or chronic bowel dysfunction. Enterocolitis can occur at any time. Treatment includes antibiotics and rectal washout. In severe cases, an ostomy may be needed. In a review of patients with HD reported by Moore (2016), 68% of HD patients had normal bowel function after postoperative repair, 10.3% had soiling, and 21.7% needed laxatives or enemas for chronic, significant constipation. Possible causes may be sphincter achalasia, ENS dysganglionosis, or other areas of aganglionosis. Some patients experience enuresis, incontinence, or dysuria and may require bowel management programs. The focus of follow-up care includes stool softeners, laxatives and enemas in addition to diet, exercise, and bowel training.

Summary

HD was historically a terminal disease for infants and children. Great progress has been made in the identification and treatment of HD. Neurobiology and genetic research is ongoing with a number of genetic expressions related to development of HD identified. Stem cell therapy is at the forefront of current research and brings hope of treatment without the need for surgical intervention. Awareness of symptoms in the early neonatal period is crucial in identifying HD and nurses play an important role in the identification, care, and family education of these infants. Close follow-up of bowel function, growth, nutrition, and early identification of enterocolitis maximizes the potential for best long-term outcomes.

Bucher, B., Pacetti, A., Lovvornb, H., & Carter, B. (2016). Neonatal surgery. In S. Gardner, B. Carter, M. Hines, & J. Hernandez (Eds.), *Merenstein & Gardener's handbook of neonatal intensive care* (pp. 786–819). St. Louis, MO: Elsevier.

Heanue, T. A., & Pachnis, V. (2007). Enteric nervous system development and Hirschsprung's disease: Advances in genetic and stem cell studies. *Nature Reviews Neuroscience, 8*(6), 466–479.

Keckler, S. J., St Peter, S. D., Spilde, T. L., Tsao, K., Ostlie, D. J., Holcomb, G. W., & Snyder, C. L. (2008). Current significance of meconium plug syndrome. *Journal of Pediatric Surgery, 43*(5), 896–898.

Malcolm, W. (2015). *Beyond the NICU: Comprehensive care of the high-risk infant* (pp. 492–494, 735). New York, NY: McGraw-Hill.

Moore, S. (2016). Hirschprung disease: Current perspectives. *Open Access Surgery, 9,* 39–50. doi:10.2147/OAS.S81552

Parry, R. (2011). Selected gastrointestinal anomalies in the neonate. In R. J. Martin, A. A. Fanaroff, & M. C. Walsh (Eds.), *Fanaroff and Martin's neonatal-perinatal medicine diseases of the fetus and newborn* (pp. 1424–1425). St. Louis, MO: Elsevier.

Sergi, C. (2015). Hirschsprung's disease: Historical notes and pathological diagnosis on the occasion of the 100(th) anniversary of Dr. Harald Hirschsprung's death. *World Journal of Clinical Pediatrics, 4*(4), 120–125.

Sulkowski, J. P., Cooper, J. N., Congeni, A., Pearson, E. G., Nwomeh, B. C., Doolin, E. J., . . . Deans, K. J. (2014). Single-stage versus multi-stage pull-through for Hirschsprung's disease: Practice trends and outcomes in infants. *Journal of Pediatric Surgery, 49*(11), 1619–1625.

■ HYDRONEPHROSIS

Charlene M. Deuber

Overview

Hydronephrosis is one of the most common fetal anomalies, detected in 1% of pregnancies. A sign rather than a diagnosis, hydronephrosis references significant dilation of the upper urinary tract. Common causes of hydronephrosis include physiologic hydronephrosis, ureteropelvic or ureterovesical junction (UVJ) obstruction, posterior urethral valves (PUVs), Eagle–Barrett (prune belly) syndrome, and vesicoureteral reflux (VUR; Martin, Fanaroff, & Walsh, 2011).

Prenatal diagnosis is highly correlated with postnatal findings (Policiano et al., 2015). The goal of prenatal ultrasound is reduction in the incidence of postnatal urinary tract infection (UTI) and prevention of acquired renal damage in asymptomatic patients. Early identification of the finding affords the opportunity for prenatal consultation with nephrology or urology specialists, facilitating postnatal care coordination. Prenatal interventions are limited in efficacy and associated with increased risk of preterm labor and chorioramnionitis. Expectant prenatal management prevails, with fetal surgical intervention rarely indicated (Liu, Armstrong, & Maizels, 2014).

Background

Occurring unilaterally or bilaterally, hydronephrosis is characterized by enlargement of the renal collecting system, including renal calyces and pelvis. The etiology is varied although it may be obstructive in origin. Prenatal hydronephrosis may be transient or secondary to clinically significant abnormalities of the kidney and urinary tract. As much as 15% of prenatally detected hydronephrosis occurs due to delayed fetal ureter maturation independently of anatomic abnormalities of the upper urinary tract (physiologic hydronephrosis) and typically resolve spontaneously before birth or by 2 years of age. The incidence of significant urinary tract disease in identified cases of hydronephrosis has been estimated at 0.2% to 0.4% (Aslan, 2005).

Ultrasound-guided prenatal grading of unilateral or bilateral hydronephrosis informs prenatal and postnatal management. The grading system of the Society of Fetal Urology (grades I–V) describes the degree of calyceal dilatation and renal parenchymal thickness.

Grading may be used as a guideline to describe the degree of hydronephrosis. Measuring the greatest dimension of the renal pelvis has also gained favor for defining hydronephrosis. An unfavorable outcome, including need for postnatal surgery, has been associated with a renal anteriorposterior (AP) diameter of 7 mm or more in the third trimester and the presence of urinary tract anomalies (Plevani et al., 2014).

Prenatal ultrasonography findings, including increased renal echogenicity, bilateral disease, and oligohydramnios may be associated with long-term renal dysfunction and deserve additional prenatal consultation with nephrology or urology specialists (Vogt & Dell, 2011). Despite improvements in technique, prenatal imaging may not detect all defects of the urinary tract.

Clinical Aspects

The majority of cases of hydronephrosis are unilateral and mild, necessitating postnatal follow-up with serial ultrasonography beginning at 7 to 10 days of age to resolution (or progression) of findings. Newborns with a normal ultrasound in the first week of life should undergo a repeated study at 4 to 6 weeks of age to eliminate an initial false-negative study owing to relative dehydration or low glomerular filtration rate (GFR). Two normal postnatal ultrasound examinations exclude the presence of significant renal disease.

Sencan et al. (2014) describe a low incidence of UTI and VUR in children with mild antenatal hydronephrosis (ANH) at 2 weeks through 3 months of age, suggesting that routine voiding cystourethrogram (VCUG) and long-term antibiotic prophylaxis should be initiated only in symptomatic children presenting with UTI. Moderate to severe unilateral hydronephrosis prompts postnatal study, including ultrasonography followed by a VCUG and a functional renal scan (diuretic renography) to identify etiology precisely.

Mild isolated bilateral hydronephrosis should similarly be followed with sequential ultrasound examination. Causes of bilateral hydronephrosis include UVJ obstruction, referring to a blockage in the region of the UVJ where the ureter meets the bladder. The obstruction impedes flow of urine down to the bladder, causing the urine to back up into and dilate the ureters and kidney, appreciated on ultrasound as megaureter (dilated ureter) and hydronephrosis. Moderate to severe bilateral hydronephrosis may indicate potential obstructive uropathy and requires prompt, detailed evaluation postnatally, particularly in male infants who have an increased risk of PUVs.

In cases of severe bilateral hydronephrosis (greater than 15-mm AP diameter in third trimester), postnatal ultrasonography should be completed in the first 48 hours of life and prophylactic antibiotic therapy initiated. A VCUG follows with the continuation of antibiotic therapy or additional renal scans to complete diagnostic evaluation and determine presence and location of obstruction.

ASSESSMENT

Trending the blood pressure is important to monitor for hypertension as well as temperature to monitor for sepsis. Strict intake and output (I&O) is crucial and need to be calculated every 4 hours. Infants may need intravenous (IV) fluids to maintain hydration and IV antibiotics to prevent infection in the bladder or kidneys. If the hydronephrosis is severe the infant may need a Foley catheter to keep the kidneys drained. Proper nutrition for growth and development is important and mothers should be encouraged to provide breast milk although there is a special commercial formula available.

NURSING INTERVENTIONS, MANAGEMENT, AND IMPLICATIONS

Treatment of all infants with hydronephrosis has the same goal, which is to preserve renal function. Nurses must be able to assess infant renal function and inform the other members of the health care team of any acute or subtle changes they observe in the infant.

In addition, nurses must understand normal and abnormal laboratory values. Serial renal function panels are performed to determine kidney function. Waste products, urea/blood urea nitrogen (BUN) and creatinine (Cr) can accumulate in the blood causing serious damage to the kidneys.

Parent education is of primary importance even if the parents are aware of the diagnosis prenatally. The different tests their infant may undergo must be reinforced to them at a level they can understand. No matter what degree of hydronephrosis, it remains a frightening experience and parents need support. An important aspect is the need for follow-up with a pediatric nephrologist and continuation of antibiotics if required.

OUTCOMES

Spontaneous resolution of mild hydronephrosis is greater than moderate or severe hydronephrosis. Infants with moderate/severe hydronephrosis are at greater risk for a UTI (Conkar, Memmedov, & Mir, 2016), but still may be treated conservatively.

Summary

Neonatal hydronephrosis is often self-limiting, but may signal obstructive pathology of the lower or upper urinary tract. Prenatal diagnosis is important in guiding postnatal follow-up and management, with the goal of amelioration of acquired renal damage. Nursing care focuses on identification of prenatal diagnosis and implementation of postnatal follow-up. Preparation for procedures necessitates parental education and support.

Aslan, A. (2005). Neonatal hydronephrosiss (UPJ obstruction) and multicystic dysplastic kidneys. In L. S. Baskin (Ed.), *Handbook of pediatric urology* (pp. 123–130). Philadelphia, PA: LWW.

Conkar, S., Memmedov, V., & Mir, S. (2016). Outcomes of antenatal hydronephrosis. *Annals of Clinical and Laboratory Research, 4*(1), 1–5.

Liu, D. B., Armstrong, W. R., & Maizels, M. (2014). Hydronephrosis: prenatal and postnatal evaluation and management. *Clinics in Perinatology, 41*(3), 661–678. doi:10.1016/j.clp.2014.05.013

Martin, R., Fanaroff, A., & Walsh, M. (2011). *Fanaroff and Martin's neonatal-perinatal medicine* (9th ed.). St. Louis, MO: Elsevier Mosby.

Plevani, C., Locatelli, A., Paterlini, G., Ghidini, A., Tagliabue, P., Pezzullo, J. C., & Vergani, P. (2014). Fetal hydronephrosis: Natural history and risk factors for postnatal surgery. *Journal of Perinatal Medicine, 42*(3), 385–391. doi:10.1515/jpm-2013-0146

Policiano, C., Djokovic, D., Carvalho, R., Monteiro, C., Melo, M. A., & Graça, L. M. (2015). Ultrasound antenatal detection of urinary tract anomalies in the last decade: Outcome and prognosis. *Journal of Maternal–Fetal & Neonatal Medicine, 28*(8), 959–963. doi:10.3109/14767058.2014.939065

Sencan, A., Carvas, F., Hekimoglu, I. C., Caf, N., Sencan, A., Chow, J., & Nguyen, H. T. (2014). Urinary tract infection and vesicoureteral reflux in children with mild antenatal hydronephrosis. *Journal of Pediatric Urology, 10*(6), 1008–1013. doi:10.1016/j.jpurol.2014.04.001

■ HYPERBILIRUBINEMIA

Donna M. Schultz
Mary F. Terhaar

Overview

Destruction of old red blood cells (RBCs) is a normal and adaptive process in newborns as it is across the life span. When RBCs die, they are lysed and bilirubin is released as a by-product. Under certain conditions, the rate of RBC destruction exceeds the body's ability to eliminate bilirubin, which results in excess levels of waste product circulating in the bloodstream. This condition is called hyperbilirubinemia, or jaundice. Jaundice is the yellow coloration of skin and sclera that results when excessive bilirubin levels accumulate in skin and mucous membranes.

During pregnancy, the placenta, attached to the fetus, removes bilirubin along with other waste from the fetal bloodstream. Once delivery is complete and the umbilical cord is cut, the newborn must activate his or her own hepatic pathways to conjugate and eliminate bilirubin along with other wastes through the gastrointestinal system. (Cohen, Wong, & Stevenson, 2010). It is the imbalance of RBC destruction and hepatic function that produces hyperbilirubinemia.

Background

Hyperbilirubinemia has two distinct presentations, physiologic and pathologic, which are distinguished by the timing, etiology, and severity of the jaundice. Approximately 60% to 85% of all term newborns develop clinical signs of hyperbilirubinemia (Azzuqa & Watchko, 2015).

Physiologic jaundice in the newborn is a normal, adaptive process; commonly self-correcting, time-limited, and lacking in clinical significance. The condition results during normal transition to extrauterine life when the newborn breaks down fetal RBCs even as the kidneys, liver, and gastrointestinal system are assuming responsibility for elimination of waste. This increase in waste-product generation precedes functional capacity for elimination. Bilirubin levels usually peak between 3 and 5 days of life and start to decrease by the end of the first week. This is the presentation of physiologic jaundice.

Pathologic jaundice occurs in a relatively small group of newborns. The jaundice presents before 24 hours of life, with total bilirubin levels rising to exceed 5 mg/dL, or greater than the 95th percentile on the Bhutani nomogram (Bhutani, Vilms, & Hamerman-Johnson, 2010). Multiple factors increase the risk for pathologic jaundice, including prematurity, polycythemia, hemolytic disease, genetic abnormalities such as G6PD or Gilbert's disease, sepsis, blood cell irregularities, extensive bruising, abnormal pooling of blood as seen in cephalohematoma, family history of jaundice, inefficient feeding, and dehydration. Newborns of Asian, Arabic, or Mediterranean ethnicity face greater risk as well. A thorough medical history from the mother is important so that health care providers can identify risk factors and monitor the baby for pathologic jaundice (Cohen et al., 2010).

The first cases of jaundice, *icterus neonatorum*, were described in the late 19th century as a benign and self-limiting yellowing of the skin and the sclera that generally disappeared by the end of the baby's stay in the hospital (which was 10–14 days in the late 19th century; Cashore, 2010). A second, more severe form of jaundice, *icterus gravis*, was associated with significant anemia, neurologic abnormalities, and increased mortality (Cashore, 2010). The acute phase of this condition is named bilirubin-induced encephalopathy (BIND) and the resultant long-term sequelae are identified as kernicterus. Bilirubin is a neurotoxin in large doses. Both BIND and kernicterus result when levels of bilirubin become too high, allowing the toxin to cross the blood–brain barrier and deposit in the basal ganglia, producing serious neurologic damage (American Academy of Pediatrics [AAP], 2004). Kernicterus has not been reported in infants with peak total serum bilirubin (TSB) levels less than 20 mg/dL. However, it has not been determined at what level kernicterus can occur.

Because length of hospital stay for the mother–baby dyad has radically decreased, careful monitoring for hyperbilirubinemia is key to newborn well-being. In the case of spontaneous vaginal delivery, mother and newborn are commonly discharged to home by 48 hours after the birth. In the case of birth by cesarean section, mother and newborn are commonly discharged to home in approximately 72 hours. In both cases, discharge takes place before bilirubin levels can be expected to peak. This discrepancy motivated The Joint Commission to issue a sentinel event detailing the rise in BIND and kernicterus. In response, the AAP revised guidelines for the management of hyperbilirubinemia and rates began to decline (2004). As a result, The Joint Commission retired its sentinel alert. Best practice now calls for all newborns to be screened for hyperbilirubinemia before discharge to home.

Clinical Aspects

ASSESSMENT

Early assessment of risk for hyperbilirubinemia is essential. Family history, maternal history, and progression of the pregnancy and labor are all relevant to risk assessment. It is important to make note of any discrepancy among maternal, paternal, and newborn blood and rH type; use of antibiotics or oxytocin during pregnancy or labor; prolonged second stage of labor; use of mechanical assistance with delivery (vacuum or forceps); any trauma or bruising to the fetus or newborn; as well as presence of cephalohematoma. Each of these findings is associated with increased risk.

A transcutaneous bilirubin (TcB) level is routinely obtained within the first 12 to 24 hours of life. TcB measurements are a noninvasive way to obtain a cutaneous bilirubin level and to determine whether a serum bilirubin level needs to be drawn (Maisels, Coffey, & Kring, 2015). Abnormal values are brought to the attention of the responsible health care provider.

Use of the Bhutani nomogram for infants of 35 or more weeks gestational age, with the four risk-zone stratification is best practice for monitoring newborns with hyperbilirubinemia (AAP Committee for Hyperbilirubinemia, 2004). Infants whose total bilirubin levels are plotted in the high-risk zone should receive phototherapy. The number of banks of lights is determined by the bilirubin level. An infant's discharge should be delayed until a pattern of declining bilirubin levels is documented (Bhutani et al., 2010).

Infants whose bilirubin levels rise to the high–intermediate risk zone should only be sent home if feeding, voiding, and stooling appropriately. A bilirubin level at discharge must be documented. A follow-up appointment should be scheduled for the following day after discharge with the family's primary care provider (PCP) to monitor the bilirubin level.

Phototherapy promotes conjugation of bilirubin, which allows it to be eliminated in urine and stool. Aside from hydration and monitoring, phototherapy is the most commonly used intervention for the jaundiced newborn (AAP, 2004). Blue to green light (wavelengths: 460–490 nm) most effectively facilitates conjugation of bilirubin and is used in treatment of the newborn (Muchowski, 2014). Fluorescent or halogen lights and light-emitting diodes (LEDs) are commonly used (Muchowski, 2014). Exposure to these lights with as much skin exposed as possible for as much time as possible maximizes effect. Eye shields are used to protect the infant and need to be placed carefully to prevent them from becoming loose, leaving the eyes unprotected. Phototherapy can lead to burns, retinal damage, temperature instability, dehydration, rashes, and loose stools.

NURSING INTERVENTIONS, MANAGEMENT, AND IMPLICATIONS

Frequent breastfeeding (or bottle feeding if the parents choose) is key. A delay in breast milk production can lead to mild dehydration in the infant. Skin-to-skin contact between mother and newborn is begun in the delivery room or birthing suite and continued unless the newborn or maternal conditions prohibits the practice. Monitoring of urine and stool output helps to determine sufficiency of intake.

Care pathways and electronic health record (EHR) documentation systems, which incorporate checklists, help ensure proper identification of all risk factors and support provision of individualized care. These approaches have been established as effective means to reduce errors of omission and promote early identification of newborns who require vigilant monitoring and careful discharge planning. Care pathways and the EHR should capture and report the initial TcB level within the first 12 to 24 hours of life. Abnormal values documented over time, measured in hours of life, should be brought to the attention of the responsible health care provider.

Educating families about hyperbilirubinemia by nursing is key. Families need to understand the need for phototherapy and to be supported as they experience separation from the infant during treatment (Muchowski, 2014). Parents should understand the importance of close primary care follow-up, because often the infant should be discharged before normal bilirubin peak levels. Families must require understanding about the effects of hyperbilirubinemia, such as sleepiness, decreased wet diapers, stooling and feeding, as well as when to call their PCP.

OUTCOMES

Parents should be given a copy of the infant's discharge summary and the bilirubin nomogram so the PCP has accurate information to transition the baby into the primary care setting and develop an appropriate plan of care. Parents should be provided with education and resources to consult after discharge to home. Many health care systems provide home-health team visits and lactation support.

Early identification of risk, early detection of rising bilirubin levels, and early treatment are key to timely resolution of the problem. These same elements of care are key to avoiding readmissions.

Summary

Hyperbilirubinemia is one of the most common complications seen in newborn infants. Hydration, monitoring, and phototherapy are usual practices. Nonetheless, the evidence to support phototherapy is based largely on consensus and expert opinion. Limited strong evidence is available to support the current practice. Research is needed to support meaningful risk assessment and to evaluate treatment options. More important, little evidence is available to predict risk for severe hyperbilirubinemia, kernicterus, or readmission.

American Academy of Pediatrics Subcommittee on Hyperbilirubinemia. (2004). Clinical practice guideline: Management of hyperbilirubinemia in the newborn infant 35 or more weeks of gestation. *Pediatrics, 114*(1), 297–316.

Azzuqa, A., & Watchko, J. F. (2015). Bilirubin concentrations in jaundiced neonates with conjunctival icterus. *Journal of Pediatrics, 167*(4), 840–844.

Bhutani, V. K., Vilms, R. J., & Hamerman-Johnson, L. (2010). Universal bilirubin screening for severe neonatal hyperbilirubinemia. *Journal of Perinatology, 30*(Suppl.), S6–S15.

Cashore, W. (2010). A brief history of neonatal jaundice. *Medicine and Health, Rhode Island, 93*(5), 154–155.

Cohen, R. S., Wong, R. J., & Stevenson, D. K. (2010). Understanding neonatal jaundice: A perspective on causation. *Pediatrics and Neonatology, 51*(3), 143–148.

Maisels, M. J., Coffey, M. P., & Kring, E. (2015). Transcutaneous bilirubin levels in newborns < 35 weeks' gestation. *Journal of Perinatology, 35*(9), 739–744.

Muchowski, K. E. (2014). Evaluation and treatment of neonatal hyperbilirubinemia. *American Family Physician, 89*(11), 873–878.

■ HYPERTENSION

Mary F. Terhaar

Overview

Hypertension in neonates may present insidiously as feeding difficulty, irritability, tachypnea, apnea, or lethargy; may be identified on routine screening; or may present more acutely as congestive heart failure or cardiogenic shock (Flynn, 2000). In infants, as in adults, hypertension is dangerous, particularly when undetected or undermanaged. Preventing organ damage, maintaining healthy function of organ systems, and promoting healthy development depend on early detection and careful management (Kaebler et al., 2016).

Background

Blood pressure (BP) in neonates increases with gestational age, neonatal age, birthweight, and time.

Evidence-based BP charts that describe ranges of pressure over time have made it possible to standardize expectations for BP values and help clinicians identify hypertension more consistently and with greater confidence (Flynn, 2000, 2010).

Normotension in the neonate is defined as a BP within the 95th percentile on the BP charts. Conversely, *hypertension* in the neonate is defined as elevation in systolic BP (on three separate occasions) higher than the 95th percentile for age, weight, and gender (Watkinson, 2002). By definition then, 5% of all neonates are hypertensive, although in practice, the incidence is closer to 0.2% to 3.0% (Dionne, Abibtol, & Flynn, 2011).

Neonatal hypertension may result from several different causes. It can develop as a result of congenital conditions, including aortic coarctation or structural defects of the renal system; as a consequence of renal disease, including parenchymal or vascular disease; as sequelae to bronchopulmonary dysplasia; as an unintended outcome of medical care following administration of certain medications; accompanying endocrine disorders such as congenital adrenal hyperplasia and hyperthyroidism; or develop from thromboembolism following umbilical catheterization (Flynn, 2002, 2010). Without proper diagnosis and management, hypertension can progress to cardiovascular disease, kidney disease, and stroke in the adult (Nickavar & Assadi, 2014).

Among 398,079 children receiving well-child care between the ages of 3 and 18 years, 3.3% met diagnostic criteria and were identified as hypertensive and another 10.1% were prehypertensive. These findings agree with prevalence projections described earlier. Regardless, the American Academy of Pediatrics recommended treatment was not initiated for the 2,813 infants diagnosed as hypertensive (Kaebler et al., 2016).

A careful history, including both the pregnancy and the neonatal period, is key to evaluating risk, detecting disease, effectively managing the condition, and preventing complications. Family history of renal disease or hypertension, in utero exposure to cocaine or other street drugs, and clinical history of bronchopulmonary dysplasia are highly correlated with development of hypertension in the newborn (Flynn & Rosenkrantz, 2016).

Clinical Aspects

ASSESSMENT

Head-to-toe assessment establishes findings to confirm or rule out hypertension. Organ systems impacted by sustained elevated BP are particularly relevant for assessment because microvascular changes in these organs lead to symptoms throughout the body (Nikavar & Assaddi, 2014). Important findings include bluish or pale coloration to the skin and rapid respirations, which indicate poor perfusion and oxygenation.

In the primary care setting, weight gain that does not correspond to postnatal age and failure to meet developmental milestones indicate compromised perfusion and oxygenation to vital organs and systems over an extended period of time. Frequent urinary tract infections point to structural or vascular abnormalities associated with hypertension. Symptoms of pronounced or advanced disease include irritability, seizures, difficulty breathing, feeding intolerance, and vomiting (Kaeber et al., 2016).

In the neonatal intensive care unit (NICU), routine assessment of respiratory rate and function, heart rate, perfusion, liver function, and oxygenation as well as systolic, diastolic, and pulse pressures provide useful information to complement BP readings. Observation of the wave formation from arterial lines, urine output, and perfusion to lower extremities provides a picture of vascular conditions. Umbilical arterial lines that are commonly used in the NICU must be discontinued at any sign of complications, including presence of blood in the urine, change in location of the catheter tip on radiography, or compromised perfusion.

Because hypertension in the neonate is defined by three discrete BP measurements that fall higher than the 95th percentile on standard BP charts, repeated measurement of BP, respiratory rate, heart rate, and pulse oximetry inform the diagnosis (Flynn, 2000, 2010). In practice, hypertension is most commonly diagnosed and treated when the BP persistently exceeds the 99th percentile. These data, in combination with the aforementioned clinical findings, indicate the need for and effectiveness of the treatment regimen, which is adjusted to the severity and responsiveness of the clinical presentation.

NURSING INTERVENTIONS, MANAGEMENT, AND IMPLICATIONS

Care for the hypertensive infant in the NICU focuses on promoting comfort, managing medications, monitoring fluid status and renal function, and parent education. Comfort is promoted through careful positioning, providing opportunities for nonnutritive sucking, clustering care to allow time for rest, administering analgesics as indicated, providing skin-to-skin experiences with parents, and maintaining a restive environment. Medications are administered as prescribed. Fluid status is assessed by checking for edema in the extremities and face; strict monitoring of intake and output; testing specific gravity; and monitoring blood urea nitrogen (BUN), creatinine levels, and hematocrit.

In the NICU, pain, agitation, renal output, underlying conditions, interventions such as ventilators and phlebotomy, and medications can influence BP. Pain can complicate assessment and exaggerate the presentation of hypertension. Meticulous pain management is an essential component of treatment, especially when hypertension is a consequence of prematurity, which requires a stay in critical care, or in the case of congenital anomalies that require surgical intervention.

BP measurements are essential for management of hypertension in the NICU and primary care. Readings can be influenced by many factors, including behavioral state, pain, hunger, and agitation. In order for data to be meaningful, it is useful to measure the BP with the infant in a quiescent state and to note any condition that may have altered the reading at any given time. Proper fit of the cuff to the size of the infant is essential (Nickavar & Assadi, 2014).

In the primary care setting, a variety of medications are prescribed to manage neonatal hypertension, which commonly resolves in the short term in the instance in which it presents as a complication of acute illness or medical management. In a meta-analysis of clinical trials conducted on hypertensive infants, angiotensin-converting enzyme (ACE) inhibitors and angiotensin receptor blockers (ARB) were most commonly prescribed (35%) followed by diuretics in 22% of the children, calcium channel blockers in 17%, and beta-blockers in another 10% (Kaebler et al., 2016). Infant weight, heart rate, respirations, and BP complete the assessment here as well. Insufficient weight gain may indicate failure to thrive as a result of hypertension and excessive weight gain that presents with edema can also indicate poor BP control.

In cases in which hypertension results from renal, vascular, or parenchymal disease, medications should focus on those disease processes. Management of hypertension that results from kidney disease commonly requires more prolonged treatment under the supervision of a renal specialist.

Lifestyle changes, including diet and exercise, which are among the most effective approaches for adults with hypertension, are ill suited for infants. Evidence supports pharmacologic interventions as most effective for this age group (Chaturvedi, Lipszyc, Licht,

Craig, & Parekh, 2014). However, until recently, few clinical trials have provided robust data to describe efficacy and long-term outcomes and to guide management. This is the reason that careful monitoring of BP and other clinical data are very important.

Medications are frequently used to manage hypertension. In a study of more than 2,000 hypertensive children and infants, angiotensin-converting enzyme inhibitors and angiotensin receptor blockers were most commonly prescribed (35%); 22% received diuretics; 17% received calcium channel blockers; and another 10% received beta-blockers (Kaebler et al., 2016).

Parents of infants with hypertension require support and education. Parents must have a clear understanding of the medications they administer, the side effects each may cause, and potential interactions between medications and foods. Parents need to understand the importance of follow-up visits, target respiratory rate, goals for growth and development, as well as the symptoms that indicate that the medications and plan of care are effective or failing. Parents must understand the nature of the disease and long-term consequences for their infants. Just as hypertension in adults is a silent disease, so, too, the negative consequences of hypertension in the infant may be advanced before signs and symptoms are recognizable. For this reason, screening and management are key.

OUTCOMES

Management of hypertension is the priority in avoiding long-term complications that result from end organ and vascular damage. Such complications include left ventricular hypertrophy, encephalopathy, and retinopathy (Nickavar & Assadi, 2014). Failure to gain weight and failure to thrive can also result when hypertension is not recognized or managed.

Summary

Effective treatment of hypertension in the NICU and in the primary care setting depends on careful assessment, early diagnosis, understanding of the disease, and a familiarity with the evidence. In the case when hypertension results from hospitalization in the NICU and associated conditions, parents need education and support to manage it. The same is true when hypertension extends beyond the NICU stay. In both cases, the goal is to prevent end organ damage, which can have lifelong negative impact. Just as hypertension is a silent disease in adults, so it is for infants. In both situations, vigilance as well as compliance with medication regimens and lifestyle modifications are associated with best outcomes.

Chaturvedi, S., Lipszyc, D. H., Licht, C., Craig, J. C., & Parekh, R. S. (2014). Cochrane in context: Pharmacological interventions for hypertension in children. *Evidence-Based Child Health: A Cochrane Review Journal, 9*(3), 581–583.

Dionne, J. M., Abitbol, C. L., & Flynn, J. T. (2012). Hypertension in infancy: Diagnosis, management and outcome. *Pediatric Nephrology, 27*(1), 17–32.

Flynn, J. T. (2000). Neonatal hypertension: Diagnosis and management. *Pediatric Nephrology, 14*(4), 332–341.

Flynn, J. T., & Rosenkrantz, T. (2016). Neonatal hypertension. Theheart.org Medscape. Retrieved from http://emedicine.medscape.com

Kaelber, D. C., Weiwei, L., Ross, M., et al.; Comparative Effectiveness Research Through Collaborative Electronic Reporting Consortium. (2016). Diagnosis and medication treatment of pediatric hypertension: A retrospective cohort study. *Pediatrics, 138*(6), e2195.

Nickavar, A., & Assadi, F. (2014). Managing hypertension in the newborn infants. *International Journal of Preventive Medicine, 5*(Suppl. 1), S39–S43.

Watkinson, M. (2002). Hypertension in the newborn baby. *Archives of Disease in Childhood. Fetal and Neonatal Edition, 86*(2), F78–F81.

■ HYPOGLYCEMIA

Tina Di Fiore

Overview

Hypoglycemia is the most common metabolic problem seen in newborn infants. The overall incidence of neonatal hypoglycemia varies from 1.3 to three per 1,000 live births (American Academy of Pediatrics, 2011). This variability is seen due in part to the controversial definition of neonatal hypoglycemia in addition to the different populations, different method and timing of feeding, and different types of glucose testing. For example, serum glucose levels are higher than whole-blood values. The controversial definition is reinforced by The American Academy of Pediatrics (2011) statement, which notes that "there has been no substantial evidence-based progress in defining what constitutes clinically important neonatal hypoglycemia particularly regarding how it relates to brain injury, and that monitoring for, preventing, and treating neonatal hypoglycemia remain largely empirical" (p. 575). In other words, the level or duration of hypoglycemia

that is harmful to an infant's developing brain is not known.

Background

The laboratory value used to define neonatal hypoglycemia varies in part due to the normal physiologic changes a newborn experiences as they transition to extrauterine life. The healthy neonate demonstrates a drop in the blood glucose concentrations to approximately 30 mg/dL within 1 to 2 hours after birth, and typically returns to more than 45 mg/dL with normal feeding within 12 hours (Cornblath et al., 2000).

Neonatal hypoglycemia is a result of an imbalance between glucose supply and the metabolic needs of the neonate, which may be due to inadequate glycogen stores, inappropriate changes in insulin secretion, inadequate muscle stores as a source of amino acids for gluconeogenesis, or inadequate lipid stores for the release of fatty acids or increased glucose utilization from sepsis or other illnesses (Deshpande & Platt, 2005). Excluding infants who are receiving insulin therapy, almost all hypoglycemia in neonates occurs during fasting. Postprandial hypoglycemia is rare in neonates but may be seen with hyperinsulinism, or persistent hyperinsulinemic hypoglycemia of infancy (PHHI). PHHI is the most common cause of hypoglycemia in the first 3 months of life. It is well recognized in infants of mothers with diabetes. The etiology for hyperinsulinism is the fetal response to elevated maternal glucose by producing elevated levels of insulin. Following birth the insulin concentrations are inappropriately elevated and lead to neonatal hypoglycemia. Most cases of hyperinsulinism are transient; however, prolonged neonatal hyperinsulinism, also known as *congenital hyperinsulinism* is most commonly associated with an abnormality of beta-cell regulation throughout the pancreas. In rare cases, surgical treatment is necessary for the neonate who is unresponsive to conventional therapy. Surgical treatment involves resection of 80% to 90% of the pancreas (Garg & Devaskar, 2006).

Clinical Aspects

ASSESSMENT

The clinical presentation of neonatal hypoglycemia is nonspecific and can vary from infant to infant. In addition, infants in the first or second day of life may be asymptomatic or may have life-threatening central nervous system (CNS) or cardiopulmonary disturbances. The most common clinical manifestations include lethargy, hypotonia, poor feeding, weak or high-pitched cry, tachypnea or respiratory distress, and hypothermia or temperature instability. Other symptoms may also be seen, including tremors, jitteriness, cyanosis, apnea, irritability, and exaggerated Moro reflex or seizures, a serious sign that usually occurs late in severe neonatal hypoglycemia (Jain, 2008).

To assist with the identification of the high-risk infant, a review of the maternal history should be obtained on all infants. The history review should focus on identifying at-risk infants. Assessment with frequent and vigilant monitoring of infants with known risk factors remains key in the diagnosis, management, and treatment of neonatal hypoglycemia. High-risk groups that need screening for hypoglycemia in the first hour of life include newborns who weigh more than 4 kg or less than 2 kg; large-for-gestational-age (LGA) infants who are above the 90th percentile in weight for their gestational age. Small-for-gestational-age (SGA) infants below the 10th percentile for their gestational age, infants with intrauterine growth restriction (IUGR), and infants less than 37-week gestation are at a higher risk of hypoglycemia due to decreased glycogen stores and larger brain size.

Infants at high risk for hypoglycemia include newborns suspected of having sepsis or born to a mother suspected of having chorioramnionitis; newborns with symptoms suggestive of hypoglycemia, including jitteriness, tachypnea, hypotonia, poor feeding, apnea, temperature instability, seizures, and lethargy; infants with respiratory distress due to their increased glucose utilization; discordant twins with weight differences greater than 20%; perinatal stress; significant hypoxia; asphyxia; hypoxic–ischemic encephalopathy; infants with hypothermia (cold stress); infants with hyperviscosity syndrome/polycythemia (central hematocrit greater than 70%); mothers who have received terbutaline or infant born to a mother with type 1, type 2, or gestational diabetes (Straussman & Levitsky, 2010).

NURSING INTERVENTIONS, MANAGEMENT, AND IMPLICATIONS

If neonatal hypoglycemia is suspected, the plasma or blood glucose level should be determined by laboratory method. However, a long delay in processing the specimen can result in a falsely low concentration as erythrocytes in the sample metabolize the glucose in the plasma. This problem can be avoided by transporting the blood in tubes that contain a glycolytic inhibitor such as fluoride. If recurrent hypoglycemia occurs, then further laboratory testing needs to be done, including obtaining serum insulin levels, evaluating for urine ketones, analyzing the urine for organic acid abnormalities, and screening for metabolic errors.

Management efforts are directed toward the immediate normalization of glucose levels and the identification and treatment of the various causes. It is important to note that feeding infants early decreases the incidence of hypoglycemia. Therefore, the nurse should identify the at-risk neonate and focus on early feeding in the newborn. Infants at high risk for hypoglycemia should be treated as soon as possible to prevent long-term complications. In the breastfed infant, early feeding may be problematic due to decreased breast milk supply and difficulty with breastfeeding initiation. Supplementation with infant formula or oral glucose gel may be used.

If the mother wishes to exclusively breastfeed, glucose gel has been demonstrated to safely treat hypoglycemia while decreasing the separation of the mother and infant. Using a dose of 0.2 g of glucose per kilogram administered orally, using the commercially available 40% oral glucose gel in the buccal mucosa in combination with feedings has been demonstrated as another treatment for neonatal hypoglycemia (Harris, Weston, Signal, Chase, & Harding, 2013). In the newborn with respiratory distress or other suspected illness, treatment should focus on the use of intravenous (IV) glucose administration. IV fluids should be started with a solution containing 10% dextrose and administered at a rate of 60 to 80 mL/kg/day. Frequent monitoring of blood glucoses with adjustment in the IV rate or an increase in dextrose concentration should occur if needed.

It is nursing's responsibility to be vigilant in monitoring infants with hypoglycemia. Most newborn nurseries and neonatal intensive care units (NICUs) have specific hypoglycemia protocols to follow. Encourage mothers to breastfeed frequently (every 1–2 hours). Education of parents is extremely important, especially if the infant is being monitored in the NICU, which increases parental stress and anxiety.

OUTCOMES

Sustained or repetitive hypoglycemia in infants has a major impact on normal brain development and function. Evidence suggests that hypoxemia and ischemia potentiate hypoglycemia, causing brain damage that may permanently impair neurologic development.

Therefore, neonates who have comorbidities should be monitored closely for hypoglycemia even when they are out of the immediate newborn period (Deshpande & Platt, 2005).

Summary

Neonatal hypoglycemia can lead to major long-term sequelae, including neurologic injury resulting in mental retardation, recurrent seizure activity, developmental delay, and possibly impaired cardiovascular function. It is imperative for nurses to monitor infants closely and to be able to recognize and promptly treat hypoglycemia.

American Academy of Pediatrics, Committee on Fetus and Newborn. (2011). Postnatal glucose homeostasis in late-preterm and term infants. *Pediatrics, 127,* 575–579.

Cornblath, M., Hawdon, J. M., Williams, A. F., Aynsley-Green, A., Ward-Platt, M. P., Schwartz, R., & Kalhan, S. C. (2000). Controversies regarding definition of neonatal hypoglycemia: Suggested operational thresholds. *Pediatrics, 105*(5), 1141–1145.

Deshpande, S., & Platt, M. (2005). The investigation and management of neonatal hypoglycemia. *Seminars in Fetal and Neonatal Medicine, 10*(4), 351–361. doi:/10.1016/j.clp.2006.10.001

Garg, M., & Devaskar, S. (2006). Glucose metabolism in the late preterm infant. *Clinics in Perinatology, 33*(40). Retrieved from https://www.ncbi.nlm.nih.gov/pubmed/17148009

Harris, D. L., Weston, P. J., Signal, M., Chase, J. G., & Harding, J. E. (2013). Dextrose gel for neonatal hypoglycemia (the Sugar Babies Study): A randomised, double-blind, placebo-controlled trial. *Lancet, 382*(9910), 2077–2083. doi:10.1016/S0140-6736(13)61645-1

Jain, A. (2008). Hypoglycemia in the newborn. *Indian Journal of Pediatrics, 75*(1), 63–66. doi:10.1007/s12098-008-0009-6

Straussman, S., & Levitsky, L. (2010). Neonatal hypoglycemia. *Current Opinion in Endocrinology, Diabetes & Obesity, 17,* 20–24.

■ HYPOXIC ISCHEMIC ENCEPHALOPATHY

Ke-Ni Niko Tien

Overview

Hypoxic ischemic encephalopathy (HIE) is impaired gas exchange caused by a decrease in cerebral blood flow that results in hypoxemia (low blood oxygen levels), hypercarbia (elevated CO_2 levels), and the severe consequence of global cerebral ischemia (Karlsen, 2013; Zanelli et al., 2016). HIE can also lead to neurologic injuries, seizures, and death. Intrauterine asphyxia, such as clotting of placental arteries, placental abruption, and inflammatory process or perinatal infarction are the most common mechanisms of hypoxic injury in term infants (Fatemi, Willson, & Johnston, 2009). Evidence has shown that providing advanced quality care may reduce the incidence and severity of the outcome of neonatal encephalopathy by half (Graham, Ruis, Hartman, Northington, & Fox, 2008).

Currently, the most promising therapy is neuroprotective/therapeutic hypothermia as indicated by intentional head or body cooling (Karlsen, 2013; Price-Douglas & Fernandes, 2015). However, cooling is primarily limited to level III and level IV neonatal intensive care units (NICUs), due to complex care issues that the infant may have. The infant may need to be transported to a tertiary care center (Barks, 2008; Price-Douglas & Fernandes, 2015). At delivery, it is critical for health care providers to recognize newborns with HIE who may be candidates for cooling.

Background

The incidence of HIE is one to four cases per 1,000 live births in the United States (Wayock et al., 2014; Zanelli et al., 2016). Worldwide, there are approximately 840,000 neonatal deaths as a result of perinatal asphyxia (Zanelli et al., 2016). Severe hypoxemia may lead to the production of lactic acid during anaerobic glycolysis that results in metabolic acidosis (a low pH and an elevated base deficit), which is the most objective assessment of perinatal HIE (Graham et al., 2008; Karlsen, 2013). In addition, studies have shown an increase in seizures if the umbilical arterial pH is less than 7.0, as well as a significant increase in neurologic morbidities (Fatemi et al., 2009; Graham et al., 2008).

The criteria identified in determining intrapartum asphyxia in an infant are late decelerations on fetal monitoring or meconium/meconium-stained fluid at delivery, delayed respiratory effort after birth, arterial cord blood pH less than 7.1, Apgar score less than 7 at 5 minutes of age, and multiorgan injury (Graham et al., 2008). However, studies have shown that numerous factors can contribute to low Apgar scores, such as intrapartum maternal sedation or anesthesia, congenital malformation, the appearance of infection, and the effectiveness of resuscitation. Therefore, the Apgar score alone is not the most reliable predictor for perinatal hypoxemia (Graham et al., 2008).

Severe HIE can lead to clinical seizures, epileptic activity seen on EEG, hypotonia, lack of gag reflex, poor feeding, and a prolonged depressed-consciousness status. Infants who survive a birth asphyxia insult may develop neurologic sequelae such as cerebral palsy, mental retardation, learning difficulties, cognitive and motor deficits as well as other disabilities (Karlsen, 2013; Zanelli et al., 2016).

Several clinical trials have shown the promising results of intentional hypothermia therapy (Fatemi et al., 2009). Clinical investigations have demonstrated an overall reduction in mortality and disability for infants who received hypothermia therapy (cooling) within the first 24 hours of life. Hypothermia therapy reduces cerebral metabolism and the inflammation process triggered by ischemic events (Fatemi et al., 2009). Currently, hypothermia therapy has become a standard of care in moderate to severe HIE treatment.

Accurately predicting the prognosis and severity of long-term complications of HIE is difficult. The lack of spontaneous respiratory effort for 20 to 30 minutes after birth; presence of frequent and uncontrollable seizure activity; prolonged abnormal clinical neurologic findings, including abnormal muscle tone and posture; abnormal background activity on EEG; persistent feeding difficulties due to abnormal sucking and swallowing and poor head growth are the most helpful indicators in determining the possible long-term outcomes of HIE (Zanelli et al., 2016).

Clinical Aspects

ASSESSMENT

There are three levels of HIE: mild, moderately severe, and severe (Zanelli et al., 2016). Mild hypertonia, poor feeding, and irritability present during the first few days of life are categorized as mild HIE. Hypotonia, diminished grasp and gag, decreased Moro reflex and sucking, seizure activity, and apneic episodes may be seen when HIE is moderately severe. These symptoms may resolve within 1 to 2 weeks and lead to a better long-term outcome. In infants with severe HIE, seizures can be delayed, severe, and show resistance to conventional anticonvulsant therapy. Other symptoms of severe HIE may also include stupor or coma, respiratory failure requiring mechanical ventilation,

generalized hypotonia and depressed reflexes, abnormal ocular motion such as nystagmus, dilated or fixed pupils, and arrhythmia as well as hypotension. These symptoms may worsen during the rewarming period and even cause death.

Therapeutic hypothermia/cooling therapy is the most promising treatment for HIE. The gold standard is to initiate cooling within 6 hours of birth to maximize an optimal outcome (Karlsen, 2013). Once cooling therapy is determined, passive (turning off the radiant warmer) or active cooling (placing an infant on a cooling blanket or head cooling) should be implemented.

All neonates who qualify for cooling therapy are cooled to a rectal temperature of 33.5°C or 92.3°F for 72 hours (Burton et al., 2015; Wayock et al., 2014; Zanelli et al., 2016). The criteria to determine whether or not to initiate cooling are a gestational age greater than or equal to 36 weeks and a birth weight greater than or equal to 1,800 g; umbilical cord blood gas or arterial blood gas obtained in the first hour of life with a pH less than or equal to 7.0; or base deficit greater than 16 mmol/L. Cooling also requires a neurologic examination denoting seizures, level of consciousness, spontaneous activity when awake or aroused, posture, tone, primitive reflexes, heart rate, respiratory rate, and reaction of pupils to light.

Seventy-two hours after being placed on a cooling blanket or cooling hat, a slow and controlled rewarming process should be cautiously performed and monitored. At present, there is limited evidence to indicate the safest way and speed to use to rewarm severely hypothermic infants. Based on the recommendation, rewarming speed should not exceed 0.5°C per hour to prevent sudden vasodilation, hypotension, and other clinical deterioration (Holton, 2014; Karlsen, 2013). During the rewarming period, vital signs, level of consciousness, neurologic exam, and blood gases should be closely monitored.

NURSING INTERVENTIONS, MANAGEMENT, AND IMPLICATIONS

It is critical for the nurse to closely monitor heart rate and rhythm, blood pressure, pulses, perfusion, respiratory rate and effort, oxygen saturation, acid/base status, and blood glucoses during both cooling and rewarming phases. Monitoring the rectal temperature is helpful because the skin temperature of the infant is higher than the rectal temperature during the rewarming period. If an infant deteriorates rapidly during either the cooling or rewarming period, the nurse must be prepared to perform a full cardiopulmonary resuscitation.

It is important to monitor closely for any seizure activity. Continuous EEG monitoring is normally placed during the duration of cooling. A full-montage EEG and an MRI should be obtained after an infant is rewarmed and stable.

It is essential to perform a complete neurologic exam with hands-on care, including checking pupils, level of consciousness, and any signs or symptoms of increased intracranial pressure. It is important to ensure appropriate sedation during cooling therapy to optimize comfort and efficacy of the cooling. Inadequate sedation increases the metabolic rate and decreases the effectiveness of cooling.

It is critical to monitor intake and output closely as fluid is normally restricted to avoid fluid overload and cerebral edema. Infants who undergo cooling therapy are at risk for renal impairment and electrolyte imbalance, which requires frequent monitoring and correction of any imbalance.

Infants who receive cooling often are treated with antibiotics for possible infection. It is vital to monitor any signs and symptoms of infection. It is also important to monitor for any signs of coagulopathy such as petechiae. Infants may require transfusions due to coagulopathy induced by hypothermia and decreased platelet function.

It is critical to frequently assess the skin for possible subcutaneous fat necrosis. Erythematous nodules and plaques over boney areas, such as the back, arms, buttocks, and thighs, are the characteristic areas of subcutaneous fat necrosis that may worsen during cooling and can be very painful.

Families are an integral part of care for an infant admitted to the NICU. Continuous updates and support are essential to families while their babies undergo cooling therapy. It is important to encourage bonding by allowing parents to touch their baby and help with care.

OUTCOMES

Perinatal HIE is a major health issue globally. It can lead to neurologic deficits, neurodevelopmental disabilities, long-term functional impairments, and significant learning difficulties later on in a child's life. Although there are no effective pharmacologic therapies to treat HIE currently, intentional cooling therapy has been the most promising and has become the standard of care for moderate to severe HIE.

Close monitoring of an infant, including thorough frequent assessments, is critical during the cooling and rewarming phase. It is important to understand and recognize any potential side effects. It is also vital to include parents and family in nursing care. Families must understand the reasons behind cooling therapy, the expected length of treatment, and the potential for long-term morbidities.

Summary

Current research supports the efficacy of intentional cooling treatment for infants who are equal to or more than 36-weeks gestation and more than or equal to 1,800 g. However, there has been significant research in HIE for multimodal therapeutic approaches, and many clinical trials are in process to prove that cooling used on infants who are younger than 36 weeks is applicable and effective as well.

Barks, J. (2008). Technical aspects of starting a neonatal cooling program. *Clinics in Perinatology*, 35(4), 765–775. doi:10.1016/j.clp.2008.07.009

Fatemi, A., Wilson, M. A. & Johnston, M. V. (2009). Hypoxic ischemic encephalopathy in the term infant. *Clinical Perinatology*, 36(4), 835–858. doi:10.1016/j.clp.2009.07.011

Graham, E. M., Ruis, K. A., Hartman, A. L., Northington, F. J., & Fox, H. E. (2008). A systematic review of the role of intrapartum hypoxia-ischemia in the causation of neonatal encephalopathy. *American Journal of Obstetrics & Gynecology*, 199(6), 587–595. doi:10.1016/j.ajog.2008.06.094

Holton, T. (2014). Clinical guidelines (nursing): Therapeutic hypothermia in the neonate. The Royal Children's Hospital Melbourne. Retrieved from http://www.rch.org.au/rchcpg/hospital_clinical_guideline_index/Therapeutic_hypothermia_in_the_neonate

Karlsen, K. A. (2013). *The S.T.A.B.L.E. program: Pretransport/ post-resuscitation stabilization care of sick infants guidelines for neonatal healthcare providers* (6th ed.). Salt Lake City: UT: The S.T.A.B.L.E. Program.

Price-Douglas, W., & Fernandes, C. J. (2015). Infants with hypoxic-ischemic encephalopathy may need to be transported for therapeutic cooling. *AAP News*, 35(10). doi:10.1542/aapnews.20153610-15.

Wayock, C. P., Meserole, R. L., Saria, S., Jennings, J. M., Huisman, T. A. G. M., Northington, F. J. & Graham, E. M. (2014). Perinatal risk factors for severe injury in neonates treated with whole-body hypothermia for encephalopathy. *American Journal of Obstetrics & Gynecology*, 211(1), 41.e1–41.e8. doi:10.1016/j.ajog.2014.03.033

Zanelli, S. A., Kaufman, D. A., Stanley, D. P., Windle, M. L., Carter, B. S., & Rosenkrantz, T. (2016). Hypoxic-ischemic encephalopathy. *Medscape*. Retrieved from http://emedicine.medscape.com/article/973501-overview

■ INCREASED PULMONARY BLOOD FLOW

Jennifer Johntony
Jodi Zalewski

Overview

Increased pulmonary blood flow may result in leakage of fluids into the interstitial space with subsequent pulmonary edema due to increased pulmonary pressures and congestion (Capozzi & Santoro, 2011). In patients with acyanotic congenital heart disease, this increase in pulmonary blood flow occurs in heart defects with left-to-right shunts. Cardiac shunting occurs when there is a diversion of normal blood flow. The type and location of the shunt, as well as the pathophysiology of the defect, determine the risk of potential complications from increased pulmonary blood blow. These complications include pulmonary bleeding, pulmonary hypertension, and eventually irreversible parenchymal lung disease. The most common congenital cardiac lesions related to increased pulmonary blood flow are patent ductus arteriosus (PDA), atrial septal defect (ASD), ventricular septal defect (VSD), and atrioventricular canal (AVC) defect also known as *endocardial cushion defect*.

Background

The PDA accounts for approximately 10% of newborns with cardiac defects, and is a normal part of fetal circulation (Park, 2016). In utero, oxygenated blood from the placental circulation bypasses the nonaerated fetal lungs and is delivered directly to the fetus' lower body organs (Capozzi & Santoro, 2011). The PDA is a vascular communication between the main pulmonary artery and the descending aorta. The degree of left-to-right shunting is determined by the size of the PDA, which includes measurement of the diameter, length, and level of pulmonary vascular resistance (Park, 2016). The PDA functionally closes within 48 hours after birth and by 2 weeks of age will close anatomically (Delaney, Baker, Bastardi, & O'Brien, 2015).

Isolated ASD accounts for 5% to 10% of all congenital heart defects and is most common in females (Park,

2016). ASDs are openings in the atrial septum that allow blood flow to shunt from the left side of the heart to the right side, leading to right atrial dilatation, right ventricular volume overload, and increased pulmonary blood flow (Jone, Darst, Collins, & Miyamoto, 2016).

There are four types of ASDs that can be distinguished by their location within the atrial septum: ostium secundum, sinus venosus, ostium primum, and coronary sinus. The type and location of the defect and/or enlargement of the right heart chambers determine what intervention is needed.

VSDs are the most common form of congenital heart disease, accounting for 15% to 20% of all pediatric heart surgeries (Park, 2016). VSDs are openings in the ventricular septum that allow for blood flow to shunt from the left side of the heart to the right side, leading to left atrial dilation, left ventricular volume overload, and increased pulmonary blood flow. If left-to-right shunting is significant at the ventricular level, there will be excessive pulmonary blood flow leading to pulmonary edema and tachypnea (Nelson, Hirsch-Romano, Ohye, & Bove, 2015). The effects of increased pulmonary blood flow depend on the size and number of defects and resistance to flow through the lungs.

There are three types of VSDs that can be distinguished by their location within the ventricular septum: perimembraneous, infundibular, and muscular defects. Infants with small VSDs usually do not require surgery. Infants with a large VSD usually have surgical repair by 1 year of age.

AVC defects account for 2% of all congenital heart diseases and 30% of this defect occurs in children with Trisomy 21 (Park, 2016). AVC consists of three components: ostium primum ASD, an inlet VSD, and clefts in the mitral valve leaflet and the septal leaflet of the tricuspid valve (Park, 2016). AVC defects can be delineated into two categories: complete or partial. A complete AVC consists of an ASD, large VSD, and single atrioventricular valve; infants may have ventricular asymmetry, which is categorized as an unbalanced AVC (Nelson et al., 2015). A partial AVC consists of an ASD with a cleft in the anterior leaflet of the left atrioventricular valve, no VSD, and the presence of two atrioventricular valves (Nelson et al., 2015). The level of left-to-right shunting depends on several factors: the shunt can be interatrial and/or interventricular; if there is atrioventricular (AV) valve regurgitation present or if there is a left ventricular to right atrial (LV–RA) shunt. The increase in left-to-right shunting increases atrial and ventricular volume overload with resultant increased pulmonary blood flow, leading to congestive heart failure (CHF; Park, 2016).

Clinical Aspects

ASSESSMENT

The size and degree of shunting of the PDA determines symptoms (Delaney et al., 2015). Patients with a small ductus usually are asymptomatic. However, if the defect is large with significant left-to-right shunting, infants can show signs of CHF (Park, 2016). Typical symptoms are tachypnea, tachycardia, and poor feeding. A widened pulse pressure and bounding pulses are also present due to extra blood flow from the aorta to the pulmonary arteries (Delaney, et al., 2015). The classic murmur of a PDA is a continuous "machinery" murmur heard best along the left upper sternal border (Nelson, et al., 2015). Indications for surgical closure of a PDA are hemodynamic instability. PDAs can be closed by surgical repair or transcatheter closure in the cardiac catheterization laboratory (Park, 2016).

Patients with ASDs are usually asymptomatic but can develop signs of heart failure later in life if the ASD is undiagnosed (Delaney, et al., 2015). The majority of ASDs can close spontaneously, but, if left untreated, infants are at risk for atrial dysrhythmias, pulmonary vascular obstructive disease, and emboli formation due to increased pulmonary blood flow (Delaney, et al., 2015). The classic physical findings in infants with ASDs include widely split and fixed S2 and a grade 2–3/6 systolic ejection murmur heard best at the left upper sternal border. This occurs due to increased flow across a normal pulmonary valve (Park, 2016). The three main interventions of choice are no therapy, if the right side of the heart is not enlarged; surgical closure; or transcatheter device closure, which has become the treatment of choice.

Patients with small VSDs are asymptomatic and the defect usually closes within the first 2 years of life. A VSD typically has a grade 2–5/6 holosystolic murmur that is best heard at the left lower sternal border. Small VSDs have louder murmurs due to restrictive blood flow (Park, 2016). Larger VSDs can cause symptoms of CHF, which include tachypnea, hepatomegaly, poor feeding, and failure to thrive (Nelson, et al., 2015). If the infant has significant heart failure, diuretics as well as digoxin and beta blockers may be initiated until surgical closure of the VSD can be performed.

Patients with AVC present early in infancy with signs and symptoms of CHF when there is both atrial-level and ventricular-level shunting (Nelson, et al., 2015). Infants, on physical examination, have a hyperactive precordium with a prominent thrill. A grade 3-4/6 holosystolic murmur can be heard best at the left sternal border (Park, 2016). Infants can be optimized on heart failure medications until they are ready for surgical repair (Nelson, et al., 2015).

NURSING INTERVENTIONS, MANAGEMENT, AND IMPLICATIONS

Nursing-related problems specific to infants with increased pulmonary blood flow focus on the management of pulmonary overcirculation and CHF. Infants with increased pulmonary blood flow can experience impaired myocardial function, pulmonary congestion, and systemic venous congestion (Delaney, et al., 2015).

Due diligence by nurses with respect to the infant's cardiac anatomy and baseline clinical presentation is vital in order to intervene when changes occur. The nurse must assess and record heart rate, respiratory rate, breath sounds, blood pressure, and pulse oximetry readings. Infants with myocardial dysfunction present with tachycardia, diaphoresis, and irritability. Improvement in cardiac function includes the administration of digitalis glycosides (digoxin) and angiotensin-converting enzyme (ACE) inhibitors (Delaney et al., 2015). Prescribed cardiac medications needs to be given at the scheduled time and any side effects or signs and symptoms of toxicity should be reported and documented (Delaney et al., 2015). Nurses must assess and document signs of pulmonary overcirculation, such as tachypnea, retractions, nasal flaring, grunting, and wheezing, due to decreased lung compliance. Administration of oxygen may assist in improving gas exchange. Increased blood flow to the heart and lungs may result in orthopnea, which can be alleviated by placing the infant in the recumbent position. Increased pressure and pooling of blood in the venous circulation are caused by systemic venous congestion due to right-sided heart failure and may result in hepatomegaly, edema, and fluid retention (Delaney, et al., 2015). The nurse must monitor laboratory results, document frequent intake and output measurements, and assess for clinical signs of fluid overload, including periorbital and peripheral edema and increased work of breathing. The administration of diuretics is the standard treatment to eliminate excess water and salt from the body. The most commonly used diuretic for treatment of right-sided heart failure in infants is furosemide.

In any infant born with a cardiac defect, alteration in parenting related to the perception of the infant as vulnerable may be present. Clear communication between all members of the health care team and the family is paramount. In addition, it is the nurse's responsibility to provide knowledge and skills to these families. This includes newborn care and adequate nutrition; safe administration of medications; learning signs of heart failure, possible complications, and when to call the primary care provider.

OUTCOMES

Infants with congenital heart disease that results in an increase in pulmonary blood flow have outcomes specific to evidence-based nursing practice that focuses on assisting the infant in improved cardiac function, reduction in accumulated fluid and sodium, a decrease in cardiac demands, improvement in tissue oxygenation, and a decrease in oxygen consumption (Delaney et al., 2015).

Improvement in cardiac function occurs when there is a decrease in the afterload of the heart, thereby increasing the overall cardiac output. ACE inhibitors reduce afterload on the heart, allowing for it to pump more easily and its ability to contract is improved with the administration of digoxin. In infants with increased pulmonary blood flow and right-sided heart failure, management of fluid and sodium retention consists of diuretic therapy. The overall goal for infants with pulmonary overcirculation is to decrease cardiac demands. The nurse can facilitate this by performing interventions that decrease the workload of the heart. Examples of these interventions include minimizing metabolic needs by providing a neutral thermal environment to avoid stress to the infant, treating infections, reducing the infant's efforts or breathing, administering sedative medication if extremely irritable, decreasing external stimuli, decreasing environmental stimuli, and providing uninterrupted rest (Delaney et al., 2015). Improving the function of the myocardium and lessening the tissue oxygen demand result in improved tissue oxygenation. Oxygen administration helps improve respiratory function and gas exchange.

Summary

Infants born with cardiac defects resulting in an increased pulmonary blood flow include PDA, ASD, VSD, and AV canal. Sustained pulmonary congestion from pulmonary overcirculation in the infant can lead to serious complications, including pulmonary hemorrhage, elevated pulmonary pressures, and irreversible lung damage. Patients are at risk for right-sided heart failure and poor weight gain. Understanding the anatomy and physiology of each specific patient's cardiac anatomy is imperative to caring for the infant effectively. Providing efficient and holistic nursing care to hospitalized infants with congenital heart disease can result in increased survival and quality of life in this vulnerable patient population.

Capozzi, G., & Santoro, G. (2011). Patent ductus arteriosus: Patho-physiology, hemodynamic effects and clinical complications. *Journal of Maternal–Fetal and Neonatal Medicine, 24*(1), 15–16.

Delaney, A., Baker, A., Bastardi, H., & O'Brien, P. (2015). The child with cardiovascular dysfunction. In M. Hockenberry, D. Wilson, & C. Rodgers (Eds.), *Wong's nursing care of infants and children* (10th ed., pp. 738–744). St. Louis, MO: Elsevier Mosby.

Jone, P., Darst, J., Collins, K., & Miyamoto, S. (2016). Cardiovascular diseases. In W. Hay, M. Levin, R. Deterding, & M. Abzug (Eds.), *Current diagnosis & treatment pediatrics* (23rd ed., pp. 550–610). New York, NY: McGraw-Hill. Retrieved from http://accessmedicine.mhmedical.com/content.aspx?bookid=1795&Sectionid=125741666

Nelson, J., Hirsch-Romano, J., Ohye, R., & Bove, E. (2015). Congenital heart disease. In G. M. Doherty (Ed.), *Current diagnosis & treatment: Surgery* (14th ed., pp. 423–454). New York, NY: McGraw-Hill.

Park, M. (2016). *The pediatric cardiology handbook* (5th ed., pp. 99–115). Philadelphia, PA: Elsevier Saunders.

■ INFANT OF A DIABETIC MOTHER

Mary F. Terhaar

Overview

Globally, the number of people living with diabetes mellitus is expected to rise to 592 million by 2035 (Guariguata et al., 2014). Many mothers and infants will be impacted because every pregnancy complicated by maternal diabetes is a pregnancy at risk. Despite a benign history, insulin deficiency or resistance develops during pregnancy in some women. The prevalence of this condition, called *gestational diabetes*, is approximately 2% to 6% globally and as high as 9.2% in the United States (DeSisto, Kim, & Sharma, 2014; Mitanchez, Burguet, & Simeoni, 2014). In both diabetes mellitus and gestational diabetes, unstable and often excessive glucose levels are a defining characteristic and may be linked to adverse fetal and neonatal outcomes.

Background

The infant of a diabetic mother (IDM) is at risk for numerous complications and requires careful monitoring during the early neonatal period. Two distinct clinical pictures present: The first is associated with overnutrition and the second with teratogenesis.

Gestational diabetes is a frequent clinical presentation in the pregnant woman and occurs when maternal glucose intolerance develops. The mother lacks sufficient functioning insulin and develops a persistent excess of her own serum glucose. The glucose-rich serum is perfused to the fetus, which results in fetal hyperglycemia. The fetus adapts by producing higher-than-normal levels of insulin to maintain fetal glucose levels within normal range. The fetus then converts and stores excess glucose as fat. The result is an overnourished, hyperinsulinemic, macrosomic infant. Complications associated with overnutrition and macrosomia include difficult labor, cephalopelvic disproportion, possible cesarean section, shoulder dystocia, birth trauma, hemorrhage, glucose instability, temperature instability, and respiratory distress in the first few days of life. For these neonates, unstable maternal insulin and glucose levels are associated with increased rates of perinatal asphyxia (Riskin & Garcia-Prats, 2016).

The second clinical presentation occurs when unrecognized or poorly controlled diabetes precedes pregnancy or complicates the early weeks of pregnancy. High serum glucose levels can be teratogenic during early fetal development and result in cardiovascular and neural malformations. These defects can lead to first trimester loss, fetal demise, or serious congenital anomalies. Referred to as *diabetic embryopathy*, these complications are the direct result of pregestational diabetes (Hay, 2012; Riskin & Garcia-Prats, 2016). Pregnancy complicated by diabetes can lead to intrapartum complications, preterm birth, altered glucose metabolism, respiratory problems, and difficulty transitioning to extrauterine life (Mitanchez et al., 2015).

Clinical Aspects

A careful history, including family history of diabetes, mother's health before and during this pregnancy as well as previous pregnancies (including birth weight of infants) are key to interpreting the clinical picture, evaluating risks, stabilizing glucose levels, and preventing complications.

ASSESSMENT

Head-to-toe assessment by the bedside nurse aids in identifying risks for complications in the IDM. Any infant with a birth weight more than 90% on the growth chart for gestational age or more than 4,000 g birth weight is classified as macrosomic and at risk for potential complications as an IDM (Hay, 2012; Riskin & Garcia-Prats, 2016).

NURSING INTERVENTIONS, MANAGEMENT, AND IMPLICATIONS

IDMs who present as macrosomic, overnourished, or hyperinsulinemic face many challenges requiring careful monitoring and support by nursing. Chief among these are low serum glucose concentrations; respiratory distress; electrolyte imbalances; polycythemia, cardiomegaly, and hyperbilirubinemia; temperature instability; feeding difficulties; and poor state regulation (Riskin & Garcia-Prats, 2016; Mitanchez, Burguet, & Simeoni, 2014).

Low blood glucose levels are an issue in the IDM. Accustomed to high circulating serum glucose levels provided by the mother through the placenta, the IDM has become efficient in producing insulin to normalize blood glucose. After cutting the umbilical cord, the glucose supply from the mother is terminated, resulting in glucose levels that fall precipitously in the newborn. As a result, the formerly adaptive elevated insulin levels also cause glucose levels to drop. Frequent glucose monitoring starting between 1 and 3 hours of life is necessary until levels stabilize. Serum glucose levels below 47 mg/dL are considered hypoglycemic and require intervention. However, thresholds vary by institution (Sweet, Grayson, & Polak, 2013).

Early feedings help prevent or attenuate low-serum glucose levels. Breastfeeding can be initiated in the delivery room and sustained through the early neonatal period. However, robust research to support this practice is not available (East, Dolan, & Forster, 2014). Some infants will be jittery, lethargic, or too unstable to breastfeed or take oral fluids. For this group of infants, providing intravenous glucose fluids at 4 to 6 mg/kg/minute will meet metabolic demands and will not stimulate insulin responses that further decrease serum glucose (Riskin & Garcia-Prats, 2016).

Fetal hyperinsulinemia can have two diametrically opposed outcomes on the lungs. In some cases, hyperinsulinemia acts as a stressor, which may cause fetal steroid levels to rise and trigger lung maturation. Therefore, the pulmonary development may be more advanced than expected for gestational age. However, hyperinsulinemia may inhibit maturation of airways and production of surfactant, resulting in respiratory distress (Riskin & Garcia-Prats, 2016).

Careful monitoring of pulse oximetry and respiratory assessment are required. Supplemental oxygen, artificial surfactant, and ventilator support may be needed.

Hyperinsulinemia may lead to hypoparathyroidism, hypomagnesemia, and hypocalcemia, which may result in acidosis due to release of intracellular phosphorous. The hypocalcemic IDM will present as jittery and irritable and may develop myocardial hypocontractility (Hay, 2012). When serum levels are found to be low, breast milk or formula feedings are indicated. Recalcitrant hypocalcemia may indicate underlying hypomagnesemia and require correction with IV replacement (Mimouni, Mimouni, & Bental, 2013).

Elevated maternal glucose levels and resultant glycation of hemoglobin can reduce the oxygen-carrying capacity of fetal hemoglobin, which then stimulates erythropoiesis and results in polycythemia (Mitanchez, et al., 2015). Simultaneously, fetal hyperglycemia and hyperinsulinemia increase metabolic demands of the placenta and fetus, leading to increased oxygen consumption by both (Hay, 2012). Diminished capacity accompanies increased demand. Although polycythemia increases the oxygen-carrying capacity of fetal blood and is adaptive for the hyperinsulinemic fetus, it can lead to both cardiomyopathy and hyperbilirubinemia. In IDMs with cardiomyopathy, the heart muscle of the fetus hypertrophies as a result of generating increased cardiac output to compensate for the low oxygen-carrying capacity of the blood, and from increased effort of pumping blood that is high in hemoglobin. This infant requires careful monitoring of heart rate, blood pressure (BP), cardiac output, and fluid status.

Hyperbilirubinemia develops when the IDM breaks down the surplus red blood cells that characterize polycythemia, conjugates the waste as bilirubin, and then eliminates the bilirubin in urine and stool. Hyperbilirubinemia is also exaggerated by macrosomia, which can contribute to difficult labor and result in bruising of the head and face. As bruising resolves, blood is resorbed and broken down, producing bilirubin that exceeds the capacity of the liver to conjugate and the capacity of kidneys and gastrointestinal track to eliminate. The result is elevated serum bilirubin levels, which present as jaundice to the skin, conjunctiva, and mucous membranes; reduced alertness in the infant, and may cause feeding difficulties. The jaundiced infant requires assessment of serum bilirubin levels at intervals, frequent feedings to facilitate elimination of bilirubin in urine and stool, and phototherapy to increase transepithelial elimination of bilirubin (Wong & Bhutani, 2016). Phototherapy is commonly required and in severe cases exchange transfusions may be indicated.

Thermoregulation may be an issue for the distressed IDM. Gestational diabetes and macrosomia predispose the IDM to intrapartum complications, which result in a fatigued infant with little reserve to maintain body temperature. Careful monitoring by nursing is key. The infant benefits from skin-to-skin care or from external heat sources. Maintaining the newborn in a neutral thermal environment decreases oxygen requirements and reduces the likelihood of chemical thermogenesis.

Low-serum glucose levels, a stressful delivery, and immaturity of the infant can result in poor state regulation, decreased alert time for feeding and socializing, and feeding difficulties. Until insulin levels normalize, infants require frequent small feedings (as frequently as every 2 hours). Colostrum is most precisely suited for metabolic needs and is thought to minimize rebound hyperinsulinemia following feedings. Formula feedings are initiated if breastfeeding is not planned and for infants whose glucose levels fall below 40 mg/dL, intravenous fluids with glucose are initiated (Riskin & Garcia-Prats, 2016).

Shoulder dystocia may result when a macrosomic infant is delivered to a mother with cephalopelvic disproportion. A difficult and prolonged second phase of labor may occur in which forceps or vacuum extraction may be used to facilitate delivery. This places infants at increased risk for complications, including fractured clavicle, Erb's palsy, Klumpke's paralysis, diaphragmatic nerve paralysis, or laryngeal nerve damage (Hay, 2012). The affected infant presents with asymmetrical tone and flexion in the arms and shoulders, asymmetry in the face, or abnormal cry. Nursing care is performed to maintain and support the arm and shoulder in good alignment. The infant is positioned for comfort and support in the affected limb (Mitanchez, Burguet, & Simeoni, 2014). Pediatric neurology follow-up is recommended.

The macrosomic infant who experiences a difficult labor and delivery can be fatigued and distressed at birth. This infant requires supportive care and may have little energy for feeding and bonding with the mother. Skin-to-skin care can help promote thermal stability and facilitate frequent feedings. Surveillance of pulse oximetry, glucose levels, respiratory status, temperature, and nutritional intake are important (Hay, 2012).

The infant may have bruising, especially of the head and face, and may have a cephalohematoma, or other bruising from assisted delivery. The infant may experience pain or discomfort, fatigue, and may develop hyperbilirubinemia. Observation, supportive care, and management of hyperbilirubinemia should begin as soon as laboratory values are confirmed (Hay, 2012).

Every newborn must make many complex adaptations in the first few minutes and hours of life. The adaptation for an IDM depends on vigilant nursing care and monitoring of cardiovascular, respiratory, metabolic, and thermoregulatory functions, as well as behavior and infant bonding. Preventing complications and long-term sequelae are the goals.

OUTCOMES

In the short term, the weight of the IDM normalizes because surplus insulin levels normalize allowing clearance of excess fluid and fat stores. As a consequence, burden on the heart and lungs is reduced and the infant can capably assume the work of respiration, circulation, and perfusion. As polycythemia resolves, the liver, kidneys, and intestines are better able to remove waste, process bilirubin, and resolve jaundice.

Long-term implications of overnutrition include increased risk for diabetes mellitus, heart disease, and renal problems (Mitanchez et al., 2014). The best treatment is prevention, and the best care for the newborn is management of the pregnancy and care for the mother.

The optimal treatment is obstetrical care of a woman who is planning a pregnancy. The best treatment is early obstetrical care for a pregnant diabetic woman.

Summary

The IDM presents as a fatigued, distressed, and fragile newborn. The IDM's large size may create the impression of a robust newborn. In reality, these babies are not robust and require careful attention as they transition to extrauterine life. Careful management of all the complexities of the disease can contribute to resolving the imbalances in many interrelated body systems. Best practices include preventive care; frequent assessment; monitoring of all systems affected; and skin-to-skin care to keep the infant in a supportive, comfortable environment with easy and timely access to breast milk or nutrition.

DeSisto, C. L., Kim, S. Y., & Sharma, A. J. (2014). Prevalence estimates of gestational diabetes mellitus in the United States, Pregnancy Risk Assessment Monitoring System (PRAMS), 2007–2010. *Preventing Chronic Disease, 11*, 1.

East, C. E., Dolan, W. J., & Forster, D. A. (2014). Antenatal breast milk expression by women with diabetes for improving infant outcomes [Review]. *Cochrane Database of Systematic Reviews, 2014*(7). CD010408. doi:10.1002/14651858.CD010408.pub2

Guariguata, L., Whiting, D. R., Hambleton, I., Beagley, J., Linnenkamp, U., & Shaw, J. E. (2014). Global estimates of diabetes prevalence for 2013 and projections for 2035. *Diabetes Research and Clinical Practice, 103*, 137–149.

Hay, W. W. (2012). Care of the infant of a diabetic mother. *Current Diabetes Reports, 12*(1), 4–15.

Mimouni, F., Mimouni, G., & Bental, Y. (2013). Neonatal management of infant of diabetic mother. *Pediatrics and Therapeutics, 4*(1), 1–4. doi:10.4172/2161-0665.1000186

Mitanchez, D., Burguet, A., & Simeoni, U. (2014). Infants born to mothers with gestational diabetes mellitus: Mild neonatal effects, a long-term threat to global health. *Journal of Pediatrics, 164*(3), 445–450.

Mitanchez, D., Yzydorczyk, C., Siddeek, B., Boubred, F., Benahmed, M., & Simeoni U. (2015). The offspring of the diabetic mother: Short- and long-term implications. *Best Practice & Research Clinical Obstetrics & Gynaecology, 29*, 256–269.

Riskin, A., & Garcia-Prats, J. A. (2016). Infant of a diabetic mother. *UpToDate*. Retrieved from https://www.upto date.com/contents/infant-of-a-diabetic-mother#H12

Sweet, C. B., Grayson, S., & Polak, M. (2013). Management strategies for neonatal hypoglycemia. *Journal of Pediatric Pharmacologic Therapy, 18*(3), 199–208.

Wong, R. J., & Bhutani, V. K. (2016). Treatment of unconjugated hyperbilirubinemia in term and late preterm infants. *UpToDate*. Retrieved from https://www.upto date.com/contents/treatment-of-unconjugated-hyperbili rubinemia-in-term-and-late-preterm-infants?source=see_ link

■ INTRAVENTRICULAR HEMORRHAGE

Helene M. Lannon

Overview

Neonatal intracranial hemorrhage is a complication of premature birth. Intraventricular hemorrhage (IVH) is defined as bleeding in or around the ventricles of the brain with potential for extended bleeding into the white matter of the brain. Periventricular leukomalacia (PVL) is defined as injury and death of areas of white matter tissue around fluid-filled ventricles and usually results from an extension of IVH (Annibale, 2014). The incidence of IVH/PVL increases as birth weight and gestation decreases. Full-term infants rarely experience IVH, but may develop a subarachnoid hemorrhage related to pregnancy risk factors or a complication of delivery. The most vulnerable infants are those born prematurely less than 34-week gestation, with a threefold risk for very-low-birth-weight (VLBW) infants born between 28 and 32 weeks of gestation and a VLBW of 1,001 to 1,500 g (Blackburn, 2015). IVH may cause serious disabilities involving cognitive and motor deficits, vision, and hearing. The onset of IVH occurs the majority of the time by 72 hours of life and 99.5% of IVH occurs by day 7 of life (Annibale, 2014). Although the incidence of IVH has started to decline in recent years, IVH remains a significant cause of morbidity and mortality in premature infants (Annibale, 2014). Prevention of preterm birth is not always possible. Treatment after delivery depends on early diagnosis and demonstration of meticulous supportive nursing care.

Background

Brain formation and cerebral blood flow are factors that influence the incidence of IVH. Volpe (2009) notes that preterm infants are at risk for IVH because birth occurs during the time of peak brain synaptogenesis and developmental differentiation, with migration of cells to match with specific receptor sites and organize the central nervous system. The subependymal germinal matrix (SEGM) is the prominent area of cell growth. It is an extremely vascularized area with high-oxygen needs to nourish glial cell growth that strengthen membranes. It matures by 36 weeks of gestation (Blackburn, 2015).

After birth, cerebral blood flow increases to meet oxygen demands. A steady blood flow is maintained by the mechanism of autoregulation. Autoregulation is the ability to maintain cerebral blood flow regardless of changes in cerebral perfusion pressure from physiologic changes; cerebral vessels constrict when pressure increases and dilate when pressure decreases (Elser & Brandon, 2011). This mechanism is mature at term. However, in prematurity, flow is pressure passive, and

systemic blood pressure becomes the primary determinant of cerebral blood flow and pressure (Annibale, 2014). Absence of autoregulation or severe changes in cerebral blood flow are hypothesized to cause central nervous system IVH (Elser & Brandon, 2011).

Papile (2006) established the first grading system to define IVH, which is used today. Classified as a small IVH are grades I and II. Grade I IVH is limited to the SEGM, often localized at the foramen of Monroe. Grade II IVH has partial filling of the lateral ventricle(s) without ventricular dilation. Grade III IVH includes ventricular hemorrhage with dilation and severe grade IV IVH includes ventricular dilation with parenchymal extension of blood into the cerebral tissue. Extension into the white matter of the brain is PVL that consists of ischemic lesions and multicystic encephalomalacia (Scher, 2013).

Mortality from severe IVH/PVL ranges from 27% to 50%. Low-grade I IVH usually resolves with only a 5% mortality rate, and grade II IVH has a 10% mortality rate (Annibale, 2014). Morbidity depends on the extension of the bleed. Approximately 25% to 30% of premature infants with grades I to II IVH will be discharged without major sequelae.

Clinical Aspects

Optimal screening is done by cranial ultrasound because of its easy availability, relatively low cost, and of high resolution to identify bleeding. The study is performed at the bedside at day 7 of life as most IVH occurs by this time. For those infants who are of VLBW and unstable after birth, the ultrasound may be done within the first 72 hours of life. Serial ultrasounds are warranted based on clinical course; however, some institutions do routine screening for IVH at 30 to 60 and 90 days of age as PVL may appear as late as 6 to 10 weeks (Volpe, 2008). Additional radiologic studies include MRI to help detect slowly progressing hemorrhage, as well as extracerebral or infratentorial hemorrhages (Hawkins, 2015). CT scan is not an appropriate screening tool for PVL due to exposure of radiation and transfer of a fragile, preterm infant to the radiology department. It is typically used for diagnosing subarachnoid hemorrhage in full-term infants.

ASSESSMENT

IVH results from premature birth, therefore, assessment begins antenatally with good prenatal care. Identification of a high-risk pregnancy with potential for premature birth, such as pregnancy-induced hypertension, maternal drug use, sepsis, or clotting disorders must be noted in the maternal history. Transporting the mother–fetus dyad to deliver at a tertiary care center is essential.

Scar formation at the initial site of bleeding is seen on cranial ultrasound as porencephalic cysts. Cerebral infarction may initiate the fibrinolytic cascade causing bleeding that extends into the white matter of the brain, leading to PVL. However, IVH may also be asymptomatic and found on routine ultrasound.

NURSING INTERVENTIONS, MANAGEMENT, AND IMPLICATIONS

Assessment of clinical signs that indicate potential IVH may be subtle, dramatic, or asymptomatic. Subtle symptoms are evidenced by changes in tone, movement, or changes in respirations. However, IVH may have a catastrophic presentation with sudden-onset hypotension, apnea/bradycardia, desaturation, full or bulging fontanel, decerebrate posturing, or a sudden drop in hematocrit. Sudden desaturation, bradycardia, hypotonia, and metabolic acidosis on blood sampling may precede dramatic changes of apnea; increased ventilator support; a decrease in hematocrit; decreased level of consciousness/activity; full, tense fontanel; and possible seizures. Nursing care is based on prevention and correction of any of these signs.

Evidence-based nursing research is limited for interventions specific to IVH because signs and outcomes are limited to retrospective studies that are complicated by other morbidities associated with prematurity. Major components of nursing care are aimed to reduce activities that can lead to hypoxia or asphyxia events, or rapid alterations and fluctuations in systemic blood pressure (Blackburn, 2015).

Oxygenation and perfusion are assessed by vital signs, oxygen saturation, and blood gases to maintain acid–base balance and perfusion pressures (Ditzenberger & Blackburn, 2014). Coagulopathies are corrected to prevent shock, and infusions of blood products or fluid boluses are administered slowly.

Comfort measures to avoid rapid swings in blood pressure that also promote physiologic support include clustering care to decrease periods of stimulation; limiting crying; positioning the VLBW infant in a neutral position with head midline and supine, avoiding neck flexion, and swaddling. Also, raising the head of the bed slightly, avoiding raising legs above head level as with a diaper change; avoiding the use of constrictive head bands and constrictive bilirubin eye shields as well as

good nutritional support and maintaining the neutral thermal environment are important (Ditzenberger & Blackburn, 2014).

Parental bonding is facilitated by including the family in the plan of care and teaching the family developmentally supportive care of handling and positioning techniques to reduce environmental stress for their infant (Blackburn, 2015). Neurology and/or neurosurgical consultations are necessary to monitor the progression of IVH/PVL, which may be lifelong. A social service referral is made for family emotional and financial support, with identification of available intervention programs in the family's community to facilitate the infant's growth and development.

OUTCOMES

Outcomes from neurological sequelae of IVH/PVL cannot be predicted. Studies rely on results from retrospective studies and reports from clinic follow-up data. Outcome depends on the extent and location of injury. Severe hemorrhage accompanies an 80% chance for neurodevelopmental disabilities along with potential seizures, hydrocephalus, and cerebral palsy (Scher, 2013). Cognitive dysfunction in learning, memory and language, attention and socialization; as well as vision, hearing, motor and behavioral issues can continue into school age and adulthood. These sequelae occur in 15% to 25% of those born weighing less than 1,500 g and more than 50% of those weighing less than 750 g at birth (Blackburn, 2015).

Summary

The primary risk for IVH/PVL is prematurity. Multiple interventions needed to support premature organ function and environmental factors of handling, sound, and temperature change affect cerebral blood flow and pressure and place the infant at risk for IVH. Once an IVH occurs, the treatment is to prevent extension through supportive nursing care. There is no cure for IVH. The incidence of IVH/PVL has decreased over the years due to improved prenatal care with treatment to prevent preterm birth. Retrospective studies and data from clinical follow-up reports show promising outcomes for those infants with a small IVH; however, severe IVH holds a high risk for neurodevelopment morbidities that can extend into adulthood. Therefore, nursing education in understanding the risks for developing IVH and subsequent bedside care are key in preventing IVH.

Annibale, D. (2014, March). Periventricular hemorrhage-intraventricular hemorrhage. *Medscape*. Retrieved from http://emedicine.medscape.com/article/976654

Blackburn, S. (2015). Brain injury in preterm infants: Pathogenesis and nursing implications. *Newborn and Infant Nursing Reviews, 16*(1), 8–12.

Ditzenberger, G. R., & Blackburn, S. T. (2014). Neurologic system. In C. Kenner & J. W. Lott (Eds.), *Comprehensive neonatal nursing care* (5th ed., pp. 392–437). New York, NY: Springer Publishing.

Elser, H. E., & Brandon, D. H. (2011). Cerebral oxygenation monitoring: A strategy to detect IVH and PVL. *Newborn and Infant Nursing Reviews, 11*(3), 153–159.

Hawkins, C. E. (2015, December). Perinatal intracranial hemorrhages: Pathology. *Medscape*. Retrieved from http://emedicine.medscape.com/article/2059564

Papile, L. (2006). Intracranial hemorrhage and vascular lesions. In A. A. Fanaroff, R. J. Martin, & M. C. Walsh (Eds.), *Fanaroff and Martin's neonatal perinatal medicine: Diseases of the fetus and infant* (8th ed.). Philadelphia, PA: Elsevier Mosby.

Scher, M. S. (2013). Brain disorders of the fetus and neonate. In A. A. Fanaroff & J. M. Fanaroff (Eds.), *Klaus and Fanaroff's care of the high-risk neonate* (6th ed., pp. 476–524). Philadelphia, PA: Elsevier Saunders.

Volpe, J. J. (2008). *Neurology of the newborn* (5th ed.). Philadelphia, PA: Elsevier Saunders.

Volpe, J. J. (2009). Cerebellum of the premature infant: Rapidly developing, vulnerable, clinically important. *Journal of Child Neurology, 24*, 1085–1104.

■ LATE PRETERM INFANT

Donna A. Dowling

Overview

Over the past 10 years, the specific needs of infants born late preterm, between 34 0/7 and 36 6/7 weeks of gestation, have been identified. These infants, who constitute more than 70% of all preterm births, have increased morbidity and mortality when compared to infants born at term. This entry provides an overview of current assessment and management approaches for this unique group of infants.

Background

Until 2005, the late preterm infant (LPI), born between 34 and 36 6/7 weeks of gestation, was not recognized as a unique subset of preterm infants (Raju, Higgins, Stark, & Leveno, 2006). In 2014, LPIs constituted 72% of all preterm infants born before 37 weeks of gestation (Hamilton, Martin, Osterman, Curtin, & Mathews, 2015). These infants, who due to their weight and appearance can seem to be full term, have increased risk for morbidities and mortalities when compared to term infants (Barfield & Lee, 2016). These risks include sepsis, respiratory (transient tachypnea and respiratory distress syndrome [RDS]), metabolic (thermoregulation and hypoglycemia), and gastrointestinal (hyperbilirubinemia and feeding issues) problems, as well as the long-term risk of developmental delay (Vohr, 2013). Consequently, approximately 50% of LPIs require admission to the neonatal intensive care unit (NICU), which results in significant family stress and increased health care cost. It is essential that health care providers be proactive in the identification and management of this group of high-risk neonates.

Clinical Aspects

ASSESSMENT

The morbidities associated with late preterm birth, which increase with decreasing gestational age (Horgan, 2015), reflect the critical phase of development of the fetus that is interrupted when the infant is required to transition to extrauterine life. Due to a decreased store of heat-generating brown adipose tissue, increased body surface-to-weight ratio, less white adipose tissue for insulation, as well as an underdeveloped hormonal response to cold, LPIs cannot conserve heat or respond adequately to heat loss (Phillips et al., 2013). The subsequent cold stress can impact transition to extrauterine life by increasing oxygen and glucose requirements, which, in turn, contribute to the development of respiratory distress and hypoglycemia.

LPIs are at risk for respiratory morbidities such as transient tachypnea of the newborn (TTN) and RDS. These morbidities reflect functional immaturity of lung structures, resulting in inadequate reabsorption of intrapulmonary fluid that predisposes the infant to TTN and inadequate surfactant production that predisposes the infant to RDS (Horgan, 2015). Both TTN and RDS increase oxygen and glucose requirements and possibly the need for assisted ventilation. In addition, due to immature development of brain stem function, including upper airway control and chemical control of breathing, LPIs are at increased risk for apnea of prematurity.

LPIs are 2 to 3 times more likely to have an episode of hypoglycemia in the neonatal period (Horgan, 2015). All infants respond to the loss of the glucose supply through glucogenolysis that occurs with cord clamping. However, LPIs have low glycogen stores and reduced function of gluconeogenic and glycolytic enzymes (Barfield & Lee, 2016), putting them at risk for hypoglycemia, especially if the first feeding is delayed.

LPIs are at twice the risk for hyperbilirubinemia at 5 days of age compared to term infants due to poor elimination of bilirubin and an increased bilirubin load related to red blood cell break down (Barfield & Lee, 2016). Poor elimination of bilirubin is related to low intestinal motility and inadequate or delayed feeding and the resulting increase in bilirubin puts the infant at risk for kernicterus (bilirubin neurotoxicity) (Horgan, 2015).

LPIs have poor muscle tone, fatigue easily and have difficulty coordinating sucking, swallowing, and breathing (Horgan, 2015), putting them at risk for poor-feeding outcomes. This is of particular concern for infants who are breastfeeding, as good muscle strength and stamina are needed to latch correctly onto the breast and suck adequately to initiate and maintain milk transfer. Failure to adequately empty the breast results in poor milk production, putting the infant at risk for dehydration and suboptimal weight gain, which can delay discharge or be a reason for rehospitalization (Baker, 2015). Consequently, mothers may discontinue breastfeeding prematurely, citing an inadequate milk supply and breastfeeding difficulty as the reasons (Kair & Colaizy, 2016).

A significant increase in brain growth occurs between 34 and 40 weeks of gestation (Horgan, 2015), making the brain of the LPIs more vulnerable to increased stress and at increased risk for long-term injury (Barfield & Lee, 2016). LPIs have been found to have developmental delays, emotional and behavioral problems, and less optimal school outcomes at preschool and kindergarten (Vohr, 2013) compared to term infants.

The assessment of the LPI begins before birth with the recognition that gestational age assessment can have an error of ±2 weeks (Medoff-Cooper et al., 2012) except for women who have conceived following reproductive technology. Therefore, health care providers should assess all infants born before 37 weeks of gestation every 30 minutes until stable for 2 hours, then every 4 hours for the first 24 hours, and then routinely until discharge using a risk assessment plan (Phillips et al., 2013). As cold stress, glucose metabolism, and respiratory distress are interrelated, a proactive approach to the prevention or immediate identification of problems can reduce short-term morbidities. It is essential

that nurseries develop their own evidence-based protocols or use the guidelines from the National Perinatal Association. Baker (2015) provides an example of a clinical practice guideline for the management of LPI.

NURSING INTERVENTIONS, MANAGEMENT, AND IMPLICATIONS

The thermoregulation of the neonate is a primary responsibility of the nurse. The initial action is drying and putting a hat on the infant. Infants placed in birth kangaroo care (KC) are covered with a warmed blanket and carefully monitored. When not in KC, the infant should be swaddled. The infant's temperature should be monitored with routine assessments; if the infant's temperature is less than 36.0°C, warming approaches should be initiated (increasing the ambient temperature, swaddling) and the temperature should be monitored every 30 minutes until returning to normal. If the temperature remains less than 36.0°C after 30 minutes, the infant should be placed in a radiant warmer (Horgan, 2015) and monitoring should continue.

Nursing must observe the infant for signs of respiratory distress such as grunting, retracting, nasal flaring, retractions, and cyanosis. For infants in KC the SpO_2 can be monitored (Tourneux et al., 2015). Glucose levels should be monitored following the unit policy. Breastfeeding should be initiated within the first hour of life and the infant should be fed frequently thereafter. Observe the infant for symptoms of hypoglycemia, including jitteriness, tremors, and tachypnea (Phillips et al., 2013). The infant's oral intake and urine output should be monitored closely. The infant should have the bilirubin level measured according to unit policy and should be assessed for jaundice.

The nurse or lactation consultant should be present at initial breastfeeding sessions to assess the infant's ability to latch onto the breast and maintain sucking to promote milk transfer. Mothers should be taught to understand and respond to the infant's feeding cues and feed the infant every 2 hours. Infants should be weighed daily to monitor for excessive loss of birth weight.

The immature immune system of LPIs put them at higher risk for infection compared to term infants. Maternal risk factors include Group B *Streptococcus* positive or unknown status, prolonged rupture of membranes, and fever during labor. LPIs should be monitored closely for signs of infection, which can be nonspecific (temperature instability, lethargy, and feeding problems) and septic workups should be initiated when symptoms appear (Phillips et al., 2013).

Detailed discharge teaching by the nursing staff is essential to promote family adaptation after discharge and to reduce the possibility of rehospitalization. In addition to standard discharge teaching for all preterm infants, parents need to understand the specific risks for the LPI, particularly concerning inadequate feeding, dehydration, and hyperbilirubinemia, as these are the most common problems that lead to rehospitalization shortly after discharge (Baker, 2015). It is essential that parents be taught to assess the adequacy of the infant's feeding, including urine and stool output, and to assess for jaundice.

OUTCOMES

The anticipation of the birth of an LPI, which allows for the determination of the adequacy of the resources available, especially in terms of well-trained health care providers, is the first step in preventing or minimizing risks for these infants. Evidence-based multidisciplinary guidelines developed by the National Perinatal Association (www.nationalperinatal.org/Resources/Late PretermGuidelinesNPA.pdf) provide a foundation for providing safe care. An international collaborative organization, The Vermont Oxford Network, has the mission to improve the quality, safety, and efficiency of health care for newborns and has developed regional perinatal quality initiatives so that the focus of the groups can reflect the health care systems in the region (Trembath, Iams, & Walsh, 2013). Projects have been aimed at reducing preterm births and reducing the morbidity and mortality related to preterm birth. However, quality initiatives focusing on care of LPIs have been impacted by both the lack of evidence-based practices and the wide variation in care practices among hospitals (Trembath et al., 2013), such as the definition and management of hypoglycemia.

Summary

The focus on the increased risk of morbidity and mortality for LPIs has recently expanded to the identification of the increased risk for moderately preterm (born between 31 and 33 6/7 weeks of gestation) and early term (born between 37 and 38 6/7 weeks of gestation) (Baker, 2015). The recognition and proactive management of the ongoing risks of LPIs by nursing and other health care providers are essential to improve short- and long-term outcomes for these infants and their families.

Baker, B. (2015). Evidence-based practice to improve outcomes for late preterm infants. *Journal of Obstetric, Gynecologic, and Neonatal Nursing, 44*(1), 127–133.

Barfield, W. D., & Lee, K. G. (2016). Late preterm infants. *UpToDate*. Retrieved from http://www.uptodate.com/contents/late-preterm-infants?

Hamilton, B. E., Martin, J. A., Osterman, M. J., Curtin, S. C., & Mathews, T. J. (2015). Births: Final data for 2014. *National Vital Statistics Report, 64*(12), 1–64.

Horgan, M. J. (2015). Management of the late preterm infant. *Pediatric Clinics of North America, 62*, 439–451.

Kair, L. R., & Colaizy, T. T. (2016). Breastfeeding continuation among late preterm infants: Barriers, facilitators, and any association with NICU admission. *Hospital Pediatrics, 6*(5), 261–268.

Medoff-Cooper, B., Holditch-Davis, M., Verklan, M. T., Fraser-Askin, D., Lamp, J., Santaonato, A., . . . Bingham, D. (2012). Newborn clinical outcomes of the AWHONN later preterm infant research-based practice project. *Journal of Obstetrics, Gynecologic and Neonatal Nursing, 41*(6), 774–785.

Phillips, R. M., Goldstein, M., Hougland, K., Nandyal, R., Pizzica, A., Santa-Donato, A., . . . Yost, E. (2013). Multidisciplinary guidelines for the care of the late preterm infant. *Journal of Perinatology, 33*, S5–S22.

Raju, T., Higgins, R. D., Stark, A. R., & Leveno, K. J. (2006). Optimizing care and outcome for late-preterm (near-term) infants: A summary of the workshop sponsored by the National Institute of Child Health and Human Development. *Pediatrics, 118*(2), 1207–1214.

Trembath, A. N., Iams, J. D., & Walsh, M. (2013). Quality initiatives related to moderately preterm, late preterm, and early term births. *Clinics in Perinatology, 40*, 777–789.

Tourneux, P., Dubruque, E., Baumert, A., Carpentier, E., Caron-Lesenechal, E., Barcat, L., . . . Fontaine, C. (2015). Skin-to-skin care in the delivery room: Impact of SpO_2 monitoring. *Archives of Pediatrics, 22*(2), 166–170.

Vohr, B. (2013). Long-term outcomes of moderately preterm, late preterm, and early term infants. *Clinics in Perinatology, 40*, 739–751.

■ MECONIUM ASPIRATION SYNDROME

Rae Jean Hemway

Overview

Meconium represents the early passage of stool in the fetus. It is a material that accumulates in the intestines of a fetus and forms the first stools of an infant in the first few days after birth. Meconium is thick, sticky, odorless, and greenish to black in color (Mosby, 2009).

Water is the major component constituting 85% to 95% of meconium; the remaining 5% to 15% primarily includes secretions of the intestinal glands, amniotic fluid, and intrauterine debris, such as bile pigments, fatty acids, epithelial cells, mucus, lanugo, and blood. Meconium is sterile and free of bacteria, differentiating it from subsequent postnatal stools (Geis, 2017). Meconium is found in the intestinal tract as early as the 12th week of gestation (Meerkov & Weiner, 2016). Because meconium is seldom found in the amniotic fluid before the 34th week of gestation, aspiration into the airways before, during labor, and/or at the time of delivery, generally affects term and postterm infants. Intrauterine distress may facilitate the passage of meconium into the amniotic fluid and increase the potential for meconium aspiration syndrome (MAS).

Background

MAS is defined as respiratory distress in an infant, usually term, born through meconium-stained amniotic fluid (MSAF) with symptoms that cannot otherwise be attributed to other causes such as infection or retained lung fluid (Fanaroff, 2008). MSAF occurs in 8% to 10% of term deliveries and approximately 2% to 3% of meconium-stained infants develop MAS, translating to an incidence of one to two per 1,000 live term births per year (Meerkov & Weiner, 2016). Infants born depressed through thick MSAF are more likely to develop MAS (Chettri, Adhisivam, & Bhat, 2015). There is a significant correlation in the incidence of MSAF with gestational age, increasing almost linearly from 37 to 42 weeks of gestation (Fischer, Rybakowski, Ferdynus, Sagot, & Gouyon, 2012). Thus, MAS continues to remain a major clinical concern for obstetricians and neonatologists. The presence of meconium in the amniotic fluid under normal circumstances is thought to be a result of increased peristalsis associated with maturation of fetal intestinal function. However, there is enhanced passage of meconium in utero under certain high-risk conditions. Although the mechanisms affecting meconium passage are not fully explained, animal studies have demonstrated increased parasympathetic activity resulting in increased peristalsis and relaxation of the anal sphincter following episodes of cord compression and fetal hypoxia (Meerkov & Weiner, 2016).

Factors that increase the passage of meconium in utero, often as a consequence of interruption of placental blood flow, include placental insufficiency; maternal hypertension; preeclampsia; oligohydramnios; infection; acidosis; and maternal drug abuse, particularly tobacco and cocaine (Geis, 2017). Irrespective of the mechanism whereby meconium reaches the amniotic fluid, the presence of MSAF poses the threat of aspiration. The majority of infants who pass meconium are either term or postterm, with the latter exhibiting peeling skin, overgrown fingernails, and a decrease in the amount of vernix. MAS is a common cause of severe respiratory distress in this population and is associated with significant morbidity and mortality. The pathophysiology will vary to a large degree on the amount of meconium aspirated as well as the newborn's underlying pulmonary vascular development. For example, in the postmature infant there is the potential for smooth muscle hypertrophy and pulmonary artery hypertension independent of the effects of the aspirated meconium. Meconium, when aspirated into the lungs of an infant, may result in mechanical obstruction of the small airways during the first few breaths and, in addition, may stimulate the release of cytokines (Swarnam, Soraisham, & Sivanandan, 2012). As a result, aspirated meconium interferes with normal breathing in a number of ways, including acute airway obstruction (partial or complete) dependent on the quantity and consistency of the aspirated meconium; inactivation or dysfunction of endogenous surfactant, particularly proteins A and B; alters compliance, functional residual capacity, and induces alveolar edema; induces chemical pneumonitis, which may potentiate the release of cytokines and other vasoactive substances leading to cardiovascular and inflammatory responses and persistent pulmonary hypertension of the newborn (PPHN) with left-to-right shunting (Swarnam et al., 2012). These effects, singularly or in combination, can result in hypoxia, hypercarbia, and acidosis (Crowley, 2015).

Clinical Aspects

ASSESSMENT

Clinical signs and symptoms include tachypnea; nasal flaring; grunting; subcostal and intercostal retractions; cyanosis or desaturation; rhonchi on auscultation; and meconium staining of the umbilical cord, nails, and/or skin. Meconium staining may be noted in the oropharynx. Infants with air trapping secondary to obstruction in the alveoli may have a barrel-shaped chest due to trapped gas in the lungs, which may result in a pneumothorax, pneumopericardium and/or pneumomediastinum. Green urine may be noted in some newborns with MAS less than 24 hours after birth, related to meconium pigments that can be absorbed by the lung and then excreted in urine.

NURSING INTERVENTIONS, MANAGEMENT, AND IMPLICATIONS

About 10% of all infants require some assistance to begin breathing after birth, and approximately 1% require extensive resuscitation (Wyckoff et al., 2015). Knowledge of potential high-risk situations and providers skilled in the Neonatal Resuscitation Program (NRP) guidelines are critical to the successful resuscitation of infants. Collaboration between obstetric and neonatal teams is also essential, particularly when a history reveals MSAF with a potential risk for MAS. Availability of a neonatal resuscitation team (where possible) before the delivery is vital, and allows the team to prebrief and discuss potential problems and potential corrective actions, as well as defining the role of each team member. The key to management of labor complicated by MSAF lies in the early identification of fetal distress, often indicated by changes in fetal heart rate patterns and/or whether the meconium is thin or thick. This should be identified immediately, and corrective actions taken, which may include delivering the infant in a timely manner, if warranted.

Initial interventions are targeted at preventing aspiration by assisting in removing the meconium from the infant's oropharynx and nasopharynx before the initial breath. Recent evidence suggests that routine tracheal suctioning of neonates delivered through MSAF has not been shown to improve outcome (Wyckoff et al., 2015). However, if the neonate's breathing appears obstructed, endotracheal suctioning should be done immediately. Early identification and treatment of meconium aspiration are critical. When this occurs, the primary goals of therapy are to maintain appropriate gas exchange and minimize complications.

Specific treatment strategies include judicious ventilator management, surfactant for mechanically ventilated neonates with high O_2 requirements, and inhaled nitric oxide. High-frequency ventilation may be required if refractory hypoxemia develops, and extracorporeal membrane oxygenation (ECMO) may be needed if medical management fails.

Nursing strategies following resuscitation should include maintaining adequate oxygenation, maintaining temperature, monitoring glucose levels to avoid hypoglycemia, closely observing intravenous fluids administration, and administering intravenous antibiotic therapy. Signs of recovery include resolving respiratory distress and achieving metabolic homeostasis. There should be a focused strategy on providing parental support that includes allowing parents to verbalize concerns regarding their infant's health and explanation of the usual progression and resolution of MAS.

OUTCOMES

Outcomes have greatly improved in recent years due to improved obstetric and neonatal care, including the use of high-frequency ventilation, use of nitric oxide, and ECMO as indicated. The risk for death is increased in the presence of early thick meconium (Meis, Hall, Marshall, & Hobel, 1978).

Summary

Management of infants with MAS has evolved over the years such that infants who were routinely suctioned in the presence of MSAF are now only suctioned, even when depressed, when there are signs of airway obstruction. The management includes a team approach involving both the obstetrician and the neonatal providers coupled with a targeted neonatal management approach; the overwhelming majority of infants survive with a normal long-term outcome.

Chettri, S., Adhisivam, B., & Bhat, B. V. (2015). Endotracheal suction for nonvigorous neonates born through meconium stained amniotic fluid: A randomized controlled trial. *Journal of Pediatrics, 166,* 1208–1213.

Crowley, M. (2015). Neonatal respiratory disorders. In R. J. Martin, A. A. Fanaroff, M. C. Walsh (Eds.), *Fanaroff and Martin's neonatal–perinatal medicine* (10th ed.). St. Louis, MO: Elsevier Saunders.

Fanaroff, A. A. (2008). Meconium aspiration syndrome: Historical aspects. *Journal of Perinatology, 28,* S3–S7.

Fischer, C., Rybakowski, C., Ferdynus, C., Sagot, P., & Gouyon, J. (2012). A population-based study of meconium aspiration syndrome in neonates born between 37 and 43 weeks of gestation. *International Journal of Pediatrics, 321545.* doi:10.1155/2012/321545

Geis, G. M. (2017). Meconium aspiration syndrome treatment & management. Retrieved from http://emedicine.medscape.com/article/974110-treatment

Meerkov, M., & Weiner, G. (2016). Management of the Meconium stained newborn. *NeoReviews, 17,* e471.

Meis, P. J., Hall, M., III., Marshall, J. R., & Hobel, C. J. (1978). Meconium passage: A new classification for risk assessment during labor. *American Journal of Obstetrics and Gynecology, 131*(5), 509–513.

Mosby. (2009). *Mosby's medical dictionary* (9th ed.). St. Louis, MO, Philadelphia, PA: Elsevier Mosby.

Swarnam, K., Soraisham, A. S., & Sivanandan, S. (2012). Advances in the management of meconium aspiration syndrome. *International Journal of Pediatrics.* doi:10.1155/2012/359571

Wyckoff, M. H., Aziz, K., Escobedo, M. B., Kapadia, V. S., Kattwinkel, J., Perlman, J. M., . . . Zaichkin J. G. (2015). Part 13: Neonatal resuscitation: 2015 American Heart Association guidelines update for cardiopulmonary resuscitation and emergency cardiovascular care. *Circulation, 132*(18, Suppl. 2), S543–S560. doi:10.1161/CIR.0000000000000267

■ NECROTIZING ENTEROCOLITIS

Charlene M. Deuber

Overview

Necrotizing enterocolitis (NEC) is the most common gastrointestinal emergency in the neonatal period. Involving ischemic necrosis of the bowel wall, or intestinal mucosa, gas-producing enteric organisms invade the mucosal lining of the intestine (pneumatosis intestinalis) potentially resulting in focal or widespread bowel perforation.

NEC occurs in one to three per 1,000 live births and predominantly occurs in preterm infants, with an incidence of approximately 6% to 7% in very-low-birth-weight (VLBW) infants (birth weight less than 1,500 g) (Stoll et al., 2015). Secondary disease is most often seen in full-term infants with comorbid conditions, including birth asphyxia, Trisomy 21, congenital heart disease, rotavirus infection, and Hirschsprung's disease. In neonatal intensive care units (NICUs) alone, NEC occurs in 1% to 5% of patients, accounting for nearly 20% of NICU costs annually (Gephart, McGrath, Effken, & Halpern, 2012). The overall incidence in the United States is approximately 3,000 infants annually with 1,000 infants succumbing to the disease.

Variations in the severity of this disorder occurs, but all cases result in substantial short- and long-term morbidity in survivors. Morbidity and mortality rates associated with NEC have not improved in decades despite other substantial advances in neonatal care. The average mortality from NEC is 20% to 30%, with mortality as high as 50% for those infants requiring surgical intervention (Fitzgibbons et al., 2009). Characterized by host intestinal immaturity and multifactorial influences, reduction in the incidence and severity of NEC

has focused on the identification and elimination of risk factors.

Background

The Centers for Disease Control and Prevention (CDC) defines NEC as a condition occurring in infants less than or equal to 1 year of age and meeting one of two criteria: (a) at least one clinical sign (bilious aspirate, vomiting, abdominal distension, or occult/gross blood in stools without rectal fissure) and one imaging test finding (pneumatosis intestinalis, portal venous gas, or pneumoperitoneum, or (b) one surgical finding (surgical evidence of extensive bowel necrosis, more than 2 cm of bowel affected, or surgical evidence of pneumatosis intestinalis with or without intestinal perforation; CDC, 2016).

Although the pathogenesis of NEC is complex and multifactorial, three major risk factors have been implicated in its development: prematurity, bacterial colonization of the gut, and formula feeding (Hackam, Afrazi, Good, & Sodhi, 2013). NEC is characterized by inflammation and initiated by impaired mesenteric perfusion with loss of mucosal integrity followed by necrosis. Disrupted, abnormal colonization of the intestine, mucosal barrier dysfunction, and an exaggerated, immune response contribute to the potential devastating consequences of the disease. Subsequent perforation of the bowel may occur at any location, allowing free air to migrate beyond the intestinal lumen to the peritoneum or venous portal system, progressing to peritonitis, sepsis, and death. The terminal ileum and colon are often affected, and, in its most severe form, the entire intestine may be involved.

Clinical manifestations vary and can be insidious or catastrophic in presentation. Commonly, the infant who presents with NEC has been thriving and suddenly presents with clinical instability. Symptoms are typically nonspecific and suggestive of general instability, including temperature instability, apnea and bradycardia, hypotension, thrombocytopenia, abdominal tenderness or distension, abdominal wall erythema or discoloration, gastric residuals, absent bowel sounds, emesis, or blood in the stool.

Although NEC may occur as late as 3 months of age in VLBW infants, it typically presents in the second or third week of life. The greatest single risk factor for NEC is prematurity, with the rate of NEC decreasing after 32 weeks postmenstrual age. The majority of patients have received enteral feedings before diagnosis. Additional risk factors for the development of

NEC include immaturity of the host immunologic system, luminal factors, intestinal epithelial barrier, and gut motility. Bacterial overgrowth in the context of low gastric-hydrogen ion output in the neonate contributes to the colonization of enteric pathogens (Carrion & Egan, 1990).

Effective treatment depends on a multisystem approach, including bowel rest; gastric decompression; supportive hydration; and correction of hypotension, hyponatremia, and metabolic acidosis. Antibiotic surveillance is warranted for potential overwhelming sepsis, with concurrent antifungal therapy if bowel perforation is suspected. Surgical consultation should be initiated when NEC is suspected and there are concerning findings of fixed dilated loops of bowel or evidence of pneumoperitoneum (free peritoneal air or portal venous gas) present on abdominal radiographs. Surgical management may include placement of a peritoneal drain or laparotomy with bowel resection for the removal of necrotic bowel.

Clinical Aspects

ASSESSMENT

NEC is a progressive disease necessitating serial laboratory testing, radiographic surveillance, and keen clinical assessment. The most significant single predictor of outcome following NEC is gestational age. When controlled for gestational age, whether or not the infant needs surgery is predictive of outcome; however, mortality and morbidity rates are highest in those infants requiring surgical intervention (Henry & Moss, 2008). There are also poorer long-term developmental outcomes in infants requiring surgical intervention versus medical management of NEC.

NURSING INTERVENTIONS, MANAGEMENT, AND IMPLICATIONS

Nursing care focuses on surveillance for NEC in populations at risk, with early recognition of clinical symptoms, serial clinical assessments, and preparation for surgery or transport to a tertiary care center. A high index of suspicion in any infant meeting the identified risk factors during the prenatal, intrapartum, or postpartum course should prompt intensive surveillance of signs and symptoms; serial radiographs, measurement of abdominal girth, analysis of blood pressure, intake, output, and acid–base balance are important indicators of severity of disease. Optimal outcome following the

diagnosis of NEC rests upon early recognition, treatment, and access to a tertiary care center when progressive disease or bowel perforation is suspected.

Research has identified strategies to reduce the incidence of NEC. Prenatal strategies for prevention include maternal administration of antenatal corticosteroids (ANCS). A Cochrane review has suggested that maternal treatment with a single course of antenatal steroids reduced NEC by 46% (Brownfoot, Gagliardi, Bain, Middleton, & Crowther, 2013).

The use of human milk has been shown to be protective against NEC in multiple randomized controlled trials. Donor breast milk for enteral feedings is protective when maternal breast milk is not available (Quigley & McGuire, 2014). Nursing support of maternal breastfeeding or pumping of breast milk is influential in the prevention of NEC, especially in preterm infants.

Standardized, unit-specific feeding protocols guiding slow advancement of feeding volume and caloric density, avoidance of hypertonic formulas and medications, and prompt treatment of polycythemia are additional preventive measures suggested in the literature, although these have less scientific rigor. In a recent meta-analysis (Morgan, 2015), the slow advancement of enteral feedings delays the establishment of full enteral feedings, but did not show a statistically significant effect on the risk of NEC in very preterm or VLBW infants.

Ibuprofen treatment as an alternative to indomethacin for closure of a patent ductus arteriosus, which is a common complication in very preterm infants, has been associated with a reduction in the incidence of NEC (Ohlsson, Walia, & Shah, 2015). Also of note, probiotics have been cited as having a protective effect in the prevention of NEC in premature infants, and in the reduction of severity as well as mortality (Neu, 2014). Ongoing research is focused on the safest preparation and administration of probiotics.

OUTCOMES

Early recognition and aggressive treatment of this disorder have improved clinical outcomes, yet NEC accounts for substantial mortality and long-term morbidity especially in the VLBW infant. Infants with NEC, especially those who require any type of surgical intervention, have prolonged periods of hospitalization and, as a result, have extraordinary high health care costs. Long-term, infants with NEC who require surgery have very slow growing patterns and adverse neurodevelopmental outcomes.

Summary

Nurses play a critical role in recognizing signs and symptoms of NEC to facilitate early diagnosis and treatment in infants at highest risk, and in encouraging mothers to provide breast milk.

Brownfoot F. C., Gagliardi, D., Bain, E., Middleton, P., & Crowther, C. (2013). Different corticosteroids and regimens for accelerating fetal lung maturation for women at risk of preterm birth. *Cochrane Database of Systematic Reviews, 2013*(8), 1–90. doi:10.1002/14651858.CD006764.pub3

Carrion, V., & Egan, E. (1990). Prevention of necrotizing enterocolitis. *Journal of Pediatric Gastroenterology and Nutrition, 11*, 317.

Centers for Disease Control and Prevention. (2016). NEC—Necrotizing enterocolitis. Surveillance definitions. Retrieved from https://www.cdc.gov/nhsn/pdfs/psc manual/17pscnosinfdef_current.pdf

Fitzgibbons, S., Ching, Y., Yu, D., Carpenter, J., Kenny, M., Weldon, C., & Jaksic, T. (2009). Mortality of necrotizing enterocolitis expressed by birth weight categories. *Journal of Pediatric Surgery, 44*, 1072–1075. doi:10.1016/j.jpedsurg.2009.02.013

Gephart, S., McGrath, J., Effken, J., & Halpern, M. (2012). Necrotizing enterocolitis risk: State of the science. *Advances in Neonatal Care, 12*(2), 77–89.

Hackam, D., Afrazi, A., Good, M., & Sodhi, C. (2013). Innate immune signaling in the pathogenesis of necrotizing enterocolitis. *Clinical and Developmental Immunology, 2013*. doi:10.1155/2013/475415

Henry, M., & Moss R. (2008). Neonatal necrotizing enterocolitis. *Seminars in Pediatric Surgery, 17*(2), 98–109.

Morgan, J. (2015). Slow advancement of enteral feed volumes to prevent necrotizing enterocolitis in very low birth weight infants. *Cochrane Database of Systematic Reviews, 2015*(10), CD001241. doi:10.1002/14651858.CD001241.pub6

Neu, J. (2014). Probiotics and necrotizing enterocolitis. *Clinics in Perinatology, 41*, 967–978.

Ohlsson A., Walia R., & Shah S. S. (2015). Ibuprofen for the treatment of patent ductus arteriosus in preterm or low birth weight (or both) infants. *Cochrane Database of Systematic Reviews, 2*, CD003481. doi:10.1002/14651858.CD003481

Quigley, M., & McGuire, W. (2014). Formula versus donor breastmilk for feeding preterm or low birth weight infants. *Cochrane Database of Systematic Reviews, 2014*, CD002971. doi:10.1002/14651858.CD002971.pub3

Stoll, B. J., Hansen, N., Bell, E., Walsh, M., Carlo, W., Shankaran, S., & Higgins, R.; The Eunice Kennedy Shriver National Institute of Child Health and Human Development Neonatal Research Network. (2015). Trends in care practices, morbidity and mortality of extremely preterm neonates, 1993–2012. *Journal of the American Medical Association, 314*(10), 1039–1051. doi:10.1001/jama.2015.10244

■ RESPIRATORY DISTRESS SYNDROME

Mary Ann Blatz

Overview

Respiratory distress is the most common diagnosis for infants admitted to the neonatal intensive care unit (NICU; Stoll et al., 2010). The term "neonatal respiratory distress" refers to hypoventilation and/ or hypoxia in the neonate (Reuter, Moser, & Baack, 2014). Neonatal respiratory distress syndrome (RDS) is a surfactant-deficient state that is most frequently associated with infants born prematurely (Lozano & Newnam, 2016). However, RDS occurs much less frequently in term infants related to inactivation of surfactant in a variety of other conditions, including asphyxia, history of maternal diabetes, infection, and/ or meconium aspiration (Reuter et al., 2014). Increased incidence of RDS has been noted if there was a sibling who had RDS, cesarean delivery or induction of labor before 37 weeks of gestation, a compromised infant at delivery with decreasing adequate circulation, a multiple pregnancy or a precipitous delivery, a history of gestational or chronic diabetes, chorioamnionitis, or being of European descent (Newman, 2016; Wambach & Hamvas, 2015). Neonatal nurses are essential to the immediate and ongoing collaborative care for the infant with RDS, who requires continuous, meticulous monitoring as well as management and support to attain and maintain physiologic stability.

Background

RDS was previously called *hyaline membrane disease* (Wambach & Hamvas, 2015). It is difficult to analyze statistics related to incidence, mortality, and neonatal outcomes since a consensus definition of RDS has not been agreed upon by clinical experts (Wambach & Hamvas, 2015). RDS is a broad term that generally includes respiratory symptoms that appear at birth or shortly thereafter, primarily in preterm neonates. RDS encompasses worsening atelectasis, hypoventilation, and/or hypoxia (Newman, 2016; Polin & Carlo, 2014).

In the United States, almost 40,000 infants are diagnosed with RDS every year. Males are affected twice as often as females. There is an inverse relationship between the gestational age of the infant and the incidence of RDS. It is found in almost 98% of 23-week infants, 86% of 28-week infants, 29% of 35-week infants, and 7% of term infants (Newman, 2016). Approximately one out of every 100 infants born suffers from RDS (Coe, Jamie, & Baskerville, 2014).

It is essential for nurses to have a basic understanding of fetal lung structure, function, and development to appreciate the impact of prematurity on the respiratory system and to collaborate with members of the health care team in providing optimally effective ventilation management and nursing care for neonates. At approximately 4 to 5 weeks of gestation, lung development begins to advance in a sequential predetermined order. Lung maturation is finished in late childhood. The stages of fetal lung development are embryonic, or formation of the proximal airway (gestational age of weeks 4–6); psuedoglandular, or formation of conducting airways (gestational age of weeks 7–16); canalicular, or formation of acini (gestational age of weeks 17–28); secular, or development of gas-exchange sites (gestational age of weeks 29–35); and alveolar, which allows expansion of surface area (gestational age of weeks 36–childhood; Lozano & Newnam, 2016; Newman, 2016). Neonatal survival becomes possible in the canalicular stage as gas-exchanging acinar units emerge. At approximately 23 to 24 weeks of gestation, surfactant is evident in amniotic fluid, with gas exchange and surfactant production starting (Lozano & Newnam, 2016).

RDS starts with compromised or delayed production and secretion of surfactant, which increases surface tension in alveoli to allow alveolar expansion thus enabling adequate oxygenation and ventilation (Wambach & Hamvas, 2015). Insufficient surfactant causes diffuse atelectasis, cell injury, and pulmonary edema. Surfactant is a complex liquid composed of lipids and proteins in the lining of the alveoli of the lungs that inhibits alveolar collapse and allows bronchioles to remain open during respiration. Surfactant also protects the lungs from injuries and infections from inhaled particles and microorganisms (Griese, 1999). Surfactant production is an active process influenced by pH, temperature, and perfusion and negatively affected by cold stress, hypovolemia, hypoxia, and acidosis (Wambach & Hamvas, 2015).

Upon microscopic examination in neonates with RDS, the most prominent characteristic is diffuse atelectasis, or collapse of alveoli (Wambach & Hamvas, 2015). Pulmonary edema contributes to the pathogenesis of RDS. In premature infants, extra lung fluid causes epithelial injury, changes in the lung epithelium,

and subsequently, oliguria in the first 2 days after birth. Generally, by the fourth day of life, premature infants get better after normal physiologic diuresis (Reuter et al., 2014).

Efforts to prevent RDS and its consequences include prevention of premature birth. Antenatal corticosteroid administration is another preventative measure that pharmacologically accelerates pulmonary maturation. Antenatal corticosteroids administered to the expectant mother at least 24 to 48 hours before delivery decrease the incidence and severity of RDS most effectively for infants between 24 weeks and 34 weeks of gestation or with a birth weight of less than 1,250 g, as well as the occurrence of comorbidities linked to prematurity (Polin & Carlo, 2014; Wambach & Hamvas, 2015).

Clinical Aspects

ASSESSMENT

Clinical indications that lead to the diagnosis of RDS include physical examination findings, laboratory data, blood gas analysis, and radiographic findings (Newman, 2016). Comprehensive assessment of the neonate's condition includes evaluating work of breathing; vital signs; oxygen needs; pulse oximetry readings; a detailed maternal; prenatal, and birth history; and the course of respiratory illness (Coe et al., 2014; Newman, 2016). Symptoms usually appear immediately after birth, but sometimes they may not be evident for several hours after delivery. Symptoms may include cyanosis; apnea; decreased urinary output; nasal flaring; rapid (tachypnea is more than 60 breaths per minute), irregular, and/or shallow breathing; shortness of breath; grunting; retractions; and increased oxygen requirement (Newman, 2016; Wambach & Hamvas, 2015). If RDS progresses, the neonate may experience alterations in central nervous system status such as lethargy, decreased responsiveness and decreased muscle tone. If RDS advances, changes in cardiac function may lead to decreased perfusion, pallor, tachycardia, and bradycardia (Newman, 2016). Nurses need to observe for possible complications such as pneumothorax, pneumomediastinum, or pneumopericardium (Wambach & Hamvas, 2015).

Tests that help to diagnose and manage RDS include blood gas analysis, which may indicate high carbon dioxide levels, low oxygen levels, low pH, and increased lactic acid levels related to altered cardiac function; complete blood count to test for anemia or polycythemia; blood typing and screen; and a blood culture to rule out infection (Newman, 2016). Chest radiograph, preferably the anterior–posterior view, may reveal a "ground glass" appearance in the lung fields typically associated with RDS and generally evident about 6 to 12 hours after birth (Newman, 2016; Wambach & Hamvas, 2015).

NURSING INTERVENTIONS, MANAGEMENT, AND IMPLICATIONS

Collaboration is essential among nurses, neonatologists, and respiratory therapists to optimize health outcomes for neonates diagnosed with RDS. Neonatal nurses are in a strategic position to monitor infant status and response to administered therapies thereby optimizing neonatal short- and long-term health outcomes. Infants with RDS require continuous monitoring and meticulous attention to care and treatment to avoid complications or sequelae such as chronic lung disease (CLD) or retinopathy of prematurity (ROP; Newman, 2016). Nursing actions include provision of vital sign monitoring, physical assessment, a quiet atmosphere, gentle handling, a neutral thermal environment, adequate fluid and nutrition, prescribed medications, venous and/or arterial access, and parental support and education.

Treatments include respiratory support such as surfactant administration, warmed humidified oxygen, continuous positive airway pressure, synchronized intermittent airway pressure, or noninvasive positive pressure ventilation or mechanical ventilation. However, assisted ventilation may harm lung tissue, so usage should be judicious. Nurses need to monitor oxygen levels and maintain levels in a therapeutic range to avoid potentially harmful side effects (Newman, 2016; Wambach & Hamvas, 2015). Nurses should monitor and collaborate to manage comorbidities such as patent ductus arteriosus, sepsis and apnea of prematurity. Nurses must be familiar with pharmacologic treatments such as caffeine and antibiotic use (Newman, 2016). The innovative practice of selective use of animal-derived or synthetic surfactants has been the most influential intervention to decrease severity, mortality rates, and comorbidities associated with RDS (Polin & Carlo, 2014; Wambach & Hamvas, 2015).

OUTCOMES

Nurses may employ interventions to minimize effects and complications of RDS by monitoring neonatal status and trends in neonatal oxygenation, assuring administration of recommended treatments, providing infant comfort measures, and educating families. Nurses can also participate in multidisciplinary systematic reviews, randomized controlled trials, or nursing research that may yield new information to optimize neonatal health outcomes related to RDS.

Summary

RDS is a pathologic disease process that involves decreased or lack of surfactant production and primarily affects premature infants. New treatments have evolved that have decreased the incidence, severity, occurrence of complications, and long-term sequelae. Neonatal nurses can offer important interventions and prescribed treatments that enhance neonatal health outcomes as well as support and educate for families in the NICU.

Coe, K. L., Jamie, S. F., & Baskerville, R. M. (2014). Managing common neonatal respiratory conditions during transport, *Advances in Neonatal Care, 14*, S3–S10.

Griese, M. (1999). Pulmonary surfactant in health and human lung diseases: State of the art. *European Respiratory Journal, 13*(6), 1455–1476.

Lozano, S. M., & Newnam, K. M. (2016). Modalities of mechanical ventilation volume-targeted versus pressure-limited. *Advances in Neonatal Care, 16*(2), 99–107.

Newman, K. (2016). Respiratory system. In C. Kenner & J. W. Lott (Eds.), *Neonatal nursing care handbook* (2nd ed., pp. 3–54). New York, NY: Springer Publishing.

Polin, R. A., & Carlo, W. A. (2014). Surfactant replacement therapy for preterm and term neonates with respiratory distress. *Pediatrics, 133*(1), 156–163. doi:10.1542/peds.2013-3443

Reuter, S., Moser, C., & Baack, M. (2014). Respiratory distress in the newborn. *Pediatric Reviews, 35*(10), 417–428.

Stoll, B. J., Hansen, N. I., Bell, E. F., Shankaran, S., Laptook, A. R., Walsh, M. C., . . . Higgins, R. D. (2010). Neonatal outcomes of extremely preterm infants from the NICHD Neonatal Research Network. *Pediatrics, 126*(3), 443–456. doi:10.1542/peds.2009-2959

Wambach J. A., & Hamvas A. (2015). Respiratory distress syndrome in the neonate. In R. J. Martin, A. A. Fanaroff, & M. C. Walsh (Eds.), *Fanaroff and Martin's neonatal–perinatal medicine* (10th ed., pp. 1072–1086). Philadelphia, PA: Elsevier Saunders.

■ RETINOPATHY OF PREMATURITY

Mary Ann Blatz

Overview

Retinopathy of prematurity (ROP) results from aberrant growth of retinal blood vessels that may cause blindness in premature infants. ROP generally resolves without producing permanent retinal injury. However, severe ROP may force the retina to separate from the edge of the eye and potentially produce blindness. Infants who are born weighing 1,250 g or less and are less than 31 weeks of gestation are at greatest risk for developing ROP (American Association for Pediatric Ophthalmology and Strabismus, 2016). Nurses play a critical role in the monitoring, management, and screening of premature infants in the neonatal intensive care unit (NICU), thereby directly impacting the occurrence of ROP (Jeffries & Canadian Paediatric Society, Fetus and Newborn Committee, 2016).

Background

It is estimated that 15 million babies are born prematurely, before 37 completed weeks of gestation, throughout the world annually (World Health Organization, 2016). Approximately 3.9 million infants are born in the United States annually, with 28,000 of these infants weighing 1,250 g or less. Approximately 14,000 to 16,000 of these infants develop ROP (National Eye Institute, 2014). ROP contributes to visual damage in 1,300 children and significant visual loss in 500 children in the United States yearly. The rate of ROP for premature infants is almost 16% (Ozsurekci & Aykac, 2016). Minor cases of ROP resolve without residual damage and 90% of infants with ROP are in the milder category and do not need treatment. However, infants with more severe disease may develop impaired vision or even blindness. About 1,100 to 1,500 infants annually develop ROP that is severe enough to require medical treatment. Each year in the United States 400 to 600 infants are diagnosed as legally blind from ROP (National Eye Institute, 2014).

The incidence of ROP is higher in preterm infants with lower birth weights and decreased gestational age. Premature infants who are born before retinal vessels complete normal growth may develop ROP. Ischemia in the ocular region contributes to this disease. In the underdeveloped retina, hyperoxia leads to obliteration of the tiny blood vessels in the eye. Research has found that maintaining oxygen saturation at lower levels from birth decreases the occurrence of the severe form of this disease (American Academy of Ophthalmology, 2015).

Hyperoxia is a significant contributing factor to retinal changes and ROP. Extremely preterm infants generally require long-term mechanical ventilation and high levels of oxygen, which may lead to inflammation and oxidative stress that contributes to an increased risk of incurring lung, brain, and retinal injury (Poon et al., 2016). ROP occurs as blood vessels grow abnormally and proliferate throughout the retina. These blood vessels are delicate and may bleed, damaging and shifting alignment of the retina, which results in retinal detachment, the chief cause of visual loss and blindness from ROP.

The eye begins to grow at approximately 16 weeks of gestation, and retinal blood vessels emerge from the optic nerve in the posterior ocular region. Oxygen and nutrients are delivered by the neovascularization that develops and stretches toward the periphery of the developing retina. The eye matures quickly in the last 12 weeks of gestation and is almost complete when a full-term infant is born. Retinal maturation is completed within the first month after delivery. However, if an infant is born prematurely, before the blood vessels have extended to the retinal edge, abnormal blood vessel development may occur (National Eye Institute, 2014). These new blood vessels are fragile and may bleed, contributing to retinal scarring. As the scars contract, they pull on the retina, causing it to separate from the back of the eye (National Eye Institute, 2014).

Numerous factors contribute to the onset of ROP. Factors that influence the development of ROP in addition to prematurity and lower birth weight include anemia, blood transfusions, respiratory distress, neonatal infections, and general neonatal health status (National Eye Institute, 2014). Additional ROP triggers include depression of retinal vascularization; placental nutrients and growth factor deficiencies; interrupted vascularization with ensuing hypoxia because of retinal growth and increasing metabolic requirements; hypoxic retina stimulating structure of the oxygen-regulated components that drive retinal vascularization by utilizing erythropoietin and vascular endothelial growth factor (VEGF); and variations in oxygen stimulating cells to cause endothelial cell death, which causes avascular retinal development (Ozsurekci & Aykac, 2016).

Clinical Aspects

ASSESSMENT

The International Committee for Classification of Retinopathy of Prematurity created a diagnostic classification system. ROP is evaluated by location or concentric zones of retinal vascularization, incomplete or immature stage, and extent of the disease. A qualified ophthalmologist should provide an indirect ophthalmoscopic examination based on gestational age of the premature infant. Examinations may need to be repeated at intervals or surgical treatment with argon or diode lasers may need to be utilized based on findings (National Eye Institute, 2014). Neonatal nurses need to be familiar with screening protocols, treatment modalities, and pathogenesis of the diagnosis.

The American Academy of Pediatrics issued a policy statement (Fierson et al., 2013) to guide screening practices to detect the presence and severity of ROP in premature infants. These guidelines remain the current standard to drive screening protocols. The Canadian Paediatric Society released an update on screening and management to minimize visual losses in preterm infants (Jeffries & Canadian Paediatric Society, Fetus and Newborn Committee, 2016). Classification of stages of ROP is necessary for consistency of treatment, so interventions can be provided at designated stages when visual loss is likely. Researchers evaluated ROP screening guidelines for extremely premature infants and concluded that additional research is essential to identify the best time frame for ROP screening for infants born at less than 24 weeks or more than 27 weeks of gestation (Kennedy et al., 2014). Nurses and other health care professionals should be familiar with ROP screening and management guidelines as well as treatment options for severe ROP in this high-risk neonatal population.

NURSING INTERVENTIONS, MANAGEMENT, AND IMPLICATIONS

Nurses can collaborate with neonatologists, respiratory therapists, and ophthalmologists to optimize results for infants who require treatment. Neonatal nurses are in a key position to minimize ROP in the NICU population. Continuous monitoring of administered oxygen to ensure that infant oxygen saturation levels remain within prescribed therapeutic ranges may reduce the risk and severity of ROP. As premature infants are screened for ROP, nurses must carefully administer prescribed dilating ophthalmic and topical anesthetic drops before the examination and monitor for side effects such as apnea. As the ROP examination begins, the nurse needs to ensure the infant is comfortable using techniques, such as swaddling, and offering 24% sucrose with a pacifier. Cardiorespiratory monitoring and pulse oximetry should continue to ensure an immediate response if physiologic instability occurs (Jeffries & Canadian Paediatric Society, Fetus and Newborn Committee, 2016). The neonatal nurse is the first link to providing increased assistance, as well as additional interventions and support to the infant as necessary during the ROP examination. Nurses can provide education to parents by explaining ROP in terms that parents can understand as well offering education-appropriate reading materials or directing them to suitable Internet resources. Nurses can give support related to ROP screening and treatment if needed, by linking families to social workers, early childhood intervention programs, financial assistance, and support groups. Therapeutic management for severe ROP includes laser ablation; cryotherapy; bevacizumab injection, which is a monoclonal antibody for VEGF; scleral buckle, which is a procedure to repair a retinal detachment; or vitrectomy in which there is removal of small portions of the vitreous humor from the front structures of the eye (Kennedy et al., 2014).

OUTCOMES

Strategies nurses may utilize to minimize the incidence and severity of ROP include monitoring trends in neonatal oxygenation, ensuring compliance with standardized screening recommendations, observing physiologic stability during ROP screening examinations and treatments, providing infant comfort measures, and educating families. Nurses can also participate in multidisciplinary large-scale research activities or nursing studies that may produce new information to enhance neonatal health outcomes related to ROP.

Summary

ROP is a pathologic disease process that affects premature infants and may lead to permanent visual loss. Many factors interact to stimulate abnormal retinal blood vessel growth. Improved screening guidelines and treatments have helped to reduce permanent visual losses. Neonatal nurses can provide important interventions that enhance neonatal health outcomes.

American Academy of Ophthalmology. (2015). Retinopathy of prematurity. *EyeWiki*. Retrieved from http://eyewiki.aao.org/Retinopathy_of_Prematurity

American Association for Pediatric Ophthalmology and Strabismus. (2016). Retinopathy of prematurity. Retrieved from https://www.aapos.org/terms/conditions/94

Fierson, W. M., Saunders, R. A., Good, W., Palmer, E. A., Phelps, D., Reynolds, J., . . . Riefe, J. G.; American Academy of Pediatrics. (2013). Policy statement: Screening examination of premature infants for retinopathy of prematurity. *Pediatrics, 131*(1), 189–195. doi:10.1542/peds.2012-2996

Jeffries, A. L., & Canadian Paediatric Society, Fetus and Newborn Committee. (2016). Retinopathy of prematurity: An update on screening and management. *Paediatrics and Child Health*, *21*(2), 101–104.

Kennedy, K. A., Wrage, L. A., Higgins, R. D., Finer, N. N., Carlo, W. A., Walsh, M. C., & Phelps, D. L. (2014). Evaluating retinopathy of prematurity screening guidelines for 24 to 27-week gestational age infants. *Journal of Perinatology*, *34*, 311–318. doi:10.1038/jp.2014.12

National Eye Institute. (2014). Facts about retinopathy of prematurity (ROP). Retrieved from https://nei.nih.gov/health/rop/rop

Ozsurekci Y., & Aykac, K. (2016). Oxidative stress related diseases in newborns. *Oxidative Medicine and Cellular Longevity*, *2016*, 1–9. doi:10.1155/2016/2768365

Poon, A. W. H., Ma, E. X. H., Vadivel, A., Jung, S., Khoja, Z., Stephens, L., & Wintermark, P. (2016). Impact of bronchopulmonary dysplasia on brain and retina. *Biology Open*, *15*(4), 475–483. doi:10.1242/bio.017665

World Health Organization. (2016). Preterm birth fact sheet. Retrieved from http://www.who.int/mediacentre/factsheets/fs363/en

■ SEPSIS

Karla Phipps

Overview

Neonatal sepsis is a systemic infection with a positive blood or spinal fluid culture, occurring in the first 28 days of life that is either early onset or late onset in the neonatal population. This differentiation is based on the timing of the infection and likely mode of transmission. Most often caused by bacteria, both fungi and some viruses can also lead to sepsis with the infection in the blood and or spinal fluid. Early-onset sepsis (EOS) is variably defined by bacteremia occurring in the first 3 days of life in preterm infants and before 7 days of life in full-term infants. EOS usually has multisystem involvement and has a rapid onset, often fulminate, with a high mortality rate. Late-onset sepsis (LOS) occurs after 3 days in preterm or hospitalized infants and after 7 days in term infants. LOS can be acute but often has a slower onset and is usually focal with meningitis being common (Fanaroff & Fanaroff, 2013). Nurses must have the critical knowledge and skills to identify the patient with developing sepsis and provide competent care to prevent complications.

Background

Historically, before treatment with antibiotics, sepsis was almost always fatal. Mortality has decreased over the last two decades due to advancements in technology and specific preventative measures. Before antibiotics, the predominant organism was *Streptococcus*, which decreased after the introduction of antibiotics and gram-negative organisms became prominent. In the 1960s, Group B *Streptococcus* (GBS) replaced *Staphylococcus aureus* as the most common cause of neonatal sepsis. A study done by the National Institute of Child Health and Human Development (NICHD) Neonatal Research Network (NRN) estimates the overall incidence of EOS to be 0.98 cases per 1,000 live births, with increased rates in premature infants (Camacho-Gonzalez, Spearman, & Stoll, 2013). GBS and *Escherichia coli* have been associated with approximately 70% of all EOS infections combined, and the most common cause of mortality is from *E. coli* sepsis (Bizzarro et al., 2015; Simonsen, Anderson-Berry, Delair, & Davies, 2014). EOS is often seen with preterm delivery, premature rupture of membranes, maternal peripartum infection, infants of low birth weight, or asphyxia (Fanaroff & Fanaroff, 2013). In the early 1990s, it was estimated that EOS caused by GBS infection was 1.7 cases per 1,000 live births.

In 1996, the Centers for Disease Control and Prevention (CDC) published the first set of guidelines for the prevention of perinatal GBS infection, by using intrapartum antibiotic (IPA) treatment for maternal GBS colonization. After IPA, a reduction in the incidence of EOS with GBS was evident; however, by 2001 the rate had plateaued. With the adoption of universal screening of mothers for GBS and the use of IPA treatment in 2002, the incidence of EOS–GBS decreased to 0.3 per 1,000 live births. The prevalence of GBS has declined dramatically over the past 15 years. However, as a result of screening and early IPA, there has been an increase in the rate of Gram-negative infections. *E. coli* is the second leading cause of EOS accounting for 24% of all cases (Simonsen, et al., 2014).

LOS is a significant cause of morbidity and mortality due to the longer survival of very-low-birth-weight, lower gestational age infants. LOS is an important cause of neurodevelopmental delays and bronchopulmonnary dysplasia (BPD) in preterm infants (Shah, Jefferies, Yoon, Lee, & Shah, 2015). The pathogens most commonly seen are those that colonize the skin and mucous membranes: coagulase negative

Staphylococcus (CONS), *S. aureus*, *E. coli*, *Klebsiella*, and *Candida* species, each of which are transmitted from the environment or vertically transmitted during the peripartum period. IPA prophylaxis has not impacted LOS. Instead, LOS is often seen with prolonged hospitalization, use of indwelling catheters and endotracheal tubes as well as other invasive procedures (Fanaroff & Fanaroff, 2013). CONS is the most common cause of LOS with death occurring in 0.9%. *S. aureus* accounts for approximately 17% of LOS cases (Bizzarro et al., 2015), with methicillin-resistant *S. aureus* seen in 28% of all infections in preterm infants (Camacho-Gonzalez, Spearman, & Stoll, 2013).

Clinical Aspects

One of the most common neonatal problems when observing for infection or suspected sepsis is that the symptoms are often nonspecific. The clinician's ability to identify neonates with sepsis is difficult. Because various maternal, neonatal, and environmental factors are associated with risk for infection, it is important to recognize them early in order to identify high-risk neonates.

ASSESSMENT

Manifestations for sepsis may include respiratory distress, apnea, decreased level of activity, abdominal distention, vomiting, diarrhea, temperature instability, jaundice, loss of muscle tone, and seizures. These symptoms are associated with other inflammatory diseases seen in the neonatal population, which makes identifying infants with sepsis challenging. When the diagnosis is obvious, the infant is usually very ill (Polin & the Committee on Fetus and Newborn, 2012). It is the nurse at the bedside who is often the first to observe these signs and symptoms and will identify changes in a newborn's examination. As the first professional to note these changes, the nurse can ensure timely diagnostic testing and the start of empiric antimicrobials that are essential in saving lives. With supportive care, the majority of infants with suspected sepsis will recover.

Maternal risk factors are most commonly associated with EOS. Because the infant is maintained in a relatively sterile environment in utero, infection usually occurs when pathogens reach the fetus or neonate after birth. Maternal chorioamnionitis and GBS colonization are associated with high rates of EOS. Nurses can identify infants at risk by reviewing maternal labor and delivery history with attention to these key factors.

NURSING INTERVENTIONS, MANAGEMENT, AND IMPLICATIONS

The neonatal risk factor most commonly associated with neonatal sepsis is preterm birth and is linked with both EOS and LOS. An infant's birth weight is inversely related to risk of EOS with lower birth weight infants at higher risk for sepsis (Camacho-Gonzalez et al., 2013). A preterm infant's skin is underdeveloped and therefore more susceptible to nosocomial pathogens. Preterm infants have a large body mass-to-surface ratio, which plays a role in hydration, temperature stability, and as a barrier against infection. Preventing hypothermia in preterm infants is a major nursing focus with direct impact on mortality. Due to evaporative loss, humidity is maintained by placing infants in incubators. Nurses are responsible for maintaining and monitoring the neutral thermal environment and are aware of the tiny changes in status that can reflect temperature instability and early sepsis.

Skin care in neonates is essential in preventing skin breakdown. Nurses can individualize bathing and care to prevent infections. Studies show daily bathing with soap and water is important; however, bathing with antiseptics like chlorhexidine can affect the skin's normal microflora (Dong & Speer, 2015). Frequent exposure to skin-disrupting procedures, such as heel sticks and intravenous (IV) placements, increases the risk for LOS. It is the nurse who can cluster blood draws, prevent multiple blood sampling, and suggest long-term intravascular access for infants, thus preventing skin breakdown where pathogens can enter.

The preterm infant's gut is essential in the development of the innate immune defenses against infection. Term infants are colonized with anaerobes after breastfeeding is initiated. Many premature infants may not receive breast milk for the first few days after birth, leading to abnormal gut microflora and delayed colonization. This may then promote bacterial translocation into the bloodstream causing LOS (Dong & Speer, 2015).

The need for slow-feeding advances and use of intravascular access devices for parenteral nutrition put infants at higher risk for LOS. Attention must be paid to feeding intolerance. The nurse must monitor the abdominal girth, residuals, emesis, and weight closely for any subtle sign of sepsis. Initiation of small-volume feeds within the first few days of life has shown to be beneficial in prevention of nosocomial infection (Dong & Speer, 2015).

The two principal influences in LOS are the hospital setting and invasive procedures. Neonates are prone to being colonized by organisms in their environment. Meticulous cleaning of equipment and handwashing helps keep colonization risk low. Continued invasive interventions, such as mechanical ventilation and intravascular catheterization, lead to the disruption of the normal neonatal flora and allow hospital-acquired pathogens to colonize infants (Dong & Speer, 2015). By following ventilator-associated and central-line related bacterial bundles (grouping of evidence-based, high-impact interventions), nurses play the most important role in minimizing the incidence of pneumonia and central line associated infections.

Many clinicians use the Centers for Disease Control and Prevention (CDC, 2010) and Mukhopadhyay, Dukhovny, Mao, Eichenwald, and Puopplo (2014) algorithms for the evaluation and management of infants at risk for EOS (Polin & the Committee on Fetus and Newborn, 2012). The neonatal EOS calculator, a means for predicating risk of EOS combining both maternal risk factors with objective measures of a newborn's clinical exam, is being adopted in many NICUs and has been shown to be beneficial (Escobar et al., 2014). This has resulted in a decrease of prolonged hospitalizations and antibiotic exposure in infants.

Complete blood counts (CBCs) and acute phase reactants, such as C reactive protein, provide diagnostic markers that help determine the length of antibiotic therapy. Other laboratory studies, such as lumbar puncture for evaluation of cerebrospinal fluid (CSF), urine culture, and blood culture, may be indicated to determine a specific pathogen. A limitation for early diagnosis of sepsis is the length of time it may take for a culture to be read as positive. However, treatment with antimicrobials needs to begin immediately after the sepsis evaluation is completed.

OUTCOMES

Mortality rates are lower in term infants compared to preterm infants in both early and late onset sepsis. Mortality estimates vary depending on gestational age of the infant and if there is a defined pathogen.

Prevention, rather than treatment, improves clinical outcomes. With the implementation of bundles, there are reduced episodes of LOS. Bundles available include hand hygiene, full-barrier precautions, prompt removal of central lines, and avoidance of femoral route for IV access.

Summary

EOS and LOS continue to be an issue for neonates. Diagnostic tests help with the decisions to begin and to stop treatment, but do not have the high diagnostic

accuracy or validity that can aid in early detection of sepsis in neonates. Antibiotic awareness and stewardship are important in preventing issues in the future. Standard contact precautions and care with good hand hygiene are essential in keeping sepsis risks low. The use of bundles for intravascular lines and tubes is now vital in the prevention of LOS.

It is the astute nurse at the bedside who can be the guide to early detection. With strict adherence to assessment skills, infection control polices, such as strict handwashing and catheter and ventilator management, nurses can reduce and possibly eliminate infections in neonates, thus improving morbidity and mortality.

Nursing can mandate best practices to prevent infections. Nurses need to understand causes, clinical manifestations, and the risk factors for neonatal sepsis. With this knowledge and with continued assessment of interventions, nurses can play a vital role in preventing mortality and limit morbidity from neonatal sepsis.

Bizzarro, M., Shabanova, V., Baltimore, R., Dembry, L. M., Ehrenkranz, R., & Gallagher, P. (2015). Neonatal sepsis 2004–2013: The rise and fall of coagulase-negative staphylococci. *Journal of Pediatrics*, 166(5), 1193–1199. doi:10.1016/j.jpeds.2015.02.009

Camacho-Gonzalez, A., Spearman, P., & Stoll, B. (2013). Neonatal infectious diseases: Evaluation of neonatal sepsis. *Pediatric Clinics of North America*, 60(2), 367–389.

Centers for Disease Control and Prevention. (2010). Trends in perinatal group B *Streptococcal* disease–United States, 2000–2006. *Morbidity and Mortality Weekly Report*, 58,109–112.

Dong, Y., & Speer, C. (2015). Late-onset neonatal sepsis: Recent developments. archives of disease in childhood. *Archives of Disease in Childhood—Fetal and Neonatal Edition*, 100, F257–F263. doi:10.1136/archdischild-2014-306213

Escobar, G., Puopolo, K., Wi, S., Turk, B., Kuzniewicz, M., Walsh, E., . . . Draper, D. (2014). Stratification of risk of early-onset sepsis in newborns ≥ 34 weeks gestation. *Pediatrics*, 133(1), 30–36. doi:10.1542/peds.2013-1689

Fanaroff, A., & Fanaroff, J. (2013). *Klaus and Fanaroff's care of the high risk neonate* (6th ed., pp. 346–367). Philadelphia, PA: Elsevier Saunders.

Mukhopadhyay, S., Dukhovny, D., Mao, W., Eichenwald, E., & Puopplo, K. (2014). 2010 Perinatal GBS Prevention Guideline and Resource Utilization. *Pediatrics*, 133(2). Retrieved from http://pediatrics.aappublications.org/content/133/2/196

Polin, R., & the Committee on Fetus and Newborn. (2012). The Committee on Fetus and Newborn: Management of neonates with suspected or proven early-onset bacterial sepsis. *Pediatrics*, 129(5), 1006–1015. doi:10.1542/peds.2012-0541

Shah J., Jefferies A. L., Yoon, E. W., Lee, S. K., & Shah, P. S. (2015). Canadian Neonatal Network. Risk factors and outcomes of late-onset bacterial sepsis in preterm neonates born at < 32 weeks gestation. *American Journal of Perinatology, 32*(7), 675–682. doi:10.1055/s-0034-1393936

Simonsen, K., Anderson-Berry, A., Delair, S., & Davies, H. D. (2014). Early-onset neonatal sepsis. *Clinical Microbiology Reviews, 27*(1), 21–47. doi:10.1128/CMR.00031-13

■ SUBSTANCE ABUSE/OPIOID WITHDRAWAL

Helene M. Lannon

Overview

Substance abuse during pregnancy has increased substantially over the past 10 years and has reached epidemic proportions. In the United States, approximately 225,000 infants yearly are exposed to illicit substances (MacMullen, Dulski, & Blobaum, 2014). Retrospectively, by 2011, 1.1% of pregnant women abused opioids, pain relievers, and heroin; 12.9% were dispensed an opioid at some time during the pregnancy, and the incidence of infant withdrawal rose from 1.2 to 5.8 per 1,000 births (Hall et al., 2014). From the years 2000 to 2009, the number of infants in the United States diagnosed with neonatal abstinence syndrome (NAS) grew threefold, accounting for $720 million in national health care expenditures (Patrick et al., 2015). In response to the growth of the problem and variable treatment for addicted infants, the American Academy of Pediatrics requested the medical community standardize care delivered to infants withdrawing from opioids (Patrick et al., 2016).

Background

NAS is a drug-withdrawal syndrome experienced by opioid-exposed infants shortly after birth (Patrick et al., 2016), with clinical signs that affect the central nervous system, as well as the autonomic, gastrointestinal, and respiratory systems. Legal use of tobacco and alcohol are harmful to the growing fetus, yet, when coupled with illicit drugs or opiates, it is difficult to extrapolate what substance or drug combinations are causing withdrawal. Because of the potential for multiple exposures, the data outcomes for infants are not conclusive and may be impossible to predict. In response to the increased incidence of infants experiencing NAS and a desire to optimize infant outcomes, collaborative neonatal groups combined strategies to develop evidence-based guidelines to treat NAS pharmacologically (Hall et al., 2014, 2016).

The health care team can anticipate withdrawal signs in the newborn if the mother is enrolled in a methadone clinic or substance abuse program and is receiving methadone or buprenorphine to treat her own withdrawal. However, it is difficult to anticipate infant withdrawal when there is no prenatal care or a poor maternal history. Pregnancy may be the first time a woman finds help for her addiction. Despite these challenges, most drugs and substances are known to cross the placenta and affect the fetus.

The effects of infant exposure to chemical substances was recognized more than 50 years ago, but fetal development has only been seriously studied in the past 30 years. Nicotine has been studied since 1960, alcohol since 1970, and illicit drugs since 1980. Marijuana is the most commonly used illicit substance during pregnancy, with approximately 2.5% of women using during pregnancy, often concurrent with tobacco and alcohol use. Therefore, isolated effects alone are difficult to study (Jaques et al., 2014). It is unknown whether the long-term effects of prenatal exposure to medicinal cannabis used in a controlled manner differs from the effects of cannabis used as a legal, recreational drug during pregnancy. However, follow-up developmental growth data report school-age children exposed to in utero marijuana exhibited decreased attention, hyperactivity, and impulsivity. Reading, spelling, and math skills were lacking, particularly for those children who were heavily exposed to marijuana during the first trimester of pregnancy (Metz & Stickrath, 2015).

The exact mechanism by which nicotine produces adverse effects is unknown, but it is believed that the vasoconstrictive effects on the placenta and umbilical vessels lead to fetal hypoxia resulting in poor infant growth and brain development (Behnke & Smith, 2013). Excessive maternal ingestion of alcohol during pregnancy may cause fetal alcohol syndrome. Infants may demonstrate neurodevelopmental deficits of poor habituation, subtle language delays, low levels of arousal with motor abnormalities, growth restriction, and potential for congenital anomalies (Behnke & Smith, 2013). Long-term effects of methamphetamine and cocaine, as potent vasoconstriction agents, are unclear but suggest an association with prematurity and intrauterine-growth restriction. Animal studies have shown disruptions in neural and glial cell organization, migration, and altered nucleic acid and protein production in the brain, suggestive of overall compromise in brain growth (Behnke & Smith, 2013).

Of critical concern is maternal substance use on the developing fetal brain. During the embryonic stage, drugs can have significant teratogenic effects that persist as subtle effects of abnormal growth and maturation. Jaques et al. (2014) studied cannabis-exposed animal models and suggested that during the embryonic stage, neurotransmitter pathways and receptors, particularly dopamine receptors, were disrupted. Disturbances in dopamine function have been associated with an increased risk of neuropsychiatric disorders such as drug addiction, schizophrenia, and depression. However, whether these changes are implicated in the future risk of addictive behaviors in the human is yet unknown (Jaques et al., 2014).

Acute narcotic withdrawal usually begins 24 to 48 hours after birth; however, symptoms may not appear until 3 to 4 days after birth. Methadone exposure symptoms may appear within 48 to 72 hours or may not be exhibited until 3 weeks of age. Readmission is common as infants are often discharged before symptoms appear. Opiate withdrawal develops in 55% to 94% of exposed infants (Hall et al., 2014). The infant with opiate NAS may exhibit hyperactivity, irritability, sleep disturbances, hypertonia and tremors, potential seizures, exaggerated Moro reflex, increased muscle tone, exaggerated sucking, high-pitched cry, diaphoresis, poor feeding, diarrhea, vomiting, poor weight gain, and overall poor orientation for self-regulation with autonomic signs of yawning, sneezing, nasal stuffiness, mottling of skin and fever (Hudak & Tan, 2012). Nursing interventions for these symptoms alone are often not adequate treatment. The most commonly used therapeutic opioid treatment for withdrawal is morphine, although some centers use methadone with emerging use of buprenorphine and clonidine as an adjunct therapy (Kraft & van den Anker, 2012).

Clinical Aspects

The Finnegan Neonatal Abstinence Scoring System (NASS) is a tool initially established by Finnegan in 1975, modified, published in standardized form, and used by nursing staff to assess an infant's withdrawal symptoms and need for pharmacologic intervention (Asti, Magers, Keels, Wispe, & McClead, 2015). It is an easy, comprehensive scoring system composed of 21 items relating to signs of neonatal withdrawal; it is the predominant tool used in NAS in the United States.

ASSESSMENT

The nursing assessment of interventions for nonpharmacologic therapy were gathered from systematic reviews of literature based on nursing case reports, descriptive or retrospective studies, nursing articles and reviews, or are sometimes based on the tradition of what seems to work. A systematic literature review published by MacMullen et al. (2014) lists nursing interventions based on a level-of-evidence scale. Level I–II has high-level evidence based on randomized control trials, level III evidence is based on retrospective cohort studies, and level IV evidence is based on case studies or observational reports.

The nursing assessment begins with a thorough maternal history to identify infants at risk. Maternal drug history and screening should be conducted for all pregnant women. Nurses use their center's NAS scoring tool to identify infant signs and symptoms of withdrawal and closely monitor scores per protocol to determine initiation, escalation, weaning, or discontinuation of pharmacological therapy.

NURSING INTERVENTIONS, MANAGEMENT, AND IMPLICATIONS

Nonpharmacologic nursing therapies based on level of evidence are as follows: supportive care measures of swaddling, decreased stimulation, low-lighted environment, limiting noise; cluster care, sucrose pacifier, and cuddling or infant massage. Auditory and eye-to-eye contact in a randomized control trial received a high level of evidence, level I–II. Rooming-in as a retrospective, cohort study scored a level III. Nutritional deficiencies from increased energy expenditure, or vomiting, diarrhea, or loose stools require a high-calorie formula; poor oral skills, which may require intravenous therapy or gavage feedings, received an evidence level IV.

Nurses must record intake and output and serum electrolytes to indicate dehydration and/or deficiencies. Daily weight is important indicators of nutritional status. Breastfeeding may be contraindicated in some instances; however, breastfeeding provides an optimal nutrition and promotes maternal–infant bonding. Mothers on methadone therapy may breastfeed, which is supported by the American Academy of Pediatrics and per most institutions, as evidence level III–IV. Skin care for any breakdown areas may require topical ointments;

barrier shields of clear, transparent dressings over reddened areas; and positioning for comfort, as evidence level IV. Pharmacologic therapy is indicated for moderate to severe signs of NAS and is used to prevent complications of fever, weight loss, and seizures or if the infant is not responding to nonpharmacologic therapies.

OUTCOMES

An infant born to a mother on a low-dose prescription opiate with a short half-life may be safely discharged if there are no signs of withdrawal by 3 days of age, whereas an infant born to a mother on an opiate with a prolonged half-life should be observed for a minimum of 5 to 7 days after cessation of pharmacologic therapy. Methadone withdrawal signs may continue for months, but late signs are often subtle and only require comfort measures as treatment. Since initiation of the 2012 American Academy of Pediatrics call for an evidence-based protocol for NAS, outcomes to date are favorable. Use of a stringent protocol for pharmacological therapy has reduced the duration of opioid exposure and the length of hospital stay, with continued research to refine the pharmacological weaning protocol in progress (Hall et al., 2014).

Nursing protocols based on evidence-based research versus systematic reviews are valuable in refining nonpharmacological therapies to treat NAS. Family-centered, rooming-in models of care are showing favorable outcomes in shortening opioid treatment for NAS and thus decreasing the length of stay. Nurses must continue to be active participants in NAS protocol development through participation in committees to evaluate literature, and to create policies and procedures to refine nonpharmacologic treatment for NAS. Therapy for NAS begins at the bedside with the nursing assessment and is the integral component that determines therapy and ultimately, the outcome.

Summary

There is a need to disentangle the many variables of substances and drugs associated with newborn exposure, withdrawal, and follow-up care. The harmful effects of any substance or drug use upon the fetus and newborn are well documented. The short- and long-term effects of drug use on infant growth and development are uncertain. Health care has responded by researching pharmacological and nonpharmacological interventions to minimize withdrawal, minimize the risk of adverse outcomes, and shorten the length of hospital stay to minimize health care costs. Until there is a significant decrease in drug abuse during pregnancy, hopeful outcomes rely on health care's dedication for research that results in effective methods and therapies to treat NAS.

Asti, L., Magers, J., Keels, E., Wispe, J., & McClead, R. (2015). A quality improvement project to reduce length of stay for neonatal abstinence syndrome. *Pediatrics, 135*(6), 1494–1500.

Behnke, M., & Smith, V. C. (2013). Prenatal substance: Short- and long-term effects on the exposed fetus. *Pediatrics, 131*(3), 1009–1024.

Hall, E., Wexelblatt, S., Crowley, M., Grow, J., Jasin, J., Klebanoff, M., . . . Walsh, M. (2014). A multicenter cohort study of treatments and hospital outcomes in neonatal abstinence syndrome. *Pediatrics, 134*(2), 527–534.

Hall, E., Wexelblatt, S., Crowley, M., Grow, J., Jasin, J., Klebanoff, M., . . . Walsh, M. on behalf of the OCHNAS Consortium. (2016). Implementation of a neonatal abstinence syndrome weaning protocol: A multicenter cohort study. *Pediatrics, 136*(4), 803–810.

Hudak, M., & Tan, R. (2012). Committee on drugs, and committee on fetus and newborn, neonatal drug withdrawal. *Pediatrics, 129*(2), 540–560.

Jaques, S., Kingsbury, A., Henshcke, P., Chomchai, C., Clews, S., Falconer, J., . . . Oej, J. (2014). Cannabis, the pregnant woman and her child: Weeding out the myths. *Journal of Perinatology, 34*(6), 417–424.

Kraft, W. K., & van den Anker, J. N. (2012). Pharmacologic management of the opioid neonatal abstinence syndrome. *Pediatric Clinics of North America, 59*(5), 1147–1165.

MacMullen, N. J., Dulski, L. A., & Blobaum, P. (2014). Evidence-based interventions for neonatal abstinence syndrome. *Pediatric Nursing, 40*(4), 165–203.

Metz, T. D., & Stickrath, E. H. (2015). Marijuana use in pregnancy and lactation: A review of evidence. *American Journal of Obstetrics and Gynecology, 213*(6), 761–778.

Patrick, S. W., Dudley J., Martin, P., Harrell, F., Warren, M., Hartmann, K., . . . Cooper, W. (2015). Prescription opioid epidemic and infant outcomes. *Pediatrics, 135*(5), 842–850.

Patrick, S. W., Schumacher, R. E., Horbar, J., Buus-Frank, M., Edwards, E., Morrow, F. K., . . . Soll, R. (2016). Improving care for neonatal abstinence syndrome. *Pediatrics, 137*(5), 1–8.

■ THERMOREGULATION

Paula Forsythe

Overview

In utero, the fetus is dependent on the mother as the source of heat. At birth, the neonate transitions from a warm environment to one that is much colder. After delivery, the neonate must assume self-regulation of body temperature. This is one of the most significant challenges faced by every newborn. Failure to regulate temperature has serious implications for many body systems and may cause even healthy newborns to experience respiratory, metabolic, and cardiovascular complications, all of which can be prevented by diligent nursing care.

Background

Thermoregulation is the ability to regulate heat production and loss to maintain normal body temperature between 36.5°C and 37.5°C (American Heart Association and American Academy of Pediatrics, 2015; Brand & Boyd, 2015; Knobel Robin, 2014). It is a key physiologic requirement for survival. In utero, fetal body heat is generated by the infant's rapid metabolic rate and heat transferred from the mother via the placenta and uterus. The result is a body temperature 0.3°C to 0.5°C higher than the mother's (Asakura, 2004; Knobel Robin, 2014). Heat loss and cold stress, which often occurs during delivery and in the minutes that follow, stimulates the newborn's skin and thermal receptors, especially the trigeminal area of the face, to signal the hypothalamus to conserve or produce heat (Brand & Boyd, 2015; Karlson, 2013). The hypothalamus activates the sympathetic nervous system and norepinephrine is released triggering several adaptations vital to maintaining body temperature (Brand & Boyd, 2015; Chaplain Maternal Newborn Regional Program [CMNRP], 2013; Karlson, 2013). Norepinephrine increases metabolism, respiratory rate, oxygen consumption, and the utilization of glucose. Norepinephrine also vasoconstricts peripheral blood vessels to minimize environmental heat loss and retain core body heat; vasoconstricts pulmonary vessels, increases pulmonary vascular pressure and shunts deoxygenated blood away from the lungs, through the ductus arteriosus to the aorta. It also stimulates brown fat metabolism (Brand & Boyd, 2015; Karlson, 2013). This constellation of physiologic reactions places the newborn, especially those born premature and/or ill at risk for hypoxemia, hypoxia, hypoglycemia, anaerobic metabolism, and acidosis which can lead to cell damage and even death (Brand & Boyd, 2015; CMNRP, 2013; Karlson, 2013).

Neonates rely on nonshivering thermogenesis to metabolize brown adipose fat (BAT) and release energy. BAT contains mitochondria, fat vacuoles, sympathetic nerve endings, and an abundant blood supply (Asakura, 2004; Brand & Boyd, 2015). BAT develops primarily during the third trimester of pregnancy and is deposited around the kidneys, adrenal glands, mediastinum, scapulae, and axilla. BAT serves as the primary source for heat generation during the perinatal and postnatal periods. Metabolism of brown fat requires oxygen and glucose and is stimulated by nerve endings that activate lipase, resulting in lipolysis, fatty acid oxidation and the generation of heat which warms circulating blood, transferring heat throughout the body (Brand & Boyd, 2015; CMNRP, 2013; Karlson, 2013).

Although central thermoregulatory mechanisms are present at birth, they are developmentally deficient and not well differentiated (Asakura, 2004; Knobel Robin, 2014) placing neonates, particularly the smallest and most critically ill, at great risk for heat loss or hypothermia. Heat loss occurs by evaporation, conduction, convection, and radiation. Factors that impact the rate of body heat transfer or loss in the neonate include a large surface area to body mass ratio; decreased amounts of subcutaneous fat and BAT; high body water content; immature, nonkeratinized skin that allows transepidermal water and heat loss; vasoconstrictive, motor and metabolic function; and differences in temperature between the neonate and environment. Without appropriate environmental modifications and nursing care interventions, the newborn loses body heat at a rate of up to 1°C per minute (Brand & Boyd, 2015; Karlson, 2013).

Hyperthermia, a body temperature higher than 37.5°C (Karlson, 2013), is less common in the neonatal period but can result in deleterious effects. Neonates are at high risk for hyperthermia due to their inability to dissipate heat (Brand & Boyd, 2015). The most frequent causes are environmental such as overheating from incubators, radiant warmers or high room temperatures, phototherapy, or excessive clothing or bundling. Hyperthermia may, however, be a sign of infection, dehydration, narcotic withdrawal, or central nervous system disorders such as asphyxia and neonatal encephalopathy. Efficient differentiation between environmental causes and illness related causality is required for appropriate care and interventions (Brand & Boyd, 2015; CMNRP, 2013).

Clinical Aspects

ASSESSMENT

Thermal regulation begins at delivery. Gestational age and risk factors for both newborn and mother determine what is needed for a safe delivery. The delivery room temperature should be set at 25°C to 26°C (75°–77°F) and a radiant warmer, preheated should be available. Immediately following delivery, the infant is evaluated by Apgar (appearance, pulse, grimace, activity, and respiration) scoring. A stable newborn with Apgar scores greater than 6, showing no signs of complications, is dried, the head is covered with a hat, and is placed on mother's chest for warmth and bonding. Both are covered with a warmed blanket (Brand & Boyd, 2015; CMNRP, 2013). A very ill, immature or compromised newborn with Apgar scores less than or equal to 6 is stabilized, resuscitated if needed, and transferred to the neonatal intensive care unit (NICU) in a transport incubator. A polyethylene body wrap or thermal mattress is used to promote thermal stability (Brand & Boyd, 2015; Knobel Robin, 2014).

Assessment for signs of hypothermia includes frequent, continuous monitoring of body temperature and respiratory status; observing for signs of distress such as apnea, bradycardia, tachypnea, or irregular breathing patterns; acrocyanosis; cool, mottled or pale skin; hypoglycemia; lethargy; and poor feeding (CMNRP, 2013). Axillary temperatures are utilized for assessment as they correlate well with core temperatures and are noninvasive. Rectal temperatures are not recommended due to the risk for intestinal trauma or injury (Brand & Boyd, 2015).

NURSING INTERVENTIONS, MANAGEMENT, AND IMPLICATIONS

Temperature control is a primary concern for nursing. Nursing care must focus on preventing temperature instability, as well as resultant metabolic and respiratory acidosis. The goal is to manage the newborn in an environment that does not expend calories and oxygen to maintain a normal body temperature.

Interventions to prevent heat loss begin at birth. Healthy, normothermic newborns should be lightly dressed. If an axillary temperature falls below 36.3°C the head is covered with a hat, and skin-to-skin contact with the mother in a warm room, covered with blankets is practiced (CMNRP, 2013; Knobel Robin, 2014).

A care bundle, a set of interventions used together to improve patient outcomes, is initiated to maintain body warmth for newborns who are premature, ill, or require resuscitation. This includes increasing the delivery room air temperature to 25°C to 26°C; head coverings and body wraps for the neonate; a thermal mattress if needed; heated, humidified respiratory gases; and skin–skin care when feasible (CMNRP, 2013; Karlson, 2013; Knobel Robin, 2014). Applying polyethylene body wraps immediately after birth while neonates are wet with amniotic fluids creates a warm, humid environment, which improves body temperatures in the immediate postnatal period. Covering the head with a hat or plastic wrap minimizes heat loss associated with the neonate's large head-to-body size ratio. A thermal mattress placed under the infant provides a source of heat for short periods of time (Karlson, 2013; Knobel Robin, 2014). Caution must be used when combining interventions to avoid idiopathic hyperthermia (Knobel Robin, 2014).

A radiant warmer is preferred during the admission, stabilization, and procedure process before the infant is placed in an incubator. Hybrid incubators provide both environments without moving the neonate (Brand & Boyd, 2015; Knobel Robin, 2014). The temperature of the radiant warmer or incubator is regulated by feedback from a probe placed on the neonate's abdomen in the right upper quadrant, avoiding the liver or any bone. Temperature is either regulated by automatic feedback from the probe to maintain a set skin temperature (servo-control mode) or regulated by caregivers controlling the desired environmental temperature (manual, air control mode). Skin temperature monitoring is continuous and correlates well with axillary core temperatures.

Heated humidity is added to incubators of very-low-birth-weight neonates to prevent transepidermal water loss. High humidity (greater than 70%) is used during the first week of life, then decreased to standard humidity levels to minimize bacterial growth and the risk of infection (Brand & Boyd, 2015; Knobel Robin, 2014). Humid environments also minimize weight loss and hypernatremia, but delay maturation of the skin barrier (Knobel Robin, 2014). Neonates are undressed, servo-control mode is used, and oxygen, if required, is heated and humidified to minimize insensible water loss (Karlson, 2013; Knobel Robin, 2014).

Transitioning neonates to open cribs occurs sequentially with continuous monitoring of body temperature and weight. Humidity is removed incrementally, guided by the neonate's weight progression. The neonate remains in the incubator to gain weight, is lightly dressed, head covered, and managed in air-control mode. The incubator temperature is then incrementally decreased until 28°C (room temperature) has been reached in the incubator and the neonate's temperature has stabilized. Neonates are transitioned to an open crib at approximately 1,500 to 1,600 g if feeding enterally and demonstrating consistent weight gain over several days (Brand & Boyd, 2015). Additional layers of blankets are applied the first day to maintain temperature stability.

Transitioning medically stable neonates who are approximately 32 weeks gestational age and 1,500 g to open cribs, can begin with a thermal challenge (applying a blanket and decreasing the incubator temperature by 1.5°C). Early transition to open cribs is associated with higher weight accrual and shortened hospital stays (CMNRP, 2013; Knobel Robin, 2014).

Rewarming hypothermic neonates occurs slowly in an incubator, increasing the neonate's temperature 0.5°C per hour to avoid physiologic instability such as apnea. However, significant hypothermia, less than 35°C, requires rapid rewarming: the incubator temperature is set 1°C to 1.5°C greater than the body temperature, readjusting the set temperature as the neonate warms, until 36.5°C is attained. Careful monitoring of the neonate's respiratory and cardiac status, blood pressure, oxygen requirement and blood glucose levels provides evidence as to whether the neonate is successfully managing the warming process or deteriorating, requiring an escalation of physiologic management (CMNRP, 2013; Karlson, 2013).

Neonates who are hyperthermic require cooling measures: adjustment of environment temperature, removal of clothing, and provision of fluids to prevent dehydration. With severe hyperthermia, the focus is on identification and management of the cause (CMNRP, 2013).

OUTCOMES

Quality and safety issues focus on successful temperature management of the newborn during the perinatal and postnatal processes. Through the implementation of evidence-based practice, delivery room temperatures have risen and skin-to-skin contact has increased for stable newborns. Polyethylene body wraps and thermal, chemical mattresses are standard practice and Neonatal Resuscitation Protocol guidelines include

temperature management as an integral part of resuscitation (American Heart Association and American Academy of Pediatrics, 2015; Brand & Boyd, 2015). Golden Hour protocols implemented in NICU settings to improve the efficiencies of admitting and stabilizing a newborn within 60 minutes of arrival, stress the importance of temperature management (Brand & Boyd, 2015).

Summary

Successful thermoregulation is based on identification of neonates at risk for temperature instability, rigorous control of environmental factors, utilization of additional heat sources, and vigilant nursing care to detect and manage hypothermia and hyperthermia. Prevention is preferable to management for successful newborn transitions and eliminates the incidence of associated sequelae and morbidities.

American Heart Association and American Academy of Pediatrics. (2015). Summary AAP/AHA guidelines for cardiopulmonary resuscitation and emergency cardiovascular care of the neonate. Retrieved from http://www2.aap.org/NRP/docs/15535 NRP Guidelines Flyer_English_Final PDF

Asakura, H. (2004). Fetal and neonatal thermoregulation. *Journal of Nippon Medical School, 71*(6), 360–370. doi:10.1272/jnms.71.360

Brand, M. C., & Boyd, H. A. (2015). Thermoregulation. In M. T. Verklan & M. Walden (Eds.), *Core curriculum for neonatal intensive care nursing* (5th ed., pp. 95–109). St. Louis, MO: Elsevier Sanders.

Chaplain Maternal Newborn Regional Program. (2013). Newborn thermoregulation: Self-learning module. Retrieved from http://www.CMNRP/ca/uploads/documents/NEWBORN_THERMOREGULATION_SLM_20

Karlson, K. (2013). *The S.T.A.B.L.E. program: Learner/provider manual* (6th ed., pp. 63–93). Park City, UT: American Academy of Pediatrics.

Knobel Robin, B. (2014). Role of effective thermoregulation in premature neonates. *Dovepress, 4*, 147–156. doi:10.2147/RRN.S52377

Nurse Anesthesia

Anesthesia care delivered by a nurse anesthetist takes place across varied health care settings, such as hospitals, ambulatory surgery centers, physician offices, and dental offices. Regardless of the health care setting, the nurse anesthetist works in an interprofessional team to deliver the highest quality health care, and utilizes evidence-based strategies to optimize the quality of care and patient-centered outcomes (American Association of Nurse Anesthetists [AANA], 2013). Nurse anesthetists are highly skilled and educated for providing high-quality, cost-effective, and safe anesthesia care (AANA, 2013). The rigorous admission and extensive curriculum enable the nurse anesthetist to develop the academic and technical skills necessary to provide highly effective acute care. A nurse anesthetist may perform these skills autonomously, collaboratively, or from medical direction according to the practitioner's state's nurse practice act (Foster, 2011).

The content of this section is focused on the clinical aspects of nurse anesthesia care. The topics include a wide range of emerging clinical areas associated with surgical and clinical procedures, as well as comorbid conditions that influence the perianesthesia care of patients. The nurse anesthetist provides care in four general areas: preanesthetic preparation and evaluation; anesthesia induction, maintenance, and emergence; postanesthesia care; and perianesthetic and clinical support functions (Foster, 2011). Given the broad scope of practice of the nurse anesthetist across the perianethesia continuum, the focus of this section is to provide novice- and intermediate-level nurse anesthetists with a resource that provides an evidence-based compendium of emerging clinical topics, novel surgical and clinical procedures, and management strategies for high-acuity patients planned to receive anesthesia.

American Association of Nurse Anesthetists. (2013). Scope of nurse anesthesia practice. Retrieved from http://www.aana.com

Foster, S. D., & Faut-Callahan, M. (2011). *A professional study and resource guide for the CRNA* (2nd ed.). Park Ridge, IL: American Association of Nurse Anesthetists.

■ Adult Difficult Airway Management *Jennifer Nicholson and Ronald L. Hickman, Jr.*

■ Anesthesia for Preeclampsia *Kerry L. Quisenberry*

■ Anesthesia in Remote Locations *Angela Milosh*

■ Anesthesia and Robotic Surgery *Angela Milosh*

■ Anticoagulation and Anesthesia *Natalie Butchko and Aimee Dickman*

■ Awake Craniotomy *Rafiu Adeniji, Christopher Bibro, and Natalie A. Slenkovich*

■ Cardiac Anesthesia *Christopher K. Ferguson*

■ Enhanced Recovery After Anesthesia *Danielle T. Winch and Brian Garrett*

■ Evoked Potentials *Melanie M. Stipp*

■ Fluid and Transfusion Management in Anesthesia Care *Andrew D. Lorenzoni and Justin R. Stegman*

■ Liver Transplant and Anesthesia *Kimberly M. Choudhary, Sonya D. Moore, and Ronald L. Hickman, Jr.*

■ Malignant Hyperthermia *Colleen Thaxton Spencer and Elizabeth Demko*

■ Morbid Obesity and Anesthesia *Elizabeth Demko, Colleen Thaxton Spencer, and Sonya D. Moore*

■ Neuromuscular Blockade Reversal: Sugammadex *Britney A. Leonardi*

■ One-Lung Ventilation *Monica M. Bitner, Brittany Hosler, and Jessica M. Tripi*

■ Peripheral Nerve Blocks *Scott M. Urigel and Jeffrey E. Molter*

■ Postoperative Nausea and Vomiting *Kimberly Kimble*

■ Respiratory Depression and Patient-Controlled Analgesia *Sonya D. Moore*

■ Sickle Cell Disease and Anesthesia *Mark A. Caldwell, Sonya D. Moore, and Ronald L. Hickman, Jr.*

■ ADULT DIFFICULT AIRWAY MANAGEMENT

Jennifer Nicholson
Ronald L. Hickman, Jr.

Overview

Airway management is a crucial skill for any health care provider. A patient with a compromised airway deteriorates rapidly, thus making it necessary for all nurses to have appropriate airway management skills (Higginson, Parry, & Williams, 2016). The ability to assess and provide care for an airway is essential to adequate ventilation and tissue respiration. The nurse anesthetist is required to be proficient in the assessment of a patient's airway and effectively implement airway maneuvers, such as head tilt/chin lift, to ensure the patient's safety.

Background

The airway anatomically comprises the nasal and oral cavities, pharynx, larynx, trachea, and principal bronchi (Barash, Cullen, Stoelting, Cahalan, & Stock, 2009). The need for airway support measures arises for a variety of reasons across clinical populations and ages. The primary driver for airway management is central respiratory drive failure or an obstructed airway (Davies, Costa, & Asciutto, 2014). Central respiratory drive failure is often the result of intrinsic factors, such as brain injury, or extrinsic factors, such as excessive sedation or drug overdose, and affects the central nervous system (Davies et al., 2014). In contrast, airway obstruction is often the result of obstruction caused by the compression of the soft tissue or a foreign body introduced into the airway.

Early recognition of a difficult airway and impaired ventilation is lifesaving. An initial airway assessment should consist of the determination of the patency of the airway. Typically, this assessment includes the appraisal of snoring, edema, trauma, or burns, which could impact the patency of the airway. In most cases, airway management is necessary because of airway obstruction. In these cases, the head-tilt, chin-lift maneuver, which places the patient's head into the sniffing position, is recommended. However, hyperextension of the neck is contraindicated for patients with suspected or diagnosed cervical spine injury. For patients with an obstructed airway or central respiratory failure, a definitive artificial airway should be placed to provide sufficient ventilation and airway protection. There are numerous airway devices that are available for use.

Clinical Aspects

After the need for support or intervention has been identified, the nurse must have a working knowledge of how to support the patient's airway and breathing. If the patient's condition necessitates the administration of oxygen, this should be carried out as quickly as possible. Although technically and legally oxygen must be prescribed by a licensed health care practitioner, in an emergency situation, the absence of a prescription should not delay the administration of this essential intervention (Higginson et al., 2016).

ASSESSMENT

An objective evaluation of the airway is pertinent to airway management of a patient with a difficult airway or experiencing respiratory failure. If the patient is able to verbally respond to the nurse's questions, then it is likely that the patient's airway is sufficiently patent to promote the ventilation. If the patient can only speak in short sentences or one or two words, the patient is experiencing respiratory distress and a history and physical examination are needed to determine the etiology of the airway compromise or respiratory failure (Higginson et al., 2016).

During the physical assessment of a patient with airway compromise or respiratory failure, the nurse should judiciously inspect the head, neck, and chest wall. While inspecting the head, neck, and chest wall, the nurse should look for bilateral chest wall expansion that is equal and without paradoxical movements (Higginson et al., 2016). Use of accessory muscles, nasal flaring, retractions of the intercostal muscles,

ventilation rate, and ventilator patterns (rhythmicity and depth of breathing) should be documented (Higginson et al., 2016). A thorough physical should also include assessment of the vital signs (i.e., heart rate, blood pressure, pulse oximetry). Indicators of acute changes in heart rate (i.e., tachycardia or bradycardia), hypotension, and decreased oxygen saturation should be frequently assessed and the appropriate licensed health care practitioner notified for airway management as well as sequelae of respiratory distress or failure. Further clinical values may be needed, such as hemoglobin and hematocrit, and arterial blood gas analysis.

NURSING INTERVENTIONS, MANAGEMENT, AND IMPLICATIONS

The most commonly used technique to remedy an obstructed airway include airway maneuvers: sniffing position, the head tilt/chin lift, and jaw thrust maneuvers (Davies et al., 2014). The sniffing position is achieved by elevating the head 15° and extending the neck 35° in the supine position. The head tilt/chin lift is one of the most common active maneuvers used to open a patient's airway. The maneuver should only be used if the clinician is confident that there is no risk of cervical spine injury. The nurse places one hand on the patient's forehead while placing the fingers of the other hand under the mandible. The head is then tilted backward while lifting the mandible forward, extending the neck (Davies et al., 2014). The jaw thrust is the preferred method in known or suspected cases of cervical spine injury because the head and neck remain in a more neutral position when applied. The jaw thrust maneuver is applied using both hands. The fingers are placed under the angle of the jaw on both sides and then used to displace the jaw upward and forward.

If a patient with airway compromise or respiratory failure requires ventilatory support, the use of bag-mask ventilation (BMV) is recommended. BMV requires proper mask size selection, effective hand placement, and coordinated manual compression of the ventilation bag (Davies et al., 2014). To initiate BMV, the mask is placed on the bridge of the patient's nose with the use of the thumb and first finger, making a "C" shape around the valve of the mask. The middle, ring, and small fingers are placed on the mandible in an "E" formation and the chin should be brought up to meet the face mask to create a seal. If possible, the small finger should be placed under the angle of the jaw to facilitate a jaw thrust during BMV. This may not be possible with obese patients. A breath should be delivered by squeezing the bag with a constant steady pressure until chest rise is observed. Effective BMV can be identified by the absence of an auditory leak, chest rise, and subsequent presence of end tidal carbon dioxide or condensation on the interior surface of the mask.

Airway equipment may be needed to keep an airway open or assist in opening an airway that cannot be opened with the aforementioned techniques. Oropharyngeal airways (OPAs) and nasopharyngeal airways (NPAs) are the two most commonly used. Proper sizing of both are imperative for successful use as airway placement may actually worsen an obstruction if improperly sized. To size an OPA, place the airway against the side of the patient's face with the flange at the corner of the mouth. The tip of the OPA should just reach the angle of the patient's mandible (Davies et al., 2014). The OPA can be inserted two ways: place the OPA at a 90° angle from the mouth, and when the OPA is past the tongue, rotate 90° so that the curve displaces the tongue forward and opens the airway. The flange should rest laterally to the patient's teeth. The second technique is to use a tongue blade. The tongue blade is used to shift the patient's tongue forward and then directly insert the airway following the natural curve of the airway until the flange rests against the teeth.

NPAs are sized by placing the flange at the tip of the patient's nose and the beveled angle of the airway at the meatus of the ear. To place the NPA, lubricate the surface with a water-soluble jelly and inspect each of the nares to observe for patency. Hold the NPA perpendicular to the face and insert straight down with a slow steady pressure until the flange rests against the nare. Do not rotate during insertion or use excessive force as this can cause bleeding. Contraindications to NPA insertion include nasal fractures, coagulopathy, cerebrospinal rhinorrhea related to basal skull fractur,e and adenoid hypertrophy (in pediatric patients; Davies et al., 2014).

For prolonged airway management, tracheal intubation may be required. Although this does not fall into the scope of practice for the registered nurse, an understanding of the required equipment is essential to assist the intubating practitioner. Endotracheal tubes come in a variety of sizes. In the adult setting, size 7 is the most common for women and size 8 for men. The number refers to the internal diameter of the tube and can be located near the end of the tube. When preparing to intubate, certain equipment must be available for the practitioner. Common laryngoscope blades are the Macintosh (a curved blade) and Miller (a straight blade). Both laryngoscope blade types come in a variety of sizes that are indicated on the blade. Another device used for intubation is the Glidescope. This device uses fiber optic technology to transmit video from the laryngoscope blade onto a screen. This is often employed in difficult airway and emergency situations.

OUTCOMES

Having a working knowledge of interventions to open the airway is a critical skill every nurse should possess. The nurse should also be prepared to intervene further if the situation requires. Practicing these skills in simulation and nonemergent situations is crucial to being prepared to apply them in practice. Nurses who have a working knowledge of airway equipment and how to properly use it will be invaluable.

Summary

Airway management is a dynamic skill that requires a thorough knowledge of how to perform an airway assessment. At times, this assessment will need to be expeditious based on the patient's current state. Early recognition and intervention of airway obstruction and inadequate ventilation are paramount to preventing further respiratory compromise and respiratory arrest.

Barash, P., Cullen, B., Stoelting, R., Cahalan, M., & Stock, M. (2009). *Clinical anesthesia* (6th ed.). Philadelphia, PA: Lippincott Williams & Wilkins.

Davies, J., Costa, B., & Asciutto, A. (2014). Approaches to manual ventilation. *Respiratory Care*, 59(6), 810–824.

Higginson, R., Parry, A., & Williams, M. (2016). Airway management in the hospital environment. *British Journal of Nursing*, 25(2), 94–100.

■ ANESTHESIA FOR PREECLAMPSIA

Kerry L. Quisenberry

Overview

Hypertensive disorders are one of the most common medical disorders of pregnancy, occurring in 12% to 22% of pregnancies (California Pregnancy-Associated Mortality Review, 2011). These disorders are responsible for approximately 17% of maternal mortality in the United States (American Congress of Obstetricians and Gynecologists [ACOG], 2002). The incidence of preeclampsia typically occurs in 3% to

10% of all pregnancies in the United States and 3% to 5% in other industrialized nations. The term "pre-eclampsia" is used to describe a period during which delivery could be induced to prevent the progression to eclampsia. Preeclampsia is defined as hypertension with proteinuria occurring approximately 20 weeks after gestation (Suresh, Segal, Preston, Fernando, & Mason, 2013).

Anesthesia for preeclampsia is challenging. The disease itself involves a multitude of pathophysiologic changes and can progress from a mild form to a more severe form rapidly. Even in its mild form, the disease may occur in the presence of medical problems, such as diabetes, morbid obesity, and chronic hypertension, to name a few. In its more severe form, the disease can challenge the anesthesia provider by deteriorating into hypertensive crisis, eclampsia or HELLP syndrome, which is a clinical condition that entails hemolysis, elevated liver enzymes, and low platelets, pressing the necessity of immediate delivery.

Background

The exact etiology of preeclampsia is still unknown. Although preeclampsia is considered a disease of the young primigravida, it can occur in older parturients. Preeclampsia may be considered even in the absence of proteinuria if any of the following exist: gestational hypertension in the parturient with persistent epigastric or right upper quadrant pain, persistent cerebral symptoms, fetal growth restriction, thrombocytopenia, or elevated serum liver enzymes (Chestnut et al., 2014). Preeclampsia can be classified as mild or severe. Preeclampsia classification criteria are as follows:

1. Mild preeclampsia: systolic blood pressure (BP) greater than or equal to 140 to 160 mmHg or diastolic BP greater than or equal to 90 to 110 mmHg with mild proteinuria greater than or equal to 1+ on dipstick and less than 5g/24-hour urine

2. Severe preeclampsia:
   a. Severe hypertension and severe proteinuria: Systolic BP greater than or equal to 160 mmHg or diastolic BP greater than or equal to 110 mmHg with severe proteinuria greater than or equal to 5g/24-hour urine
   b. Mild hypertension with severe proteinuria: Systolic BP greater than or equal to 140 to 160 mmHg or diastolic BP greater than or equal to 90 to 110 mmHg with greater than or equal to 5g/24-hour urine

   c. Hypertension with proteinuria with onset after 20 weeks gestation + any of the following: oliguria, cerebral symptoms, pulmonary edema, right upper quadrant pain, thrombocytopenia, impaired liver function, or fetal growth restriction

The anesthetic plans of care are dynamic and responsive to the needs of the parturient. The preanesthetic evaluation of the parturient, independent of the severity of preeclampsia, should focus on airway assessment and maternal hemodynamics. Seizure prophylaxis should be in place and fluid balance should be assessed, and, if needed, optimized.

Clinical Aspects

ASSESSMENT

The California Maternal Quality Care Collaborative (CMQCC) developed the following tool kit for assessment of the preeclamptic parturient (approved 2013):

1. The anesthesia provider should have a low threshold for considering preeclampsia when encountering a parturient with new-onset hypertension and/or proteinuria.

2. Although preeclampsia is typically encountered in the third trimester of pregnancy, when encountered before 34 weeks, it may be more severe or present as atypical.

3. If a parturient presents with vague symptoms such as headache, shortness of breath, abdominal pain, or generalized edema, that patient should be evaluated for preeclampsia.

4. If the parturient with preeclampsia presents to a center with limited resources to care for mom or infant, that patient should be transferred to a center that has the resources to deal with existing and potential complications and complexities associated with the disease.

NURSING INTERVENTIONS, MANAGEMENT, AND IMPLICATIONS

1. *Communication*: The nurse may encounter different expectations and opinions regarding mild and severe preeclampsia. Team training on the unit is essential to management of preeclampsia. The nurse should routinely ask about the plan and restate any concerns. Standardized protocols for magnesium sulfate administration and complications should be developed.

2. *Identification of potential risks to the preeclamptic patient*: Stroke, pulmonary edema, generalized

edema of the upper airway leading to a difficult tracheal intubation for the anesthesia provider, eclamptic seizures, coagulation abnormalities, HELLP syndrome, and placental abruption are possible complications (Suresh, Segal, Preston, Fernando, & Mason, 2013).

3. *Immediate delivery regardless of gestational age*: The nurse should be prepared for immediate delivery. Anesthesia may proceed with a neuraxial block in the absence of thrombocytopenia or in the presence of thrombocytopenia with caution. General anesthesia may be indicated as a result of patient refusal of neuraxial anesthesia, emergency cesarean delivery for fetal compromise, coagulopathy, and hemorrhagic hypovolemia.

4. *Prevention and control of seizures*: Intravenous magnesium sulfate is the gold standard of seizure prophylaxis. Magnesium sulfate works by depressing the central nervous system. In cases of severe preeclampsia, magnesium sulfate has been shown effective in reducing the rate to progression of eclampsia. It's effectiveness in mild preeclampsia is in debate. ACOG does not recommend the administration of magnesium sulfate for women with preeclamspia universally, for prevention of preeclampsia, nor in women with a systolic BP less than 160 mmHg and a diastolic BP less than 110 mmHg and no maternal symptoms (CMQCC, 2013).

5. *Airway considerations*: Meticulous airway examination in this patient population is a must. Generalized edema is common in the parturient with preeclampsia and often involves the upper airway. The nurse should make preparations to have immediate access to difficult airway equipment. Repeated attempts at tracheal intubation may also result in severe hypertension and tachycardia. Vasodilators should be readily available.

6. *Control of hypertension*: Maternal blood pressure control is imperative. Medications include direct-acting vasodilators, *B*-adrenergic blocking agents, and calcium channel blockers. The nurse should take care not to allow the blood pressure to decrease rapidly as a rapid decrease may result in reduced renal and placental perfusion.

OUTCOMES

The CMQCC has identified the need for a preeclampsia tool kit. It proposes the need for an algorithm to identify, evaluate, and treat the preeclamptic antepartum as well as the postpartum patient. The algorithm includes nursing assessment, obstetric management, and anesthetic concerns. Anesthesia for the preeclamptic patient continues to evaluate evidence-based practice and perform studies to evaluate the lowest platelet count considered safe for a neuraxial block so as to avoid general anesthesia. To date, no data exists to show the lowest platelet count considered safe enough to perform regional anesthesia (Suresh, Segal, Preston, Fernando, & Mason, 2013).

Summary

Nurse anesthetists play an integral role in the relationship, satisfaction, and adherence to medical treatment, and they are an integral part of the anesthesia team. One of the major quality-improvement items was identified by the CMQCC after data analysis was that despite presenting identifiers indicating preeclampsia was rapidly progressing, the health care team failed to recognize and respond accordingly. In addition, the Preeclampsia Task Force emphasized the need for clinician education on the importance of BP measurement in an effort to promote initiation of antihypertensive medications and progression in the severity of preeclampsia (California Department of Health Care Services Maternal Child and Adolescent Health Branch, 2011).

Severe preeclampsia is a leading cause of death in the pregnant population. Outcomes are directly related to complications. Etiology remains unknown with the only cure being delivery of the infant. Anesthesia providers should direct its management to prevention of seizures and control of hypertension.

American Congress of Obstetricians and Gynecologists. (2002). Diagnosis and management of preeclampsia and eclampsia #33. American Congress of Obstetricians and Gynecologists Practice Bulletin Number 33.

California Department of Health Care Services Maternal Child and Adolescent Health Branch. (2011). MCAH Bulletin California: The California Pregnancy-Associated Mortality Review (CA-PAMR) report from 2002 to 2004 maternal death reviews. Retrieved from http://www.cdph.ca.gov/data/statistics/Documents/MO-°©-CA-°© -PAMR-°©-MaternalDeathReview-°©-2002-°© -04.pdf

California Maternal Quality Care Collaborative Preeclampsia Toolkit. (2013). Retrieved from https://www.cmqcc.org/ resources-tool-kits/toolkits/preeclampsia-toolkit

Chestnut, D., Wong, C., Tsen, L., Kee, W., Beilin, Y., Mhyre, J., & Nathan, N. (2014). *Chestnut's obstetric anesthesia: Principles and practice*. Philadelphia: PA: Elsevier Saunders.

Suresh, M., Segal, B., Preston, R., Fernando, R., & Mason, C. (2013). *Shnider and Levinson's anesthesia for obstetrics*. Baltimore, MD: Lippincott Williams & Wilkins.

■ ANESTHESIA IN REMOTE LOCATIONS

Angela Milosh

Overview

Anesthesia in remote locations, referred to as *nonoperating room anesthesia (NORA)*, involves the provision of anesthesia care for patients undergoing diagnostic or therapeutic procedures outside of the traditional operating room settings. Surgical and diagnostic procedures outside of the operating room are increasing in prevalence, led by both advances in medical technology, and an increased demand for minimally invasive procedures (Chang & Urman, 2016). Due to differences in the patient population, procedure, and environment of care, NORA presents a number of unique challenges to the certified registered nurse anesthetist (CRNA).

Background

The areas in which anesthesia care is delivered is expanding rapidly outside the traditional operating room setting. NORA accounts for nearly 28% to 40% of anesthesia care provided (Nagrebetsky, Gabriel, Dutton, & Urman, 2017). The factors influencing patient outcomes of NORA focus around three main areas: complexity of the procedure, acuity of patients, and environment of care. Each of these aspects may require an adjustment in the approach to anesthesia care.

As medical technologies have advanced, many patients are receiving less invasive diagnostic and therapeutic interventions instead of traditional surgical procedures. These procedures often include diagnostic or interventional radiology, radiation therapy, interventional cardiology, cardioversion, gastroenterology, psychiatry, and dentistry. The procedures are also increasing in both length and complexity, potentially requiring surgical conditions (patient immobility, precise hemodynamic control, or airway protection) in order to optimize the patient outcome.

The patient's status contributes greatly to the need for anesthesia services outside of the operating room. Certain patient populations may need sedation or general anesthesia for even the most minor of procedures. Pediatric patients, developmentally delayed patients, and patients with severe psychiatric disorders are often unable to tolerate procedures typically performed without any sedation. Other comorbidities may also influence the need for anesthesia: chronic pain syndromes, neuromuscular diseases or movement disorders, or severe systemic disease. In addition, some patients are only candidates for certain therapeutic procedures because of their acuity, having been deemed "too sick" for traditional surgery.

The environment in which these procedures are performed also presents unique challenges to the delivery of anesthesia. Many of the procedure locations were not designed to accommodate the equipment and monitoring devices that are used when anesthesia is administered. Space is often constrained, and supplies are frequently limited to what is reasonably expected to be used. Access to the patient may be restricted, forcing the patient to be monitored from a distance. The proximity of the procedure location to the operating room may also present a challenge. The proceduralist or other staff may be unaware of how to assist the anesthesia provider in case of difficulty and immediate assistance from anesthesia colleagues may not be available. Recovery from anesthesia may take place outside of a traditional postanesthesia care unit (PACU), leaving the patient to be monitored by staff unfamiliar with common side effects or complications of anesthesia care. There are also hazards to the anesthesia provider that are unique to these remote environments. These may include ionizing radiation from fluoroscopy and computed tomography, or magnetic field exposure in the MRI suite.

The quality of anesthesia care provided to patients outside of the operating room environment is subjected to influences from these factors. This is an area that is infrequently studied and inadequately described in the literature. Most analyses of complications demonstrate an increase in morbidity and mortality in certain NORA procedures, as compared to operating room procedures, especially cardiologic and radiologic procedures (Chang et al., 2015; Metzner, Posner, & Domino, 2009; Youn, Ko, & Kim, 2015). Patients undergoing NORA tend to be older, sicker, and with more emergent disease processes, leading to the need for anesthesia outside the operating room. The most frequent complication is related to inadequate oxygenation and ventilation, occurring with the administration of moderate or deep sedation (Metzner et al., 2009). These complications most often occur with inappropriate or inadequate monitoring techniques, suggesting that they may be preventable through better monitoring (Rosero & Joshi, 2016).

Clinical Aspects

ASSESSMENT

The combination of procedure complexity, patient acuity, and an unfamiliar environment of care in NORA presents an opportunity for quality improvement in the delivery of anesthesia care. Addressing each of these factors individually, with particular emphasis on vigilant patient monitoring, may promote better outcomes for patients as a whole.

Appropriate, continuous communication with the practitioner performing the procedure is necessary. The CRNA must be familiar with the extent and duration of the procedure as well as the backup plan in case of procedural complications. In addition, the patient's position, location in the room, and level of sedation required by the proceduralist should be discussed to optimize patient safety and facilitate the procedure. The availability of additional equipment, including blood products, emergency medications, and invasive monitoring modalities, should be available as indicated by the procedure.

OUTCOMES

A complete preanesthesia assessment prior to the procedure is essential and is a standard of care (American Association of Nurse Anesthetists [AANA], 2013). With the exception of relatively healthy pediatric patients, most NORA patients tend to be older and sicker, and are often not surgical candidates due to the extent of their disease. A thorough preanesthesia assessment may identify potential concerns that will better inform the CRNA to develop the most appropriate anesthetic plan. Specific attention should be paid to comorbidities, fasting status, a thorough airway examination, and monitoring needs as indicated. A procedure that typically does not warrant anesthesia care may require it, depending on the patient's medical status or ability to tolerate the procedure. This information will assist in the development of both an anesthesia plan as well as an appropriate plan for postprocedure recovery.

Finally, the environment of care must be considered. The CRNA should identify and obtain the necessary equipment that is expected to be used as well as any equipment that may be needed in case of an emergency. The equipment should be set up such that it is easily accessible, and other personnel can easily fit into the procedure location to assist if the need should arise. Monitors should be equivalent to those used in a traditional operating room suite, as the AANA Standards of Care apply to all anesthetizing locations (AANA, 2013). Discussion with the procedure staff regarding the plan of care, as well as identification of roles in the event of a complication, should take place prior to the initiation of anesthesia care. Identification of a secondary anesthesia colleague to assist, when available, should be considered. After the procedure, patient care should only be assumed by someone who is knowledgeable about the common side effects and complications of anesthesia care. Personal protective equipment (lead apron, thyroid shield, radiation safety glasses, etc.) should be worn, as appropriate.

Summary

Anesthesia care provided outside of the operating room has its own unique set of challenges. As diagnostic and therapeutic techniques undergo innovative changes, it is expected that more procedures will move out of the traditional operating room suite and into more remote procedural areas. Complex procedures, higher patient acuity, and unfamiliar environments may contribute to an increase in anesthesia-related morbidity and mortality. Careful attention to these factors, including meticulous preoperative assessment, vigilance in monitoring, and appropriate communication with the procedure team, will promote positive patient outcomes.

American Association of Nurse Anesthetists. (2013). *Standards for nurse anesthesia practice*. Park Ridge, IL: Author.

Chang, B., Kaye, A. D., Diaz, J. H., Westlake, B., Dutton, R. P., & Urman, R. D. (2015). Complications of non-operating room procedures: Outcomes from the National Anesthesia Clinical Outcomes Registry. *Journal of Patient Safety*. Epub ahead of print.

Chang, B., & Urman, R. D. (2016). Non-operating room anesthesia: The principles of patient assessment and preparation. *Anesthesiology Clinics, 34*(1), 223–240.

Metzner J., Posner K. L., & Domino K. B. (2009). The risk and safety of anesthesia at remote locations: The U.S. closed claims analysis. *Current Opinion in Anaesthesiology, 22*, 502–508.

Nagrebetsky, A., Gabriel, R. A., Dutton, R. P., & Urman, R. D. (2017). Growth of nonoperating room anesthesia care in the United States: A contemporary trends analysis. *Anesthesia & Analgesia, 124*(4), 1261–1267. doi:10.1213/ANE.0000000000001734

Rosero, E. B., & Joshi, G. P. (2016). Ambulatory anesthesia in remote locations. *Current Anesthesiology Reports, 6*(4), 412–419. doi:10.1007/s40140-016-0181-6

Youn, A. M., Ko, Y- K., & Kim, Y- H. (2015). Anesthesia and sedation outside of the operating room. *Korean Journal of Anesthesiology, 68*(4), 323–331. doi:10.4097/kjae.2015.68.4.323

■ ANESTHESIA AND ROBOTIC SURGERY

Angela Milosh

Overview

Advances in surgical techniques over the past 30 years have led to significant improvements in patient outcomes. Robot-assisted surgical techniques are performed for a variety of procedures, in many different surgical specialties: cardiology, general surgery, gynecology, neurology, urology, and orthopedics. The traditional *open* approach, involving large incisions and tissue trauma, is often associated with higher states of postoperative pain, prolonged hospital stays, longer recoveries, and extensive scarring. Minimally invasive techniques using laparoscopy have demonstrated better outcomes: less pain, faster recovery, shorter hospital stays, and a better cosmetic result (Lee, 2014). As laparoscopic techniques have evolved, a new technique has emerged: robotic surgery. The introduction of remotely controlled surgical robots has added a new dimension to the delivery of safe, effective anesthesia care.

Background

Traditional open surgical techniques often require large incisions to facilitate adequate surgical exposure. Larger incisions are associated with more tissue trauma, postoperative pain, postoperative pulmonary complications, prolonged postoperative recovery, longer hospital stays, larger scars, and increased health care costs when compared with minimally invasive techniques (Lee, 2014). As surgical techniques evolved, the use of laparoscopy in the 1980s provided a significant advance in positive patient outcomes. Patients undergoing laparoscopic procedures report less pain, undergo a faster recovery, have shorter hospital stays, and experience less surgical scarring (Gala et al., 2014; Spinelli, Vargas, Aprea, Cortese, & Servillo, 2016). There are some limitations of the laparoscopic technique, including two-dimensional video, requirement for significant hand–eye coordination, and small visual fields. As a result, the introduction of remote-controlled robotic surgical devices has aimed to alleviate these shortcomings.

Current robotic systems in use involve a surgeon-controlled console that is separate from the patient, but electronically connected to four robotic *arms*. The arms function as conduits for surgical tools and an endoscope. The internal view of the patient is transmitted to the console, where the surgeon is able to view it in three dimensions. The surgeon uses hand controls on the console to manipulate the arms in real time. The advantages to robotic surgery include less intraoperative blood loss, a short learning curve for the surgeon, better imaging, and more freedom of movement (Xiong, Ma, & Zhang, 2012). Patients also report higher levels of satisfaction with robotic surgery. Limitations to robotic surgery include longer operating time and potentially higher costs (Miller, 2015).

As surgical techniques evolve, the anesthesia care also evolves. The introduction of laparoscopy, and then robotic surgery, has drastically changed the anesthetic management of patients in the perioperative period. The choice of anesthetic technique, monitoring modalities, medications, and postoperative care is influenced by the surgical approach.

Clinical Aspects

ASSESSMENT

Both laparoscopic and robotic procedures present unique challenges in the delivery of anesthesia. Access to the patient is often limited due to the amount of equipment involved with the surgical robot. The robotic arms are mounted on a sidecar that is placed directly adjacent to the operating table, usually requiring the patient's arms to be tucked under and inaccessible during the procedure. Depending on the type of surgery, the sidecar may be placed very close to the patient's head, limiting access to the patient's airway and neck. Once the robot sidecar is placed, the patient's position cannot be changed. Although the surgical instruments are inside the patient, unintentional movement must be avoided. This is most often accomplished by the use of neuromuscular blocking medications. In the case of a surgical or anesthetic emergency, the robot would need to be rapidly disengaged to facilitate access to the patient. Robotic surgery usually necessitates general endotracheal anesthesia due to extreme positioning, length of procedure, and avoidance of unexpected movement.

NURSING INTERVENTIONS, MANAGEMENT, AND IMPLICATIONS

Patients are often placed in steep Trendelenberg or reverse Trendelenberg to facilitate surgical exposure of the relevant anatomy. The robotic arms are often located close to the patient's head, and there is a risk of collision between the patient's head and the arms of the robot. Ventilation may be quite challenging, especially if the duration of the case is lengthy, position is extreme, or the surgical procedure requires single-lung ventilation. Careful attention is paid to the patient positioning to ensure optimal ventilation and circulation, as well as to ensure that there is no unnecessary pressure on the patient's body from the surgical equipment.

The use of carbon dioxide for abdominal or pelvic insufflation to facilitate optimal visualization of the surgical field presents its own set of challenges. During initiation of the pneumoperitoneum, the patient undergoes a number of physiologic changes. The potential risks and side effects of the pneumoperitoneum or pneumothorax include carbon dioxide embolus, reduced cardiac output, and increased pulmonary vascular resistance (Wang & Gao, 2014). As the body cavity is insufflated with carbon dioxide, the gas diffuses into the bloodstream. The intraperitoneal or intrathoracic pressure from insufflation may cause the development of subcutaneous, or surgical emphysema. This may cause edema in the head, face, and neck, and may be severe enough to prevent extubation at the end of the procedure. Insufflation may also prevent expansion of the pulmonary alveoli. As a result, peak airway pressures often increase, increasing the risk of barotrauma, and potentially causing inadequate gas exchange. The combination of inadequate ventilation and insufflation with carbon dioxide frequently leads to the development of respiratory acidosis. Ventilator adjustments are often required to normalize the exhaled carbon dioxide. In some cases, insufflation may need to be temporarily stopped to allow the acid–base balance to return to an acceptable level. If ventilation continues to be inadequate, the surgical procedure may need to be converted to an open technique.

OUTCOMES

Because robotic surgery is a relatively new innovation, an adjustment period is needed while the surgical team becomes skilled at the technique. This adjustment period often increases the duration of the surgical procedure and the anesthetic, until expertise is gained. Advanced clinical monitoring and vascular access, including invasive monitors and access lines, may be appropriate.

Summary

The introduction of robot-assisted surgical techniques is a positive development in surgical innovation. Anesthesia management for patients undergoing minimally invasive robotic procedures can be a challenge due to the significant differences in surgical technique. As surgeons gain more experience with the use of surgical robots, patient outcomes will likely improve through shorter surgical times, less tissue trauma, less postoperative pain, and less blood loss. The implications for anesthetic management will focus on maintenance of physiologic homeostasis, optimal pain control, and an efficient recovery from the anesthetic.

Gala, R. B., Margulies, R., Steinberg, A., Murphy, M., Lukban, J., Jeppson, P.,…Sung, V. (2014). Systematic review of robotic surgery in gynecology: Robotic techniques compared with laparoscopy and laparotomy. *Journal of Minimally Invasive Gynecology, 21*(3), 353–361.

Lee, J. R. (2014). Anesthetic considerations for robotic surgery. *Korean Journal of Anesthesiology, 66*(1), 3–11.

Miller, R. D. (2015). *Miller's anesthesia* (8th ed.). Philadelphia, PA: Churchill Livingstone/Elsevier.

Spinelli, G., Vargas, M., Aprea, G., Cortese, G., & Servillo, G. (2016). Pediatric anesthesia for minimally invasive surgery in pediatric urology. *Translational Pediatrics, 5*(4), 214.

Wang, G., & Gao, C. (2014). Anesthesia for robotic cardiac surgery. In C. Gao (Ed.), *Robotic cardiac surgery* (pp. 15–32). Dordrecht, The Netherlands: Springer.

Xiong, B., Ma, L., & Zhang, C. (2012). Robotic versus laparoscopic gastrectomy for gastric cancer: A meta-analysis of short outcomes. *Surgical Oncology, 21*(4), 274–280.

■ ANTICOAGULATION AND ANESTHESIA

Natalie Butchko
Aimee Dickman

Overview

Anticoagulation is the use of medication to directly or indirectly inhibit one or more coagulation factors in the human body, preventing the formation of a thrombus or clot. Many people take anticoagulation medications as treatment or as prophylaxis for a venothrombus embolus. Certified registered nurse anesthetists (CRNAs) must be aware of the implications that anticoagulation agents have on the anesthetics they administer, specifically, the anticoagulation effects of safely performing a regional anesthetic, and how anticoagulation affects a patient's bleeding and clotting risk during the perioperative period. Guidelines for anticoagulation have been revised many times due to development of new medication and new techniques in surgical and pain management procedures.

Background

Venous thromboembolism (VTE) is a significant risk to patient morbidity and mortality. Risk factors for the development of a VTE include immobility, advanced age, malignancy, vascular disease, chronic kidney disease, genetic predisposition, and major surgery, of which 40% of the patient population has three or more risk factors (Elisha, Heiner, Nagelhout, & Gabot, 2015). Prophylactic or therapeutic use of anticoagulation therapy has been on the rise due to an increase in the aging population's prevalence of coronary artery disease and atrial fibrillation (Oprea, Noto, & Halaszynski, 2016). The number of patients on anticoagulation therapy is on the incline, and the types of anticoagulation medications are increasing as well. Anticoagulant medications have increased in number throughout the recent decade due to new advancements in therapies for different pathologies and the need for a reduction in unwanted side effects. Providers should consider the etiology for thrombus formation, the location of the thrombus, and the composition of the thrombus, in terms of platelet-to-fibrin ratio, when selecting antithrombotic therapy (Elisha et al., 2015). Thus, there are a multitude of anticoagulant medications that a CRNA may encounter in practice that are used for a variety of different patient conditions.

Warfarin (Coumadin) is a commonly prescribed anticoagulant that interferes with the vitamin K-dependent clotting factors, factors III, VII, IX, and X (Belil, 2014). Another typical anticoagulant utilized in practice is unfractionated heparin, which is an antithrombin III catalyst that inactivates factors II, IX, XI, and XII (Franco & Gabot, 2014). Low molecular weight heparin, such as enoxaparin (Lovenox), has a mechanism that is similar to unfractionated heparin; however, it specifically inactivates factors II and X, and is irreversible with protamine (Belil, 2014). Fondaparinux is an antithrombin III catalyst as well and works by inhibiting factor Xa. Oral direct thrombin inhibitors work by directly inhibiting thrombin and include argatroban (Hirudin), bivalirudin (Angiomax), and dabigatran (Pradaxa). Factor Xa inhibitors, such as rivaroxaban (Xarelto) and apixaban (Eliquis), work by inhibiting factor Xa (Oprea et al., 2016). There are specific agents that are used to reverse the effects of some of these anticoagulants; however, some anticoagulants do not currently have reversal agents.

Clinical Aspects

ASSESSMENT

Perioperative management of anticoagulation regimens has become the task of anesthesia providers (Oprea, Noto, & Halaszynski, 2016). The CRNA is required to both assess the patient's anticoagulation regimen as well as discuss any potential perioperative complications with the patient's primary physician and surgical team (Oprea et al., 2016). The clinical judgment of the CRNA is essential in the assessment of continuation, discontinuation, bridging, and resuming anticoagulation during the perioperative period (Oprea et al., 2016). This requires an understanding of the clinical implication for therapy and the drug pharmacology as well as the evaluation of the risk of thromboembolic and hemorrhagic complications involved with interrupting or continuing therapy. Situational and patient-specific considerations must be integrated into the clinical management of patients on anticoagulation during the perioperative period (Franco & Gabot 2014).

The CRNA's management of anticoagulation involves the risk stratification of thrombosis associated with the risk of discontinuing anticoagulants versus the risk of bleeding complications related to the procedure (Oprea et al., 2016). This management becomes challenging when attempting to achieve a balance between thrombosis and bleeding, and a general approach to assessing risk may be beneficial to management.

A risk-benefit analysis during perioperative management with anticoagulant medications must include the following: (1) risk of bleeding during the surgical procedure; (2) type of surgical procedure; (3) pharmacologic profile of the agent; (4) patient comorbidities (eg, hepatic or renal insufficiency); and (5) patient risk factors for development of a VTE. (Elisha et al., 2015)

Following the proposed analysis, the CRNA may develop a plan to present to the patient, anesthesiologist, surgical team, and any other members concerned with the perioperative medical management of the patient.

Assessment of a patient's bleeding risk involves both the patient's comorbidities and the invasiveness of the planned procedure. Currently, there are no validated predictors for the perioperative risk of bleeding; however, evidence does show increased risk linked to active cancer, thrombocytopenia, presence of a mechanical mitral valve, and a history of bleeding (Oprea, Noto, & Halaszynski, 2016). Low bleeding risk (less than 1.5%)

has been associated with procedures such as endotracheal intubation, tooth extractions, endoscopy, and cataract surgery. Procedures associated with a higher bleeding risk (greater than or equal to 1.5%) may include spinal and epidural anesthesia, coronary intervention, ablation of tumors and vascular lesions, bowel resections, and hysterectomy (Oprea et al., 2016). The patient's comorbidities, indication for anticoagulation, as well as planned surgical procedure should be considered when determining the patient's surgical risk for bleeding.

An increased bleeding risk may require a longer period of anticoagulation interruption (Lip & Douketis, 2016). When determining the timing of anticoagulation interruption, the specific agent that the patient is taking must be considered. Current recommendations are to stop warfarin 4 to 5 days before a planned procedure, and international normalized ratio (INR) should be normalized before a planned neuraxial block (Belil, 2014). Intravenous unfractionated heparin should be stopped 1 hour before the placement of neuraxial anesthesia, and consultation with the surgery team is necessary regarding procedural stop time, taking the type of procedure into consideration (Franco & Gabot, 2014). A subcutaneous heparin dose of 5,000 units twice daily requires no interruption. If intraoperative intravenous heparin will be utilized for a specific surgery that can include a neuraxial block, heparin administration should be delayed for 1 hour after neuraxial block placement (Belil, 2014). The recommendation for low molecular weight heparin is to wait 12 hours before neuraxial placement if the dose is a prophylactic dose or 24 hours if the dose is a high dose such as 1.5mg/kg (Belil, 2014). Fondaparinux should be stopped 4 days before a procedure, but no guidelines are currently available for neuraxial anesthesia other than an atraumatic, one-attempt needle placement with no indwelling catheters (Oprea et al., 2016). Direct thrombin inhibitor recommendations are as follows: argatroban 4–6 hours, hirudin 8 hours, bivalirudin or Angiomax 2 to 3 hours, and dabigatran or Pradaxa 1 to 4 days (Franco & Gabot, 2014). Rivaroxaban and apixaban should be stopped 24 to 48 hours before a surgical procedure and 72 hours before a neuraxial procedure (Douketis, Syed, & Schulman, 2016).

OUTCOMES

Each year, approximately 10% of patients will require anticoagulant interruption for an elective procedure (Douketis et al., 2016). The interruption of any of these agents proposes an increased risk in developing thromboembolism. Estimating thromboembolic risk for patients diagnosed with atrial fibrillation may be based on age, comorbidities, how recently the deep vein thrombosis occurred, pulmonary embolism, or stroke as well as the number of conditions that predisposes the patient to thromboembolism (Lip & Douketis, 2016). Risk of thromboembolism is increased if therapy is stopped, and bleeding risk is increased if anticoagulation is continued throughout the perioperative period, both of which increase the mortality rate (Lip & Douketis, 2016). These considerations are important when determining whether the benefit of an interruption in therapy outweighs the risk in order to provide safe, competent care.

Summary

The use of anticoagulation therapies is an evolving area of perioperative management for the CRNA. New medications and guideline therapies influence the decision and preventative measures utilized to balance bleeding and thromboembolic risk throughout the surgical period. It is the duty of the CRNA to have up-to-date knowledge regarding anticoagulation medications and their surgical implications, and to use this knowledge to perform a safe and effective anesthetic for his or her patient.

Bellil, L. (2014). American Society of Regional Anesthesia and Pain Medicine (ASRA) guidelines: Neuraxial anesthesia and anticoagulation. In B. S. Freeman & J. S. Berger (Eds.), *Anesthesiology core review: Part one basic exam* (Chapter 76). New York, NY: McGraw-Hill. Retrieved from http://accessanesthesiology.mhmedical.com/content.aspx?bookid=974&sectionid=61588451

Douketis, J. D., Syed, S. M., & Schulman, S. M. (2016). Periprocedural management of direct oral anticoagulants. *Regional Anesthesia and Pain Medicine, 41*(2), 127–129.

Elisha, S., Heiner, J. C., Nagelhout, J., & Gabot, M. (2015). Venous Thromboembolism: New concepts in perioperative management. *American Association of Nurse Anesthetists, 83*(3), 211–221.

Franco, J. A., & Gabot, M. H. (2014). Hematology and anesthesia. In J. J. Nagelhout, & K. L. Plaus (Eds.), *Nurse anesthesia* (pp. 880–899). St. Louis, MO: Elsevier Saunders.

Lip, G. Y., & Douketis, J. D. (2016, Nov 30). Perioperative management of patients receiving anticoagulants. In L. L. Leung (Ed.), *UpToDate*. Retrieved from https://www.uptodate.com/contents/perioperative-management-of-patients-receiving-anticoagulants

Oprea, A. D., Noto, C. J., & Halaszynski, T. M. (2016). Risk stratification perioperative and periprocedural management of the patient receiving anticoagulant therapy. *Journal of Clinical Anesthesia, 34,* 586–599. doi:10.1016/j.jclinane.2016.06.016

■ AWAKE CRANIOTOMY

Rafiu Adeniji
Christopher Bibro
Natalie A. Slenkovich

Overview

Awake craniotomy uses anesthesia techniques that keep patients conscious during open brain surgery and enable surgeons to receive continuous, real-time feedback from the patient during surgery (Hill, Severgnini, & McKintosh, 2017). It is used for tumor resection, treatment of epilepsy, and deep brain stimulation. The procedure helps surgeons detect interference with critical areas of the brain and avoids damaging them (Hill et al., 2017). Awake craniotomy has been shown to have significant benefits for patients, such as shorter hospital stays, fewer postoperative complications, and improved survival (Hill et al., 2017).

Background

The history of awake craniotomy can be traced back to 19th-century studies of human brain function that utilized direct electrical stimulation (DES). Even in the early days of modern neurological surgery, the risks of using general anesthesia were recognized. This resulted in increased use of regional anesthesia with awake patients who could report the sensations they experienced during cortical stimulation (Surbeck, Hildebrandt, & Duffau, 2015).

Otfrid Foerster was instrumental in promoting the use of awake surgery in the early 20th century, initially for patients with epilepsy. During the 1990s, Mitchel Berger and George Ojemann advanced the use of awake procedures for tumor surgeries (Surbeck et al., 2015). Today, awake craniotomy is used for tumor resection, epilepsy surgery, and deep brain stimulation for Parkinson's and other conditions (Surbeck et al, 2015).

It is estimated that each year in the United States, there are approximately 60,000 new cases of Parkinson's disease and 150,000 news cases of epilepsy (Parkinson, 2017; Epilepsy, 2017). According to the Central Brain Tumor Registry of the United States (CBTRUS), there will be over 79,000 new cases of brain and other central nervous system (CNS) tumors in 2017 (CBTRUS, 2017). Although all of these cases will not require awake craniotomy, it is clear that the procedure will continue to be commonly used.

Anesthesia protocols often used in awake craniotomies are monitored anesthesia care (MAC), regional anesthesia, and asleep–awake–asleep (AAA) techniques with airway instrumentation (Surbeck et al., 2015). Typically, a scalp block is the regional anesthesia technique utilized. A scalp block involves the application of a long-acting agent, such as ropivacaine or levobupivacaine, on seven nerves—the zygamticotemporal, supraorbital, supratrochlear, auriculotemporal, lesser occipital, great auricular, and occipital. Epinephrine can be added to reduce bleeding and maximize the duration of efficacy (Ishida & Kawamata, 2015). The AAA technique requires general anesthesia and airway control using either laryngeal mask or endotracheal intubation (Surbeck et al., 2015). Dexmedetomidine, an alpha 2-agonist, is the commonly used sedation agent (Surbeck et al, 2015).

Patient's full cooperation and participation are very crucial to the success of anesthesia and the surgical procedure. Patients with mental confusion or severe dysphasia must be excluded from awake craniotomy. Adequate and thorough preanesthetic assessment must be completed to determine possible exclusion in patients, especially those with obstructive sleep apnea, gastroesophageal reflux disease (GERD), uncontrollable seizures, and intracranial pressure (ICP) concerns (Ishida & Kawamata, 2015).

Clinical Aspects

ASSESSMENT

Advantages of the awake craniotomy include significantly reduced intensive care unit (ICU) time and decreased duration of overall admission time (Hoosein, 2006). The reduced length of hospital stay dictates the paramount importance of vigilant nursing care throughout the perioperative period. Nursing assessment during the preoperative and intraoperative phase is primarily focused on patient anxiety and comfort (Hoosein, 2006). Initially, following the procedure, patients are managed in an ICU consistent with other neurosurgical procedures (Brooks, 2015; Hanak et al., 2014).

On admission to the ICU, an initial baseline neurologic examination is vital to providing continuity of care as well as a benchmark against which future assessments may be evaluated (Brooks, 2015). Hourly neurologic examinations are critical in the ongoing assessment for potential deterioration in patient condition (Brooks, 2015). Vital components of the neurologic assessment include a determination of the Glasgow Coma Scale (GCS) score, pupil appearance and reactivity, and limb strength and mobility. In addition to ongoing assessment of the level of consciousness (LOC), patients must be acutely monitored for vital sign changes, pain control, development of nausea and vomiting, and surgical site integrity (Brooks, 2015; Hoosein, 2006).

Assessment findings that indicate the presence of neurologic deterioration may necessitate radiologic evaluation. CT provides for rapid assessment, whereas MRI may provide a more comprehensive depiction of the clinical course (Brooks, 2015). Nurses must remain alert to the potential that patients with neurologic decline may require airway protection and possible mechanical ventilation for diagnostic procedures (Brooks, 2015).

NURSING INTERVENTIONS, MANAGEMENT, AND IMPLICATIONS

Patients preparing for awake craniotomy may experience anxiety and lack of knowledge regarding the procedure. Nurses in the preoperative setting may address preprocedural angst and begin the process of discharge teaching (Hoosein, 2006). Intraoperatively, patients may experience discomfort and stress from the operative environment (Hoosein, 2006). Following awake craniotomy, the most dreaded complication is neurologic deterioration, which may be facilitated by blood pressure changes that compromise cerebral perfusion. In addition, the patient may experience pain, nausea, and vomiting as well as complications with surgical-site healing (Brooks, 2015; Hoosein, 2006).

OUTCOMES

The expected outcome of evidence-based management for the patient following awake craniotomy is a safe discharge from the ICU and hospital, and prevention of complications at home (Hoosein, 2006). Vigilant nursing care is essential in realizing these outcomes. Preoperatively, nursing care is focused on anxiety management and education regarding the procedure (Hoosein, 2006). Intraoperatively, nurses may promote patient ease by assessing for causes of discomfort, providing measures, such as warm blankets, and maintaining a soothing environment through noise reduction (Hoosein, 2006).

Nursing care of the patient following awake craniotomy is focused on prevention of neurologic deterioration

(Hoosein, 2006). Change in LOC or discrepancy with the baseline examination may indicate the development of intracranial hemorrhage, cerebral edema, hematoma, or seizures (Hoosein, 2006), and must be promptly reported to the medical team (Brooks, 2015). Clinical indicators, such as heart rate and fluid volume status, should guide adequate resuscitation to maintain adequate cerebral perfusion (Brooks, 2015; Hanak et al., 2014; Hoosein, 2006). It is vital that blood pressure be maintained within 20% to 30% of baseline to ensure adequate cerebral perfusion and prevent complication (Brooks, 2015). Pain should be promptly addressed with a focus on minimizing opiate administration to prevent oversedation (Brooks, 2015). Nausea and vomiting may indicate changes in intracranial pressure and deteriorating neurologic status. Neurologic procedures also carry a heightened risk of postoperative nausea and vomiting (PONV). Thus, astute nursing care dictates determination of the cause of PONV as well as anticipation for the possible requirement of antiemetic medication (Brooks, 2015). Finally, effective teaching regarding surgical wound care, medications, and signs and symptoms of infection may aid in preventing complications following discharge from the hospital (Hoosein, 2006).

Summary

Awake craniotomy is an efficacious procedure utilized for brain tumor resection, epilepsy treatment, and deep brain stimulation for a variety of neurologic disorders. The primary advantages of the awake craniotomy include avoidance of damage to functionally important regions of the brain as well as a substantially shorter ICU and hospital admission. With attentive monitoring and through the application of evidence-based practice, nursing care is vital in supporting the realization of the expected outcomes of safe perioperative course and expedient discharge to home.

Brooks, C. (2015). Critical care nursing in acute postoperative neurosurgical patients. *Critical Care Nursing Clinics of North America, 27*(1), 33–45.

Central Brain Tumor Registry of the United States. (2017). 2016 CBTRUS fact sheet. Retrieved from http://www.cbtrus.org/factsheet/factsheet.html

Epilepsy Foundation. (2017). Epilepsy statistics. Retrieved from http://www.epilepsy.com/learn/epilepsy-statistics

Hanak, B. W., Walcott, B. P., Nahed, B. V., Muzikansky, A., Mian, M. K., Kimberly, W. T., & Curry, W. T. (2014). Postoperative intensive care unit requirements after elective craniotomy. *World Neurosurgery, 81*(1), 165–172.

Hill, C. S., Severgnini, F., & McKintosh, E. (2017). How I do it: Awake craniotomy. *Acta Neurochirurgica, 159*, 173–176.

Hoosein, S. (2006). Eyes wide open: The awake craniotomy for tumor resection: A review. *Axon/l'Axone, 28*(1), 15–18. Retrieved from http://search.ebscohost.com/login .aspx?direct=true&db=rzh&AN=106253815&site=eh ost-live

Ishida, T., & Kawamata, M. (2015). Anesthesia in awake craniotomy. In H. Uchino, K. Ushijima, & Y. Ikeda (Eds.), *Neuroanesthesia and cerebrospinal protection* (pp. 371–379). Tokyo, Japan: Springer.

Parkinson's Disease Foundation. (2017). Statistics on Parkinson's. Retrieved from http://www.pdf.org/en/ parkinson_statistics

Surbeck, W., Hildebrandt, G., & Duffau, H. (2015). The evolution of brain surgery on awake patients. *Acta Neurochirurgica, 157*, 77–84.

■ CARDIAC ANESTHESIA

Christopher K. Ferguson

Overview

The development and advancement of cardiac anesthesia has been closely tied to the ongoing advancements in science and also the field of cardiac surgery. The evolution of intraoperative transesophageal echocardiography along with a movement toward minimally invasive surgical techniques has given rise to new areas of opportunity and research for the cardiac anesthetist. Advanced understanding of cardiac anatomy and physiology, cardiac surgical techniques, and placement of invasive monitoring devices are vital to the success in the operative theater.

Background

From 1996 to 2011, coronary artery bypass grafting procedures steadily declined (from 366,000 cases in 2006 to 252,000 cases in 2011; Etzioni & Starnes, 2011). This drastic decrease in surgical cases can be attributed to the scientific and technologic growth of the noninvasive management of coronary artery disease in the cardiac cath lab. However, it was noted that during this same time, an increase in the number of cardiac valve surgeries and pneumonectomy operations both increased by 26% and 19%, respectively (Etzioni & Starnes, 2011).

Anesthetic techniques have varied greatly over the past century with respect to the cardiac surgery patient. An extreme example of an anesthetic choice can be noted in the late 1950s at the Cleveland Clinic. Dr. C. E. Wasmuth administered an 80% to 50% mix of nitrous oxide and oxygen supplemented with small amounts of thiopental, morphine or Demerol, and local anesthetic infiltration into the intercostal incision. He further insisted that the patients respond appropriately to questions during the operation (Kaplan, 2006). Anesthetic techniques continue to adapt to changing patient populations and advanced surgical techniques. Improvement in invasive monitoring and transesophageal echocardiography have driven anesthetics toward minimal drugs and early-extubation protocols. Cost-effective care drives the anesthetic choices in the operative setting to set the patient up for decreased intensive care unit (ICU) and overall hospital length of stay.

Clinical Aspects

ASSESSMENT

Vital to the operative care of the cardiac surgery patient is a complete history, physical assessment, necessary laboratory tests, and cardiac diagnostic testing. A solid understanding of any comorbid conditions that affect the patient is also important for development of an intraoperative plan. Assessment of the functional status of the patient prior to surgery can help modify techniques as well as set attainable goals for the patient and family members in the postoperative period.

The physical assessment of the patient needs to focus on all body systems to understand the magnitude of the surgical insult. Monitoring the heart rate, blood pressure, and pulse oximetry in the preoperative setting is important and adheres to the American Association of Nurse Anesthetists (AANA) standards. Interventions to optimize patient status before surgery should be taken to improve patient outcomes. Laboratory data, such as hemoglobin, hematocrit, platelet count, coagulation screen, and renal function, are all important assessment tools. Chest radiography, arterial blood gases as well as pulmonary function tests are important to the management of the respiratory system. Review of the cardiac catheterization, transthoracic echocardiography, and vascular studies of carotid arteries is also necessary.

The anesthetic plan for the surgical course of the cardiac surgery patient must be modified given the aforementioned assessment data. A thorough review of systems is necessary to develop a precise plan of care that will seek to improve overall patient outcome from surgery. With changing health care, the assessment data should be integrated with a desire to provide cost-effective care with the best possible patient outcome to develop the plan of care preoperatively.

NURSING INTERVENTIONS, MANAGEMENT, AND IMPLICATIONS

Between 2010 and 2025, the U.S. population is expected to increase by 40.5 million (13.1% increase; Etzioni & Starnes, 2011). To cater to this continued increase and the disproportional increase in the elderly population, techniques of care will have to adapt to higher levels of acuity of patient status. With the advancement of transesophageal echocardiography in the operative setting, the cardiac nurse anesthetist is becoming fully responsible for intraoperative patient care. Also, with a shift to provide cost-effective care to both the patient and maximize the financial situation of health care institutions, anesthesiologists are required to provide care for multiple patients at any given time while overseeing up to four certified registered nurse anesthetists (CRNAs).

The nurse anesthesia care starts during the preoperative period. Developing an understanding of cardiac anatomy and physiology will help the nurse anesthetist develop an optimal plan of care. Assessment of the functional status of the patient is important to modify the anesthetic technique that will be used in the operative setting. Understanding the use of echocardiography and being able to adapt a plan based on the pathology of the disease as well as cardiac function (ejection fraction) is vital. Advanced monitoring skills are necessary for the care of the cardiac surgical patient. The nurse anesthetist must be able to insert arterial and central venous lines as well as Swanz–Ganz catheter and interpret the data.

OUTCOMES

Postoperative outcomes of cardiac surgical patients have garnered a considerable amount of research in the past decade, which has been motivated by health care policy and emphasized the need for health care organizations to decrease the lengths of hospital stays to maintain their financial prosperity. A concept termed *fast track cardiac recovery* (FTCA) is currently being evaluated to determine the effective evidence-based plan for the delivery of anesthetic agents that may reduce the length of hospital stay, while minimizing the occurrence of adverse health events. Several randomized trials have addressed this question and have found no differences in outcomes in multiple FTCA techniques versus conventional anesthetic techniques (Kaplan, 2006). The primary goal of the nurse anesthetist should

be to maximize patient outcomes while utilizing a technique that will allow for early extubation in the ICU setting. Early extubation has been defined as a key factor in improving patient outcomes in the cardiac surgery patient (Hensley, Martin, & Gravlee, 2008).

Summary

Nurse anesthesia plays a vital role in the care of the cardiac surgical patient today. Sound assessment skills are key to providing care to this subset of patients. Development of an understanding of cardiac anatomy and physiology is also vital for the success of both the anesthetist and the patient in the operative setting. The shift toward continued cost-cutting and the expectation of improved patient outcomes provides a huge opportunity for the field of nurse anesthesia to advance in the operative setting. It is to be hoped that opportunities for invasive skills and echocardiography skills will exist in the future and become a standard practice of the advanced practice nurse.

Etzioni D. A., & Starnes V. A. (2011). The epidemiology and economics of cardiothoracic surgery in the elderly. In M. Katlic (Ed.), *Cardiothoracic surgery in the elderly* (pp. 5–24). New York, NY: Springer.

Hensley, F. A., Martin, D. E., & Gravlee, G. P. (2008). *A practical approach to cardiac anesthesia* (4th ed.). Philadelphia PA: Lippincott Williams & Wilkins.

Kaplan, J. A. (2006). *Kaplan's cardiac anesthesia*. Philadelphia PA: Saunders Elsevier.

■ ENHANCED RECOVERY AFTER ANESTHESIA

Danielle T. Winch
Brian Garrett

Overview

Enhanced recovery after anesthesia (ERAA) is a multimodal approach to developing protocols to address patients' physiological and psychological factors, and aid the recovery and timely discharge of patients after an exposure to anesthesia. ERAA is branch of a related clinical approach, enhanced recovery after surgery (ERAS), which was first introduced in the 1900s by Henrik Kehlet (Kehlet, 1997; Melnyk, Casey, Black, & Koupparis, 2011). Kehlet hypothesized that multimodal interventions, such as preoperative education and information, stress management, pain relief, physical exercise, enteral nutrition, and attention to growth factors, when initiated across the perioperative period, could effectively shorten postoperative recovery time, and reduce a patient's morbidity and mortality risk (Kehlet, 1997). This section is a review of the ERAA and the evidence-based strategies that facilitate an enhanced recovery for patients who underwent anesthesia.

Background

Delayed recovery from anesthesia can prove both costly to the institution and decrease overall patient satisfaction. A study by Geltzeiler et al. demonstrated that after implementation of an enhanced recovery protocol in their community hospital, their findings demonstrated a decreased length of hospital stay from 6.7 days versus 3.7 days, without an increase in the 30-day readmission rate (Greltzeiler et al., 2014). This resulted in an estimated hospital cost savings of $3,202 per patient in 2011 and approximately $4,803 per patient in 2012 (Greltzeiler et al., 2014). Because anesthesia providers continually follow and treat patients throughout the entire perioperative period, these clinicians are often the most influential individuals for the development and implementation of ERAA protocols.

Within the specialty of anesthesia, providers must first assess patients for the most appropriate risk category and determine anesthesia delivery that is best suited for the surgical procedure. There are three main categories or types of anesthesia delivery: general anesthesia, regional anesthesia, and monitored anesthesia care (a form of sedation) with local anesthetic supplementation near the surgical site. Each of the anesthesia types can be used either independently or in combination. The American Association of Nurse Anesthetists (AANA) defines *general anesthesia* as the loss of sensation throughout the entire body (AANA, 2017). This can be accomplished through the use of inhalational agents (gases) or intravenous infusions or boluses of anesthesia medications, both with or without the concurrent use of muscle paralytic medications (neuromuscular blockers). Regional anesthesia is classified as "the loss of sensation to a specific region of the body," which is accomplished through the use of peripheral nerve blocks (blocking impulses to a specific body part such as the arm or leg), spinal anesthesia (blocking sensation at the level of the spinal cord) or epidural analgesia (similar to spinal anesthesia; AANA, 2017, p. 1). Finally, AANA defines *monitored anesthesia care with local anesthesia* as "the loss of sensation to a small specific part of the body" (AANA, 2017, p. 1). This category of anesthesia is accomplished through the use of drugs (local anesthetics) that can numb tissue by blocking local neurons from sending signals to the brain while giving intravenous sedation during the injection of the local anesthetics and during the procedure. The category or type of anesthesia delivery can influence the ERAA.

Clinical Aspects

ASSESSMENT

General anesthesia is a nonspecific form of anesthesia delivery causing a full loss of sensation to the whole body by depressing central nervous system (brain) activity. Because of its site of action, this may result in longer recovery times compared to other categories or types of anesthesia that affect only a specific part of the body. In general, when providing a more site-specific anesthetic that bypasses or limits exposure of anesthesia to the brain, the recovery from anesthesia is faster. This is a reason why practitioners choose to employ regional and local techniques whenever possible, based on the patient's risk profile.

In certain situations, patients are not optimal candidates for regional or local anesthesia (site specific) due to their pathology, physiology, or type of surgical procedure required. In these situations, it is important for anesthesia providers to have multimodal enhanced recovery protocols in place to optimize enhanced postoperative recovery. According to Melnyk et al., the major elements of an effective protocol include preoperative counseling and education, optimization of nutrition, standardized analgesics and anesthetic regimens, and early mobilization (Melnyk et al., 2011). These are all essential components when considering implementing an ERAA protocol.

NURSING INTERVENTIONS, MANAGEMENT, AND IMPLICATIONS

Preoperatively, it is an essential requirement for anesthesia providers to conduct a thorough assessment and optimize patients based on their risk stratification. Providers must educate both patients and family members on the perioperative experience and set realistic expectations. According to Lukyanova and Reede (2015), setting realistic preoperative expectations for anesthesia, surgery, and recovery may help decrease patient anxiety and improve safety even after discharge, because it allows patients to be active participants in their care. Lukyanova and Reede also stress the importance of following the new American Society of Anesthesiologists

Preoperative Fasting guidelines, shortening fasting times for patients preoperatively and providing fluid and carbohydrate loading to decrease preoperative hunger, thirst, and insulin resistance (Lukyanova & Reede, 2015). They further stress having antibiotic prophylaxis to prevent infection and thromboprophylaxis, eliminating bowel preparation, and avoiding premedication when possible to allow for a faster emergence from anesthesia (Lukyanova & Reede, 2015).

Intraoperatively, anesthesia providers want to utilize short-acting anesthesia drugs and employ regional techniques whenever possible in order to decrease opioid usage (Bakan et al., 2015). Opioid usage intraoperatively can lead to postoperative hyperalgesia and increased analgesic consumption as well as increase the incidence of postoperative nausea and vomiting (Bakan et al., 2015). A multimodal drug regimen given preoperatively, including but not limited to, nonsteroidals, acetaminophen, gabapentin, and/or tramadol may help to limit the need for opioids intra- and postoperatively (Lukyanova & Reede, 2015). It is also beneficial intraoperatively to maintain normothermia to attenuate perioperative release of catecholamines and loss of body nitrogen, and to maintain euvolemia to avoid excess salt and water in order to prevent delayed anesthesia emergence and increased recovery stay times (Carli, 2015; Miller, Roche, & Mythen, 2015).

At the end of the procedure (and before the patient regains or returns to consciousness), the recovery process begins. This process is referred to as *emergence from anesthesia*. Neurological, immune, pain pathway, and cardiovascular functions are just a few of the systems that were affected during the procedure. The ability to emerge and recover the patient with minimal disruption of these body systems is vital to enhanced recovery. Factors that affect recovery from anesthesia in the short term are preoperative and intraoperative medications, self-medicating by the patient (over-the-counter drugs, illicit drug use, etc.), hypothermia, metabolic disturbances, and neurologic changes (Stoelting, 2015). Successful planning for emergence from anesthesia to reduce these changes begins in the preoperative phase.

Summary

Enhanced recovery after anesthesia can be a successful, multimodal approach to delivering anesthesia using research, evidence-based practice, and multidisciplinary stakeholder input. Planning and execution of ERAA must encompass the entire perioperative period with keen attention to communication in the preoperative period. Nursing is an integral part of this process and can lead by utilizing quality and patient satisfaction metrics to drive enhanced recovery for the patient.

American Association of Nurse Anesthetists. (2017). All about anesthesia. Retrieved from http://www.aana.com/forpatients/Pages/All-About-Anesthesia.aspx

Bakan, M., Umutoglu, T., Topuz, U., Uysal, H., Bayram, M., Kadioglu, H., & Salihoglu, Z. (2015). Opioid-free total intravenous anesthesia with propofol, dexmedetomidine and lidocaine infusions for laparoscopic cholecystectomy: A prospective, randomized, double-blinded study. *Revista Brasileira de Anestesiologia, 65*, 191–199. doi:10.1016/j.bjane.2014.05.001

Carli, F. (2015). Physiologic considerations of enhanced recovery after surgery (ERAS) programs: Implications of the stress response. *Canadian Journal of Anesthesia, 62*, 110–119. doi:10.1007/s12630-014-0264-0

Greltzeiler, C. B., Rotramel, A., Wilson, C., Deng, L., Whiteford, M. H., & Frankhouse, J. (2014, September). Prospective study of colorectal enhanced recovery after surgery in a community hospital. *JAMA Surgery, 149*, 955–961. doi:10.1001/jamasurg.2014.675

Kehlet, H. (1997, May). Multimodal approach to control postoperative pathophysiology and rehabilitation. *British Journal of Anaesthesia, 78*, 606–617. doi:10.1093/bja/78.5.606

Lukyanova, V., & Reede, L. (2015, May). Perioperative care pathways for enhanced recovery and anesthesia. *AANA News Bulletin*, pp. 17–19. Retrieved from http://www.aana.com/resources2/professionalpractice/Documents/Perioperative%20Care%20Pathways%20for%20Enhanced%20Recovery%20and%20Anesthesia.pdf

Melnyk, M., Casey, R., Black, P., & Koupparis, A. (2011, October). Enhanced recovery after surgery (ERAS) protocols: Time to change practice? *Canadian Urological Association Journal, 5*, 342–348. doi:10.5489/cuaj.11002

Miller, T. E., Roche, A. M., & Mythen, M. (2015). Fluid management and goal-directed therapy as an adjunct to Enhanced Recovery After Surgery (ERAS). *Canadian Journal of Anesthesia, 62*, 110–119. doi:10.1007/s12630-014-0266-y

Stoelting, R. (2015). *Stoelting's anesthesia and co-existing disease* (6th ed.). Philadelphia, PA: Saunders/Elsevier

■ EVOKED POTENTIALS

Melanie M. Stipp

Overview

Intraoperative electrophysiologic monitoring of evoked potentials (EPs) is utilized as an adjunct during surgical procedures that pose risk for iatrogenic neurologic injury. EPs are electrostatic potentials that can be measured in response to an induced stimulus (Koht, Sloan, & Hemmer, 2017). The latency and amplitude of the resultant evoked potential can provide insight to the integrity of neural pathways (Koht et al., 2017). Through the utilization of intraoperative electrophysiologic monitoring, motor evoked potentials (MEPs) and sensory evoked potentials (SEPs) can be monitored while a patient is anesthetized (Koht et al., 2017). This is advantageous in that the integrity of neural pathways may be assessed during general anesthesia, without the active participation of the patient (Bithal, 2014). Vigilance must be employed in planning and executing these procedures to optimize evoked potential monitoring, which can be affected by physiological factors and anesthetic agents that alter the evoked potential response (Koht et al., 2017; Nagelhout & Plaus, 2014).

Background

MOTOR EVOKED POTENTIALS

MEPs are the gold standard for monitoring the integrity of the corticospinal tract through direct or indirect electrical or magnetic stimuli to the cerebral cortex (Koht et al., 2017; Nagelhout & Plaus, 2014). Stimulation of the internunical and pyramidal cells of the motor cortex results in an MEP that descends via the corticospinal tract, synapses in the anterior horn of the spinal cord, and travels through a peripheral motor neuron to the neuromuscular junction (Mackey, Butterworth, Mikhail, Morgan, & Wasnick, 2013). The muscle response that is elicited can be subsequently measured by direct epidural D waves, indirect epidural I waves, or as a compound muscle action potential (CMAP; Koht et al., 2017; Nagelhout & Plaus, 2014). Evoked CMAPs are most frequently monitored in the adductor pollicus brevis to assess the integrity of the upper extremity corticospinal tracts (Koht et al., 2017). The lateral gastroscnemius, adductor hallucis, or the tibialis anterior are used to assess the integrity of the lower extremity corticospinal tracts (Koht et al., 2017). Magnetic MEP monitoring is contraindicated in patients with cranial skull defects, pacemakers, epilepsy, recent cerebral ischemia or infarct, prior craniotomy, and metallic implants or devices (Mackey et al., 2013; Nagelhout & Plaus, 2014). Factors that increase the difficulty of MEP monitoring include extremes of age, preexisting neuromuscular deficits, neuropathy, and hypertension (Koht et al., 2017).

SENSORY EVOKED POTENTIALS

There are three types of SEPs utilized clinically: somatosensory evoked potentials (SSEPs), visual evoked potentials (VEPs), and brainstem auditory evoked potentials (BAEPs) (Nagelhout & Plaus, 2014). SSEPs are the most frequently monitored evoked potential and are utilized to monitor the integrity of somatosensory pathways via mechanical or electrical stimuli of sensory or mixed peripheral nerves (Koht et al., 2017; Mackey et al., 2013; Nagelhout & Plaus, 2014). Once the peripheral nerve is stimulated, the SSEP enters the spinal cord through the posterior root of the spinal nerve and ascends to the cervicomedullary junction via the dorsal column pathway. The SSEP synapses, crosses midline, and ascends to the thalamus via the medial leminiscus (Koht et al., 2017). Within the thalamus, the SSEP synapses in the ventral posterolateral nucleus and travels to the sensory cerebral cortex (Koht et al., 2017). Stimulation of the median nerve is most commonly utilized for upper extremity SSEP monitoring, whereas stimulation of the posterior tibial nerve is most frequently utilized for SSEP monitoring of the lower extremities (Nagelhout & Plaus, 2014). SSEP recordings may be made anywhere along the aforementioned neural pathway (at the peripheral nerve, the level of the spinal cord, or in the sensory cortex), albeit they are most commonly recorded at the sensory cortex (via electroencephalography [EEG] electrodes), at the cervical spine (utilizing a pair of electrodes at C2, C3, and C4 for cortical SSEPs or C7 for subcortical SSEPS), at Erb's point, and at the popliteal fossa (Koht et al., 2017; Miller, 2015; Nagelhout & Plaus, 2014).

BRAINSTEM AUDITORY EVOKED POTENTIALS

BAEPs are monitored to assess the integrity of the auditory pathway during surgeries on the posterior fossa (Koht et al., 2017). A 10 Hz, 65 to 70 decibel acoustic stimuli, such as a loud repetitive clicking noise, is delivered through an earphone placed in the internal auditory canal and transmitted to the brain stem via the cochlear nerve (Koht et al., 2017; Nagelhout & Plaus, 2014). BAEPs are recorded utilizing electrodes that are most commonly placed at the mastoid (Koht et al., 2017). Five peaks are produced, correlating to various segments of the auditory pathway (Nagelhout & Plaus, 2014).

VISUAL EVOKED POTENTIALS

VEPs are monitored to assess the integrity of the visual pathway, including the retina, the optic nerve, the optic chiasm, and the occipital cortex (Miller, 2015; Nagelhout & Plaus, 2014). A patterned or unpatterned visual stimuli is transmitted to the patient, and the cerebral response is measured (Nagelhout & Plaus, 2014). A luminescence stimuli may be utilized in the anesthetized patient (Nagelhout & Plaus, 2014). VEPs are recorded by placing an active electrode over the visual cortex, a reference electrode, and a ground electrode (Nagelhout & Plaus, 2014). The VEP action potential measurement consists of three positive and three negative deflections that are labeled as P1–P3 and N1–N3, respectively (Nagelhout & Plaus, 2014).

Surgical procedures necessitating evoked potential monitoring include procedures that manipulate structures within the central nervous system (Bithal, 2014). Procedures utilizing electrophysiology monitoring of EPs include, but are not limited to spinal fusion, spinal instrumentation, spinal fracture repair, spinal and intracranial tumor resections, brachial plexus surgery, surgery involving the brain stem or posterior fossa, thoracoabdominal aortic aneurysm repair, acute aortic dissections, aneurysm repair, vascular surgery of the brain or spinal cord, epilepsy surgery, carotid endarterectomy, cortical mapping, stereotactic neurosurgery, acoustic neuroma resection, arteriovenous malformation embolization, and peripheral nerve surgery (Jaffe, Schmiesing, & Golianu, 2014; Nagelhout & Plaus, 2014).

Clinical Aspects

ASSESSMENT

Intraoperative neurologic injury may occur due to surgical retraction, electrocautery, vessel damage, nerve transection, or from stretching a nerve to greater than 20% of its original size (Nagelhout & Plaus, 2014). The neurophysiologist, the anesthetist, and the surgeon must work together to recognize early signs of neurologic injury (Nagelhout & Plaus, 2014). Thus, a sound understanding of EPs and the factors that affect them is essential in preventing irrecoverable neurological damage. When analyzing the evoked potential waveform, in the absence of other causes, a reduction in latency and amplitude of greater than 10% and 50%, respectively, should alert the team of potential neurological injury (Nagelhout & Plaus, 2014).

NURSING INTERVENTIONS, MANAGEMENT, AND IMPLICATIONS

When administering volatile anesthetic agents at higher concentrations, a reduction of frequency, amplitude, and an increase in the latency of EPs is observed (Koht et al., 2017). At a minimum alveolar concen-

tration (MAC) of 1.5, burst suppression occurs (Koht et al., 2017). When monitoring SSEPs in patients without preexisting neurological deficits, up to 1 MAC of volatile agent may be utilized (Koht et al., 2017). When monitoring MEPs, up to 0.5 MAC of volatile agent may be utilized (Koht et al., 2017). Exceptions to these guidelines include the use of halothane and also when monitoring BAEPs, which are unaffected by volatile anesthetics (Koht et al., 2017). Nitrous oxide acts synergistically with volatile anesthetics, eliciting a 50% reduction of cortical SSEP amplitude; consequently, it should be avoided in SSEP and MEP monitoring (Bithal, 2014; Koht et al., 2017).

Intravenous anesthetics have minimal effects on EP monitoring; thus, a total intravenous anesthetic (TIVA) is the optimal choice for monitoring (Koht et al., 2017). Benzodiazepines typically do not affect EPs (Koht et al., 2017). Propofol infusions are standard for MEP monitoring, although it should be noted that propofol does cause a reduction in MEP amplitude, particularly in the lower extremity, when administered in higher doses (Koht et al., 2017). Barbituates have a transient effect amplitude and latency when monitoring SSEPs; however, they are not an ideal choice for MEP monitoring due to a prolonged suppression of latency and amplitude (Bithal, 2014; Koht et al., 2017). Ketamine increases the cortical amplitude of SSEPs and can be utilized as a multimodal adjunct to offset the depressant effects of other anesthetic agents (Koht et al., 2017). Etomidate increases MEP and cortical SSEP amplitude, and may also be utilized to counter the depressant effects of other anesthetic agents (Bithal, 2014). Caution should be utilized when administering etomidate in patients with adrenocortical suppression, sepsis, and epilepsy (Koht et al., 2017). Opioid infusions have little depressant effect on EPs and may be used as an adjunct in a TIVA anesthetic (Koht et al., 2017).

Anesthetic maintenance for SSEP monitoring includes a low-dose infusion of propofol, an inhalation anesthetic with an MAC no greater than 0.5, and an opioid infusion of fentanyl, sufentanil, or remifentanil (Koht et al., 2017). Neuromuscular blocking agents (NMBAs) may be utilized in SSEP monitoring (Koht et al. 2017). For MEP monitoring, a TIVA consisting of a propofol infusion and an opioid infusion of fentanyl, sufentanil, or remifentanil is ideal (Bithal, 2014; Koht et al., 2017). NMBAs should either be limited to short-acting agents or completely avoided in MEP monitoring; however, if paralysis is requested by the surgeon, a train-of-four (TOF) should be used and the paralytic should be titrated to a 2/4 TOF (Koht et al., 2017).

Vigilance is required to maintain an optimal physiological profile during EP monitoring. Cortical SSEP suppression may result from the following factors: hypotension with cerebral blood flow reduction to less than 20 mL/min/100 g, severe hypoxia (end-tidal oxygen tension [PETO$_2$] <48 mmHg), hypothermia less than 35°C, hypercapnia (PETCO$_2$ >100 mmHg), and elevated intracranial pressure (Bithal, 2014). Pressure on peripheral nerves due to positioning in the prone or sitting position or any vascular compromise can also suppress evoked potential responses (Koht et al., 2017). Thus, baseline EPs should be obtained after the induction of anesthesia and prior to positioning the patient (Koht et al., 2017).

OUTCOMES

Evoked potential monitoring serves as a valuable adjunct to assess the integrity of neural pathways during various surgical procedures. To optimize the monitoring of EPs, the anesthetist must carefully select the appropriate anesthetic agents and control the aforementioned factors that alter the evoked potential response. EP monitoring has high utility in the early recognition of neurologic ischemia.

Summary

The anesthetist, the surgeon, and the neurophysiologist must work together to devise a plan, to monitor, and to make surgical and anesthetic modifications to identify signs of ischemia and prevent iatrogenic neurologic injury.

Bithal, P. (2014). Anaesthetic considerations for evoked potentials monitoring. *Journal of Neuroanaesthesiology and Critical Care, 1*(1), 2. doi:10.4103/2348-0548.124832

Jaffe, R. A., Schmiesing, C., & Golianu, B. (2014). *Anesthesiologist's manual of surgical procedures* (5th ed.). Philadelphia, PA: Lippincott Williams & Wilkins.

Koht, A., Sloan, T. B., & Hemmer, L. B. (2016). Neuromonitoring in surgery and anesthesia. Retrieved from https://www.uptodate.com/contents/neuromonitoring-in-surgery-and-anesthesia

Mackey, D. C., Butterworth, J. F., Mikhail, M. S., Morgan, G. E., & Wasnick, J. D. (2013). *Morgan & Mikhail's clinical anesthesiology* (5th ed.). New York, NY: McGraw-Hill.

Miller, R. D. (2015). *Miller's anesthesia* (8th ed.). Philadelphia, PA: Churchill Livingstone/Elsevier.

Nagelhout J. J., & Plaus K. L. (2014). *Nurse anesthesia* (5th ed.). Philadelphia, PA: Saunders.

■ FLUID AND TRANSFUSION MANAGEMENT IN ANESTHESIA CARE

Andrew D. Lorenzoni
Justin R. Stegman

Overview

The principles of fluid and transfusion management in the perioperative patient were established decades ago with medical knowledge and monitoring equipment of that time as guiding factors. As medical knowledge advanced, a better understanding of the negative consequences of these widely accepted management techniques has been discovered. Recent research is assisting practitioners in developing new management guidelines with a goal of limiting negative consequences and promoting better outcomes for patients. A comparison of the traditional fluid and transfusion management is fundamental for the provider in deciding which course of management is the best for the patient.

Background

Traditional fluid management (TFM), meaning patients are given 4 mL/kg (0–10 kg):2 mL/kg (11–20 kg):1 mL/kg (more than 21 kg) has an ambiguous beginning that can trace its roots back to the 1950s. The 4:2:1 rule evolved out of the calculations derived from children's calculated energy expenditure to provide stepped down approach to fluid management and the adult diet's equivalent caloric intake of cow's milk (Frost, 2016). Finally, this hypothesis was expanded to include other fluid losses, such as insensible loss, and estimated blood loss along with other volume-depleting causes. All of the calculated fluid loss was then to be replaced with only crystalloids (Frost, 2016). Beginning in the late 1980s and 1990s, new research was being published about the complications that arose from liberal fluid administration. Traditional perioperative fluid therapy neglected to address tissue oxygenation and metabolic demands without contributing to fluid volume impairment or metabolic derangements (Trinooson & Gold, 2013). Also, TFM did not take into account any of the patient's health problems such as impaired renal status, cardiovascular status, pulmonary status, or any other pathologic conditions (Frost, 2016). Current TFM in use today has five distinct components: hourly maintenance rate (MIV) calculated using the 4:2:1 rule, nothing per os (NPO) status (MIV × fasting hours), third spacing (based on the level of tissue trauma 0–2 mL/kg for minimal tissue trauma, 2–4 mL/kg for moderate tissue trauma and 4–8 mL/kg for severe tissue trauma), surgical blood loss replaced by 3 mL of crystalloid for 1 mL of blood loss, or 1 mL of colloid for 1 mL of blood loss, and finally a compensatory volume expansion (CVE) for the prevention of hypotension brought on by the induction dose of anesthetic drugs or effects of a neuraxial block (Miller, 2011). A one-time dose usually before administration of anesthesia is given; doses range from 10 mL/kg from neuraxial blockage to 5 to 7 mL/kg for an induction dose during general anesthesia (Gallagher, 2014). The calculated amount is given throughout the perioperative phase, depending on the patient's circumstances multiple liters of fluid could be given using this formula.

Fluid management of crystalloids is a key component in perioperative management of a patient. However, it does not aid in the increase of oxygen delivery in times of inadequate tissue perfusion or oxygenation of vital organs. It has been an age-old question for anesthetists as to when to transfuse allogeneic blood products (packed red blood cells, platelets, fresh frozen plasma, cryoprecipitate). According to The Joint Commission, the transfusion of blood products has been named one of the top five overused procedures in the United States (Thakkar et al., 2016).

The overuse of blood products places an increased burden on hospitals due to their scarcity and high cost. Not only is there a burden on the hospital, but also the use of allogeneic blood components poses serious implications for the patient and warrants careful consideration. Specifically, transfusion of blood components has been associated with hospital-acquired and transfusion-transmitted infections, transfusion-related immunomodulation (TRIM), transfusion-associated graft-versus host disease, transfusion reactions (febrile, allergic, hemolytic) as well as the leading cause of transfusion related deaths, which is transfusion-related acute lung injury (TRALI; Miller, 2012). Consideration needs to be taken as to the risk versus benefit of giving blood products. Conservative approaches have begun to gain acceptance by many clinicians. Several recent major publications have looked at the use of restrictive transfusion protocols, adjuvant therapies, substitution of blood components with pooled factor concentrates, and the use of point-of-care testing to target specific component use (Klein et al., 2016). Reducing the amount of allogeneic blood components starts in the preoperative period with the optimization of the patient and the availability of point-of-care testing. In the intraoperative

period, it is imperative to maintain a temperature above 36° C, consider cell saver and/or tranexamic acid when blood loss is anticipated to exceed 500 mL, and apply a restrictive transfusion threshold (Hgb 7–8 g/dL) dependent on the patient's characteristics and hemodynamic status (Klein et al., 2016). The exceptions to the conservative transfusion technique are cases of trauma, hemorrhage, or any clinical scenario in which infusing blood rapidly is lifesaving.

Clinical Aspects

ASSESSMENT

The clinical aspects of finding this "right" amount of fluid to give each individual patient during surgery has led to different strategies on management. Recent research has brought issue with this long-held TFM. The amount of fluid given to compensate for "third space" loss has been overinflated and should be minimized to the lower end of the range (Regenmortel, Jorens, & Malbrain, 2014). Recent strategies have been implemented to prevent significant preoperative dehydration by reducing fasting times and allowing clear fluids up to 2 hours before the operation, thus decreasing the initial NPO deficit (Trinooson & Gold, 2013). Numerous new studies have been published comparing the traditional or "liberal" therapy to a "restrictive" or goal-directed therapy. The consensus of the studies showed a reduction in pulmonary, cardiovascular, and surgical complications as well as a shortened overall hospital stay in the restrictive group (Gallagher, 2014). In contrast to the TFM, support is gaining for goal-directed therapy.

NURSING INTERVENTIONS, MANAGEMENT, AND IMPLICATIONS

The goal of intraoperative fluid management is to maintain an adequate circulating volume to ensure end-organ perfusion and oxygen delivery to the tissues (Naglehout & Plaus, 2014). Goal-directed therapy-specific endpoints, such as hourly urine output, or cardiac output, are used to guide the therapy and does not use definite volumes calculations as in traditional approach (Gallagher, 2014). The individualized goal-directed fluid therapy is based on that particular patient's response to intravenous fluid given.

The Frank–Starling Law explains the relationship between venous return and stroke volume, which is foundational knowledge for the nurse anesthetist's approach to fluid and transfusion management. A simplified explanation of the Frank–Starling curve is that as the ventricular preload increases, giving fluid leads to an increase in stretch on the ventricle and subsequent increase in force of contraction, which results in an increase in stroke volume and cardiac output. The increase in stretch only works up to a certain point. If there is too much fluid, the ventricle will overstretch and not be able to contract as efficiently, and thereby, a reduction in stroke volume and cardiac output will occur (Klabunde, 2015).

The application of the Frank–Starling Law to fluid management in perianesthesia care indicates that a patient should be given fluid until there is no longer a "response," specified as a 10% increase in stroke volume. Strategies for monitoring goal-directed therapy include pulse contour and analysis of arterial waveform, which uses a monitoring system to combine arterial waveform or pulse oximetry plethysmography data with end-tidal capnography data to determine the stroke volume response (Gallagher, 2014). Goal-directed therapy is more efficient at preventing fluid overload by stopping fluid administration when there is no longer a desirable physiological response to the volume.

OUTCOMES

The question still remains when does it become necessary to transfuse allogeneic blood products? According to Miller: "The decisions to transfuse should be based on a combination of (1) monitoring for blood loss, (2) monitoring for inadequate perfusion and oxygenation and vital organs, and (3) monitoring for transfusion indicators, especially hemoglobin concentration" (Miller & Pardo, 2011, p. 373). *Estimation of blood loss* (EBL) is a subjective measurement that looks at net suction volume as well as counting or weighing saturated sponges. The accuracy of this technique has been examined and, according to Nagelhout, on an average, blood loss was underestimated by nearly 300 mL. EBL is taken into consideration along with a calculation of maximum allowable blood loss (MABL). MABL is found by using the patient's estimated blood volume (EBV; 70 mL/kg in adults) × (starting hematocrit − target hematocrit)/(starting hematocrit) (Nagelhout & Plaus, 2014, p. 395). The MABL indicates an idea of when to consider a transfusion, but it should not be the only indicator. Clinical indicators, such as a measured hemoglobin level, are very helpful in deciding when to transfuse. As mentioned earlier, restrictive transfusion thresholds have been implemented to allow for hemoglobin to drop down to 7 to 8 g/dL; however, this is not a steadfast rule, nor is it patient specific. Exceptions include: symptomatic patients, patients with acute coronary syndromes, severe thrombocytopenia, and chronic transfusion-dependent anemia (Carson & Kleinman, 2016). In addition, thresholds cannot be used in the event of an acutely hemorrhaging patient. The decision to transfuse should be based on the pace of the bleeding, and the ability to stop the bleeding rather than hemoglobin levels due to their time sensitive requirements (Carson & Kleinman, 2016). Patient presentation is the most important indicator of whether to transfuse or not, aside from visual blood loss and lab values. The main purpose of hemoglobin is the transfer of oxygen to the tissues. Thus, anemia has the potential to decrease oxygen delivery to the tissue resulting in inadequate tissue perfusion and oxygenation of vital organs.

Clinical signs of anemia include an increase in heart rate, a decrease in blood pressure, a decrease in central venous pressure, a decrease in oxygen saturation, and a decrease in urine output. Other clinical signs to assess inadequate tissue perfusion are biochemical markers, such as elevated blood lactate concentrations, decreased pH, and increased base deficit (Gallagher, 2014). Once the decision to transfuse has been made, it is critical to monitor for adverse events or reactions during the transfusion. Monitoring should be for any signs of transfusion reaction, such as tachycardia, rash, hypotension, fever, and increased respiratory rate, that is, if spontaneously breathing or at increased peak airway pressures if mechanically ventilated (Miller & Pardo, 2011). If any reactions occur, management may include an antihistamine, steroid, or epinephrine. Diagnosis of a transfusion reaction during an ongoing hemorrhage may be difficult to distinguish and requires careful monitoring.

Summary

The commitment to update these guidelines and standards is of a growing interest in the medical community, using the latest evidence-based practice and knowledge of the human physiology as guiding factors to advance the field of medicine. The ways anesthesia providers manage a patient's fluid status must also change. No longer should providers use these outdated concepts that still persist in some hospitals. Using strict guidelines of how much fluid to give or when exactly to transfuse blood products has been a double-edged sword. Individualizing each patient's care using that patient's whole clinical picture will produce the best possible outcomes for our surgical patient population.

Carson, J. L., & Kleinman, S. (2016). Indications and hemoglobin thresholds for red blood cell transfusion in the adult. Retrieved from http://www.uptodate.com/contents/indications-and-hemoglobin-thresholds-for-red-blood-cell-transfusion-in-the-adult

Frost, E. (2016). A history of fluid management. In E. Farag & A. Kurz (Eds.), *Perioperative fluid management* (pp. 23–25). Cham, Switzerland: Springer.

Gallagher, K. (2014). Reexamining traditional intraoperative fluid administration: Evolving views in the age of goal-directed therapy. *AANA Journal, 82*(3), 235–242. Retrieved from http://www.aana.com/aanajournalonline

Klabunde, R. D. (2015) Frank–Starling mechanism. Cardiovascular physiology concepts. Retrieved from http://www.cvphysiology.com

Klein, A. A., Arnold, P., Bingham, R. M., Brohi, K., Clark, R., Collis, R., ... Walsh, T. S. (2016). AAGBI guidelines: The use of blood components and their alternatives 2016. *Anaesthesia, 71*(7), 829–842. doi:10.1111/anae.13489

Miller, R. D., & Pardo, M. (2011). *Basics of anesthesia*. Philadelphia, PA: Elsevier Saunders.

Nagelhout, J. J., & Plaus, K. L. (2014). *Nurse anesthesia*. St. Louis, MO: Elsevier Saunders.

Regenmortel, N. V., Jorens, P. G., & Malbrain, M. L. (2014). Fluid management before, during and after elective surgery. *Current Opinion in Critical Care, 20*(4), 390–395.

Thakkar, R. N., Lee, K. K., Ness, P. M., Wintermeyer, T. L., Johnson, D. J., Liu, E.,...Frank, S. M. (2016). Relative impact of a patient blood management program on utilization of all three major blood components. *Transfusion, 56*(9), 2212–2220. doi:10.1111/trf.13718

Trinooson, C. D., & Gold, M. E. (2013). Impact of goal-directed perioperative fluid management in high-risk surgical procedures: A literature review. *AANA Journal, 81*(5), 357–368. Retrieved from http://www.aana.com/aanajournalonline

■ LIVER TRANSPLANT AND ANESTHESIA

Kimberly M. Choudhary
Sonya D. Moore
Ronald L. Hickman, Jr.

Overview

The U.S. Department of Health and Human Services reports that approximately 5.5 million Americans are living with chronic liver disease (U.S. Department of Health and Human Services, National Institutes of Health, National Insitute of Diabetes and Digestive and Kidney Diseases, Subcommittee of the Digestive Diseases Interagency Coordinating Committee, 2004). Chronic liver disease, including cirrhosis, ranks as the 12th leading cause of death in the United States (Kochanek, 2016). Although liver transplantation is not a primary treatment for most patients with chronic liver disease, it does offer patients with end-stage liver disease (ESLD) an effective treatment option to attenuate the high mortality associated with ESLD. Patients with ESLD are at high risk of systemic and coagulation abnormalities that heighten the complexity of their perianesthesia management. In this section, an overview of patients with ESLD is presented and also special considerations for the perianesthesia management of patients with ESLD are highlighted.

Background

Within the United Sates, the Organ Procurement and Transplantation Network (OPTN) oversees policy development and compliance, and functions under the U.S. Department of Health and Human Services. According to a OPTN report, the liver is the second most common organ transplanted in the United States (OPTN & Scientific Registry of Transplant Recipients, 2017). The demand for liver transplants continues to grow as advances in medical technology, surgical technique, and pharmaceutical immunosuppression improve outcomes for transplant recipients. Transplantation rates, however, remain limited by the availability of donor organs. As a result of the imbalance between supply and demand, OPTN adopted the Model for End-Stage Liver Disease (MELD) in 2002. This scoring system provides a tool for prioritizing patients on the liver transplant list in the United States. A patient's MELD score is based on a combination of laboratory results, including serum creatinine, serum bilirubin, and international normalized ratio (INR). Scores range from 6 to 40, with higher scores indicating patients with a higher severity of liver disease and the likelihood of mortality if they do not receive a transplant. The implementation of this system aids with the allocation of donor livers to those patients with the greatest short-term mortality risk, regardless of the length of time they have been on the national waitlist.

Indications for liver transplant include acute liver failure, cirrhosis accompanied by portal hypertension or liver dysfunction, liver neoplasms, and liver-related metabolic disorders. Within the United States, the most frequent cause of chronic liver disease has shifted from viral hepatitis to nonalcoholic, fatty liver disease (NAFDL). The increase in NAFDL has coincided with the obesity epidemic in the United States, and this trend is expected to continue (Issa, 2015; Younossi et al., 2011). Contraindications to liver transplant include severe cardiopulmonary disease, uncontrolled HIV, history of medical noncompliance, anatomic abnormalities that preclude liver transplant, and, in most cases, extrahepatic malignancy.

Clinical Aspects

ASSESSMENT

Prior to a liver transplant, patients are recommended to undergo a comprehensive preoperative evaluation. Similar to other transplant populations, a comprehensive preoperative evaluation aims to assess a patient's readiness for surgery with respect to cardiac, pulmonary, immunologic, and nutritional status. Second, a preoperative assessment should also capture the family and social support system of the patient. During the preoperative evaluation, the nurse anesthetist should collect serum chemistry panel, coagulation studies, virology studies, arterial blood gas, chest radiograph, electrocardiogram, and pulmonary function testing. In some cases, cardiovascular studies, such as an echocardiogram, may be warranted in patients with known atherosclerosis disease or hyperdynamic circulation.

Given the often protracted length of time that patients awaiting liver transplantation experience, progressive worsening of ascites or indications of hepatic encephalopathy are clinical indicators that have been linked to poor health outcomes among patients with ESLD and should be monitored (Clayton, 2011). Reappraisals of the MELD score and the identification of deterioration in patient's general health status or liver function are recommended to promote early implementation of medical therapies and assessment of the urgency for liver transplantation.

Once an organ becomes available for a patient awaiting liver transplantation, arrangements are made for the recipient to be admitted to the hospital and operating room preparations are made. A conventional general anesthetic approach is appropriate for patients with ESLD. If the patient was unable to maintain nil per os (NPO; nothing by mouth) status, a risk for esophageal bleeding or impaired gastric emptying, rapid sequence induction with cricoid pressure should be used. Once an artificial airway device is successfully introduced, the insertion of large-bore intravenous catheters, pulmonary artery, and invasive blood pressure measurement (i.e., arterial line catheters) to monitor hemodynamic instability are taken care of. The cardiac output and volume status monitoring should be evaluated intra- and postoperatively to quell hemodynamic instability and fluid replacement management (Hall, 2013).

NURSING INTERVENTIONS, MANAGEMENT, AND IMPLICATIONS

Intraoperative phases of liver transplantation require special considerations by anesthesia providers. Liver transplantation consists of three distinct phases. The first stage, the time from skin incision until removal of the native liver (hepatectomy), is referred to as the preanhepatic phase. It is during the preanhepatic phase that the patient is at greatest risk for surgical bleeding and hypotension due to surgical manipulation. The administration of cystralloid fluids is indicated, and infusion of colloids should be administered cautiously. The second phase is referred to as the *anhepatic phase*—from the time that the portacaval cross-clamp is placed until anastomosis and reperfusion of the donor graft takes place. In the anhepatic phases, risk for acidosis, hemodynamic instability, and arrhythmias are heightened. The neohepatic phase is the last phase of the liver transplantation procedure, in which the hemostasis is achieved, and surgical closure is completed. Coagulopathies, electrolyte imbalances, and possible hypothermia that can develop at any point intraoperatively should also be addressed in the neohepatic phase of the surgical procedure (Ramsay, 2015).

A number of clinical factors may contribute to the transplant recipient's hospital course in the postoperative period. The patient's quantity and severity of comorbid conditions, the severity of liver failure, and the quality of the donor liver may all impact the success of the transplant procedure. Throughout the postoperative period, the patient is monitored closely for an indication of graft dysfunction, which may indicate thrombosis of the hepatic artery.

Postoperative liver transplant patients are at risk of several clinical conditions. Of these clinical conditions, alterations in the synthesis of clotting proteins predisposes liver transplant patients at risk for impaired hemostasis and bleeding. The transfusion of blood products and clotting factors should be judiciously considered. Acute renal insufficiency can occur as a result of hypovolemia. Monitoring urine output, blood urea nitrogen, and creatinine is recommended for the surveillance of renal function. An acid–base imbalance can result from varied etiologic mechanisms, and arterial blood gas profiles along with lactate levels should be conducted to identify pathologic mechanism of an acid–base imbalance and guide the clinical management for correction.

OUTCOMES

The initiation and maintenance of immunosuppressive therapy is a key facet of liver transplantation. Medication schedules must be closely adhered to and serum drug levels should be monitored frequently to assess for possible toxicity and ensure adequate serum concentrations. Patient education stresses the importance of immunosuppressive therapy in maintaining donor organ function. Side effects of these medications are common and must be managed in an ongoing fashion. Severity may range from changes in hair growth, loss of energy, joint pain to nephrotoxicity, diabetes, hypertension, thrombocytopenia, and leukocytosis (Cupples, Lerret, McCalmont, & Ohler, 2016).

Liver transplant recipients must manage the side effects of lifelong immunosuppression and face a number of potential long-term complications. Hypertension, cardiovascular disease, diabetes, chronic renal insufficiency, hyperlipidemia, metabolic bone disorders, and posttransplant malignancy are all potential long-term complications of immunosuppression therapy. Nurses, along with the other members of the interdisciplinary transplant team, play an important role in optimizing the health of patients with ESLD who require a liver transplantation procedure.

Summary

Liver transplantation is a cure for patient's suffering from ESLD. As a result of surgical and pharmaceutical advancements, liver transplantation now has excellent long-term outcomes. Nurses play a vital role in helping patients with ESLD to optimally recover after liver transplantation. Emotional and social support are essential to the transplant recipient's psychosocial well-being. Each successful transplant is achieved as a result of multidisciplinary teamwork and communication. Nurses who provide direct patient care are often the first to identify clinical changes that reduce the impact of numerous complications related to the surgical procedure or its medical management.

Clayton, M. (2011). Assessing patients before and after a liver transplant. *Practical Nursing, 22*(5), 236–241.

Cupples, S. A., Lerret, S., McCalmont, V., & Ohler, L. (Eds.). (2016). *Core curriculum for transplant nurses* (2nd ed.). Philadelphia, PA: Lippincott Williams & Wilkins.

Issa, D. H., & Alkhouri, N. (2015). Long-term management of liver transplant recipients: A review for the internist. *Cleveland Clinic Journal of Medicine, 82*(6), 361–372.

Kochanek, K. D., Murphy, S. L., Xu, J., & Tejada-Vera, B. (2016). Deaths: Final data for 2014. Retrieved from https://www.cdc.gov/nchs/data/nvsr/nvsr65/nvsr65_04.pdf

Organ Procurement and Transplantation Network & Scientific Registry of Transplant Recipients. (2017). 2015 annual data report: Introduction. *American Journal of Transplant, 17*(Suppl. 1), 11–20. doi:10.1111/ajt.14123

Ramsay, M. A. (2015). Anesthesia for liver transplantation. In G. B. Ronald & W. Busuttil (Eds.), *Transplantation of the liver* (3rd ed., pp. 589–606). Philadelphia, PA: Elsevier Saunders.

U.S. Department of Health and Human Services, National Institutes of Health, National Insitute of Diabetes and Digestive and Kidney Diseases, Subcommittee of the Digestive Diseases Interagency Coordinating Committee. (2004). Action plan for liver disease research. Retrieved from https://www.niddk.nih.gov/about-niddk/strategic-plans-reports/Pages/action-plan-for-liver-disease-research.aspx

Younossi, Z. M., Stepanova, M., Afendy, M., Fang, Y., Younossi, Y., Mir, H., & Srishord, M. (2011). Changes in the prevalence of the most common causes of chronic liver disease in the United States from 1988 to 2008. *Clinical Gastroenterology and Hepatology, 9*(6), 524–530.

■ MALIGNANT HYPERTHERMIA

Colleen Thaxton Spencer
Elizabeth Demko

Overview

Malignant hyperthermia (MH) is an inherited genetic disorder of skeletal muscle hypermetabolism (Rosenberg, Malhotra, & Gurvitch, 2008). This clinical syndrome occurs with exposure to volatile anesthetic agents and an anticholinergic drug, succinylcholine. Physical and emotional stressors have been associated with the manifestation of MH. Sinus tachycardia, tachypnea, hypercarbia, hyperthermia, masseter spasm, acidosis, and hyperkalemia are clinical manifestations of MH (Rosenberg et al., 2008). Because a MH episode can be life-threatening, it is imperative that all heath care providers are knowledgeable about the condition and rapid interventions that are necessary during a suspected occurrence.

Background

Malignant hyperthermia is a life-threatening condition that has an autosomal dominant pattern of inheritance

(Diu & Mancuso, 2012). MH can happen in one in 100,000 adult surgeries and one in 30,000 pediatric surgeries. Approximately, one in 2,000 people has the genetic disposition that places the individual at risk for MH. A history of a first-degree relative with MH under anesthesia should raise suspicion for MH susceptibility during preoperative evaluation. Children and siblings with a relative with known MH susceptibility can have up to a 50% chance of inheriting the gene defect for MH. In addition, children with central core disease, King–Denborough syndrome, Duchenne's muscular dystrophy, and other myopathies are at increased risk (Van Tassel & Schulman, 2007). MH does not discriminate across gender or race. However, adolescents have the highest incidence rate compared to all other age cohorts.

Patients with MH are likely to express defective calcium channel receptors of the sarcoplasmic reticulum (SR) of skeletal muscle. The SR is the storage site for calcium in a muscle. A constant leak of calcium from the SR of skeletal muscle causes calcium to be depleted resulting in muscle weakness results (Diu & Mancuso, 2012). During an MH episode, the calcium channel is locked in an open position and uncontrolled release of calcium results in continuous muscle activation. This causes abnormal increase in metabolism and heat production. As adenosine triphosphate (ATP) is depleted, the cells release potassium into the bloodstream, leading to hyperkalemia. This can cause cardiac arrhythmias and possibly death (Rosenberg et al., 2008).

Malignant hyperthermia can have profound tissue and organ dysfunction. Typical clinical features of MH include hypermetabolism, acid–base imbalance related to tissue respiration and serum lactate, generalized muscle rigidity, masseter muscle rigidity, and an increase in core temperature higher than 40°C. Stimulation of the sympathetic nervous system causes sinus tachycardia, tachypnea, arrhythmias, skin mottling, profuse sweating, hypertension, arterial hypoxemia, metabolic and respiratory acidosis as well as hyperkalemia, hypercalcemia, hyperphosphatemia, and myoglobinuria (Din & Mancusso, 2008). Acute hypercarbia while receiving mechanical ventilation under anesthesia and masseter spasm, or jaw rigidity, is often mentioned as the signs of a potential MH episode.

Malignant hyperthermia that is recognized late or ineffectively treated substantially impacts the patient's postoperative health status. When MH is not identified early or treated effectively, it can lead to kidney failure, internal hemorrhage, liver failure, brain injury, and ultimately cardiac arrest. The mortality rate of an untreated episode is 70%, whereas treatment with dantrolene decreases the mortality rate to 4% (Van Tassel & Schulman, 2007).

Clinical Aspects

ASSESSMENT

To identify patients planned for a surgical procedure under general anesthesia, a careful preoperative interview should be conducted. Questions regarding past anesthetic complications and family history of MH should be asked of every patient. It is prudent for the nurse anesthetist to have a treatment plan in the event of an unsuspected episode of MH occuring. Early recognition and treatment of the signs of MH are important. Monitoring a patient's exhaled CO_2, minute ventilation, and temperature during surgery is vital for the early recognition and management of MH (Din & Mancuso, 2008).

In the event of MH in an unsuspected patient, all triggering anesthetic agents should be discontinued and a plan made to abort or expeditiously complete the surgical procedure. The patient should be hyperventilated with 100% oxygen. Dantrolene should be intravenously administered. Dantrolene is suspected to inhibit calcium transport through the ryanodine receptor channel and enhance skeletal muscle relaxation (Diu & Mancuso, 2012). In addition to the administration of dantrolene, therapeutic hypothermia, and the use of evidence-based practices to prevent respiratory failure, acid–base imbalances, and renal dysfunction are recommended (Van Tassel & Schulman, 2007). Once stabilized in the operating room, the patient with MH should be transferred to the intensive care unit (Rosenberg et al., 2008).

NURSING INTERVENTIONS, MANAGEMENT, AND IMPLICATIONS

While administering anesthesia and preparing for surgery for a patient with known MH, a critical aspect of the anesthesia care plan should strictly avoid potent inhalation agents and succinylcholine. Anesthetic agents that are safe for administration include benzodiazepines, etomidate, ketamine, brevital, propofol, nitrous oxide, opioids, and nondepolarizing muscle relaxants (Van Tassel & Schulman, 2007).

In addition to careful selection of pharmacologic agents, attention to modifying the anesthesia equipment should be considered for patients known to have MH. A fresh circuit, a new reservoir bag, and soda lime canister should be applied to the anesthesia machine. An activated charcoal filter can be placed on the inspiratory and expiratory limbs of the anesthesia machine to remove additional volatile anesthetics (Diu & Mancuso, 2012). Also, the anesthesia ventilator must be flushed by flowing 10 liters of oxygen through it for at least 10 minutes, and vaporizers should be taped or removed from the anesthesia machine. Although no special monitoring equipment is necessary in the operating room, the anesthesia provider should ensure that end-title carbon dioxide and temperature are monitored closely throughout the surgical procedure.

OUTCOMES

The presentation of the clinical features of MH often do not occur in operating room. In fact, an MH event can occur up to 1 hour after surgery is completed. Therefore, anesthesia providers and postanesthesia nurses should diligently monitor for the manifestation of MH during the recovery period after exposure to general anesthesia. It is recommended that patients who underwent a surgical or diagnostic procedure with general anesthesia should recover for about 4 hours in a postanesthesia care unit (PACU), and, if the recovery phase is uneventful, the patient should be discharged from the PACU to an appropriate disposition. As a result, the patient should be monitored diligently for a minimum of 4 hours postoperatively and should be discharged to the floor or home if the PACU course is uneventful (Van Tassel & Schulman, 2007).

Summary

A thorough assessment of a patient's risk for MH is to inform the perianesthesia care plan. Nurses who care for patients who receive inhalation anesthetic agents or succinylcholine should be vigilant in their evaluation of the signs and symptoms of MH. If clinical features of MH present, nurses must contact the patient's health care team to provide prompt treatment. As an anesthesia provider, preparedness is the key to preventing complications associated with MH.

Diu, M. W., & Mancuso, T. J. (2012). Pediatric diseases. In R. Hines & K. Marschall (Eds.), *Stoelting's anesthesia and co existing disease* (6th ed., pp. 636–640). Philadelphia, PA: Saunders.

Rosenberg, H., Malhotra, V., & Gurvitch, D. L. (2008). Malignant hyperthermia. In F.-S. F. Yao, M. L. Fontes, & V. Malhotra (Eds.), *Yao & Artusio's anesthesiology* (6th ed., pp. 1091–1104). Philadelphia, PA: Lippincott Williams & Williams.

Van Tassel, K. M., & Schulman, S. R. (2007). Malignant hyperthermia. In J. L. Atlee (Ed.), *Complications in anesthesia* (2nd ed., pp. 654–656). Philadelphia, PA: Saunders.

■ MORBID OBESITY AND ANESTHESIA

Elizabeth Demko
Colleen Thaxton Spencer
Sonya D. Moore

Overview

Morbid obesity is defined as a weight greater than 20% over ideal body weight (Albright & Popescu, 2012). Obesity continues to be a growing public health concern. According to data from the National Health and Nutrition Examination Survey from 2011 to 2014, just over 36% of adults and 17% of youth meet the criteria for obesity (Ogden, Carroll, Fryar, & Flegal, 2015). Body mass index (BMI) is a classification system used to stratify individuals as normal (18.5–24.9 kg/m²), overweight (25–29.9 kg/m²), obese (30–39.9 kg/m²), morbidly obese (40–49.9 kg/m²), and super morbidly obese (greater than 50 kg/m²; Hyman & Furman, 2011). Individuals who are classified as obese have increased likelihood of multimorbidity that heightens the risks of complications across the perioperative continuum. In this section, evidence for evaluation and perianesthesia management of the patient with morbid obesity is presented.

Background

Morbid obesity is a significant public health concern that is steadily on the rise among Americans across the life span. From 1992 to 2012, rates of overweight and obesity have increased from 63% to 75% for men and from 55% to 67% for women (Yang, 2015). The prevalence of obesity is highest in the non-Hispanic Black population at 48.1% and the Hispanic population at 42.5% (Ogden et al., 2015). Asian adults and non-Hispanic White populations have the lowest incidence of obesity at 11.7% and 34.5%, respectively (Ogden et al., 2015). Among these four groups, the only difference in obesity between genders is seen in the non-Hispanic Black (men: 37.5% and women: 56.9%) and Hispanic (men: 39% and women: 45.7%) populations.

Changes in the American diet and lifestyle have been linked to the increase in obesity rates. In 2000, the number of calories Americans consumed had increased by 20% compared to 1983 ("Public Awareness," n.d). Since 1970, Americans have consumed 45% percent more grain. The amount of meat and processed hydrogenated oil, sugar, and fast-food ingested has also increased. The

Centers for Disease Control and Prevention estimates that 80% of Americans fail to exercise enough ("Public Awareness," n.d). Consumption of minimally processed food, including fresh fruits and vegetables, is expensive. Cost and availably of healthier food choices can limit their consumption in populations with lower socioeconomic status. In addition, the time and out-of-pocket costs of health care services, and the rise in the number of bariatric surgery cases per year are all recognized barriers to a healthy lifestyle for many Americans.

Obesity has substantial impact on the individual and society. For patients who are obese or morbidly obese, the life spans is significantly shortened and health-related quality of life is diminished due to multimorbidity (Malchow, 2014). From the vantage point of the economic burden of obesity, the associated costs of treatment for cardiovascular disease and diabetes, is projected to be $60 billion in 2030 (Endocrine Society, 2015).

Clinical Aspects

ASSESSMENT

There are many things to consider when providing anesthesia for a morbidly obese patient, as obesity affects all organ systems. Obesity is associated with restrictive lung disease, obstructive sleep apnea (OSA), hypertension, coronary artery disease (CAD), right-sided heart failure, stroke, gastroesopageal reflux (GERD), endocrine abnormalities, and increased risk of cancer. The preoperative assessment should focus on optimizing each of the patient's comorbid conditions.

A thorough cardiac assessment should be completed prior to anesthesia administration. The morbidly obese patient should be assessed for hypertension, CAD, and heart failure. Basic testing should include a review of vital signs and electrocardiography. For uncontrolled hypertension, a referral should be made to a primary care provider in order to optimize the patient's medication regimen prior to anesthesia. Patients who endorse chest pain, shortness of breath, intolerance to activity, palpitations, fatigue, syncope, or signs of heart failure should be referred for a cardiac stress test, and possibly, a transthoracic echocardiography. Additional testing may be indicated to rule out CAD in patients with diabetes, very limited levels of activity due to body habitus, or limited mobility that results from degenerative joint disease. Intraoperatively, the patient's vital signs should be maintained within 20% of baseline and fluid resuscitation should be based on trends in vital signs and lab values (Hyman & Furman, 2011).

NURSING INTERVENTIONS, MANAGEMENT, AND IMPLICATIONS

Patients with morbid obesity are at risk of difficult intubation, airway obstruction, and impaired gas exchange. A thorough airway examination should be performed prior to administering anesthesia and should include a Mallampati score (a score greater than 3 is indicative of increased risk for difficult intubation), assessment of thyromental distance, mouth opening, neck range of motion, dentition, and inquiry about history of difficult intubation. If general anesthesia is required for a case, the patient should be adequately preoxygenated and positioned to optimize success for intubation. Ramping the patient (placing folded blankets behind the patient's shoulders and neck) is usually required in order to align the airway for intubation (sniffing position). Elevating the head of the bed by 30° and ramping the patient also help to optimize the body mechanics of breathing. The presence of additional adipose tissue around the chest causes restrictive airway disease. Increased airway resistance and decreased lung compliance results in a decreased functional residual capacity (FRC) that is even more pronounced when the patient is supine (Albright & Popescu, 2012). This causes rapid desaturation during periods of hypoventilation or apnea. It can also make it difficult to adequately mechanically ventilate these patients. Additional airway equipment, such as nasal trumpets, oral airways, laryngeal mask airway, and fiber optic scope, should be available in case a difficult airway is encountered. The anesthetist should be knowledgeable about the American Society of Anesthesiologist (ASA) difficult airway algorithm.

As increased BMI (greater than 30 kg/m^2) is a risk factor for OSA, morbidly obese patients should be screened. As respiratory centers become desensitized to nocturnal hypercarbia, obesity hypoventilation syndrome (OHS) develops. OHS is characterized as nocturnal episodes of central apnea and can develop into pickwickian syndrome (Albright & Popescu, 2012). Signs of pickwickian syndrome include obesity, daytime hypersomnolence, arterial hypoxemia, hypercarbia, polycythemia, respiratory acidosis, pulmonary hypertension, and right-sided heart failure (Albright & Popescu, 2012).

OSA occurs in 70% of morbidly obese patients. The preoperative assessment of the patient with OSA is critical. Care must be taken when providing anesthesia to these patients as respiratory arrest can result from minimal sedation. Patients with OSA should be advised to bring their CPAP or BiPAP machine with them on the day of surgery to ensure that it is available for postoperative use.

Renal function, hemoglobin A1C, and blood glucose levels should be evaluated preoperatively to assess for renal failure and diabetes mellitus (DM). It is also prudent to premedicate morbidly obese patients for GERD prior to anesthesia (Malchow, 2014). Nonparticulate antacids, proton pump inhibitors, and metoclopramide are commonly used for gastric prophylaxis. Body habitus and gastroporesis associated with DM increases the risk for aspiration. For this reason, rapid sequence induction should be used during general anesthesia.

Any patient undergoing anesthesia requires intravenous (IV) access. Even with much experience in IV placement, IV access is often difficult to obtain and maintain in morbidly obese patients because of body habitus. Use of a vein viewer or central intravenous catheter may be necessary.

OUTCOMES

When choosing an anesthetic for a morbidly obese patient, one should take into consideration the location of the operative field, patient positioning, and duration of the surgery as well as postoperative pain management. The American Society of Anesthesiologist practice guidelines recommend local or regional anesthesia over general anesthesia for obese patients (Albright & Popescu, 2012). Use of regional anesthesia or peripheral nerve blocks with sedation are beneficial for postoperative pain control while minimizing potential for respiratory depression associated with high doses of narcotic. The patient also benefits from more stable intraoperative hemodynamics, which decreases the risk for ischemic events. Although the use of regional anesthesia allows the anesthetist to avoid airway manipulation, vigilance is required when sedating morbidly obese patients to avoid hypoventilation, aspiration, and possible loss of a patient airway. Though regional anesthesia and peripheral nerve blocks may be the preferred anesthetic technique for morbidly obese patients, it is important to note that there is a higher rate of complications and failure. Thus, general anesthesia with an endotracheal tube is always a possibility.

If general anesthesia is required, short-acting medications should be used and narcotics avoided. The patient should also be warmed during the procedure to aid in metabolism of the anesthetic agents used. Morbidly obese patients should be completely awake with neuromuscular blocking agents completely reversed prior to extubation. Finally, a multimodal approach to pain management should be employed in order to avoid respiratory depression and obstruction postoperatively. Acetaminophen, nonsteroidal anti-inflammatory drugs, low-dose ketamine, dexamethasone, clonidine, lidocaine, and gabapentin are a few examples of medications utilized for multimodal analgesia.

Vigilance in positioning is required by the perioperative team when caring for morbidly obese patients. These patients are at increased risk of pressure sores and nerve injuries such as brachial plexus, ulnar and sciatic nerves (Albright & Popescu, 2012). The team should be knowledgeable about the weight limitations for equipment and be educated on ancillary equipment such as specific beds for the morbidly obese, table extenders, HoverMatts, and Hoyer lifts. Care should be taken to ensure both patient and perioperative team safety.

Summary

A thorough preoperative evaluation is necessary for the morbidly obese patient. For any comorbidity, the patient has to be medically optimized before he or she is anesthetized. The anesthesia plan should utilize peripheral nerve block or regional anesthesia with minimal sedation and narcotic, if possible. If general anesthesia is indicated, the patient should be intubated and medication that is short-acting should be utilized. Extra care should be taken with the positioning of morbidly obese patients to avoid injury to the patient and members of the perioperative team.

Albright, B. E., & Popescu, W. M. (2012). Nutritional diseases: Obesity and malnutrition. In R. L. Hines & K. E. Marschall (Eds.), *Stoelting's anesthesia and co-existing disease* (6th ed., pp. 314, 326). Philadelphia, PA: Saunders.

Hyman, S. A., & Furman, W. R. (2011). Nutritional and gastrointestinal disease. In R. D. Miller & M. C. Pardo (Eds.), *Basics of anesthesia* (6th ed., pp. 389, 463). Philadelphia, PA: Saunders.

Malchow, R. J. (2014). Morbid obesity in the free-standing ambulatory surgery center. *Current Reviews Nurse Anesthesia, 37*(5), 49–60.

Public awareness obesity in America. (n.d). *The Endocrine Society. Endocrine facts and figures: Obesity* (1st ed.). Hyattsville, MD: National Center for Heath Statistics. Retrieved from http://www.publichealth.org/public-awearness/obesity

Ogden C. L., Carroll M. D., Fryar C. D., & Flegal K. M. (2015). *Prevalence of obesity among adults and youth: United States, 2011–2014.* NCHS data brief, no 219. Hyattsville, MD: National Center for Health Statistics.

Yang, C. (2015). Prevalence of overweight and obesity in the United States, 2007–2012. *JAMA Internal Medicine*, *175*(8), 1412–1413.

■ NEUROMUSCULAR BLOCKADE REVERSAL: SUGAMMADEX

Britney A. Leonardi

Overview

Neuromuscular blocking drugs (NMBDs) are defined as drugs that prevent the ability of nerves to transmit impulses at the neuromuscular junction (NMJ), producing temporary paralysis of skeletal muscles (Miller & Pardo, 2011). Multiple indications for neuromuscular blockade exist: the need for a motionless surgical field, vocal cord paralysis for intubation, and mechanical ventilation for patients with underlying lung pathology (Miller & Pardo, 2011). Although the administration of NMBDs in the surgical setting is frequently required, reversal of the effect of these NMBDs is often indicated to terminate skeletal muscle paralysis. This entry reviews the clinical indications and pertinent characteristics of sugammadex, an NMBD reversal agent newly approved in the United States.

Background

An ideal reversal agent for an NMBD is expected to have a fast onset, minimal side effects, provide complete reversal for mild or significant motor blockade, and have a longer half-life than the NMBD (Nag et al., 2013). In an effort to mimic these characteristics, sugammadex was created to compete with current reversal agents utilized in anesthesia, such as neostigmine, pyridostigmine, and edrophonium. Sugammadex has been approved for use across the world in countries, such as Australia, Iceland, New Zealand, and Norway, for several years (Yang & Keam, 2012). According to the U.S. Food and Drug Administration (2015), sugammadex was approved for use in the United States in late 2015 after sufficient data were generated on the drug safety and efficacy was confirmed across three phase-III clinical trials. When used as the NMBD reversal agent in healthy adults, sugammadex provided quicker reversal of rocuronium bromide and vecuronium bromide-induced motor blockade with limited recurrent neuromuscular blockade, proving itself clinically superior to alternative reversal agents (Blobner et al., 2010; Yang & Keam, 2012).

Clinical Aspects

MECHANISM OF ACTION

Sugammadex is a γ-cyclodextrin molecule, which exhibits greater bioavailability, water solubility, and internal molecular cavity size than the other two naturally occurring cyclodextrins, α- and β-cyclodextrin (Nag et al., 2013). This enhances sugammadex's ability to chelate the aminosteroid NMBD molecule. It has a hydrophobic inner cavity and a hydrophilic exterior, forming tight complexes with aminosteroid NMBDs using van der Waals forces (Nag et al., 2013). Sugammadex has greatest affinity for rocuronium bromide, followed by vecuronium bromide, and least with pancuronium bromide (Nag et al., 2013). Because there is a high attraction between the NMBD and reversal agent coupled with a low dissociation rate, there is a plasma reduction of free NMBD and reduced occupancy at the nicitonic receptor in the NMJ (Nag et al., 2013). Thus, as the free plasma NMBD becomes bound to sugammadex to form a neutral compound, a gradient between the NMBD plasma concentration and NMBD nicotinic receptor concentration increases. This leads to the movement of NMBD from tissue to plasma, reducing occupancy at the nicotinic receptor, further reversing neuromuscular blockade (Nag et al., 2013). Sugammadex has a large volume of distribution and is not plasma-protein bound. No metabolites are produced and it is renally excreted within 24 hours.

EFFICACY

The therapeutic efficacy of sugammadex has been evaluated in both the adult and pediatric populations; however, in the United States, the drug is only approved for adults. A standard dose of sugammadex is 2 mg/kg. Sugammadex 4 mg/kg provided faster onset of blockade reversal than a maximum dose of neostigmine 70 μg/kg paired with glycopyrrolate 14 μg/kg with 1–2 posttetanic count twitches (Yang & Keam, 2009). These results were consistent across multiple studies. Blobner et al. (2010) found that "time to recovery of the TOF ratio of 0.9 after sugammadex compared with neostigmine was significantly shorter (p <0.00001), being 1.5 versus 18.6 minutes" (p. 874).

CONTRAINDICATIONS

Sugammadex is contraindicated for patients with known hypersensitivity to the drug after exposure and renal impairment. Although the complex binding between sugammadex and the aminosteroid NMBD is irreversible, safety of using this drug in patients with decreased ability to renally excrete the complexes has not been studied (Welliver, Cheek, Osterbrink, & McDonough, 2015). It is not designed for reversal of NMBDs other than rocuronium bromide or vecuronium bromide. Caution should be exercised for patients with known coagulopathies or patients receiving blood thinners. The maximum dose of sugammadex (16 mg/kg) may increase the risk of coagulopathy by prolonging the activated partial thromboplastin time and prothrombin time/international normalized ratio (Merck & Company, Incorporated, 2016).

SIDE-EFFECT PROFILE

The side-effect profile for sugammadex is constrained. Rare occurrences of bradycardia have been reported in studies (Merck & Company, Incorporated, 2016). Recurrence of neuromuscular blockade has occurred secondarily due to underdosing of sugammadex (Merck & Company, Incorporated, 2016). Reduced efficacy of contraceptive agents for up to 7 days has been reported when the reversal agent was administered to women of reproductive age (Merck & Company, Incorporated, 2016). If elected for use in this population, women of childbearing years should be made aware of its administration.

Summary

The approval of sugammadex by the U.S. Food and Drug Administration has benefitted anesthesia practices in two ways. First, it allows for complete and immediate reversal of nondepolarizing NMBDs in the event of a failed airway. Second, it allows for complete and immediate reversal of NMBDs in the event of an unanticipated or abrupt cessation of surgery in which complete immobility was required for the duration. Its use in the clinical arena is organization dependent, but it should be recognized, at minimum, as a rescue reversal agent for clinical situations in which abrupt termination of neuromuscular blockade is indicated.

Blobner, M., Eriksoon, L., Scholz, J., Motsch, J., Della Rocca, G., & Prins, M. (2010). Reversal of rocuronium-induced neuromuscular blockade with sugammadex compared with neostigmine during sevoflurane anaesthesia: Results of a randomised, controlled trial. *European Journal of Anasthesiology, 27*(10), 874–881. doi:10.1097/EJA.0b013e32833d56b7

Merck & Company, Incorporated. (2016). Selected safety information about BRIDION (sugammadex). Retrieved from https://www.merckconnect.com/bridion/overview.html

Miller, R., & Pardo, M. (2011). *Basics of anesthesia.* Philadelphia, PA: Saunders.

Nag, K., Roshan Singh, D., Shetti, A., Kumar, H., Sivashanmugam, T., & Parthasarathy, S. (2013). Sugammadex: A revolutionary drug in neuromuscular pharmacology. *Anesthesia Essays and Researches, 7*(3), 302–306. doi:10.4103/0259-1162.123211

U.S. Food and Drug Administration. (2015). FDA approves Bridion to reverse effects of neuromuscular blocking drugs used during surgery. Retrieved from https://www.fda.gov/NewsEvents/Newsroom/PressAnnouncements/ucm477512.htm

Welliver, M., Cheek, D., Osterbrink, J., & McDonough, J. (2015). Worldwide experience with sugammadex sodium: Implications for the United States. *AANA Journal, 83*(2), 107–114.

Yang, L. P. H., & Keam, S. J. (2009). Sugammadex: A review of its use in anaesthetic practice. *Drugs, 69*(7), 919–942. doi:10.2165/00003495-200969070-00008

■ ONE-LUNG VENTILATION

Monica M. Bitner
Brittany Hosler
Jessica M. Tripi

Overview

One-lung ventilation (OLV) is often used for thoracic and cardiac procedures. It refers to the process of isolating one lung from the nondependent lung (Miller & Pardo, 2011). OLV allows for improved visualization and access of the operating area while also preventing damage to healthy lung tissue. Delivering ventilation to one lung can be done with double-lumen tubes (DLT), bronchial blockers, or single lumen tubes (SLT). The most commonly used tube for OLV is the DLT. Most patients undergoing thoracic surgery have preexisting pulmonary diseases and should have preoperative assessments as well as lung function tests (Butterworth, Mackey, & Wasnick, 2013). The anesthetic goal during OLV is to maintain stability as well as adequate gas exchange (Miller & Pardo, 2011). Prevention of complications, such as acute lung injury, hypoxemia, and worsening of right-to-left shunt, is crucial in the management of these patients.

Background

Thoracic surgery patients have difficult airways due to pathological changes of the upper and lower airway anatomy, such as lung carcinomas of the pharynx or epiglottis or scar tissue formation due to radiation therapy (Miller et al., 2015). Placing a DLT can be difficult in these patients. An SLT with the use of a bronchial blocker to isolate one lung may be the preferred technique in patients with previous neck or oral surgery and distorted anatomy. Thoracic surgery patients also have underlying pulmonary diseases that increase their risk for respiratory complications. Respiratory complications are the leading cause of morbidity and mortality among this surgical population. Complications, such as atelectasis, pneumonia, and respiratory failure, occur in 15% to 20% of thoracic surgery patients (Miller et al., 2015). Acute lung injury (ALI) during OLV has a 40% mortality and morbidity risk (Butterworth et al., 2013).

Although only one lung is being ventilated, both lungs are perfused. Perfusion of the nonventilated lung results in shunting, in which blood passing through does not participate in gas exchange. Atelectasis contributes to this impaired oxygenation. A drop in PaO_2 and a low ventilation-to-perfusion ratio (V/Q) lead to hypoxemia (Miller et al., 2015). Low V/Q ratio indicates inadequate ventilation and inability to oxygenate blood. The hypoxemia rate during OLV is 5% to 10% (Waheedullah & Schwarzkopf, 2009). Hypoxemia usually occurs with the mixing of shunted, nonoxygenated blood from the nondependent lung with blood from the dependent lung. As a protective measure, hypoxic pulmonary vasoconstriction (HPV) occurs, causing a decrease in blood flow to the nonventilated lung (Butterworth et al., 2013). Lateral positioning can also stimulate HPV, and ventilation-perfusion mismatching further increases with use of the lateral decubitus position. The onset of HPV can occur as quickly as 20 to 30 minutes and decrease blood flow to the nondependent lung by as much as 50% (Reed & Yudkowitz, 2013). However, HPV can be altered by vasodilators, which can cause an increase in hypoxemia (Miller et al., 2015). Patient populations at an increased risk for hypoxemia include those with poor PaO_2 during two-lung ventilation, high perfusion to the operative lung, restrictive lung disease, and supine position during OLV (Miller et al., 2015). Identifying specific techniques

to decrease lung injury, especially after resection procedures, can help improve patient stability and safety. Using lower tidal volumes, positive end-expiratory pressure (PEEP), pressure-controlled ventilation, permissive hypercapnia, and maintaining Fio2 above 90% are a few of the ventilation techniques that can reduce ALI (Butterworth et al., 2013).

Clinical Aspects

ASSESSMENT

Assessment of a patient undergoing OLV needs to be completed prior to, during, and after the surgery. An initial thorough preoperative history and physical of the patient are required to estimate the patient's ability to tolerate OLV. The patient's history should include any preexisting comorbidities, new-onset diagnoses associated with the current condition, a review of any pulmonary function tests, prior radiology reports, as well as any specific respiratory signs and symptoms the patient may be experiencing, such as shortness of breath, orthopnea, dyspnea, presence of a cough and whether or not it is productive. Many patients undergoing lung procedures have a long history of smoking and a reduced pulmonary function (Barash et al., 2013). A cardiac- and respiratory-focused assessment should be completed prior to inducing anesthesia. Lung and heart sounds should be auscultated before intubation to establish a baseline for the patient. Respiratory effort and oxygen saturation should also be noted. Body habitus, specifically patient's height, should be documented to approximate the appropriate tube sizing. It is imperative to have a proper-fitting to tube to successfully isolate one lung for ventilation (Purohit, Bhargava, Mangal, & Parashar, 2015).

Confirmation of correct placement of a DLT or bronchial blocker is completed immediately after placement. Assessment of bilateral breath sounds with only the tracheal cuff inflated indicates successful placement of the DLT through the vocal cords and indicates that the tube is not too far down the right or the left main stem bronchus (Barash et al., 2013). Positive $ETCO_2$ is a standard of care indicating successful intubation. Inflating both tracheal and bronchial cuffs, and clamping the right side (tracheal lumen), and then auscultating only left side breath sounds confirms correct placement. Standard of care for assessment of correct placement is the utilization of a pediatric flexible fiberoptic bronchoscope. This allows for visualization of correct placement (Barash et al., 2013). Continued ongoing assessment of tube placement during the surgical procedure is needed to promote adequate ventilation and oxygenation. Assessment of the patient's respiratory status should continue after extubation through the postoperative phase. Respiratory rate, rhythm, effort, and oxygenation should be evaluated to ensure proper recovery from lung isolation and the surgical procedure.

NURSING INTERVENTIONS, MANAGEMENT, AND IMPLICATIONS

One of the commonly encountered problems with OLV is hypoxia. The first intervention to be performed at this time includes ensuring an FiO_2 of 1 and to check the placement of the DLT with the fiberoptic bronchoscope. Once correct placement is verified, continuous positive airway pressure (CPAP) of 10 cm H_2O should be applied to the nondependent lung, except in the case of video-assisted thoracoscopic surgery (VATS) as this will restrict the surgeon's view. If hypoxemia is still present, the next intervention would be to add 5 to 10 cm H_2O of PEEP to the ventilated lung. Using frequent recruitment maneuvers can also help to prevent atelectasis, and therefore, improve hypoxia (Barash et al., 2013). Suction tubing may also be used to deliver O_2 to the nondependent lung without inflating it. If hypoxia is still present despite these interventions, then intermittent double-lung ventilation may need to be implemented (Purohit et al., 2015).

The routine approach during OLV has been to use the same tidal volumes used during two-lung ventilation, which would be around 10 to 12 mL/kg (Barash et al., 2013). With the recent concern for lung protective ventilation, there is not a lot of research surrounding the application of this to OLV. A large tidal volume could potentially overdistend and stretch the lung parenchyma, whereas a small tidal volume (6 mL/kg) could lead to atelectasis in the dependent lung (Barash et al., 2013; Blank et al., 2016). A recent study suggests that the benefits of low tidal volume may have a place in OLV, but it must be done in the presence of adequate PEEP and further studies are needed to investigate lung-protective ventilation's place in OLV (Blank et al., 2016).

OUTCOMES

The expected outcomes of evidence-based nursing care focus on adequate oxygenation during OLV and facilitation of the earliest possible extubation to prevent pulmonary complications. Preoperative optimization of lung function with bronchodilators, mucolytic agents, and decreasing irritant exposure will help minimize hypoxemia during OLV (Purohit et al., 2015). Adequate oxygenation and prevention of atelectasis in the dependent lung can be optimized through the use of CPAP, PEEP, and recruitment maneuvers during OLV (Barash, 2013; Purohit et al., 2015). Promoting early extubation can be accomplished with conservative fluid administration, adequate neuromuscular blockade reversal, and correction for blood loss or fluid shifts (Barash et al., 2013). Despite these efforts, ventilatory support postoperatively may be necessary, and it is imperative for the clinician to plan for this possibility in advance. Transition to an SLT is the most favorable option, but in the situation of a difficult airway and/or facial swelling from fluid shifts, it would be prudent to leave the DLT or use a tube exchanger (Barash et al., 2013).

Summary

OLV is a useful technique used to isolate each lung in order to optimize the surgical field for thoracic procedures. Assessing and optimizing patients preoperatively provides the best conditions for successful OLV. It is necessary to continuously monitor the position of the DLT, oxygenation, and effective ventilation throughout the OLV period. Identifying and understanding complications that can occur during OLV allows the nurse to troubleshoot and provide focused care to optimize a patient's respiratory status. Effective nursing care involves thorough assessment, planning, and implementation of all of these factors.

Barash, P. G., Cullen, B. F., Stoelting, R. K., Cahalan, M. K., Stock, M. C., & Ortega, R. (2013). *Clinical anesthesia* (7th ed., pp. 1041–1054). Philadelphia, PA: Lippincott Williams & Wilkins.

Blank, R. S., Colquhoun, D. A., Durieux, M. E., Kozower, B. D., McMurry, T. L., Bender, S. P., & Naik, B. I. (2016). Management of one-lung ventilation: Impact of tidal volume on complications after thoracic surgery. *Anesthesiology, 124*(6), 1286–1295. doi:10.1097/ALN.0000000000001100

Butterworth, J., Mackey, D., & Wasnick, J. (2013). *Morgan and Mikhail's clinical anesthesiology* (5th ed.). New Delhi, India: McGraw-Hill.

Miller, R., Eriksson, L., Fleisher, L., Wiener-Kronish, J., Cohen, N., & Young, W. (2015). *Miller's anesthesia* (8th ed.). Philadelphia, PA: Saunders.

Miller, R., & Pardo, M. (2011). *Basics of anesthesia* (6th ed.). Philadelphia, PA: Saunders.

Purohit, A., Bhargava, S., Mangal, V., & Parashar, V. K. (2015). Lung isolation, one-lung ventilation and hypoxaemia during lung isolation. *Indian Journal of Anaesthesia, 59*(9), 606–617. doi:10.4103/0019-5049.165

Reed, A., & Yudkowitz, F. (2013). *Clinical cases in anesthesia* (4th ed.). Philadelphia, PA: Saunders.

Waheedullah, K., & Schwarzkopf, K. (2009). Hypoxemia during One-lung Ventilation: Prediction, Prevention, and Treatment. *Anesthesiology, 110*(6), 1402–1411

■ PERIPHERAL NERVE BLOCKS

Scott M. Urigel
Jeffrey E. Molter

Overview

Peripheral nerve blocks are a type of regional anesthesia used for surgical anesthesia, postoperative analgesia, or chronic pain management. Local anesthetics are injected or infused around a specific nerve or group of nerves, thereby blocking nerve conduction and inhibiting the transmission of pain stimuli through nerves. These blocks can target specific regions of the body, including the neck, upper extremity, chest, abdomen, and lower extremity.

Background

The inception of peripheral nerve blocks originates with the work of American surgeon William Stewart Halsted, who performed the first peripheral nerve block in 1884 (Lopez-Valverde, De Vicente, & Cutando, 2011). Throughout the late nineteenth and early twentieth centuries, the field of regional anesthesia flourished with the development of new local anesthetics and nerve block techniques. Initial blocks were placed by surgeons utilizing a landmark technique in which a paresthesia was elicited from direct needle contact with the nerve. Following the paresthesia, local anesthetic was injected and the needle was withdrawn. This technique was advanced in 1912 by German surgeon, Georg Clemen Perthes, who demonstrated the location of peripheral nerves through nerve stimulation (Klein, Melton, Grill, & Nielsen, 2012). Nerve simulation techniques were further developed by Greenblatt and Denson in 1962, when they constructed the first mobile peripheral nerve stimulator (Klein, Melton, Grill, & Nielsen, 2012). By the 1980s, nerve stimulators and block needles were widely used in peripheral nerve blocks (Marhofer & Harrop-Griffiths, 2011). This method applies a low electrical current to the block needle to elicit muscle twitching as the needle is advanced toward the nerve. Utilization of the nerve stimulator was intended to locate nerves and indicate the proximity of the needle tip to nerve tissue. Early users of this method believed this would improve the block success rate while decreasing the incidence of nerve injury. Despite this claim, evidence shows there is no statistical difference in the success rate, block onset, or incidence of nerve injury when comparing the paresthesia-seeking and nerve stimulator techniques (Neal et al., 2009).

Clinical Aspects

ASSESSMENT

The performance of peripheral nerve blocks continues to evolve and now includes the use of ultrasound guidance. The first use of this technique in anesthesiology was reported by La Grange, Foster, and Pretorius (1978). Doppler ultrasound was used to detect blood flow in the subclavian artery to assist in the placement of a supraclavicular brachial plexus block. This technology was limited and prevented anesthesia providers from directly visualizing the nerves. The first use of ultrasound guidance to observe needle placement and the spread of local anesthetic was by Ting and Sivagnanaratnam (1989) during placement of axillary blocks. The performance of ultrasound-guided peripheral nerve blocks continue to expand with the development of new approaches and techniques.

The use of ultrasound guidance when performing peripheral nerve blocks allows nurse anesthetists to directly visualize in real time, neurovascular structures, fascial planes, surrounding anatomic structures, needle advancement, and the spread of local anesthetic during injection. Several advantages associated with the use of ultrasound guidance with or without the use of a peripheral nerve stimulator have emerged in recent literature (Lewis, Price, Walker, McGrattan, & Smith, 2015). Block performance times are shorter, while the rate of pain experienced during the block significantly reduced. Ultrasound guidance also leads to higher block success rates with improved sensory and motor blockade. As a result, patients are less likely to require supplemental or rescue blockade postoperatively (Lewis et al., 2015). A significant advantage has been a reduction in the incidence of intravascular injections and subsequent local anesthetic systemic toxicity. Early supporters of ultrasound guidance claimed that the risk of nerve injury would be lower; however, recent data suggests there is no difference in the postoperative neurological side effects when comparing ultrasound-guided versus peripheral nerve stimulation techniques

(Munirama & McCleod, 2015). The use of ultrasound guidance has improved the efficacy and reduced the risk of performing a peripheral nerve blockade.

NURSING INTERVENTIONS, MANAGEMENT, AND IMPLICATIONS

Whether used as a surgical anesthetic or for postoperative analgesia, peripheral nerve blocks provide numerous benefits to surgical patients, including a decrease in anesthetic requirements and a reduction in postoperative pain. Patients report lower visual analogue scale ratings, greater satisfaction, and reduced opioid consumption during the recovery phase (Jakobson & Johnson, 2016). This reduction in opioids leads to a lower incidence in nausea and vomiting, respiratory depression, sedation, urinary retention, constipation, and pruritus. Peripheral nerve blocks may be used in conjunction with nonopioid medications as part of multimodal analgesia to help reduce pain and shorten the recovery period.

The duration of action of nerve blocks varies, depending on the type of peripheral nerve block performed, the local anesthetic chosen, and whether the block is performed as a single injection or as a continuous infusion with an indwelling catheter. Local anesthetics can be classified as being short, intermediate, or long acting. These medications are available in various concentrations and have a duration of action that can last from a few hours up to 3 days. The local anesthetic can be administered either as a single injection or as a continuous infusion. The single-injection technique involves a one-time administration of a local anesthetic around the target structure. The continuous infusion method includes the placement of a flexible indwelling catheter adjacent to the target structure. Local anesthetic is continuously administered through the catheter via an electronic or elastomeric pump to provide patients with postoperative analgesia for up to 3 days after surgery.

In today's health care delivery model, there is increasing pressure placed on health care providers to decrease hospital lengths of stay, surgical complications, and costs. Surgical procedures that previously required multiple days in a hospital are now being performed on an outpatient basis with the assistance of peripheral nerve blocks. Utilization of ultrasound guidance has also led to the development of peripheral nerve blocks that provide sensory blockade while preserving motor function. Patients are able to ambulate earlier after surgery with improved pain control. This can reduce the incidence of respiratory complications and deep vein thrombosis while also shortening the length of hospital stay (Epstein, 2014).

OUTCOMES

The implementation of ultrasound-guided peripheral nerve blocks into clinical practice can be challenging. Many anesthesia providers lack the training and knowledge required to operate ultrasound equipment. There is a steep learning curve for acquiring an image, identifying anatomical structures, guiding the needle, and recognizing the spread of local anesthetic. In addition, the initial cost associated with establishing an ultrasound-guided peripheral nerve block practice can be high. This includes the cost of additional education as well as the purchase of ultrasound equipment.

Summary

Peripheral nerve blocks have been refined over the years with the development of new technology and techniques. The placement of peripheral nerve blocks with anatomical landmarks has been replaced by the use of peripheral nerve stimulation and ultrasound technology. The combination of ultrasound guidance with the advent of safer and longer acting local anesthetics has improved anesthesia care and increased the demand for peripheral nerve blocks. Although there are barriers to implementing this anesthetic modality into the clinical practice, the benefits to patients should be considered by nurse anesthetists.

Epstein, N. E. (2014). A review article on the benefits of early mobilization following spinal surgery and other medical/surgical procedures. *Surgical Neurology International*, 5(Suppl. 3), S66–S73.

Jakobson, J., & Johnson, M. Z. (2016). Perioperative regional anesthesia and postoperative longer-term outcomes. *F1000Research*, 5(F1000), 2501. doi:10.12688/f1000research.9100.1

Klein, S. M., Melton, M. S., Grill, W., & Nielsen, K. C. (2012). Peripheral nerve stimulation in regional anesthesia. *Regional Anesthesia and Pain Medicine*, 37(4), 383–392.

La Grange, P., Foster, P. A., & Pretorius, L. K. (1978). Application of ultrasound blood flow detector in supraclavicular brachial plexus block. *British Journal of Anaesthesia*, 50(9), 965–967.

Lewis, S. R., Price, A., Walker, K. J., McGrattan, K., & Smith, A. F. (2015). Ultrasound guidance for upper and lower limb blocks. *Cochrane Database of Systematic Reviews*, 9, 1–108. doi:10.1002/14651858

Lopez-Valverde, A., De Vicente, J., & Cutando, A. (2011). The surgeons Halsted and Hall, cocaine and the discovery of dental anesthesia by nerve blocking. *British Dental Journal*, 211(10), 485–487.

Marhofer, P., & Harrop-Griffiths, W. (2011). Nerve locations in regional anesthesia: finding what lies beneath the skin. *British Journal of Anaesthesia*, 106(1), 3–5.

Munirama, S., & McCleod, G. (2015). A systematic review and meta-analysis of ultrasound versus electrical stimulation for peripheral nerve location and blockade. *Anaesthesia*, 70(9), 1084–1091.

Neal, J. M., Garancher, J. C., Heble, J. R., Ilfeld, B. M., McCartney, C. J., Franco, C. D., & Hogan, Q. H. (2009). Upper extremity regional anesthesia: Essentials of our current understanding. *Regional Anesthesia and Pain Medicine*, 34(2), 134–170.

Ting, P. C., & Sivagnanaratnam, V. (1989). Ultrasonographic study of the spread of local anaesthetic during axillary brachial plexus block. *British Journal of Anaesthesia*, 63(3), 326–329.

■ POSTOPERATIVE NAUSEA AND VOMITING

Kimberly Kimble

Overview

Postoperative nausea and vomiting (PONV) is a common, yet distressing side effect of general surgery and is a leading cause of patient dissatisfaction after anesthesia. Despite advances in treatment modalities and the implementation of evidence-based prevention protocols, the incidence of PONV remains 30% in postsurgical patients and up to 80% in high-risk patients (Hooper, 2015). PONV has untowardly effects on both adult and pediatric patients, resulting in increased utilization of health care resources. The Anesthesia Quality Institute has listed PONV as a quality indicator requiring documentation for each patient. Consequently, perioperative guidelines providing current and comprehensive information are continuously being revised in an attempt to curtail the occurrence of PONV (American Society of Anesthesiology, 2014).

Background

Postoperative nausea and vomiting is defined as nausea, retching, or vomiting that occurs 24 to 48 hours after surgery (Berkun, Khechen, & Berkun, 2016). The etiology behind PONV is not fully understood, as there is no anatomically defined "vomiting center" in the brain. The chemoreceptor trigger zone (CRTZ) and nucleus tractus solitarius (NTS), implicated in the pathophysiology of vomiting, are distributed throughout the medulla oblongata of the brainstem and communicate through dopamine-2 (D2) receptors. There are also neurotransmitter pathways between the brainstem and gastrointestinal tract, including serotonin, which communicates with the CRTZ via serotonin 5-HT3 receptors. The vestibular system, responsible for detecting changes in equilibrium, communicates with the NTS via histamine-1 (H1) and acetylcholine (mACh) receptors (Berkun, et al., 2016). Complications associated with PONV include pulmonary aspiration of gastric content, esophageal perforation, bleeding, and wound dehiscence (Stoicea et al., 2015). Though these complications are rare, their prevention requires reducing the incidence of PONV through identification of high-risk patients.

Risk factors for PONV in adult patients can be categorized into three groups: patient specific, anesthetic-related, and surgically related. Patient-specific risk factors include female gender, history of PONV, younger age, nonsmoker, and obesity. Female gender is considered to be the greatest risk factor for postoperative nausea, prevailing in women three to four times more than men (Stoicea et al., 2015). Anesthetic risk factors include the use of volatile anesthetics, nitrous oxide, and perioperative opioid administration. Postoperative opioid administration is considered one of the most likely predictors of PONV. Incidence was decreased by 6% when postoperative opioid administration was reduced by half (Stoicea et al., 2016). Duration and type of surgery are surgically related risk factors. Abdominal, ear, nose, throat, and longer duration procedures have higher incidences of PONV. For children, risk factors are as follows: surgeries lasting longer than 30 minutes, patients older than 3 years, those receiving strabismus surgery, and patients with a history of postoperative vomiting (POV) or family history of PONV (Hooper, 2015). With the exception of patient-specific risk factors, all others can be modified to reduce the chance of patients developing nausea and vomiting (Berkun et al., 2016).

Though relatively common and short-lived, patients list PONV as one of the most dreaded postoperative side effects of anesthesia causing more distress than postoperative pain (Stoicea et al., 2015). Protracted nausea and vomiting can lead to extended postanesthesia care unit (PACU) length of stay, unplanned admissions, and increased health care costs. Nausea and vomiting not relieved after discharge have been associated with inability to return to work, impaired performance of activities of daily living, and are often associated with emergency room visits and hospital readmission (Hooper, 2015). The goal in treating PONV involves reducing patient distress through prophylaxis, thus reducing health care cost and resource consumption.

Clinical Aspects

The high prevalence of PONV in adults and children undergoing general anesthesia has prompted the development of multidisciplinary, evidence-based guidelines to aid in prophylactic management for PONV. The American Society of Anesthesiologists (2014) adopted PONV guidelines from the Society for Ambulatory Anesthesia (SAMBA) recommendations. SAMBA convened a multidisciplinary group of health care professionals to create PONV guidelines based on scientific evidence of clinical effectiveness. The guidelines define risk factors, have demonstrated effective prophylaxis, and are adaptable to different surgical settings (Hooper, 2015).

ASSESSMENT

Assessment of each patient in the preoperative period is crucial to identifying those at risk for developing nausea and vomiting postoperatively. According to SAMBA, there are four risk factors shown to cause increased incidence of nausea and vomiting when present in adult patients. Female gender, history of PONV, patients younger than 50 years of age, and use of opioids are all individually given one point based on the SAMBA risk factor scoring system. For every factor present in an adult patient, one point is assessed, and the risk for PONV increases by 20%. For instance, a patient with zero risk factors has a 10% to 20% chance of developing nausea and vomiting, whereas a patient with all four risk factors has an 80% chance (Berkun et al., 2016). Similarly, SAMBA risk factors for children include: those older than 3 years of age, surgery lasting longer than 30 minutes, patients receiving strabismus surgery, and patients with history of POV or family history of PONV. If no risk factors are present in a child, his or her risk of developing POV is 10%. Risk remains at 10% for one risk factor and increases to 30%, 50%, and 70% for each additional risk factor (Hooper, 2015).

Clinical practice guidelines for PONV have been established for over a decade; however, there continues

to be poor provider compliance (Kolanek et al., 2014). Perianesthesia nurses must advocate for guideline adherence. By including SAMBA risk assessment in the preoperative setting, results can be communicated to the interdisciplinary team responsible for patient care (Hooper, 2015).

NURSING INTERVENTIONS, MANAGEMENT, AND IMPLICATIONS

The SAMBA guidelines also suggest reducing baseline risk factors for PONV by incorporating specific interventions: using regional anesthesia instead of general anesthesia, using propofol intraoperatively, avoiding nitrous oxide and volatile anesthetics, minimizing opioid administration, and hydrating adequately (Hooper, 2015). Certified registered nurse anesthetists (CRNA) are responsible for developing a patient-tailored anesthetic plan. For a patient with increased risk of PONV, the CRNA can minimize opioid administration by using multimodal pain management techniques. Total intravenous anesthetic (TIVA) techniques can be incorporated to reduce the use of volatile anesthetics. CRNAs can also ensure adequate hydration by collaborating with preoperative providers to ensure that hydration starts preoperatively and is continued intraoperatively and postoperatively.

Additional SAMBA recommendations involve the administration of prophylactic medications, using one to two antiemetics for moderate-risk patients and more than two for high-risk patients (Hooper, 2015). The use of multiple antiemetics from different pharmacological classes has been proven more effective and causes fewer side effects than multiple doses of a single antiemetic (Berkun et al., 2016). The recommended first- and second-line classes of pharmacologic antiemetics are 5-HT3 receptor antagonist, corticosteroids, NK-1 receptor antagonist, phenothiazines, phenylethylamines, butyrophenones, antihistamines, and anticholinergics (American Society of Anesthesiologists, 2014). Although the perioperative nurse is not directly responsible for the ordering of prophylactic antiemetics, communication of the risk with the surgical and anesthetic team is critical to identify patients at risk. Nurses can also implement nonpharmacologic interventions to supplement the pharmacologic plan. Examples include music therapy, aromatherapy, and supplemental oxygen (Hooper, 2015).

OUTCOMES

After at-risk patients are identified and an appropriate PONV prophylactic plan of action is determined, the final SAMBA guidelines suggest ensuring that treatment and prevention methods are implemented and assessing the postoperative needs of patients to identify those who did not receive treatment or in whom prophylaxis failed (Hooper, 2015). Assessment and treatment of PONV should be routinely documented and communicated throughout the perioperative setting. Hooper (2015) suggests quantifying nausea and vomiting in a fashion similar to the pain assessment scale, ranging from 0 to 10. Nausea and vomiting occurring postoperatively should be treated with an antiemetic from a different class than the one used intraoperatively. If no antiemetic was given, the initial recommended and gold standard treatment would be a 5-HT3 receptor antagonist like ondansetron (Berkun et al., 2016).

Summary

Although rarely life-threatening, PONV continues to be a leading cause of patient dissatisfaction. Prophylactic guidelines provide insight on evidence-based multimodal treatment. However, guideline utilization continues to be poor among the medical and nursing professions. Routine implementation of guideline recommendations like SAMBA and others is key to improving patient outcomes and overall satisfaction. Nursing implications include assessment of risk factors, advocating for patients by ensuring implementation of prophylactic regimens, and evaluation of institutional roadblocks that cause reduced compliance.

American Society of Anesthesiologists. (2014). Prevention of postoperative nausea and vomiting-combination therapy. Retrieved from https://www.asahq.org/~/media/sites/asahq/files/public/resources/quality%20improvement/measures-clearinghouse/ponv-combination-therapy-for-adults-at-high-risk-for-ponv-oct-2015.pdf?la=en

Berkun R., Khechen B., & Berkun R. (2016). Incident reduction of postoperative nausea and vomiting (PONV) following office-based surgery: A retrospective chart analysis. *Journal of Anesthesia & Critical Care Open Access*, 5(4). doi:10.15406/jaccoa.2016.05.00197

Hooper, V. D. (2015). SAMBA consensus guidelines for the management of postoperative nausea and vomiting: An executive summary for perianesthesia nurses. *Journal of Perianesthesia Nurses*, 30(5), 377–382.

Kolanek, B., Svartz, L., Robin, F., Boutin, F., Beylacq, L., Lasserre, M.-C.,...Nouette-Gaulain, K. (2014). Management program decreases postoperative nausea and vomiting in high-risk and general surgical patients: A quality improvement cycle. *Minerva Anesthesiologica*, 80(3), 337–346.

Stoicea, N., Gan, T. J., Joseph, N., Uribe, A., Pandya, J., Dalal, R., & Bergese, S. D. (2015). Alternate therapies for the prevention of postoperative nausea and vomiting. *Frontiers in Medicine*, 2(87). doi:10.3389/fmed.2015.00087

■ RESPIRATORY DEPRESSION AND PATIENT-CONTROLLED ANALGESIA

Sonya D. Moore

Overview

In the United States, more than 43 million Americans receive anesthesia for surgical procedures per year and require postoperative pain management (American Association of Nurse Anesthetists, 2016). Intravenous patient-controlled analgesia (IVPCA) is commonly used for postoperative patients with acute pain. It is important to acknowledge that patient-controlled analgesia (PCA) may not always be administered intravenously. PCA administration also includes oral, transdermal, subcutaneous, intramuscular, and epidural routes when the patient is expected to manage the administration of an analgesic medication. However, the focus of this entry is on the evidence base between respiratory depression and PCA. For nurse anesthetists and health care providers managing postoperative or procedural pain, there has been a long-standing concern about which patients to prescribe IVPCA and the pharmcotherapeutic agents that optimize pain control without inducing respiratory depression.

Background

Patient-controlled analgesia (PCA) is a widely used strategy to manage pain among postoperative and procedural patients. The concept of PCA was studied and developed in the 1960s by Dr. Philip Sechzer. Patients could push a button and receive a 1-mL injection of intravenous solution containing small doses of morphine or meperidine per the reinforcement schedule. Sechzer postulated that the patient-controlled analgesic demand system is an efficient and satisfactory means of providing analgesia (Sechzer, 1971).

The orientation to permit patients to receive as-needed doses of analgesic medications was initially supported by evidence of inadequate pain control among patients with acute, postoperative pain (Golembiewski, Dasta, & Palmer, 2016). Conventional techniques of the time principally used opioid administration (oral and intramuscular routes) but did not provide sufficient pain relief. However, studies of patients controlling their own analgesia allow for lower dosing and greater efficacy than when administered by another individual, such as a nurse. (Golembiewski, et al., 2016).

As PCA devices have evolved, a greater ease of programming and more sophisticated programing have allowed for easier use. The advent of several modes and variables aided in PCA's ability to manage pain (Golembiewski et al., 2016; Grass, 2005). A demand dose and continuous infusion with a demand dose are the most frequently used methods. All PCA devices have the ability to deliver an initial loading dose, demand dose, lockout interval, background infusion, and dose limits (Grass, 2005). The lock-out variable is designed to prevent overdosage by monitoring the amount of time after a demand dose. All parenteral opioids have been used in for PCAs, with morphine being the most utilized. Opioids are mu receptor agonists. The ligand binds with the mu receptor and activates the G protein. This effect results in primarily inhibitory actions. Adenylate cyclase and voltage-dependent calcium channels are depressed (Hemmings & Egan, 2013). Morphine is considered the "gold standard" for opiates. The active metabolite of morphine M6G has similar effects as morphine, causing a delayed onset of respiratory depression (Grass, 2005 & Hemmings & Egan, 2013).

Respiratory depression has been quantified in most studies by the observed changes in respiratory frequency and alterations in oxygen saturation (Dahan, Aarts, & Smith, 2010). Prolonged alterations in respiratory status can lead to a multitude of adverse outcomes: compromised wound healing, brain dysfunction, arrhythmias, and myocardial ischemia (Belcher et al., 2016). The mu agonist (opioids) depresses the ventilatory control center in the medulla, altering the response to arterial carbon dioxide (Hemmings & Egan, 2013). This alteration results in hypoxemic hypoxia from hypoventilation. The decrease in respiratory rate and tidal volume results in increased arterial carbon dioxide and decreased oxygen tension at the tissues (Samuel & Franklin 2008). The literature is insufficient to determine whether supplemental oxygen decreases the incidence of respiratory depression or masks it (Horlocker et al., 2016).

Clinical Aspects

ASSESSMENT

When considering whether an IVPCA is the best technique to use to manage an individual's postoperative pain, the anesthetist must decide whether the candidate is suitable. Numerous factors play a role in patient selection. The question to the provider should be whether the patient is susceptible or has any of the factors that predispose the patient to hypoxia. These factors include age, type of surgery, type and duration of anesthesia, obesity, and obstructive sleep apnea (Belcher et al., 2016). One must keep in mind that opioid-induced hypoventilation is the major cause of respiratory depression in the patient receiving an IVPCA. Adequate monitoring techniques and opioid titration are highly recommended by the Anesthesia Safety Foundation (Belcher et al., 2016).

The literature is consistent that the first 24 hours are when vigilance should be at its greatest and sedation scales should be used and no further monitoring detail noted. The respiratory assessment should include the frequency, depth, and quality of respiration. Respirations of 8 to 10 per minute (for a full minute count), and/or shallow in nature is considered respiratory depression (Dahan, Aarts and Smith, 2010).

NURSING INTERVENTIONS, MANAGEMENT, AND IMPLICATIONS

The American Society of Anesthesiologists created guidelines for The prevention, detection, and management of respiratory depression associated with neuraxial opioid administration (spinal or epidural administration of opioids; Horlocker et al., 2016):

■ Monitor during the entire time infusion is in place

■ Monitor continually for the first 20 minutes after initiation

■ Monitor at least once per hour until 12 hours have passed

■ For first 12 to 24 hours, monitor at least once every 2 to 4 hours

Electronic monitoring is used as an adjunct to the physical assessment to determine adequate respiration and ventilation. The pulse oximeter is used as a measurement of gas exchange in the lungs. Specific measurement of hypoxemia varies in the literature. In Dahan's review, when postoperative hypoxemia is SpO_2 less than 94%, moderate hypoxemia is SpO_2 less than 90%, and severer hypoxemia is SpO_2 less than 85% for more than 6 minutes per hour, end-tidal carbon dioxide monitoring allows for the trending of ventilatory status. The Anesthesia Patient Safety Foundation discovered that by monitoring end-tidal carbon dioxide ($ETCO_2$) trends and alarms, respiratory depression can be detected as much as 2 hours earlier than SpO_2 (Horlocker et al., 2012). The $ETCO_2$ concentration rises in the presence of spontaneous breathing with adequate air exchange but decreased ventilation. Respiratory depression may occur with the most vigilant provider. Along with monitoring, safe practice must be followed. The use of the IVPCA without the continuous basal infusion has little to no incidence of respiratory depression (Grass, 2005).

OUTCOMES

Alternative routes for PCA administration also decrease the incidence of respiratory depression. Patient-controlled epidural analgesia (PCEA) is commonly practiced with less side effects and greater patient satisfaction. The use of combined opiate and local anesthetic minimize the side effects and increase the efficacy than when used singly (Grass, 2005). Peripheral nerve catheters (PCAs) have proven efficacious in minimizing the sensory and motor blockade. A smaller amount of local anesthetic can be infused with these catheters. Transdermal PCAs are available and allow for more patient control and decreased programmable errors. Patient-controlled analgesia utilizing sublingual sufentanil is showing promise. The limitation with this system is that it requires the patient to have the dexterity and cognitive ability to operate the device (Golembiewski et al., 2016; Grass, 2005; Viscusi et al., 2016).

Summary

IVPCA with opiates continues to be an integral part of postoperative pain management and has changed how the industry viewed postoperative pain management. The vigilant and prudent provider must make certain the patient is monitored and that human-based errors are minimized. Many pain and safety organizations have created guidelines or made recommendations as to how we can abolish respiratory depression with IVPCA use. The literature demonstrates a consensus that monitoring standards should be in place.

The future of PCA use is growing, as is multimodal pain management. Minimizing the use of opiates, using weak mu agonist or non-mu agonist and or alternate techniques mentioned earlier may decrease the occurrence of respiratory depression.

American Association of Nurse Anesthetists. (2016). CRNA fact sheet. Retrieved from http://www.aana.com/ceand education/becomeacrna/Pages/Nurse-Anesthetists -at-a-Glance.aspx

Belcher, A. W., Khanna, A. K., Leung, S., Naylor, A. J., Hutcherson, M. T., Nguyen, B. M., . . . Saager, L. (2016). Long-acting patient-controlled opioids are not associated with more postoperative hypoxemia than short-acting patient-controlled opioids after noncardiac surgery: A cohort analysis. *Anesthesia–Analgesia, 123*(6), 1471–1479. Retrieved from http://www.anesthesia -analgesia.org

Dahan, A., Aarts, L., & Smith, T. W. (2010). Incidence, reversal, and prevention of opioid-induced respiratory depression. *Anesthesiology, 112*(1), 226–238.

Golembiewski, J., Dasta, J., & Palmer, P. P. (2016). Evolution of patient-controlled analgesia: From intravenous to sublingual treatment. *Hospital Pharmacy, 51*(3), 214–229.

Grass, J. A. (2005). Patient-controlled analgesia. *Anesthesia & Analgesia, 101*(Suppl.), S44–S61.

Hemmings, H. C., & In Egan, T. D. (2013). *Pharmacology and physiology for anesthesia: Foundations and clinical application* (pp. 253–271). Philadelphia, PA: Elsevier Saunders.

Horlocker, T., Burton, A. W., Connis, R. T., Hughes, S. C., Nickinovich, D. G., Palmer, C. M., . . . Wu, C. L. (2016). Practice guidelines for the prevention, detection, and management of respiratory depression associated with neuraxial opioid administration. *Anesthesiology, 124*(3), 535–552.

Samuel J., & Franklin C. (2008) Hypoxemia and hypoxia. In J. A. Myers, K. W. Millikan, & T. J. Saclarides (Eds.), *Common surgical diseases* (2nd ed., pp. 391–394). New York, NY: Springer.

Sechzer, P. H. (1971). Studies in pain with the analgesic-demand system. *Anesthesia & Analgesia, 50*(1), 1–10.

Viscusi, E. R., Grond, S., Ding, L., Danesi, H., Jones, J. B., & Sinatra, R. S. (2016). A comparison of opioid-related adverse events with fentanyl iontophoretic transdermal system versus morphine intravenous patient-controlled analgesia in acute postoperative pain. *Pain Management, 6*(1), 19–24.

■ SICKLE CELL DISEASE AND ANESTHESIA

Mark A. Caldwell
Sonya D. Moore
Ronald L. Hickman, Jr.

Overview

Sickle cell disease (SCD) is a recessive autosomal disorder that disproportionately affects African Americans. It is estimated that one out of 365 African American children will be born with sickle cell disease (Centers for Disease Control and Prevention, 2016b). Individuals with sickle cell disease inherit an abnormal variant of hemoglobin, known as hemoglobin S, which is the result of a defect in the beta goblin component of hemoglobin and alters its structure. The hemoglobin S variant will form a sickle shape when encountering a deoxygenating or dehydrating environment within the body. Persons living with sickle cell trait, asymptomatic carriers, should not be confused with those diagnosed with sickle cell disease, individuals who are homozygous for the two recessive alleles and are symptomatic. Individuals with sickle cell disease have a structural defect in the hemoglobin, which predisposes them to inefficient oxygen delivery and chronic anemia. Individuals with sickle cell disease require thoughtful anesthesia care to minimize the damaging effects of sickle cell disease and maximize their recovery after a diagnostic or surgical procedure.

Background

Individuals whose ancestry originated in sub-Saharan Africa, Mediterranean countries, India, and equatorial countries are the persons most frequently affected with sickle cell disease. Sickle cell disease affects approximately 100,000 people in the United States. Sickle cell trait is present in one in 13 African American births. One percent of children born with SCD die within the first 3 years of life. Fortunately, deaths in children younger than 4 years have declined by 42% between 1999 and 2002. For SCD, $475 million for health care costs were generated within the United States between 1989 and 1993 (Centers for Disease Control and Prevention, 2016a).

Organ infarction, pain, and vasoocclusive problems occur due to the sickled cells obstructing the microcirculatory system. Sickling is intermittent with multiple triggers that include hypothermia, low plasma volume, increased hydrogen ion concentration, and hypoxemia (decreased pO_2). The level of oxygen already present at the tissue level will also affect the sickle rate as the hemoglobin will have to give up more of its oxygen to more deoxygenated tissue. A stressor to the body can also affect sickling by inducing a greater need for oxygen at the tissue level (McCance & Huether, 2014).

Acute chest syndrome (ACS) can occur in these patients as a result of the sickled erythrocytes. In ACS, the microcirculation within the pulmonary system is affected. Fever, cough, and hypoxia are the symptomatology in children. In adults, the symptoms include skeletal pain, hypoxia, chest pain, fever, cough, and dyspnea. A new pulmonary infiltrate on chest radiograph, fever, and hypoxia are features of ACS. Patients with acute chest syndrome often present with some degree of hypoxia, which can quickly progress to life-threatening states of hypoxia and hypoxemia, if not treated. For patients with sickle cell disease undergoing a surgical procedure, ACS can occur at any time during the perioperative continuum. However, ACS most commonly occurs in the postoperative period among patients with SCD. Patients at the highest risk of ACS are patients with SCD who have undergone abdominal surgery, profound volume depletion, or uncorrected anemia.

Clinical Aspects

ASSESSMENT

Pain, organ damage, anemia, and vasoocclusive events can occur as a consequence of a sickle cell crisis. The lodging of the sickled cells within the vasculature creates the vasoocclusive event. Anemia occurs as the number of red blood cells circulating decline from their decreased life span and their propensity to sickle when becoming deoxygenated. With the occlusion of smaller vessels, organ damage can be a subsequent event. Pain develops from the occlusion of these vessels in the body and the organs (McCance & Huether, 2014; Oprea, 2012). Prevention of these problems is a focus of anesthesia care provided by a nurse anesthetist.

Based on the fraction of hemoglobin S, there is significant interpersonal variation in the clinical picture of patients with sickle cell disease across the perioperative continuum. Due to patient variability, multiple recommendations for patient care have been outlined, but may differ in application depending on the extent of the patient's sickle cell disease. During any procedure involving sickle cell patients, goals include avoiding hypothermia, dehydration, and acidosis. Sickling events can occur related to these conditions (Franco & Gabot, 2014). Hypothermia causes peripheral vasoconstriction and vascular stasis; therefore, maintaining normothermia is essential. Convection thermoregulation devices and fluid warmers are used to maintain patient core temperature. Warming the operating room prior to induction also aids in maintaining normothermia (Firth, & Head, 2004). If hydration is not maintained, circulatory stasis can occur. Prudent consideration should be taken in measuring fluid intake and output among patients "at risk for" or who "have known" impaired renal or cardiac function (Miller, Eriksson, Fleisher, Wiener-Kronish, Cohen, & Young, 2015). The correction of anemia is important as it may lead to hypoxia causing increased sickling. If there are large fluid shifts and the procedure is lengthy, a method to perform acid–base analysis should be considered (Firth, & Head, 2004). Most important, correcting the underlying cause of the academia (Firth, & Head, 2004).

Elevation of normal hemoglobin through blood transfusion preoperatively has shown no benefit. However, obtaining a 30% hematocrit is a management goal for these patients, especially for procedures deemed high risk. High-risk procedures include intracranial and intrathoracic surgeries, hip surgery, and hip replacement (Oprea, 2012). A detriment to blood transfusion, blood viscosity can increase when blood is transfused, creating the environment for further occlusive events especially in the organs or the periphery of the body (Franco & Gabot, 2014). Vasoocclusive events should be avoided; thus, optimal patient positioning is encouraged for surgical procedures under anesthesia, and the use of tourniquets on the extremity to decrease blood flow to the operative site is controversial (Oprea, 2012).

NURSING INTERVENTIONS, MANAGEMENT, AND IMPLICATIONS

The choice of anesthetic technique should be made based on patient assessment. A general anesthetic may be preferred because regional anesthesia, though not contraindicated, may render the patient more susceptible to sickling in nonblocked areas. During a general anesthetic, care must be taken to avoid hypothermia, dehydration, and acidosis (Firth, & Head, 2004). Inhalation agents with neuroprotective and cardioprotective qualities should be considered during maintenance of anesthesia. If muscle relaxation is needed, depolarizers and nondepolarizes are appropriate (Firth, & Head, 2004). Postoperative management is focused on adequate analgesia, early mobilization, and oxygen supplementation (Firth & Head, 2004). High tolerance to opioids is frequent among patients with sickle cell disease due to recurrent pain crises. Pain management postoperatively may prove challenging (Oprea, 2012). Adherence to evidence-based guidelines for the administration of opioid medications should be discussed with the patient's surgical and hematology teams.

OUTCOMES

Prompt attention and recognition should be given to the risk of acute chest syndrome in these patients. Respiratory support may be needed. Oxygen-level maintenance guidelines intraoperatively and postoperatively include keeping the SaO_2 greater than or equal to 95% or within 3% of the patient's baseline. Postoperative care should involve pain relief, adequate hydration, incentive spirometry, bronchodilators, and blood transfusion. Advanced respiratory support may also be needed in some cases (Howard et al., 2015).

Summary

Patients with sickle cell disease may present a challenge to the nurse anesthetist. The nurse anesthetist must be aware of and understand the modalities of treatment for sickle cell disease, and the impact of condition and its treatment will have on the patient planned to receive anesthesia. Current medical therapy involves hydroxyurea. It increases the fraction of hemoglobin F, which has shown to reduce incidence of vasoocculsive crises, sickling, and acute chest syndrome. There is some evidence that lower levels of circulating neurtrophils may be beneficial and aid in minimizing the likelihood of a vasoocculsive crisis (Agrawal, Patel, Shah, Nainiwal, & Trivedi, 2014). Avoiding hypothermia, hypovolemia, acidosis, and occlusion of vessels is the goal of anesthesia for the sickle cell patient. Ensuring optimal oxygen saturation throughout any procedure helps prevent sickling events and promote an uneventful recovery for the patient with sickle cell disease.

Agrawal, R. K., Patel, R. K., Shah, V., Nainiwal, L., & Trivedi, B. (2014). Hydroxyurea in sickle cell disease: Drug review. *Indian Journal Hematology Blood Transfusion, 30*(2), 91–96.

Centers for Disease Control and Prevention. (2016a). Data and statistics. Retrieved from https://www.cdc.gov/ncbddd/sicklecell/data.html

Centers for Disease Control and Prevention. (2016b). Sickle cell trait. Retrieved from https://www.cdc.gov/ncbddd/sicklecell/traits.html

Firth, P. G., & Head, A. (2004). Sickle cell disease and anesthesia. *Anesthesiology, 101*(3), 766–785.

Franco, J. & Gabot, M. (2014). Hematology and anesthesia. In J. Nagelhout & K. Plaus (Eds.), *Nurse anesthesia* (5th ed., pp. 896–898). St. Louis, MO: Elsevier.

Howard, J., Hart, N., Roberts-Harewood, M., Cummins, M., Awogbade, M., & Davis, B. (2015) Guideline on the management of acute chest syndrome in sickle cell disease. *British Journal of Haematology, 169*(4), 492–505. doi:10.1111/bjh.13348

McCance, K. L., & Huether, S. E. (2014) *Pathophysiology: The biologic basis for disease in adults and children* (7th ed., pp. 1063–1069). St. Louis, MO: Elsevier.

Miller, R., Eriksson, L., Fleisher, L., Wiener- Kronish, J., Cohen, N., & Young, W. (2015). *Miller's anesthesia* (8th ed.). Philadelphia, PA: Saunders.

Oprea, A. D. (2012). Hematologic disorders. In R. L. Hines & K. E. Marschall (Eds.), *Stoelting's anesthesia and co-existing disease* (6th ed., pp. 411–413). Philadelphia, PA: Elsevier.

Obstetrics and Women's Health

Women's health covers a vast array of unique health issues and concerns for all women, beginning in adolescence, through childbirth, menopause, and on through the "golden years."

This unit enhances our understanding of the important and specialized role OB/GYN nurses play in the delivery of care to women. This specialty offers a wide range of opportunities and challenges in providing education, care, and compassion to women, such as the GYN patient struggling to get pregnant, someone dealing with ovarian cancer, intimate partner violence, or menopause. Women's health encompasses both physiological and psychological issues that require a highly knowledgeable, empathetic, and skilled nurse.

In addition to GYN, this section also describes the obstetrical aspect of women's health. Throughout pregnancy, women may face many health care issues impacting their health and that of the baby. Pregnancy can often lead to complications, including diabetes and hypertension; therefore, a wide medical knowledge base is important to a highly skilled obstetrical nurse. Working in labor and delivery is like no other place in the hospital. It resembles the emergency department (ED; as you never know what is coming in the door). You will need the operating room (OR), where clinical surgery is performed; and the delivery room, where you coach moms and provide labor support. Critical care thinking is also a major skill as this is a high-risk area, and you have two patients to care for, mother and baby. It is extremely challenging, but the satisfaction of bringing life into the world is surely the greatest reward any nurse could experience!

- Breast Cancer and *BRCA Una Hopkins*
- Cervical Cancer *Godsfavour Guillet*
- Contraception *Latina M. Brooks*
- Endometriosis *Ingrid Apryl Spears*
- Episiotomy *Loraine O'Neill*
- Home Birth *Sabrina Nitkowski-Keever*
- Infertility *Tammy M. Lampley*
- Intimate Partner Violence *Marilyn E. Smith*
- In Vitro Fertilization *Donna Lynn Rose and Mary T. Quinn Griffin*
- Labor and Delivery *Carrie Gerber*
- Lactation *Jarold T. Johnston*
- Menopause *Maryann Clark*
- Motherhood *Stacen A. Keating and Miriam J. Chickering*
- Osteoporosis *Mary Variath*
- Ovarian Cancer *Kristine Cooper and Tasina Jones*
- Pelvic Pain *Loraine O'Neill*
- Perinatal Mood Disorders *Deepika Goyal*
- Polycystic Ovary Syndrome *Latina M. Brooks*
- Postpartum *Debra Bingham and Patricia Suplee*
- Postpartum Hemorrhage *Sabrina Nitkowski-Keever and Mary Anne Gallagher*
- Pregnancy *Miriam J. Chickering and Stacen A. Keating*
- Sexually Transmitted Infections *Maryann Clark*
- Skin Aesthetics *Erin Hennessey and Mary Anne Gallagher*

■ BREAST CANCER AND *BRCA*

Una Hopkins

Overview

Breast cancer 1 (*BRCA1*) and breast cancer 2 (*BRCA2*) are human suppressor genes responsible for DNA repair. All humans have these genes. Persons have higher risk for breast cancer if there is a mutation in either or both of these genes. These genes are mutated in 0.2% to 0.3% of the general population and 3% in breast cancer patients. Breast cancer incidence and prevalence in the United States, according to American Cancer Society

(ACS; n.d.) statistics, is that one in eight women will experience breast cancer, with approximately 40,000 deaths a year from the disease. Nurses facilitate appropriate screening for patients with mammography, ultrasound, and genetic testing for the appropriate patients.

Background

According to the Patient Protection and Affordable Care Act (ACA) in 2016, 2,600 males and 246,660 females were diagnosed with breast cancer of whom 40,890 will die of the disease. Breast cancer remains the leading cancer in women despite many excellent screening tools, such as 3D mammography and ultrasound for women with dense breasts. Having a genetic mutation in *BRCA1* or *BRCA2* increases the risk of being diagnosed with for breast and ovarian cancer. Approximately 55% to 65% of women who inherit the *BRCA1* gene and 45% of those who inherit the *BRCA2* gene will develop breast cancer by age 70 years. The risk of developing ovarian cancer by age 70 years occurs in 39% of women who inherit a *BRCA1* mutation and 11% to 17% of women who inherit a harmful *BRCA2* mutation. There are other diseases that *BRCA1* and *BRCA2* carriers have higher risk of being diagnosed with and they include fallopian tube peritoneal cancer, pancreatic cancer, and prostate cancer in male carriers.

There are specific geographies as well as ethnic backgrounds that hold higher incidence of *BRCA1* and *BRCA2* mutations. The geographic locations with a higher prevalence of *BRCA1* and *BRCA2* are Norway, Netherlands, and Iceland. The Ashkenazi Jewish population also carries a higher rate of mutations. There are specific genetic tests that can be run to detect mutations in *BRCA1* and *BRCA2*. These tests can be done on a person's DNA from a blood test or saliva. The testing is generally accompanied by a genetic counseling visit and is very important part of the care of this population. The counseling session will outline for the person what is being tested and the implications of a positive result. This first step is important as this is the point at which a person who will not be doing any risk-reduction interventions may decline testing. According to the U.S. Preventive Services Task Force (USPSTF) and the National Comprehensive Cancer Network (NCCN) guidelines, there are several people who should be tested in a high-risk group. The general public, due to the small amount of variations, should not be tested. The group of people that should be tested includes those with:

- Breast cancer diagnosed before age 50 years
- Bilateral breast cancer
- Both breast and ovarian cancers in either the same woman or the same family
- Multiple breast cancers
- Two or more primary types of *BRCA1*- or *BRCA2*- related cancers in a single family member
- Cases of male breast cancer
- Ashkenazi Jewish ethnicity (National Cancer Institute, 2017)

The recommendations direct clinicians to test the person with cancer before testing family members. There are cases in which this is not possible, and with a strong family history or high level of suspicion this should be completed. The recommendations also state not to test children younger than 18 years as there are no proven risk-reduction strategies for children. Interpreting the results of genetic testing should also be completed with a dialogue with the genetic counselor. The results will come back as positive, meaning the person has inherited a mutation in the *BRCA1* and/or *BRCA2* gene, or negative, meaning no mutation has been identified or there is a variant of unknown significance. When the results come back with this unknown variant it just means this is not correlated to an increased risk in a cancer (Chen & Parmigiani, 2014).

Clinical Aspects

ASSESSMENT

The person with known *BRCA1* and/or *BRCA2* mutation can undergo risk-reduction interventions that include enhanced screening, prophylactic surgery, and/or chemoprevention with medication. Enhanced screening may include starting a screening regimen with clinical breast exam and mammography at a much younger age than the general population. Screening can begin as early as 25 years for women who are at high risk according to the NCCN guidelines. An MRI may also be added to the screening regimen as it sometimes is more sensitive in women with dense breast tissue. Currently, there are no proven screening routines for ovarian cancer, but some clinicians will order annual pelvic ultrasounds. There is no evidence to support this practice as suggestive in reducing mortality (Warner et al., 2014).

NURSING INTERVENTIONS, MANAGEMENT AND IMPLICATIONS

Women can choose to have prophylactic surgery and remove breasts with mastectomy and a bilateral salpingo-oophorectomy. This decision is one that should be made after true counseling of the risk reduction in cancer development. The evidence is suggestive of a significant risk reduction to 80% in the development of ovarian cancer, and 56% in the development of breast cancer. The counseling of a female should also include that this risk reduction is not 100%, and there remains a possibility cancer will develop, as not all of the suspected tissue at risk can be removed in either one of these surgeries (Finch et al., 2015).

OUTCOMES

In addition to surgery, there were two major studies that demonstrated risk reduction with chemoprevention. The Study of Tamoxifen and Raloxifene (STAR) trial showed that a 5-year administration of tamoxifen or raloxifene decreased the risk of developing breast cancer in high-risk patients. This information can be extrapolated to the *BRCA1* and *BRCA2* carriers but has not specifically been studied in this group. There is some evidence to suggest that the use of oral contraceptives may reduce the risk of ovarian cancer (McLaughlin et al., 2007).

Summary

Men and women who carry mutations in *BRCA1* and *BRCA2* should be vigilant in their screening for breast cancer. Nursing's role is to continue health promotion through risk-reduction activities such as eating a healthy diet, exercising, and avoiding excessive alcohol intake. Nursing teaching in health promotion is critical to these high-risk persons.

American Cancer Society. (n.d.). Cancer statistics. Retrieved from http://onlinelibrary.wiley.com/doi/10.3322/caac.21332/full

Chen, S., & Parmigiani, G. (2014). Meta-analysis of BRCA1 and BRCA2 penetrance. *Journal of Clinical Oncology 2007*, 25(11), 1329–1333.

Finch, A. P., Lubinski, J., Møller, P., Singer, C. F., Karlan, B., Senter, L., . . . Narod, S. A. (2015). Impact of oophorectomy on cancer incidence and mortality in women with a BRCA1 or BRCA2 mutation. *Journal of Clinical Oncology*, 32(15), 1547–1553.

McLaughlin, J. R., Risch, H. A., Lubinski, J., Moller, P., Ghadirian, P., Lynch, H., . . . Narod, S. A. (2007). Reproductive risk factors for ovarian cancer in carriers of BRCA1 or BRCA2 mutations: A case-control study. *Lancet Oncology*, 8(1), 26–34.

National Cancer Institute. (2017). Genetics of breast and ovarian cancer PDQ. Retrieved from http:// www.cancer.gov/ types/ breast/ hp/ breast-ovarian-genetics-pdq

Warner, E., Plewes, D. B., Hill, K. A., Causer, P. A., Zubovits, J. T., Jong, R. A., . . . Narod, S. A. (2004). Surveillance of BRCA1 and BRCA2 mutation carriers with magnetic resonance imaging, ultrasound, mammography, and clinical breast examination. *Journal of the American Medical Association*, 292(11), 1317–1325.

■ CERVICAL CANCER

Godsfavour Guillet

Overview

Cervical cancer is the fourth most common cancer among women in the world, yet it is also one of the most preventable cancers if detected early. Best practice in nursing care of cervical cancer patients focuses on patient education, professional competence of the nurse, emotional support, and individualized care of the patient. Great significance is placed on the psychological characteristics of nursing care as well as focusing on effective communication skills and supportive care training for nurses.

Background

The direct annual health care costs for screening, treating, and managing abnormalities related to cervical cancer and cervical dysplasias in the United States are estimated to be as high as $8 billion. Although the direct costs of cervical cancer (invasive disease, screening, and testing) are substantial, annual indirect costs resulting from lost productivity and loss of earnings due to premature death are also significant and are estimated to be higher than direct costs.

In 2012, 527,000 new cases were diagnosed worldwide. The vast majority were reported in Eastern Africa. Malawi and Zambia representing two of the underdeveloped countries that shared the burden of approximately 84% of these cases due to late presentation and poor access to treatment (World Cancer Research Fund International, 2013). Mortality rate of cervical cancer patients in Malawi and Zambia is more than 50% (Kingham et al., 2013). Conversely, in Finland, cervical cancer is at the bottom of the list, in 20th place, with credit going to efficient national screening programs.

Cervical cancer is vastly more common in developing nations than it is in developed nations, like the United States. Congress enacted a Gynecological Cancer Education and Awareness Act in 2005 to create a strategy for improving efforts to increase awareness and knowledge of gynecological cancers among the public and health care providers.

In 2013, the MaZaFi 3-project was established in Malawi, Zambia, and Finland to promote high-quality health care and health care education through active participation and collaboration among the partner countries. This project aimed to promote evidence-based knowledge and clinical education to students from these three countries in a multicultural environment (CIMO, 2014).

Nearly all cervical cancers are caused by the human papilloma virus (HPV), which is the most common sexually transmitted infection (STI; McCormish, 2011). Genital HPV is commonly transmitted through epithelial contact with an infected cervical, vaginal, penile, or anal area (Bedford, 2009). Infection is often asymptomatic, which increases the risk of unwitting transmission.

Because of this, women who do not regularly have a Pap test to detect abnormal changes to the cervix are at increased risk of developing the disease. However, not all women who have been infected with HPV will develop cervical cancer if the virus naturally abates and the infection resolves. Other risk factors for developing cervical cancer include smoking, age, socioeconomic status, and the number of sexual partners in one's past. Familial history is an additional risk factor.

Persistent oncogenic HPV infection is the leading cause of cervical dysplasia and neoplasia, and evidence shows that oncogenic HPV is present in 99.7% of cervical cancer specimens. Cervical cancer and cervical dysplasias are responsible for the vast majority of morbidities and deaths associated with HPV-related illness. According to Rogers and Cantu (2009), a patient's quality of life (social, emotional, and sexual functioning) is adversely affected following a diagnosis with an HPV infection or cervical cancer.

There are two main types of cervical cancer. About 80% to 90% of cases are squamous cell carcinoma (thin, flat cells that line the bottom of the cervix) and 10% to 20% are adenocarcinoma (glandular cells that line the upper portion of the cervix). Metastatic cervical cancer is cancer that has spread to other parts of the body. In most cases, cervical cancer does not cause noticeable symptoms in the early stages of the disease. To facilitate early treatment, routine yearly Pap screening and exams by a gynecologist are important to check for abnormal cells in the cervix. The Pap test is one of the most reliable and effective cancer screening methods available. The HPV test may be utilized for abnormal cells in the cervix. Diagnostic procedures include Pap test, pelvic examination, PET/CT scan, colposcopy, cone biopsy loop electrosurgical excision procedure (LEEP), MRI, CT scan, lab tests, sentinel lymph node biopsy.

Cervical cancer is staged using the TNM system, where *tumor (T)* describes the size of the original tumor, *lymph node (N)* indicates whether the cancer is present in the lymph nodes, and *metastasis (M)* refers to whether cancer has spread to other parts of the body, usually the liver, bones, or brain. Stages 0 to IVB describe how far the cancer has spread into the tissues, cervix, uterus, pelvic walls, lymph nodes, and/or other organs.

Clinical Aspects

ASSESSMENT

Common symptoms of cervical cancer may include vaginal bleeding between periods, after sexual intercourse, or postmenopausal bleeding. Unusual vaginal discharge that is watery, pink, or foul-smelling is common as is pelvic pain during intercourse or at other times. In advanced stages, symptoms include weight loss, fatigue, back pain, leg pain or swelling, leakage of urine or feces from the vagina, and bone fractures. The patient will undergo a complete array of diagnostic tests, thorough review of medical records and health history, and a physical exam, including a pelvic exam. A general health history includes history and background information, allergies, childhood diseases/immunizations, hospitalizations/surgical procedures/injuries/fractures, medications, habits (alcohol, street drugs, caffeine, and tobacco use), and family medical history. This comprehensive information allows providers to create treatment recommendations best suited to the patient.

NURSING INTERVENTIONS, MANAGEMENT, AND IMPLICATIONS

Nursing care is holistic and individualized to the patient. Goals of plans of care are to alleviate suffering, restore and promote health, and prevent illness. Nurses use clinical judgment to facilitate the healing process. A nurse's role in care of the patient with cervical cancer is to educate the patient; encourage her to attend screening programs and treatments; and provide for her psychological, social, physical, emotional, spiritual and sexual needs during treatment, and all along the continuum of care (Bedford, 2009).

Care of the patient includes patient education to guide the patients' expectations and reduce anxiety and fears. Nurses utilize the principles of adult learning when providing education. They assess patients' readiness and ability to learn. Patient education must surround the experience and be comprehensive. Women with cervical cancer need information to understand the disease, its treatment and side effects, and potential changes it may have on sexuality and gender roles. Nurses must initiate conversations about sexuality issues with patients in a sensitive matter while offering practical problem-solving methods. Open communication and clear information about sexual concerns ease anxiety and foster acceptance and healing (Rasmusson & Thomé, 2008). Communication skills training for nursing staff highlighting listening and responding to psychosocial concerns that cancer patients may have is crucial.

Patient teaching will include symptoms, pathology, side effects, and body changes so that the patient understands and accepts them. Preoperative education regarding possible complications and postoperative education regarding pain management or sexual dysfunction are fundamental. Nurses should focus their attention on all the symptoms occurring during and after treatments, to reduce the severity of these symptoms, and prevent them from occurring by assessing and caring for their patients (Phianmongkhol & Suwan, 2008). Timing of nursing interventions is described as an important feature in patient care (Cook, McIntyre, & Recoche, 2014; Rasmusson & Thomé, 2008). According to Lloyd et al. (2014), providing statistical information about treatment survival, and recurrence rates may improve the patients' experience and decision making.

When choosing a treatment for cervical cancer, the most important factor to consider is the stage of the cancer. Other factors include age, physical condition, and type and location of the cancer (American Cancer Society, 2013). Based on these factors, surgery, chemotherapy, and/or radiation therapy is chosen as treatment. Women's fertility, pregnancy, and, where pertinent, the high prevalence of HIV and AIDS are a few additional special considerations when treating and managing cervical cancer. National and international groups, such as the World Health Organization (WHO), Scottish Intercollegiate Guidelines Network (SIGN), and the National Comprehensive Cancer Network (NCCN), have developed specific practice guidelines to help determine appropriate treatment in each stage.

Surgical interventions for cervical cancer include multiple options. Options range from simple hysterectomy (removal of cervix and uterus), radical hysterectomy (removal of cervix, uterus, upper part of the vagina, and a wide area of surrounding ligaments and tissues), total hysterectomy with salpingo-oophorectomy (removal of fallopian tubes and ovaries), and pelvic exenteration (in addition to cervix, uterus, vagina, ovaries and nearby lymph nodes, lower colon, rectum, and bladder are removed). Plastic surgery may be required to reconstruct an artificial vagina for the patient after other operations (National Cancer Institute, 2014). With larger and metastasized tumors, the standard treatment is radiation along with chemotherapy. This treatment has more severe side effects for the patient, such as infection and digestive system side effects.

Approximately 40% of women diagnosed with cervical cancer are concerned about fertility. Women may have a trachelectomy or oophoropexy to preserve fertility (Schwartz, 2009). Although it is rare, sometimes cervical cancer is diagnosed in pregnant women. This can be devastating for a woman and her family to accept, especially if treatment requires termination of the pregnancy. If in the early stage of pregnancy, up to 20 weeks, radical hysterectomy or chemo radiation may be offered. After 28 weeks of pregnancy, cancer may be treated after caesarean delivery of the baby.

Women with cervical cancer need a lot of support and may require interventions from social work and psychological counseling. Sexuality and sexual function changes related to treatment of cervical cancer and the loss of fertility may be very traumatic for some women. The psychological impact includes an altered body image and loss of femininity. Overall sexual dysfunction, dyspareunia, and adverse vaginal changes may persist for 2 years after completing therapy. This may lead to the need for other treatments for ovarian function or hormone replacement therapy to prevent osteoporosis, heart disease, and cerebrovascular accident. It is imperative for the nurse to establish an integrative plan of care that involves the necessary components of the interdisciplinary care team (Schwartz, 2009). Oncology nursing care layers competence with specialized medications and treatments and a focus on end-of-life care on top of the basic nursing skills.

OUTCOMES

The early stages of cervical cancer may be successfully detected through screening programs. This helps to prevent it from developing into malignant carcinoma. Routine Pap testing is the best way to detect abnormal changes to the cervix. Women who do not regularly have a Pap test are at increased risk of developing the disease. Cervical cancer is a major cause of suffering and premature death among women in the developing world; yet, it is largely prevented in most higher income countries. Barriers to screening include increased age, non-White race/ethnicity, low educational level, low income, decreased access, insufficient funding, and unfavorable attitudes toward screening. These social disadvantages are intensified by the disease itself, with serious consequences for women, their families, and communities.

The nursing profession plays a decisive role in increasing the number of women who participate in cervical cancer screening. The goal of the Breast and Cervical Cancer Mortality Prevention Act in 2005 was to increase the access of medically underserved women to breast and cervical cancer screening. The American College of Obstetricians and Gynecologists

(ACOG) recommends routine annual pelvic examination in all women aged 21 years and older. Guidelines for cervical cancer screening are routinely updated and issued jointly by the American Cancer Society (ACS), the American Society for Colposcopy and Cervical Pathology (ASCCP), and the American Society for Clinical Pathology (ASCP). Newer prevention and treatment modalities provide answers that include vaccines against HPV, rapid HPV testing, visual inspection of the cervix with acetic acid (VIA), and cryotherapy. Early detection of cervical cancer allows fast and efficient intervention for precancerous stages such as colposcopy, conization, laser vaporization, LEEP, and even hysterectomy to prevent more invasive disease (McCormish, 2011).

Being available to a patient with cervical cancer during diagnosis, treatment, and recovery or at end of life can trigger hope and activate her inner strength and power (Hammer, Mogensen, & Hall, 2009). Patients value direct interaction with health care professionals and families. Nurses can also support and teach caregivers and family to provide more effective support for their loved ones. This psychological support improves their ability to cope. Because body image and sexuality are fragile, patients and their partners may need encouragement to maintain sexual relations and basic healthy habits of rest, diet, and exercise after treatments (Hart et al., 2011). Boosting the patients' ability to self-heal will increase positivity of the entire experience.

Summary

The most valuable and central attributes that nurses can bring to the care of patients with cervical cancer are support and education. Cervical cancer patients, as a vulnerable patient group, face fear of survival, fear of treatments and their outcomes, and the condition's eventual effect on their and their family members' future quality of life. Nursing care must focus on the nurse as an expert in relatability to facilitate patients' coping with challenges and difficulties and designing care delivery formats that create more time for the nurse to address their patients' concerns.

Cervical cancer affects the lives of women locally and globally. Nurses must use their influence to advocate for improved health outcomes by initiating and supporting interventions of vaccination, screening, and treatment anchored by education and emotional support to wipe out the social, economic, and political disadvantages that contribute to disparities in cervical cancer incidence and mortality.

American Cancer Society. (2013). Treatment options for cervical cancer by stage. Retrieved from http://www.cancer.org/cancer/cervicalcancer/detailedguide/cervical-cancer-treating-by-stage

Bakker, D., Strickland, J., MacDonald, C., Butler, L., Fitch, M., Olson, K., & Cummings, G. (2013). The context of oncology nursing practice. Cancer Nursing, 36(1), 72–88.

Bedford, S. (2009). Cervical cancer: Physiology, risk factors, vaccination and treatment. British Journal of Nursing 18(2), 80–84.

Chesson, H. W., Ekwueme, D. U., Saraiya, M., Watson, M., Lowy, D. R., & Markowitz, L. E. (2012). Estimates of the annual direct medical costs of the prevention and treatment of disease associated with human papillomavirus in the United States. Vaccine, 30(42), 6016–6019.

CIMO. (2014). Malawi–Zambia health care project, MAZAFI. Retrieved from http://www.cimo.fi/ohjel-mat/north-south-south/nss-verkostot/mazafi3

Cleary, V., Hegarty, J., & McCarthy, G. (2011). Sexuality in Irish women with gynecological cancer. Oncology Nursing Forum, 38(2), 87–96.

Cook, O., McIntyre, M., & Recoche, K. (2014). Exploration of the role of specialist nurses in the care of women with gynecological cancer: A systematic review. Journal of Clinical Nursing, 24(5–6), 683–695.

Hammer, K., Mogensen O., & Hall E. O. C. (2009). Hope as experienced in women newly diagnosed with gynaecological cancer. European Journal of Oncology Nursing, 13(2009), 274–279.

Hart L. K., Haylock P. J., & Lutgendorf S. K. (2011). The use of healing touch in integrative oncology. Clinical Journal of Oncology Nursing 15(5), 519–525.

Kingham T. P., Alatise O. I., Vanderpuye V., Casper C., Abantanga F. A., Kamara T. B., . . . Denny L. (2013). Treatment of cancer in sub-Saharan Africa. Lancet Oncology, 14, 158–167.

Lloyd P. A., Briggs E. V., Kane N., Jeyarajah A. R., & Shepher J. H. (2014). Women's experiences after a radical vaginal trachelectomy for early stage cervical cancer. A descriptive phenomenological study. European Journal of Oncology Nursing, 18, 362–271.

McCormish, E. (2011). Cervical cancer, Who's at risk? Nursing for Women's Health, 15(6), 478–483.

National Cancer Institute. (2014). Treatment option overview. Retrieved from http://www.cancer.gov/cancertopics/pdq/treatment/cervical/Patient/page4

Phianmongkhol, Y., & Suwan, N. (2008). Symptom management in patients with cancer of the female reproductive system receiving chemotherapy. Asian Pacific Journal of Cancer Prevention 9, 741–745.

Pinar, G., Kurt, A., & Gungor, T. (2011). The efficacy of preoperative instruction in reducing anxiety following gynecological surgery: A case control study. *Journal of Surgical Oncology, 9*(38), 1–8.

Rasmusson E., & Thomé B. (2008). Women's wishes and need for knowledge concerning sexuality and relationships in connection with gynecological cancer disease. *Sex Disability,* (26), 207–218.

Rogers, N. M., & Cantu, A. G. (2009). The nurse's role in the prevention of cervical cancer among underserved and minority populations. *Journal of Community Health, 34*(2), 135–143.

Schwartz, S. (2009). Young cervical cancer patients and fertility. *Seminars of Oncology Nursing, 25*(4), 259–267.

World Cancer Research Fund International. (2013). Cervical cancer statistics. Retrieved from http://www.wcrf.org/int/cancer-facts-figures/data-specific-cancers/cervical-cancer-statistics

■ CONTRACEPTION

Latina M. Brooks

Overview

Contraception is the prevention of ovulation, fertilization of an egg cell, or implantation of a fertilized egg in the uterine wall through the use of various drugs, devices, sexual practices, or surgical procedures (MedicineNet, 2012). Most sexually active women of childbearing age will use one or more method of birth control throughout their lifetime (Daniels, Mosher, & Jones, 2013). Nursing care for women of reproductive age who chose a contraceptive method should focus on education of how to safely and effectively practice the chosen method, assessment of tolerability, recognition of adverse side effects, and evaluation of success or failure.

Background

The modern contraception movement began in the early 20th century and has been credited to Margaret Sanger, a public health nurse (Centers for Disease Control and Prevention [CDC], 1999). Family planning at that time was used primarily used by married women to limit the number and space the births of children amid health concerns related to multiple back-to-back childbirths (CDC, 1999). During the early 1900s, most birth control methods had to be used at the time of intercourse and included condoms and withdrawal. In the late 1960s, more modern methods became available, including oral contraceptives (the pill) and the intrauterine device (IUD). These methods are not intercourse dependent and therefore highly effective; however, the unintended pregnancy rate in the United States remains at approximately 45% of pregnancies (Finer & Zolna, 2016). In the late 1900s and into the early 2000s, a number of additional contraceptive methods became available to women, including various combinations of the oral contraceptive pill, implantable devices, injectable patches, and vaginal rings.

Contraceptive methods have been categorized based on type, class, and how the method is used, those that contain hormones and those that do not. Broad categories include nonhormonal, hormonal, and permanent. These categories can be further delineated as barrier methods, long-acting reversible contraception (LARC), hormonal methods, emergency contraception, and sterilization.

Nonhormonal contraception includes methods of birth control that do not contain hormones or involve sexual practices to prevent pregnancy. These include barrier methods, spermicides, copper IUD, and natural family planning (NFP).

Barrier methods include the male and female condom, diaphragm, cervical cap, and the cervical sponge. Barrier methods are intercourse-dependent removable devices that prevent sperm from reaching the uterus. Spermicides in the form of cream, foam, jelly, suppository, or vaginal film contain agents, most common, nonoxynol-9, which when inserted into the vagina before intercourse can kill sperm cells. The copper intrauterine device (Cu-IUD), which is classified as an LARC, prevents pregnancy by interfering with sperm's ability to reach and fertilize an egg and can prevent an egg from attaching to the uterine wall (U.S. Food and Drug Administration [FDA], 2016). The Cu-IUD can be used continuously for up to 10 years. NFP or fertility-based awareness to prevent pregnancy do not require devices or drugs, but rely on awareness of the body's natural functions to predict the days a woman is most likely to get pregnant and during which she would therefore abstain from sexual activity. Natural family planning is used by women not only to prevent pregnancy but also to achieve it. Barrier methods, spermicides, natural family planning, or fertility-based awareness methods have a failure rate of 12% to 28% depending on the method used, whereas copper IUDs have a failure rate of less than 1% (Trussell, 2011).

Hormonal methods of contraception prevent pregnancy by suppressing ovulation, thereby preventing the release of an egg from the ovary. These methods can also work by thickening cervical mucus making it difficult for the sperm to reach an egg thus preventing fertilization (FDA, 2016) and by thinning the lining of the uterus making implantation less likely, depending on the method (American College of Obstetricians and Gynecologists [ACOG], 2016). Hormonal contraceptive methods are classified as long-acting and short-acting. Long-acting hormonal contraceptive methods, also referred to as *LARC*, include intrauterine systems (IUS), also referred to as a *hormonal IUD* and contraceptive implants. Short-acting hormonal contraceptive methods include orals, injectables, patches, and vaginal rings.

The hormonal IUD or IUS is a T-shaped device that is inserted into the uterus and releases levonorgestrel (a progestin hormone) directly into the uterus, causing cervical mucus thickening that prevents sperm from fertilizing an egg and that can also suppress ovulation, thereby preventing the release of eggs from the ovaries. The progestin hormone released from the IUS also thins the lining of the uterus to prevent implantation of a fertilized egg (ACOG, 2016). Hormonal IUDs can be used continuously for up to 3 to 5 years depending on the brand and have a failure rate of less than 0.5% (Trussell, 2011). As mentioned previously, the copper IUD is classified as an LARC; however, it is the only nonhormonal method that has this classification.

Contraceptive implants are rods that are surgically implanted beneath the skin of the upper arm and release a progestin hormone (etonogestrel). Much like other progestins, implants prevent pregnancy by suppressing ovulation, thickening cervical mucus, and thinning the uterine lining. In the United States, only a single rod implant is approved for use (CDC, 2016).

Oral contraceptives are classified as progestin-only pills (POPs) and combined oral contraceptives (COCs). POPs contain only a progestin hormone, are taken daily, and prevent pregnancy by suppressing ovulation, and thickening cervical mucus much like LARCs. Combined oral contraceptives contain both progestin and estrogen hormones, are taken daily, and prevent pregnancy in the same manner as POPs. With perfect use, oral contraceptives have a failure rate of 0.3%; however, the failure rate with typical use is 9% (Trussell, 2011).

Injectable contraception is a method of birth control in which a progestin hormone, medroxyprogesterone acetate, is injected every 3 months either intramuscularly or subcutaneously depending on the dosage (CDC, 2016). Injectables are progestin-only methods

and prevent pregnancy much in the same manner as POPs. The failure rate is 0.2% for perfect use and 6% for typical use (Trussell, 2011)

Patches, rings, and combined oral contraceptives (COCs) are all classified as combined hormonal contraceptives (CHCs). Contraceptive patches and rings like COCs contain both estrogen and progestin. The contraceptive patch is applied to the lower abdomen, buttock, outer arm or upper back, sticks to the skin, and releases a combination of progestin and estrogen hormones. A new patch is applied once weekly for 3 weeks and no patch is applied on the fourth week (CDC, 2016). A new patch is applied every 7 days. The contraceptive ring is a small ring-shaped device that is inserted into the vagina once a month, remains in place for 3 weeks, and is removed on the fourth week (CDC, 2016). Seven days later, a new l ring is inserted. Combined hormonal contraceptives (CHCs) all prevent pregnancy in the same manner and have the same failure rates.

Emergency contraception methods are used to prevent pregnancy after unprotected intercourse. Two methods are available in the United States: the copper IUD and emergency contraceptive pills (ECPs). The copper IUD is a highly effective method of emergency contraception when inserted within the first 5 days of an episode of unprotected intercourse. There are three types of ECPs: levonogestrel, combined estrogen and progestin, and ulipristal acetate. Emergency contraceptive pills are most effective if taken within 3 to 5 days of unprotected intercourse depending on the type of ECP being used (CDC, 2016).

Sterilization is considered a permanent method of contraception. There are three methods: bilateral tubal occlusion, tubal ligation, and vasectomy. Two of the methods, bilateral tubal occlusion and tubal ligation, prevent women from getting pregnant by blocking sperm from reaching the egg to fertilize it and by preventing an egg from reaching the uterus. Vasectomy is performed on the male and prevents sperm from fertilizing an egg by blocking the release of sperm from the testes (NICHD, 2016). First-year failure rates for female and male sterilization are 0.5% and 0.15%, respectively (Trussell, 2011).

Clinical Aspects

ASSESSMENT

Nursing care of women of reproductive age in need of contraceptive management begins with thorough and accurate documentation of medical history, social and family history, physical assessment findings, and laboratory results. A history should include age, menstrual cycle history, date of last menstrual period, pregnancy history taking note of any complications during pregnancy or delivery, current and prior methods of birth control and how well they were tolerated, and any current or past medical conditions such as sexually transmitted infections, hypertension, diabetes, cancers, heart attack, stroke, liver disease, or clotting disorders. Social history should include documentation of smoking, amount and frequency of alcohol use, and sexual activity. Family medical history should be documented as well, particularly first-degree relatives with a history of breast cancer, heart attack, and strokes. Patient's medical and family histories are essential for determining the most appropriate method of contraception.

Need for physical examination and laboratory testing depends on the medical history of the patient and method of contraception being considered. For the average healthy woman few if any examinations or tests will be needed prior to starting most methods of birth control (CDC, 2016). However, the physical assessment should include, at a minimum, baseline height, weight, body mass index (BMI), blood pressure, and, in some instances, a pregnancy test. Bimanual examination and cervical inspection may be indicated depending on the method of contraception chosen.

NURSING INTERVENTIONS, MANAGEMENT, AND IMPLICATIONS

Contraceptive management is a private and sensitive topic for many women. The most important first step will be to provide a comfortable and safe environment for women to share and discuss the most private and intimate details of their personal lives. Women may present with concerns related to misinformation and myths regarding birth control. There may also be concern about access to contraception, which has long been a controversial issue in the United States (CDC, 1999). The nurse should be aware of these issues, listen to any concerns women may have, and be ready to provide appropriate education, support, and referral as needed.

Nursing interventions, management, and implications for women seeking contraception focuses on education regarding the many options available and monitoring the tolerance, compliance, and effectiveness of the chosen method of contraception.

In order to effectively educate women seeking birth control, the nurse must be knowledgeable of the various methods, how they prevent pregnancy, how each is to be used, and its potential side effects. Once patients have chosen a method, follow-up is imperative. Nursing care for women using any method of birth control should focus on assessment of health status at each encounter.

OUTCOMES

Outcomes of contraception depend on the women's empowerment to care for their own health and choices about their bodies and lives. Thus, both health literacy and knowledge about the various contraceptive methods are extremely important in determining the desired outcomes for the woman and her family. The nurse should assess for and document continued and proper use, tolerability, and effectiveness of the chosen method. In addition, nursing care for all woman of childbearing age should include an assessment of need or desire for birth control and education. Not all women of childbearing age need or desire contraception at any given time; however, good nursing care involves assessing for the need and providing education as appropriate.

Summary

Most sexually active women will use some form of contraception over the course of their lifetime (Daniels, 2013). Therefore, contraception is a topic that most nurses will encounter. The care of women seeking and using contraception is complex due to the number of birth control options available and the sensitive nature of the conversation. Through listening, careful assessment, and providing appropriate and timely education, nurses can provide a safe and informative environment to assist women with making the best possible contraceptive choice. Once a contraceptive choice has been made, nursing care then centers on monitoring for adverse side effects, changes in health status, and evaluation of method of choice over time.

American College of Obstetricians and Gynecologists. (2016). Long-acting reversible contraception (LARC): IUD and implant. Retrieved from https://www.acog.org/Patients/FAQs/Long-Acting-Reversible-Contraception-LARC-IUD-and-Implant

Centers for Disease Control and Prevention. (1999). Achievements in public health, 1900–1999: Family planning. *Morbidity and Mortality Weekly Report, 48*(47),1073–1080. Retrieved from http://www.cdc.gov/mmwr/preview/mmwrhtml/mm4847a1.htm

Centers for Disease Control and Prevention. (2016). U.S. selected practice recommendations for contraceptive use, 2016. *Morbidity and Mortality Weekly Report, 65*(4), 1–66.

Daniels K., Mosher W. D., & Jones J. (2013). *Contraceptive methods women have ever used: United States, 1982–2010* (National Center for Health Statistics Reports No. 62). Hyattsville, MD: National Center for Health Statistics.

Definition of Birth Control. (2012). *MedicineNet.* Retrieved from https://www.medicinenet.com/script/main/art.asp ?articlekey=53351

Finer, L. B., & Zolna, M. R. (2016). Declines in unintended pregnancy in the United States, 2008–2011. *New England Journal of Medicine, 374*, 843–852. doi:10.1056/NEJM sa1506575

Trussell, J. (2011). Contraceptive failure in the United States. *Contraception, 83*(5), 397–404. doi:10.1016/ j.contraception.2011.01.021

U.S. Food and Drug Administration. (2016). Birth control: Medicines to help you. Retrieved from https://www.fda .gov/ forconsumers/byaudience/forwomen/freepublications/ ucm313215.htm#LARC

■ ENDOMETRIOSIS

Ingrid Apryl Spears

Overview

Endometriosis is defined as the endometrial tissue from the inside of the uterus being found outside of the uterus as superficial implants or deep implants on the peritoneum, ovaries, bowel, bladder, or other organs (Yong, Chen, Allaire, & Williams, 2013). Endometriosis is an estrogen-dependent disease predominantly affecting reproductive-age women (Schrager, Falleroni, & Edgoose, 2013). Its etiology is unknown, but can manifest as severe pelvic pain, infertility, and decreased quality of life resulting from pain and multiple surgeries. The goal of medical therapy for women suffering from endometriosis is to manage and reduce pain, reduce symptoms, preserve fertility, and prevent recurrence of the disease.

Background

One in 10 women of reproductive age (usually between the ages 15 and 49 years), are affected by endometriosis, equating to more than 176 million women worldwide. This figure encompasses 50% to 70% of women with chronic pelvic pain (CPP) and 38% of infertile women (Farrell & Garad, 2012). In the United States, endometriosis is the third leading cause of gynecologic hospitalizations, with the disease leading to an estimated $2,801 in health care costs and $1,023 in lost productivity at work per patient annually (Schrager et al., 2013).

Diagnosing endometriosis is not an easy task due to its wide array of symptoms, which may mimic other conditions. Although there is not an internationally recognized noninvasive method for diagnosis, most presurgical diagnostic methods are clinical judgment based on medical history, symptoms, and signs, with the most commonly reported symptoms being dysmenorrhea and pelvic pain (Riazi, Tehranian, Ziael, Mohammadi, & Montazeri, 2015). Pain is a prominent feature of this condition and is not related to severity of the disease, but is associated with the location of endometrial tissue and from new sprouting nerves affecting the activity of neurons in the spinal cord and brain (Farrell & Garad, 2012). Histologic confirmation is usually achieved with the detection of extra-uterine endometrial cells on laparoscopy (Schrager et al., 2013). An evaluation of symptoms combined with physical findings is insufficient to confirm or exclude the presence of the disease, and lack of non-invasive options further limits the diagnostic process; therefore, surgical evaluation with histologic confirmation is the definitive means of obtaining true diagnosis (Sinervo, 2015).

Failure to understand the causes of endometriosis creates obstacles that interfere with identification of all of the risk factors. Although the etiology of endometriosis is unknown, there are explanations that are possible and others that have been dismissed. It has been reported that the risk of endometriosis is six times higher in first-degree relatives of women with severe endometriosis. A more recent case–control study showed that familial impact on the incidence of endometriosis is not significant (Shrager et al., 2013). Risk factors associated with endometriosis are lower body weight; alcohol use; early menarche (occurring before age 11 years); shorter cycles (less than 27 days); and heavy, prolonged cycles (Farrell & Garad, 2012). Endometriosis has several impacts in overall physical, mental, and social well-being (Riazi et al., 2015). The quality of life of women suffering from endometriosis is diminished and to some extent compromised. Quality of life is diminished by features such as severe, acute, and/or incapacitating chronic pain, dysmenorrhea, painful intercourse, heavy periods, subfertility, fatigue, and on average 11 hours of lost productivity per week, which severely compromises work and educational opportunities (Farrell & Garad, 2012). Management of this chronic disease should be individualized and focused on the symptoms. Surgical therapies for endometriosis-associated pain include the removal of endometriotic implants and adhesions with restoration of normal anatomy. Laparoscopy is an effective surgical approach with the goal of excising visible endometriosis. Laparoscopic surgery is often used as an effective way to view endometriosis. Women with endometriosis may suffer from general cyclic or noncyclic pelvic pain for which medical and surgical treatments are utilized to control the pain (Bernardi & Pavone, 2013). Although management of the disease is difficult, patients have the options of surgical and pharmacological treatment outcomes.

Clinical Aspects

ASSESSMENT

The most common symptom associated with endometriosis is pain. It is believed that the endometriosis-related pain results from the effects of inflammatory cytokines within the peritoneal cavity (Bernardi & Pavone, 2013).

Astute nursing assessment of symptoms, support of medical interventions, and acknowledgment of the psychosocial effects that endometriosis has on the patient allows the nurse to provide adequate support, which will ultimately affect treatment.

NURSING INTERVENTIONS, MANAGEMENT, AND IMPLICATIONS

Although some aspects of endometriosis are still the subject of research, it is imperative that nurses have extensive knowledge regarding the disease process to include causes, symptoms, clinical presentation, management, and treatment options. Medical therapies may include use of analgesics such as nonsteroidal anti-inflammatory medication (NSAIDs) and hormone therapies to include the combined oral contraceptive pills and other hormone therapies (Farrell & Garad, 2012).

OUTCOMES

Decreased pain associated with endometriosis is experienced by women who undergo medical treatment. All medical therapy, whether administered as first-line treatment or postoperatively, is associated with high rates of disease recurrence with pain recurrence as high as 50%, 1 to 2 years after surgery for symptomatic endometriosis (Sinervo, 2015). Nursing-centered care should focus on prompt recognition of symptoms, pain management, health promotion, patient education, and close monitoring of symptoms along with medication compliance.

Summary

Although endometriosis has been defined as a complex disease, effective treatment of endometriosis requires a multidisciplinary approach. Disease management must be individualized with prompt recognition of symptoms and implementation of proactive measures.

Bernardi, L. A., & Pavone M. E. (2013). Endometriosis: An update on Management. *Women's Health*, 9(3), 233–250.

Farrell, E., & Garad, R. (2012). Endometriosis. *Australian Nursing Journal*, 20(5), 37–39.

Riazi, H., Tehranian, N., Ziael, S., Mohammadi, E., & Montazeri, A. (2015). Clinical diagnosis of pelvic endometriosis: A scoping review. *BMC Women's Health*, 15(39), 1–12. doi:10.1186/s12905-015-0196-z

Schrager, S., Falleroni, J., & Edgoose, J. (2013). Evaluation and treatment of endometriosis. *American Family Physician*, 87(2), 107–113.

Sinervo, K. (2015). The case for surgery for endometriosis. *Contemporary OB/GYN*, October 2016, 51–54.

Yong, P. J., Chen, I., Allaire, C., & Williams, C. (2013). Surgery for pelvic pain in endometriosis. In J. Merrick (Ed.), *Pain management yearbook 2013* (pp. 207–214). Hauppauge, NY: Nova Science.

■ EPISIOTOMY

Loraine O'Neill

Overview

Episiotomy is a surgical incision that is performed at the time of birth to reduce maternal perineal tearing. The perineal body is comprised of dense connective tissue that includes the superficial and deep muscles of the perineal membrane, including the transverse perineal muscles and the bulbocavernosus muscles. First described in the 18th century, episiotomy was the most common procedure performed by accoucheurs. Studies have demonstrated a downward trend in practice, with rates of 25% in 2004 reduced to 12% in 2012

(Friedman, Ananth, Prendergast, D'Alton, & Wright, 2015). The current best practice use of this technique is considered *restrictive*; nevertheless, there persists wide variation in its use, with various confounding factors that influence the prevalence (Webb & Culhane, 2002).

Background

The most recent American College of Obstetricians and Gynecologist (ACOG) Practice Bulletin Number 165 (ACOG, 2016) continues to recommend reducing the use of "routine" episiotomy and adopting practices that reduce the risk of severe perineal lacerations. This chapter also reports the increased incidences of obstetrical anal sphincter injuries (OASIS) associated with episiotomy. There are two directions of incision used when performing an episiotomy: *midline* or *mediolateral*. The former, also known as *median*, is more commonly used in the United States. There is a debate as to whether *midline* episiotomies lead to more severe lacerations (Hastings-Tolsma, Vincent, Emeis, & Francisco, 2007). Several research studies have proved that the routine use of episiotomy can actually increase the number of third- or fourth-degree lacerations at the time of birth (Hartmann, Viswanathan, Palmiere, Gartlehner, Thorp, & Lohr, 2005). Indications for use of episiotomy are dependent upon the clinical context affecting either the fetus or the mother. It is used when extra room is needed in the soft tissue to allow delivery of the fetus and/or to reduce perineal tears, in particular, third- and fourth-degree lacerations. Factors that appear to influence the need for episiotomy are varied; the most common *was* practitioner use but others include prior history, perineal anatomy, fetal position, use of operative-assisted delivery, namely, vacuum or forceps, and complicated delivery, such as shoulder dystocia. The complications and risks associated with this procedure can be observed either immediately postdelivery or in the postpartum period (generally considered 6 weeks postdelivery), but may also carry long-term sequelae. These include bleeding, tears, swelling, hematoma, infection, fecal or urinary incontinence, and pain during sex (dyspareunia).

Clinical Aspects

ANTEPARTUM

The nurse's role in providing education to the pregnant patient and her partner in preparation for labor and birth is essential. Many women use the Internet, family members, or friends to gain their information. By talking with the woman about her own understanding of the birth process, the nurse can help to alleviate anxiety and prepare the patient for her labor experience. The use of perineal massage in the prenatal period has been shown to reduce the likelihood for need of episiotomy in first-time mothers delivering vaginally (Beckmann & Stock, 2013). Use of antenatal massage has shown a decrease in serious vaginal lacerations among woman who previously had an episiotomy (Davidson, Jacoby, & Brown, 2000). If considered acceptable by the patient, perineal massage should commence around 35 to 36 weeks of gestation and involves digital massage of the perineum, by the woman or her partner, with a mild lubricant for up to 10 minutes per session, at least once or twice per week. Use of the Kegel exercise is highly recommended for all parturients as this helps to strengthen the pelvic floor muscles, which can be weakened during pregnancy and childbirth.

INTRAPARTUM

Many pregnant patients present to the labor and delivery unit with birth plans that may include position at the time of delivery and the application of mineral oil or warm soaks to the perineal area during the pushing phase. Although research is somewhat conflicting on maternal position or delay in pushing when in the second stage, the use of perineal warm compresses at the time of pushing was analyzed in a Cochrane database review (Aasheim, Nilsen, Lukasse, & Reinar, 2011). It concluded that this practice is well accepted by women. Suggested techniques for preparing perineal soaks include: immerse perineal pad in warm tap water (45–59°F), apply to perineum at pushing, presoak between contractions, and replace water every 15 minutes or continuously hold in compress in place while ensuring maintenance of adequate temperature and ensure hygiene. Caution must be taken to ensure that the patient has adequate sensation to avoid any injury from compresses that might be too hot.

During the second stage of labor, it is important that the patient listens to the instructions of the delivery provider. This person is at the perineum and able to gauge the tissue stretching as the head begins to crown. Controlled extension of the head can reduce tearing or need for surgical incision. The nurse should facilitate and aid the patient's understanding and cooperation during pushing and the birthing process.

As it is difficult to predict whether an episiotomy will be required, the nurse should assist to ensure that the delivering provider has the necessary analgesia, sutures, equipment, and added support as indicated.

POSTPARTUM

In the immediate hours after delivery, an ice pack should be provided to reduce local swelling at the episiotomy site. However, this again should be used with caution by assessing the patient's ability to feel the temperature in her perineal area. The ice pack should be changed as needed. The initial assessment of the perineal area should include bleeding from the site pain and swelling. Pain at the site can be the first indication of a hematoma that is not always visualized, and care must be taken to adequately assess for swelling before providing pain medication.

ASSESSMENT

Ongoing assessment and care of the episiotomy site are the same as for any surgical site, although the location may not be easily accessible. It is therefore important to ensure adequate visualization to determine the presence of any localized bleeding (differentiated from vaginal lochia), swelling, pain, or redness. These perineal checks should be conducted as per local institutional guidelines.

OUTCOMES

As in the antenatal period, the nurse plays a key role in postpartum patient education, including care of the incision site. The mother should be instructed to keep the area clean and dry, particularly in the presence of any fecal matter. She can be offered witch hazel pads or use of squeeze bottle for perineal care. Many new mothers are concerned about the first bowel movement after an episiotomy. They can be prescribed a stool softener and should be asked to report their bowel movements so as to help prevent constipation. Some patients may require comfort measures to assist with sitting. The sutures will dissolve; nevertheless, the patient should be aware of any pain or redness and report any concerns to her primary provider after discharge to home. Delayed episiotomy breakdown and localized infection are not unknown. All such remedies should be used only after consultation with the patient's primary provider.

Summary

The nurse plays an important role by providing the pregnant woman with education on expectations and

options for the antepartum, labor, delivery, and the postpartum periods. Choices may include the use of antenatal perineal massage and second-stage perineal compresses to reduce the need for an episiotomy. Labor support and coaching are provided by the attendant nurse to promote patient satisfaction and safe outcomes. Postpartum self-care practice for this type of surgical incision can help to reduce the likelihood of morbidity.

Aasheim, V., Nilsen, A. B., Lukasse, M., & Reinar, L. M. (2011). Perineal techniques during the second stage of labour for reducing perineal trauma. *Cochrane Database of Systematic Reviews, 2011*, CD006672. doi:10.1002/14651858.CD006672.pub3

American College of Obstetricians and Gynecologists. (2016). *Practice Bulletin No. 65*, p. 1.

Beckmann, M. M., & Stock, O. M. (2013). Antenatal perineal massage for reducing perineal trauma. *Cochrane Database of Systematic Reviews, 2013*(4), CD005123. doi:10.1002/14651858.CD005123.pub3

Davidson, K., Jacoby, S., & Brown, M. S. (2000). Prenatal perineal massage: Preventing lacerations during delivery. *Journal of Obstetric, Gynecologic, & Neonatal Nursing, 29*(5), 474–479.

Friedman, A. M., Ananth, C. V., Prendergast, E., D'Alton, M. E., & Wright, J. D. (2015). Variation in and factors associated with use of episiotomy. *Journal of the American Medical Association, 313*(2), 197–199.

Hartmann, K., Viswanathan, M., Palmieri, R., Gartlehner, G., Thorp, J., & Lohr, K. N. (2005). Outcomes of routine episiotomy: A systematic review. *Journal of the American Medical Association, 293*(17), 2141–2148.

Hastings-Tolsma, M., Vincent, D., Emeis, C., & Francisco, T. (2007). Getting through birth in one piece: Protecting the perineum. *American Journal of Maternal/Child Nursing, 32*(3), 158–164.

Webb, D. A., & Culhane, J. (2002). Hospital variation in episiotomy use and the risk of perineal trauma during childbirth. *Birth, 29*(2), 132–136.

■ HOME BIRTH

Sabrina Nitkowski-Keever

Overview

Health care models in the United States value evidenced-based practices, improved outcomes, and decreased cost. As education and services improved in the 20th century, births came out of the home and into the hospital with the thought of improving outcomes. This somewhat took the control of childbirth from the mother and gave it to the physician, who was viewed as the expert on birth. In the 21st century, dissatisfaction with previous hospital births, empowerment, privacy, and the idea that interventions harm the birth process has given rise to planned out-of-hospital births (Bernhard, et al., 2014). Planned out-of-hospital births have seen an increase of 80.2% from 2009 to 2014, home births by 77.3%, and free-standing birth centers by 79.6% (Grunebaum, 2014). This phenomenon has created much discussion on the safety of this choice and the responsibility of health care providers to understand it in order to help their patients make informed decisions concerning birth. This discussion reviews the history of home births and the need for additional studies on its impact to the health and well-being of society.

Background

Birth is a physiological experience, and as health care providers, we are obligated to educate ourselves to ensure that we provide mothers the choices to foster this physiological experience. Hospitals are inadvertently synonymous with a high number of interventions and with that comes controversy over the decision to use those interventions. High induction rates, increased surgical procedures, and decreased patient-centered decision making result in unsatisfied mothers, pushing them to think about planning an out-of-hospital birth. Home birth has been on the rise in the United States as more women are choosing to educate themselves and take control of the choices that best fit their family.

Home birth is widely accessible in countries like the Netherlands, Canada, New Zealand, and the United Kingdom. The availability of providers in all birth settings is intergraded into the medical systems of these countries that is in contrast to the United States, Australia, and much of the remaining developing world. In countries like Canada, educational requirements include attendance at both hospital and home births acknowledging that home birth is a standard of care. Outlining the attitudes of midwives across the United States and Canada, midwives in the United States noted education, time constraints, fear of lawsuits, and judgment of hospital colleagues as reasons that home birth was not favorable (Vedam, Stoll, Schummers, Rogers, & Plaine, 2013).

Home births remain controversial as studies have published conflicting results. Studies in the United States use birth certificate data as a source limiting the validation of the results related to inaccurate data entry. In his Oregon-based study, Snowden et al. (2015) found that although interventions were lower for out-of-hospital births, there was a higher rate of perinatal deaths, seizures, and admissions to the neonatal intensive care unit than hospital births. Some home births in this particular study were carried out with a certified professional and others were deemed high risk. Hutton et al. (2015) determined that low-risk women could safely plan a home birth without concern for poor outcomes. Canadian home births were done in areas that had well integrated the practice into the health care system, and outcomes were comparable to that of hospital births. Fewer cesarean sections, inductions, and interventions in home births are reported in both studies. Each study did recognize that birth-attendant education and certification played a key role in the outcomes (Goer, 2016).

One study looked at the risks of pregnancy and the culture of safety surrounding the assessment and quick actions needed for all births and deemed this as lacking in home birth. There are several outcomes that can occur without warning, and the time available when contemplating "decision to deliver" can affect the health of the mother and newborn. Preeclampsia, cord prolapse, and newborn respiratory support needs can be unexpected outcomes in any birth. In order to claim home births are safe, some feel that we must adopt the "no risk" pregnancy philosophy, which is professionally unacceptable (Grunebaum, McCullough, Arabin, Brent, Levene, & Chervenak, 2015). Conflicting data are a barrier for many health care professionals who are seeking to consult with their patients on alternative birth methods.

Clinical Aspects

ASSESSMENT

Hospital birth remains the standard place to deliver your newborn; yet, there are a growing number of women who are choosing to give birth at home. In the United States, home birth is not integrated into mainstream health care as it is in many other countries. Women who begin to consider home birth are choosing to face judgment from friends, family, and providers, and the information to assist her in the decision is inadequate.

NURSING INTERVENTIONS, MANAGEMENT, AND IMPLICATIONS

Health care professionals must recognize this trend and educate themselves on home birth in order to provide our patients with the most evidenced-based research so that they can feel comfortable about their choices. The first step in our responsibility urges us to understand why women are choosing these options.

Choice and empowerment are a common theme among women who look to alternative birth places (Bernhard, Zielinski, Ackerson, & English, 2014). Birth is often considered a rite of passage, placing women in their most vulnerable state, stripping away their autonomy and often leaving them unfilled during what should have been a life-changing experience. Exploring other options is a way for some women to gain some of that control back and feel empowered. Hospital births can be full of interruptions and interventions placing undue stress on women in their most vulnerable state, yet the most notable reason for seeking alternative birth methods is disrespect (Bernhard et al., 2014). An impersonal feel to birth and recovery as well as dismissal of opinions and choices in the hospital setting is a theme that should be studied in more depth.

American College of Nurse Midwives (ACNM) recognizes home birth as a safe and satisfying option for low-risk mothers. Clinical practice guidelines (CPGs) are a key component to an ethical home-birth practice. These guidelines are strongly encouraged to be based on the ACNM's Midwifery Provisions of Home Birth Services and based on the most current evidence. It is placing the woman and her family at the center of patient care throughout the entire process and establishing an understanding of a "normal pregnancy" for the midwife and her patient. Open discussions on the current evidence of the risks and benefits of home birth jump-start the informed-consent process, establishing the roles and responsibilities of the provider and patient (Bailes, 2016).

OUTCOMES

Responsibilities of ensuring a safe and satisfying birth experience at home begin at the first visit and continue through to the end of the postpartum period. Outlining a plan for unexpected transfer to a hospital should be included in the plan. A home-birth midwife's CPGs must outline clinical conditions that indicate a transfer to a hospital birth that can often be unexpected or develop later in pregnancy, including hypertension, gestation diabetes, and malpresentation. Postpartum indications, such as hemorrhage, retained placenta, or a laceration beyond the midwives expertise, are other indications for transfer. Newborns with unstable status may require a transfer. Clinical practice guidelines can also be used when the available evidence on certain indications is conflicting.

Attendants of home birth are held to the same standard as those who practice in the hospital. The current evidence establishes guidelines that outline and support a safe satisfying home birth. Health care professionals are obligated to understand those guidelines and discuss the risk and the benefits of home birth so that a mother and her family can make an informed choice to fit their desire without judgment.

Summary

American College of Obstetrics and Gynecologists recognizes that hospitals and birth centers are the safest places to give birth while also acknowledging that women should have the right to make an informed choice of birth options. Attempts at adequate randomized control studies are unsuccessfully related to a small sample size and little interest from women to participate. Birth certificate data is the most used source for the collection of home-birth data. Problems with accuracy are related to entry errors, insufficiencies in self-reporting, accurate accounting of transfers and identification of birth-attendant skills and certification. Currently, it has been established that standardized clinical guidelines are not broadly practiced across the United States, and yet home births that adhere to strict guidelines have better outcomes. A standardized approach to CPGs can drive research to focus on what influences a safe home delivery (ACOG, 2016).

Goer (2016) encourages us to look beyond the question of whether home birth is safe, and seek answers to what factors influence its outcomes. Home birth is a personal decision and by establishing broad guidelines and improving research, we can better understand what factors influence its positive outcome, ensuring that all women who seek this option will have more adequate evidence to make an informed decision.

American College of Obstetricians and Gynecologists. (2017). *Planned home birth* (Committee opinion number 697). Retrieved from https://www.acog.org/Resources-And-Publications/Committee-Opinions/Committee-on-Obstetric-Practice/Planned-Home-Birth

Bailes, A., (2016). *The home birth practice manual*. Silver Spring, MD: American College of Nurse Midwives.

Bernhard, C., Zielinski, R., Ackerson, K., & English, J. (2014). Home birth after hospital birth: Women's choices and reflections. *Journal of Midwifery & Women's Health*, 59(2), 160–166.

Goer, H. (2016). Dueling statistics: Is out-of-hospital birth safe? *Journal of Perinatal Education, 25*(2), 75–79.

Grunebaum, A., & Chervenak, F. (2014). Out-of-hospital births in the United States 2009–2014. *Journal of Perinatal Medicine, 44*(7), 845–849.

Grunebaum, A., McCullough, L., Arabin, B., Brent, R., Levene, M., & Chervenak. (2015). Home birth is unsafe: FOR: The safety of planned home births: A clinical fiction. *British Journal of Obstetrics and Gynaecology, 122*(9),1235.

Hutton, E. K., Cappelletti, A., Reitsma, A. H., Simioni, J., Horne, J., McGregor, C., & Ahmed, R. J. (2015). Outcomes associated with planned place of birth among women with low-risk pregnancies. *Canadian Medical Association Journal, 188*(5), 80–90.

Snowden, J., Tilden, E., Synder, J., Quigley, B., Caughey, A., & Cheng, Y. W. (2015) Planned out-of-hospital birth and birth outcomes. *New England Journal of Medicine, 373*(27), 2642–2653.

Vedam, S., Stoll, K., Schummers, L., Rogers, J., & Plaine, L. (2013). Home birth in North America: Attitudes and practices of US certified nurse midwives and Canadian registered midwives. *Journal of Midwifery & Women's Health, 59*(2), 1–12.

■ INFERTILITY

Tammy M. Lampley

Overview

Infertility is a significant health issue, impacting both men and women. Infertility crosses all cultural, social, and economic groups. Approximately 186 million people, 9% of the global reproductive population (Centers for Disease Control and Prevention [CDC], 2017) experience the condition. In general, infertility is a failure to become pregnant after trying for 12 months, or 6 months for women older than the age of 35. Along with the failure to have a child, a diagnosis of infertility has a profound psychosocial impact on the individual. In 2014, the CDC developed a national public health plan focused on promoting reproductive health and the prevention and management of infertility. Nurses provide care throughout an individual's reproductive years and are in a pivotal position to educate patients on healthy behaviors that promote fertility as well as provide holistic care during the diagnosis and treatment of infertility. Nurses must be knowledgeable and supportive to meet the complex health care needs of a socially diverse population that desires to have a child.

Background

Infertility is "a disease of the reproductive system defined by the failure to achieve a clinical pregnancy after 12 months or more of regular unprotected intercourse" (Zegers-Hochschild et al., 2009). *Impaired fecundity* describes women who are unable to conceive a pregnancy or unable to carry a pregnancy to term. In 40% of couples, the female partner is the source of (or contributing cause) infertility; in 40%, the male partner is the source (or contributing cause) of infertility; and in 20% of cases, the cause is unexplained (American Society for Reproductive Medicine [ASRM], 2015; CDC, 2017). Approximately 9% to 15% of the childbearing population is impacted by infertility (Phillips, Elander, & Montague, 2014), making it one of the most common diseases affecting people between the ages of 20 and 45 years (ASRM, 2014). In developing countries, the incidence of infertility is reported to be as high as 30% of couples (Stevenson & Hershberger, 2016). The most recent report, published from the National Survey of Family Growth on Infertility and Impaired Fecundity in the United States, collected in 2010, indicated that infertility rates have dropped in the United States, whereas the ability to carry a pregnancy to term has risen (Chandra, Copen, & Stephen, 2013).

It is estimated that about half of the women who need infertility treatment seek help. Between 1968 and 2010, the number of persons seeking infertility treatment has quadrupled (CDC, 2014).

A woman's age is a primary factor impacting infertility. After age 30, the chances of becoming pregnant gradually decrease each year until age 37 when a dramatic decrease occurs (Practice Committee ASRM, 2014). Changes in social structure over recent decades have led to an increase in the average age of educated women having their first child (Vespa, Lewis, & Kreider, 2013). Other conditions impacting female fertility include polycystic ovary syndrome (PCOS), thyroid disease, hormonal disorders, and ovarian surgery; exposure to chemotherapy or radiation can impact ovulation (CDC, 2017; Stevenson, et al., 2016). Blocked or damaged fallopian tubes can be caused by endometriosis, pelvic inflammatory disease from untreated sexually transmitted diseases (STDs), or pelvic surgery (CDC, 2017; Stevenson, et al., 2016). Uterine anomalies, such as fibroids, decrease the likelihood of carrying a successful pregnancy. Lifestyle risk factors for infertility in women include smoking, excessive alcohol use, overweight or underweight, and STDs (ASRM, 2017a).

Common contributors to male fertility involve factors affecting sperm formation or sperm transport, including diabetes, cystic fibrosis, hormone imbalance chromosomal disorders, varicocele, radiation, chemotherapy, testicular injury, and history of mumps or hernia (ASRM, 2017a; American Urological Association [AUA], n.d.; CDC, 2017). Lifestyle risk factors for male infertility include smoking, heavy alcohol use, excessive weight, drug use such as marijuana or anabolic steroids, or exposure to environmental toxins (CDC, 2017; McEleny, 2016).

Clinical Aspects

ASSESSMENT

Women may initially seek care from an obstetrician/gynecologist and men from a urologist. Individuals may also contact or be referred by a provider to a reproductive endocrinologist. Care begins with a thorough physical assessment, including a detailed family history, reproductive history, and lifestyle history. Diagnostic evaluation includes a pelvic exam and blood tests to assess ovary function and explore the presence of medical conditions. Additional tests may be performed such as ultrasound hysterosalpingography to examine the follicles or fallopian tubes or a sonohysterography to examine the uterus for anomalies (CDC, 2017). Evaluation of male fertility includes a physical assessment and a detailed medical, reproductive, and lifestyle history. The assessment focuses on issues with prostate, penis, testicles, or tubal patency. A semen analysis to evaluate the number, shape, and movement of sperm as well as other tests to evaluate hormones or genetic issues are commonly ordered (AUA, n.d.; CDC, 2017; Stevenson et al., 2016). About 85% to 90% of patients are treated with surgery or medication therapy; fewer than 3% of the population affected undergo more invasive artificial reproductive techniques such as in vitro fertilization (ASRM, 2017a).

NURSING INTERVENTIONS, MANAGEMENT, AND IMPLICATIONS

Nurses have meaningful interactions with patients throughout the reproductive years and are in an ideal position to help assess for issues with fertility and provide education to promote fertility. Nurses are pivotal members of the health care team and collaborate with other providers, including physicians and advanced practice nurses, to provide care. As the primary contact person for men and women who seek fertility care, nurses must be highly knowledgeable and skilled in communication to foster effective coordination and collaboration among the team (Leonard & Stevenson, 2016) and promote patient retention (Lesser & Hilse, 2014). Due to the high stress experienced by infertility and the complex nature of treatment, patients' communication should be clear and timely (Leonard, & Stevenson, 2016). A primary role of nurses involves providing emotional support to the couple during this highly emotional time. Specialized knowledge as well as organization and leadership are needed by nurses who are responsible for coordinating numerous appointments for exams or lab work, addressing patient concerns, educating patients on medication administration such as changes in doses, and proving emotional support. Nurses provide physical care to patients during assessment and complex treatment plans ordered by physicians or advanced practice nurses (Leonard & Stevenson, 2016). Nurses should provide holistic care that is evidence based and patient centered (den Breejen, Nelen, Schol, Kremer, & Hermens, 2013). Providing education and nonjudgmental support to help lessen the impact of infertility is another important function to ensure quality of care for these patients (Leonard & Stevenson, 2016).

OUTCOMES

When the goal of having a child is interrupted, the outcomes can be devastating, impacting biological, psychological, and social well-being. Infertility has been described as the most challenging experience faced by anyone (Phillips, Elander, & Montague, 2014). Coping with the uncertainties of infertility is stressful. Individuals affected report sexual dysfunction, depression, anxiety, isolation, guilt, grief, low self-esteem (ASRM, 2017b; Lawson, 2016; Lawson et al., 2014; Luk & Loke, 2015), diminished quality of life (Direkvand-Moghadam, Delpishes, & Direkvand-Moghadam, 2014), and loss of control (Leonard, & Stevenson, 2016). Infertility may create a spiritual crisis leaving individuals to question "Why me?" Persons suffering from infertility are constantly reminded of the diagnosis in day-to-day encounters with families, children, and pregnant women in a society that celebrates babies and parenthood.

Summary

For millions of women and men, infertility is a stressful diagnosis with complex treatments. Nurses are in a unique position to help improve patient outcomes by providing care, education, and support based on best practice. The emotional distress of infertility and complex nature of treatment requires nurses who are both educated and emotionally supportive to provide patient-centered care to this vulnerable population. Nurses are an integral part of the health care team to promote well-being and improve fertility outcomes for men and women who desire parenthood.

American Society for Reproductive Medicine. (2014). Fact sheet: Defining infertility. Retrieved from http://www.reprodsurgery.org/uploadedFiles/ASRM_Content/Resources/Patient_Resources/Fact_Sheets_and_Info_Booklets/Defining%20inertility%20FINAL%20%202-19-14.pdf

American Society for Reproductive Medicine. (2015). Infertility: An overview. Retrieved from http://www.asrm.org/Booklet_Infertility_An_Overview

American Society for Reproductive Medicine. (2017a). Quick facts about infertility. Retrieved from http://www.reproductivefacts.org/faqs/quick-facts-about-infertility

American Society for Reproductive Medicine. (2017b). What impact does infertility have on psychological well-being? Retrieved from http://www.reproductivefacts.org/faqs/faqs-about-the-psychological-component-of-infertility/q1.-what-impact-does-infertility-have-on-psychological-well-being

American Urological Association. (n.d.). The optimal evaluation of the infertile male: Best practice statement. Reviewed and validity confirmed 2011. Retrieved from https://www.auanet.org/education/guidelines/male-infertility-d.cfm

Chandra, A., Copen, C. E., & Stephen, E. H. (2013). Infertility and impaired fecundity in the United States, 1982–2010: Data from the National Survey of Family Growth (Report No. 67). Retrieved from https://www.cdc.gov/nchs/data/nhsr/nhsr073.pdf

Centers for Disease Control and Illness Prevention. (2014). National public health action plan for the detection, prevention, and management of infertility. Retrieved from https://www.cdc.gov/reproductivehealth/infertility/pdf/drh_nap_final_508.pdf

Centers for Disease Control and Prevention. (2017). Reproductive health: Infertility. Retrieved from https://www.cdc.gov/reproductivehealth/infertility

den Breejen, E. M. E., Nelen, W. L. D. M., Schol, S. F. E., Kremer, J, A, M., & Hermens, R. P. M. G. (2013). Development of guideline-based indicators for patient-centeredness in fertility care: What patients add. Human Reproduction, 27, 1073–1079. doi:10.1093/humrep/det010

Direkvand-Moghadam, A., Delpisheh, A., & Direkvand-Moghadam, A. (2014). Effect of infertility on quality of life, A cross-sectional study. Journal of Clinical and Diagnostic Research, 8(10), 1–3. Retrieved from https://www.ncbi.nlm.nih.gov/pmc/articles/PMC4253230/pdf/jcdr-8-OC13.pdf

Lawson, A. K. (2016). Psychological stress and fertility. In E. L. Stevenson & P. E. Hershberger (Eds.), Fertility and assisted reproductive technology (ART): Theory, research, policy, and practice for health care practitioners (pp. 65–87). New York, NY: Springer Publishing.

Lawson, A. K., Klock, S. C., Pavone, M. E., Hirshfeld-Cytron, J., Smith, K. N., & Kazer, R. (2014). A prospective study of depression and anxiety in female fertility preservation and infertility patients. Fertility and Sterility, 102(5), 1377–1384. doi:10.1016/j.fertnstert.2014.07.765

Leonard, J., & Stevenson, E. L. (2016). Team communication: Critical in the care of the couple with infertility challenges. In E. L. Stevenson & P. E. Hershberger (Eds.), Fertility and assisted reproductive technology (ART): Theory, research, policy, and practice for health care practitioners (pp. 295–309). New York, NY: Springer Publishing.

Lesser, C. B., & Hilse, M. (2014). The IVF nurse. Untapped resource for recruiting and retaining patients (Supplement: Best Practices in IVF Nursing, Newsletter Series). OBG Management, 26(10), 1–4. Retrieved from http://www.mdedge.com/sites/default/files/images/Actavis_1014_V2.pdf

Luk, B. H., & Loke, A. Y. (2015). The impact of infertility on the psychological well-being, marital relationships, sexual, relationships, and quality of life of couples: A systematic review. Journal of Sex and Marital Therapy, 41(6), 610–625. doi:10.1080/0092623X.2014.958789

McEleny, K. (2016). Men and infertility: Their experience with challenges in family formation. In E. L. Stevenson & P. E. Hershberger (Eds.), Fertility and assisted reproductive technology (ART): Theory, research, policy, and practice for health care practitioners (pp. 323–335). New York, NY: Springer Publishing.

Phillips, E., Elander, J., & Montague, J. (2014). Managing multiple goals during fertility treatment: An interpretive phenomenological analysis. Journal of Health Psychology, 19(4), 531–543. doi:10.1177/1359105312474915

Practice Committee ASRM. (2014). Female age related fertility decline. Fertility and Sterility, 101(3), 633–634. Retrieved from http://www.fertstert.org/article/S0015-0282(13)03464-X/pdf

Stevenson, E. L., Hershberger, P. E., & Bergh, P. A. (2016). Evidence-care for couples with infertility. Journal of Obstetric, Gynecologic, and Neonatal Nursing, 45, 100–110. doi:10.1016/j.jogn.2015.10.006

Vespa, J., Lewis, J. M., & Kreider, R. M. (2013). America's family and living arrangements: 2012 Population characteristics (Report No. P20—570). Retrieved from http://www.censud.gov/library/publications/2013/demo/p20-570.html

Zegers-Hochschild, F., Adamson, G. D., de Mouzon, J., Ishihara, O., Mansour, R., Nygren, K., . . . Vanderpoel, S. (2009). International committee for monitoring assisted reproductive technology (ICMART) and the World Health Organization (WHO) revised glossary of ART terminology. Fertility and Sterility, 92(5), 1520–1524. Retrieved from http://www.fertstert.org/article/S0015-0282(09)03688-7/pdf

■ INTIMATE PARTNER VIOLENCE

Marilyn E. Smith

Overview

Violence toward an intimate partner continues to be a serious and preventable national health problem. Intimate partner violence (IPV) is described as physical violence, sexual violence, stalking and psychological aggression (including coercive acts) by a current or former intimate partner by the Centers for Disease Control and Prevention (CDC; 2015). An intimate partner is a person with whom one has or had a close personal relationship. IPV can occur between heterosexual or same-sex couples and does not require sexual intimacy. IPV is usually a series of events starting with verbal and emotional abuse accompanied by controlling and intimidating behaviors of the perpetrator. These behaviors include, but are not limited to slapping, intimidation, shaming, forced intercourse, isolation, monitoring of behaviors, spying, showing up in places where the victim does not want him or her; harming or threatening the victim's pet; opposing or interfering with school or employment; restricting access to health care; and making decisions concerning contraception, pregnancy, and elective abortion.

Nurses play an important role in the prevention and assessment of IPV. Nursing care for victims of IPV, after establishing a trusting relationship, includes providing information, creating a safety plan, and empowering the victim.

Background

According to the CDC (2014), lifetime prevalence of physical violence by an intimate partner is 31.5% among women and 27.5% among men. It is noted that, although there is a small difference in the overall prevalence of physical violence by an intimate partner when comparing women and men, the severity, frequency, and impact is often not considered in these comparison rates. For example, from 2002 to 2011, intimate partner victimization resulted in a serious injury, such as internal injury, unconsciousness, or broken bones, in 13% of women versus 5% of males (Catalano, 2013). Thus, in this discussion, the focus will be on violence against women.

Violence against women takes many forms and is pervasive in the United States, with substantial humanitarian and economic costs. According to a report by the McKinsey Global Institute (Ellingrud et al., 2016), more than 39 million women, nearly one-third of the U.S. female population, have experienced physical violence by an intimate partner, from slapping to beating. They estimate that this type of violence costs about $4.9 billion in the United States annually. This estimate includes direct medical costs, lost productivity, and lost earnings.

There is a wide range of health problems related to IPV. Whiting, Liu, Koyuturk, and Karakurt (2016) found that chronic and acute conditions, as well as acute injuries, were prevalent among victims of IPV. These included gynecological and pregnancy-related issues as well as gastrointestinal, cardiovascular, and neurological symptoms. Poor pregnancy outcomes, low-birth-weight infants, depression, anxiety, and posttraumatic stress disorder can also be prevalent among victims of abuse. Besides the millions of women who are affected by IPV, it is estimated that each year 10 million children witness IPV within their families, putting these children at risk for developing long-term emotional problems, psychiatric disorders, developmental problems, school failures, violence against others, and low self-esteem (Hamby, Finkelhor, Turner, & Ormrod, 2011).

Often, as the duration of the relationship in which IPV is occurring increases, the abuse may become more frequent and severe. Consequently, the longer the woman maintains the abusive relationship, the more vulnerable she becomes to being severely hurt or murdered. Many female homicide victims are intimate acquaintances of their killers, including wives, common-law wives, ex-wives, and girlfriends. Catalano (2013) reports that in 2010, of the 3,032 homicide incidents involving females, 39% were committed by an intimate partner. During the same year, of the 10,878 homicide incidents involving males, an intimate partner was responsible for 3%.

Despite abuse and potential danger of homicide, many women find leaving the abusive relationship very difficult. Society, including nurses, is often confused, bewildered, impatient, and even angry that victims of IPV do not simply leave the abusive situation. Nurses may have an instant negative reaction when their patients return to or stay in an abusive relationship. As nurses, we must understand that women stay in an abusive relationship for many reasons. These may include commitment to the relationship, feeling responsible for the abuse, feeling responsible for helping the partner, economic stability, social standing, fear of reprisals, and fear for the physical safety of themselves and their children, and the universal need to be loved. Yes, the need to be loved. Some women may interpret a partner's jealousy, constant attention, or controlling behaviors as signs of love. An emotional bond with another person is a central motivating factor in the human experience. The fear of being alone is often more frightening than the physical abuse. Feeling judged, blamed, or disbelieved might cause shame in a woman and constitute a major barrier to being able to leave an abusive relationship.

Clinical Aspects

ASSESSMENT

Nurses are often the first point of contact for an abused woman and thus have an important role in assisting women and children. As nurses themselves may be victims of IPV they need to educate themselves concerning IPV as well as confront fears, biases, and beliefs concerning victims.

Assessing for IPV is very important in all health care settings. Victims may be reluctant to disclose abuse for many reasons, which include, fear of their own or their children's safety, denial, shame, or commitment to the relationship. The evidence shows that screening does increase the identification of women experiencing IPV in health care settings, significantly in antenatal settings (O'Doherty et al., 2015).

A victim must be approached in a nonjudgmental manner. One way to do this is to maintain a curiosity about the victim's experiences and allow her to tell her story. There are various recommended screening tools that your practice or institution may acquire. However, simply asking about abuse in an empathetic manner often gives the victim the feeling that someone cares and thus the courage to reveal the abuse. Nurses should be alert in identifying victims who hesitate to come forward by recognizing the telltale signs of IPV. Possible red flags include physical injuries that seem nonaccidental, presentation of the partner's point of view, partner's abuse of pets, minimization of partner's abusive behavior, and description of partner as having a bad temper.

NURSING INTERVENTIONS, MANAGEMENT, AND IMPLICATIONS

In the prevention of intimate partner violence, nurses can play a key role by advocating for legislature that holds offenders more accountable for their crimes, including prosecuting domestic violence cases. Nurses must also be knowledgeable of the services provided to victims in their area, which may include counseling, legal advice, shelter, and skills training.

After establishing a trusting and therapeutic relationship and providing the victim with knowledge of resources, the nurse needs to help the victim establish a safety plan. If she is not ready to contact domestic violence advocates, provide her with domestic violent resource brochures describing in detail a safety plan to follow during an explosive incident or when she is preparing to leave.

OUTCOMES

When working with a victim remember to empower her by allowing her to make her own decisions. She has had little control in her life while being in an abusive relationship. It is imperative that she does not experience the nurse telling her what to do. The nurse should give the woman choices and express acknowledgment of the difficult decisions the woman must make. Remember you can influence a victim's ability to leave by maintaining a nonjudgmental attitude, validating what she is feeling, remembering she is grieving the loss of what the relationship was and her dreams for it, and finally by connecting her physical/emotional abuse to her child's possible difficulties at school.

Summary

To mitigate and prevent devastating health effects resulting from IPV, it is vital that nurses push to improve screening and identification of victims. Approaching victims in an empathic nonjudgmental manner is imperative because many are reluctant to report for fear of being judged.

Catalano, S. (2013). Intimate partner violence: Attributes of victimization, 1993–2011. U.S. Department of Justice. Retrieved from https://www.bjs.gov/content/pub/pdf/ipvav9311.pdf

Centers for Disease Control and Prevention. (2014). Prevalence and characteristics of sexual violence, stalking, and intimate partner violence victimization—National intimate partner and sexual violence survey, United States, 2011. Retrieved from https://www.cdc.gov/mmwr/preview/mmwrhtml/ss6308a1.htm?s_cid=ss6308a1_e

Centers for Disease Control and Prevention. (2015). Intimate partner violence surveillance uniform definitions and recommended data elements, version 2.0. Retrieved from https://www.cdc.gov/violenceprevention/pdf/intimatepartnerviolence.pdf

Ellingrud, K., Madgavkar, A., Manyika, J., Woetzel, J., Riefberg, V., Krishnan, M., & Seoni, M. (2016). The power of parity: Advancing women's equality in the United States. Retrieved from https://www.mckinsey.com/global-themes/employment-and-growth/the-power-of-parity-advancing-womens-equality-in-the-united-states

Hamby, S., Finkelhor, D., Turner, H., & Ormrod, R. (2011). *Children's exposure to intimate partner violence and other family violence.* Juvenile Justice Bulletin – NCJ 232272. Washington, DC: U.S. Government Printing Office. Retrieved from http://www.unh.edu/ccrc/pdf/jvq/NatSCEVChildren's%20Exposure-Family%20Violence%20final.pdf

O'Doherty, L., Hegarty, K., Ramsay, J., Davidson, L. L., Feder, G., & Taft, A. (2015). Screening women for intimate partner violence in healthcare settings. *Cochrane Database of Systematic Reviews, 2015*(7), CD007007. doi:10.1002/14651858.CD007007.pub3

Whiting, K., Liu, L, Koyuturk, M., & Karakurt, G. (2016). Network map of adverse health effects among victims of intimate partner violence. *Pacific Symposium on Bio Computing, 22,* 324–335.

■ IN VITRO FERTILIZATION

Donna Lynn Rose
Mary T. Quinn Griffin

Overview

Most people consider the process of bearing children a significant and desirable experience. However, many individuals are unable to achieve pregnancy in the traditional manner and may turn to assistive reproductive therapy (ART). In vitro fertilization (IVF) is the most common and effective type of ART (CDC, 2017). IVF is a procedure that involves extracting eggs from the ovaries, fertilizing them with sperm in a laboratory dish, and implanting the fertilized egg(s) into the uterus. Nurses working in a variety of settings have the opportunity to be a part of the interprofessional team providing care for individuals with fertility issues undergoing IVF. The nurse must understand the process of fertility care and IVF, to include physiologic, psychosocial, socioeconomic, and legal and ethical considerations, in order to provide holistic, evidence-based care and support.

Background

As of 2014, approximately 1 million babies were conceived in the United States through IVF (American Society for Reproductive Medicine [ASRM], 2017). IVF is a treatment that offers hope for those who are infertile. *Infertility* is defined as being unable to conceive after 12 months of unprotected intercourse (ASRM, 2017). Statistics from the 2011 to 2013 National Survey of Family Growth (CDC, 2015) reported a continued increase in the percentage of women from 15 to 44 years of age (all marital statuses) who have impaired fecundity (this includes women having difficulty getting pregnant and those who cannot carry a pregnancy to term), increasing from 10.9% in 2006 to 2010 to 12.3% in the 2011 to 2013 survey. In addition, the CDC (2014) reports that significant disparities exist by race, ethnicity, sex, and socioeconomic status in the prevalence, diagnosis, referral, and treatment of infertility. Currently, only 15 states in the United States have some form of infertility insurance laws and, of these, three states specifically exclude IVF, and four states mandate coverage of IVF only (ASRM, 2017).

It is often thought that fertility issues occur mostly with women; however, according to the ASRM (2017) about one third of infertility cases result from an issue with the male partner, and another one third of infertility cases results from a combination of male and female problems. In approximately 20% of cases, the cause of infertility is unable to be identified (ASRM, 2017), whereas, 40% of the cases are female and 40% are male. Male fertility issues can be the result of the male not being able to produce or ejaculate sperm. Sperm quality, which takes into account the amount, movement, and shape of sperm, plays a role in fertility and can be affected by conditions such as diabetes, cystic fibrosis, obesity, and smoking (ASRM, 2017).

The most common cause of infertility in women is an ovulation disorder. Smoking, weight (being too thin or obese), and damaged or blocked fallopian tubes, often the result of endometriosis or pelvic inflammatory disease also contributes to infertility (ASRM, 2017). Advanced maternal age at the desired time of conception is a major contributor to infertility (CDC, 2017). The ASRM (2017) reports that by the time a woman is in her 40s, the chances of conceiving each month is 10% or less. Repeated miscarriages add to impaired fecundity and are sometimes attributed to congenital anomalies of the uterus and uterine fibroids (ASRM, 2017).

Clinical Aspects

ASSESSMENT

There is not a single test to confirm the diagnosis of infertility. In general, couples should seek medical care after a year of trying to conceive (ASRM, 2017) and women older than 35 should seek care if conception has not occurred within 6 months (CDC, 2017). Initial evaluation should include a medical history, physical examination, and basic blood tests. If the etiology is still undetermined, more specific testing will occur. Women will undergo ovulation testing to assess fallopian tube patency (ASRM, 2014). Invasive testing, such as a laparoscopy or hysteroscopy, may be necessary. Initial infertility testing for men will focus on semen analysis. Additional testing may include a urologic evaluation to assess for a varicocele (enlargement of a vein within the scrotum) or tumor along with more specific blood work analysis (ASRM, 2017).

Approximately 99% of the ART procedures performed are IVF (CDC, 2015). In vitro (occurring outside of the body) fertilization is a process of combining a woman's egg and a man's sperm in a laboratory dish. The success rate for couples undergoing IVF in the United States is approximately 29% (CDC, 2015). The first step in the IVF process is giving the woman medications to stimulate the ovaries to produce multiple eggs. More than one egg is required because some of the eggs will fail to develop or fertilize. There are numerous medication regimes for ovarian stimulation, and nurses must be aware of the different protocols, their actions, and side effects. The ovary stimulation is carefully monitored using transvaginal ultrasound and blood tests to assess hormone levels. The eggs are retrieved by aspirating the ovarian follicles using a hollow needle inserted vaginally into the pelvic cavity guided by transvaginal ultrasound. The male partner provides a fresh specimen of sperm. The eggs and sperm are mixed together and incubated for about 36 hours. During this period, the eggs are monitored for fertilization, quality, and growth. Approximately 48 hours after retrieval, the best quality embryos are transferred into the uterus through the cervix using a soft catheter. Embryos are transferred between days 3 to 5, day 3 when at the cleavage stage or day 5 at the blastocyst stage. Success rates are greater for more than one embryo, but there is increased risk of multiple pregnancy. The IVF cycle is typically as follows: (a) preadministration treatment as necessary (oral contraceptives to regulate the menstrual cycle) and medications to prevent premature ovulation, (b) ovarian stimulation with medications called *fertility drugs* to increase the number of mature oocytes, (c) monitoring follicle development, (d) human chorionic gonadotropin (hCG) administration to facilitate oocyte maturation, (e) transvaginal oocyte retrieval (using anesthesia

and ultrasound), (f) oocyte fertilization with semen in the laboratory, (g) embryo transfer to uterus 3 to 6 days after retrieval, (h) progesterone administration (i) pregnancy test, and (j) continued follow-up care (Stevenson, Hershberger, & Bergh, 2016).

NURSING, INTERVENTIONS, MANAGEMENT, AND IMPLICATIONS

Nurses must be able to provide evidence-based education, physical care, and psychological support when working with a patient undergoing infertility evaluation and IVF.

Patients are likely to have deficient knowledge regarding the process, side effects, and potential complications of IVF, and nurses need to provide education in these areas. Education regarding risks of multiple births is important, as women who undergo IVF are more likely to have multiple births, and this substantially increases obstetrical risks for mothers. Infants are more likely to be preterm and of low birth weight (CDC, 2015). Education regarding modifiable risk factors associated with infertility, such as smoking and being too thin or overweight, should be provided by the nurse (ASRM, 2017).

Patients need to be instructed on the side effects of fertility medications and be aware of the symptoms of ovarian hyperstimulation syndrome (OHSS), a complication causing buildup of fluid in the abdomen (ASRM, 2017). Education regarding the risks associated with the process of egg retrieval, such as complications from anesthesia, infection, bleeding, and possible damage to structures surrounding the uterus, should be provided.

The stress related to the treatment of infertility has been linked to a negative effect on psychological health and sexual relationships (Luk & Loke, 2015). The time commitment required for fertility testing and IVF treatment, often causing work absences and lost wages, along with the cost of IVF totaling more than $12,000 in the United States (CDC, 2015) may be additional stressors. Nurses must be active in health policy and engage with policy makers to work to ease the financial burden of IVF in order to reduce disparities in the use of IVF related to socioeconomic conditions.

Social support from family can have a significant positive correlation to mental health, anxiety, and depression in women with infertility issues (Hasanpour, Bani, Mirghafourvand, & Kochaksarayie, 2014). Priority psychosocial nursing interventions include assessing perceived social support and monitoring for increased levels of stress. The nurse should be able to recognize more than moderate levels of stress in women with infertility issues. Stress management strategies, such as relaxation exercises, yoga, and community resources, can be suggested, and, in some cases, pharmacotherapy may be necessary.

OUTCOMES

The nurse should also be aware of potential ethical and legal issues related to IVF so that he or she can be a source of support and work with the patient and interdisciplinary team, which often includes legal counsel. Oocyte donation and gestational surrogacy are essential for some undergoing IVF, yet they have increased legal implications. The handling of surplus embryos sometimes created during IVF has been a topic of much ethical and legal debate. IVF nurses are ethically obligated to treat all patients undergoing IVF equally regardless of marital status or sexual orientation, so they must be aware of their own personal biases.

Summary

Undergoing fertility testing and IVF treatment is very challenging to most individuals/couples. Infertility treatments often affect physical and psychological health, thus affecting overall quality of life. It is imperative that nurses assess social support and monitor for increased stress levels of these patients, and take appropriate interventions. Being engaged in health policy can allow the nurse to be aware of and contribute to ethical and legal issues surrounding IVF. Nurses are an integral part of the interprofessional team and are in a unique position to provide evidence-based education, physical care, and psychological support to individuals/couples undergoing IVF.

American Society for Reproductive Medicine. (2017). Reproductive facts. Retrieved from http://www .reproductivefacts.org/?vs=1

Centers for Disease Control and Prevention. (2014). *National public health action plan for the detection, prevention, and management of infertility*. Atlanta, GA: Author.

Centers for Disease Control and Prevention. (2015). Key statistics from the national survey of family growth. Retrieved from https://www.cdc.gov/nchs/nsfg/key_ statistics/i.htm#impaired

Centers for Disease Control and Prevention. (2017). Fertility FAQS. Retrieved from https://www.cdc.gov/reproductive health/infertility

Hasanpour, S., Bani, S., Mirghafourvand, M., & Yahyavi Kochaksarayie, F. (2014). Mental health and its personal and social predictors in infertile women. *Journal of Caring Science, 3*(1), 37–45. doi:10.5681/jcs.2014.005

Luk, B. H., & Loke, A. Y. (2015). The impact of infertility on the psychological well-being, marital relationships, sexual relationships, and quality of life of couples: A systematic review. *Journal of Sex & Marital Therapy, 41*(6), 610–625.

Stevenson, E., Hershberger, P., & Bergh, P. (2016). Evidence-based care for couples with infertility. *Journal of Obstetric, Gynecologic, & Neonatal Nursing. 45*, 100–110.

■ LABOR AND DELIVERY

Carrie Gerber

Overview

Labor is a natural part of the birthing process. It is a unique moment in time for a woman and her partner. As a labor and delivery nurse, you are privileged to be a part of this journey with a family, to guide them through it, and provide both emotional and physical support to women. Whether a woman is having a vaginal delivery or a cesarean delivery, the nursing role is crucial in providing care for the mother and her newborn.

A perinatal nurse has a profound effect on a woman's birth experience and the care she feels she receives during it. It is important for the patient to be a part of the decision-making process in the birth, this is likely a moment she has thought about for many years. Birth preparation, communication, support, and respect of a patient's wishes (Fair & Morrison, 2011) are the most common themes associated with having a feeling of satisfaction and control about one's labor and birth experience. This is a complex dynamic that requires constant, continual nursing care from a perinatal nurse.

Background

According to the Centers for Disease Control and Prevention (CDC), in the United States, there were nearly 4 million births in 2014 with 98.5% of all births occurring in hospitals (2014). From 2013 to 2014, there was a 1% increase in the number of births nationwide (CDC, 2014). With the increasing number of births in the hospital setting, the role of labor and delivery nurses continues to be at the forefront.

Hospital systems throughout the United States have begun efforts to improve quality and safety in obstetrics by standardizing care. Nursing frameworks are created to enhance patient-centered care relationships in the perinatal setting to facilitate the complex role, to include both the caring behaviors and technical skills required of the labor and delivery nurse (Glenn, Stocker-Schnieder, McCune, McClelland & King, 2013).

The role of a perinatal nurse is multidimensional: There is the caring work of patients: providing massage, therapeutic touch, coaching, and guided imagery through the many hours of painful labor. There is the "hands on" work of fetal monitoring ensuring the well-being of the fetus. Labor is a process that the entire family goes through, and the perinatal nurse provides the compassionate touch and assurance needed to the partner and family of the expectant mother. There is also a technical component related to being a modern-day bedside perinatal nurse. There are numerous technological skills and elements that are required for a perinatal nurse to master. This includes, but is not limited to, electronic fetal monitoring, scanning of medications, and intravenous placement. Paramount to this are the lifesaving skills of resuscitation for the adult and the neonate, the maneuvers needed to assist in a shoulder dystocia, or the supplies needed to manage a postpartum hemorrhage to save a woman's life. The nursing care for an intrapartum patient is all encompassing; it is the continual care of a woman, her family, and her newborn.

Communication is an essential element in a labor and delivery suite. It is of the utmost importance to keep patient safety in mind for all providers, including physicians, midwives, physician's assistants, and for nurses to all speak the same dialect and communicate with one another clearly and concisely. Ineffective communication has been implicated as a major contributor to adverse obstetrical events (Grobman et al., 2010). Both interdepartmental and intradepartmental coordination was identified as a major barrier related to communication (Grobman et al., 2010). There has been a large focus on standardizing communication through the implementation of Team Strategies and Tools to Enhance Performance and Patient Safety (STEPPS). Team STEPPS, designed by the U.S. Department of Health and Human Services is a teamwork system designed for health care professionals that is a powerful solution to improving patient safety within your organization (2016). Improved communication will continue to lead to better outcomes throughout the United States.

Clinical Aspects

ASSESSMENT

A critical component of labor and delivery nursing is fetal heart rate monitoring and assessment. The fetal heart rate can be monitored intermittently or continuously throughout labor. This decision is made based on a myriad of factors, including maternal or fetal comorbidities, the category of the fetal heart rate tracing as defined by the National Institute of Child Health and Human Development (NICHD), or if the patient's labor is spontaneous, augmented or induced. In addition, a discussion is had with the patient care team, including the nurse, physician, and patient about what is most appropriately indicated at this period. Keep in mind, labor is a dynamic process, it is possible to have intermittent monitoring at the onset and then require continuous monitoring and vice versa.

In April 2008, the NICHD, along with the American College of Obstetrics and Gynecology (ACOG) and the Society for Maternal–Fetal Medicine reviewed and defined the nomenclature, interpretation, and research recommendations for intrapartum electronic fetal heart rate monitoring (National Certification Corporation [NCC], 2010). Standardizing the terminology and the requirements to describe an electronic fetal heart tracing and the development of a three-tiered classification system have improved the ease of sharing information among all clinicians, as everyone is speaking and hearing the same language, thereby having the same understanding of the fetal status (NCC, 2010).

In addition to assessing the fetal well-being via electronic fetal monitoring, the labor and delivery nurse also provides numerous assessments of the mother. A woman's past medical, surgical, and obstetrical history can have a dramatic effect on her mode of delivery, ability to receive neuraxial analgesia, and expectations of delivery. Managing a woman's pain throughout labor is one of the many roles of a labor and delivery nurse. It is incumbent upon the nurse to inform a patient about her pain management options, which include but are not limited to neuraxial analgesia. Neuraxial analgesia, which includes an epidural, combined spinal–epidural, and continuous spinal–epidural, are the most common forms of labor analgesia (Grant, Tao, Craig, McIntire & Leveno, 2014). Approximately 60% of women in the United States receive neuraxial analgesia for labor. It is important for women to know that research has concluded that receiving an early labor analgesia, if less than 4-cm cervical dilation, does not slow the progress of labor as previously thought (Grant et al., 2014).

NURSING INTERVENTIONS, MANAGEMENT, AND IMPLICATIONS

A perinatal nurse has the responsibility to be prepared for any emergency. One of the most clinically challenging aspects of being a delivery room nurse is that the status of the mother or fetus can change in an instant. This requires the nurse to always be present, ready, and available to assist with a procedure, mobilize a patient to an operating room for an emergent delivery, and to have the situational awareness to prepare for the unexpected.

OUTCOMES

The expected outcomes of evidenced-based nursing care for all labor and delivery patients and their newborns are centered on having a healthy newborn and postpartum mother. Actively managing a patient's labor can facilitate a positive outcome.

Summary

In summary, a well-supported birth honors and respects the wishes of the patient. A perinatal nurse provides a patient with the emotional, physical, and intellectual support to endure the labor and delivery process while simultaneously managing the fetal heart rate tracing to assess fetal well-being. Labor and delivery require a multidisciplinary team, including an obstetrician, anesthesiologist, pediatricians, and nurses to be ready with the ability to provide comprehensive care for any impending situation. The role of the labor and delivery nurse is one of the most unique and rewarding opportunities because every day you have the opportunity to play an integral role in the development of a family.

About Team STEPPS. (2016). Rockville, MD: Agency for Healthcare Research and Quality. Retrieved from http://www.ahrq.gov/teamstepps/about-teamstepps/index.html

Centers for Disease Control and Prevention. (2014). Births: Final data for 2014. *National Vital Statistics Reports, 64*(12), 1–64.

Fair, C. D., & Morrison, T. (2011). I felt part of the decision-making process: A qualitative study on techniques used to enhance maternal control during labor and delivery. *International Journal of Childbirth Education, 26*, 21–25.

Glenn, L. A., Stocker-Schnieder, J., McCune, R., McClelland, M., & King, D. (2013). Caring nurse practice in the intrapartum setting: Nurses' perspectives on complexity, relationships and safety. *Journal of Advanced Nursing, 70*(9), 2019–2030. doi:10.1111/jan.12356

Grant, E. N., Tao, W., Craig, M., McIntire, D., & Leveno, K. (2014). Neuraxial analgesia effects on labour progression: Facts, fallacies, uncertainties and the future. *British Journal of Obstetrics and Gynaecology, 122*, 288–293.

Grobman, W. A., Holl, J., Woods, D., Gleason, K. M., Wassilak, B., & Sxekendi, M. K. (2010). Perspectives on communication in labor and delivery: A focus group analysis. *Journal of Perinatology, 31*, 240–245.

National Certification Corporation. (2010). NICHD definitions and classifications: Application to electronic fetal monitoring. *NCC Monograph, 3*(1), 1–20.

■ LACTATION

Jarold T. Johnston

Overview

The value of breastfeeding and human breast milk is nearly incontrovertible. The studies linking failure to breastfeed with increased morbidity and mortality are legion. A 2016 global meta-analysis evaluating data from more than 150 countries and evaluating 28 systematic reviews and meta-analyses confirmed that children who are breastfed have lower infectious morbidity and mortality, fewer dental malocclusions, and higher intelligence than those who are not breastfed (Victoria et al., 2016). The review also reported lower rates of maternal illness, including breast and ovarian cancer and diabetes, and improved child spacing. The study concluded by reporting that if 90% of the global population breastfed their children for 12 months, an estimated 823,000 child deaths and 20,000 maternal breast cancer deaths might be prevented every year (2016). There is near global uniformity regarding breastfeeding recommendations from the World Health Organization (WHO), the U.S. Surgeon General (OTSG), the American Academy of Pediatrics (AAP), The Academy of Breastfeeding Medicine (ABM), and the U.K.'s National Institute for Health and Care Excellence (NICE) that all newborn infants should be exclusively breastfed for the first 6 months at which time complementary foods may be introduced, but infants should continue to breastfeed until 1 to 2 years of age (Chantry, Eglash, & Labbock, 2015). Mothers who are not offered adequate breastfeeding support are at increased risk for shorter breastfeeding duration, thereby increasing their risk and the risks of their infant to morbidity and mortality mentioned previously (Chantry et al., 2015).

Perhaps more important than breastfeeding's global impact on the wellness of the population is the fact that some families of newborn infants want to breastfeed, but are unable to do so due to a lack of competent health care providers (Garner et al., 2016). More than 80% of childbearing women chose to breastfeed their newborns, yet according to readily available data from the Centers for Disease Control and Prevention (CDC), there is a sharp decline in breastfeeding over the first 6 weeks and by 6 months, only 37% of infants are getting breast milk. More than 80% of new mothers report at least one significant breastfeeding complication that threatens their breastfeeding success. Many nurses graduate from their training programs, residencies, and graduate schools with negligible amounts of training in human lactation, often without even a basic understanding of the known risks of formula feeding (Garner et al., 2016). This phenomenon persists despite the ready availability of evidence-based protocols and several well-written systematic reviews, and nurses continue to find themselves unprepared to offer support to the breastfeeding dyad. This entry addresses this problem by drawing from the evidence-based protocols. It is hoped that with this information at hand, the clinical nurse can begin to overcome some of the deficiencies of the health care system as they relate to human lactation.

Background

Lactation is a basic mammalian survival mechanism. Indeed, the very term *mammal* is derived from the ability of the offspring to draw milk from his mother's mammary gland (Hartmann, 2007). Cutting-edge research has begun to confirm what lactation consultants have suspected for more than 10 years, that breast milk and the act of breastfeeding form a complex biosystem involving multiple maternal and neonatal factors far beyond simple nutrition. For a preliminary review of these concepts, the reader is encouraged to review the work of Peter Hartmann, Nils Bergman, or Margaret Neville.

Sufficient lactation is the maternal–infant dyad's ability to synthesize, produce, and transfer enough human milk to support adequate growth of the infant during the first 2 to 3 years of life. As this definition suggests there are four critical and interrelated antecedents: milk synthesis, milk production, milk transfer, and infant growth. Each of these four factors is, to some degree, related to the other and yet also independent. To successfully manage and support lactation, a nurse must understand these concepts.

Milk synthesis is the creation of milk at a cellular level within the glandular tissue of the breast. The ability to synthesize milk is directly related to the overall success of the mother's breast development during puberty and pregnancy. Glandular development is affected by maternal conditions such as polycystic ovarian syndrome (PCOS), diabetes, thyroid disorders, and preterm birth (Marasco, 2014). A complete history of breast development should be part of the nurse's breastfeeding assessment.

There are two phases of milk synthesis: secretory differentiation (lactogenesis I), and secretory activation (lactogenesis II; Hartmann, 2007). Secretory differentiation produces a type of milk known as *colostrum*. This milk is low in volume with the average woman having only 37 mL available in the first day postpartum and approximately 100 mL on the second day postpartum (Kent, 2012). The low lactose level in colostrum yields only 18.7 kcal/30 mL (Hartmann, 2007). This minimal amount of available calories explains the need for babies to be born with ample amounts of brown fat, and why all newborns lose weight in the first 48 hours of life. Infants born with little brown fat (late preterm and small for gestational age) may require additional screening and close monitoring (Meier, Patel, Wright, Engstrom, 2013). Although colostrum is not intended to be a nourishing liquid, colostrum is thought to protect the newborn mucosal surfaces from the world outside of the womb. The components of human colostrum are constantly changing, but are known to contain secretory immunoglobulin A, lactoferrin, human milk oligosaccharides, growth factors, cytokines, transforming growth factors, interleukin 10, and erythropoietin, which may act to protect and promote the development of the neonatal microbiome (Bode, 2012).

Secretory activation (lactogenesis II) is the rapid and copious synthesis of "mature milk" that occurs shortly after birth. With the removal of the placenta, there is a rapid withdrawal of placental progesterone that signals the lactocyte to activate and synthesize significant amounts of lactose, which leads to a rapid increase in milk volume due to the osmotic nature of this disaccharide (Hartmann, 2007). This process usually occurs 48 to 72 hours postpartum, but is known to be delayed in women who are obese, have delivered via cesarean section, or have diabetes (Hartmann, 2007; Kent et al., 2012). The mother often is able to perceive this phenomenon known as the milk *coming in*, and describe it as a rapid onset period of breast fullness, hardness, and tenderness (Hartmann, 2007). During the period, the volume of milk synthesis rises from 30 mL/d to 100 ml/d on day 2, and 395 to 868 mL/d by day 6 postpartum (Kent, et al., 2012). The volume of milk synthesis stabilizes in the first month postpartum and averages 750 mL/d with a normal range of 440 to 1,220 mL/d for the first 6 months of life (Kent et al., 2012).

Milk production is the expression of milk to the baby or artificial collection device. It is well known that milk synthesis is related to milk production, whereas the more milk a mother is able to remove from the breast, the more milk her breasts will make. Milk production occurs primarily as a result of pulsatile surges of oxytocin that cause the myoepithelial cells of the terminal duct lobular unit (TDLU) to contract causing a rapid expression of milk from the nipple known as the *milk ejection reflex* (*MER*), colloquially known as *let down*. The work of Prime, Kent, Hepworth, Trengove, and Hartmann (2012) suggests that the average woman experiences four to five MER per pumping session, that the maximum milk removal occurs in the first or second MER, and that by the 8th minute approximately 54% ± 25% of the available milk has been removed (Prime et al., 2012). Neither the baby nor the pump are capable of emptying the breast. Although there is tremendous variability between each woman's breast and between women in general, the average pump-dependent mother is only able to successfully remove 60% (range: 20.8%–105%) of the milk available (Prime et al., 2012). Finally, there is a consensus that the amount of milk removed is inversely proportional to the time since last milk removal (Hartmann, 2007; Prime et al., 2012).

Milk transfer to the infant is rarely discussed, but is critically important to successful breastfeeding. A baby with oral motor difficulties (preterm birth, operative vaginal birth, oral anomalies) may have difficulty latching properly and transferring milk from the mother's breast (Meier et al., 2013). To enhance successful milk transfer the mother is encouraged to respond to infant stress cue (rooting, hand sucking, fussing) as infants exhibiting these signs may be having stress due to hunger. It is important to teach parents that these are not hunger signs as it is well known that infants express these stress cues for all forms of stress and that teaching these cues as "hunger signs" may lead the mother to assume hunger even though the infant has recently been well fed (Johnston, 2010). Although there is tremendous individual difference in the feeding habits of breastfed infants, well newborns attempt to nurse seven to 13 times each 24 hours if the mother offers the breasts frequently (Prime et al., 2012). The American Academy of Pediatrics recommends offering the breast eight to 12 times per day and encouraging the infant to nurse for an adequate length of time, generally 15 to 20 minutes; these findings are in alignment with studies on the feeding habits of well newborns (Prime et al., 2012).

Clinical Aspects

ASSESSMENT

Careful assessment of the breastfeeding infant is critical to assessing milk transfer. The components of adequate latch are not universally accepted; however, most authors agree to the following basic principles: the head should be aligned with the trunk and the mouth should be facing the breast at the level of the maternal areola. The mouth should be opened wide encompassing most of the areolar complex, usually at a jaw angle of more than 60° is required. The lips should flare out above and below the nipple, and the cheeks should be well rounded and full. Finally, the mother should feel a gentle tug, but not feel any pain while latching (Johnston, 2010; Mulder, 2006). The most reliable sign of adequate milk transfer is audible swallowing from the infant, an increase in pre- and postfeeding weights using an accurate digital scale, and steady infant weight gain of ½ to 1 oz/d or 5 to 7 oz/wk over the first month of life (Meier et al., 2013; Mulder, 2006).

There are several reliable and validated latch assessment tools available to the nurse to assist with breastfeeding assessment (Altuntas et al., 2014). The LATCH tool allows the nurse to assess breastfeeding techniques of the mother and infant. LATCH is an acronym representing the ability to the infant to latch, the amount of audible swallowing, the type of maternal nipple (everted, flat, or inverted), the mother's comfort regarding her breasts (no pain, some pain, severe pain), and the amount of help the mother needs to latch the infant (Altuntas et al., 2014). The tool allows for 0, 1, or 2 points in each measure for a maximum score of 10. The IBFAT is the Infant Breast Feeding Assessment Tool. The IBFAT measures the rooting, fixing, and suckling behavior of the infant during a feeding. The first item is infant's readiness to feed. Items 2 to 5 measure the infant's ability to fix, root, suckle, and feed. A maximum score of 15 can be earned. The Mother–Baby Assessment Tool (MBA) assesses the process of learning to breastfeed. The tool lists five steps: signaling, positioning, fixing, milk transfer, and ending. Considering that breastfeeding is a mutual skill, both the mother and infant are assessed in each of these behaviors and given a 0 or 1 for each. A score of 10 (five maternal and five infants) is awarded. Each of these tools is validated and reliable. They are easy to use with minimal training (Altuntas et al., 2014). Each facility caring for a breastfeeding dyad is recommended to choose one, train their nursing staff on the use and scoring of the tools, and develop a protocol for assessing infant feeding at least one time each shift (Chantry et al., 2015).

NURSING INTERVENTIONS, MANAGEMENT, AND IMPLICATIONS

No discussion of breastfeeding behavior is complete without addressing the mother's support system and follow-up plan (Mitchell-Box & Braun, 2012). All breastfeeding mothers should be assessed for the availability of breastfeeding support after discharge from the hospital and scheduled for a follow-up visit with a competent health care provider within 48 to 72 hours after discharge (Chantry et al., 2015). Support at home is crucial to success, and multiple studies have demonstrated that fathers are willing and able to provide the necessary support (Mitchell-Box & Braun, 2012). Mitchell-Box has proposed a framework for the education of fathers to prepare them for their role in breastfeeding support (2013). Finally, two authors have presented "father friendly" teaching techniques to help men prepare. Public Services of Canada has created an online resource through an organization named "Dad Central" using automotive analogies to help fathers prepare for their role in infant care, and Johnston (2010) proposed a feeding assessment and support algorithm for new fathers in *Breastfeeding in Combat Boots: A Survival Guide to Breastfeeding While Serving in the Military* by Rouche-Paule. Both of these resources offer "father friendly" methods to teach the components of adequate latching and assessment of milk transfer to provide support upon discharge when medical professionals are not available.

OUTCOMES

The success of the breastfeeding family is critical to global health. An estimated 823,000 infant lives and 20,000 maternal lives can be saved every year with this simple and natural health behavior (Victoria et al., 2016). Breastfeeding support is a basic clinical skill for the nurse generalist, and all nurses are expected to offer at least minimal support to the breastfeeding mother. Currently, more than 80% of women choose to breastfeed, and 80% experience difficulty that threatens their success. If nursing hopes to promote wellness on a public health level, nurses must promote breastfeeding as normative infant feeding behavior, and be at least marginally competent to evaluate and assess normal feeding behavior.

Summary

Several excellent reviews are readily available to help nurses educate themselves in this valuable skill. As a minimum competency, the nurse should understand the basic components of breastfeeding (milk synthesis, milk production, milk transfer, and infant growth), and possess the ability to assess normal newborn feeding behavior. A support person and close health care provider follow-up in the first 2 weeks are critical to the health and wellness of both mother and infant.

Altuntas, N., Turkyilmaz, C., Yildiz, H., Kulali, F., Hirfanoglu, I., Onal, E., . . . Atalay, Y. (2014). Validity and reliaility of the infant breastfeeding assessment tool, The mother baby assessment tool, and the LATCH scoring system. *Breastfeeding Medicine*, 9(4), 191–195.

Bode, L. (2012). Human milk oligosaccharides: Every baby needs a sugar mama. *Glycobiology*, 22(9), 1147–1162.

Chantry, C. J., Elash, A., & Labbok, M. (2015). ABM position on breastfeeding—Revised 2015. *Breastfeeding Medicine*, 10(9), 407–411.

Garner, C. D., Ratcliff, S. L., Thomburg, L. L., Wethington, E., Howard, C. R., & Rasmussen, K. M. (2016). Discontinuity of breastfeeding care: There is no captain of the ship. *Breastfeeding Medicine*, 11(1), 32–39.

Hartmann, P. E. (2007) The lactating breast: An overview from down under. *Breastfeeding Medicine*, 2(1), 3–9.

Hassiotou, F., Geddes, D. T., & Hartmann, P. E., (2015). Cells in human milk: State of the science. *Journal of Human Lactation*, 29(2), 171–182.

Johnston, J. T. (2010). Dads and breastfeeding. In R. Roche-Paull (Ed.), *Breastfeeding in combat boots: A survival guide to successful breastfeeding while serving in the military* (pp. 257–263). Amarillo, TX: Hale.

Kent, J. C., Prime, D.K., & Garbin, C. P. (2012). Principles for maintaining or increasing breast milk production. *Journal of Obstetric, Gynecologic & Neonatal Nursing*, 41, 114–121.

Marasco, L. A. (2014). Unsolved mysteries of the human mammary gland: Defining and redefining the critical questions from the lactation consultant's perspective. *Journal of Mammary Gland Biology and Neoplasia*, 19, 271–288.

Meier, P., Patel, A. L., Wright, K., & Engstrom, J. L. (2013). Management of breastfeeding during and after the maternity hospitalization for late preterm infants. *Clinics in Perinatology*, 40, 689–705.

Mitchell-Box, K., & Braun, K. L. (2012). Fathers' thoughts on breastfeeding and implications for a theory-based intervention. *Journal of Obstetric, Gynecologic, & Neonatal Nursing, 41*(6), E41–E50.

Mitchell-Box, K. M., & Braun, K. (2013). Impact of male-partner-focused interventions on breastfeeding initiation, exclusivity, and continuation. *Journal of Human Lactation, 29*(4), 473–479. doi.org/10.1177/0890334413491833

Mulder, P. J. (2006). A concept analysis of effective breastfeeding. *Journal of Obstetric, Gynecologic, & Neonatal Nursing, 35,* 332–339.

Prime, D. K., Kent, J., Hepworth, A., Trengove, N., & Hartmann, P. (2012). Dynamics of milk removal during simultaneous breast expression in women. *Breastfeeding Medicine, 7,* 100–106.

Victoria, C. G., Bahl, B., Barros, A. J. D., França, G. V. A., Horton, S., Krasevec, J., . . . Rollins, N. C. (2016). Breastfeeding in the 21st century: Epidemiology, mechanisms, and lifelong effect. *Lancet, 387,* 475–490.

■ MENOPAUSE

Maryann Clark

Overview

Menopause is the permanent cessation of menses after 1 full year without menstruation brought on by ovarian failure when follicles become less hormonally responsive (Jackson, 2011). Changing levels of estrogen and progesterone, the two female hormones made in the ovaries, will bring on such short-term symptoms such as palpitations, difficulty concentrating, hot flashes, night sweats, mood changes, and slow metabolism. According to the Mayo Clinic Foundation for Medical Education and Research, 1% of women experience menopause before the age of 40, whereas others will experience symptoms in their 50s. According to the National Institute on Aging, the average age of a woman in menopause is 51 years (National Institutes of Health, 2010).

Background

The menopausal transition is a natural stage for every woman as she ages. Signs and symptoms of menopause are significant enough that most women know their bodies are changing because of decreased hormone patterns. There are blood tests that can check hormone levels such as follicle-stimulating hormone (FSH) and estradiol, but with the cessation of menstruation as the definition, there are visual signs a woman begins to experience such as hot flashes and/or night sweats (vasomotor symptoms) that will indicate that a patient is in menopause. These episodes can happen several times an hour, few times a day, and/or occasionally at night. According to the National Institutes of Health, some studies suggest that as many as three fourths of White women and African American have hot flashes, whereas Japanese and Chinese women are least likely to report this symptom.

Other changes include drier skin and the loss of collagen, which makes skin thinner and less elastic. This generally happens in the areas near the vagina and urinary tract. Sexual intercourse may become more painful and many women in menopause may experience a decrease in sexual libido. There is also evidence that stress, history of depression, and poor general health are likely to contribute to mood changes, anxiety, and irritability during hormonal fluctuations (National Institute on Aging, 2016). Physical changes, such as weight gain in the abdominal area and loss of muscles, also occur in menopausal women. Short-term memory recall is affected. Women begin to have difficulty remembering a familiar word, a person's name, or what one was looking for. Lastly, getting a good night's sleep may become an issue. Night sweats and the need to urinate can interfere with uninterrupted sleep.

Menopause can be brought on by surgical intervention such as a total hysterectomy (removal of the uterus/ovaries) and/or bilateral oophorectomy (removal of the ovaries). This will cause immediate cessation of menstruation and ovulation, and onset of menopausal signs and symptoms will begin and often can be severe as hormonal changes occur abruptly rather than over several years. Chemotherapy and radiation therapy are cancer therapies that can induce menopause as well causing symptoms such as hot flashes and infertility during or shortly after the course of treatment. However, infertility is not always permanent, so birth control measures may still be needed. Menopause may also result from primary ovarian insufficiency when ovaries fail to produce normal levels of reproductive hormones stemming from genetic factors or autoimmune disease. Often no cause can be found. Hormone therapy is typically recommended for these women until the natural age of menopause in order to protect the brain, heart, and bones.

Clinical Aspects

ASSESSMENT

Caring for the menopausal patient as she ages and enters into the postmenopausal phase requires close monitoring of the patient. These patients are at risk for heart and blood vessel disease. Cardiovascular heart disease is the leading cause of death in women as well as men (Mayo Clinic, 2016). Changes in estrogen levels and the aging process may be part of the cause. As a woman ages, changes in weight gain and development of high blood pressure can put one at risk for heart disease. Regular blood pressure screening and blood work, such as fasting blood sugar, cholesterol, and triglycerides, are useful in the prevention of cardiovascular disease in menopausal women. Educational opportunities, such as encouraging a healthy diet and regular exercise, will help decrease weight gain and are an integral part of the care of menopausal women.

Osteoporosis is another condition that can occur with menopause. This condition causes the bones to become weak and brittle leading to increased risk of fractures. Estrogen helps control bone loss and during the first few years after menopause, bone density can be lost at a rapid rate. Often the first sign of osteoporosis is a bone that cracks when twisting or straining. Postmenopausal women with osteoporosis are especially susceptible to fractures of their hips, wrists, and spine. Half of American women older than the age of 50 years will probably have a bone break or fracture later in life because of osteoporosis (National Institutes of Health, 2010).

As the tissues in your vagina and urethra lose elasticity, many women may also experience frequent, sudden urges to have to urinate followed by an involuntary loss of urine. Stress incontinence may also occur, which is the loss of urine while laughing or coughing. Urinary tract infections can also occur more frequently after menopause. Using Kegal exercises and a topical vaginal estrogen may help relieve the problems associated with incontinence.

NURSING INTERVENTIONS, MANAGEMENT, AND IMPLICATIONS

Short-term symptoms of menopause require no medical treatment. Instead, the focus is on relieving signs and symptoms and the prevention and management of the chronic conditions that may occur with aging. The use of hormone-replacement therapy (HRT) has been vigorously debated for many years. In general, all guidelines point to how safe and efficient prescribing estrogen is to women at or around the onset of menopause for relieving symptoms. Several guidelines specifically state that HRT is efficacious for symptoms of menopause other than hot flashes (Stuenkel et al., 2015). Depending on your personal and family history, the physician may recommend estrogen in the lowest of doses in order to prevent the suspected risk of breast cancer and cardiac heart disease similar to the results of the Women's Health Initiative (WHI), which was published in the early 2000s. Estrogen is also known to prevent bone loss and is appropriate even in asymptomatic young women who are at significant risk of osteoporotic fractures (North American Menopause Society, 2012). Often progesterone may be recommended for those women who have not had a hysterectomy.

Estrogen can also be administered vaginally to relieve dryness associated with menopause. It is administered as a cream, tablet, or ring and inserted directly into the vagina. This treatment releases a small amount of estrogen that is absorbed by the vaginal tissues. It can help relieve the dryness and discomfort associated with intercourse and some urinary problems.

Low-dose antidepressants called *selective serotonin-reuptake inhibitors (SSRIs)* can also be prescribed to help decrease menopausal hot flashes especially in women who cannot take estrogen due to medical or family history. It also can help the mood changes that may occur in menopause. Cognitive behavioral therapy (CBT) and acupuncture are also known to help menopausal women to improve their sense of well-being.

Finally, lifestyle changes, such as reducing alcohol, caffeine, and smoking, can have a positive effect on hot flashes, night sweats, and sleep disturbances. Regular exercise is known to increase bone density, reduce hot flashes, and prevent coronary heart disease (Jackson, 2011). Following a healthy diet by eating foods rich in calcium and vitamin D, such as salmon, and dark green leafy vegetables, can help preserve bone density.

OUTCOMES

Fortunately, the short-term symptoms associated with menopause can be addressed with lifestyle changes and home remedies. Nurses can be instrumental in helping a woman adjust to the hormonal changes that are inevitable for every woman. Education should focus on reducing or eliminating triggers of hot flashes such as spicy foods, alcohol, hot weather, or a warm room. Dressing in layers can help alleviate this as well as drinking cold water. Menopausal women should avoid very hot temperatures outside during the summer months and doing anything that makes you feel warmer than you already are. Dietary changes, such as removing late-day caffeine and avoid drinking too much alcohol, are also helpful to reduce sleep disturbance. Promote a well-balanced diet of fruits, vegetables, whole grains, with limited sugar and saturated facts. These changes need to be encouraged as the patient begins to notice her body is changing. These steps are beneficial in helping a woman to deal with the aging process. Practicing relaxation techniques, such as deep breathing and paced respirations, are often used to help alleviate the stress of dealing with *the change of life*, as menopause is often referred to (National Institutes of Health, 2010). The goal for your patient in menopause is to try to assist her with resources that she can use to make this transitional change tolerable and to be able to enjoy her aging years.

Summary

In conclusion, menopause is a natural part of a woman's life. It is a time of change in the body whereby hormonal levels vary and unpredictably decrease. Some women experience these changes more significantly than others, but the process is inevitable and, once it begins, it lasts the rest of their lives. Having a strong knowledge base of this changing process enables a health care provider to provide assistance and empathy when caring for someone who is struggling with this change. Treatment should be chosen on what works best for the patient's symptoms and health risks. According to the National Institutes of Health, the average woman today has more than one third of her life ahead of her after menopause (National Institutes of Health, 2010). That means that the menopausal transition is a good time for lifestyle changes that can help women make the most of the coming years.

Jackson, L. (2011). Menopause. *Nursing Standard, 25*(47), 59–60.

Mayo Clinic. (2016). Mayo Foundation for Medical Education and Research. Retrieved from http://www.mayoclinic.org/diseases-conditions/menopause/home/ovc-20342324

National Institute on Aging. (2016). What are the signs and symptoms of menopause? Retrieved from https://www.nia.nih.gov/health/what-are-signs-and-symptoms-menopause

National Institutes of Health. (2010). *Mystified by menopause: A major life transition.* (USDHHS Publication No. 08-6143). Washington, DC: U.S Department of Health and Services. Retrieved from https://newsinhealth.nih.gov/2010/10/mystified-menopause

North American Menopause Society. (2012). *Menopause: The Journal of The North American Menopause Society, 24*(7), 728–753. doi:10.1097/GME.0000000000000921

Stuenkel, C., Davis, S., Gompel, A., Lumsden, M. A., Hassan Muad, M., Pinkerton, J., & Santen, R. (2015). Treatment of symptoms of the menopause: An endocrine society clinical practice guideline. *Journal of Endocrinology Metabolism, 100,* 3975–4011.

■ MOTHERHOOD

Stacen A. Keating
Miriam J. Chickering

Overview

For many women, becoming a mother is viewed as the most important role to achieve during their lifetime. Defining the concept of motherhood would at first seem straightforward but it is complex. Motherhood has been defined as a process in which the mother is competent in her role and able to successfully execute mothering behaviors such as providing proper feeding and bonding with the new baby (Mercer, 2004). In reality, each woman's experience of motherhood can be quite different given that the context of a woman's life (health, age, number of children, culture, financial resources, work status, marital status, and country of residence) will vary widely. For nurses in clinical roles, assessing and positively impacting a mother's health and, by extension, the health of her family, can be both rewarding and challenging. The focus of this present discussion is on the concept of becoming a new mother. This period often signals profound changes for a woman. Changes can come in the form of physical, emotional, social, and financial factors. New mothers may experience feelings of extremely good health, joy, and creativity after having a child. Alternatively, some new mothers may end up with feelings of isolation, frustration, and/or fatigue (Cheng, Fowles & Walker, 2006). It is important for nurses working with new mothers to effectively assess and support women entering into this profoundly important life role.

Background

According to the Pew Research Center study of U.S. women done in 2007, "Most women (71%) say it is more difficult to be a mother today than it was 20 or 30 years ago" (p. 1, para 6). The reasons for this often relate to difficulties of balancing work and family life. Current trends in society also play a large role in the experience of motherhood. There are many factors—biological, social, and structural—that impact a woman's experience with new motherhood.

Becoming a competent mother is an extremely important developmental accomplishment that affects not only one individual (the mother) but also the child and the entire family structure. Infants rely on their mothers for nurturing, and to grow and develop into adults over the course of many years. The commitment to become a new mother carries with it tremendous responsibilities and life changes for the woman. For example, the arrival of a first baby alters the relationship between a mother and her partner if she is co-parenting. (For some mothers caring for other children or stepchildren, in addition to the new baby, compounds the responsibilities and demands of motherhood.)

A number of researchers have conducted studies to identify factors in the successful transition to the role of mother. Some key factors that influence the successful role attainment of a new mother include the "mother's age, relationship with the father, socioeconomic status, birth experience, experienced stress, available support, personality traits, self-concept, childrearing attitudes, role strain, health status, preparation during pregnancy, relationships with own mother, depression and anxiety" (Mercer & Walker, 2006, p. 580). Other contributing factors for successfully transitioning to role attainment are related to characteristics of the infant. These include the infant's "appearance, responsiveness, temperament, and health status" (Mercer & Walker, 2006, p. 580).

Recent research has been conducted to add more to our understanding of what women view as the most important factors in achieving successful maternal role attainment. Jenkins, Ford, Morris, and Roberts (2014) found that women valued a supportive environment where important information, continuity of care, and a focus on the mother and her family are conducted by caring staff. Mercer (2004) conducted a review of research involving transitional experiences of becoming a mother and noted new mothers can feel overwhelmed, exhausted, resentful, ambivalent, and even angry.

Gaboury, Capaday, Somera, and Purden (2017) conducted a study to understand how mothers and fathers prioritized goals for support after the baby was born. The researchers noted how the hospital can add to or detract from achieving goals is important to the mother and father. The study noted that both parents valued education and information on how to become competent parents and wanted help with meeting their personal needs. Some further findings included that responsive nursing was highly valued by both mother and father. However, hospital nursing routines and schedules and lack of privacy could detract from optimal role attainment immediately after the baby was born (Gaboury et al., 2017). In general, a mother wants to know that she can successfully feed her baby as well as keep her child healthy and safe from harm. Nurses can have a significant impact on the successful achievement of the new mother's role attainment. If the woman is successful in her attainment of the motherhood role, this will have a reverberating effect and positively impact the functioning of the family unit to achieve high levels of health and wellness.

Clinical Aspects

ASSESSMENT

Assessment during the first 24 hours involves physical examination of the mother and her baby. The nurse wants to assess for any abnormalities in vital signs, bleeding, edema, infection, or pain for the new mother. Other key assessments focus on understanding aspects of the family profile, especially as it relates to involving the father or partner in the care of the baby. Understanding aspects of the pregnancy in terms of whether or not it was planned or unplanned is also helpful regarding initial mother–baby bonding.

NURSING INTERVENTIONS, MANAGEMENT AND IMPLICATIONS

Nursing care of the new mother is critical to help foster a healthy transition to becoming a confident and competent mother. Meeting the nutritional needs of the newborn is of paramount importance to new mothers whether the woman decides to breastfeed or not (Gaboury et al., 2017). Women can become anxious when trying to get the newborn to latch on to the breast. Understanding whether the baby is taking in enough nutrition is a key concern for mothers. Mothers want to be supported and educated on how to determine this key goal of providing nutrition to ensure adequate health of their baby.

Nurses can teach mothers how to properly care for newborns. Mothers express the desire to learn general baby care such as how to feed, bathe, and change diapers for a small infant. A mother wants to be able to recognize when her baby may be ill and in need of medical attention. Nurses can demonstrate proper newborn care and also watch and support mothers when providing this care to her baby in the hospital. Nurses can provide education on how to note whether the baby is ill by showing how to properly take a newborn's temperature and to assess for changes in activity, hydration, and temperament. Mothers want to know that they are doing things correctly, and nurses can provide positive education, support, and feedback in this regard leading to enhanced self-efficacy of the mother caring for her newborn child (Cheng et al., 2006; Gaboury et al., 2017).

Nursing interventions for a woman after she has given birth also involve providing education on aspects of maternal self-care. According to Gaboury et al. (2017), a woman should make herself a priority during the transition to motherhood. Especially important are instructions on nutrition, physical activity, positive body image, and adequate rest/sleep (Gabour et al., 2017). Other physical factors that nurses should ask new mothers about include feelings of fatigue or tiredness, backaches and headaches, gastrointestinal issues such as constipation, problems with urination, decrease in sexual desire, and pain during intercourse (Cheng et al., 2006). Mothers may need management and nursing care in one or more of these areas.

OUTCOMES

In general, mothers are anxious to return to their earlier level of health and want to heal quickly after giving birth. Sometimes new mothers will have to confront feelings of pain and how to care for possible stitches, wounds, and other physical changes they are encountering in their postbirth bodies. In addition, nurses will want to accurately assess the mother for any signs or symptoms of depression or anxiety as this will affect all members of the family unit. Along this line, nurses should educate mothers on the avoidance of excessive alcohol and tobacco use as this can contribute to worsening feelings of depression and isolation. Cheng et al. (2006) have recommended that national health objectives should include the collection of data on postpartum maternal health status, and nursing care should be given well beyond the first 6 or 8 weeks after giving birth. Nurses can be health advocates for actively assuming a key role in improvements in maternal care during early and ongoing phases of motherhood.

Summary

Overall, the transition to motherhood for women is a life-altering change that most will anticipate with great joy and enthusiasm. Nurses can play a pivotal role in helping women achieve success in motherhood. The role of the hospital nurse is to be responsive to the needs of the new mother and that responsive nursing was critical to parents' achievement of their goals, and included providing information, answering questions, demonstrating skills, providing support and reassurance, and responding promptly (Gaboury et al., 2017). Providing information and meeting the educational needs of mothers is of paramount importance to help a woman gain the skills and self-confidence she need to care for her children (Beake et al., 2010). Nurses are in a key position to help mothers begin their important journey to fulfill the motherhood role.

Beake, S., Rose, V., Bick, D., Weavers, A., & Wray, J. (2010). A qualitative study of the expectations of women receiving in-patient postnatal care in one English maternity unit. *BMC Pregnancy and Childbirth, 10,* 70. doi:10.1186/1471-2393-10-70

Cheng, C., Fowles, E. R., & Walker, L. O. (2006). Postpartum maternal health care in the United States: A critical review. *Journal of Perinatal Education, 15*(3), 34–42.

Gaboury, J., Capaday, S., Somera, J., & Purden, M. (2017). Effect of the postpartum hospital environment on the attainment of mothers' and fathers' goals. *Journal of Obstetric, Gynecologic & Neonatal Nursing, 46,* 40–50.

Jenkins, M. G., Ford, J. B., Morris, J. M., & Roberts, C. L. (2014). Women's expectations and experiences of maternity care in NSW: What women highlight as most important. *Women and Birth, 27*(3), 214–219.

Mercer, R. T. (2004). Becoming a mother versus maternal role attainment. *Journal of Nursing Scholarship, 36,* 226–332.

Mercer, R. T., & Walker, L. O. (2006). A review of nursing interventions to foster becoming a mother. *Journal of Obstetric, Gynecologic & Neonatal Nursing, 35*(5), 568–582.

Pew Research Center: Social and Demographic Trends. (2007). Motherhood today: Tougher challenges, less success. Retrieved from http://www.pewsocialtrends.org/2007/05/02/motherhood-today-tougher-challenges-less-success

■ OSTEOPOROSIS

Mary Variath

Overview

The word "osteoporosis" (OP) literally means "porous bones" (Dickinson, 2014). Porousness of the bone occurs due to the excessive loss of protein and minerals. OP is a progressive, systemic skeletal disease, characterized by low bone density due to microarchitectural deterioration of bone tissue. Continuous bone tissue deterioration leads to reduced bone mass and decreased bone strength, which result in increased bone fragility and mechanical fractures (Bell et al., 2017; Nichols, 2016). Repeated fractures and the resulting hospital admissions can negatively influence affected individual's self-confidence, body image, and mental status, resulting in loss of independence and quality of life (Korkmaz, Tutoglu, Korkmaz, & Boyaci, 2014). Furthermore, OP can have devastating effects on the lives of families, communities, and the nation at large, due to repeated hospitalization, increased long-term care facility admissions, and the associated cost. Therefore, prevention and efficient management of the condition are necessary, which include pharmaceutical as well as nonpharmaceutical interventions, such as bisphosphonates and exercises, smoking cessation, and alcohol consumption reduction.

Background

OP is often considered a "women's disease" because women are two to three times more likely to be affected. An estimated 10 million people in the United States are affected with OP and 80% of them are women (Dickinson, 2014). Approximately half of all of women older than the age of 50 years will experience a fracture of hip, wrist, or vertebrae due to OP (Dickinson, 2014; Edmonds et al., 2017; Nichols, 2016). Although OP is seen in young adults, older adults are more affected. After menopause, women have a much higher chance of getting OP-related fractures. Usually, the age-related fractures signal the presence of OP in women.

Genetic factors play an important role, as OP is more likely in women with family members who have the disease as well as in White and Asian women. Other risk factors include late onset of puberty and attaining early menopause either naturally or through removal of ovaries, which results in low levels of estrogen. In addition, certain health conditions, including a variety of endocrine, gastrointestinal, hematologic, rheumatologic, autoimmune disorders, along with sickle cell disease, and some cancers are associated with an increased risk for OP (Dickinson, 2014). The projected economic impact from OP treatment is estimated to be more than $25 billion a year over the next 10 years (Nichols, 2016). The incidence of osteoporotic fractures is greater than the incidence of breast cancer, stroke, and heart attack combined.

Clinical Aspects

ASSESSMENT

OP can be divided into different stages: primary and secondary, the primary stage has two substages: type I and type II. Type I is otherwise called *postmenopausal OP*, in which excessive loss of trabecular bone occurs due to a low level of estrogen. Type II OP is known as the *senile OP*, in which both trabecular and cortical bone loss occur due to progressive age. OP is categorized into a secondary stage if the bone loss is due to an existing previous inflammatory condition, and/or the result of the use of medication (Dickinson, 2014).

Bone health depends on nutritional status, physical activity, genetics, age, and age-related hormonal changes. Thus, a complete assessment of all these factors needs to be considered (Bell et al., 2017). Diet assessment for sufficient calcium and vitamin D intake is a crucial factor because bone health depends on calcium and vitamin D intake from food as vitamins taken in through food last longer than supplements. Assessing lifestyle for sufficient exercise is another important factor as lack of exercise can contribute to bone mass reduction and leads to development of OP. Prolonged corticosteroid therapy and age-related hormonal changes can either put individuals at high risk or aggravate the existing osteoporotic condition. While assessing these, it is important to focus on the types of fractures, especially fragility fractures, which are fractures that result from mechanical forces that would not ordinarily result in a fracture otherwise. Fragility fractures occur due to low bone mineral density in the spine, forearm, hip, and shoulder (Bell et al., 2017). Low bone mineral and the resulting decreased bone mass lead to easy fractures from mechanical pressure. Further, genetic factors predispose individuals to increased risk for OP. For example, studies show that microRNAs play important roles in bone physiology and disease. Particularly, miR-34a is a key factor that acts as an osteoclast suppressor, the absence of which results in bone mass reduction (Krzeszinski et al., 2014).

In addition, rising age is one of the major contributing factors. OP is four times more likely for women after attaining menopause. Therefore, OP can be a threat to the health and quality of life of postmenopausal women because with menopause, the estrogen level, an essential factor for bone health, is reduced considerably, triggering an increase in bone loss and bone deterioration. Estrogen is essential for bone-forming osteoblasts used in the bone-formation process. The loss of estrogen shortens the osteoblast's life span, increasing bone fragility, and leading to high-risk fracture conditions (Nichols, 2016). In addition to age and factors related to female gender, smoking, increased caffeine intake, increased sodium consumption, and chronic corticosteroid usage are documented as contributing factors (Nichols, 2016).

Menopausal women can experience a 1% to 5% loss of bone mineral density per year (Nichols, 2016). It is imperative that women at risk of developing OP be made aware of those risks and of preventive strategies; consider frequent bone mineral density tests and the available complementary, alternative, and pharmaceutical management options.

The gold standard screening tool for OP is dual-energy x-ray absorptiometry, quantitative-computed tomography, peripheral quantitative-computed tomography, quantitative ultrasonography, or MRI, all of which are noninvasive, inexpensive, and effective at identifying individuals with high risk of fracture (Bell et al., 2017; Edmonds et al., 2017). Annual evaluation for estradiol level is important for menopausal women. Bone health instruction for women should include a discussion of the link between the loss of estrogen that occurs with menopause and increased bone deterioration, fragility, and fracture risks (Nichols, 2016). Members of the health care team need to commit to bone health education initiatives to improve the quality of life of premenopausal women. The effects of OP can be a long-term burden for the families of the affected individuals. In addition, health care providers have a professional responsibility to communicate with women about osteoporotic fracture risks to facilitate their understanding of preventive behaviors.

NURSING INTERVENTIONS, MANAGEMENT, AND IMPLICATIONS

A multidisciplinary evidence-based bone health education program, including nutrition, calcium, vitamin D, exercise, and pharmaceuticals is an important component in the management of OP (Nichols, 2016). In addition, weight-bearing exercises; smoking cessation; and caffeine, sodium, and alcohol consumption reduction are considered beneficial. The use of bisphosphonates and selective estrogen receptor modulators are believed to be effective in the treatment and prevention of OP by reducing bone resorption and decreasing bone turnover (Bell et al., 2017; Nichols, 2016). Bisphosphonates are drugs that inhibit bone resorption

by causing apoptosis of osteoclasts. There are two groups of bisphosphonates: nonnitrogen-containing and nitrogen-containing bisphosphonates. The presence of a nitrogen or amino group in the chemical structure of bisphosphonates increases the potency of the drugs for osteoclastic activity (Bell et al., 2017).

Increased calcium intake promotes bone mineralization by improving bone matrix formation. Contrarily, decreased calcium leads to reduced blood calcium level, which leads to decreased calcium storage in the bone, resulting in osteoclasts and poor bone health (Bell et al., 2017). Thus, a diet filled with sufficient calcium is necessary. Calcium intake needs to be accompanied by vitamin D, as vitamin D is vital for improved calcium absorption in the intestine. The major source of vitamin D is sunlight although there are some foods that contain vitamin D such as whole milk. Moreover, regular and low-intensity weight-bearing exercise improves osteoblasts and promotes bone health considerably (Bell et al., 2017).

Prevention and management measures include counseling on the risk of OP and related fractures. A diet with adequate calcium of 1,000 mg/d for men and 1,200 mg/d for women older than 50 years, vitamin D intake of 800 to 1,000 IU/d, and weight-bearing and muscle strengthening exercises are also recommended. Cessation of alcohol consumption, tobacco smoking for at-risk individuals, and assessment for medications that include steroids (Cosman et al., 2014) as prolonged steroid intake affects bone mass. Furthermore, prolonged use of heparin, lithium, proton pump inhibitors, chemotherapeutic agents, selective serotonin-reuptake inhibitors, and some antiepileptic drugs results in loss of bone mass that leads to OP (Dickinson, 2014).

OUTCOMES

Various organizations, such as *Healthy People 2020* (Office of Disease Prevention and Health Promotion, 2016) and the National Osteoporosis Foundation are focusing on preventing the incidence of OP. The two objectives of *Healthy People 2020* that are noteworthy are the reduction of the percentage of adults with OP from 5.9% to 5.3% and a reduction in the number of female, osteoporotic fracture-related hospitalizations from 823.5 per 100,000 to 741.2 (Nichols, 2016). With good assessment and appropriate interventions of nursing care, it is possible to achieve the goals of controlling disease progression, alerting the individuals at risk, and adapting effective treatment protocol.

Summary

OP is a progressive, systemic skeletal disorder, characterized by decreased bone density, resulting in reduced bone mass, reduced bone strength, and increased bone fragility, and microarchitectural deterioration of bone tissue. OP is considered a "women's disease" as more women are affected by OP, especially after menopausal age. OP is a condition in which the total bone mass is decreased as a result of poor osteoblast or bone formation. OP results in an increased number of fractures that occur even with mild pressure on the bone. Therefore, assessing the individuals at risk for OP can help prevent fractures and reduce the risk of illness. Increased calcium and vitamin D intake, either through diet or supplements, is highly recommended. In addition, annual diagnostic assessment would also help women to stay healthy.

Bell, J. M., Shields, M. D., Watters, J., Hamilton, A., Beringer, T., Elliott, M., . . . Blackwood, B. (2017). Interventions to prevent and treat corticosteroid-induced osteoporosis and prevent osteoporotic fractures in Duchenne muscular dystrophy. *Cochrane Database of Systematic Reviews*, 2017(1), CD010899. doi:10.1002/14651858 .CD010899.pub2

Cosman, F., De Beur, S. J., LeBoff, M. S., Lewiecki, E. M., Tanner, B., Randall, S., & Lindsay, R. (2014). Clinician's guide to prevention and treatment of osteoporosis. *Osteoporosis International*, 25(10), 2359–2381.

Dickinson, E. (2014). Osteoporosis, fragility fractures, and associated surgeries. *OR Nurse*, 8(2), 16–24.

Edmonds, S. W., Solimeo, S. L., Nguyen, V. T., Wright, N. C., Roblin, D. W., Saag, K. G., & Cram, P. (2017). Understanding preferences for osteoporosis information to develop an osteoporosis patient education brochure. *Permanente Journal*, 21, 16–24.

Korkmaz, N., Tutoğlu, A., Korkmaz, İ., & Boyacı, A. (2014). The relationships among vitamin D level, balance, muscle strength, and quality of life in postmenopausal patients with osteoporosis. *Journal of Physical Therapy Science*, 26(10), 1521–1526.

Krzeszinski, J. Y., Wei, W., Huynh, H., Jin, Z., Wang, X., Chang, T. C., . . . Sood, A. K. (2014). MiR-34a blocks osteoporosis and bone metastasis by inhibiting osteoclastogenesis and Tgif2. *Nature*, 512(7515), 431–435.

Nichols, G. N. (2016). Bone health education for osteoporosis risk reduction in premenopausal women: A quality improvement project. Retrieved from http://scholarworks.waldenu.edu/cgi/viewcontent.cgi?article=3779&context=dissertations

Office of Disease Prevention and Health Promotion. (2016). *Healthy People 2020*. Retrieved from https://www .healthypeople.gov

■ OVARIAN CANCER

Kristine Cooper
Tasina Jones

Overview

Ovarian cancer begins in the ovaries, which are the female reproductive glands (American Cancer Society, 2016). Ovarian cancer occurs when malignant cells form around the tissue of the ovaries (American Cancer Society, 2016). The majority of ovarian cancer cases are epithelial and diagnosed at an advanced stage. Women older than 65 years account for 50% of these cases (National Cancer Institute, 2017). It is estimated that in 2017 there will be 22,400 new cases and 14,080 deaths from ovarian cancer (National Cancer Institute, 2017). It is the ninth most common cancer and the fifth most deadly disease in women in the United States, partly because it is most commonly diagnosed at an advanced stage (National Cancer Institute, 2017).

Background

There are various types of ovarian cancer, each classified by the cell that it is derived from. There are three main types of ovarian cells. These three types of cells are: surface epithelium, germ cell, and stromal cell (Memorial Sloan Kettering Cancer Center, 2017b). Other types of tumors include clear cell, germ, endometrioid and low malignant potential tumors (National Cancer Institute, 2017). Epithelial ovarian tumors are one of the most common types of ovarian cancer. Epithelial tumors can be benign or cancerous. Brenner and serous adenomas are a type of benign tumor. The cancerous tumors begin in the tissue lining the ovaries (National Ovarian Cancer Coalition, n.d.).

Germ cell tumors involve the reproductive cells that form the eggs. The most common tumors are dysgerminomas, mature teratomas, and endodermal sinus (National Ovarian Cancer Coalition). These tumors are usually unilateral; uncommon and mostly diagnosed in adolescent girls or younger women (National Cancer Institute, 2017). Germ cell tumors can be aggressive but curable if diagnosed and treated early. Mature teratomas are benign and can contain different types of tissue, including teeth and bone (American Cancer Society, 2016). Immature tumors are cancerous and contain cells that bear a resemblance to fetal tissue.

Stromal tumors account for about 1% of ovarian cancer and develop in the connective tissue cells that produce the female hormones and the ovaries (American Cancer Society, 2016). *Sertoli-Leydgi* is a rare type of stromal tumor, yet one of the most common of the rare tumors (National Ovarian Cancer Coalition). Low malignant or borderline tumors account for 15% of all epithelial tumors (National Cancer Institute, 2015).

There are four stages of ovarian cancer, each stage ranging from stage I to II. Stage I is considered an early stage and stage II is an advanced stage of the disease (Memorial Sloan Kettering Cancer Center, 2017b).

The number of lifetime ovulations is comparative to the risk of ovarian cancer. Factors associated with suppression of ovulation are associated with a decrease in ovarian cancer. Such factors are multiparity, oral contraceptive use, and lactating (Jelovac & Armstrong, 2011). Greater estrogen exposure and/or lifetime ovulation, for example, nulliparity, late menopause, and hormone replacement therapy increase risk. Inflammatory diseases, such as endometriosis, can increase a woman's risk as well (Jelovac & Armstrong, 2011).

Certain ethnic backgrounds may have an increase in the risk of ovarian cancer. The incidence is higher in Caucasian women in comparison to African Americans. Women over the age of 50 are at risk for developing ovarian cancer (Jelovac & Armstrong, 2011). Family history is an important risk factor for ovarian cancer. A history of ovarian cancer in first-degree relatives is considered a risk and is higher if there are two or more first-degree relatives with ovarian cancer (National Cancer Institute, 2017).

According to the National Cancer Institute (2017), "approximately 20% of ovarian cancers are familial and although most of these are linked to mutations in either the Breast Cancer 1 (*BRCA1*) or breast cancer 2 (*BRCA2*) gene, several other genes have been implicated" (p. 2 of website, para 8). These mutations vary within populations. For example, the Ashkenazi Jewish populations has a higher *BRCA* mutation carrier rate than average (Jelovac & Armstrong, 2011). Lynch syndrome has also been associated with early onset and higher incidence of gastrointestinal tract, ovarian, uterine, and colon cancer (Jelovac & Armstrong, 2011).

Clinical Aspects

ASSESSMENT

In many women diagnosed with ovarian cancer the disease presents late. The most characteristic sign of ovarian cancer is persistent pelvic and abdominal pain, increased abdominal size, and persistent bloating (Jayson et al., 2014). At present, there are no routine screening mechanisms. The diagnosis of ovarian cancer is suggested by the presence of abnormal pelvic exam, abnormal findings on a transvaginal ultrasound, and an elevated CA-125 (Memorial Sloan Kettering Cancer Center, 2017a). Pelvic examination often does not detect early ovarian cancer, and pelvic imaging techniques are not always definitive. The CA-125 blood test, a tumor marker test, may be helpful in determining follow-up care after diagnosis but not in early screening.

Surgical exploration is performed first to determine the diagnosis and to evaluate the extent of disease. Surgical staging and exploration, reduction of tumor mass, chemotherapy, and radiation are the basis of treatment. Staging the tumor by the Federation of International Gynecologists and Obstetricians (FIGO) system is performed to guide treatment choice. Chemotherapy modalities greatly increase the likelihood of remission but do not prevent recurrence. Radiation therapy is given to treat any remaining local disease. The aim of treatment in women with early disease is to maximize the cure rate while minimizing treatment toxicity. In advanced disease, the aim is to maximize the quality of life and reduce the side effects (Gibbs & Gore 2001).

NURSING INTERVENTIONS, MANAGEMENT, AND IMPLICATIONS

Many women diagnosed with ovarian cancer experience major challenges associated with day-to-day life. As a result of its late presentation and aggressive treatment regimens, ovarian cancer is associated with a greater level of uncertainty, anxiety, and depression (McCorkle, Pasacreta & Tand, 2003). Most women experience symptoms of a nonspecific nature, and the lack of preparation for the detection of cancer may make the diagnosis more difficult and shocking. Many women experience numerous symptoms, including fatigue and change in appetite, sleep, and sexual relationships, as well as the side effects of treatment (McCorkle et al., 2003). Nurses manage both physical and psychological factors.

Nurses play a vital role in the patient's quality of life relative to treatment. Failure to meet the patient's information needs could lead to women making less well-informed decisions regarding their treatment. Good communication and allowing patients to express their feelings are essential to aid in coping with this devastating diagnosis. Nurses have an important role in providing patients with information to aid in decision making. Nurses advise women about the aim of treatment, expected outcomes, and side effects to enable them to make an informed decision.

The Institute of Medicine (IOM) developed a conceptual framework in 2013 to improve the quality of cancer care (Nekhlyudov, Levit, Hurria, & Ganz, 2014). The framework recommends to engage the patient in making informed medical decisions; have an adequately staffed, trained, and coordinated workforce; provide evidence-based cancer care; use advances in information technology (IT) to enhance the quality and delivery of cancer care; incorporate new medical knowledge into clinical practice guidelines; and provide accessible affordable cancer care (Nekhlyudov et al., 2014). Nurses play a role in implementing the recommendation of the IOM specifically in regard to decision making. It is important that information be given in various formats to assist with the retention of details. Information needs may change with time, and this has to be continually assessed by skilled health care professionals.

OUTCOMES

Nurses should use sources of quality information and increase their knowledge so that they can offer patients and their relatives an up-to-date guidance. The IOM laid out a guiding framework for improving the quality of cancer care. Implementation of improved care coordination, better patient–clinician communication, targeted clinician training, effective dissemination of evidence-based guidelines and strategies for eliminating waste, and continuous quality assessment can improve patient outcomes (Nekhlyudov et al., 2014). Nurses are well placed to suggest ways of managing difficult symptoms and to act as advocates for patients. Nurses can offer support by being present and assist in decision making.

Summary

Ovarian cancer has both physical and psychological effects on patients and their families. Knowledge of the signs and symptoms, specific tests, and disease staging will allow nurses to support women. Following diagnosis, having an understanding of treatment options and their rationales allows nurses to act as advocates when difficult decisions are being made. Nurses should provide patient-centered evidence-based information to allaying patient's fear.

American Cancer Society. (2016). What is cancer? Retrieved from https://www.cancer.org/cancer/ovarian-cancer/about/what-is-ovarian-cancer.html

Gibbs, D. D., & Gore, M. E. (2001). Pursuit of optimum outcomes in ovarian cancer: methodological approaches to therapy. *Drugs, 61*(8), 1103–1120.

Jayson, G. C., Kohn, E. C., Kitchener, H. C., & Ledermann, J. A. (2014). Ovarian cancer. *Lancet, 384*(9951), 1376–1388.

Jelovac, D., & Armstrong, D. K. (2011). Recent progress in the diagnosis and treatment of ovarian cancer. *A Cancer Journal for Clinicians, 61*(3), 183–203.

McCorkle R., Pasacreta J. T., & Tand, S. T. (2003). The silent killer: Psychological issues in ovarian cancer. *Holistic Nursing Practice, 17*(6), 300–308.

Memorial Sloan Kettering Cancer Center. (2017a). Ovarian cancer diagnosis. Retrieved from https://www.mskcc.org/cancer-care/types/ovarian/diagnosis

Memorial Sloan Kettering Cancer Center. (2017b). Stages of ovarian cancer. Retrieved from https://www.mskcc.org/cancer-care/types/ovarian/diagnosis/stages

National Cancer Institute. (2015). Ovarian low malignant tumor treatment. Retrieved from https://www.cancer.gov/types/ovarian/hp/ovarian-low-malignant-treatment-pdq

National Cancer Institute. (2017). Ovarian epithelial, fallopian tube, and primary peritoneal cancer treatment. Retrieved from https://www.cancer.gov/types/ovarian/hp/ovarian-epithelial-treatment-pdq#link/_416_toc

National Ovarian Cancer Coalition. (n.d.). Types & stages of ovarian cancer. Retrieved from http://ovarian.org/about-ovarian-cancer/what-is-ovarian-cancer/types-a-stages

Nekhlyudov, L., Levit, L., Hurria, A., & Ganz, P. A. (2014). Patient-centered, evidence-based, and cost-conscious cancer care across the continuum: Translating the institute of medicine report into clinical practice. *A Cancer Journal for Clinicians, 64*(6), 408–421.

■ PELVIC PAIN

Loraine O'Neill

Overview

Pain is a common complaint and symptom that is often underreported. It is estimated that chronic pain affects 37% of the U.S. population, with a cost, due to lost productivity and health care dollars of greater than $600 billion annually in the United States (Abercrombie & Learman, 2012). Pelvic pain can affect both sexes. For the purposes of this text, however, we review its effects on women and, in particular, a condition known as chronic pelvic pain (CPP). Estimates on the prevalence of CPP vary from 6% to 27% (Speer, Mushkbar, &

Erbele, 2016). By creating a supportive and trusting relationship with a patient suffering from CPP, the nurse can play an essential role in the disease management.

Background

"Pain" is defined as an unpleasant sensation that can range from mild, localized discomfort to agony. It has both physical and emotional components (Toye, Seers, & Barker, 2014). Pain may be characterized as nociceptive and nonnociceptive. Nociceptive pain originates from stimulation of the nociceptors in the nervous system, which leads to the feeling of pain. This type of pain can also be described as visceral or somatic. Nonnociceptive pain involves damage to the pain-signaling pathway and can be described as sympathetic or neuropathic. Pain can also be further classified as cyclic or noncyclic. If cyclic, it may be associated with such conditions such as menstrual cramps, sexual activity, and postdelivery (as in a vaginal hematoma) and therefore may be treatable. The noncyclic type, which persists for more than 6 months, is commonly known as CPP. Myofascial pelvic pain refers to pain experienced in the musculature of the pelvic floor and surrounding fascia (Pastore & Katzman, 2012). Pain in this region is often elicited by a stimulus, such as a cotton swab, that would not normally cause pain. This type of pain is known as *allodynia* (Hickey, 2013).

The clinical dilemma in providing care to a woman with CPP is to establish a cause for the pain, thereby leading to a diagnosis and tailored treatment. However, there are many systems that can be involved and a definitive cause is often difficult to establish. The source of pelvic pain might be found in one or more of the following systems: gynecological, urological, gastrointestinal, musculoskeletal, neurological, or psychological (Tu & As-Sanie, 2017). Benign causes of pain for females include endometriosis, adenomyosis, chronic pelvic infection, irritable bowel syndrome, postsurgical adhesions, and musculoskeletal conditions (Howard, 2003). Psychological conditions can include depression and posttraumatic stress syndrome.

It is essential to take a full medical and social history, conduct a physical examination, and perform diagnostic testing. Time should be taken to create a trusting environment in which the woman can feel comfortable recalling and revealing any traumatic experiences that she might have endured. Depending on the etiology, there are various approaches to treating CPP. After a full review of all examinations and test results, providers may order further testing, medications, surgery, or other therapies. If a known disease is found to be the source of a woman's pain, then she will be treated according to the guidelines specific to that illness. As a first-line therapy, often while waiting for test results, the provider may start anti-inflammatory medication and/or analgesia. If this does not provide adequate relief, then a patient with cyclic pain may be prescribed hormonal therapy. If neuropathic pain is suspected, the patient can be considered for a variety of pharmacological treatments, including antidepressants or opioids (Speer et al., 2016). Surgical interventions can range from local steroid injections to laparoscopy and sometimes hysterectomy. Studies indicate that women with CPP have lower general health scores and report a lower quality of life (Daniels & Khan, 2010). Due to the decrease in access to care, cultural attitudes, and language barriers, several authors have suggested that this condition goes underreported in ethnic minorities.

Clinical Aspects

ASSESSMENT

As part of the routine gynecological yearly exam, a woman should be asked about any pain she is experiencing. Time should be taken to elicit the exact location, type, quality, and severity of pain (Howard, 2003). To further evaluate a woman's pain she may be instructed to maintain a pain diary and to map the pain location. There are technical devices today that support this daily record keeping. Often quality-of-life questionnaires or screening tools are used to fully explore the extent to which pain is affecting aspects of daily living. Further investigation would include full sexual history, including any traumatic events such as rape.

A detailed medication profile is required, including over-the-counter medicines and any herbal or complementary medicine being used. A full screening, including blood work and urine, vaginal, and cervical swabs for microscopy culture, and sexually transmitted disease (STD) detection is usually performed. Imaging studies ordered may include ultrasound, CT, or MRI and can help to rule our pelvic masses, either benign or cancerous.

NURSING INTERVENTIONS, MANAGEMENT, AND IMPLICATIONS

Patients may require a review and/or explanation of the tests, results, and treatments as prescribed by the provider, and in such cases, the nurse can act as a listener, educator, and advocate. Nursing care of the patient undergoing a surgical procedure is dependent upon the type of anesthesia used and the type of surgery performed. Vital signs and concerns for increased bleeding are relevant after laparoscopy and hysterectomy. Adequate pain medication will ensure early ambulation and reduce the risk of thromboembolic disorders. Local standards should be followed.

Women with CPP may opt for alternative treatment methods. These should be thoroughly understood by the care team. Physical therapy is often used in the cases of myofascial pelvic pain (Pastore & Katzman, 2012). Certain vitamin deficiencies, such as D or B$_{12}$, have been noted in women with CPP in which cases review of supplements and dietary intake may be warranted (Pastore & Katzman, 2012). There is limited evidence that cognitive therapies or complementary medicines benefit these patients, but each woman is an individual and as such may find relief by the use of such modalities. The nurse should be familiar with local services that can be utilized.

OUTCOMES

There is a large body of literature dealing with the issues women face with CPP and, in particular, in the cases for which there is no obvious diagnosis or cause. This does not mean that the pain is any less debilitating; in fact, the opposite may be true. These women describe feeling alienated, isolated, and left out. In the face of such feelings, the patient often distrusts the medical profession. As a nurse, it is important to help the patient feel that her concerns are heard. Nurses as frontline caregivers can assess the varied aspects of their patient's status—namely physically, mentally, and socially—thus helping to ensure a comprehensive care plan.

Summary

Pelvic pain is a symptom, and CPP can be a complex syndrome. This condition may not easily be diagnosed leading the patient to feel to frustration and to have diminishing confidence in her health care team. The nurse should act as an advocate for the patient and ensure that trust and empathy prevail. The management of a woman with CPP requires a team effort.

Abercrombie, P. D., & Learman, L. A. (2012). Providing holistic care for women with chronic pelvic pain. *Journal of Obstetric, Gynecologic, & Neonatal Nursing, 41*(5), 668–679.

Daniels, P., & Khan, K. S. (2010). Chronic pelvic pain in women. *British Medical Journal, 341*(10), c4834.

Hickey, J. (2013). *Clinical practice of neurological & neurosurgical nursing.* Philadelphia, PA: Lippincott Williams & Wilkins.

Howard, F. M. (2003). Chronic pelvic pain. *Obstetrics & Gynecology, 101*(3), 594–611.

Pastore, E. A., & Katzman, W. B. (2012). Recognizing myofascial pelvic pain in the female patient with chronic pelvic pain. *Journal of Obstetric, Gynecologic, & Neonatal Nursing, 41*(5), 680–691.

Speer, L. M., Mushkbar, S. A. U. D. I. A., & Erbele, T. A. R. A. (2016). Chronic pelvic pain in women. *American Family Physician, 93*(5), 380–387.

Toye, F., Seers, K., & Barker, K. (2014). A meta-ethnography of patients' experiences of chronic pelvic pain: Struggling to construct chronic pelvic pain as "real." *Journal of Advanced Nursing, 70*(12), 2713–2727. Retrieved from http://www.medicinenet.com/script/main/art.asp?articlekey=4723

Tu, F. F., & As-Sanie, S. (2017). Evaluation of chronic pelvic pain in women. In H. T. Sharp (Ed.), *UpToDate.* Retrieved from https://www.uptodate.com/contents/evaluation-of-chronic-pelvic-pain-in-women

■ PERINATAL MOOD DISORDERS

Deepika Goyal

Overview

Although the perinatal period is a time of joy for families, pregnancy-related hormonal changes are associated with an increased risk for developing perinatal mood disorders (PMD; Iliadis et al., 2016). PMDs include affective depressive disorders that can occur any time during the pregnancy or the first 12 months after the birth of a new infant (O'Hara & Wisner, 2014). Common PMD includes antenatal depression, maternity blues, postpartum depression (PPD), and postpartum psychosis. When left untreated PMD can lead to poor maternal–infant bonding, lower breastfeeding rates, contributes to poor infant medical care and safety (e.g., immunizations, car seat use), and increases suicide and infanticide risk (Kingston, McDonald, Austin, & Tough, 2015; Sockol, Epperson, & Barber, 2013; Wouk, Stuebe, & Meltzer-Brody, 2017). Women left unidentified and untreated for PMD are at risk for poor prenatal and postpartum maternal–infant well-being outcomes. Nursing care for women with PMD is focused on early recognition of signs and symptoms, identification of risk factors, and timely referral to promote optimal maternal–infant well-being outcomes.

Background

Perinatal mood disorders present with unique signs, symptoms, and follow-up needs. Antenatal depression describes the onset of depressive symptoms during the pregnancy. Rates range widely depending on country and population studied. A recent meta-analysis indicates that 10% of women will experience antenatal depressive symptoms (Falah-Hassani, Shiri, & Dennis, 2017). Antenatal depressive symptoms are the same as major depressive disorder and include poor sleep and appetite, anxiety, loss of interest, and feelings of guilt. Antenatal depression has been associated with fetal abnormalities (premature birth, low birth weight, low Apgar scores, congenital anomalies) and stillbirth (Raisanen et al., 2014).

Maternity or baby blues is the most common PMD, affecting up to 80% of new mothers (Centers for Disease Control and Prevention [CDC], 2017). Symptoms include anxiety, crying, labile mood, insomnia, loss of appetite, and irritability that present within the first few days after childbirth and often resolve on their own without medical intervention.

Defined as the onset of an affective mood disorder within the first 12 months after childbirth, PPD affects up to 20% of women (CDC, 2017). Again, symptoms are the same as major depression, including irritability, sleep disturbance, fatigue, impaired memory, anhedonia, and persistent low mood. Postpartum depression can be well managed when identified; however, when left untreated, PPD is associated with poor maternal–infant bonding, lower breastfeeding rates, and delayed infant cognitive and language development (Kingston et al., 2015; Wouk et al., 2017). The most significant risk factors for developing PPD are antenatal depression and anxiety (Norhayati, Hazlina, Asrenee, & Emilin, 2015).

The rarest of all PMD, postpartum psychosis affects one to two per 1,000 women but this tends to be the illness most likely reported in the news and media (e.g., Andrea Yates, Susan Smith). Symptoms present within 2 to 4 weeks after childbirth and include rapid mood swings, hallucinations, and mania present within the first few days postpartum and require immediate hospitalization, and psychiatric intervention and treatment (Wisner et al., 2013). In 40% of the women studied, symptoms presented by 4 weeks postpartum, one third reported symptoms began during pregnancy, and one fourth had onset before pregnancy.

Risk factors for all of PMD includes previous history of mood disorders, sleep disturbance (Stremler, Sharkey, & Wolfson, 2017), low socioeconomic status (Goyal, Gay, & Lee, 2010), and a lack of social support.

Clinical Aspects

ASSESSMENT

As with any illness, the cornerstone of effective nursing care begins with a thorough patient history, physical examination, psychosocial assessment, and examination of available laboratory tests. The history for any childbearing woman should include previous history of depressive disorders, obstetric history (previous pregnancy, miscarriage, stillbirth, pregnancy loss), and past or current medication use (antidepressants, mood stabilizers). Physical assessment should include vital signs, postpartum fundus assessment, appetite changes, fatigue level, sleep disturbance, maternal effect, and observation of maternal–infant bonding. Psychosocial assessment should include observation of family interaction. If available, thyroid and hemoglobin/hematocrit levels should be reviewed to identify hypothyroidism and anemia, which are known to contribute to depressive symptoms. In addition, a self-report depression screening questionnaire should be completed when PMD is suspected or for baseline assessment any time during the pregnancy through the first 12 months postpartum.

NURSING INTERVENTIONS, MANAGEMENT, AND IMPLICATIONS

Nursing care of the childbearing woman should focus on timely identification of depressive symptoms. Evidence-based PMD screening as outlined by the Association of Women's Health, Obstetric and Neonatal Nurses (AWHONN; AWHONN Position Statement, 2015) and the U.S. Preventive Services Task Force (USPSTF; Siu et al., 2016) should be incorporated into patient care. The well-validated, self-report, 10-item Edinburgh Postnatal Depression Screening Scale (Cox, Holden, & Sagovsky, 1987) provides an objective measure of severity of depressive symptoms over the past week. If time is short, nurses can use the Patient Health Questionnaire—2 (PHQ-2; Bennett et al., 2008), which asks two questions, "Over the past 2 weeks, how often have you been bothered by any of the following problems? Little interest or pleasure in doing things or feeling down, depressed, or hopeless?" Using Likert-type scoring, a "yes" answer to either question warrants referral for further evaluation.

Other interventions for nurses caring for childbearing women include careful history taking, encouraging new mothers to share negative emotions, staying current with evidence regarding medication use during pregnancy and lactation, and developing a list of current community resources (AWHONN Position Statement, 2015). Along with screening and being vigilant for signs and symptoms of PMD, preventative interventions include rescheduling medication administration, vital signs, and other nursing duties to allow new mothers to sleep without interruption as much as possible. Also, discharge teaching should provide a comprehensive overview of the common postpartum mood disorders with an emphasis on onset and severity of symptoms, managing sleep, and early mental health help seeking if any PMD is suspected.

OUTCOMES

The expected outcomes of evidence-based nursing care are centered on promoting optimal perinatal maternal health, postpartum maternal–infant bonding, and maternal–infant safety, all of which contribute to long-term maternal–infant well-being outcomes.

Summary

When left unidentified, PMD can impact prenatal growth and development, postpartum maternal–infant bonding, infant cognitive and language development, and contribute to poor family functioning, which places women at higher risk of suicide and infanticide. Early recognition of symptoms and the initiation of evidence-based screening and early referral are critical to promote maternal–infant well-being outcomes.

AWHONN Position Statement. (2015). Mood and anxiety disorders in pregnant and postpartum women. *Journal of Obstetric, Gynecologic, & Neonatal Nursing, 44*(5), 687–689. doi:10.1111/1552-6909.12734

Bennett, I. M., Coco, A., Coyne, J. C., Mitchell, A. J., Nicholson, J., Johnson, E., . . . Ratcliffe, S. (2008). Efficiency of a two-item pre-screen to reduce the burden of depression screening in pregnancy and postpartum: An IMPLICIT network study. *Journal of the American Board of Family Medicine, 21*(4), 317–325. doi:10.3122/jabfm.2008.04.080048

Centers for Disease Control and Prevention. (2017). Depression among women. Division of Reproductive Health, National Center for Chronic Disease Prevention and Health Promotion. Retrieved from https://www.cdc.gov/reproductivehealth/depression/index.htm

Cox, J. L., Holden, J. M., & Sagovsky, R. (1987). Detection of postnatal depression. Development of the 10-item Edinburgh Postnatal Depression Scale. *British Journal of Psychiatry, 150*, 782–786.

Falah-Hassani, K., Shiri, R., & Dennis, C. L. (2017). The prevalence of antenatal and postnatal co-morbid anxiety and depression: a meta-analysis. *Psychological Medicine, 47*, 1–13. doi:10.1017/s0033291717000617

Goyal, D., Gay, C., & Lee, K. A. (2010). How much does low socioeconomic status increase the risk of prenatal and postpartum depressive symptoms in first-time mothers? *Womens Health Issues, 20*(2), 96–104. doi:10.1016/j.whi.2009.11.003

Iliadis, S. I., Sylven, S., Hellgren, C., Olivier, J. D., Schijven, D., Comasco, E., . . . Skalkidou, A. (2016). Mid-pregnancy corticotropin-releasing hormone levels in association with postpartum depressive symptoms. *Depression and Anxiety, 33*, 1023–1030. doi:10.1002/da.22529

Kingston, D., McDonald, S., Austin, M.-P., & Tough, S. (2015). Association between prenatal and postnatal psychological distress and toddler cognitive development: A systematic review. *PLOS ONE, 10*(5), e0126929. doi:10.1371/journal.pone.0126929

Norhayati, M. N., Hazlina, N. H., Asrenee, A. R., & Emilin, W. M. (2015). Magnitude and risk factors for postpartum symptoms: A literature review. *Journal of Affective Disorders, 175*, 34–52. doi:10.1016/j.jad.2014.12.041

O'Hara, M. W., & Wisner, K. L. (2014). Perinatal mental illness: Definition, description and aetiology. *Best Practice & Research Clinical Obstetrics & Gynaecology, 28*(1), 3–12. doi:10.1016/j.bpobgyn.2013.09.002

Raisanen, S., Lehto, S. M., Nielsen, H. S., Gissler, M., Kramer, M. R., & Heinonen, S. (2014). Risk factors for and perinatal outcomes of major depression during pregnancy: A population-based analysis during 2002–2010 in Finland. *BMJ Open, 4*(11), e004883. doi:10.1136/bmjopen-2014-004883

Siu, A. L., Bibbins-Domingo, K., Grossman, D. C., Baumann, L. C., Davidson, K. W., Ebell, M., . . . Pignone, M. P. (2016). Screening for depression in adults: US Preventive Services Task Force recommendation statement. *Journal of the American Medical Association, 315*(4), 380–387. doi:10.1001/jama.2015.18392

Sockol, L. E., Epperson, C. N., & Barber, J. P. (2013). Preventing postpartum depression: A meta-analytic review. *Clinical Psychology Review, 33*(8), 1205–1217. doi:10.1016/j.cpr.2013.10.004

Stremler, R., Sharkey, K., & Wolfson, A. (2017). Postpartum period and early motherhood. In M. Kryger, T. Roth, & W. C. Dement (Eds.), *Principles and practice of sleep medicine* (6th ed., pp. 1547–1552). Philadelphia, PA: Elsevier.

Wisner, K. L., Sit, D. K., McShea, M. C., Rizzo, D. M., Zoretich, R. A., Hughes, C. L., . . . Hanusa, B. H. (2013). Onset timing, thoughts of self-harm, and diagnoses in postpartum women with screen-positive depression findings. *JAMA Psychiatry, 70*(5), 490–498. doi:10.1001/jamapsychiatry.2013.87

Wouk, K., Stuebe, A. M., & Meltzer-Brody, S. (2017). Postpartum mental health and breastfeeding practices: An analysis using the 2010–2011 Pregnancy Risk Assessment Monitoring System. *Maternal and Child Health Journal, 21*(3), 636–647. doi:10.1007/s10995-016-2150-6

■ POLYCYSTIC OVARY SYNDROME

Latina M. Brooks

Overview

Polycystic ovary syndrome (PCOS) is a common endocrine disorder affecting women of reproductive age. PCOS is the result of a hormonal imbalance primarily characterized by anovulation leading to irregular menstrual cycles or amenorrhea, high levels of androgens, and cysts on the ovaries (American College of Obstetricians and Gynecologists, 2015). The hormonal imbalance associated with PCOS may also produce other symptoms, including hirsutism, acne, weight gain, and infertility. Nursing care for all women with PCOS is focused on being aware of and identifying symptoms attributed to PCOS, monitoring treatment effectiveness over time, and providing education and support of symptom management.

Background

PCOS was first characterized in 1935 by Irving Stein, Sr. and Michael Leventhal from whom the original name of PCOS was derived (Stein & Leventhal, 1935). Currently, PCOS is the most common endocrine disorder among women of reproductive age worldwide (Goodman et al., 2015). The exact cause of PCOS is unknown, but is believed to be caused by both genetic and environmental factors. Depending on the criteria used for diagnosis, the prevalence rate of PCOS has been reported from between 5% and 10% of women of childbearing age (Office of Women's Health, U.S. Department of Health & Human Services, 2016) to as high as 15% to 20% (Sirmans & Pate, 2014). Women with PCOS are at increased risk for obesity, insulin resistance, development of type 2 diabetes, cardiovascular disease, and infertility. Women of all races and ethnicities are at risk for PCOS, but the risk increases with obesity or having a first-degree female relative with PCOS (Shannon & Wang, 2012). There is no cure for PCOS, so as women move beyond childbearing years they may continue to have increased levels of androgen hormone and insulin resistance making continued surveillance for related comorbid conditions imperative.

Clinical Aspects

ASSESSMENT

Guidelines have varied slightly on the criteria for diagnosis of PCOS. However, there is a general consensus that a diagnosis of PCOS must include at least two of the three criteria of chronic anovulation, elevated androgen levels, and polycystic ovaries (Goodman et al., 2015). Although these three features are used to diagnose PCOS, women with PCOS may present with many different signs and symptoms most of which are related to increased levels of androgen, including hirsutism, alopecia, acne, obesity, menstrual irregularities, pelvic pain, and infertility (American College of Obstetricians and Gynecologists, 2015).

Nursing care of the woman with suspected PCOS includes accurate and thorough documentation of medical history, physical assessment findings, and laboratory results. A detailed medical and family history should include age, age at onset of menses, and menstrual cycle history. Particular attention should be given to menstrual irregularities, pelvic pain, issues with infertility, weight gain, and other medical conditions such as diabetes, hypertension, and family history of PCOS or symptoms related to PCOS, particularly in a mother or sister. The physical assessment should focus on signs associated with elevated androgen hormone, including facial hair growth, acne, and dark thick patches on the skin (acanthosis nigricans), as well as measurement of blood pressure, waist circumference, and body mass index (BMI). An accurate detailed history and physical assessment can provide strong evidence for a diagnosis of PCOS. Laboratory data should also be used to assess glucose levels, lipid levels, and the level of androgen hormone, although androgen hormone levels can be normal in a woman with PCOS (Sterling, 2015). Findings from a pelvic exam and pelvic ultrasound will be useful to rule out other conditions that might cause menstrual cycle irregularities, such as endometrial hyperplasia, cervical polyps or uterine fibroids, and aid in a diagnosis of PCOS.

NURSING INTERVENTIONS, MANAGEMENT, AND IMPLICATIONS

Nursing interventions and management for women with PCOS centers around monitoring symptom management, assessing for symptoms of comorbid conditions, education on prevention measures for conditions related to PCOS, and long-term patient support. Women with PCOS are primarily managed clinically based on presenting symptoms that include most notably menstrual and reproductive problems related to elevated androgen levels and anovulation. However, women with PCOS are also at increased risk for the metabolic syndrome that can include elevated fasting glucose, dyslipidemia, hypertension, and abdominal obesity (NCEP, 2002). Due to the additional risks of comorbid conditions, nursing care of the women with PCOS requires long-term monitoring of signs and symptoms, continual review, and assessment of medical and family history. The nurse should also be aware of infertility issues that women with PCOS may face. Infertility and the subsequent treatments involved can be very complex and stressful for women and their partners. Nursing care in the case of women with PCOS with menstrual or reproductive issues should include supporting the individual through the referral process to appropriate specialties, including obstetrics and gynecology or reproductive endocrinology. Also, the nurse should assess the need for and identify resources to provide emotional support that is often needed in cases of infertility. Nurses can be of great support by not only identifying resources that meet emotional needs but also assisting with coordination of these resources.

Treatment for PCOS is primarily centered around lifestyle modification and treatment of the signs and symptoms associated with PCOS. Treatment generally includes education, diet, exercise, and medication. Referral to specialists for surgical procedures, alternative treatments, counseling, or any combination of these will depend on the individual patient's needs.

Diet and exercise are often recommended for weight reduction and maintaining a normal weight in women with PCOS. Maintenance of a healthy weight can help minimize symptoms related to insulin resistance often seen in PCOS (Goodman et al., 2015). Nursing care includes educating the patient on a prescribed diet and exercise plan, including how adhering to the plan can positively impact symptoms of PCOS.

Medication treatment is centered around presenting symptoms in PCOS. Hormonal contraception is used to suppress overproduction of androgen hormone and assist with regulation of menstrual cycles, improvement of acne, and hirsutism (Ndefo, Eaton, & Green, 2013). Other medications may be prescribed to help address insulin resistance and infertility issues. Nursing care for the individual treated with medication for symptoms of PCOS would include reinforcing the need to take medications as prescribed, assessing that the patient understands the symptoms or medications prescribed,

educating patients about the side effects, and how and when to report any adverse effects. Nursing care would also include monitoring treatment effectiveness by assessing whether the patient reports continuance or resolution of symptoms.

OUTCOMES

The outcomes of nursing care are primarily focused on identifying signs and symptoms, monitoring for treatment effectiveness, and prevention of comorbid conditions related to PCOS. Thorough history taking and physical assessment are essential to identifying intervention needs for women with PCOS. Nursing care should also encompass evaluation of psychosocial needs of a woman with PCOS. PCOS is the leading cause of anovulatory infertility (Sirmans & Pate, 2014). In addition to infertility, other symptoms associated with PCOS, such as hirsutism, alopecia, and acne, can be very emotionally distressing for women. The expected outcome of effective nursing care as it relates to PCOS is to relieve symptoms, prevent the development of secondary comorbidities, and provide psychosocial support as needed. Lifestyle modifications, including diet and exercise, can be effective treatments for prevention of insulin resistance, type 2 diabetes, hypertension, and hyperlipidemia (Shannon & Wang, 2012). This also includes educating and supporting women's success with lifestyle modifications and symptoms before and after treatment, as well as assessing for the development of comorbid conditions and patient education.

Summary

PCOS is a chronic condition affecting multiple systems in women potentially over the course of one's entire life. The care of women with PCOS is multifaceted, long term, and a collaborative effort between the patient and the health care team. Nurses, through systematic monitoring and assessment, can identify ongoing physical, social, and psychosocial needs over a lifetime for women with PCOS.

American College of Obstetricians and Gynecologists. (2015). Polycystic ovary syndrome. Retrieved from http://www.acog.org/~/media/For%20Patients/faq121 .pdf?dmc=1&ts=20120510T1116545699

Goodman, F. N., Cobin, H. R., Futterweit. W., Glueck, S. J., Legro, S. R., & Carmina, E. (2015). American Association of Clinical Endocrinologists, American College of Endocrinology, and androgen excess and PCOS Society disease state clinical review: Guide to the best practices in the evaluation and treatment of polycystic ovary syndrome—Part 2. *Endocrine Practice, 21*(12), 1415–1426.

National Cholesterol Education Program. (2002). National Heart, Lung, and Blood Institute National Institutes of Health (NIH Publication No. 02-5215). Third Report of the National Cholesterol Education Program (NCEP) Expert Panel on Detection, Evaluation, and Treatment of High Blood Cholesterol in Adults (Adult Treatment Panel III) Final Report. Bethesda, MD: National Institutes of Health.

Ndefo, U. A., Eaton, A., & Green, M. R. (2013). Polycystic ovary syndrome: A review of treatment options with a focus on pharmacological approaches. *Pharmacy and Therapeutics, 38*(6), 336–355.

Office of Women's Health, U.S. Department of Health and Human Services. (2016). Polycystic ovarian syndrome fact sheet. Retrieved from http://www.womenshealth .gov/publications/our-publications/fact-sheet/polycystic -ovary-syndrome.html

Shannon, M., & Wang, Y. (2012), Polycystic ovary syndrome: A common but often unrecognized condition. *Journal of Midwifery & Women's Health, 57,* 221–230.

Sirmans, S. M., & Pate, K. A. (2014). Epidemiology, diagnosis, and management of polycystic ovary syndrome. *Clinical Epidemiology, 6,* 1–13. doi:10.2147/CLEP .S37559

Stein, I. F., & Leventhal, M. L. (1935). Amenorrhea associated with bilateral polycystic ovaries. *American Journal of Obstetrics and Gynecology, 29*(2), 181–191. doi:10.1016/S0002-9378(15)30642-6

Sterling, E. (2015). Hormone levels and PCOS. Contemporary OB/GYN. Retrieved from http://contemporary obgyn.modernmedicine.com/contemporary-obgyn/ news/hormone-levels-and-pcos?page=0,1

■ POSTPARTUM

Debra Bingham
Patricia Suplee

Overview

The *postpartum period* begins immediately after the birth of an infant and delivery of the placenta and is usually defined as ending 6 weeks, or 42 days later. There are approximately 4 million women who give birth each year in the United States. Women go through major physiologic and psychological adjustments during the postpartum period. This transition period is more challenging for women who give birth surgically, which encompasses a little more than one third of women. The postpartum period is a time in a woman's life when she is vulnerable and in need of both physical and emotional support from family, friends, clinicians, public health leaders, insurers, and government agencies. Although most women in the United States adapt well during this period, morbidity rates have been on the rise and approximately 61% of all maternal deaths occur during the postpartum period (Creanga et al., 2015).

Background

During the postpartum period, there are myriad physiologic and psychological adaptations that occur. Although most women transition into this period without complications, some women are more at risk and may experience issues at various times such as immediately following delivery or within the first few days or weeks thereafter.

Actual physiologic changes occur in almost all body systems, including hormone adjustments. Uterine involution begins immediately after giving birth with the uterus descending back into the pelvis by day 10 (Ladewig, London, & Davidson, 2017). During this time, the fundus (top of the uterus) is assessed for position and placement. Lochia (vaginal discharge) is also assessed and can be affected by several factors such as parity of the woman, type of delivery, and breastfeeding practices. Lochia is described as rubra (2–3 days), serosa (3–10 days), and alba (up to 2 weeks). The cervix almost completely closes by the first week, and the vagina decreases in size within a month. Any perineal changes, including repairs of episiotomies or lacerations usually heal within the first few weeks after giving birth. Ovulation and menstruation return at different time frames for the lactating (up to 3 years) versus nonlactating (up to 12 weeks) woman. Women are advised to practice birth control because ovulation may occur prior to the first menstrual period. There is a fluctuation of several hormones in the postpartum period. Progesterone and estrogen levels decrease significantly leading to physiologic changes and may contribute to psychiatric-related disorders.

Breast changes begin in early pregnancy and, following the delivery of the placenta, a surge of hormones leads to an increase in milk production and filling of the breasts. Prolactin, produced in the pituitary, aids in milk production and is elevated after birth as is oxytocin, produced in the hypothalamus, which stimulates the uterus to contract after birth and assists in lactation.

The gastrointestinal system may be slow at first related to the effects of progesterone, decreased muscle tone, pain medications, or decreased food intake during the birth process (Ladewig et al., 2017). Postpartum women may have difficulty voiding related to swelling and bruising of the urethra, a decreased sensation of bladder filling, use of pitocin (antidiuretic effect), or inhibited neural functioning related to anesthesia (Ladewig et al., 2017). Diuresis occurs within the first 24 hours postbirth, and an increase in diuresis may be seen with certain medical conditions.

Cardiovascular (CV) changes, such as a decrease in cardiac output, and a slight rise in blood pressure are normal; however, women can experience a drop in blood pressure related to hypovolemia or orthostatic hypotension due to blood loss. Other CV changes include a slight drop in pulse, a decrease in blood volume and cardiac effort, and increase in stroke volume (Ladewig et al., 2017). Blood values, such as hemoglobin, hematocrit, and platelets, are monitored during the postpartum period due to blood loss during the delivery. Blood loss values of up to 500 mL for a vaginal delivery and 1000 mL for a cesarean section delivery are considered normal. A weight loss of approximately 10 to 12 pounds is expected following the birth of a singleton pregnancy, and additional loss is expected with multiple gestations. This weight includes the baby, placenta, amniotic fluid, and shifting of fluids with diuresis. Additional potential physiologic changes that women may experience are related to the actual care of the newborn that can lead to sleep deprivation, nutritional imbalance with lactation, and challenges with activities of daily living. How women adjust to all of these changes may be based on delivery type (vaginal versus cesarean section birth), parity, chronic or acute conditions, and their social supports.

There are several psychologic adaptations that may affect women postbirth. The idea of becoming a mother, perceptions of self in this new mothering role, and familial interactions can contribute to the adjustment phase of motherhood. Postpartum psychiatric disorders are characterized as postpartum blues, postpartum depression, postpartum psychosis, postpartum posttraumatic stress disorder, and anxiety disorders specific to the puerperium (Rai, Pathak, & Sharma, 2015). Women may also have additional psychiatric diagnoses that will also need to be readdressed and followed during the postpartum period. Postpartum blues occur during the first few days of giving birth and usually resolve within 2 weeks. Postpartum depression (PPD) occurs in 5% to 25% of all postpartum women (American College of Obstetricians and Gynecologists [ACOG], n.d.), can be diagnosed days to weeks after giving birth, and is usually underdiagnosed and treated. Several risk factors for PPD exist, including but not limited to, hormone level fluctuations, stress, low social support, difficulty getting pregnant, pregnancy and birth complications, and having a baby or infant who has been hospitalized (Centers for Disease Control and Prevention [CDC], 2017b). Combination therapy of individual/group counseling and antidepressants has shown the best success.

In the United States, *maternal mortality* or a *pregnancy-related death* is defined as

The death of a woman while pregnant or within 1 year of pregnancy termination—regardless of the duration or site of the pregnancy—from any cause related to or aggravated by the pregnancy or its management, but not from accidental or incidental causes. (CDC, 2017a)

This definition is different from what most countries use, which is a cut-off period of 42 days postbirth. Maternal mortality rates have been on the rise since 1987, with the most current reported rate of 17.3 deaths per 100,000 births in 2013 (CDC, 2017a). How much of this rise is related to improved reporting or coding mechanisms is not known. During this same time period, there has been a 75% rise in severe maternal morbidity, which is further evidence that maternal outcomes have worsened (Callaghan, Creanga, & Kuklina, 2012). Leading causes of maternal deaths from most common to least common include cardiovascular diseases, noncardiovascular diseases, infection/sepsis, hemorrhage, cardiomyopathy, thrombotic pulmonary embolism, hypertensive disorders, cerebrovascular accidents, amniotic fluid embolism, and anesthesia complications (CDC, 2017a). Racial disparities in maternal mortality exist whereby Black women are three to four times more likely to die during the childbearing period than women of all other races or ethnicities.

Clinical Aspects

ASSESSMENT

RNs are responsible for assessing the physical and emotional health of women, their adjustment to parenthood and bonding with their newborn, and for providing the majority of education on self-care and caring for a newborn. The physical assessments RNs perform should include evaluation of the fundus, lochia, and perineum as well as whether the new mother is urinating adequately, and whether or not she has had a bowel movement. Some women will have more difficulty with urination and bowel movements depending on the type and severity of any urethral or perineal tears they may have experienced when giving birth. Preventive care in the form of dietary counseling to inform her that she should eat a diet high in fiber and to increase their fluid intake is helpful for all postpartum women. Some women may also benefit from taking stool softeners. Vital signs are monitored to detect subtle changes in body system functions, which may require nursing or medical interventions.

NURSING INTERVENTIONS, MANAGEMENT, AND IMPLICATIONS

Postpartum education begins prior to birth and extends into the postpartum period. Although maternal self-care and infant care teaching are a priority, education should also include information about what are normal and abnormal postpartum symptoms. This education should include recommendations for a plan of action should the woman experience any of the most concerning symptoms such as chest pain, shortness of breath or obstructed breathing, seizures, or thoughts of hurting herself or her baby (Suplee, Kleppel, Santa-Donato, & Bingham, 2016). These authors also recommend to call her health care provider or go to the nearest emergency department if she cannot reach her health care provider if she has bleeding where she is soaking through a pad per hour, has blood clots with the size of an egg or bigger, an incision that is not healing, a red or swollen leg that is painful or warm to touch, a temperature of 100.4°F or higher, a headache that does not get better even after taking medicine, or a bad headache with vision changes.

All women should be screened and receive care for all types of peripartum psychiatric disorders. Ideally, all women should be screened for depression during pregnancy; however, screening for postpartum depression should occur within a few days of giving birth and then repeated a few weeks later. Women who show signs of postpartum depression should be referred for ongoing counseling and support. Women with a known history of mental illness should receive additional support and be connected to services during the postpartum period.

All women should receive at least one postpartum follow-up. Women with a high-risk pregnancy or birth may need to be evaluated within the first 2 weeks after giving birth such as those who had hypertension issues.

Women who do not have any complications can wait until 5 to 6 weeks postbirth to be evaluated. Women who had gestational diabetes during pregnancy should receive a postpartum glucose screening test at the 6-week postpartum checkup.

During the immediate postpartum period, a woman's breasts will go through several changes while she is initiating breastfeeding. The first food her breasts produce will be colostrum, and she will then begin to produce milk. During the initial weeks, it is particularly important that the woman does not introduce pacifiers and formula. The addition of these artificial devices and food substitutes interrupt the intricate feedback system and make it more difficult for her body to know how much food to make in order to meet the needs of the infant.

Ideally, pregnant women should be vaccinated against tetanus, diphtheria, pertussis (Tdap) and influenza during pregnancy. If she did not receive these vaccinations during pregnancy, then she should receive them during the postpartum period. If a pregnant woman is not immune to rubella, she should receive the rubella vaccine in the postpartum period.

Maternal–infant bonding experiences and parental adaptation should also be part of the RN's postpartum assessment. Bonding is enhanced when newborns are immediately placed skin-to-skin with their mothers and remain skin-to-skin for at least an hour (Feldman-Winter, 2016). Skin-to-skin and liberal rooming-in policies are particularly needed for the women with fewer social supports and more social challenges. These more vulnerable women also can benefit from home visits during which the RN can perform periodic assessments, provide these new mothers with additional education, and support the new mother as she and other family members assume the demanding role of caring for a newborn.

OUTCOMES

A postpartum plan can be developed in partnership with the woman during her pregnancy. Postpartum care can be improved by anticipatory guidance during the prenatal period. Involving the woman in her care decisions will lead to a plan that the woman will find easier to comply with and improve care and outcomes for herself, her newborn, and her family.

Routine postpartum visits are 6 weeks postnatal. Women with a preexisting condition, medical or psychological, should be seen earlier. The visit includes a full physical and psychosocial assessment. The woman's nutritional status and physical and sexual activity are reviewed. This is an opportune time to discuss family planning. Maternal–infant bonding and infant feeding are assessed. The woman adjusts to physical, psychological, and social changes; recovers from childbirth; becomes a new mother or a mother to an expanded family; and experiences hormonal fluctuations while caring for a newborn and family. The woman may be experiencing lack of sleep, pain or discomfort, fatigue, and lack of sexual desire. The provider and patient should discuss a plan for ongoing care.

Discussing the importance of the postpartum visit and scheduling her appointment before discharge may help improve visit attendance. The use of technology—texting or emailing an appointment reminder—may help improve attendance at the postpartum visit.

Summary

RNs have a primary role in educating and supporting women before and during the postpartum period. This role includes providing prenatal and postpartum education, performing thorough physical assessments, identifying abnormal signs and symptoms, providing necessary treatments, facilitating routine and emergent treatment, and helping the new mother develop a plan for obtaining the physical and psychological support that she needs.

American College of Obstetricians and Gynecologists. (n.d.). Depression and postpartum depression: Resource overview. Retrieved from http://www.acog.org/Womens-Health/Depression-and-Postpartum-Depression

Callaghan, W. M., Creanga, A. A., & Kuklina, E. V. (2012). Severe maternal morbidity among delivery and postpartum hospitalizations in the United States. *Obstetrics and Gynecology, 120*(5), 1029–1036. doi:10.1097/AOG.0b013e31826d60c5

Centers for Disease Control and Prevention. (2017a). Pregnancy mortality surveillance system. Retrieved from https://www.cdc.gov/reproductivehealth/maternalinfanthealth/pmss.html

Centers for Disease Control and Prevention. (2017b). Reproductive health: Depression among women. Retrieved from https://www.cdc.gov/reproductivehealth/depression

Creanga, A. A., Berg , C. J., Syverson, C., Seed, K., Bruce, F. C., & Callaghan, W. M. (2015). Pregnancy-related mortality in the United States, 2006–2010. *Obstetrics & Gynecology, 125*(1), 5–12. doi:10.1097/AOG.0000000000000564

Feldman-Winter L., & Goldsmith J. P. (2016). AAP Committee on Fetus and Newborn, AAP Task Force on Sudden Infant Death Syndrome. Safe sleep and skin-to-skin care in the neonatal period for healthy term newborns. *Pediatrics, 138*(3), e1–e10, doi:10.1542/peds.2016-1889

Ladewig, P. A. W., London, M. L., & Davidson, M. R. (2017). *Contemporary maternal–newborn nursing care.* New York, NY: Pearson.

Rai, S., Pathak, A., & Sharma, I. (2015). Postpartum psychiatric disorders: Early diagnosis and management. *Indian Journal of Psychiatry, 57*(Suppl. 2), S216–S221. doi:10.4103/0019-5545.161481

Suplee, P. D., Kleppel, L., Santa-Donato, A., & Bingham, D. (2016). Improving postpartum education about warning signs of maternal morbidity and mortality. *Nursing for Women's Health, 20*(6), 552–567. doi:10.1016/j.nwh.2016.10.009

■ POSTPARTUM HEMORRHAGE

Sabrina Nitkowski-Keever
Mary Anne Gallagher

Overview

Postpartum hemorrhage (PPH) can be a devastating event in what can be considered one of the most treasured experiences, childbirth. As a widely recognized risk of childbirth, postpartum hemorrhage is the most preventable cause of maternal morbidity and mortality. Despite all the advances in health care, PPH is on the rise in developed countries and remains one of the most serious complications of pregnancy and childbirth (Main, 2015). Much effort has been put into studying PPH and developing tools for quick recognition and action with the hope to decrease its devastating and permanent effects. A woman can experience a hemorrhage any time after delivery up to 12 weeks postpartum. This trend requires that all health care providers become familiar with the signs of PPH in order to act quickly and decrease adverse outcomes.

Background

PPH occurs in 2.9% of all childbirth deliveries in the United States and is defined as blood loss of more than 500 mL in a vaginal birth and 1,000 mL or more in a cesarean section, remaining the number one cause of maternal morbidity and mortality, despite the advances in medical care. If occurring within 24 hours of birth, the hemorrhage will be considered primary. Causes of primary hemorrhage can include uterine atony, lacerations, or birth trauma.

Hemorrhage occurring any time after 24 hours postdelivery is considered secondary hemorrhage. Secondary PPH can be linked to retained products of conception (Ekin et al., 2015).

Although rare, PPH can lead to severe hemorrhage that has been identified as a leading characteristic in maternal mortality in the United States. Severe PPH is identified as a blood loss of 1,500 to 2,500 mL. Rates of severe PPH have increased from 1.9% per 1,000 births to 4.2%. This change can either be associated with increased incidences or increased attention and identification of PPH. Active management of the third stage of labor (AMTSL), which includes cord traction, fundal massage, and uterotonic use, is not practiced consistently, although it is recommended to prevent severe PPH (Schorn, Dietrich, Donaghey, & Minnick, 2017).

Failure to recognize PPH quickly can lead to maternal death. Bingham (2016) noted that Black women experienced more fatalities related to PPH than their White counterparts although they did not have increased incidences of the diagnosis. The responsibility falls on the clinicians to be prepared in identifying risks and developing protocols that address hemorrhage. A human body has a unique way to prepare for impeding birth. Maternal blood volume increases with pregnancy to prepare the body for increased blood loss. Blood volume increases by 45% creating a hypovolemic state while vascular resistance decreases to assist with perfusion of the uterus. Coagulation factors move to a hyper state in order to assist with returning the body to hemostasis after placental expulsion. Changes in the maternal body assist with compensating for increased blood loss, yet impact the quick identification of PPH, therefore delaying imperative treatment. In 2014, 14% of maternal deaths related to childbirth were found to be secondary to PPH (Schorn & Phillippi, 2014).

PPH can cause inadequate tissue perfusion leading to a catecholamine response, releasing epinephrine and norepinephrine. This response causes an increase in heart rate, vascular tone, and myocardial contractibility. Once PPH becomes severe, a patient will experience tissue hypoxia, acidosis, and depletion of factors needed to have effective coagulation leading to disseminated intravascular coagulation (Schorn, 2014). Massive PPH and resuscitative efforts can cause disseminated intravascular coagulation (DIC), a widespread depletion of clotting factors and end organ damage leading to massive transfusions, hysterectomy, and/or death (Jelks, 2014).

Advances in medical care have not been able to prevent maternal death related to PPH. Clinicians must learn to be better prepared in recognizing the risks and the signs of PPH in order to prevent its devastating outcomes. Tools to identify risk and protocols should be established for management in all birth facilities.

Clinical Aspects

Identifying risk is a key first step in preventing the severity of PPH. Women presenting with singleton pregnancy, no prior uterine incisions, and less than four vaginal births can be considered at low risk for postpartum hemorrhage. Previous uterine surgery, multiple gestations, multipara, and history of PPH and/or fibroids put women at moderate risk. Women who experience any of the following: placenta previa, low-lying placenta, hemoglobin greater than 30% with other risk factors, platelets greater than 100,000, or antenatal hypertension should also be considered high risk (Schorn & Phillippi, 2014). Bottom line, all women must be considered at risk for PPH, and, by identifying risk categories you can be prepared to identify signs quickly and have protocols in place to then treat without delay.

ASSESSMENT

As previously reviewed, PPH causes a catecholamine response. Most women may experience a 20% to 25% blood loss before signs can be detected, making it even more important to identify and treat without delay. This early response to increased blood loss can be identified as tachycardia and hypotension, followed by tachypnea, altered mental status, cool skin, and hypothermia (Schorn & Phillippi, 2014). Closer monitoring of vital signs and accurate measurement of blood loss during the entire postpartum period are important in identifying the early signs of PPH.

Visual estimate of blood loss has been the standard for measurement until recently. Inaccurate estimations have contributed to the delay in implementing effective treatments to prevent severe implications. Standard of care now includes weighing all items to accurately determine blood loss. Recommendations include calibrated drapes, scales in each labor room, and formulas in the electronic medical record that can determine accurate blood loss (Association of Women's Health, Obstetric and Neonatal Nurses, 2015).

NURSING INTERVENTIONS, MANAGEMENT, AND IMPLICATIONS

Identifying the PPH risk should be completed on admission. Know your patient's risks so you can be prepared. There has also been much discussion on active management of third-stage labor (AMTSL) and its role in preventing adverse outcomes. Cord traction, fundal massage, and uterotonics, all steps in AMTSL, are recommended for every delivery. If these processes fail to prevent PPH, additional intravenous (IV) access should be initiated while uterotonics are administered. A uterine tamponade balloon is another tool available to prevent further blood loss. The Bakri balloon is an invasive procedure used to manage PPH quickly and without complications (Katsinis, 2015).

In conjunction with these treatments, fluid replacement must be considered. Replacement of fluid loss can be done with crystalloid fluids, such as lactated Ringer's. Crystalloids can be used for small amounts of blood loss but can contribute to hemodilution if used excessively, affecting clotting factors and causing third spacing. If bleeding continues, hemostatic resuscitation should be activated to restore intravascular blood volume and enhance coagulation factors in order for oxygen to reach the tissues. Oxygen administered through a nonrebreather mask at 10 mL should be used in combination with the preceding treatment.

OUTCOMES

PPH increases maternal morbidity and mortality. PPH occurs on average in 3% of deliveries (Marshall et al., 2017). Two percent of women after post partum hemorrhage die (Shakur et al., 2010). Worldwide 3.5% of women with post partum hemorrhage undergo a hysterectomy and in the United States 2.5% of women with PPH undergo a hysterectomy (WOMAN Trial Collaborators, 2017). Per 1,000 deliveries, four to seven women receive a transfusion in the United States.

There is impact on length of stay and cost of hospitalization related to additional treatments, transfusion of blood and blood products, and need for higher level of care.

Summary

The National Partnership for Maternal Safety, Council on Patient Safety in Women's Health Care has developed an obstetrical hemorrhage safety bundle, outlining a comprehensive plan that focuses on readiness, recognition, response, and reporting. Although plans may vary from facility to facility based on individual needs, each plan should minimally include the establishment of a risk assessment tool for every admission and hemorrhage carts with PPH medications and supplies at each delivery. Preparing staff by reviewing protocols and policies and holding drills will improve communication among the team and facilitate quick response and treatment. Some hospitals will also institute a response team of experts, to be called when needed. Daily briefings on cases provide the staff with feedback on strengths and opportunities to improve response time and teamwork (Main, 2015).

PPH can have devastating outcomes that are preventable with early detection and treatment. Postpartum vital signs, accurate blood loss measurements, and lab results should be monitored closely and discussed within the health care team to determine the plan of care for every patient despite established risk. Establishing consistent evidenced-based protocols and improving communication among the health care team will enhance the patient experience and improve outcomes.

Association of Women's Health, Obstetric and Neonatal Nurses. (2015). Quantification of blood loss: AWHONN practice brief number one. *Journal of Obstetric, Gynecologic, & Neonatal Nursing, 44*, 158–160.

Bingham, D., Scheich, B., Byfeild, R., Wilson, B., & Bateman (2016). Postpartum hemorrhage. Preparedness element vary among hospitals in New Jersey and Georgia. *Journal of Obstetric, Gynecologic, & Neonatal Nursing, 45*, 227–238.

Ekin, A., Gezer, C., Solmaz, U., Taner, C., & Dogan, A. (2015). Predictors of severity in primary postpartum hemorrhage. *Archives of Gynecology and Obstetrics, 292*, 1247–1254.

Jelks A., Berletti, M., Hamlett, L., & Hugin, M. (2014). Nonpneumatic antishock garment combined with Bakri balloon as a nonoperative "uterine sandwich" for temporization of massive postpartum hemorrhage from disseminated intravascular coagulation. *Case Reports in Obstetrics and Gynecology, 2015*, 1–3.

Katsinis, B. (2015). Bakri balloon displacement in the uterus: Sonographic demonstrations. *Journal of Diagnostic Medical Sonography, 3*(6), 386–389.

Main, E., Goffman, D., Scavone, B., Low, L., Bingham, D., Fontane P., . . . Levy, B. (2015). National partnership for maternal safet: Consensus bundle on obstetric hemorrhage. *Journal of Obstetric, Gynecologic, & Neonatal Nursing, 44*(4), 462–470.

Marshall, A. L., Durani, U., Bartley, A., Hagen, C. E., Ashrani, A., Rose, C., . . . Pruthi, R. K. (2017, September). The impact of postpartum hemorrhage on hospital length of stay and inpatient mortality: A National Inpatient Sample–based analysis. *American Journal of Obstetrics and Gynecology, 217*(3), 344.e1–344e.6. doi:10.1016/j.ajog.2017.05.004

Schorn., M., Dietrich, M., Donaghey, B., & Minnick, A. (2017). U.S. physician and midwives adherence to active management in third stage of labor. International recommendations. *Journal of Midwifery and Women's Health, 62*(1), 58–67.

Schorn, M., & Phillippi, J. (2014). Volume replacement following severe postpartum hemorrhage. *Journal of Midwifery and Women's Health, 10*, 336–343.

Shakur, H., Elbourne, D., Gulmezoglu, M., Alfirevic, Z., Ronsmans, C., Allen, E., & Roberts, I. (2010). The WOMAN Trial (World Maternal Antifibrinolytic Trial): Tranexamic acid for the treatment of postpartum haemorrhage: An international randomised, double blind placebo controlled trial. *Trials, 11*, 40. doi:10.1186/1745-6215-11-40

WOMAN Trial Collaborators. (2017, May 27–June 2). Effect of early tranexamic acid administration on mortality, hysterectomy, and other morbidities in women with post-partum haemorrhage (WOMAN): An international, randomised, double-blind, placebo-controlled trial. *Lancet, 389*, 2105–2116. doi:10.1016/S0140-6736(17)30638-4

■ PREGNANCY

Miriam J. Chickering
Stacen A. Keating

Overview

Pregnancy begins when the male's sperm unites with the female egg creating a new life and terminates with the birth of the baby and placenta. Gender, eye color, and many other characteristics are determined at conception. Supporting structures for the fetus develop and include the fetal membranes, the placenta, the umbilical cord, and amniotic fluid. The amniotic membranes surround the fetus. The placenta provides transfer of substances, protects the fetus from unwanted substances, and produces hormones. The umbilical cord both removes deoxygenated blood through the umbilical arteries and provides oxygenated blood through the umbilical vein. The amniotic fluid regulates fetal temperature, allows for unrestricted movement, provides protection, and promotes symmetrical growth.

Nursing care for pregnant women includes prenatal care that monitors fetal development and maternal adaptation to pregnancy, and provides opportunities for early intervention if problems occur: education for the expectant family regarding pregnancy changes, preparing for labor and delivery, breastfeeding, and the care of the newborn, and management of common clinical conditions associated with pregnancy.

Background

The World Health Organization lists the childbearing years as ages 15 to 49 years (World Health Organization, n.d.-b). Worldwide, there are 133 pregnancies per every 1,000 women of childbearing age (Sedgh, Singh, & Hussain, 2014). Pregnancy is a natural function of the female reproductive system and is not considered a disease state; however, there are several populations that experience increased risk of poor pregnancy outcomes: adolescents, women of advanced maternal age, and women with comorbidities.

Optimal childbearing age is 20 to 35 years, with increased risks to the mother and fetus when pregnancies occur outside of this range (Bewley, Davies, & Braude, 2005). Increased risks during adolescence are due to the mother's needs to continue her physical, social, and psychological development along with the increased demands of maintaining a pregnancy and preparing to mother a newborn. Adolescent pregnancies make up about 11% of all births worldwide (World Health Organization, n.d.-a). Pregnant adolescents drop out of school more frequently and are less likely to attain a high school diploma or college degree resulting in lower incomes over a life span. Not only this, but children born to teen parents have a higher incarceration rate than the general public. There is an estimated taxpayer cost of $9 billion in the United States alone (Centers for Disease Control and Prevention, 2016).

Pregnancies in women older than 35 years carry additional risks, including increased risk of gestational diabetes, hypertensive disorders, stillbirth, miscarriage, ectopic pregnancy, and increased maternal mortality (Laopaiboon et al., 2014). Delayed childbearing is a trend in developing countries as some women choose to obtain advanced education and establish a career before having babies.

Nurses should be aware of comorbid conditions that can complicate pregnancy. Maternal organ injury or death is most likely in pregnant women with the following: severe preeclampsia/eclampsia, chronic congestive heart failure, congenital heart disease, and pulmonary hypertension (Bateman et al., 2013). The use of a comorbidity index like that developed by Bateman et al. can be extremely useful in guiding the care of high-risk obstetric patients. Comorbid conditions, particularly nongestational diabetes and hypertension, contribute significantly to the cost of care (Law et al., 2014).

Clinical Aspects

ASSESSMENT

Nursing care of the pregnant individual at first presentation to a health care provider should include a complete medical and reproductive history, including family medical and reproductive history, a social assessment, laboratory data, and physical assessment findings. The following specific data should be obtained: age; weight; date of the first day of the last menstrual cycle; desirability of the pregnancy; comorbid conditions (congenital heart defects, diabetes mellitus, hypertension, etc.); recent medical or surgical procedures; prescription drugs; exposure to alcohol and illicit drugs; environmental hazards; workplace, domestic, and social support; incidence of domestic violence; and access to food, water, shelter, and transportation.

The physical exam includes a complete head-to-toe assessment, including a breast exam and an exam of the vagina and cervix with a speculum as well as a bimanual exam. A Pap smear will be obtained and the practitioner may elicit Hegar sign, a softening of the cervix and uterine isthmus, or note Chadwick's sign, a bluish discoloration of the cervix, vagina, and labia.

Laboratory tests include human chorionic gonadotropin (HCG) levels, urinalysis, complete blood count, possibly a hemoglobin electrophoresis test if the woman is at risk for sickle cell anemia or thalassemia, and thyroid levels. A blood type and antibody screen are performed to assess for A, B, O, and Rho(D) incompatibilities between the mother and baby. Other tests are completed to rule out infections and/or check for immunity: hepatitis B, HIV, gonorrhea and chlamydia, syphilis, and rubella. Depending on the individual's ethnicity, specific genetic screens may be ordered for the following conditions: sickle cell anemia, thalassemia, Tay-Sacks disease, and cystic fibrosis. A transvaginal or abdominal ultrasound may be ordered to diagnose pregnancy. The nurse may use Doppler radar to assess fetal heart tones.

Some assessments will be the same at all points in the pregnancy, whereas other assessment points are specific to a certain point in the gestation. Pregnant individuals will be asked at each prenatal appointment about a headache, blurred vision, epigastric pain, and assessed for edema of the hands and face to assess for preeclampsia. There will be other questions regarding vaginal bleeding, leaking or gushing fluid from the vagina, vaginal bleeding, and amount of fetal movement. Preterm labor will be assessed through questions regarding uterine contractions (no more than four per hour), pelvic pressure, low backache, and menstrual-like cramps.

Between 18 and 32 weeks, fundal height is measured in centimeters, and the value is expected to correlate with the gestation (e.g., a fundal height of 20 cm should indicate a pregnancy of 20 weeks). Discrepancies between fundal height and weeks of gestation should be investigated to rule out incorrect dates, multiple pregnancy, a problem with fetal growth or amount of amniotic fluid, or molar pregnancy.

Between 15 and 20 weeks, maternal serum alpha-fetoprotein screening (MSAFP) may be ordered to check for genetic abnormalities. Gestational diabetes screening occurs between 24 and 28 weeks unless there are risk factors in which case screening may occur earlier. Women who are Rho(D) negative should be screened for antibodies and given RhoGAM if indicated between 24 and 28 weeks. Between 35 and 37 weeks, screening is performed for group B *Streptococcus*. If positive, antibiotics should be administered during labor and the newborn should be closely observed for 48 hours following birth.

Other tests to assess fetal well-being include ultrasound for fetal abnormalities, fetal kick counts (10 movements in 2 hours beginning at 28 weeks), Doppler flow studies to measure fetal blood flow, multiple marker screening, amniocentesis, chorionic villus sampling, and percutaneous umbilical blood sampling. Nonstress tests, contraction stress tests, and vibroacoustic stimulation are tests for fetal well-being that are often performed by the nurse. The nurse assesses fetal heart rate, including variability, accelerations, and presence of decelerations as an overall measure of fetal well-being. The biophysical profile combines a nonstress test with an ultrasound to measure fetal breathing and body movements, tone, and amniotic fluid volume.

NURSING INTERVENTIONS, MANAGEMENT, AND IMPLICATIONS

Nursing care of pregnant individuals should focus on maintenance of a healthy pregnancy and proactive management of comorbidities if present. Priority nursing-related problems include ongoing monitoring of the pregnancy, psychological support for the mother and family, preventative teaching for illnesses related to pregnancy such as urinary tract infection (UTI), candida infection, and other common aches and pains. The nurse provides prenatal education related to pregnancy, delivery, and the postpartum period.

OUTCOMES

Evidenced-based nursing care is focused on preventing poor pregnancy outcomes, particularly maternal–infant morbidity, and mortality. Studies confirm that consistent prenatal care that allows for ongoing assessment of the mother and fetus, education, and attended births result in improved pregnancy outcomes. Effective nursing care during pregnancy should prevent poor pregnancy outcomes for mothers and babies.

Summary

Individuals experiencing pregnancy require access to early and ongoing prenatal care as well as patient education related to pregnancy, delivery, and the postpartum period. Early intervention when problems arise can prevent poor maternal–child outcomes and help mothers and newborns retain health and vibrancy.

Bateman, B., Mhyre, J., Hernandez-Diaz, S. Huybrechts, K. Fischer, M., Creanga, A., . . . Gagne, J. (2013) Development of a comorbidity index for use in obstetric patients. *Obstetrics and Gynecology, 122*(5). Retrieved from https://www.ncbi.nlm.nih.gov/pmc/articles/PMC 3829199

Bewley, S., Davies, M., & Braude, P. (2005). Which career first? *British Medical Journal, 331*, 558. Retreived from http://www.bmj.com/content/331/7517/588

Centers for Disease Control and Prevention. (2016). Teen pregnancy in the United States. Retrieved from https://www.cdc.gov/teenpregnancy/about

Laopaiboon, M., Lumbiganon, P., Intarut, N., Mori, R., Ganchimeg, T., Vogel, J., . . . Gulmezoglu, A. (2014). Advanced maternal age and pregnancy outcomes: A multilcountry assessment. *British Journal of Obstetrics and Gynaecology, 121*. Retrieved from https://www.ncbi.nlm.nih.gov/pubmed/24641535

Law, A. McCoy, M., Lynen, R. Curkendall, S., Shevrin, M., Juneau, P., & Landsman-Blumberg, P. (2014) The impact of maternal comorbidities on the costs of care for pregnant women and newborns [Abstract]. The Association of Women's Health, Obstetric and Neonatal Nurses. Retrieved from https://awhonn.confex.com/awhonn/2014/webprogram/Paper9940.html

Sedgh, G., Singh, S., & Hussain, R. (2014). Intended and unintended pregnancies worldwide in 2012 and recent trends. *Studies in Family Planning, 45*(3), 301–314. Retrieved from https://www.ncbi.nlm.nih.gov/pmc/articles/PMC4727534

World Health Organization. (n.d.-a). Adolescent pregnancy. Retrieved from http://www.who.int/maternal_child_adolescent/topics/maternal/adolescent_pregnancy/en

World Health Organization. (n.d.-b). Infertility definitions and terminology. Retrieved from http://www.who.int/reproductivehealth/topics/infertility/definitions/en

■ SEXUALLY TRANSMITTED INFECTIONS

Maryann Clark

Overview

The term "sexually transmitted infections" (STIs) is used to refer to a variety of clinical syndromes caused by pathogens that can be acquired and transmitted through sexual contact. STIs are the most common infectious diseases in the United States. According to the Centers for Disease Control and Prevention (CDC), they have a nationwide prevalence of more than 110 million cases; nearly 20 million new cases are reported every year (CDC, 2013). STIs have numerous health implications, including infertility, increased risk of HIV transmission, and cervical cancer. They also have enormous consequences in pregnancy and can cause neonatal injury and death. In addition, they are also associated with social stigma and can have a substantial psychological impact on many lives. Nurses play a critical role in educating patients on STIs, screening for the disease, and providing treatment. Nurses can also help minimize the impact of social stigma by providing informed, confidential, and sensitive care, and by promoting sexual health. Establishing a trusting, nonjudgmental relationship with the patient is crucial for the nurse working with patients who acquire an STI. Nurses can help minimize the impact of social stigma by providing an environment conducive to sensitivity, trust, and confidentiality. Due to the numerous sexually transmitted diseases that exist, the focus of the information provided concentrates on those STIs requiring mandatory reporting to the CDC. These include syphilis, gonorrhea, and chlamydia.

Background

STIs disproportionately affect young people, racial and ethnic minorities, and men who have sex with men. According to the CDC, young people between the ages of 15 and 24 years account for 50% of all new cases each year (CDC, 2014). The economic consequences are enormous. It is estimated that STIs cost the nation $16 billion in health care costs (Owusu-Edusei, 2013). As frontline providers with frequent contact with the patients and knowledge of the community, nurses are well positioned to help treat and prevent STIs.

Syphilis is a serious, highly contagious transmitted disease caused by the organism *Treponema pallidum*. The rates of syphilis vary widely across the country with higher rates in women who are prostitutes and those women with multiple random partners (Leveno, 2013). In the clinical diagnosis, syphilis is divided into stages, which can overlap. Primary infection is characterized by an ulcer or chancre at the infection site. If left untreated, secondary syphilis develops and includes a systemic infection that can be disseminated throughout the body by the bloodstream. This often presents with a fever and a rash on the trunk, limbs, palms, and soles of the feet. Tertiary infection may include cardiac or granulomatous lesions. Latent infections may be characterized by cranial nerve dysfunction and altered mental status. Untreated syphilis can eventually lead to blindness, central nervous damage, and death. There is no immunity from prior infection and reinfection is not uncommon (CDC, 2014).

Those at risk for acquiring syphilis include a substantial majority of the population. Any sexually active person can get syphilis through unprotected anal, vaginal, or oral sex. Direct contact with a person known to have a syphilis sore is often the mode of transmission. Sores can be found on the penis, vagina, anus, in the rectum, or on the lips, and in the mouth. Diagnosis includes serology testing for *T. pallidum* through the quantity of bacteria (treponemes) in the blood. Nontreponemal antigen screening, including rapid plasma regain (RPR) and Venereal Disease Research Laboratory (VDRL) is also used in the screening process. Some providers diagnose syphilis by culturing any fluid draining from the actual sore.

Gonorrhea is caused by the bacterium *Neisseria gonorrhoeae*, which grows and multiplies in the mucosa and can infect the cervix, uterus, fallopian tubes, urethra, mouth, throat, and anus. According to the CDC, as of 2013, 106.1 cases per 100,000 people have been reported with more than 80% occurring in 15- to 29-year-olds. It is the second most commonly reportable communicable disease in the United States (Bolan, Sparling & Wasserheit, 2012). It often presents without symptoms. However, dysuria, urethral or vaginal discharge, and bleeding from the site of the infection can occur in the female population. Men can experience burning upon urination, discharge from the penis or painful, swollen testicles. Rectal infections that both women and men experience may include anal itching, soreness, bleeding, and painful bowel movements.

Diagnosis of gonorrhea can be confirmed by urinalysis, pharyngeal screening for those participating in oral sex, rectal cultures as well as cervical cultures used for pregnant women.

Undiagnosed and untreated, this STI can result in significant complications, particularly for women in childbearing years. Evidence has consistently demonstrated the effects of *Neissena gonorrhea* as pathogenic bacteria involved in reproductive tract morbidities, including tubal factor infertility and pelvic inflammatory disease (Tsevat, Wiesenfeld, Parks & Peipert, 2017) Some of the complications associated with pelvic inflammatory disease (PID) include ectopic pregnancy, long-term pelvic and abdominal pain, as well as the formation of scar tissue blocking the fallopian tubes. In men, gonorrhea can cause a painful condition in the tubes attached to the testicles. In rare cases, this may cause sterility and prevent him from fathering a child. For both men and women, untreated gonorrhea can also spread to blood or joints and can cause life-threatening conditions. Finally, gonorrhea, like some other STIs, can increase your chances of getting or giving HIV that causes AIDS.

Chlamydia is caused by the bacterium *Chlamydia trachomatis* and is the most common reportable communicable disease in the United States (CDC, 2014). It is a major cause of genital tract and ocular infections worldwide. More than 4 million infections occur annually. The highest rates of infection are seen in adolescents and young adults between the ages of 15 to 24 years. High-risk groups include inner-city women, particularly African Americans. It is transmitted through vaginal, oral, or anal sex with someone who is already infected and can be transmitted to a neonate as it passes through the birth canal. Most cases are asymptomatic making difficult to seek treatment if you are not experiencing any symptoms. However, some clinical manifestations in women can include cervicitis, urethritis, and pelvic inflammatory disease. Men are more likely to be symptomatic and exhibit urethritis, epididymitis, prostatis, and proctitis (Sing &

Marrazzo, 2013). However, complications in men are unusual and rarely result in reproductive problems. As in the case of other STIs, untreated infection increases the risk of acquiring HIV.

Historically, cultures were considered the standard testing in diagnosing for chlamydia. Now nucleic acid amplification tests (NAAT) provide superior sensitivity and specificity for diagnosing chlamydia (Sing & Marrazzo, 2013). In testing for men, urine is the preferred specimen for NAATs; for women, it is the vaginal/cervical swab. Self-collected rectal swabs are also shown to be highly acceptable to both men and women.

Clinical Aspects

ASSESSMENT

Effective nursing assessment for those who are suspected of having an STI requires a detailed history, intake and risk assessment, physical examination, and laboratory specimens to identify those who need prevention, education, and/or early treatment to prevent long-term sequelae. Patient education regarding screening is an important intervention in preventing complications. As some of the STIs are asymptomatic, both the CDC and the U.S. Preventive Services Task Force recommend annual screening for all sexually active women younger than 25 years, as well as older women with risk factors such as multiple partners or a new sexual partner (U.S. Preventive Services Task Force, 2014). Also recommended by the CDC is "at least" annual urethral screening for men having sex with men who have insertive intercourse and rectal screening for those having anal intercourse (Workowski & Berman, 2010). Routine annual screening is recommended for all sexually active gay, bisexual, and men having sex with men to prevent the spread of all STIs.

NURSING INTERVENTIONS, MANAGEMENT, AND IMPLICATIONS

Providing education and counseling to those at risk are other components of nursing care that are required when dealing with this population to prevent STIs. Nurses need to inquire about sexual behavior and feel comfortable in obtaining a complete sexual assessment history and physical examination, especially when caring for an asymptomatic patient. Discussion needs to take place regarding noncompliance in using barrier protection, multiple partners, and the social stigma associated with STIs. Sexual health discussions should be appropriate for the patient's developmental level and aimed at identifying risk behaviors. Recommendation of serology testing and cultures should be included in their clinical examination. As no state requires parental consent when dealing with STIs, there should be no reason to refuse.

Sexually active adolescents have high rates of STIs and many barriers to prevention and treatment because of developmental immaturity, difficulty accessing health care, lack of knowledge, and the need for confidential care, which requires trust. Serious health consequences of STIs may occur many years after the infection, further compounding the adolescent's ability to link cause and effect.

Nurses who are committed to the challenge of providing services for this population to treat and prevent STIs can help by providing access to confidential care and promoting sexual health. High-risk youth require intensive preventive efforts. Nurses are in an ideal position to meet this challenge in their roles as providers, counselors, educators for all patients requiring care of sexually transmitted diseases in such areas as prevention clinics, community centers, and schools. Effective STI care and prevention should apply theories of behavior change, and incorporate attitudes, beliefs, and input of the patient.

The implications of nursing interventions of patient education, providing timely access to care, confidentially, psychosocial support leads to a safe, healthy sexual lifestyle. A lack of interventions can lead to long-term serious complications. Failure to develop a trusting relationship may deter patients from being open of their concerns, sexual activity and symptoms.

OUTCOMES

The expected outcomes for those who are at risk or who acquire syphilis, gonorrhea, or chlamydia is to provide immediate treatment which generally requires antibiotics. Education and compliance in being in a monogamous relationship with a partner tested who has been negative will help alleviate the complications and transmission of untreated STIs. The use of the partner notification process in which the partners involved are treated without previous medical evaluation or prevention counseling may enhance the compliance of treatment and prevent the continuance of STIs. Consistently using latex condoms remains highly effective in preventing transmission of STIs. Routine annual screening for chlamydia for women younger than 25 and older women with risk factor as well as annual screening for all sexually active patients would be a huge benefit in identifying those infected and would help decrease transmission to another person. Having an open, honest, and caring dialogue with your patient to gain his or her trust will also allow the proper nursing care required to decrease STIs.

Summary

In conclusion, caring for a patient diagnosed with an STI includes many aspects of nursing care. It incorporates prevention as well as treatment. Limiting the spread of disease requires behavior change. Strategies include education, counseling, identification, and treatment of infected individuals (whether symptomatic or not), evaluation and counseling of sexual partners. It begins with providing a therapeutic environment for your patient to feel comfortable discussing a topic that may be quite uncomfortable and one that is extremely personal.

Bolan, G. A., Sparling, P. F., & Wasserheit, J. N. (2012). The emerging threat of untreatable gonococcal infection. *New England Journal of Medicine, 366*(6), 485–487.

Centers for Disease Control and Prevention. (2013). *Incidence prevalence and cost of sexually transmitted infections in the United States.* Atlanta, GA: Author. Retrieved from http://www.cdc.gov./std/stats/sti-estimates-factsheet-feb -2013.pdf

Centers for Disease Control and Prevention. (2014). *Sexually transmitted disease surveillance 2013.* Atlanta, GA: Centers for Disease Control, National Center for HIV/AIDS, Viral Hepatitis, STD and TB Prevention, Division of STD Prevention.

Leveno, K. J. (2013). *William's manual of pregnancy complications* (23rd ed.). New York, NY: McGraw-Hill Medical.

Owusu-Edusei, K. (2013). The estimated direct medical cost of selected transmitted infections in the United States. *Sexual Transmitted Disease, 40*(3), 197–201.

Sing, D., & Marrazzo, J. M. (2013). Screening and management of genital chlamydial infections. *Infectious Disease Clinical North America, 27*(4), 739–753.

Tsevat, D. G., Wiesenfeld, H. C., Parks, C., & Peipert, J. F. (2017). Sexual transmitted diseases and infertility. *American Journal Obstetrics and Gynecology, 216*(1), 1–9. doi:10.1016/j.ajog.2016.08.008

U.S. Preventive Services Task Force. (2014). *Final recommendation statement. Gonorrhea and chlamydia: Screening.* Rockville, MD: Author. Retrieved from http://www.uspreventiveservicestaskforce.org/Page/ Document/ RecommendationStatementFinal/ chlamydia-andgonorrhea-screening#Pod2

Workowski, K. A., & Berman, S. (2010). Sexually transmitted diseases treatment guidelines, 2010. *MMWR Recommendations and Reports: Morbidity and Mortality Weekly Report Recommendations and Reports/Centers for Disease Control, 59,* 1–110.

■ SKIN AESTHETICS

Erin Hennessey
Mary Anne Gallagher

Overview

Skin aesthetics is a broad topic inclusive of many different cosmetic appearance concerns, including scars, skin laxity, facial volume loss, dyschromia of the skin, rhytides, cellulite, unwanted hair, cellulite, erythema, and visible skin vasculature. In recent years, the field of surgical and nonsurgical aesthetics has grown exponentially. According to the American Society for Aesthetic Plastic Surgery's (ASAPS) 2014 statistics, nonsurgical procedures totaled 740,751 in 1997. In 2016, there were 11,674,754 nonsurgical cosmetic procedures performed (ASAPS, 2017). The most often performed skin procedures are BOTOX injections, chemical peels, laser skin resurfacing and rejuvenation, microdermabrasion, and dermal filler injections. It is critical that nurses are aware of these procedures, understand how to evaluate potential cosmetic patients, evaluate for possible complications, and deliver patient education regarding the procedures.

Over the course of skin aging, visible changes can be observed. These changes are often a combination of physiologic and environmental factors. Overexposure to ultraviolet radiation is a large contributing factor to photo aging or sun damage. Other extrinsic factors to photo aging include smoking, diet, poor sleep habits, and alcohol consumption (Small & Hoang, 2012a). As the skin ages, visible changes can be seen in the form of fat and bone atrophy, changing the appearance of the face and skin. Common changes that occur with the aging process include textural changes (wrinkles, dilated pores, dry and rough skin, solar elastosis), structural changes, (sagging and laxity), pigmentary changes (sallow discoloration, hypopigmentation, hyperpigmentation, poikiloderma of civatte), and vascular changes (telangiectasia, cherry angioma formation, and erythema). Aesthetic interventions are aimed at improving the appearance of aging and natural skin imperfections.

Skin aesthetic procedures can be broken down into four categories: topical agents, exfoliation procedures, injectable agents, and laser procedures.

Topical agents are applied to the skin with the intent of improving the appearance of the skin and promoting healthy skin in patients. Topical agents can be over-the-counter or prescription, and they are drugs or cosmeceuticals that affect both the structure and the function of the skin. A topical skin care regimen can be developed by providers with input from the patient regarding specific skin concerns (sensitivity, erythema or rosacea, acne or hyper/hypopigmentation). Medical-grade topical creams and gels typically contain one or more of the following ingredients:

Retinol is a vitamin A derivative that may be used in nonprescription creams, but at higher concentrations, it can be found in prescription or medical-grade products. It is considered an antioxidant. Within the context of topical skin care products, antioxidants work to neutralize free radicals in the skin that would otherwise break down skin cells and cause wrinkles.

Vitamin C is an antioxidant that is thought to protect the skin from sun damage and solar lentigo. Vitamin C breaks down very quickly in sunlight and is usually stored in a dark container to protect the integrity of the product.

In addition to salicylic acid, alpha, beta, and poly hydroxyl acids can be found in aesthetic topical products and act as chemical exfoliants to the skin. They assist to break down aged, dead skin that tends to sit on the top of the stratum corneum and stimulate the growth of healthy skin.

Niacinamide is another potent antioxidant that is related to vitamin B-3. It assists in reducing insensible water loss and improves skin elasticity.

Growth factors used within the context of topical skin care aim to bind to the cell surface and repair damaged epidermal cells that help to provide support, firmness, and elasticity. Growth factors can come from both human sources (i.e., fibroblasts and platetet-rich plasma [PRP]) and animal/plant sources.

Many times, a combination of the aforementioned ingredients are the active change agents in topical skin care products like serums, gels, lotions, or creams.

Chemical peels, microdermabrasion, and derma-planing fall under the category of exfoliation. The goal of these procedures is to regulate the skin's epidermal renewal process, stimulate the production of collagen, glycosaminoglycans, even melanin distribution, and improve epidermal barrier function (Small, Hoang, & Linder, 2012). Chemical peels contain primarily acids and are classified based on the depth of the skin they penetrate (Small et al., 2012a). These are categorically superficial, medium, and deep. Ideal patients for exfoliation procedures are patients who would like to see improvement in skin texture, fine lines, pore size, active acne, superficial acne scars, and hyperpigmentation.

The first described use of the neuromodulator for aesthetic use was by Clark and Berris in 1989 to correct facial asymmetry due to facial nerve paralysis after rhytidectomy (Clark & Berris, 1989). The use of neuromodulators in facial rejuvenation have since grown, despite that most procedures are considered off-label use. On April 15, 2002, the use of botulinum toxin type A to ameliorate moderate to severe glabellar rhytides was approved by the U.S. Food and Drug Administration (Rohrich, Janis, Fagien, & Stuzin, 2003). Neuromodulators are currently approved to treat glabellar lines and crow's feet. These were the most popular of all provider-administered cosmetic procedures (surgical and nonsurgical combined) in 2016. The ASAPS estimates that over 6.7 million people were treated with BOTOX, a neuromodulator, for cosmetic purposes in 2015 alone (ASAPS, 2017). Dermal fillers are materials injected into the skin that fill in wrinkles or areas of volume lost within the face. The following are approved by the FDA for use in the face: collagen injections (made of highly purified cow or human collagen), hyaluronic acid gel (a protective lubricating gel, produced naturally by the body), calcium hydroxylapatite (a mineral and a major component of bone), and poly-L-lactic acid (PLLA; a biodegradable, biocompatible, synthetic material; FDA, 2017). Microneedling is another injection procedure that has become quite popular. It is the process by which small-gauge needles are inserted into the skin creating microchannels. After a numbing agent is applied to the skin, this procedure aims to stimulate the skin's natural ability to heal itself as well as producing collagen and elastin (Widgerow et al., 2016).

Laser technology has come a very long way since its inception, both in speed and efficacy. "LASER" is an acronym and stands for "light amplification by stimulated emission of radiation." Laser and light treatments include intense pulsed light (IPL), broad band light (BBL), Co_2, erbium-YAG (Erbium-doped yttrium aluminum garnet laser), Q-switched, and hybrid combination lasers. The first laser was produced by Theodore H. Maiman in 1960 using ruby as a lasing medium that was stimulated using high-energy flashes of intense light (Chang et al., 2013). Laser light is monochromatic, bright, unidirectional, and coherent. In cosmetic uses, laser-light technology usually focuses on three chromophores—melanin, oxyhemoglobin, or water. If there is no chromophore, then all the photons will pass through the tissue without producing any effect (Chang et al., 2013). This is total transmission. Therefore, selection of a proper chromophore in or near the target tissue is the first important step in laser therapy. The conditions with clinical indications for laser treatment are:

- Skin rejuvenation with both ablative and nonablative resurfacing
- Vascular lesions, acne, birthmarks, and scarring
- Pigmented lesions and unwanted tattoos
- Varicosities of the legs

Clinical Aspects

ASSESSMENT

In general, assessment includes age, medical history including allergies, any previous skin treatments, medications, sun exposure history and a physical assessment of skin. Specific interventions based on chosen aesthetic method follow.

Patient assessment for topical skin therapies includes previous hypersensitivity to any ingredients or preservatives. Patients with erythema, irritation, sunburn, eczema, pregnancy, or those who are breastfeeding should use topical agents with caution and avoid any retinol derivatives.

Before the administration of injectable neurotoxins, the patient must be evaluated for previous hypersensitivity to neurotoxin, hyperrsensitivity to albumin, preexisting neuromuscular disease, inflammation of skin at the injection site, facial asymmetry, deep dermal scarring, and thick sebaceous skin. These are contraindications to neurotoxin injection. Dermal-filler patients are evaluated for severe allergies, marked by a history of anaphylaxis or history or presence of multiple severe allergies, and fillers should not be used in patients with a history of allergies to gram-positive bacterial proteins or lidocaine. Contraindications to microneedling include keloid scars, eczema, psoriasis, a history of actinic keratosis, a history of herpes simplex injection, a history of diabetes, or the presence of raised moles or warts. Microneedling should not be performed in patients who have scleroderma, collagen vascular diseases, active bacterial or fungal infections, active acne breakouts, individuals with cardiac abnormalities, or immunosuppression.

For patients who would like to engage in a laser treatment, typing of the skin is necessary as is documentation of a history of surgical procedures to the area being treated and a history of melanoma, nonmelanoma skin cancers, and pigmented lesions (Small & Hoang, 2016). Contraindications to laser therapy, including laser hair removal may include Accutane use in the past 6 months, pregnancy, use of medication that increases photosensitivity, diabetes, use of anticoagulants, a history of keloid scarring or a history of seizures, recent sun exposure, or use of or topical skin-darkening agents. The skin should be inspected for any open areas, nonhealing sores, or pigmented lesions before laser treatments.

NURSING INTERVENTIONS, MANAGEMENT, AND IMPLICATIONS

- Conduct a though medical history
- Ascertain patient's expected outcome clarify misconceptions. Communicate to provider any unrealistic expectations to clarify.
- Establish a therapeutic relationship
- Patient education
  - Any preprocedure care—may include prescribed cleansing, refrain from using certain products
  - Overview of procedure
  - Healing process
  - Postprocedure care
    - Topical agents: Careful discussion of the propensity for sun sensitivity with certain products and the proper storage of topical agents.
    - Injectable: May include not laying down for a period of time, not wearing a head covering, and avoiding massage of the area injected.
    - Laser: Advise to engage in the use of sun avoidance or covering their skin depending on the procedure due to the high risk of burns and sun damage.
  - Signs and symptoms to notify provider
- During procedure
  - May include eye protection or surrounding areas, assessment for local or systemic allergic reaction to product.
  - Topical anesthetics or nerve blocks may be used to lessen pain from injections and fillers. Injectable may include lidocaine to decrease pain during injection (Wollina, 2013).
- Postprocedure
  - Pain management
    - Medication as prescribed
    - Adjunct therapy as prescribed, may include cold or warm compress, elevation of treated area, massage
    - Care of treated area

Possible risks of injectable include tissue necrosis, vascular impingement, granuloma formulation, bruising, bleeding, and infection (U.S. Food and Drug Administration, 2017).

Complications of laser therapies include but are not limited to scarring, keloid formation, blistering, hyperpigmentation, and hypopigmentation. Most adverse effects are temporary and consist of bruising, swelling and pain. Patients should be informed of the expected immediate appearance. There may be change in a person's body image. The care team should be alert to this and provide anticipatory guidance and support.

OUTCOMES

Open communication among care team members and the patient will establish realistic outcomes. Patient compliance with postprocedure care influences.

Summary

Understanding the patient's desires for cosmetic outcome is very important in the assessment of what procedures will attain the appropriate clinical endpoints for patients. Traditionally, skin aesthetic procedures were primarily performed on and marketed to women, but they are becoming increasingly popular with men as well. Proper assessment of past skin aesthetic procedures, current skin conditions and treatments, skin malignancies, and chronic health conditions that affect the healing process are imperative. Discussion with the patient as to how his or her past medical, surgical, family, and medication history affect treatment and healing will help reduce complications and assist the patient in understanding his or her individualized healing process. Proper documentation and communication with all members of the care team are paramount. Lifestyle details with regard to career, regular exercise, and sun exposure must be discussed to educate the patient on the potential healing process and downtime of a skin aesthetic application or procedure.

American Society for Aesthetic Plastic Surgery. (2017). 2016 cosmetic surgery national data bank statistics. Retrieved from https://www.surgery.org/sites/default/files/ASAPS-Stats2016.pdf

Chang, A. L. S., Bitter, P. H., Qu, K., Lin, M., Rapicavoli, N. A., & Chang, H. Y. (2013). Rejuvenation of gene expression pattern of aged human skin by broadband light treatment: A pilot study. *Journal of Investigative Dermatology*, 133(2), 394–402. doi:10.1038/jid.2012.287

Clark, R. P., & Berris, C. E. (1989). Botulinum toxin: A treatment for facial asymmetry caused by facial nerve paralysis. *Plastic Reconstructive Surgery, 84*, 353.

Rohrich, R. J., Janis, J. E., Fagien, S., & Stuzin, J. M. (2003, October). The cosmetic use of botulinum toxin. *Plastic Reconstructive Surgery, 112*(5), 177S–188S. doi:10.1097/01.PRS.0000082208.37239.5B

Small, R., & Hoang, D. (2012a). *A practical guide to botulinum toxin procedures.* Philadelphia, PA: Wolters Kluwer/Lippincott Williams & Wilkins.

Small, R., & Hoang, D. (2012b). *A practical guide to dermal filler procedures.* Philadelphia, PA: Wolters Kluwer/Lippincott Williams & Wilkins.

Small, R., & Hoang, D. (2016). *A practical guide to laser procedures.* Philadelphia, PA: Wolters Kluwer/Lippincott Williams & Wilkins.

Small, R., Hoang, D., & Linder, J. (2012). *A practical guide to chemical peels, microdermabrasion & topical products.* Philadelphia, PA: Lippincott Williams & Wilkins.

U.S. Food and Drug Administration. (2017). Filling in wrinkles safely. Retrieved from https://www.fda.gov/ForConsumers/ConsumerUpdates/ucm049349.htm

Widgerow, A. D., Fabi, S. G., Palestine, R. F., Rivkin, A., Ortiz, A., Bucay, V. W., . . . Chasan, P. E. (2016). Extracellular matrix modulation: Optimizing skin care and rejuvenation procedures. *Journal of Drugs in Dermatology*, 15(4), 63–71. Retrieved from http://jddonline.com/articles/dermatology/S1545961616S0063X

Wollina, U. (2013). Perioral rejuvenation: Restoration of attractiveness in aging females by minimally invasive procedures. *Clinical Interventions in Aging, 8*, 1149–1155. doi:10.2147/CIA.S48102

Palliative Care Nursing

The nursing process involves assessing, planning, implementing, and evaluating plans of care, often with a goal of identifying and reducing bothersome patient symptoms. In this role, all nurses deliver palliative care at the generalist level. The provision of caring, patient-centered care is at the heart of the nursing profession.

Palliative care uses a holistic approach devoted to caring for the person and family facing serious illness and encompasses physical, social, psychological, and spiritual domains (Coyle, 2010). Originally associated with care for patients at the end of life, palliative care is now a recognized specialty, with board certification available for registered nurses, advanced practice registered nurses, physicians, social workers, and chaplains (Center to Advance Palliative Care [CAPC], 2017). Hospitals that demonstrate excellence in palliative care can be certified by The Joint Commission as advanced providers of palliative care (CAPC, 2017).

Palliative care can be integrated into any serious illness at any stage. Clinical practice guidelines have been established to promote high-quality palliative care (National Consensus Project, 2013). Specialty palliative care can be delivered in hospitals, outpatient clinics, long-term care facilities, and in homes (Wiencek & Coyne, 2014). This care is focused on relieving distressing symptoms, facilitating patient-directed goals of care, and improving the quality of life for both patient and families.

This section focuses on nursing strategies to help patients who are suffering with a high symptom burden related to chronic and advanced illness. As nurses communicate effectively with their patients and advocate for them, suffering can be reduced, even when an illness cannot be cured. The nurse's contribution as a member of the interdisciplinary team is vital in promoting effective palliative care.

Center to Advance Palliative Care. (2017). Certification and licensing. Retrieved from https://www.capc.org/providers/palliative-care-resources/palliative-care-resources-certification-licensing

Coyle, N. (2010). Introduction to palliative nursing care. In B. Ferrell & N. Coyle (Eds.), *Oxford textbook of palliative care* (3rd ed., pp. 3–9). New York, NY: Oxford University Press.

National Consensus Project for Quality Palliative Care. (2013). Promoting quality and excellence. In *Clinical practice guidelines for quality palliative care* (pp. 30–32). Pittsburgh, PA: Author. Retrieved from https://www.hpna.org/multimedia/NCP_Clinical_Practice_Guidelines_3rd_Edition.pdf

Wiencek, C., & Coyne, P. (2014). Palliative care delivery models. *Seminars in Oncology Nursing, 30*(4), 277–233. doi:10.1016/j.soncn.2014.08.004

- Advance Directives in Palliative Care *Marilyn Bookbinder, Joyce Palmieri, and Molly J. Jackson*
- Anorexia and Weight Loss *Janine Stage Galeski and Molly J. Jackson*
- Anxiety in Advanced Illness *Lori A. Fusco*
- Bowel Obstruction *Hilary Applequist*
- Communication *Anne M. Kolenic*
- Constipation *Angela M. Johnson*
- Delirium *Colleen Kurzawa*
- Diarrhea *Sheila Blank*
- Dysphagia *Marianna K. Sunderlin*
- Dyspnea *Katharine K. Cirino*
- Ethics *Laura Caramanica and Molly J. Jackson*
- Grief and Bereavement *Kathleen Leask Capitulo*
- Mucositis *Petique Oeflein*
- Persistent Pain *Brendon Bowers and Molly J. Jackson*
- Urinary Incontinence *Kathy J. Meyers and Molly J. Jackson*

■ ADVANCE DIRECTIVES IN PALLIATIVE CARE

Marilyn Bookbinder
Joyce Palmieri
Molly J. Jackson

Overview

Advance directives are legal documents that a person may complete to provide the family and providers with guidance regarding expressed wishes for treatment and limitations to treatment if the patient cannot speak for himself or herself. All patients, but especially those receiving palliative care for end-stage disease progression, can benefit by communicating their care goals to the health care team, as well as the family decision makers. Advance directives have been linked to cost savings; with them there is less Medicare spending at the end of life, a lower likelihood of dying in a hospital, and higher usage of hospice care (Detering & Silveira, 2016; Rao, Anderson, Lin, & Laux, 2014). Nurses are well positioned to support and advocate for patients' preferences across all health care settings, they spend more time with patients than other health care team members, and have repeatedly been acclaimed by the U.S. public as being the most trusted profession.

Background

In the United States, the enactment of the Patient Self-Determination Act (PSDA) in 1991 drove social change as it mandated that all federally funded hospitals, nursing homes, and home health agencies give competent adult patients written information about advance directives. Since the passage of the PDSA, population-based prevalence estimates of completed advance directives among American adults range from 5% to 26.3% (Rao et al., 2014). The patient characteristics associated with higher advance directives completion include older age, Caucasian race, history of chronic illness, high disease burden, higher socioeconomic and education levels, and knowledge about advance directives (Rao et al., 2014). Black care recipients were less likely than White care recipients to have any advance directive. The factors contributing to lower advance directive completion rates in the Black population may include greater preferences for life-sustaining therapies, less comfort discussing death, and greater distrust of the health care system, suggesting the need for more culturally sensitive approaches to implementing the PSDA (Rao et al., 2014).

Advance care planning (ACP) discussions, typically completed with primary providers or in family meetings, have been shown to increase compliance by the clinicians (and families) in adhering to a patient's expressed preferences at the end of life. Nurses, as key members of the health care team, typically have early interaction with patients; this enables opportunities to start discussions about an advance directive, advocate for, and document patient and family wishes.

ACP is an ongoing process in which patients, their families, and their health care providers reflect on the patient's goals, values, and beliefs; discuss how they should inform current and future medical care, and ultimately, use this information to accurately document their future health care choices, if the patient cannot speak for himself or herself (Hospice & Palliative Nurses Association, 2013). ACP ideally includes completion of advance directives after an exploration of the patient and caregiver's knowledge, fears, hopes, consideration of the patient's relationships, and culture. Advance directives need to be consistent with state laws and regulations. The facilitators of ACP discussions try to answer key questions, such as "Who would the patient want to act as his or her agent when medical decisions must be made?" and "Does the patient have specific preferences for care that should be respected if he or she becomes unable to communicate them?"

Advance directives are used when a patient is found to lack decisional *capacity* (as opposed to *competence*, a legal term that requires a review by a court). *Capacity* is a clinical judgment based on the assessment of an attending physician and his or her evaluation of the patient's ability to understand the details of the health care proposal, possible risks and benefits, alternatives to treatment, and the consequences of different decisions.

One type of advance directive is the health care proxy (HCP) or the durable power of attorney for health care (DPOAHC), which specifically authorizes an agent to speak on behalf of a patient who has lost the capacity for decision making in a short- or long-term situation. States have specific legal requirements for this document. If an agent is designated, the person who is selected by the patient as his or her agent should be able to make decisions on behalf of the patient based on his or her knowledge of the patient's values and preferences ("substituted judgment"), or in the event that these are not known, based on the best interests of the patient. If no agent is designated, and the patient loses capacity, the health care team may seek guidance about medical decisions from others (typically family members) who know the patient. This person is called a *surrogate*. States have regulations that govern the process by which surrogates are selected based on blood relationship (spouse, adult children, etc.).

Living wills are documents or witnessed oral statements through which a patient spells out wishes regarding life-sustaining interventions in the event of a terminal illness or significant clinical change. These documents are considering binding and cannot be changed by a surrogate. Another specific type of advance directive is a do-not-resuscitate (DNR) form (NIA, 2016). This documentation of the decision to forego cardiopulmonary resuscitation can be completed for any treatment venue, including hospitals and home. In some states, a home DNR form, which is legally recognized by the emergency service staff, can be completed by the patient's physician or an advanced practice nurse.

Clinical Aspects

ASSESSMENT

Protection of patient autonomy and advocacy for individual rights are core values for nurses, thus perfectly positioning them to assist in the initiation and completion of ACP discussions and advanced directives. The nursing process, a systematic critical thinking method, provides nurses with opportunities to participate in ACP discussions and obtain advanced directives. Each interaction with patients and families during the episodes of care is a chance to perform a comprehensive assessment and build on a relationship to secure an advanced directive. By using open-ended questions during admission, for example, nurses can invite the patient to discuss his or her current condition and future medical care goals. They can assess the patient's comfort level and how active he or she wants to be in the discussion.

Research indicates that most elderly patients would welcome a discussion about advanced directives but are not being asked. Astute nurses can also judge whether others should be involved in the conversation, and with the patient's permission, invite them. If the nurse identifies a problem, such as a discrepancy between what the patient "says" he knows, and what he "should" know, it is important to get a sense of how much information he or she is seeking and share this with the health care team. The more specific and relevant the information is, the more likely the patient will engage in the process.

NURSING INTERVENTIONS, MANAGEMENT, AND IMPLICATIONS

Older adults especially, may describe situations with friends or family that upset them, such as someone who needed cardiopulmonary resuscitation (CPR) and died in an emergency room or who were placed on mechanical ventilation in a nursing home. These shared experiences can be used by the nurse to invite a conversation about the patient's end-of-life wishes, and explore values and beliefs around death. Asking what it means to "have a good life," and what hopes and goals he or she seeks in the subsequent month can provide insight. As the nurse–patient relationship grows and trust develops, nurses can assess the patient's readiness to elicit advanced directives preferences. Specific interventions can be discussed, depending on the patient's health history, such as hemodialysis in a patient with renal failure. Most important, nurses need to document when such conversations occur, as the documentation may be the only discoverable narrative describing the patient's wishes.

A patient should be encouraged to name an agent who would be willing to serve as a surrogate decision maker. If more than one surrogate is named, asking how disagreements among surrogates should be reconciled is the key; should the surrogate follow the documented wishes exactly, or be free to use her or his judgment? Ideally, health care professionals should trust that the agent can serve in this role, is available for discussions when needed, and has no conflicts of interest. If there are questions about the ability of the agent to represent the patient, a referral should be made to someone representing ethics.

Obtaining of an advanced directive, conducting an interactive dialogue about wishes and goals, and identifying a durable power of attorney for health care (DPOAHC) are evidence-based nursing interventions. The research indicates that a multimodal educational approach using face-to-face discussion, brochures, and decision aides has the greatest impact on completion of advanced directives. Once the advanced directive is complete, the document is signed, witnessed, and dated, copies are given to the family, primary physician, and placed in the patient's record. If patients and surrogates change their minds, particularly as the illness progresses, nurses can help them revise the care plan and advanced directives and revoke either with a simple oral declaration. The nurses need to routinely perform a self-assessment of their competencies in ACP and end-of-life care, the laws, and how to facilitate difficult conversations. They need to continually educate themselves about how cultural differences affect the grieving process and help those of all ethnicities experience death with dignity. The novice nurses report discomfort initiating advanced directive conversations and a need for more education regarding communication

strategies (Hospice and Palliative Nurses Association, 2013). There are online courses and increasing numbers of resources to assist nurses in gaining competency (The Conversation Project, 2017).

OUTCOMES

ACP is an ongoing process in which patients and families and health care providers reflect on the patient's goals, values, and beliefs, and accurately document the patients' future health care choices in advanced directives, the legal documents outlining one's wishes. Nurses, by profession and proximity to patients and families, are accountable for the translation of information about prognosis, treatment options, and ascertaining patient care preferences. Interdisciplinary collaboration and communication are important elements in achieving effective, patient-centered outcomes.

One population reaching "epidemic" proportions is those with dementia, especially Alzheimer's type, with cases expected to triple from 5.2 million to 13.8 million by 2050 (Compassion and Choice, 2016). It is critical that nurses caring for this vulnerable population receive advanced education to identify the early stages of dementia and ensure high-quality care and advocacy.

Summary

Nurses, as frontline clinicians in many settings, can share in the responsibility to initiate advanced directives, inform the patient and family about options, and engage in the periodic discussions that yield legal and accessible documentation of the results (Fried, Zenoni, & Iannone, 2017). To make significant contributions in advanced directive communication, the nurse needs to become comfortable with end-of-life conversations and bring best practices into care. Informed and skilled nurses today need to have a seat at the table to help shape policy and practice changes for tomorrow and ensure that all patients receive compassionate and patient-directed care at the end of life.

Compassion and Choice. (2016). Care and choice at end of life. Retrieved from https://www.compassionandchoices.org/userfiles/Dementia_Provision.pdf

The Conversation Project. (2017). Retrieved from http://theconversationproject.org

Detering, K., & Silveira, M. J. (2016). Advance care planning and advance directives. In R. M. Arnold (Ed.), *UpToDate*. Retrieved from http://www.uptodate.com/contents/advance-care-planning-and-advance-directives

Fried, T., Zenoni, M., & Iannone, L. (2017). A dyadic perspective on engagement in advance care planning. *Journal of American Geriatrics Society*, 65(1), 172–178.

Hospice & Palliative Nurses Association. (2013). HPNA position statement: The nurse's role in advance care planning. Retrieved from http://hpna.advancingexpertcare.org/wp-content/uploads/2015/08/The-Nurses-Role-in-Advance-Care-Planning.pdf

National Hospice and Palliative Care Organization. (2013). Lack of awareness continues to be a barrier for Americans in making medical wishes known. Retrieved from http://www.nhpco.org/press-room/press-releases/new-study-advance-directives

National Institute on Aging. (2016). Advance care planning. Retrieved from https://www.nia.nih.gov/health/publication/advance-care-planning

Rao, J. K., Anderson, L. A., Lin, F. C., & Laux, J. P. (2014, January). Completion of advance directives among U.S. consumers. *American Journal of Preventative Medicine*, 46(1), 65–70.

■ ANOREXIA AND WEIGHT LOSS

Janine Stage Galeski
Molly J. Jackson

Overview

Anorexia, loss of appetite, and weight loss are common occurrences that develop with advancing age, in certain disease trajectories, and at the end of life (Plonk & Arnold, 2005; Sanford, 2017). If unresolved, anorexia contributes to weakness, physical decline, sarcopenia, and cachexia as death approaches. A decreased desire to eat and an undesired weight loss are distinct entities in assessment and diagnosis, yet should be managed as a unit when possible. Treatment may include pharmacologic and nonpharmacologic interventions or even surgical placement of feeding tubes. Both anorexia and weight loss, however, are often a natural development during the dying process (Plonk & Arnold, 2005). Palliative care nursing must, then, include patient and family education and support for decisions regarding nutritional intake that align with the stated goals of care, even if death occurs as a natural consequence.

Background

Anorexia is an involuntary loss of appetite and a decrease in either desire or willingness to eat. Anorexia of aging alone is a syndrome that affects about 20% to 30% of the elderly (Sanford, 2017). General changes in taste and smell occur with aging; older adults frequently have a diminished taste sensitivity for sweet and salty foods (Jensen, 2015). Changes in hormones, cytokines, and metabolism, as well as mood disorders, can also contribute to appetite loss. However, this does not make anorexia a normal part of aging; instead, it is a complicated geriatric syndrome involving multiple causes (Sanford, 2017).

Anorexia can affect patients of any age and can be a sign of serious underlying illness, either acute or chronic. Patients with gastrointestinal infections (such as norovirus) often develop nausea, vomiting, diarrhea, abdominal pain, and loss of appetite (Kirby, Streby, & Moe, 2016). In these acute cases, the loss of appetite is temporary and will resolve with time and treatment. Clinically, a short duration of decreased food intake does not have lasting consequences; any weight loss is usually regained within a reasonable time.

Chronic anorexia, however, leads to persistent weight loss, sarcopenia, and cachexia, and usually increases as the underlying pathological process worsens. Anorexia may occur as a complication of the underlying disease, such as in Alzheimer's dementia, where the urge to eat diminishes as cognitive function deteriorates. Alternatively, chronic anorexia in cancer may be related to nausea and vomiting associated with chemotherapeutic agents, or with the disease progression itself (Vanhoutte et al., 2016). Cancer should always be suspected when a patient has unintentional weight loss without anorexia.

Loss of appetite is common in the terminal stages of illness or the very aged, yet a decreased drive to eat, in itself, is not always perceived as uncomfortable to the patient (Plonk & Arnold, 2005). In fact, a patient being urged to eat who is not experiencing hunger may become angry, resulting in a conflict between the patient and family. Frequently, family and caregivers are distressed by the lack of food intake on the part of the patient, recognizing that food is necessary for survival. As a patient weakens and approaches the last days or weeks of life, the gastric tract slows, and digestion comes to a permanent halt. There is no evidence that this process can be altered or stopped (Plonk & Arnold, 2005).

Clinical Aspects

ASSESSMENT

Nursing assessment of anorexia or weight loss should begin with a careful history and physical examination.

The discovery of weight loss might precede the diagnosis of anorexia in situations in which there is limited access to health care providers; the location where the patient resides also plays a role. A downward trend in weight or loose-fitting clothes should always be investigated. Monitoring patient weight is necessary to notice the decline—even if it is subtle. Weight loss should always be addressed with the patient when possible, to determine whether the loss was intentional or unintentional. In institutionalized settings, such as hospitals, skilled nursing facilities or long-term care facilities, close observation of eating habits can reveal a decline in oral intake even before weight loss becomes noticeable. Patient verbalizations of a loss of appetite should also trigger further investigation.

A comprehensive assessment should include noting both the composition and amount of food and fluid ingested. The estimates of caloric and nutrient intake are helpful, as are identifying social and environmental factors that can contribute to a suboptimal diet (Jensen, 2015). Assessment tools include a 24-hour intake recall, food-frequency questionnaire, patient food diaries, or recorded fluid intake and percentage of meals eaten (D'Amico & Barbarito, 2016). Weight recordings for patients should occur at the same time of day using the same scale and wearing similar clothing. In the case of a nonambulatory patient, it is important to account accurately for the weight of pillows and linens, and assistive devices used to access the scale. The nurse can also calculate the body mass index, and measure waist circumference or triceps skin-fold thickness (Jensen, 2015).

Underlying illness may be identified and treated, if present. For example, thrush (oral candida) infection often alters taste perception and produces pain with swallowing. Thrush presents as a white coating of the mouth and throat and is frequently accompanied by swollen lymph nodes of the neck. If untreated, the fungal infection can extend into the esophagus. Treatments include the topical antifungal agent mycostatin ("swish and swallow"); in immunocompromised patients, systemic antifungals may be required (Denning et al., 2017). The use of antibiotics is a risk factor that predisposes patients to fungal infections, as is hyposalivation (Billings, Dye, Iafolla, Grisius, & Alevizos, 2016). Poor oral hygiene places patients at risk for infection (Millsop & Fazel, 2016). It is the nurse's responsibility to assess and direct the oral hygiene plan of care.

Dysphagia, the inability to swallow, can also be an underlying cause of weight loss. It is often associated with brain pathologies, including stroke, traumatic brain injury, and dementia (Kimura, Ohno, & Honjyo, 2015). Nurses and other caregivers may observe an affected patient taking a longer time to chew and swallow, pocketing food, or choking when eating or drinking. A speech therapist formally diagnoses dysphagia; treatments can include speech therapy as well as dietary recommendations.

In dementia, anorexia and dysphagia often develop simultaneously and should be considered a normal progression of the disease (Takagi et al., 2016). As such, they can be attenuated in the early stages but ultimately cannot be cured. As weight loss and dysphagia progress, family decision makers may consent to, or request that a provider insert a feeding tube. Despite the short-term emotional satisfaction of being able to "feed" the patient, the use of gastrostomy tubes in Alzheimer dementia patients has been shown not to prolong life and instead adds to discomfort and care burden (Goldberg & Altman, 2014). As benefits are only short term and run counter to the principles of patient comfort in palliative care, the use of feeding tubes for the sole purpose of providing nutritional intake should be discussed in detail and aligned with the overall expectations and desires of the patient.

NURSING INTERVENTIONS, MANAGEMENT, AND IMPLICATIONS

Medications can provide appetite stimulation and weight gain in some patient populations, although the drugs used were not originally developed for this purpose. Mirtazapine, an antidepressant, is often recommended as a first-line choice to stimulate appetite (Hilas & Avena-Woods, 2014). Low doses of this medication have been shown to improve appetite, whereas higher doses do not achieve the same benefit. Owing to its original indication for depression, patients taking mirtazapine should be monitored for mood and behavior changes.

Although mirtazapine use for appetite stimulation is widely accepted in the United States, the use of megestrol, a hormonal oncologic agent, is more controversial. Its main indication is for use as a palliative adjunct in advanced breast and endometrial cancer. However, in the treatment of AIDS and cancer-related cachexia, it has been prescribed as an appetite stimulant; off-label use for dementia-related anorexia is reported as well. There is no strong evidence to support this use, and it is currently not recommended for noncancer cachexia (Taylor & Pendleton, 2016).

Other medications occasionally prescribed for appetite stimulation include cannabinoids, the antihistamine cyproheptadine, and dexamethasone. Cannabinoids are scheduled substances and are primarily used for nausea treatment in cancer therapy; they have been found to be helpful for AIDS- and Alzheimer-related anorexia and cachexia as well (van den Elsen et al., 2014). Their relation to cannabis makes their use, at times, controversial, and multiple central nervous system (CNS) effects require strict monitoring. Dexamethasone has been used successfully in treating anorexia associated with cancer (Yennurajalingam, Williams, Chisholm, & Bruera, 2016). However, strong evidence is lacking regarding long-term benefits for this population.

Nursing strategies that focus on optimizing nutrition and promoting a positive social climate for the patient should be encouraged. The small amounts of food the patient is able and willing to ingest should be high in nutrients; empty-calorie foods should be discouraged. Personal preferences for taste and food consistency need to be explored and matched to physiological abilities and needs. Dieticians and nutritionists can assist in developing meal plans and recommending appropriate supplements such as multivitamins or protein add-ons (Pouyssegur et al., 2015). The ability to self-feed and have access to healthy food should be part of the nursing assessment, and interventions should be tailored to the individual.

OUTCOMES

Anorexia and weight loss go hand-in-hand. They are best prevented and treated by addressing the underlying causes. Nurses play crucial roles in preventing, detecting, and treating both conditions by thorough assessment, as well as by assisting with activities of daily living. In addition, nurses can assist by providing education. Optimal care can be achieved through collaboration with the interdisciplinary team of physicians, speech therapists, and dieticians.

Summary

Overall, the most crucial element of managing anorexia and weight loss in advanced illness is to optimize nutrition and align medical and pharmacological treatment options with the wishes and desires of the patient and family. The benefits and burdens of each must be carefully considered.

Billings, M., Dye, B. A., Iafolla, T., Grisius, M., & Alevizos, I. (2017). Elucidating the role of hyposalivation and autoimmunity in oral candidiasis. *Oral Diseases*, 23(3), 387–394. doi:10.1111/odi.12626

D'Amico, D., & Barbarito, C. (2016). *Health & physical assessment in nursing.* Hoboken, NJ: Pearson.

Denning, D. W., Perlin, D. S., Muldoon, E. G., Colombo, A. L., Chakrabarti, A., Richardson, M. D., & Sorrell, T. C. (2017). Delivering on antimicrobial resistance agenda not possible without improving fungal diagnostic capabilities. *Emerging Infectious Diseases*, 23(2), 177–183. doi:10.3201/eid2302.152042

Goldberg, L. S., & Altman, K. W. (2014). The role of gastrostomy tube placement in advanced dementia with dysphagia: A critical review. *Clinical Interventions in Aging*, 9, 1733–1739. doi:10.2147/CIA.S53153

Hilas, O., & Avena-Woods, C. (2014). Potential role of mirtazapine in underweight older adults. *Consultant Pharmacist*, 29(2), 124–130. doi:10.4140/TCP.n.2014.124

Jensen, S. (2015). *Nursing health assessment: A best practice approach.* Philadelphia, PA: Wolters Kluwer.

Kimura, Y., Ohno, K., & Honjyo, M. (2015). Clinical analysis of evaluation of the swallowing function before gastrostomy in an acute-care hospital for elderly people. *Nihon Jibiinkoka Gakkai Kaiho*, 118(12), 1422–1428.

Kirby, A. E., Streby, A., & Moe, C. L. (2016). Vomiting as a symptom and transmission risk in norovirus illness: Evidence from human challenge studies. *PLOS ONE*, 11(4), e0143759. doi:10.1371/journal.pone.0143759

Millsop, J. W., & Fazel, N. (2016). Oral candidiasis. *Clinics in Dermatology*, 34(4), 487–494. doi:10.1016/j.clindermatol.2016.02.022

Plonk, W. M., Jr., & Arnold, R. M. (2005). Terminal care: The last weeks of life. *Journal of Palliative Medicine*, 8(5), 1042–1054. doi:10.1089/jpm.2005.8.1042

Pouyssegur, V., Brocker, P., Schneider, S. M., Philip, J. L., Barat, P., Reichert, E., . . . Lupi-Pegurier, L. (2015). An innovative solid oral nutritional supplement to fight weight loss and anorexia: Open, randomised controlled trial of efficacy in institutionalised, malnourished older adults. *Age Ageing*, 44(2), 245–251. doi:10.1093/ageing/afu150

Sanford, A. M. (2017). Anorexia of aging and its role for frailty. *Current Opinion Clinical Nutrition and Metabolic Care*, 20(1), 54–60. doi:10.1097/MCO.0000000000000336

Takagi, D., Hirano, H., Watanabe, Y., Edahiro, A., Ohara, Y., Yoshida, H., . . . Hironaka, S. (2016). Relationship between skeletal muscle mass and swallowing function in patients with Alzheimer's disease. *Geriatrics and Gerontology International.* doi:10.1111/ggi.12728

Taylor, J. K., & Pendleton, N. (2016). Progesterone therapy for the treatment of non-cancer cachexia: A systematic review. *BMJ Support Palliative Care, 6*(3), 276–286. doi:10.1136/bmjspcare-2015-001041

van den Elsen, G. A., Ahmed, A. I., Lammers, M., Kramers, C., Verkes, R. J., van der Marck, M. A., & Rikkert, M. G. (2014). Efficacy and safety of medical cannabinoids in older subjects: A systematic review. *Ageing Research Reviews, 14*, 56–64. doi:10.1016/j.arr.2014.01.007

Vanhoutte, G., van de Wiel, M., Wouters, K., Sels, M., Bartolomeeussen, L., De Keersmaecker, S., . . . Peeters, M. (2016). Cachexia in cancer: What is in the definition? *BMJ Open Gastroenterology, 3*(1), e000097. doi:10.1136/bmjgast-2016-000097

Yennurajalingam, S., Williams, J. L., Chisholm, G., & Bruera, E. (2016). Effects of dexamethasone and placebo on symptom clusters in advanced cancer patients: A preliminary report. *Oncologist, 21*(3), 384–390. doi:10.1634/theoncologist.2014-0260

■ ANXIETY IN ADVANCED ILLNESS

Lori A. Fusco

Overview

Anxiety disorders involve persistent, excessive worry and fear often interfering with routine life, and can worsen over time (National Institute of Mental Health [NIMH], 2016). Anxiety disorders are common mental illnesses that affect women more than men, and are believed to originate from an interaction of genetic, psychosocial, and neurobiological factors (Bandelow, Lichte, Rudolf, Wiltink, & Beutel, 2014). Early detection and treatment are the keys to help reduce the severity and persistence of symptoms, especially in adolescents and young adults (Baxter, Vos, Scott, Ferrari, & Whiteford, 2014). For patients of all ages with advanced illnesses, anxiety can be exacerbated by many physical and existential factors. Evidence-based nursing support for patients and their families is vital to reducing suffering related to anxiety.

Background

Anxiety disorders are some of the most common psychiatric illnesses in the Western world, causing excessive worry, fear, and distress, negatively affecting an individual's coping and productivity in his or her day-to-day life (Baxter et al., 2014). In the United States alone, the incidence of anxiety disorders is estimated to affect 18%

of the population, with annual costs approaching $42 billion (Remes, Brayne, Linde, & Lafortune, 2016). In 2016, the World Health Organization (WHO) reported a global increase of nearly 50% in people suffering from depression or anxiety, from 416 million to 615 million. During times of crisis and emergencies, the incidence increases, with as many as one in five people affected by depression and anxiety (WHO, 2016). For those battling life-threatening illnesses, at least 25% of cancer patients and 50% of patients with heart failure and chronic obstructive pulmonary disease (COPD) experience significant anxiety (Stoklosa, Patterson, & Rosielle, 2015).

Blanco et al. identified several risk factors for anxiety and major depressive disorders (MDD), often occurring together, from a large, national representative sample in the United States. The risk of anxiety disorders and MDD is higher in persons with low self-esteem, female gender, family history of depression, White race, childhood sexual abuse, history of traumatic experiences, lower education level, or a troubled family environment (Blanco et al., 2014). Anxiety and depression are among the most common mental disorders in the United States, causing burden not only on the individual but also on public health and society as a whole (Blanco et al., 2014).

Globally, anxiety disorders are reported as the sixth leading cause of disability in 2010 throughout high-, middle-, and low-income countries (Baxter et al., 2014). Anxiety disorders are chronic, disabling conditions contributing to an estimated 26.8 million disability adjusted life years globally (Remes et al., 2016), with the highest burden in both males and females between the ages of 15 and 34 years (Baxter et al., 2014). Women are almost twice as likely to be affected by anxiety disorders as men (Remes et al., 2016). Remes et al. reported that in 2010 the prevalence of anxiety disorders was highest in North America (7.7%) and the North African/Middle East Region (7.7%), and lowest in East Asia (2.8%).

Anxiety disorders start at an early age, recur, and have lifelong negative effects on health, income, education, and relationships (Baxter et al., 2014). For individuals with advanced illnesses, existing comorbidities, such as multiple sclerosis, cardiovascular disease, and diabetes, may intensify anxiety (Remes et al., 2016). Remes et al. (2016) note that the elderly and their caregivers are both disproportionately affected by anxiety, especially when older dependents have cognitive dysfunction. In addition, patients at the end of life may experience anxiety related to dyspnea, pain, spiritual distress, or existential suffering related to death. As symptoms worsen, the patient's perceived quality of life may diminish, resulting in an increase in psychological distress (Pasacreta, Minarik, & Nield-Anderson, 2010).

Clinical Aspects

ASSESSMENT

Recognition and diagnosis of patients suffering from anxiety can be difficult. Patients often seek medical care with complaints of muscle tension, difficulty sleeping, fatigue, palpitations, difficulty concentrating, nervousness, constant worry, and other somatic problems (Bandelow et al., 2014). Psychological symptoms that the nurse may note include apprehension, worry, fear, nervousness, and vigilance. The patient may report diarrhea, shortness of breath, diaphoresis, nausea, abdominal pain, insomnia, or paresthesias (Chai, Meier, Morris, & Goldhirsch, 2014). Vital signs may reveal tachycardia or tachypnea.

A comprehensive patient history should be obtained to ascertain whether previous episodes of anxiety have occurred and, if so, what treatments were recommended. The lab testing may reveal iatrogenic causes that can lead to anxiety such as undiagnosed hyperthyroidism. Prescribed or discontinued medications may be implicated in anxiety, and a complete medication reconciliation should be obtained. Medications associated with anxiety include hormones, antiviral agents, psychostimulants, corticosteroids, and chemotherapeutic agents (Chai et al., 2014).

NURSING INTERVENTIONS, MANAGEMENT, AND IMPLICATIONS

Ensuring early detection and prompt access to evidence-based treatments is challenging but critical in reducing anxiety-related health loss (Baxter et al., 2014). Unfortunately, surveys indicate most people with milder cases of anxiety do not seek treatment (Baxter et al., 2014). Research by Baxter et al. (2014) explains the early recognition and treatment of mild and moderate anxiety can reduce the persistence of symptoms and incidence of more severe cases.

Nursing, physician, and health care team interventions and recommendations should include the administration of targeted anxiety screenings and treatments as appropriate (Remes et al., 2016). Anxiety disorders are treatable with psychotherapy and drug treatment and other interventions, with a positive response rate of 45% to 65% (Bandelow et al., 2014). The treatment

plan should be selected carefully and individually for the patient, taking into account treatment preferences, previous treatment modalities, the severity of the anxiety, and comorbidities (Bandelow et al., 2014). Bandelow et al. (2014) stress the importance of the development of therapeutic relationships among the patient, physician, psychologist, nurse, and health care team; this ensures that the patient is aware of the treatment options, risks, and chances of improvement.

When considering psychotherapeutic techniques, cognitive behavioral therapy (CBT) is supported by the highest level evidence (Bandelow et al., 2014). CBT teaches people how to think, behave, and react differently to anxiety-producing and fearful situations (NIMH, 2016). CBT can be conducted individually or as group therapy (NIMH, 2016). Spiritual and social work support may be helpful if existential distress is reported.

Medications may be prescribed to relieve the symptoms of anxiety, but are not curative. The research studies show better outcomes for patients treated with a combination of psychotherapy and medication instead of treatment with only one or the other (NIMH, 2016). First-line recommendations for treating anxiety disorders include antidepressants, such as selective serotonin-reuptake inhibitors and serotonin-norepinephrine-reuptake inhibitors. Although benzodiazepines are effective in reducing anxiety, they are not recommended as initial treatment for general anxiety states because of the risk of dependence (Bandelow et al., 2014). In the palliative care patient, however, anxiolytics, such as benzodiazepines, are sometimes prescribed when benefit outweighs the risks in a terminal state (Chai et al., 2014).

Other treatment modalities for anxiety include self-help or support groups, talking with a trusted friend or clergy, stress management techniques and meditation, and nutrition modifications and exercise (NIMH, 2016). Research by Yang et al. (2016) supports the benefit of music therapy in alleviating patient anxiety in clinical settings.

OUTCOMES

Diagnosis and treatment of patient anxiety by health care professionals result in positive individual health, societal, and financial outcomes. Economically, a study by the WHO (2016) estimates every dollar spent in the United States for better treatment of depression and anxiety results in a return of $4 in improved health and ability to work. The benefits outweigh the cost for treatment, resulting in both improved health and greater numbers of productive individuals in the labor force (WHO, 2016).

Summary

Anxiety disorders are common, chronic, disabling conditions across the world, with onset usually in young people, particularly women younger than 35 years (Baxter et al., 2014). The resulting burden can be experienced individually, publicly, and financially as a result of substantial work and social difficulties (Blanco et al., 2014). The palliative care patient often has multifactorial causes of anxiety, including existential distress related to the approach of death. For this patient, early detection, diagnosis, and treatment can help alleviate suffering and improve the quality of life.

Bandelow, B., Lichte, T., Rudolf, S., Wiltink, J., & Beutel, M. E. (2014). Clinical practice guideline: The diagnosis of and treatment recommendations for anxiety disorders. *Deutsches Arzteblatt International, 111,* 473–480. doi:10.3238/arztebl.2014.0473

Baxter, A. J., Vos, T., Scott, K. M., Ferrari, A. J., & Whiteford, H. A. (2014). The global burden of anxiety disorders in 2010. *Psychological Medicine, 44,* 2363–2374. doi:10.1017/S0033291713003243

Blanco, C., Rubio, J., Wall, M., Wang, S., Jiu, C. J., & Kendler, K. S. (2014). Risk factors for anxiety disorders: Common and specific effects in a national sample. *Depression and Anxiety, 31,* 756–764. doi:10.1002/da.22247

Chai, E., Meier, D., Morris, J., & Goldhirsch, S. (2014). *Geriatric palliative care: A practical guide for clinicians.* New York, NY: Oxford University Press.

National Institute of Mental Health. (2016). Anxiety disorders. Retrieved from https://www.nimh.nih.gov/health/topics/anxiety-disorders/index.shtml

Pasacreta, J., Minarik, P., & Nield-Anderson, L. (2010). Anxiety and depression. In B. Ferrell & N. Coyle (Eds.), *Oxford textbook of palliative care* (3rd ed., pp. 425–448). New York, NY: Oxford University Press.

Remes, O., Brayne, C., Linde, R., & Lafortune, L. (2016). A systematic review of reviews on the prevalence of anxiety disorders in adult populations. *Brain and Behavior, 6*(7), 1–33. doi:10.1002/brb3.497

Stoklosa, J., Patterson, K., & Rosielle, D. (2015). Fast facts and concepts #186. *Anxiety in Palliative Care-Causes and Diagnosis.* Retrieved from https://www.mypcnow.org/blank-zh5tm

World Health Organization. (2016). Investing in treatment for depression and anxiety leads to fourfold return. Retrieved from http://www.who.int/mediacentre/news/releases/2016/depression-anxiety-treatment/en

Yang, C., Miao, N., Lee, T., Tsai, J., Yang, H., Chen, W., . . . Chou, K. (2016). The effect of a researcher designated music intervention on hospitalized psychiatric patients with different levels of anxiety. *Journal of Clinical Nursing, 25,* 777–787. doi.org/10.1111/jocn.13098

■ BOWEL OBSTRUCTION

Hilary Applequist

Overview

Bowel obstruction is a partial or complete blockage of material through the lumen of the small or large intestine (McCance & Huether, 2014). It can represent a surgical emergency. The causes of bowel obstruction include adhesions, hernias, malignancy, irritable bowel syndrome, intussusception, volvulus, foreign bodies, fecal impaction, and paralytic ileus (Paulson & Thompson, 2015; Serrano Falcón, Barceló López, Mateos Muñoz, Álvarez Sánchez, & Rey, 2016). Adults with bowel obstruction may present with abdominal pain, distention, nausea, vomiting, and constipation. Palliative nursing care of the patient with a bowel obstruction focuses on symptom control and relief, as well as following a treatment plan consistent with the patient's goals of care.

Background

Approximately 2 million cases of bowel obstruction are reported yearly in the United States. Small bowel obstructions (SBO) account for 350,000 cases, or roughly 15% of all surgical admissions (Coe, Chang, & Sicklick, 2015; O'Malley et al., 2015). SBO accounts for more than $1 billion in care annually with mortality of 2% to 8%, increasing to 25% if ischemia is present and surgical intervention is delayed (Lombardo, Baum, Filho, & Nirula, 2014; Paulson & Thompson, 2015). The risk factors include gastric, bowel, and ovarian malignancy; carcinomatosis; and previous abdominal surgery or radiation (Krielen et al., 2016; Paul Olson, Pinkerton, Brasel, & Schwarze, 2014; Protus, Kimbrel, & Grauer, 2015). Multidetector computed tomography is the standard imaging used to diagnose bowel obstruction, although abdominal x-ray can be used if a large bowel obstruction is suspected (Jaffe & Thompson, 2015).

Extrinsic or intrinsic compression of the bowel prevents contents from moving through the lumen with resulting accumulation of gas and fluids proximal to the obstruction or narrowing. Colicky pain results as the peristaltic activity of the bowel continues to move chyme through the lumen; severe nausea and vomiting often develop as fluids and gases meet resistance at the obstruction. Nausea and vomiting may be delayed if the obstruction is in the large bowel (Protus et al., 2015). Subsequent distension leads to a cascade of events resulting in a hypertensive situation within the lumen that triggers an inflammatory response (Protus et al., 2015). Increased pressure in the lumen of the bowel diminishes venous return, causing ischemia, possibly accompanied by gangrene, perforation, and systemic hypovolemia (McCance & Huether, 2014; Protus et al., 2015). If treatment is not promptly initiated, the hypovolemia can result in multiorgan failure (Protus et al., 2015).

Depending on the clinical presentation, treatment ranges from conservative measures to immediate surgery (Springer, Bailey, Davis, & Johnson, 2014). Conservative treatment comprises drainage via nasogastric tube, hydration, and bowel rest as well as medications to combat symptoms. Surgical treatment is reserved for an infarcted or strangulated bowel, gangrene, adhesiolysis, an internal hernia, or irritable bowel, and can be performed as an open procedure or laparoscopically (O'Leary et al., 2014). Palliative treatments include drainage via a nasogastric tube, aggressive pain management, antiemetics and antisecretory agents, steroids, placement of a venting percutaneous endoscopic gastrostomy tube (PEG), or palliative surgery (Paul Olson et al., 2014).

Clinical Aspects

ASSESSMENT

Obtaining a thorough patient history is imperative when a bowel obstruction is suspected. Determination of medical history, as well as documentation of past surgeries or radiation involving the abdomen, is vital. If the bowel obstruction is believed to be malignancy-related, the patient's oncologic history, treatment course, and complications need to be assessed. If the patient has a history of previous bowel obstructions, past treatments and effectiveness should be noted.

Physical assessment may reveal a distended, tender abdomen. Bowel sounds may be absent or hyperactive with a tinkly sound (McCance & Huether, 2014). Diaphoresis and tachycardia may be present because of severe pain and the presence of hypotension. The appearance of the emesis varies depending on the site of obstruction, ranging from clear (pylorus), bile colored (proximal intestine) to fecal (small intestine or colon).

If perforation occurs, fever and leukocytosis result. Assessment of bowel history is imperative, including the date of last bowel movement, bowel consistency to check whether any seepage was noted. In addition, acidosis or alkalosis may be present if vomiting has been severe or dehydration has developed as a result of fluid accumulation in the gut (McCance & Huether, 2014).

NURSING INTERVENTIONS, MANAGEMENT, AND IMPLICATIONS

A palliative approach to bowel obstruction focuses on symptom relief in the least invasive manner possible. The evidence suggests that outcomes and survival are not improved via surgical intervention if the obstruction is malignant (Protus et al., 2015). A palliative stent or venting PEG tube may be placed for comfort and resumption of some oral intake, but the benefits and burdens associated with the procedure must be considered in advance. A nasogastric tube (NGT) may be inserted to determine whether discomfort is reduced. If the patient's prognosis is days to weeks, the NGT may further contribute to discomfort and social isolation (Protus et al., 2015). Hydration needs should be balanced with the potential risk of increasing peristalsis and abdominal pain. Increasing edema or prolongation of the dying process through intravenous fluid administration would be deleterious in a palliative situation. Patient and family education regarding nutrition and fluid intake are necessary.

Pain and emesis associated with bowel obstruction can be difficult to manage. A cadre of pharmacological approaches can be used to control pain or vomiting while slowing secretions into the bowel (2015). Parenteral opioids are used for pain relief, whereas anticholinergic medications, such as glycopyrrolate or hyoscyamine, can help reduce associated colicky pain. Careful assessment for deleterious effects of anticholinergics should be a priority, as delirium can occur or worsen with these drugs (2015). Corticosteroids, such as dexamethasone, can combat the inflammation associated with obstruction as well as aid in nausea control. Small doses of haloperidol scheduled or given as needed combat nausea as well.

OUTCOMES

Evidence-based interventions for bowel obstruction can help control pain, nausea, and vomiting. A palliative approach always keep the patient's goals of care at the forefront and interventions are selected with those goals in mind. If the bowel obstruction is likely to recur or expected to cause significant suffering, a hospice discussion should be initiated.

Summary

Bowel obstruction in adults can cause severe symptoms that require thorough assessment and prompt intervention. Treatment approaches should be guided by the patient's expressed goals of care in a palliative situation. Strong nurse advocacy and evidence-based interventions enhance symptom control and improve the quality of life for patients experiencing distress from a bowel obstruction.

Coe, T. M., Chang, D. C., & Sicklick, J. K. (2015). Small bowel volvulus in the adult populace of the United States: Results from a population-based study. *American Journal of Surgery*, *210*(2), 201–210. doi:10.1016/j.amjsurg.2014.12.048

Jaffe, T., & Thompson, W. M. (2015). Large-bowel obstruction in the adult: Classic radiographic and CT findings, etiology, and mimics. *Radiology*, *275*(3), 651–663. doi:10.1148/radiol.2015140916

Krielen, P., van den Beukel, B. A., Stommel, M. W. J., van Goor, H., Strik, C., & ten Broek, R. P. G. (2016). In-hospital costs of an admission for adhesive small bowel obstruction. *World Journal of Emergency Surgery*, *11*, 1–8. doi:10.1186/s13017-016-0109

Lombardo, S., Baum, K., Filho, J. D., & Nirula, R. (2014). Should adhesive small bowel obstruction be managed laparoscopically? A National Surgical Quality Improvement Program propensity score analysis. *Journal of Trauma and Acute Care Surgery*, *76*(3), 696–703. doi:10.1097/TA.0000000000000156

McCance, K. L., & Huether, S. E. (Eds.). (2014). *Pathophysiology: The biologic basis for disease in adults and children* (7th ed.). St. Louis, MO: Mosby.

O'Leary, E. A., Desale, S. Y., Yi, W. S., Fujita, K. A., Hynes, C. F., Chandra, S. K., & Sava, J. A. (2014). Letting the sun set on small bowel obstruction: Can a simple risk score tell us when nonoperative care is inappropriate? *American Surgeon*, *80*(6), 572–579.

O'Malley, R., Al-Hawary, M., Kaza, R., Wasnik, A., Platt, J., Francis, I., . . . Francis, I. R. (2015). MDCT findings in small bowel obstruction: Implications of the cause and presence of complications on treatment decisions. *Abdominal Imaging*, *40*(7), 2248–2262. doi:10.1007/s00261-015-0477-x

Paul Olson, T. J., Pinkerton, C., Brasel, K. J., & Schwarze, M. L. (2014). Palliative surgery for malignant bowel obstruction from carcinomatosis: A systematic review. *JAMA Surgery*, *149*(4), 383–392. doi:10.1001/jamasurg.2013.4059

Paulson, E. K., & Thompson, W. M. (2015). Review of small-bowel obstruction: The diagnosis and when to worry. *Radiology*, *275*(2), 332–342. doi:10.1148/radiol.15131519

Protus, B. M., Kimbrel, J. M., & Grauer, P. A. (2015). *Palliative care consultant: Guidelines for effective management of symptoms* (4th ed.). Mongomery, AL: HospiScript Services.

Serrano Falcón, B., Barceló López, M., Mateos Muñoz, B., Álvarez Sánchez, A., & Rey, E. (2016). Fecal impaction: A systematic review of its medical complications. *BMC Geriatrics*, *16*, 4. doi:10.1186/s12877-015-0162-5

Springer, J. E., Bailey, J. G., Davis, P. J. B., & Johnson, P. M. (2014). Management and outcomes of small bowel obstruction in older adult patients: A prospective cohort study. *Canadian Journal of Surgery*, *57*(6), 379–384.

■ COMMUNICATION

Anne M. Kolenic

Overview

Communication is a fundamental part of providing high-quality nursing care. It is the essential aspect of good nursing practice, and studies suggest that communication training is mandatory for any nurse working in palliative care (Dahlin, 2010). Nurses spend more time with patients and families facing end-of-life issues than any other health care professional and are often the ones whom the patients and families turn to for help and guidance (Caton & Klemm, 2006; Peereboom & Coyle, 2012). Palliative care encompasses all aspects of physical, psychosocial, social, and spiritual needs and requires specialized skills (Caton & Klemm, 2006). These domains require the nurse to demonstrate competence not only in medical knowledge and assessment skills but in communication and advocacy as well.

Background

All exchanges between nurses and their patients are facilitated through communication. Communication is central to nursing care, and with good communication skills, the nurse can assess various domains related to the patient's illness (Dahlin, 2010). The American Association of Colleges of Nursing's (AACN) document titled, "*Peaceful Death Competencies*," outlines competencies for nurses who are providing end-of-life care (AACN, 2002). The third competency states that a nurse should communicate compassionately and effectively with the patient, family, and members of the health care team about issues surrounding end of life (AACN, 2002). In 2006, a consortium of leading palliative care organizations developed clinical practice guidelines to establish quality standards in palliative care titled the National Consensus Project (NCP) for Quality Palliative Care (2013). The importance of communication is emphasized throughout the document and is addressed in all eight domains (Dahlin, 2010; Peereboom & Coyle, 2012). The revised third edition of the NCP guidelines states that patients, families, and all health care providers should collaborate and communicate regarding patient care needs (NCP, 2013). However, even before these competencies and guidelines were developed, the principles of effective communication were exemplified in nursing practice (Dahlin, 2010). It is critical to realize that no aspect of expert palliative nursing practice can be executed without proficiency in communication (Wittenberg-Lyles et al., 2013).

Therapeutic communication involves the essential skills of effective listening, appropriate nonverbal and verbal communication, counseling skills, reflection, clarification, empathy, and supportiveness (Dahlin, 2010; Peereboom & Coyle, 2012). These skills come naturally to some, but others must learn them through coaching, mentoring, and modeling. Developing skills at all levels of communication can assist the nurse to establish trusting relationships with patients and families and allow for accurate assessment of all dimensions of palliative care (Dahlin, 2010). As a member of the interdisciplinary team, the nurse plays a vital role in the exchange of information among patients, families, and other disciplines. Nurses are often the "constant" team members engaged with patients and families battling life-limiting illnesses, which results in the development of strong, trusting relationships (Dahlin, 2010; Peereboom & Coyle, 2012). Patients consider communication skills to be very important and good communication allows for optimal palliative care (Dahlin, 2010).

Clinical Aspects

ASSESSMENT

There are many roles and responsibilities for the nurse when providing palliative care. Effective communication skills enable the nurse to build relationships with patients and families, and it is through these relationships that data and vital information regarding what is relevant to the patient are gathered. Often the nurse's role in palliative care communication is inaccurately depicted as a supportive role (Wittenberg-Lyles et al., 2013), but in reality, it is so much more than that. The nurse's role requires flexibility and attention to both the task and relational dimensions of communication during interactions with patients and families (Wittenberg-Lyles et al., 2013).

Initial communication occurs when the nurse and patient first meet and learn about each other (Dahlin, 2010). During this time the nurse can explore the patient's understanding of his or her illness, elicit personality and coping styles, and identify any existing advanced care planning (Dahlin, 2010). The nurse must be able to assess the patient's information and communication needs. To gather information from the patients, the use of open-ended questions is most effective (Dahlin, 2010).

Wittenberg-Lyles et al. (2013) describe a communication technique entitled "narrative clinical practice," which reveals who people are and where they are headed. To engage in the narrative clinical practice, the nurse must allow herself or himself to witness, which involves being with and relating to others while honoring her or his voice, and lived experience (Wittenberg-Lyles et al., 2013). Allowing the patient to tell his or her story in narrative provides the opportunity to hear the patient's own words, expressions, and nonverbal cues, which may then express issues of importance and priorities of care (Dahlin, 2010; Wittenberg-Lyles et al., 2013).

NURSING INTERVENTIONS, MANAGEMENT, AND IMPLICATIONS

Despite the knowledge that the nurse is well positioned to elicit goals of care from patients by using communication skills, there are many barriers to the nursing facilitation of these discussions. These barriers may include lack of experience, fear of saying the wrong thing, fear of eliciting strong emotions (patient, family, or their own), feelings of guilt, disagreement with patient or family's decisions for goals of care, or moral distress (Peereboom & Coyle, 2012). These barriers combined with a lack of training, education, and confidence can leave nurses ill prepared to engage in these discussions (Dahlin, 2010; Peereboom & Coyle, 2012).

Nurses can use specific strategies to assist in engaging their patients in goals-of-care conversations. One strategy is the usage of nonverbal expressions of empathy, such as facing the patient squarely, sitting at eye level, maintaining an open body posture, using eye contact when appropriate, and maintaining a relaxed posture (Peereboom & Coyle, 2012). Another strategy is *ask–tell–ask,* which helps to assess how much the patient knows, how much he or she wants to know, and whether he or she wants to discuss it (Back, Arnold, & Tulsky, 2009; Peereboom & Coyle, 2012). Using the phrase "tell me more" allows the nurse to explore the patient's world and can be very helpful at the beginning of an encounter, functioning as an invitation (Back et al., 2009). The acronym NURSE is helpful in responding to and addressing emotions when a patient has received bad news. *Naming* (N) the emotion, using words to communicate *understanding* (U), communicating *respect* (R) and *support* (S), and using words to *explore* (E) the patient's world all communicate empathy and align the nurse with patient (Back et al, 2009; Peereboom & Coyle, 2012). Another phrase that can be used when discussing the possibility of a poor outcome is to suggest the approach as "hoping for the best, but preparing for the worst" (Peereboom & Coyle, 2012).

OUTCOMES

Studies have shown that patients who have conversations about their wishes for end-of -life care are more likely to receive care consistent with their preferences (Peereboom & Coyle, 2012). Initiating end-of-life discussions earlier and more systematically can allow patients to make informed choices, achieve better palliative care, and have more opportunity to work on issues for closure (Peereboom & Coyle, 2012).

Summary

Communication is a complex, continual transaction process and it is central to nursing care, especially in the setting of palliative care. It is the foundation for the nurse–patient relationship and the cornerstone of palliative care, hence making communication skills an essential competency for all nurses (Dahlin, 2010). Nurses must embrace the vital role that they play in communication with patients, families, and the interdisciplinary team members.

American Association of Colleges of Nursing. (2002). *Peaceful death competencies: Recommended competencies and curricular guidelines for end-of-life nursing care.* Washington, DC: Author.

Back, A., Arnold, R., & Tulsky, J. (2009). *Mastering communication with seriously ill patients: Balancing honesty with empathy and hope.* New York, NY: Cambridge University Press.

Caton, A., & Klemm, P. (2006). The introduction of novice oncology nurses to end-of-life care. *Clinical Journal of Oncology Nursing, 10*(5), 604–608.

Dahlin, C. (2010). Communication in palliative care: An essential competency for nurses. In B. Ferrell, & N. Coyle (Eds.), *Oxford textbook of palliative nursing* (3rd ed., pp. 107–133). Oxford, UK: Oxford University Press.

National Consensus Project for Quality Palliative Care. (2013). In *Clinical practice guidelines for quality palliative care* (3rd ed.). Pittsburgh, PA: Author. Retrieved from https://www.hpna.org/multimedia/NCP_Clinical_Practice_Guidelines_3rd_Edition.pdf

Peereboom, K., & Coyle, N. (2012). Facilitating goals-of-care discussions for patients with life-limiting disease-communication strategies for nurses. *Journal of Hospice & Palliative Nursing, 14,* 251–258.

Wittenberg-Lyles, E., Goldsmith, J., Ferrell, B., & Ragan, S. (2013). *Communication in palliative nursing.* New York, NY: Oxford University Press.

▪ CONSTIPATION

Angela M. Johnson

Overview

Constipation at the end of life is a common complication that can be a challenge to manage. Constipation is defined as three or fewer bowel movements in a week or hard small bowel movements that may be painful to pass (National Institute of Diabetes Digestive and Kidney Disease, 2017). Patient descriptions and perception of the problem vary widely, which often leads to undiagnosed or untreated constipation (National Clinic Effectiveness Committee [NCEC], 2015). Constipation at the end of life may cause abdominal discomfort and pain, yet it is overlooked in light of more distressing symptoms. The common contributing factors include medications, immobility, dehydration, and malnutrition. It is more likely to affect the elderly but can affect anyone at the end of life. Constipation is common among healthy children, but is not frequently reported at the end of life. In patients with advanced cancer, constipation is a commonly reported distressing symptom, along with pain and anorexia (Tai et al., 2016). The condition is associated with nearly 50,000 hospitalizations per year and an estimated $851 million in health care costs across the life span (Sethi et al., 2014).

Background

A number of factors contribute to constipation in advanced illness. Immobility at the end of life can lead to constipation as a result of decreased peristaltic stimulation. Walking stimulates peristalsis and is the first recommended intervention for a patient suffering from constipation or ileus, if feasible. Opioid analgesic use contributes to constipation if not managed properly. As many as 81% of patients are suffering from opioid-induced constipation (Sonu, Triadafilopoulos, & Gardner, 2016). Opioids decrease pain signals by blocking mu receptors in the brain but also affect the same receptors in the gastrointestinal tract, resulting in slowed peristalsis. Many patients are prescribed opioids at the end of life to treat pain and dyspnea. If opioids are indicated, a bowel regimen, including a stimulant laxative, is recommended to prevent constipation.

Another medication class frequently used near the end of life are anticholinergics. These drugs are commonly prescribed to help decrease salivary and respiratory secretions but are also associated with constipation. As the patient grows weaker, dehydration and malnutrition often develop as a result of decreased oral intake. This exacerbates constipation, resulting in the stool that is hard and difficult to expel.

Cognitive impairment and altered mental status also play a role in constipation. Owing to an altered mental status, patients may instinctually hold their stool to prevent incontinence when unable to communicate their need to defecate. Untreated constipation can lead to serious complications and symptoms such as pain, anorexia, nausea, bowel impaction, and bowel perforation (National Clinic Effectiveness Committee, 2015; Zhe, 2016). Constipation may also be misdiagnosed as malignant bowel obstruction. A malignant bowel obstruction occurs when a tumor has grown large enough to block part of the small or large intestine. Symptoms of bowel obstruction are an absence of flatus, severe abdominal pain with distention, absent bowel sounds, nausea, and vomiting. When this occurs, laxatives may cause increased pain and should not be used.

Clinical Aspects

ASSESSMENT

As a patient nears the end of life, communication becomes more difficult, and the patient may only show nonverbal signs of discomfort. He or she may exhibit abdominal guarding on the examination, which could easily be mistaken for pain from disease progression, rather than constipation. The nurse's assessment plays a key role in finding and interpreting constipation as a source of the discomfort.

Pertinent history of constipation and understanding of how a patient treats constipation is important when managing this symptom at the end of life. It is also imperative to discuss bowel frequency with the patient and family as this topic is often not mentioned until the symptoms become severe. Physical assessment findings may include abdominal pain, back pain, bloating, nausea, and vomiting. Patients may have diarrhea from overflow, and they can still be suffering from constipation. A digital rectal exam may be required, for those properly trained. On exam, the nurse may detect small, hard stool or rectal vault impaction.

NURSING INTERVENTIONS, MANAGEMENT, AND IMPLICATIONS

Nursing interventions are focused on promoting comfort and alleviation of symptoms. Instruction regarding prevention of constipation through maintaining adequate hydration, the initiation of a bowel regimen while on opioids, and knowledge deficits related to constipation. Ongoing communication regarding the effectiveness of interventions is important.

The nurse assesses for signs and symptoms of constipation, bowel obstruction, and fecal impaction. It is imperative that members of the team communicate bowel elimination concerns to ensure that constipation is managed. Constipation can be prevented and treated with nursing interventions along with medications. Walking and mobility should also be encouraged, if possible. Many patients may not be able to verbalize their need to eliminate their bowels and should be placed on a toilet after breakfast as the gastrocolic reflex is the strongest in the morning (NCEC, 2015). If the patient is unable to use the toilet and must use a bedpan, a high Fowler's position should be maintained if possible with feet supported on a hard surface to encourage abdominal muscle use. In addition, patients should always be offered privacy during toilet times (NCEC, 2015). Feedback from family members in identifying their loved one's patterns of behavior and habits should be elicited.

The nurse should collaborate with the provider regarding appropriate medication for treatment if indicated. Information regarding history, symptoms, and physical assessment findings should be communicated to the provider to ensure that an appropriate treatment plan is in place for the patient. Treatment for constipation starts with fiber and bulk-forming laxatives, but it is recommended that patients drink at least 1.5 liters of water per day to prevent worsening constipation from these medications (NCEC, 2015). To treat and prevent opioid-induced constipation, recommendations are to use stimulant laxatives. All patients on opioids should be on a bowel regimen to prevent constipation as a standard of care as recommended by the World Health Organization (NCEC, 2015). Opioid-induced constipation can be relieved by methylnaltrexone (Relistor) if laxative therapy has failed; this drug is also approved for use in noncancer patients.

OUTCOMES

Expected nursing outcomes are to relieve and prevent constipation. If the patient has easily eliminated stools, the nurse relieved the discomfort caused by constipation and assisted the patient in elimination. Ultimately, at the end of life, the patient experiences less discomfort.

Summary

Constipation is one of the most common symptoms in patients at the end of life. It is also often untreated and underdiagnosed. Untreated constipation can cause intense pain, bowel perforation, nausea, and vomiting, and should be considered a priority during the nursing assessment. Prevention is imperative and starts with a discussion with the patient and family. All patients on opioids should have a bowel regimen in place with a stimulant laxative. Collaboration among the provider, nursing, family, and the patient is crucial in keeping the patient comfortable at the end of life and controlling this very common symptom.

National Clinic Effectiveness Committee. (2015). National clinical guideline no. 10: Management of constipation in adult patients receiving palliative care. Retrieved from http://health.gov.ie/wp-content/uploads/2015/11/Mgmt-of-Constipation-Guideline.pdf

National Institute of Diabetes Digestive and Kidney Disease. (2017). Constipation. Retrieved from https://www.niddk.nih.gov/health-information/digestive-diseases/constipation

Sethi, S., Mikami, S., LeClair, J., Park, R., Jones, M., Wadhwa, V., . . . Lembo, A. (2014). Inpatient burden of constipation in the United States: An analysis of national trends in the United States from 1997 to 2010. American Journal of Gastroenterology, 109(2), 250–256. doi:10.1038/ajg.2013.423

Sonu, I., Triadafilopoulos, G., & Gardner, J. D. (2016). Persistent constipation and abdominal adverse events with newer treatments for constipation. BMJ Open Gastroenterology 3(1), e000094. doi:10.1136/bmjgast-2016-000094

Tai, S., Lee, C., Wu, C., Hsieh, H., Huang, J., Huang, C., & Chien, C. (2016). Symptom severity of patients with advanced cancer in palliative care unit: Longitudinal assessments of symptoms improvement. BMC Palliative Care, 15(1), 1–7. doi:10.1186/s12904-016-0105-8

Zhe, H. (2016). The assessment and management of constipation among patients with advanced cancer in a palliative care ward in China. JBI Database of Systematic Reviews and Implementation Reports, 14(5), 295–309. doi:10.11124/jbisrir-2016-002631

■ DELIRIUM

Colleen Kurzawa

Overview

Delirium is an acute change in attention and cognition accompanied by changes in behavior (Cohen, 2015). The prevalence of delirium in palliative care accounts for 2% to 68% of the patient population (Moens, Higginson, & Harding, 2014). Delirium in palliative care patients is common, frequently not recognized, and may be inadequately treated (Finucane, Lugton, Kennedy, & Spiller, 2016). The management and prevention of delirium are cost-effective in this population, with a possible decrease of 30% in hospital admission rates (Lawlor & Bush, 2015). Therefore, it is important to identify, assess, and treat delirium in palliative care patients (Lawlor & Bush, 2015).

Background

Delirium is defined as a serious, distressing, and common neuropsychiatric syndrome across many health care settings, including palliative care (Finucane et al., 2016; Hosie, Davidson, Agar, Sanderson, & Philips, 2012), and is associated with significant morbidity and mortality (Grassi & Riba, 2014). It is characterized by disordered awareness, attention, cognition, behavioral manifestations (Finucane et al., 2016), sleep disturbances, delusions, and emotional fluctuations (PDQ Supportive and Palliative Care Editorial Board, 2016). When delirium occurs in the palliative care patient, considerations must include the vulnerability of the patient, cognitive status and the implications for care, potential for reversibility, medications and side effects, and life expectancy (Bush et al., 2014). Delirium is considered a complication in palliative care patients and even more so at the end of life (Bush et al., 2014).

According to the *Diagnostic and Statistical Manual of Mental Disorders;* (DSM-5; American Psychiatric Association, 2013; Lawlor & Bush, 2015), the clinical criteria for a diagnosis of delirium include the following: a disturbance of consciousness with reduced awareness and attention deficit; changed cognitive and perceptual disturbances; onset of hours to days with fluctuations during a 24-hour period; and underlying comorbidities, medications, and a combination of etiologies. Delirium is classified into three subtypes: hyperactive, hypoactive, and mixed or a combination of hyperactive and hyperactive (Bush et al., 2014; Cohen, 2015; PDQ Supportive and Palliative Care Editorial Board, 2016). Hyperactive delirium is described as a state of increased arousal and restlessness with excessive verbal and motor activity (Cohen, 2015) accompanied by possible physical aggressiveness (Cohen, 2015; Grassi & Riba, 2014). Hypoactive delirium is less obvious with decreased cognitive status and motor activity such as sleepiness, withdrawal, and pleasant confusion (Cohen, 2015). Hypoactive delirium is underrecognized, misdiagnosed, and undertreated in palliative care populations (Grassi & Riba, 2014). All patients who develop delirium have an increased mortality and morbidity (Hey, Hosker, Ward, Kite, & Speechley, 2015).

In patients with advanced illnesses, the prevalence of delirium is 85% (Cohen, 2015). Anywhere from 30% to 50% of palliative care patients and 88% of patients with advanced cancer are affected by delirium (Hey et al., 2015), although Moens et al. (2014) suggested that the prevalence of delirium in palliative care patients ranges from 2% to 68%. A retrospective study conducted by Hey et al. (2015) suggested that the prevalence documented with a diagnosis of delirium ranged from 0% to 8.4%, yet climbed to 35.7% to 39.2% when both documentation and described synonyms of delirium were considered. In palliative care patients, 30% to 50% of delirium is reversible (Grassi et al., 2015). The prevalence of hypoactive delirium is 20% to 86% and hyperactive is 40% to 50% (Grassi et al., 2015).

Delirium is multifactorial and includes a combination of baseline precipitating risk factors that are modifiable (Bush et al., 2014). Precipitating factors vary and include infection, constipation, enteral feedings, medications, and electrolyte abnormalities (Cohen, 2015). Persons who are at an increased risk for delirium are hospitalized patients with the following risk factors: severe illness, the level of comorbidity, advanced age, previous dementia, hypoalbuminemia, infection, azotemia, and psychoactive medications (PDQ Supportive and Palliative Care Editorial Board, 2016). The etiology of delirium in palliative care is caused by several different factors and varies per person. The presence of multiple comorbidities, metabolic imbalances, organ failure, prescribed medications, and withdrawal of opioids may contribute to acute disorientation (Grassi et al., 2015). The underlying causes of the delirium should be investigated and treated (Grassi et al., 2015). The other potential causes include infection, sepsis, trauma, central nervous system pathology, hypoxia, urinary and fecal retention, myocardial causes, dehydration, nutritional deficiencies, and drug toxicity (Grassi et al., 2015).

Clinical Aspects

ASSESSMENT

The diagnosis of delirium is frequently missed (PDQ Supportive and Palliative Care Editorial Board, 2016) or misdiagnosed as depression or dementia (PDQ Supportive and Palliative Care Editorial Board, 2016). Nursing assessments should include observation and the use of screening tools to detect delirium (PDQ Supportive and Palliative Care Editorial Board, 2016). A diagnosis of hyperactive, hypoactive, or mixed delirium should be considered if a patient shows any signs or symptoms of delirium no matter how minor, such as agitation and uncooperative behavior, personality changes, impaired cognitive functioning, fluctuation in the level of consciousness, and anxiety or depression (PDQ Supportive and Palliative Care Editorial Board, 2016). The assessment of palliative care patients should be ongoing as goals of care change, with the involvement of psychiatry and pharmacy disciplines (Cohen, 2015).

Semistructured interviews are essential to assist in the recognition and diagnosis of delirium in palliative care (Lawlor & Bush, 2015) and should also be conducted at the end of life, if possible (Lawlor & Bush, 2015). Interventions are influenced by both the prognosis and agreed on goals of care (Lawlor & Bush, 2015). There are screening and rating instruments that may be used to diagnose delirium in palliative care. The Confusion Assessment Method (CAM) is designed to screen for cognitive impairment and does not require formal patient participation (Lawlor & Bush, 2015). The Memorial Delirium Assessment Scale (MDAS) is used to rate the severity of delirium symptoms occurring over the course of a day (Lawlor & Bush, 2015). Other validated instruments include the Mini-Mental

State Examination (MMSE), the Blessed Orientation Memory and Concentration Test (BOMC), and the Delirium Scale-Revised-98 (PDQ Supportive and Palliative Care Editorial Board, 2016).

The underlying causes of delirium include modifying predisposing factors such as discontinuing or reducing the dose of psychoactive medications, administering of fluid to treat dehydration, treating hypercalcemia and other electrolyte imbalances, and prescribing antibiotics to treat infections (PDQ Supportive and Palliative Care Editorial Board, 2016). Visual or hearing impairments and protein–calorie nutrition should also be considered as contributing factors (Grassi & Riba, 2014). The interventions should be individualized to treat signs and symptoms, and, if sedation is used, monitoring and reassessment are required (PDQ Supportive and Palliative Care Editorial Board, 2016).

NURSING INTERVENTIONS, MANAGEMENT, AND IMPLICATIONS

The plan of care should include management of a structured environment, using an appropriate amount of stimulation for the individual (Cohen, 2015). Nonpharmacological interventions include reorientation, providing adequate room lighting, having familiar objects in the room, maintaining continuity of care and caregivers, promoting a calm environment (decreased noise and stimulation), and encouraging family presence (PDQ Supportive and Palliative Care Editorial Board, 2016). The principles of good sleep hygiene should be incorporated into the care (Cohen, 2015). If a patient becomes aggressive, safety principles should be reviewed (Cohen, 2015). Physical restraints should be avoided or discontinued as soon as possible; a bedside companion is also suggested (Cohen, 2015; PDQ Supportive and Palliative Care Editorial Board, 2016).

Pharmacological interventions include medication to control delirium and treat underlying comorbidities such as infection and electrolyte imbalances (Cohen, 2015). The medications that are frequently prescribed include opioids, antipsychotics, benzodiazepines, and psychostimulants (Cohen, 2015; Grassi et al., 2015). Other medications that may be helpful include ondansetron, melatonin, modafinil, gabapentin, and valproate (Grassi et al., 2015; Lawlor & Bush, 2015). For patients in whom deep sedation is appropriate, he or she should be monitored and evaluated, and sedation should be discontinued when appropriate (PDQ Supportive and Palliative Care Editorial Board, 2016). The general

responsibilities of monitoring should include knowledge of medication side effects such as Q-T prolongation, arrhythmias, and metabolic changes (Cohen, 2015).

OUTCOMES

Clear communication and goal setting are necessary when caring for people with delirium in palliative care across all settings (Lawlor & Bush, 2015). Education is necessary to help family members understand symptoms and participate in the plan of care (Cohen, 2015). Interdisciplinary communication in the development of patient goals of care should be established, and a care plan developed to assist in planning treatment and interventions (Cohen, 2015). Lawlor and Bush (2015) have suggested that patients (when able) should be offered opportunities to talk about their episodes of delirium, although this has not been studied. Early detection and control of hallucinations and delirium are important, as delirium may be reversible; therefore, it should be treated as soon as possible (Lawlor & Bush, 2015).

Summary

Delirium in palliative care patients may go unrecognized or even misdiagnosed in all palliative care settings. Nurses must take a good history, be observant, and screen palliative care patients for delirium. Early recognition and treatment (pharmacologic and nonpharmacologic) are important as 50% of cases may be reversible. Individualized goals of care aid in preventing and managing delirium. Care and treatment should be evaluated on an ongoing basis and changed as needed to provide comfort and symptom management (Grassi & Riba, 2014).

American Psychiatric Association. (2013). *Diagnostic and statistical manual of mental disorders* (5th ed.). Arlington, VA: American Psychiatric Publishing.

Bush, S. H., Pereira, J. L., Currow, D. C., Rabheru, K., Wright, D. K., Agar, M., . . . Lawlor, P. W. (2014). Treating an established episode of delirium in palliative care: Expert opinion and review of the current evidence base with recommendations for future development. *Journal of Pain and Symptom Management, 48*(2), 231–248. doi:10.1016/j.jpainsymman.2013.07.018

Cohen, C. L. (2015). Refectory delirium in a hospice patient. *Journal of Hospice & Palliative Nursing, 17*(2), 98–201. doi:10.1097/NJH.0000000000000112

Finucane, A. M., Lugton, J., Kennedy, C., & Spiller, J. A. (2016). The experiences of caregivers of patients with delirium, and their role in its management in palliative care settings: An integrative literature review. *Psycho-Oncology* 26(3), 291–300. doi:10.1002/pon.4140

Grassi, L., Caraceni, A., Mitchell, A. J., Nanni, M. G., Berardi, M. A., Caruso, R., & Riba, M. (2015). Management of delirium in palliative care: A review. *Current Psychiatry Rep*, 17(3), 1–9. doi:10.1007/s11920-015-0550-8

Grassi, L., & Riba, M. (2014). *Psychopharmacology in oncology and palliative care: A practical manual.* New York, NY: Springer Publishing.

Hey, J., Hosker, C., Ward., J., Kite, K., & Speechley, H. (2015). Delirium in palliative care: Detection, documentation, and management in the setting. *Palliative and Supportive Care*, 13(6), 1541–1545. doi:10.1017/S1478951513000813

Hosie, A., Davidson, P. M., Sanderson, C. R., & Phillips, J. (2012). Delirium prevalence, incidence, and implications for screening in specialist palliative care inpatients settings: A systematic review. *Palliative Medicine*, 27(6), 486–498. doi:10.1177/02692163124557214

Lawlor, P. G., & Bush, S. H. (2015). Delirium in patients with cancer: Assessment, impact, mechanisms, and management. *Clinical Oncology*, 12, 77–92. doi:10.1038/nrclinonc.2014.147

Moens, K., Higginson, I. J., & Harding, R. (2014). Are there differences in the prevalence of palliative care-related problems in people living with advanced cancer and eight non-cancer conditions? A systematic review. *Journal of Pain and Symptom Management*, 48(4), 660–677. doi:10.1016/j.painsymman.2013.11.009

PDQ Supportive and Palliative Care Editorial Board. (2016). *PDQ delirium.* Bethesda, MD: National Cancer Institute. Retrieved from http://www.cancer.gov/about-cancer/treatment/side-effects/memory/delirium-hp-pdq

■ DIARRHEA

Sheila Blank

Overview

Diarrhea is a worldwide problem, and, in acute cases, it is considered one of the top five leading causes of death (Chai, Meier, Morris, & Goldhirsch, 2014). Children, the elderly, and immunocompromised patients are at an increased risk of death from the condition. The major causes of diarrhea include ingestion of contaminated food and water, allergies, medications, bacterial or parasitic infection, and stress. For patients dealing with advanced illness, diarrhea causes social embarrassment and isolation and increases caregiver burden (Chai et al., 2014). Supportive nursing care is vital to managing the symptoms of diarrhea, preventing further complications, and promoting a good quality of life.

Background

The definition of diarrhea involves two elements: frequency and consistency. Both components need to be present to diagnose diarrhea. By contrast, pseudo-diarrhea (or hyperdefecation) is the presence of frequent stool but with normal consistency. Diarrhea can be simply defined as a high frequency (more than four times in 1 day) of loose stool. Chronic diarrhea describes a pattern of loose stools occurring for 3 to 4 weeks, or persistent loose stools at least three times daily (Chai et al., 2014; Schiller, Pardi, & Sellin, 2017).

Diarrhea is one of the leading causes of death in the world in elderly people. Death from diarrhea occurs most commonly as a result of dehydration and electrolyte imbalance. It can be caused by a number of factors, including stress, anxiety, depression, and hypochondriasis. A life-changing event, for example, the death of a loved one, divorce, or poor health prognosis, can lead to short-term diarrhea because of an increased stress level to the body (Camilleri, Sellin, & Barrett, 2017). Diarrhea in the elderly is most commonly caused by impaired absorption, with poorly absorbed carbohydrates often a contributing factor. Another cause of diarrhea is overactive motility in the gastrointestinal tract. Conversely, diarrhea can also be caused by slow motility in the gastrointestinal tract, which leads to bacterial growth, causing infection (Camilleri et al., 2017).

Many medications result ingastrointestinal upset, including diarrhea; more than 700 medications are associated with the condition (Schiller et al., 2017). Laxative abuse in the elderly may also contribute to frequent loose stools. Diarrhea is prevalent in patients undergoing radiation therapy for malignancy. Gastrointestinal surgeries can also result in postsurgical diarrhea, and constipation can produce frequent loose stool leakage around the hard stool—known as *overflow diarrhea* (Schiller et al., 2017).

In palliative care patients, diarrhea may be caused by partial intestinal obstruction, pancreatic insufficiency, fecal impaction, *Clostridium difficile* infection, HIV infection, radiation enteritis, and chemotherapeutic agents (Alderman, 2015). In advanced cancer, the incidence of diarrhea may be as high as 60% (Alderman, 2015).

Clinical Aspects

ASSESSMENT

The diagnosis of diarrhea focuses on the symptoms experienced, patient history, and serology. A complete patient history is essential when diagnosing diarrhea (Camilleri et al., 2017). The history should include detailed information on recent travels, current medications, daily stress level, pain or injuries, and allergies. Any history of inflammatory bowel disease, irritable bowel syndrome (IBS), or other gastrointestinal diseases should be noted. A complete diet history may reveal a relationship between certain foods and diarrhea. A complete blood count can point to infection as a cause. A stool sample may be ordered to check for the presence of *Clostridium difficile* or other infectious agents. Any fever or blood in the stool should warrant a prompt investigation. Medical imaging may also detect inflammation, pancreatitis, diverticulitis, or anatomical defects that could be the cause of diarrhea (Schiller et al., 2017). A colonoscopy may reveal useful information; however, the benefit versus burden of the procedure must be considered in palliative care patients before proceeding.

NURSING INTERVENTIONS, MANAGEMENT, AND IMPLICATIONS

As electrolyte imbalance and dehydration are common problems associated with diarrhea, primary treatment involves the replacement of lost electrolytes before further complications develop. Passive or oral rehydration therapy (ORT) is indicated to replace lost electrolytes and is often initiated in children with diarrhea. This solution can be easily made using water, salt, and glucose in proper proportions. The use of ORT in early diarrhea may help prevent hospitalization (Chai et al., 2014; Schiller et al., 2017). Other treatments include dietary changes and medications, both over-the-counter and prescription. Dietary modifications are used to remove foods that may cause diarrhea. Counseling the patient to avoid sugar alcohols (mannitol, sorbitol, xylitol, maltitol, and erythritol) found in some sugar-free candy and gums, lactose in dairy, and caffeine may help. Patients should also reduce intake of fatty, fried, and gas-producing foods like beans and cabbage (Soleimani, Foroozanfard,& Tamadon, 2017). Over-the-counter medications that may help decrease the occurrence of diarrhea include bismuth subsalicylate, oral calcium, and probiotics to supplement the body's natural bacteria. Dietary fiber and bulking agents like Metamucil and Benefiber are commonly used for people experiencing small-volume diarrhea (Lacy & Moreau, 2016).

When nonpharmacological and over-the-counter remedies do not curb diarrhea, prescription medications are the subsequent alternative. Providers may order anticholinergic agents, diphenoxylate, amitriptyline, or antispasmodics to slow gastrointestinal motility to control diarrhea (Soleimani et al., 2017). Loperamide works directly in the intestine to decrease stool frequency and increase the stool consistency. It is usually administered 30 minutes before meals, and its normal dose is 2 to 4 mg given by mouth (Lacy & Moreau, 2016). Clonidine in small doses (0.1 mg twice daily) can be administered to help with fluid and electrolyte absorption (Soleimani et al., 2017). In 2015, the Food and Drug Administration (FDA) approved eluxadoline (Viberzi), a mu-receptor opioid agonist for use in patients with IBS with diarrhea (IBS-D; Lacy & Moreau, 2016). Aspirin and cholestyramine can reduce enteritis associated with radiation. Mesalamine is frequently prescribed for inflammatory bowel disease (Alderman, 2015). Overall, treatments are aimed at eliminating the cause of diarrhea and preventing further complications.

OUTCOMES

Diarrhea is one of the most common illnesses seen in individuals across the life span. An individual's quality of life is adversely affected, as bathroom access and availability control the individual's daily schedule. Diarrhea can also lead to anxiety, social isolation, shame, and relationship difficulties (Lacy & Moreau, 2016). Affected individuals often experience frustration and feelings of abandonment because of difficulties in determining an underlying cause and initiation of effective treatment. Patient outcomes can be improved through the development of trusting relationships with nurses and other members of the health care team.

Summary

Nursing care for patients who are experiencing acute or chronic diarrhea must include promoting comfort, privacy, and evidence-based interventions. Support must also be offered to caregivers of palliative care patients through providing resources, education, and compassionate care.

Alderman, J. (2015). Diarrhea in palliative care [Fast Facts and Concepts #96]. Retrieved from https://www.mypc now.org/blank-reuft

Camilleri, M., Sellin, J. H., Barrett, K. E. (2017). Pathophysiology, evaluation, and management of chronic watery diarrhea. *Gastroenterology, 152*(3), 515–532.

Chai, E., Meier, D., Morris, J., & Goldhirsch, S. (2014). *Geriatric palliative care: A practical guide for clinicians.* New York, NY: Oxford University Press.

Lacy, B. E., & Moreau, J. C. (2016). Diarrhea-predominant irritable bowel syndrome: Diagnosis, etiology, and new treatment considerations. *Journal of the American Association of Nurse Practitioners, 28,* 393–404.

Schiller, L. R., Pardi, D. S., & Sellin, J. H. (2017). Chronic diarrhea: Diagnosis and management. *Clinical Gastroenterology and Hepatology, 15,* 182–193.

Soleimani, A., Foroozanfard, F., & Tamadon, M. R. (2017). Evaluation of water and electrolytes disorders in severe acute diarrhea patients treated by WHO protocol in eight large hospitals in Tehran: A nephrology viewpoint. *Journal of Renal Injury Prevention, 6*(2), 109–112. doi:10.15171/jrip.2017.21

■ DYSPHAGIA

Marianna K. Sunderlin

Overview

Dysphagia is an impaired swallow, or the inability to protect the airway during swallowing, either because of a mechanical obstruction or neurological disorder. An impaired swallow increases the risk of aspiration during eating and drinking and can lead to pneumonia and death. Diagnosis is made via a swallow evaluation, which can be done at the bedside by a registered nurse or speech therapist (Weinhardt et al., 2008), or by a video fluoroscopic swallow study. Often the treatment of choice is to provide food, fluids, and medications via a nasogastric tube (NG) for short-term therapy, or by percutaneous endoscopic gastrostomy tube (PEG) for continued therapy. Patients and families who choose palliative care over aggressive treatment may continue oral feeding for enjoyment despite the risk of aspiration or decide to forego artificial nutrition and hydration completely.

Background

Dysphagia is a common sequela of stroke, which is recognized as a leading cause of disability worldwide (Mahoney, Rowat, Macmillan, & Dennis, 2015). Swallowing difficulties are also commonly present in cancers of the head or neck, neurological diseases, such as amyotrophic lateral sclerosis, and dementia. Aspiration pneumonia is often the cause of death in the late stages of dementia regardless of the particular type (Schwartz et al., 2014). The signs of impaired swallowing include coughing with food or fluids, choking, wet speech following fluids, or identified aspiration pneumonia. In a systematic review of published research regarding PEG placement, findings were consistent that 1-year mortality was 50% or more in patients with dementia, and higher for those aged 80 years and older. There was no evidence of an increased survival time for those who underwent PEG placement (Goldberg & Altman, 2014). It should be understood that late-stage dementia is considered a terminal illness, and remains without a cure at this time.

Clinical Aspects

ASSESSMENT

Swallowing ability should be assessed in all patients with a new diagnosis of stroke or after a head or neck surgery before the initiation of fluids or solid foods; this may be performed either by a speech pathologist or a nurse trained in dysphagia assessment. A bedside swallow evaluation is inexpensive, 90% accurate for determining dysphagia and aspiration risk, and able to be performed without delay. In all cases, it is necessary that the patient is alert enough to cooperate with instruction and has an intact gag reflex. With the patient sitting in the high Fowler's position and the head midline, small amounts (3–10 mL) of water are given. The nurse evaluates whether there is a delay in the swallow or choking/coughing during or immediately after a swallow. Evaluation of voice quality for wetness or a noted decrease in pulse oximetry readings immediately after swallow increases the accuracy of the test (Festic et al., 2016). If the results are negative, this can be repeated with a small amount of pudding to further evaluate feeding safety. The results can be confirmed by video fluoroscopy swallow evaluation if needed.

NURSING INTERVENTIONS, MANAGEMENT, AND IMPLICATIONS

If the patient is unable to swallow without difficulty or aspiration, patients or their surrogate decision makers need to have the benefits and burdens of treatment options explained in plain language; this will promote a patient-centered approach to decision making. In addition, prognosis should be discussed related to underlying disease progression. Placement of a PEG tube should not be a rushed decision, especially if the underlying cause of dysphagia is related to a terminal disease. Although survival requires adequate nutritional intake, studies demonstrate that artificial feeding does not guarantee survival. Mahoney et al. (2015) note that tube feeding offers little in survival and may result in physical discomfort, distress, and use of restraints to prevent dislodgment. Often people who choose to proceed with PEG placement die in 30 days of insertion despite enhanced nutrition efforts. An Aspen report (Schwartz et al., 2014) revealed that PEG placement did not decrease decubitus ulcer development, disease progression, or aspiration risk. It is often the palliative care nurse who discusses the benefits of continued feeding in the face of life-limiting illness, as well as the burden that continued feeding places on the patient. This conversation must be conducted with an understanding that feeding is tied to culture, as well as positive social rituals. The nurse employing palliative care principles provides clear information regarding artificial nutrition to aid the patient and family in determining the goals of care (San Luis, Staff, Fortunato, & McCullough, 2013).

In some cases, oral feeding can continue with diet modifications; use of thickened liquids and chopped or pureed solids may enable a controlled swallow without aspiration. Speech therapists can teach exercises of chin tuck during the swallow, attention to swallowing, supraglottic swallow, and proper positioning, which may provide some benefit. The family should be included in any feeding instruction session. Thickeners for food include xanthan gum or cornstarch, which provide nutrition without changing the taste of the food. There are commercially prepared prethickened food items that are readily available in grocery or drug stores (Samargia, 2016).

Ullrich and Crichton (2015) discuss the social value of eating and its loss when elders are placed on dysphagia diets. This usually occurs with little communication or buy-in from the patient, who is then expected to be compliant with meals that offer little in taste and cultural acceptability. Patients report that modified diets lead to eating "out of necessity and hunger," without pleasure (Ullrich & Crichton, 2015). The authors suggest support for a patient-directed approach to care in which communication precedes a change in diet, and focuses on choice rather than authoritarian talk of what the patient must do to avoid aspiration, illness, and death.

Medication administration for patients who have dysphagia requires altering the route or the drug formulation. If the patient has a PEG or NG tube, then medications can be given via this route in liquid form, or by crushing oral medications and mixing them in solution with water. Check pharmacy recommendations to determine whether pills can be crushed before opening the capsules. Giving one medication at a time with a 10-mL water flush before and after can be time-consuming, but is likely to prevent clogging of the feeding tube. If the patient is receiving an oral diet with a modified texture, small pills can be given one at a time in a pudding or applesauce base. Larger pills can be halved if scored. If crushing the medication is necessary, it should be well mixed with, rather than sprinkled on top of, a food item (Bennett, 2013). In palliative care situations medications for symptom management can be administered via drops placed under the tongue, or by subcutaneous routes.

For dysphagia related to tumor obstruction, the current focus of medical research has been on the use of stents in the esophagus to treat dysphagia related to head and neck malignancies (Mezes et al., 2014). Radiation is also used for palliative reduction of tumor burden in neck cancer with a noted increase in comfort. Although guided swallowing exercises are thought to have some benefit following radiation treatment of neck cancer, studies show that patients tend to discontinue exercises because of fatigue and benefits were minimal (Mortensen et al., 2015). Electrical stimulation has shown promise in improving swallow in stroke patients, with a noted decrease in aspiration by fluoroscopy (Suntrup et al., 2015). Research continues using retroesophageal hypopharyngeal suction to prevent aspiration but is not currently available as a treatment (Belafsky, Mehdizadeh, Ledgerwood, & Kuhn, 2015).

OUTCOMES

The nurse supports the patient by providing frequent mouth care, which eases the discomfort caused by a dry mouth. Commercial products are available that simulate saliva that can relieve dry mouth and lessen the frequency of sores of the mouth and lips because of of dryness. A lip balm should be kept at the bedside for use as well. Secretions in the mouth can be controlled with the use of hyoscine transdermal patch or atropine drops placed under the tongue. In the dying patient, continued feeding either orally or via tube feed may cause abdominal pain, bloating, nausea, or constipation as peristalsis slows. As a result of the underlying physiological changes in terminal illness, it is unlikely that the dying patient experiences hunger; conveying this information to families promotes understanding and helps allay concerns regarding "starving" a patient to death.

Summary

Artificial feeding and hydration can prolong suffering in a terminal illness. The occurrence of dysphagia is a predictor of mortality in many cases. Research does not support artificial feeding in the face of terminal illness, as it often leads to discomfort and does not slow disease progression. Decisions about feeding or not feeding can cause feelings of helplessness, anger, or guilt on the part of family decision makers. The nurse's provision of education and support is the key to informed, compassionate, care for the patient and family at the end of life.

Belafsky, P., Mehdizadeh, O. B., Ledgerwood, L., & Kuhn, M. (2015). Evaluation of hypopharyngeal suction to eliminate aspiration: The retro esophageal suction (REScue) catheter. *Dysphagia, 30*, 74–79.

Bennett, B. (2013). Medication management in patients with dysphagia: A service evaluation. *Nursing Standard, 27*(41), 41–48.

Festic, E., Soto, J., Pitre, L., Leveton, M., Ramsey, D., Freeman, W., . . . Lee, A. (2016). Novel bedside phonetic evaluation to identify dysphagia and aspiration risk. *Chest, 149*(3), 649–659.

Goldberg, L., & Altman, K. (2014). The role of gastrostomy tube placement in advanced dementia with dysphagia: A critical review. *Clinical Interventions in Aging, 9*, 1733–1739.

Mahoney, C., Rowat, A., Macmillan, M., & Dennis, M. (2015). Nasogastric feeding for stroke patients: Practice and education. *British Journal of Nursing, 24*(6), 319–325.

Mezes, P., Krokidis, M., Katsanos, K., Spiliopoulos, S., Sabharwal, T., & Adam, A. (2014). Palliation of esophageal cancer with a double-layered covered nitinol stent: Long-term outcomes and predictors of stent migration and patient survival. *Cardiovascular Interventional Radiology, 37*, 1444–1449.

Mortensen, H. R., Jensen, K., Aksglaede, K., Lambertsen, K., Eriksen, E., & Grau, C. (2015). Prophylactic swallowing exercises in head and neck cancer radiotherapy. *Dysphagia, 30*, 304–314.

San Luis, C., Staff, I., Fortunato, G., & McCullough, L. (2013). Dysphagia as a predictor of outcome and transition to palliative care among middle cerebral artery ischemic stroke patients. *BMC Palliative Care, 12*(21), 1–7.

Samargia, S. (2016). Clinical nutrition: Improve compliance in dysphagia patients. *Todays Dietitian, 18*(4), 12.

Schwartz, D. B., Barrocas, A., Wesley, J. R., Kliger G., Pontes-Arruda, A., Marquez, H. A., . . . DiTucci, A. (2014). Gastrostomy tube placement in patients with advanced dementia or near end of life. *Nutrition in Clinical Practice, 29*(6), 829–840.

Suntrup, S., Marian, T., Schroder, J., Suttrup, I., Muhle, P., Olenberg, S., ... Dziewas, R. (2015). Electrical pharyngeal stimulation for dysphagia treatment in tracheotomized stroke patients: a randomized control trial. *Intensive Care Medicine, 41*, 1629–1637.

Ullrich, S., & Crichton, J. (2015). Older people with dysphagia: Transitioning to texture-modified food. *British Journal of Nursing, 24*(13), 686–692.

Weinhardt, J., Hazelett, S., Barrett, D., Lada, R., Enos, T., & Keleman R. (2008). Accuracy of a bedside dysphagia screening: A comparison of registered nurses and speech therapists. *Rehabilitation Nursing, 33*(6), 247–252.

■ DYSPNEA

Katharine K. Cirino

Overview

Dyspnea, or breathlessness as it is sometimes called, has been defined by the American Thoracic Society as "a subjective experience of breathing discomfort that consists of qualitatively distinct sensations that vary in intensity. The experience derives from the interaction between multiple physiologic, psychological, social, and environmental factors, and may induce secondary physiologic and behavioral responses" (Myers & Dudgeon, 2016, p. 172).

A commonly reported symptom in advanced illness, it is often accompanied by anxiety and necessitates compassionate and timely interventions on the part of the nurse. A knowledge of the precipitating cause can help the nurse determine which treatment(s) may be most beneficial.

Nursing care of patients with dyspnea involves a thorough physical examination, assessment, and employment of both pharmaceutical and nonpharmaceutical interventions.

Background

Dyspnea is a common symptom experienced at the end of life involving multiple diseases, including pulmonary and nonpulmonary malignancy, chronic obstructive pulmonary disease (COPD), congestive heart failure (CHF), and respiratory muscle weakness (Quill et al.,

2014). It is estimated that 60% to 90% of those individuals with advanced CHF and COPD experience shortness of breath. In the last 6 weeks of life, 70% of cancer patients report dyspnea as a burdensome symptom (Myers & Dudgeon, 2016).

Dyspnea can negatively impact a person's quality of life. Mobility is decreased, with even minimal exertion, leading to dyspnea. It also contributes to insufficient nutritional intake, as eating worsens the sensation of breathlessness. Functional status is impacted, and the ability to perform activities of daily living becomes increasingly difficult (Balkstra, 2015). Patients with dyspnea use descriptive terms such as "air hunger, choking, smothering, congestion, tightness, suffocation, and strangling" (Balkstra, 2015, p. 488). In the terminal stage of illness, a patient may have a fear of suffocation. Increased dyspneic episodes are associated with disease progression, and may signal that death is imminent. Dyspnea is considered a prognostic indicator of decreased life expectancy in patients with advanced cancer (Balkstra, 2015).

Dyspnea may be classified as acute, in the case of bronchospasm or pulmonary embolism, or chronic, which is seen in progressive conditions such as COPD or lung cancers (Balkstra, 2015). Acute symptoms typically occur over a period of hours to days, whereas chronic symptoms are experienced over a period of days to weeks (Myers & Dudgeon, 2016).

Physical, psychosocial, and spiritual factors all contribute to dyspnea. Physical factors include fluid overload, edema, tumor burden, weakness, injury, or obesity. Psychosocial and spiritual factors include fear of loss of function, fear of death, and fear of suffocation (Protus, Kimbrel, & Grauer, 2015). Known social and environmental factors associated with dyspnea include smoking, chemotherapy, radiation, and environmental exposures (Balkstra, 2015).

The pathophysiological alterations that cause dyspnea can be quite complex. For this section, mechanisms are classified as nonreversible and reversible. A palliative care provider is likely to treat patients who have nonreversible mechanisms of dyspnea. Broad categories of nonreversible sources of dyspnea include airway obstruction, cardiac etiologies, muscle weakness, and parenchymal failure (Protus et al., 2015). Heart failure, pulmonary hypertension, cachexia, degenerative neuromuscular conditions (amyotrophic lateral sclerosis, multiple sclerosis, myasthenia gravis), cystic fibrosis, pneumonia, or interstitial lung disease (pulmonary fibrosis) would be thus considered nonreversible disease processes.

Palliative care patients often experience potentially reversible causes of breathlessness, including anxiety or fear of suffocation, cough, respiratory secretions, pain, abdominal pressure, and pneumothorax or effusion (Protus et al., 2015). The other contributing conditions that may be reversible are infections (i.e., pneumonia), COPD exacerbation, ascites, rib pain (secondary to malignant fractures or metastasis), inflammation, dehydration, or even medications (Protus et al., 2015).

Clinical Aspects

ASSESSMENT

Dyspnea is a highly subjective experience that requires a careful and detailed assessment. Conducting a thorough medical history of the current illness is important. A patient's self-report of dyspnea is considered the gold standard in assessment (Myers & Dudgeon, 2016). Information should be obtained regarding timing or onset, the frequency of episodes, precipitating factors, associated symptoms, alleviating factors, physical examination, and any recent diagnostic testing (Balkstra, 2015).

The identification of precipitating factors can help pinpoint the underlying cause of dyspnea. For example, patients with COPD or CHF often experience dyspnea when lying supine because of redistribution of fluid. A patient with ascites from cirrhosis may feel dyspneic when sitting upright. Certain triggers, such as environmental allergens, smoke, or fumes, may cause dyspnea symptoms in a patient with COPD (Balkstra, 2015). Symptoms, such as chest pain, wheezing, increased cough, or change in color or amount of sputum, hemoptysis or even weight loss, can help clinicians identify the reason for the dyspnea. The causes may include myocardial infarction, pneumothorax, COPD, CHF, lung cancer, or pulmonary embolism, to name a few. It is also important to assess for any psychological symptoms such as anxiety (Balkstra, 2015).

The alleviating factors of dyspnea can include both pharmaceutical and nonpharmaceutical interventions. Pharmaceutical interventions are often based on the cause of dyspnea (i.e., bronchodilators for COPD). However, low-dose opioids are the preferred treatment for systemically treating dyspnea. These can be used in isolation or combined with other treatments for reversible etiologies and work by suppressing awareness of the sensation of dyspnea (Quill et al., 2014). Opioids also cause vasodilation in the lungs, which improves the ventilation/perfusion ratio (Protus et al., 2015).

Some clinicians may be hesitant to prescribe opioids for fear of respiratory depression. However, respiratory depression is uncommon in patients who do not have preexisting carbon dioxide retention. In these patients, it is best to start with small doses of opioids until the effects are known (Quill et al., 2014). Benzodiazepines may be useful if anxiety is a significant component of a patient's dyspnea. Oxygen can be used to help reverse hypoxemia and can help relieve dyspnea in certain conditions and is well tolerated (Protus et al., 2015).

Nonpharmacological treatments can also be helpful in the management of dyspnea. These interventions include sitting upright, using a fan or opening a window to promote air circulation, using a humidifier or air conditioner, avoiding strong odors or perfumes, and determining and avoiding triggers that exacerbate dyspnea (Quill et al., 2014). It is also helpful for patients to practice relaxation techniques such as quiet meditation; reduction in noise or stimuli helps to promote a calm environment. Relaxation can be promoted through the use of music, massage, pet therapy, or hydrotherapy (Protus et al., 2015).

A physical assessment can help provide information about the patient's condition as well as the possible treatment options. Balkstra (2015) recommends that physical inspection should include the "color of skin, nails, lips, nutritional state, sternal/spinal deformities, chest shape and movement, breathing rate rhythm (full minute), capillary refill, the presence/absence of nasal flaring, tracheal deviation, jugular venous distention, costal retractions, accessory muscle use, and clubbing" (p. 491).

Palpation should be performed to determine the presence of crepitus, masses, tenderness, and enlarged nodes. Chest percussion can yield evidence of tissue consolidation (dullness) or presence of air (tympany). Auscultation of the lungs determines whether there are any adventitious lung sounds, diminished breath sounds, or pleural friction rubs (Balkstra, 2015).

In advanced illness, decisions regarding whether to order diagnostic tests should be determined only after considering the patient's goals of care. Such diagnostic tests may include chest x-ray, EKG, pulmonary function tests, arterial blood gas analysis, complete blood count, or complete metabolic panel (Balkstra, 2015).

NURSING INTERVENTIONS, MANAGEMENT, AND IMPLICATIONS

Nursing interventions include conducting a thorough history and physical examination to determine the underlying etiology, interpretation of appropriate diagnostic tests, administration of opioids, and instruction of nonpharmacological techniques for the management of dyspnea.

OUTCOMES

Collaboration with the interdisciplinary team is essential. Patient-directed goals of care should be established when the patient is not experiencing extreme dyspnea, if possible. Finally, life-sustaining measures, such as intubation, should be specifically addressed and documented. Nursing measures should focus on promoting comfort and alleviating the symptoms of dyspnea whenever possible. A hospice referral may be appropriate if the causes are nonreversible or progressing. Patient and family education by the nurse is essential when difficult decisions are being contemplated.

Summary

Dyspnea is a very distressing symptom that is experienced by patients both during periods of exacerbation and at the end of life. Compassionate, evidence-based nursing assessment and care can lead to improvement of symptoms and overall increased quality of life.

Balkstra, C. (2015). Dyspnea. In M. Matzo & D. W. Sherman (Eds.), *Palliative care nursing: Quality care to the end of life* (pp. 487–507). New York, NY: Springer Publishing.

Myers, J., & Dudgeon, D. (2016). Breathlessness. In S. Yennurajalingam & E. Bruera (Eds.), *Oxford American handbook of hospice and palliative medicine and supportive care* (2nd ed., pp. 171–183). New York, NY: Oxford University Press.

Protus, B. M., Kimbrel, J. M., & Grauer, P. A. (2015). *Palliative care consultant: Guidelines for effective management of symptoms* (4th ed.). Mongomery, AL: Hospiscript Services.

Quill, T. E., Bower, K. A., Holloway, R. G., Shah, M. S., Caprio, T. V., Olden, A., & Storey Jr., C. P. (2014). *Primer of palliative care*. Chicago, IL: American Academy of Hospice and Palliative Medicine.

■ ETHICS

Laura Caramanica
Molly J. Jackson

Overview

The traditional and current practice of nursing is exemplified by the therapeutic role of the nurse who makes ethical decisions shaped by morals and values (Fry & Johnstone, 2008). In the palliative care patient, ethical issues often arise concerning advance directives, patient decision-making capacity, and the benefits versus burdens of instituting life-prolonging treatments (Griggins, 2017). The nurse should be knowledgeable and able to apply ethical principles to serve as an advocate for patients and their families in increasingly complex health care settings.

Background

Professional nurses face ethical decisions regularly in almost every practice setting. Today, nurses are aided in the process by two essential documents: *The International Code of Ethics for Nurses,* developed and adopted by the International Council of Nurses (ICN; 2012) and the American Nurses Association's (ANA) *Code of Ethics and Its Interpretative Statements* (ANA, 2015). These documents serve as ethical guides as nurses perform their fundamental responsibilities, which include the promotion of health, prevention of illness, restoration of health, and alleviation of suffering.

Four overarching principles in *The International Code of Ethics* serve to guide the practice of nursing. The first precept is that the nurse's primary professional responsibility is to the people who require nursing care (ICN, 2012). The three other focus areas delineate the nurse's responsibility to maintain competence by continuing to learn; the requirement that the nurse determine and implement acceptable standards of clinical nursing practice, management, research, and education; and that the nurse collaborates in respectful relationships with coworkers in nursing and other fields (ICN, 2012). Through discussion, reflection, and collaboration with peers in conducting their professional roles and responsibilities, nurses are aided by ICN's standards for ethical practice and decision making.

The ANA *Code of Ethics and Its Interpretative Statements* (ANA, 2015) serves as a foundation for nursing theory, practice, and expresses the values and obligations that shape, guide, and inform nursing as a profession. Originally penned in 1950, the nine provisions emphasize that the practice of nursing is to advocate for and to protect the right to health and safety for all people. Core tenets emphasize the primacy of the nurse–patient relationship, compassion, respect for all persons, patient safety, duty to self, social justice, health policy engagement, and a responsibility to impact global health (ANA, 2015).

For the nurse to practice in a way that demonstrates the full understanding and enactment of these two important codes, the nurse must first understand nursing's values and moral framework. *Value* is defined as a measure of worth held by an individual or a group, whereas morals are rules of conduct held by the culture of a group one belongs to. An individual or a group can change values or morals because of the lived experience, the influence of education, and change in social norms of the group culture. One way that nurses can understand their values and morals and how these influence their practice is by engaging in reflective practice.

Reflection is a process whereby an individual retrospectively thinks about a series of actions or decisions taken to determine what contributed to such decisions and actions, as well as their relative merit. Bulman and Schutz (2013) maintain that some describe the practice of reflection as a means to focus on "actions to be reflected on," others expand reflection to include the "feeling and emotions" exhibited while those actions were taken. The use of reflective practice can enable the nurse to understand one's values and morals.

Ethical dilemmas are described as situations occurring in which there are conflicting moral claims (Burkhardt & Nathaniel, 2014). Two opposing approaches may each have a sense of inherent "rightness," which creates uncertainty when selecting a single "best" option. In patients facing advanced illness, treatment choices may be debated as to their likely beneficial or nonbeneficial outcomes. Employing an ethical decision-making model in these situations can assist nurses. One method suggested by Daly (2017) is to identify the problem, differentiate facts from assumptions, list possible courses of action, consider bioethical principles in light of possible actions, choose a course of action, and evaluate the outcome.

Key bioethical principles that nurses should be familiar with include autonomy, beneficence, nonmaleficence, and justice (Butts & Rich, 2016; Marquis & Huston, 2015). Autonomy implies that self-determination and freedom of choice regarding treatment decisions are a primary right of the patient. It is considered a "negative right," such as the right to say *no* to unwanted interventions. Daly (2016) cautions, however, that the principle of autonomy does not compel health care providers to offer treatments that, in their professional judgment likely cause more harm than good. Beneficence implies that actions should be taken to promote good, although nonmaleficence is the ethical obligation to do no harm. Justice implies that general fairness and equality should extend to all people (Butts & Rich, 2016).

Clinical Aspects

ASSESSMENT

Nursing assessments related to ethics start with understanding a patient's medical history and current bothersome symptoms. In advanced illness, the nurse should ask the patient and family what their understanding of the illness is, and what treatments or plans are being considered. Does the patient have advance directives in place? Who are the decision makers, or who does the patient look to for guidance? What is most important to the patient and the family now? Spiritual and cultural values are also important to assess and note. Eliciting patient goals of care and careful documentation on the part of the nurse prove helpful if there is a change in patient condition and such communication is no longer possible.

NURSING INTERVENTIONS, MANAGEMENT, AND IMPLICATIONS

Ethical nursing practice should entail communicating with the interdisciplinary team, engaging in therapeutic communication with patient and family members, and advocating for the patient in all situations. If there is a conflict among the family members, or between the health care team and patient or family, an ethics consultation may be helpful in providing recommendations. The Joint Commission on the Accreditation of Healthcare Organizations (JCAHO) mandated in 1992 that all JCAHO-approved hospitals must have a process in place to address ethical concerns (Butts & Rich, 2016).

OUTCOMES

Nurses who care for patients with advanced illness are involved in increasingly challenging roles, serving as patient and family advocates. In the United States, technology advances mean that patients can live longer than before. As the nurse develops competency in recognizing and responding to ethical concerns raised in this environment, he or she can help facilitate patient-driven treatment plans that best reflect their values. The nurse serves as an important interdisciplinary team member in providing education and compassionate care.

Summary

Ethical complexities of advanced illness and at the end of life can be overwhelming to patients and families. In some settings and situations, patients may not have an identified proxy to speak for them at the end of life. When the nurse advocates for patients and families in establishing and honoring goals of care or in voicing concern about potentially nonbeneficial treatments or procedures, suffering can be reduced, and a peaceful end of life facilitated.

American Nurses Association. (2015). *Code of ethics for nurses with interpretive statements*. Silver Spring, MD: Author.

Bulman, C., & Schulz, S. (2013). *Reflective practice in nursing* (5th ed.). Oxford, UK: Blackwell.

Burkhardt, M. A., & Nathaniel, A. K. (2014) *Ethics & issues in contemporary nursing* (4th ed.). Clifton Park, NY: Cengage.

Butts, J. B., & Rich, K. L. (2016). *Nursing ethics: Across the curriculum and into practice* (4th ed.). Burlington, Ontario, Canada: Jones & Bartlett.

Fry, S., & Johnstone, M. (2008). *Ethics in nursing practice: A guide to ethical decision making* (3rd ed.). Oxford UK: Wiley-Blackwell.

Griggins, C. (2017). Lecture: Common ethical dilemmas at the end of life [PowerPoint slides]. Retrieved from https://blackboard.case.edu/webapps/blackboard/content/listContentEditable.jsp?content_id=_1452897_1&course_id=_85284_1&mode=reset

International Council of Nurses. (2012). *The ICN code of ethics for nurses*. Geneva, Switzerland: Author.

Marquis, B. L., & Huston, C. J. (2015). *Leadership roles and management functions in nursing: Theory and application*. Philadelphia, PA: Wolters Kluwer.

■ GRIEF AND BEREAVEMENT

Kathleen Leask Capitulo

Overview

Grief is a universal experience after a loss. As people journey through life, there are many loss experiences, the loss of a job, home, marriage, pet, and loved ones, to name a few. Of these, the loss of a loved one is among the most painful, precipitating a myriad of physiological, psychological, and social responses. Grief is a healthy process that promotes healing by incorporating the loss into oneself. Bereavement is the experience of those who are grieving (Arnold, 1995). Expressions of grief are framed in culture, which guides mourning rituals. Grief work is the experience of bereavement. It includes the remembrance and attachment to the loved one throughout life, considered to be a healthy bereavement adaptation (Schuchter & Zisnook, 1999). To implement a plan of care for families experiencing grief, nurses should understand the normal grieving process as well as identify circumstances that may contribute to complicated grief.

Background

Freud was the first to describe the concept of grief as a normal process of mourning after suffering a loss, which eventually does enable the person to enjoy other things or people. Freud's concept of grief had three aspects. The first is survivor's grief, feelings of those left behind that can include guilt at experiencing happiness. The next is anniversary grief reactions, which is an expected exacerbation of grief on special days on which the deceased person is remembered, such as birthdays, death days, and holidays. A seminal study of survivor's grief by Lindemann (1944) identified survivor's grief as a syndrome resulting from a crisis or loss, and its attributes, including guilt, hostility, physical ailments, changes in behavior, and preoccupation with thoughts of the deceased.

The spectrum of what a person experiences in normal grief is very broad. Arnold (1995) described grief as a mosaic depicting feelings, including, shock, bewilderment, anger, disbelief, depression, and disrupted sleep. Freud (1917) described the grief that was excessive as pathological. Today, this grief is termed *complicated* and can manifest as an inability to function in daily life. The risk factors associated with complicated grief include a history of previous significant losses, maladaptive coping skills, concurrent stressors and burdens, and traumatic or unexpected death (Zhang, El-Jawahri, & Prigerson, 2009).

The death of a child or infant (born or unborn) is one of the most painful grief experiences. When a child dies, there are feelings of emptiness, guilt, loss of identity as a parent, accompanied by unbearable pain and suffering. Dias, Docherty, and Brandon (2017) studied bereaved parents and found that bereavement challenges included sadness and adaptation to the absence of the child and changed relationships with family, friends, and caregivers. They further identified that bereaved parents were at a risk of higher morbidity and mortality than those not bereaved, with contributing diagnoses, including hypertension, diabetes, cardiac diseases, and cancer. Milic et al. (2017) studied older adults experiencing complicated grief following the death of a spouse or child. They found that 15% of grievers experienced complicated grief. Those with both normal and complicated grief often reported sleep disturbances associated with depressive symptoms (Milic et al., 2017).

Children also experience grief but may express it differently, depending on the relationship and their developmental age. Preschool children think of death as temporary, as with cartoon characters who have died and quickly come back to life. As children age, they understand that death is permanent. Bereavement during childhood is very traumatic. Attributes of childhood grief include fear, anger, apathy, regression, difficulty sleeping, depression, and psychosomatic expressions (Lytje, 2017).

Anticipatory grief is a term used to describe the grief felt by a patient who has been diagnosed with an incurable or terminal illness (Chai, Meier, Morris, & Goldhirsch, 2014). In addition to sadness, depression, and guilt, some patients react to serious illness by withdrawing from loved ones. Conversely, some family members withdraw emotionally from the patient (Chai et al., 2014).

Clinical Aspects

ASSESSMENT

As a patient approaches the end of life, it is important for the nurse to address patient and family concerns related to the dying process. Observation of family dynamics, as well as verbal communication with all involved, can help determine readiness and preparation for death. An awareness of the risk factors predisposing loved ones to complicated grief should also be noted. Other interdisciplinary team members, for example, social workers or child-life specialists can assess and provide recommendations. It is important to ascertain the cultural practices and spiritual beliefs of the family to facilitate any rituals or support before and immediately following death. Ensuring that family cultural and religious rituals are observed validates the importance of the individual and conveys respect for the family.

NURSING INTERVENTIONS, MANAGEMENT, AND IMPLICATIONS

When a patient is actively dying, a calm and peaceful atmosphere should be maintained when possible, even in busy inpatient hospital units. Suggestions to facilitate a peaceful environment include placing a small lamp in the patient room, placing a symbol (such as a dove) on the door to signify that a patient is dying, requesting snacks and drinks for the family, and reminding staff to keep noise levels down.

Simply being present at the time of death and providing active listening are important nursing interventions. It is appropriate to ask family members whether they would like a nurse present with them at the time of death, or simply prefer to be together as a family. Some hospitals have rituals offered to families when a loved one dies. For example, in Veterans Affairs Medical Centers, when a military veteran who has died is transported off the nursing floor, an honorary tribute ("The Final Salute") is conducted. Staff stand at attention and salute or cover their hearts; a flag-like cloth covers the body while taps are played. Families and staff find this ritual comforting and respectful.

Notification of families not present at death is best done by a provider who has a relationship with the family. When preparing the deceased for viewing, tubes and medical equipment should be removed whenever possible. The body should be cleaned and covered with a gown and blanket before viewing, with the face and hands exposed to permit the family to touch them. Viewing should take place in a pleasant room, never in the morgue. In the case of babies and children, families should be given time to see, hold, touch, and photograph the child. Allowing the family to stay with the deceased, calling a chaplain or clergy if requested, and supporting them with kind and caring presence make the experience less painful.

In conversing with the newly bereaved, acknowledging the death validates the significance of the deceased. Simple phrases such as, "I'm so sorry Joe died" or "It was a privilege to care for Lois" are most appropriate. Trite statements should be avoided, for example, "It's better that she died, she was so sick." Although there may be some relief for a close family when they see an end to the suffering of their loved one, that statement connotes a meaning that the individual's life was not valued. Simply being with and listening is a gift, allowing the bereaved to vent if he or she desires (Capitulo, 2005).

OUTCOMES

The family should be provided with resources related to grief support. If a patient was enrolled in hospice before death, bereavement counseling is provided for up to a year following death. Names and contacts for grief counselors and psychologists should be provided when appropriate, especially if there is a concern for complicated grief.

Although recognizing that older bereaved loved ones may have no interest or background in the use of technology, newer expressions of grief support are available through the use of social media for those inclined. There are listservs and blogs in which the bereaved write about their feelings and receive support from around the world in a socially equalizing Internet culture. Facebook has also changed the way people communicate, grieve, and mourn. On notification of death,

an active page is converted by Facebook to a memorial page, where family and friends may continue to post messages to the site and tag photos of the deceased person. Willis and Ferrucci (2017) studied motivations for interacting with the deceased on Facebook. They found that people post on the deceased's site to get and give information. Some post the death to inform family and friends, whereas others inquire about what happened to the person. Facebook also provides a place to post messages to the deceased, for example, "I miss you." Social support and validation are perceived when others acknowledge the posting with a "like" or a comment. The researchers found that the posts were motivated by an emotional release to mourn publicly. Although traditional mourning in Western cultures has been short, social media links have significantly extended the period of public mourning.

Summary

Grief is an experience that no one chooses but that is inevitable. The nursing role in assessing, facilitating, and acknowledging expressions of grief and loss help lay a foundation for the bereaved to cope with the loss. The use of therapeutic communication and listening skills assists the bereaved to find meaning in the loss. Palliative care nurses can assist in this process through providing compassionate interventions based on knowledge of the grieving process.

Arnold, J. (1995). *A reconceptualization of the concept of grief for nursing: A philosophical analysis*. New York, NY: New York University.

Capitulo, K. (2005). Evidence for healing interventions with perinatal bereavement. *American Journal of Maternal Child Nursing, 30*(6), 389–396.

Chai, E., Meier, D., Morris, J., & Goldhirsch, S. (2014). *Geriatric palliative care: A practical guide for clinicians*. New York, NY: Oxford University Press.

Dias, N., Docherty, S., & Brandon, D. (2017). Parental bereavement: Looking beyond grief. *Journal of Death Studies, 41*(5), 318–327. doi:10.1080/07481187.2017.1279239

Freud, S. (1917). Mourning and melancholia. In J. Starcey (Ed. and Trans.), *Basic works of Sigmund Freud*. Franklin Center, PA: Franklin Library.

Lindemann, E. (1944). Symptomatology and management of acute grief. *American Journal of Psychiatry, 101*(September), 361–381.

Lytje, M. (2017). Towards a model of loss navigation in adolescence. *Journal of Death Studies, 41*(5), 291–302. doi:10.1080/07481187.2016.1276488

Milic, J., Perez, H. S., Zuurbier, L. A., Boelen, P. A., Rietjens, J. A., Hofman, A., & Tiemeier, H. (2017). The longitudinal and cross-sectional associations of grief and complicated grief with sleep quality in older adults. *Behavioral Sleep Medicine*, 1–12. doi:10.1080/15402002.2016 .1276016

Schuchter, S., & Zisnook, S. (1999). The course of normal grief. In M. Stroebe, W. Stroebe, & R. Hansson (Eds.), *Handbook of bereavement*. New York, NY: Cambridge University Press.

Willis, E., & Ferrucci, P. (2017). Mourning and grief on Facebook: An examination of motivations for interacting with the deceased. *Omega, Journal of Death and Dying*, 1–19. First Published January 11, 2017. doi:10.1177/ 0030222816688284

Zhang, B., El-Jawahri, A., & Prigerson, H. G. (2006). Update on bereavement research: Evidence-based guidelines for the diagnosis and treatment of complicated bereavement. *Journal of Palliative Medicine*, 9(5), 1188–1203.

■ MUCOSITIS

Petique Oeflein

Overview

Mucositis is the inflammation of the oral mucosa and presents as erythema and swollen gums, mouth ulcerations, and increased mucus. Mucositis occurs when the cells of the mucosal epithelial and subepithelial tissue are destroyed, leaving the mucosal lining exposed; ulceration and infection often develop as a result. (Majdaeen, Babaei, & Rahimi, 2015; Radvansky, Pace, & Siddiqui, 2013). When the immune system is compromised from disease or treatments, such as chemotherapy and radiation, quickly dividing epithelial cells in the oral mucosa are most susceptible to early injury. The oral mucosa is one of the most sensitive parts of the body and often breaks down first before traveling down the mucosal lining into the gastrointestinal tract. Mucositis often significantly impacts the affected individual's quality of life making it difficult to eat, increasing the person's susceptibility to infection, and causing nutritional deficiencies. Nursing care in this painful condition is focused on developing strategies to decrease oral discomfort and optimize nutritional intake.

Background

Development of mucositis depends on patient-associated factors and therapy regimens. Mucositis is commonly associated with neutropenic patients who are prone to developing a cellular injury. Other predisposing factors include age, body mass index, gender, alterations in saliva production, oral health, and mucosal trauma (Raber-Durlacher, Elad, & Barasch, 2010; Radvansky et al., 2013) that contribute to the development of mucositis in patients. Mucositis is a common adverse effect of high-dose chemotherapy (Salvador, Azusano, Wang, & Howell, 2012) and is seen virtually in all patients treated for head and neck cancer (Raber-Durlacker et al., 2010). More than 40% of all patients who receive chemotherapy develop mucositis (Raber-Durlacker et al., 2010), whereas more than half of the patients who receive radiotherapy of the abdomen or pelvis develop the condition (Radvansky et al., 2013). Severity depends on nutritional factors, class of chemotherapeutic agent, length, and the amount of radiation therapy. Symptoms often begin 2 to 3 weeks after the start of radiation therapy for the affected patients (Radvansky et al., 2013).

Clinical Aspects

ASSESSMENT

Assessment of the oral cavity is a key nursing intervention because it facilitates early detection of inflammation or breakdown. One common method of consistently assessing mucositis is by use of the World Health Organization (WHO) Oral Toxicity Scale (Gussgard, Hope, Jokstad, Tenenbaum, & Wood, 2014; Radvansky et al., 2013; Worthington et al., 2011). Another clinician-based scoring tool is the National Cancer Institute Common Terminology Criteria of for Adverse Events version 3 (NCI-CTCAE v.3). Both of these scoring tools grade oral mucosa findings. The Oral Toxicity Scale ranges oral assessment from no oral mucositis (grade 0) to severe mucositis (grades 3 and 4). The National Cancer Institute recommends using a visual analog scale ranging from 0 to 100 mm to assess erythema and ulcerations (Gussgard et al., 2014). The initial symptom of mucositis is pain and local redness (grade 1). Mucositis tends to be present in the mucosa of the cheek, tongue, or lips. Mucositis worsens as the mucosa becomes milky white and degrades into single erosions (grade 2) and eventually develops into massive ulcers (grades 3 and 4). As mucositis worsens, pain increases, which leads to difficulty in swallowing and subsequent poor nutrition and hydration (Pels, 2012).

Mucositis impacts nutritional status, making it hard for a patient to swallow and eat as the result of pain and open sores. Infection of the open sores also impacts the immunity of an already weakened patient. Therefore, preventing the mouth sores and protecting sores from infection is paramount. Radvansky et al. (2013) maintain that basic oral care is the key to reducing both pain and risk for infection. Worthington et al. (2011), and Salvadore et al. (2012), recommend treatment for mucositis, including cryotherapy in addition to oral care. Both of these treatments appear to reduce the severity of mucositis (Pels, 2012; Salvador et al., 2012).

Nursing interventions include keeping the oral cavity moist, brushing teeth and cleaning oral tissue to prevent decay and bacterial growth (Pels, 2012). Cryotherapy, or applying ice chips, alleviates symptoms, making it easier to improve nutrition and quality of life (Pels, 2012; Worthington et al., 2013). Additional treatment interventions used for mucositis include chlorhexidine, sucralfate, keratinocyte growth factor, antibiotic paste or lozenge, and benzydamine. In general, however, there is a lack of evidence that these agents are clinically beneficial (Radvansky et al., 2013).

NURSING INTERVENTIONS, MANAGEMENT, AND IMPLICATIONS

Providing comfort care to patients with mucositis can be a challenge. Managing pain is part of the palliative treatment plan for mucositis. Viscous lidocaine helps to numb the throat and mouth, aiding in managing pain. Promoting hydration to the mucous membranes provides comfort as well. Oral care using simple saline rinses hydrates the oral mucous membrane and aids in mucositis prevention and pain management (Majdaeen et al., 2015; Radvansky et al., 2013; Worthington et al., 2011). Additional compounded mouthwashes sometimes referred to as *magic mouthwash*, include diphenhydramine, milk of magnesia, aluminum hydroxide, nystatin, lidocaine, and occasionally corticosteroids (Radvansky et al., 2013). These mouthwashes do not have significant evidence proving their effectiveness; however, they continue to be recommended as an aid for decreasing discomfort (Radvansky et al., 2013; Worthington, et al., 2011).

OUTCOMES

The priority for treating mucositis is to support proper hydration and nourishment to prevent infection. Ensuring patient comfort and utilizing prevention strategies allow patients to continue to eat and hydrate without pain and discomfort while treating mucositis.

Summary

Patients with cancer who are undergoing chemotherapy and radiotherapy are at risk for developing gastrointestinal mucositis. The development of difficult, painful swallowing in the oral cavity can severely impact a patient's quality of life. Palliation of this symptom consists of oral care interventions that promote hydration and help prevent bacterial colonization of the mucosa.

Gussgard, A. M., Hope, A. J., Jokstad, A., Tenenbaum, H., & Wood, R. (2014). Assessment of cancer therapy-induced oral mucositis using a patient-reported oral mucositis experience questionnaire. *PLOS ONE, 9*(3), 1–9. doi:10.1371/journal.pone.0091733

Majdaeen, M., Babaei, M., & Rahimi, A. (2015). Sodium bicarbonate containing mouthwash for preventing radiotherapy-induced oral mucositis in patients with locally advanced head and neck cancer. *Reports of Radiotherapy and Oncology, 2*, 5–7. doi:10.17795/rro-3721

Pels, E. (2012). Oral mucositis in children suffering from acute lymphoblastic leukaemia. *Wspolczesna Onkolpgia (Contemporary Oncology), 16*(1), 12–15. doi:10.5114/wo.2012.27331

Raber-Durlacker, J. E., Elad, S., & Barasch, A. (2010). Oral Mucositis. *Oral Oncology, 46*, 452–456.

Radvansky L. J., Pace, M. B., & Siddiqui, A. (2013). Prevention and management of radiation-induced dermatitis, mucositis, and xerostomia. *American Journal of Health-System Pharmacists, 70*, 1025–1032.

Salvador, P., Azusano, C., Wang, L., & Howell, D. (2012). A pilot randomized controlled trial of an oral care intervention to reduce mucositis severity in stem cell transplant patients. *Journal of Pain and Symptom Management, 44*(1), 64–73.

Sonis, S. T., Elting, L. S., Keefe, D., Peterson, D. E., Schubert, M., Jensen-Hauer, M., . . . Rubenstein, E. B. (2004). Perspectives on cancer therapy-induced mucosal injury. *Cancer, 100*(9), 1995–2025.

Worthington, H. V., Clarkson, J. E., Furness, B. G., Glenny, A. M., Littlewood, A., McCabe, M. G., . . . Khalid, T. (2011). Interventions for preventing oral mucositis for patients with cancer receiving treatment. *Cochrane Database of Systematic Reviews, 2011*(4), 1–35. doi:10.1002/14651858

■ PERSISTENT PAIN

Brendon Bowers
Molly J. Jackson

Overview

Chronic or persistent pain is a condition that plagues nearly 100 million Americans (Institute of Medicine, 2011). Owing to the stigma attached to the term "chronic pain," newer recommendations suggest using "persistent pain" when describing this condition (American Geriatrics Society [AGS], 2009). Persistent pain is defined as pain that lasts for more than 3 months after the usual course of an acute illness or procedure (American Chronic Pain Association). It may or may not be attributed to an underlying disease process (AGS, 2009). This section discuss persistent pain in its many facets, treatment modalities for affected individuals, and nursing strategies to assist palliative care patients in coping and living with such pain.

Background

Persistent pain is a complex condition associated with many underlying factors, especially in older adults (AGS, 2009). Preexisting comorbid conditions, musculoskeletal conditions associated with aging, and acute illness all may contribute to persistent pain. Adverse complications often accompany the diagnosis, including depression, falls, reduced functional ability, decreased socialization, and sleep disturbances (Nicholas et al., 2013). Persistent pain is common in the elderly and is underreported and undertreated (AGS, 2009). In elderly patients with cancer, 80% experience pain either related to the illness itself or from the treatments initiated (AGS, 2009). In addition, persistent pain is reported as a long-term sequela of cancer-related treatment; chemotherapy-induced neuropathies are one example (AGS, 2009). In advanced illness, patients with end-stage HIV infection, Parkinson's disease, renal or hepatic failure, also report significant pain.

Persistent pain in some instances is associated with previous traumatic experiences, including sexual abuse and posttraumatic stress disorder (PTSD; Outcalt et al., 2015; Spiegel et al., 2016). Conversely, persistent pain that developed as a result of a traumatic injury may worsen PTSD (Spiegel et al., 2016). It is often reported in patients diagnosed with major depressive disorder as well (Outcalt et al., 2015).

The physiological mechanisms producing pain are complex, but in general, two main types of pain are described: nociceptive and neuropathic pain (Chai, Meier, Morris, & Goldhirsch, 2014). Nociceptive pain is created via transmission of pain signals along nerve fibers. It is subdivided into two types: somatic (musculoskeletal) and visceral pain, arising from the abdominal or thoracic region. The common conditions associated with somatic pain include acute injuries such as fractures, surgeries, and osteoarthritis (Chai et al., 2014). Visceral pain often arises from conditions that produce organ distension or inflammation; examples include bowel obstruction, pancreatitis, and renal colic (Chai et al., 2014).

Neuropathic pain originates from damage to or diseases affecting the peripheral or central nervous system. Patient descriptors of the pain include tingling, numbness, or electric shocks. Common etiologies include diabetic or chemotherapy-related neuropathies, poststroke pain, and postherpetic neuralgia (AGS, 2009; Chai et al., 2014).

Clinical Aspects

ASSESSMENT

Nursing assessment should begin with reviewing the medical and surgical history of the patient. Whenever possible, the patient's self-report of pain is most helpful. In older patients or the cognitively impaired, the family provide needed insight into behavioral aspects related to pain. The elements in a comprehensive pain assessment should include location, intensity, quality, onset, duration, pattern, exacerbating and alleviating factors, and impact on physical and social function (Chai et al., 2014). A cognitively impaired person may be able to point to a pain location despite being unable to report verbally. A complete medical history, including prescription and over-the-counter drugs should be obtained. A history of substance abuse or misuse should be documented (Chai et al., 2014).

The treatment options for persistent pain depend on the individual, the type of pain he or she is experiencing, and provider preference. Nonpharmacological treatments that may be helpful include physical exercise, acupuncture, hot and cold compresses, physical and occupational therapy, transcutaneous electrical nerve stimulation (TENS), and cognitive behavioral therapy (Chai et al., 2014).

The initial recommendations for pharmacological treatment of persistent pain include scheduled acetaminophen for mild pain, and nonsteroidal anti-inflammatory drugs (NSAIDs) for mild to moderate pain. Liver and renal function should be assessed before initiating a scheduled analgesic regimen. NSAIDs are not recommended long term in the elderly because of an increased risk of gastrointestinal bleeding, renal failure, and cardiovascular complications (AGS, 2009).

The other classes of nonopioids, which can be helpful, include antidepressants and antiseizure medications. Antidepressants can have a twofold effect through directly blocking pain receptors while also treating the depression frequently associated with the pain. Selective norepinephrine reuptake inhibitors such as duloxetine (Cymbalta) and venlafaxine (Effexor), may be efficacious. Antiseizure drugs, such as gabapentin, pregabalin, and carbamazepine, have been used effectively to decrease neuropathic pain. With both antidepressants and antiseizure therapy, dosing is started low and gradually titrated up, with careful attention paid to patient response and any adverse effects.

Opioid analgesics remain a good option for treating chronic pain. Drugs like morphine, oxycodone, fentanyl, hydromorphone, and others have some of the highest potentials for addiction when used long term, but may be used when combined with risk screening, monitoring, and documentation. If the prognosis is short, the benefits may outweigh the risks in initiating opioid therapy. Short-acting opioids should be prescribed for patients initially, and the patient or caregiver is instructed to record the number of doses along with pain intensity rating. Long-acting opioids may be appropriate to avoid peaks and valleys in pain intensity in advanced illness, and also decrease the pill burden. All patients on opioids should have a bowel regimen instituted at the start of the therapy.

OUTCOMES

Although the goal of assessing and managing pain is always to provide optimum comfort, it is often not possible to entirely relieve persistent pain at the end of life. Priority nursing problems include careful assessment of pain, reassessment after pharmacological and nonpharmacological therapies are initiated, maintaining patient safety and comfort, and providing emotional support to the patients. Caregiver support and education are essential as well.

Summary

Nurses play an important role in assessing, managing and advocating for the patient experiencing persistent pain in advanced illness. Compassionate nursing care is vital to help alleviate pain, lessen suffering, and promote a peaceful death while experiencing the best quality of life possible.

American Chronic Pain Association. (n.d.). Retrieved from https://theacpa.org/condition/Chronic-Pain

American Geriatrics Society. (2009). AGS panel on pharmcological management of persistent pain in older persons. *Journal of American Geriatrics Society, 57*(8), 1331–1346.

Chai, E., Meier, D., Morris, J., & Goldhirsch, S. (2014). *Geriatric palliative care: A practical guide for clinicians.* New York, NY: Oxford University Press.

Institute of Medicine Committee on Advancing Pain Research, Care and Education. (2011). *Relieving pain in America: A blueprint for transforming prevention, care, education, and research.* Washington, DC: National Academies Press.

Nicholas M. K., Asghari A., Blyth, F. M., Wood, B. M., Murray, R., McCabe, R., . . . Overton, S. (2013). Self-management intervention for chronic pain in older adults: A randomized controlled trial. *Pain, 154*(6), 824–835. doi:10.1016/j.pain.2013.02.009

Outcalt, S. D., Kroenke, K., Krebs, E. E., Chumbler, N. R., Wu, J., Yu, Z., & Bair, M. J. (2015). Chronic pain and comorbid mental health conditions: Independent associations of posttraumatic stress disorder and depression with pain, disability, and quality of life. *Journal of Behavioral Medicine, 38*(3), 535–543. doi:10.1007/s10865-015-9628-3

Spiegel, D., Shaukat, A., McCroskey, A., Chatterjee, T., Simmelink, D., Oldfield, E., . . . Raulli, O. (2016). Conceptualizing a subtype of patients with chronic pain: The necessity of obtaining a history of sexual abuse. *International Journal of Psychiatry in Medicine, 51*(1)84-103. doi:10.1177/0091217415621268

■ URINARY INCONTINENCE

Kathy J. Meyers
Molly J. Jackson

Overview

Urinary incontinence is common, distressing, and in many cases life altering for people who experience this condition. Palliative care consists of a multidisciplinary approach focused on the relief of symptoms; incontinence impacts human dignity and requires careful assessment and treatment. This entry address the clinical aspects of urinary incontinence, as well as the nursing implications for treatment in the palliative care patient.

Background

According to the National Hospice and Palliative Care Organization [NHPCO] (2015), there were approximately 1.6 to 1.7 million patients who received palliative care in the United States in 2014. Although cancer remains a primary palliative care diagnosis, in 2014 more than 63% had a noncancer diagnosis (NHPCO, 2015). Patients with cardiac disease, pulmonary disease, dementias, hepatic disease, stroke, renal disease, HIV, and neurological disorders each present with a multitude of symptoms. Urinary incontinence is prevalent in this population and requires careful management to maintain quality of life (Worldwide Palliative Care Alliance, 2014).

Incontinence is caused by an overactive bladder and affects approximately 33 million people in the United States, or an average of one in six adults (National Association for Continence [NAFC], 2015). According to the NAFC (2015), incontinence directly affects the individual through loss of confidence (54%), self-esteem (49%), and intimacy (45%). Furthermore, the overall quality of life is diminished in patients and their caregivers when dealing with urinary incontinence (Baker & Ward-Smith, 2011). Economically, care for incontinence is projected to exceed $82 million per year in the United States by the year 2020 (Coyne et al., 2014).

Physiologically, muscles inside the bladder along with spinal nerves work together to sense fullness in the bladder. As the bladder muscles contract, the nerve signal allows the sphincters to open and release urine to the ureters to be expelled. It is the combination of nerve signals from the spinal cord and brain, along with muscle contraction that allows for urination (Gray & Sims, 2015). Any process that interferes with nerve impulses to the bladder can result in incontinence, such as nerve trauma, spinal cord cancers, multiple sclerosis, and Parkinson's disease. Irritation of the bladder commonly occurs when constipation is present or when caffeine or alcohol is ingested, leading to bladder spasms and a sense of urgency. Cancers of the bladder, abdomen, or pelvis and treatments for such cancers can obstruct the flow of urine as well (Baker & Ward-Smith, 2011; American Society of Clinical Oncology, 2016).

The four major types of incontinence include stress, overflow, urge, and functional categories. Stress incontinence is most prevalent in women aged 30 years and older (45%), and is related to sphincter weakness; leakage of urine occurs when engaging in certain activities such as coughing, sneezing, and exercising. Urge incontinence is prevalent in older men (42%) and older women (31%) and is related to uninhibited muscle contractions creating a sensation of urinary urgency. Overflow incontinence is prevalent in men and women who have an overextended bladder or outflow obstruction that results in continual leakage because of muscle control loss. Functional incontinence is referred to as *leakage* because of environmental or physical inability to urinate (Khandelwal & Kistler, 2013).

Clinical Aspects

ASSESSMENT

Effective nursing care, grounded in the nursing process, begins with obtaining a comprehensive medical history and performing a careful assessment. Information should be gathered about the onset of symptoms (i.e., leakage, urgency), and history of abdominal or spinal traumas (including surgeries or diagnostic procedures). Any history of cancer (including treatments), and other comorbid conditions, such as diabetes, renal disease, cardiac disease, Alzheimer's dementia, and multiple sclerosis, should be noted. All prescribed and over-the-counter medications should be documented. Drugs, such as diuretics, are often implicated in incontinence. Laboratory and radiographic results along with postvoid residuals and voiding journal can further assist with the focused assessment (Gray & Sims, 2015; Khandelwal & Kistler, 2013).

The physical assessment should include a careful examination and documentation of the abdominal system (distention, bladder, or kidney pain on palpation), musculoskeletal system (presence of low back pain or decreased movement) and neurological system (paralysis, seizure activity, tremors, paresthesia, or changes in levels of consciousness). A physical examination that yields palpable bladder distention or results in bladder discomfort should lead to a laboratory urinalysis to determine the presence of an infectious agent. Other forms of noninvasive and invasive testing, such as CT, ultrasound, cystogram, and cystoscopy, may be necessary to determine the cause of incontinence (American Society of Clinical Oncology, 2016). Together, the focused interview, physical assessment, laboratory, and radiographic findings can confirm both the type and potential cause of the incontinence.

NURSING INTERVENTIONS, MANAGEMENT, AND IMPLICATIONS

Nursing care of the person with incontinence should focus on the reversal of the cause whenever possible.

Fluid volume restriction is a simple start, but caution is advised as this may lead to dehydration. Reduction or elimination of bladder irritants, such as caffeine and alcohol, may prove useful (Baker & Ward-Smith, 2011; Gray & Sims, 2015). Patient education regarding exercises to strengthen the pelvic floor muscles, such as Kegal exercises or biofeedback, can assist with stress leakage. Scheduled voiding may assist in bladder training and urine retention. Dietary changes to decrease bladder and bowel irritation and management of constipation through increased fiber intake and exercise are recommended (NAFC, 2015). In advanced illness, medications that contribute to incontinence should be reduced or discontinued whenever possible. If other measures are unsuccessful, diapers or barrier pads may be used. Careful attention to skin care is required to avoid irritation and prevent a breakdown in the presence of increased bacteria and moisture.

A catheterization is an invasive option that can be employed either short term to empty the bladder, or long term to assist with obstruction. Bladder retraining through the use of intermittent self-catheterization may help reduce incontinence related to nerve injury. However, catheterization is associated with urinary tract infection, renal calculi formation, inflammation, and ureteral trauma, and should not be routinely performed unless necessary. Medications are also widely employed, with anticholinergic drugs often prescribed as first-line agents. Such medications can cause dry mouth, constipation, urinary retention, blurred vision, tachycardia, and weakness. In addition, anticholinergics are linked to increased falls in the elderly. Surgical interventions may include the implantation of sacral nerve stimulators, cystoplasty, or bladder enlargement procedures.

OUTCOMES

Some types of incontinence may be able to be reversed. Noninvasive treatment recommendations, such as scheduled toileting, dietary modifications, pelvic floor exercises, and fluid management strategies, may lead to a decrease or reversal of incontinence. Medication regimens along with other noninvasive therapies can provide a complete respite. Invasive treatments, such as catheterization and surgery, may be required but can lead to complications such as infection. Until the cause of incontinence can be determined, use of incontinence pads or diapers are an option but also require patient education to maintain skin integrity.

In patients with advanced illness, bladder incontinence frequently develops owing to cognitive decline, fatigue, and weakness. Nursing interventions should promote patient privacy, respect, and comfort.

Summary

Urinary incontinence is a common symptom that is often associated with the aging process, as well as with underlying comorbid conditions. In some cases, incontinence can be corrected by determination of the cause and institution of evidence-based treatments. In palliative patients, the nurse's compassionate and knowledgeable care helps to ease the symptom burden and promote patient dignity.

American Society of Clinical Oncology. (2016). Urinary incontinence. Retrieved from http://www.cancer.net/navigating-cancer-care/side-effects/urinary-incontinence

Baker, B., & Ward-Smith, P. (2011). Urinary incontinence nursing considerations at the end of life. *Urologic Nursing*, 31(3), 169–172.

Coyne, K., Wein, A., Nicholson, S., Kvasz, M., Chen, C., & Milsom, I. (2014). Economic burden of urgency urinary incontinence in the United States: A systematic review. *Journal of Managed Care Pharmacy*, 20(2), 130–140.

Gray, M., & Sims, T. (2015). Urinary tract disorders. *Oxford textbook of palliative nursing* (5th ed., pp. 262–278). Madison, NY: Oxford University Press.

National Association for Continence. (n.d.). Retrieved from https://www.nafc.org/conditions

National Hospice and Palliative Care Organization. (2015). Facts and figures. Retrieved from http://www.nhpco.org/sites/default/files/public/Statistics_Research/2015_Facts_Figures.pdf

Worldwide Palliative Care Alliance. (2014). In S. R. Connor & M. C. S. Bermedo (Eds.), Global atlas of palliative care at the end of life. Retrieved from http://www.who.int/nmh/Global_Atlas_of_Palliative_Care.pdf

Pediatric Nursing

Pediatric nursing care is highly specialized and requires specific education, including knowledge of growth and development, anticipatory guidance, developmentally appropriate communication, and creating a relaxed atmosphere. Pediatric health care is delivered to children in a variety of settings, including inpatient units, outpatient clinics, home-health programs, and school settings. Family-centered care is the hallmark of pediatric nursing and the patient should be viewed as the whole family, not just the child.

Topics selected for this section are those illnesses that most commonly require hospitalization of the child. Each entry provides details for the professional nursing staff on the disease process, the required nursing interventions, and references to encourage the search for an in-depth understanding of the disease process. The entry on developmental communication presents the standard of care, which guides nurses in caring for the child and family during hospitalization and in the community care setting.

Regardless of the disease, every child and family deserves a nurse who understands and utilizes communication skills built upon the principles of growth and development. Our wish is that each entry educates, stimulates, and motivates pediatric nurses to provide safe, efficient, and comforting care.

- Acute Renal Failure *Christine Horvat Davey*
- Appendicitis *Kerry D. Christy*
- Asthma *Laurine Gajkowski*
- Autism Spectrum Disorder *Sheila Blank and Celeste M. Alfes*
- Bronchiolitis Respiratory Syncytial Virus *Shannon Courtney Wong*
- Cancers of Childhood *Breanne M. Roche*
- Cerebral Palsy *Rachael Weigand*
- Cystic Fibrosis *Karen Vosper*
- Developmentally Appropriate Communication *Nanci M. Berman*
- Diabetes *Julia E. Blanchette*
- Failure to Thrive *Mary Alice Dombrowski*
- Inflammatory Bowel Disease *Sharon Perry*
- Obesity *Rosanna P. Watowicz*
- Oral Health *Marguerite DiMarco*
- Orthopedics *Michelle Calabretta, Emily Canitia, and Michelle A. Janas*
- Seizure Disorder *Kathleen Maxwell*
- Sickle Cell Disease *Valerie Cachat*

■ ACUTE RENAL FAILURE

Christine Horvat Davey

Overview

Acute renal failure (ARF) also known as *acute kidney injury* is a reversible acute decline in renal function with rapid onset (Devarajan, 2017). The most extensively used and standardized definitions for pediatric ARF are pediatric RIFLE (pRIFLE; R for risk for renal dysfunction, I for injury to the kidney, F for failure of kidney function, L for loss of kidney function, and E for end-stage renal disease), Acute Kidney Injury Network (AKIN), and kidney disease improving global outcomes (KDIGO) classifications (Sutherland et al., 2015). ARF is marked by a decrease in glomerular filtration rate, an inability of the kidneys to regulate fluid and electrolyte homeostasis as well as an increase in serum creatinine and blood urea nitrogen levels (Andreoli, 2009). The exact incidence of pediatric ARF is unknown. Nursing care of pediatric patients

with ARF focuses on determination and treatment of the underlying cause of ARF along with early medical management.

Background

The incidence of ARF is rising in relation to increased use of advanced medical technology for children who are critically ill or experience chronic conditions (Devarajan, 2017). Worldwide, one in three children experience ARF during an occurrence of hospitalization (Susantitaphong et al., 2013). Pediatric ARF can arise from multiple causes with clinical manifestations that range from minimal elevation in serum creatinine to anuric renal failure (Devarajan, 2017).

The pathophysiology behind an acute kidney insult is classified into three phases, which include development, extension, and resolution phase. During the development phase, a kidney insult leads to injury and may be subclinical (Hayes, 2017). Repair processes commence during the extension phase. Adaptive repair results in correction of the renal structure without long-term consequence (Hayes, 2017). Maladaptive repair often results in change of renal structure and, in turn, reduced kidney function (Hayes, 2017). Net result of renal injury and repair are represented in the extension phase (Hayes, 2017). Overall, renal recovery results from adaptive repair, whereas progression leads to change in kidney function and/or structure that can be detected by histopathology, imaging studies, or biomarkers (Basile et al., 2016).

Diagnosis of ARF is based on characteristic signs and symptoms; edema, decreased urine output, hematuria, hypertension, and laboratory results. Diagnosis of ARF by laboratory results is based on serum creatinine levels. Normal serum creatinine level for an infant is 0.2 to 0.4 mg/dL, 18 to 35 µmol/L (Devarajan, 2017). Diagnostic use of serum creatinine levels can present issues. ARF serum creatinine is an insensitive and delayed measure of decreased kidney function as serum creatinine may not increase until a 50% or higher reduction in glomerular filtration rate is present (Andreoli, 2009; Devarajan, 2017). In addition, if dialysis is initiated as a treatment, serum creatinine levels cannot be measured accurately. An abnormal urinalysis can also indicate ARF. Although individuals with prerenal ARF may display a normal urinalysis, urinalysis is most often utilized to determine the underlying cause of ARF. Regardless of the limitations posed by serum creatinine levels in the diagnosis of ARF, it is presently the best laboratory test for diagnosis in pediatrics.

The risk of ARF is highest among children cared for in an intensive care unit (Devarajan, 2017). Pediatric patients requiring critical care or dialysis have the highest ARF mortality rates (Sutherland et al., 2015). Several key factors can contribute to ARF in pediatrics. These factors include: hypoxia, ischemia, acute injury, or illness. Nephrotoxic-induced ARF is often related to hospitalization as hospitalization poses increased risk for exposure to medications that are nephrotoxic (Sutherland et al., 2013). In addition to the environmental factors, there may be genetic risk factors for ARF. Several candidate polymorphisms have shown an association with ARF (Andreoli, 2009).

ARF causes can be classified in several ways. The most widely used mechanisms for classification are the three major categories based on anatomic location of the primary injury. The three major categories include: prerenal, intrinsic renal, and postrenal disease. Prerenal disease is caused by reduced renal perfusion due to hypovolemia (bleeding, gastrointestinal, urinary,

or cutaneous losses), or decline of effective circulation (septic shock, heart failure, or cirrhosis; Devarajan, 2017). Prerenal is considered the most common form of pediatric ARF. In prerenal, glomerular filtration rate is reduced, but renal tubular function remains intact in prerenal disease (Devarajan, 2017). Intrinsic renal or, intrarenal disease, is most commonly caused by sepsis, nephrotoxins, prolonged hypoperfusion, or severe glomerular diseases. Structural damage to the renal parenchyma occurs in intrinsic renal disease. Postrenal disease or obstructive ARF is most commonly a result of congenital or acquired anatomic obstructions of the lower urinary tract (Devarajan, 2017).

A less used approach to classify ARF is based on clinical setting or circumstance and urine output. Hospital-acquired ARF is often multifactorial and often associated with multiple organ failure (Devarajan, 2017). Hospital-acquired ARF greatly complicates clinical outcomes. Community-acquired ARF is often the result of a single primary insult, most often volume depletion, but is regularly reversible (Devarajan, 2017). Measurement of urine output can be used, but presence of normal urine output does not exclude ARF. The ability to classify the cause of ARF can lead to early and targeted medical interventions.

Clinical Aspects

ASSESSMENT

As soon as the diagnosis of ARF is suspected or determined, further assessment is dedicated to identifying the underlying cause. This evaluation includes an accurate record of an individual's physical assessment, medical history, and laboratory data. The physical assessment should focus on signs and symptoms related to alterations in renal function. These assessment findings include decreased or no urine output, edema, hematuria, and/or hypertension (Devarajan, 2017).

NURSING INTERVENTIONS, MANAGEMENT, AND IMPLICATIONS

Nursing responsibilities include accurate blood pressure measurement and assessment for edema or volume depletion, which is indicated by dry mucous membranes, decreased skin turgor, tachycardia, orthostatic falls in blood pressure, and decreased peripheral perfusion. Assessment of recent weight gain; signs of systemic disease such as rash or joint disease; palpation of enlarged kidneys, an indication of renal vein thrombosis, and an enlarged bladder, which may indicate urethral obstruction, are also important (Devarajan, 2017).

An accurate medical history is essential, as there is often a known etiologic factor that predisposes the child to ARF. These factors include heart failure, shock, or a preceding streptococcal infection seen in patients with poststreptococcal glomerulonephritis (Devarajan, 2017). Laboratory data to monitor when assessing for alterations in renal function include elevation of serum creatinine and\or blood urea nitrogen levels, abnormal urinalysis, hyperkalemia, hyponatremia, or less often hypernatremia, high anion gap (metabolic acidosis), hypocalcemia and\or hyperphosphatemia. Renal imaging can also be performed or, on rare occasions, a kidney biopsy may be conducted to determine the underlying cause. Utilization of an accurate physical assessment, medical history, and laboratory data can facilitate initiation of proper and timely nursing care that can positively impact patient outcomes.

Nursing care of pediatric patients with ARF should focus on treatment of ARF and prevention of long-term sequelae. Priority nursing care includes monitoring of vital signs, maintenance of proper blood pressure, accurate measurement of intake and output, maintenance of electrolyte and nutrition balance, and determination of the underlying cause of ARF. If necessary, initiation of hemodialysis, peritoneal dialysis, continuous renal reperfusion therapy (CRRT), monitoring of laboratory data, and psychological support for the family unit should be initiated.

OUTCOMES

Evidence-based nursing practice should focus on treatment of ARF and prevention of long-term sequelae. Early determination of ARF based on signs, symptoms, and laboratory data as well as prompt correction of the underlying cause facilitate positive outcomes. In addition to correction of the underlying cause of ARF, effective management of signs, symptoms, and treatment options, which can include hemodialysis, peritoneal dialysis, and CRRT, are required. Effective nursing care outcomes should result in correction of ARF without long-term sequelae (Hayes, 2017).

Summary

The incidence of pediatric ARF is expected to increase, and therefore, it is important to recognize the early signs and symptoms of the condition. Early detection

and medical management can facilitate positive outcomes and decreased incidence of long-term sequelae.

Andreoli, S. P. (2009). Acute kidney injury in children. *Pediatric Nephrology, 24*(2), 253–263. doi:10.1007/s00467-008-1074-9

Basile, D., Bonventre, J., Mehta, R., Nangau, M., Unwin, R., Rosner, M., & Ronco, C. (2016). Progression after AKI: Understanding maladaptive repair processes to predict and identify therapeutic treatments. *Journal of the American Society of Nephrology, 27*(3), 687–697. doi:10.1681/ASN.2015030309

Devarajan, P. (2017). Acute kidney injury in children: Clinical features, etiology, evaluation, and diagnosis. In T. Mattoo (Ed.), *UpToDate*. Retrieved from https://www.uptodate.com/contents/acute-kidney-injury-in-children-clinical-features-etiology-evaluation-and-diagnosis

Hayes, W. (2017). Stop adding insult to injury—identifying and managing risk factors for the progression of acute kidney injury in children. *Pediatric Nephrology, 32*(2), 1–9. doi:10.1007/s00467-017-3598-3

Susantitaphong, P., Cruz, D., Cerda, J., Abulfaraj, M., Alqahtani, F., Koulouridis, I., & Jaber, B. L. (2013). World incidence of AKI: A meta-analysis. *Clinical Journal of the American Society of Nephrology, 8*(9), 1482–1493. doi:10.2215/CJN.00710113

Sutherland, S., Byrnes, J., Kothari, M., Longhurst, C., Dutta, S., Garcia, P., & Goldstein, S. (2015). AKI in hospitalized children: Comparing the pRIFLE, AKIN, and KDIGO definitions. *Clinical Journal of the American Society of Nephrology, 10*(4), 554–561. doi:10.2215/CJN.01900214

Sutherland, S. M., Ji, J., Sheikhi, F. H., Widen, E., Tian, L., Alexander, S., & Xuefeng, L. (2013). AKI in hospitalized children: Epidemiology and clinical associations in a national cohort. *Clinical Journal of the American Society of Nephrology, 8*(10), 1661–1669. doi:10.2215/CJN.00270113

■ APPENDICITIS

Kerry D. Christy

Overview

Acute appendicitis is one of the primary causes of abdominal pain in children and a leading contributor to the emergency department visits worldwide. A thorough assessment and exam must be conducted to distinguish appendicitis from other diseases that could cause acute abdominal pain. Once identified, attentive monitoring for potential complications preoperatively and postoperatively will ensure patient safety.

Background

Butler (2015) defines "acute appendicitis" as the inflammation of the appendix, which is a blind-ending pouch that arises where the small and large intestine meet (cecum). Although appendicitis has been treated for more than 300 years, the cause is still not entirely known (Rentea, St. Peter, & Snyder, 2017). In most cases, it is presumed that luminal obstruction by stool may incite the process; alternatively, a neoplasm, parasite, or lymphocyte proliferation may induce the appendix to swell (Rentea et al., 2017). The obstruction leads to inflammation and decreased blood flow to the appendix with subsequent bacterial overgrowth (Brown, 2014). This progression generates an inflammatory exudate on the surface of the appendix, which locally irritates the perineum (peritonitis) causing symptoms classic to appendicitis (Butler, 2015). Appendicitis can be described in three categories: simple acute appendicitis, gangrenous appendicitis, or complicated perforated appendicitis. Acute appendicitis is the inflammation of the appendix, whereas gangrene suggests a microscopic perforation or discoloration of the appendix (Pennington & Burke, 2015). Appendiceal perforation is described by Butler (2015) as having generalized peritonitis and formation of an abscess or phlegmon.

The lifetime risk of getting appendicitis in the Western world is about 7% (Pennington & Burke, 2015). The U.S. incidence is one per 1,000 (Rentea et al., 2017), but geographical differences have been reported (Bhangu, Soreide, Di Saverio, Assarsson, & Drake, 2015). The incidence of acute appendicitis typically peaks in the summer months. It most often occurs between the ages of 10 and 19 years, and males have a slightly higher prevalence (Bhangu et al., 2015). It has been found that up to 40% of children who present with appendicitis have a perforated appendix (Tian, Heiss, Wulkan, & Raval, 2015). Children are often unable to specify their symptoms or location of pain when it occurs, delaying the evaluation and allowing time for perforation to occur. Fortunately, overall mortality with appendicitis is low in the United States and only slightly higher in low- and middle-income countries (Bhangu et al., 2015). The key to treating appendicitis is to have an accurate assessment and timely intervention. This is how nursing plays a large role in the management of appendicitis.

Clinical Aspects

ASSESSMENT

Nurses are most often the first line of evaluation both preoperatively and postoperatively, so knowing the pertinent symptoms, risk factors, and complications of appendicitis are key for a positive outcome. Beginning with a thorough primary assessment in triage and asking the relevant questions to both the patient and his or her caregiver leads to an accurate diagnosis. The assessment of symptoms, including timing and location, as well as nausea, vomiting, anorexia, diarrhea or constipation, fevers, chills, or sepsis is critical. A hallmark symptom of appendicitis is the gradual onset of diffuse abdominal pain most often starting around the umbilicus (Bishop & Carter, 2013). With time, often just a few hours, the diffused abdominal pain will worsen and localize to the right lower quadrant where the appendix is located. Any moving, walking, jumping, and even riding in the car may exacerbate the pain. Patients with acute appendicitis will be in pain, but they often do not appear ill, and the pain will not improve with time until perforation occurs. Following the perforation, peritonitis develops, and patients may become febrile, tachycardic, hypotensive, and septic (Brown, 2014).

A thorough assessment rules out other conditions that can mimic appendicitis. Make sure to assess any signs of a streptococcal infection as well as flank or urinary pain that could be caused by a urinary tract infection (Bishop & Carter, 2013). A primary indicator of appendicitis during physical examination is tenderness at McBurney's point—tenderness on the right side of the abdomen one third of the distance along a line between the superior iliac spine and umbilicus. Involuntary guarding is often associated with palpation of this area. Three other key findings that suggest peritoneal and pelvic irritation are a positive Rovsing sign, psoas sign, and obturator sign. All of these findings support a diagnosis that there is peritoneal and pelvic irritation, but do not definitively diagnose appendicitis.

Although physical findings can be helpful in pinpointing a diagnosis, laboratory tests as well as imaging will confirm appendicitis. A complete blood count (CBC) with differential and C-reactive protein (CRP) are most often drawn and an elevated white blood cell count with a left shift and elevated CRP are found to be associated with appendicitis (Bishop & Carter, 2013). These labs are also important for postoperative monitoring of perforated appendicitis and also for antibiotic management (Brown, 2014). Radiographic tests used to diagnose appendicitis include ultrasound and CT. Ultrasound, although useful, is often operator specific as well as limited by the location of the appendix (Bishop & Carter, 2013). A CT scan with intravenous and oral contrast is much more accurate and can identify the location of the appendix as well as findings of appendicitis such as inflammation, wall thickening, fat stranding, or abscess formation.

NURSING INTERVENTIONS, MANAGEMENT, AND IMPLICATIONS

Once a diagnosis of appendicitis has been made, there are four main nursing diagnoses that correlate with appendicitis that must be considered both pre- and postoperatively. Those are deficient fluid volume, acute pain, risk for infection, and deficient knowledge of the parent and/or patient. Preoperatively, these patients should have nothing by mouth (NPO) and be given intravenous (IV) fluids as they are frequently dehydrated. Resuscitation is vital prior to administration of anesthesia and can be given with a fluid bolus of an isotonic solution followed by the maintenance of IV fluids. If children do not have appendicitis, but rather have viral gastroenteritis, these fluids will often improve their symptoms and again help confirm a diagnosis (Bishop & Carter, 2013). Postoperatively, it is important to continue intravenous hydration while awaiting return of bowel function. Adequate hydration can be evaluated by monitoring urine output. If urine output is around 1 mL/kg/hr with a normal specific gravity, there is adequate hydration.

Administration of pain medication before definitive diagnosis will not completely mask the symptoms of appendicitis and, if a thorough exam is done, the diagnosis can still be made. Postoperatively, pain assessment is the key as it can mark the progression of healing and alert to a complication, such as the formation of an abscess, if pain is not improving or new pain is noted. Pain control can be managed by distraction techniques, ice, or analgesics such as morphine sulfate or Toradol while NPO, and oral pain meds when taking a diet (Bishop & Carter, 2013).

If the decision is made to go to the operating room, broad-spectrum antibiotics should also be administered preoperatively. Antibiotics administered prior to surgery have shown a reduction in wound infections as well as abscess formation (Bishop & Carter, 2013). Postoperatively, antibiotics are often given for 24 hours for acute appendicitis, however, perforated appendicitis often requires a longer duration of broad-spectrum antibiotics to prevent wound infections and abscess formation (Brown, 2014). The American Pediatric Surgical Association is now recommending that antibiotic therapy be based on clinical criteria, such as down trending labs and no fever, rather than a set, standard time frame (Brown, 2014). The surgery may be done either laparoscopically or open, however, frequent inspection of the wounds must be performed. Identifying any erythema, drainage, or tenderness could indicate a wound infection and may warrant prolonged antibiotic coverage (Bishop & Carter, 2013).

Lastly, families can be overwhelmed with the abundance of information they receive from medical teams. As a nurse, it is important to identify whether there is deficient knowledge or lack of recall of information received and help to relieve any anxiety or answer questions the family may have. Postoperatively, nurses must educate the family about wound care, management of surgical wound dressings, appropriate bathing time frame, and symptoms to look for at home that warrant a call to the surgeon.

OUTCOMES

From preoperative to postoperative care, nursing plays a role in preventing potential complications, promoting overall comfort, and reducing anxiety through patient and family education. Through the team efforts of both the nursing staff and the surgical team, patients with appendicitis can have shorter hospitalizations with positive outcomes.

Summary

Acute appendicitis is one of the most common pediatric conditions that require emergent surgery. Signs and symptoms of appendicitis often mimic those of other conditions so it is vital that the nursing staff is educated on hallmark signs, such as fevers, nausea, vomiting, and right lower quadrant pain, to diagnose appendicitis.

Bhangu, A., Soreide, K., Di Saverio, S., Assarsson, J. H., & Drake, F. T. (2015). Acute appendicitis: Modern understanding of pathogenesis, diagnosis, and management. *Lancet, 386*(10000), 1278–1287. doi:10.1016/s0140-6736(15)00275-5

Bishop, C. A., & Carter, M. E. (2013). Appendicitis. In N. T. Browne, L. M. Flanigan, C. A. McComiskey, & P. Pieper (Eds.), *Nursing care of the pediatric surgical patient, third edition* (pp. 407–415). Burlington, MA: Jones & Bartlett.

Brown, R. L. (2014). Appendicitis. In M. M. Ziegler, R. G. Azizkhan, D. von Allmen, & T. R. Weber (Eds.), *Operative pediatric surgery* (2nd ed., pp. 613–631). New York, NY: McGraw-Hill.

Butler, K. L. (2015). Acute appendicitis. In K. L. Butler & M. Harisinghani (Eds.), *Acute care surgery: Imaging essentials for rapid diagnosis* (pp. 79–86). New York, NY: McGraw-Hill.

Pennington, E. C., & Burke, P. A. (2015). Appendix. In G. M. Doherty (Ed.), *Current diagnosis & treatment: Surgery* (14th ed., pp. 651–656). New York, NY: McGraw-Hill.

Rentea, R. M., St. Peter, S. D., & Snyder, C. L. (2017). Pediatric appendicitis: State of the art review. *Pediatric Surgery International*, 33(3), 269–283. doi:10.1007/s00383-016-3990-2

Tian, Y., Heiss, K. F., Wulkan, M. L., & Raval, M. V. (2015). Assessment of variation in care and outcomes for pediatric appendicitis at children's and non-children's hospitals. *Journal of Pediatric Surgery*, 50, 1185–1892. doi:10.1016/J.JPEDSURG.2015.06.012

■ ASTHMA

Laurine Gajkowski

Overview

Asthma is a common chronic inflammatory disorder of the large and small airways. Varying degrees of airflow obstruction occur due to bronchial muscle constriction, edema of the tracheobronchial mucosa, and increased mucus secretions. Susceptible children have intermittent respiratory symptoms, such as wheezing, dyspnea, and cough, especially at night. In the United States, 6.3 million children or 8.6% of those under the age of 18 years have a diagnosis of asthma (National Center for Health Statistics [NCHS], 2016). It poses a burden on the affected child, the parents, and the community. Children with asthma can experience a decreased quality of life due to impairment of daily activities, emergency department visits, and school absences (Miadich, Everhart, Borschuk, Winter, & Fiese, 2015). Childhood asthma is associated with high rates of school absenteeism (Cicutto, Gleason, & Szefler, 2014), and exacerbations or "flare-ups" of symptoms are the leading cause of pediatric hospital admissions in the United States (Sylvester & George, 2014). Nurses provide acute care to these children in hospitals when the level of respiratory compromise is too severe to be managed at home. Nursing interventions in outpatient settings, such as schools and clinics, are aimed at assisting the child and family to assume responsibility for asthma management.

Background

According to Global Initiative for Asthma (GINA), asthma is characterized by chronic airway inflammation. This condition is defined by the history of respiratory symptoms, including shortness of breath, wheezing, chest tightness, and cough, that vary in intensity and expiratory airflow limitation over time (GINA, 2016). Asthma is a complex disease caused by an interplay of many genetic and environmental factors. "Atopy, the genetic predisposition for the development of an immunoglobulin E (IgE)-mediated response to common aeroallergens, is the strongest identifiable predisposing factor for developing asthma" (NAEPP, 2007, p. 11). Other risk factors include intrauterine exposures (cigarette smoke, inadequate nutrition, and stress), prematurity, viral respiratory infections in early childhood, early antibiotic use, obesity, acetaminophen use, emotional stress, and air pollution (Woodruff, Bhakta, & Fahy, 2016). A hygiene hypothesis suggests that the increasing prevalence of allergies and asthma may be related to modern society's emphasis on cleanliness, which leads to reduced early exposure to pathogens in children. There have been many theories about possible primary prevention strategies for the development of asthma, but none of them has been proven by existing evidence (Beasley, Semprini, & Mitchell, 2015).

The prevalence and severity of asthma are highest in certain vulnerable populations. According to the National Health Interview Survey, "For children under age 15 years, the sex-adjusted percentage by race and ethnicity (of children) who had an asthma episode in the past 12 months was 3.7% for Hispanic children, 3.5% for non-Hispanic White children, and 9.1% for non-Hispanic Black children" (National Center for Health Statistics, 2016, p. 99). This variability in prevalence, morbidity, and mortality may be attributable to many factors, including access to culturally competent health care, exposure to inflammatory agents such as air pollution in urban environments, coping with psychosocial stress, and exposure to substandard housing problems such as mold and roaches (Gruber et al., 2016).

Ongoing research in genetics and immunology is increasing our knowledge about the development of asthma. Once a child has developed this condition, ongoing inflammatory exposures seem to increase the risk of exacerbations and lead to progressive loss of pulmonary function. A range of indoor and outdoor allergens, as well as viral infections, food, medicine (beta-blockers, aspirin, or other nonsteroidal anti-inflammatory drugs [NSAIDs]), exercise, psychological stress, and weather changes may trigger a child's asthma symptoms. Common indoor triggers include secondhand smoke, dust mites, mold, rodents, cockroaches, fragrances, chemical particulate matter, and pet dander. Common outdoor allergens include ozone, pollen, and air pollution (U.S. Environmental Protection Agency (EPA), Indoor Environments Division, Office of Air and Radiation, 2015).

Initially, the diagnosis of asthma is based on the child's physical exam, history of respiratory symptoms, and pulmonary function test (spirometry). The most common spirometry measurement is the child's forced expiratory volume in 1 second (FEV_1), and it is reported as a percentage of the predicted value for the child's height and age. This measurement can demonstrate impaired airflow and airway hyperresponsiveness. The child's clinical response to inhaled and oral medications is also considered in classifying the child's asthma severity. The "Classification of Asthma Severity in Children" was written in the *2007 National Asthma Education and Prevention Program (NAEPP)* by the National Heart, Lung, and Blood Institute of the National Institutes of Health (2007). Symptom-based definitions are used to classify the severity as intermittent, mild persistent, moderate persistent, or severe persistent. A child classified with the mildest form, "intermittent asthma," has symptoms 2 or fewer days per week, has no nighttime awakenings, requires use of a rescue inhaler 2 or fewer days per week for symptom control, and has a normal (FEV_1) between exacerbations. By contrast, a child with the most severe form, "severe persistent asthma," has symptoms throughout the day, nighttime awakenings every night, uses a rescue inhaler several times daily, has extremely limited activity, uses oral corticosteroids two or more times per year, and has an FEV_1 less than 60% predicted.

Clinical Aspects

The typical presentation of a child during an acute asthma episode is ill and uncomfortable, with rapid, labored respirations and a fatigued look from an ongoing struggle to breathe. Coughing, nasal flaring, intercostal retractions, and accessory muscle use may be observed along with complaints of chest tightness. The expiratory phase is prolonged. On auscultation, wheezing is heard on expiration and/or inspiration unless the episode is so severe that a "silent chest" develops because of extremely poor air exchange. The child prefers to sit in an upright position, leaning forward in the tripod position. If the episode progresses to hypoxia, the child becomes wide-eyed, agitated, and confused or suddenly quiet as ventilation becomes

ineffective. Episodes that fail to respond to medications, oxygen therapy, and hydration (acute severe asthma, also called *status asthmaticus*) can lead to death from respiratory failure, so the child must be immediately moved to and treated in the intensive care unit.

ASSESSMENT

The pediatric nurse begins with a respiratory assessment, which includes color, respiratory rate, heart rate, level of consciousness, quality of breath sounds, ability to speak in sentences rather than single words, presence of abnormal findings that indicate impaired gas exchange (wheezing, nasal flaring, retractions, grunting, accessory muscle use, head bobbing), and pulse oximetry measurement. The pediatric nurse must compare the child's heart and respiratory rate to the normal ranges based on the child's age. Tachypnea, tachycardia, and SpO_2 below 92% indicate hypoxemia. In addition to a respiratory assessment, the nurse must determine the child's fluid status based on the child's weight, intake and output, and skin turgor. Once the child's condition is stable, the nurse can assess the child's developmental and psychosocial concerns, as well as the family's home asthma management history, using the Childhood Asthma Control Test (C-ACT) and the GINA (2016) guidelines.

NURSING INTERVENTIONS, MANAGEMENT, AND IMPLICATIONS

During the acute phase of an asthma exacerbation, the pediatric nurse focuses on the child's risk for respiratory failure. Nursing interventions that eliminate the risk for respiratory failure include ongoing monitoring of breathing, supporting respiratory functioning (positioning, oxygen administration, hydration), and medication administration. Two categories of medications are commonly used to treat asthma: control and quick relief. Control medications are used on a daily basis to prevent an exacerbation. These include inhaled long-acting beta$_2$-agonists (LABAs), inhaled corticosteroids (ICSs), oral leukotriene receptor antagonists (LTRAs), and others. Quick-relief medications are used when needed for asthma flare-ups. These include inhaled short-acting beta$_2$-agonists (SABAs), oral corticosteroids, and inhaled anticholinergics. These medications are ordered according to the child's asthma-severity classification. Nursing care often follows a standardized asthma care pathway that outlines a sequence for assessments and interventions to be used for hospitalized children. Studies have shown that the use of clinical pathways has decreased the patient length of stay and lowered the cost of treatment. Unfortunately, pathway use has not been shown to reduce hospital readmission rates (Sylvester & George, 2014). Support of parental participation in the hospitalized child's care is often essential for the child's overall sense of well-being.

At every health encounter, asthma education for self-management is a priority. Each member of the interprofessional team, including the bedside nurse, hospitalist, respiratory therapist, primary care provider, asthma specialist, and school nurse, develops a partnership with the patient and family. Supportive, open communication among all team members helps to build trust and alleviate misconceptions. Parents may be instructed to keep a symptom diary to help identify triggers. Asthma control is achieved through avoidance of triggers, adherence to prescribed controller and maintenance therapy, and the family's ability to recognize symptoms and respond appropriately to them. Families may need help to view asthma management from a prevention perspective instead of viewing it from a crisis perspective (Archibald, Caine, Ali, Hartling, & Scott, 2015). Any child diagnosed with asthma should be provided with an individualized written asthma action plan that spells out specific guidelines for daily management when the child is symptom free (green zone), when the child's symptoms begin to increase (yellow zone), and when emergency care is indicated (red zone; GINA, 2016). The pediatric nurse ensures that the child and/or caregivers have a clear understanding of their asthma home management plan. When caring for a child, it is especially important to educate about the correct use of inhaler devices and give the child an opportunity to perform a return demonstration. Parents need information about ways to reduce allergens at home, such as encasing the child's mattress and pillow to control dust mites, or reducing molds by lowering humidity.

OUTCOMES

The expected outcome of quality nursing care for the child asthma patient is successful self-management through avoidance of triggers, early recognition and treatment with rescue medications, and compliance with an individualized asthma action plan that maintains daily control of symptoms.

Summary

Because there is no cure for asthma, the care of children with asthma should focus on successful home management in order to control symptoms. Nurses must be knowledgeable about the pathophysiology of asthma, prevention and management of exacerbations, and principles of health-maintenance education, and play a critical role in providing comprehensive family-centered asthma education that promotes a sense of shared responsibility.

Archibald, M. M., Caine, V., Ali, S., Hartling, L., & Scott, S. D. (2015). What is left unsaid: An interpretive description of the information needs of parents of children with asthma. *Research in Nursing & Health*, 28(1), 19–28.

Beasley, R., Semprini, A., & Mitchell, E. A. (2015). Risk factors for asthma: Is prevention possible? *Lancet*, 386(9998), 1075–1085.

Cicutto, L., Gleason, M., & Szefler, S. J. (2014). Establishing school-centered asthma programs. *Journal of Allergy and Clinical Immunology*, 134(6), 1223–1230. doi:10.1016/j.jaci.2014.10.004

Global Initiative for Asthma. (2016). The 2016 update of the global strategy for asthma management and prevention. Retrieved from http://ginasthma.org/2017

Gruber, K. J., McKee-Huger, B., Richard, A., Byerly, B., Raczkowski, J. L., & Wall, T. C. (2016). Removing asthma triggers and improving children's health: The asthma partnership demonstration project. *Annals of Allergy, Asthma & Immunology*, 116(5), 408–414.

Miadich, S. A., Everhart, R. S., Borschuk, A. P., Winter, M. A., & Fiese, B. H. (2015). Quality of life in children with asthma: A developmental perspective. *Journal of Pediatric Psychology*, 40(7) 672–679. doi:10.1093/jpepsy/jsv002

National Center for Health Statistics. (2016). Early release of selected estimates based on data from the National Health Interview Survey, January–March 2016. Retrieved from https://www.cdc.gov/nchs/nhis/releases/released201611

National Institutes of Health: National Heart, Lung, and Blood Institute. (2007). National Asthma Education Prevention Program: Guidelines for the diagnosis and management of asthma: Expert panel report 3. Retrieved from http://www.nhlbi.nih.gov/files/docs/guidelines/asthgdln.pdf

Sylvester, A. M., & George, M. (2014). Effect of a clinical pathway on length of stay and cost of pediatric inpatient asthma admissions: An integrative review. *Clinical Nursing Research*, 23(4), 384–401. doi:10.1177/1054773813487373

United States Environmental Protection Agency, Indoor Environments Division, Office of Air and Radiation. (2015). Asthma facts. EPA-402-F-04-019. Retrieved from https://www.epa.gov/sites/production/files/2015-10/documents/asthma_fact_sheet_eng_july_30_2015_v2.pdf

Woodruff, P. G., Bhakta, N. R., & Fahy, J. V. (2016). Asthma: Pathogenesis and phenotypes. In V. C. Broaddus (Ed.), *Murray and Nadel's textbook of respiratory medicine* (pp. 713–730). Philadelphia, PA: Elsevier Saunders.

■ AUTISM SPECTRUM DISORDER

Sheila Blank
Celeste M. Alfes

Overview

Autism spectrum disorder (ASD) is a neurodevelopmental disorder that can affect a child developmentally, neurologically, and socially. Children with ASD may communicate, interact, behave, and learn in ways that are different from others. ASD has a wide range of symptoms, behaviors, developmental, and social delays that can range from gifted to severely challenged. Some people with ASD require a lot of help in their daily lives; others require less, for this reason, autism truly is an individual disorder.

ASD has been affecting children for the past century but within the past 10 years at an increasingly rapid rate, increasing 123% from 2002 to 2010 (Centers for Disease Control and Prevention [CDC], 2016). Autism does not discriminate based on race, ethnicity, or socioeconomic groups. Autism is gender-specific, affecting males 4.5 times more often (one in 42) than females. Children who have a sibling with ASD are at a higher risk of being diagnosed with ASD. In 2013, the *Diagnostic and Statistical Manual of Mental Disorders, fifth edition* (*DSM-5*) grouped the diagnosis of autism together with pervasive developmental disorders not otherwise specified (PDD-NOS; American Psychiatric Association, 2013). Asperger syndrome is a higher functioning form of autism. Childhood disintegrative disorder is seen when the child begins to develop normally, meeting each developmental milestone on time until the age of 3 or 4; then the child begins regressing, losing language and motor or social skills they may have previously learned. Rett syndrome is a severe brain disorder in which a child begins to develop normally in early life, but between 6 and 18 months of age, changes in the normal patterns of mental and social development begin. Pervasive developmental disorder is a developmental disorder affecting communication and socialization.

Background

ASD is a neurodevelopmental disorder that affects intellect, communication, and socialization with an unknown cause. Much research has been done in the search for a cause and the only common theme is that much more research needs to be conducted. Research in a variety of areas indicates that the cause of ASD is multifaceted. Researchers have alluded to genetics and environmental factors having a possible connection to ASD but nothing concrete has emerged (National Institute of Neurological Disorders and Stroke, 2016).

The CDC established red-flag indicators, which can be detected in children with ASD as early as infancy and up to about the age of 3 years. Red-flag indicators focus on areas of socialization, communication, development, and behaviors. Some indicators include lack of meeting developmental milestones at the appropriate age such as head lagging, delay of speech, and no cooing or babbling within the first 6 months of age. Infants are usually social through gesturing, smiling, or turning of the head when their name is called, however, if ASD is suspected, infants develop a flat affect and lack socialization (CDC, 2016). As the child grows, other indicators can include aggression, tantrums, social isolation, lack of eye contact, and speech delays. About 25% to 30% of children with ASD have some words at 12 to 18 months of age but may lose them as they grow older. By the age of 3 or 4, a child with ASD may demonstrate no eye contact, very noticeable speech delays, employ repetitive words or phrases (echolalia), or total lack of speech. About 40% of the children with ASD do not talk at all. These children may demonstrate developmental delays as well as gross motor or fine motor movement delays. Children with ASD may become socially isolated and use self-play, which leads to inappropriate play. They do not understand or use pretend play. Repetitive movements, such as hand flapping, turning, bouncing, spinning, and toe-walking, are seen. Aggression and injurious behaviors may increase as the child grows.

Clinical Aspects

ASSESSMENT

ASD can be diagnosed as early as 18 months of age but more commonly by the age of 3 or 4 years. Diagnosis is difficult as not all children develop at the same pace. If delays are noticed, children with delays will be monitored more closely than a normally developing child and may be referred for further testing. Physicians can perform a modified checklist for autism in toddlers as early as 16 to 30 months. The checklist is a screening tool that can indicate whether further testing is necessary. The checklist is a series of questions about developmental growth. If a child fails two or more of the critical items, then a referral should be made for further testing. The referral is made to a developmental specialist and a multidisciplinary team is formed. The team includes a psychologist, neurologist, psychiatrist, and speech therapist who perform a variety of neurological assessments, in-depth cognitive testing, language testing, and hearing testing. Direct observation of the child in a variety of settings and a thorough history provided by the parents is crucial in the diagnosis process.

Sensory disturbances can affect behaviors and increase anxiety in an individual with ASD, which will cause difficulty in gathering necessary health information to provide appropriate care. Touch, increased sounds, textures, smells, and overly bright rooms are all sensory stimuli that can affect individuals with ASD. Nurses are taught the art of compassion and the appropriate use of touch when caring for any patient, but nurses need to realize when caring for a patient with ASD that this art may have negative effects. The best way to approach a patient with ASD is to take it slow, with no time restraints, but persistence is needed. The nurse will need to establish a working rapport with the patient before gathering assessment information. A brief preference assessment is a tool used to find individual favorites that can be used as reinforcers. A reinforcer is an object, food, computer game, movie, or television show that the patient likes and should be used to reinforce positive behavior (Cooper, Heron, & Heward, 2006). By reinforcing positive behavior, the nurse is beginning to establish a comfort level with the patient.

NURSING INTERVENTIONS, MANAGEMENT, AND IMPLICATIONS

Providing nursing care for children with ASD can be a difficult task. Children with ASD communicate, learn, and socialize differently than typically developing children. The lack of understanding of verbal and nonverbal language makes it difficult for children to communicate effectively and may lead to increased stress (Prelock & Nelson 2012). Children with ASD are easily distracted, therefore, communication needs to be concise and focused directly on the individual. Effective communication needs to be delivered slowly, softly, and in short sentences. This method allows time for the patient to understand and process information. A communication board or picture exchange communication system (PECS) can be used to express an individual's needs and wants during a hospital stay or

physician visit and can be customized for each patient to promote individual communication.

Health care visits or hospital stays can be difficult for individuals with ASD due to ineffective communication, sensory issues, understanding expectations, and general feelings of fear and anxiety (Prelock & Nelson, 2012). Children with ASD are very rigid in their daily routines and do not handle change well. Caregivers need to plan for health care visits and explain to individuals with ASD what to expect at each visit. Picture books or storybooks can be developed and read to the individual to promote understanding of what will be done at each visit and increase the comfort level that can produce more accurate results during each visit. Role modeling is another technique that can be used to demonstrate what to expect at physician appointments and hospital stays, and the testing that needs to be done.

OUTCOMES

As shown throughout literature, children diagnosed with ASD grow up and transition into adulthood. Numerous schools are available for children with ASD up until the middle school years. A smaller number of high schools are available as the children grow and then education seems to drift off. Children with ASD need continued education to manage behaviors, learn, socialize, and communicate appropriately, and we need to continue that into high school and into young adult and adulthood.

Summary

Children with ASD lack socialization and communication, and have cognitive and developmental delays. Research has found that early diagnosis, by age 3 or 4, and intervention will help some children with ASD better manage their behaviors and learn ways to cope with their deficits in an attempt to live a more typical life. To date, researchers have not been able to determine a concrete cause for ASD. With the increased numbers of children being diagnosed, efforts to improve the lives of children affected with ASD are needed.

American Psychiatric Association. (2013). *Diagnostic and statistical manual of mental disorders* (5th ed.). Arlington, VA: American Psychiatric Publishing.

Centers for Disease Control and Prevention. (2016). Autism data and statistics. Retrieved from http://www.cdc.gov/ncbddd/autism/data.html

Cooper, J. O., Heron, T. E., & Heward W. L. (2006). *Applied behavior analysis* (2nd ed.). Upper Saddle River, NJ: Prentice Hall.

National Institute of Neurological Disorders and Stroke. (2016). Autism spectrum disorder fact sheet. Retrieved from http:// www.ninds.nih.gov/disorders/autism/detail_autism.htm

Prelock, P. J., & Nelson N. W. (2012). Language and communication in autism: An integrated view. *Pediatric Clinics of North America Journal, 59*(1), 129–145.

■ BRONCHIOLITIS RESPIRATORY SYNCYTIAL VIRUS

Shannon Courtney Wong

Overview

Bronchiolitis occurs when a viral or bacterial infection invades the lower respiratory tract, causing inflammation and obstruction of the bronchioles (Ball, Bindler, Cowen, & Shaw, 2017). Although there are a variety of viruses that can cause bronchiolitis, respiratory syncytial virus (RSV) is the leading cause of bronchiolitis, and the leading cause of severe lower respiratory tract infections in young children (Walsh, 2016). Bronchiolitis occurs when a viral or bacterial infection invades the lower respiratory tract, causing inflammation and obstruction of the bronchioles (Ball et al., 2017). The RSV virus attacks and kills the mucosal cells lining the small bronchi and bronchioles, obstructing the bronchioles and irritating the airway (Ball et al., 2017). This irritation leads to excessive mucus production, cough, wheezing, hyperexpansion of the lungs, hypoxia, and respiratory distress (Zhou et al., 2015). Current nursing care for infants and young children with RSV bronchiolitis focuses on supporting the child, maintaining respiratory function, and supporting fluid balance and rest.

Background

According to the Centers for Disease Control and Prevention (CDC), RSV infections lead to 57,527 hospitalizations and 2.1 million outpatient visits among children younger than 5 years old in the United States each year (CDC, 2016). In fact, RSV is the most important reason previously healthy infants are admitted to the hospital, predominantly due to an immature immune system and smaller dimensions of the airways of the lungs of infants and young children (Pickles & DeVincenzo, 2015). Infants who were born prematurely are at an even higher risk for an RSV infection causing hospitalization than infants born at term (Figueras-Aloy et al., 2016).

RSV is an extremely common infection, and by the age of 2 years, almost all children have been infected with RSV at least once (Figueras-Aloy et al., 2016). The transmission of RSV happens most effectively through contact of nasal secretions; the RSV virus can survive for several hours on hard surfaces and hands, so the virus is transmitted via direct contact with objects that have been contaminated (Walsh, 2016). The season for RSV infections in the United States starts in October, peaks in December through February, and finishes in March or April (Bont et al., 2016).

Although all people contract the RSV virus several times throughout their lifetime, infants and young children are at the greatest risk for severe complications from the virus. Risk factors for severe bronchiolitis are: age younger than 3 months of age, premature birth, immunodeficiency, and cardiopulmonary disease (Pickles & DiVincenzo, 2015). These risk factors are all important, but the age of infection seems to be the most significant risk factor. In fact, 80% of infants hospitalized with an RSV infection under the age of 2 months had no significant past medical history (Pickles & DiVincenzo, 2015). In addition, studies have shown that the disease can impact a child long after hospital discharge. In fact, children who were hospitalized as infants with RSV bronchiolitis have a higher prevalence of asthma when compared to matched control infants (Mejias & Ramillo, 2015).

RSV bronchiolitis should be considered in any infant presenting with acute symptoms of lower respiratory tract infection, especially during the winter months (Pickles & DiVincenzo, 2015). A conclusive diagnosis is made by taking a posterior nasopharyngeal wash or swab specimen and conducting an enzyme-linked immunoabsorbent assay (ELISA) or a immunofluorescent assay to identify the specific virus causing the symptoms (Ball et al., 2017). Also, a chest radiograph should be obtained. A child with bronchiolitis will have a chest x-ray showing hyperinflation, patchy atelectasis, and signs of inflammation (Ball et al., 2017). Clinical manifestations can also support a diagnosis of RSV. Children with an RSV infection will present with nasal congestion, cough, intermittent low-grade fever, wheezing, tachypnea, and poor feeding, with possible vomiting or diarrhea (Ball et al., 2017; Pickles & DiVincenzo, 2015). A child with a more significant infection will present with increased tachypnea, significant wheezing and coughing, poor fluid intake, and a distended abdomen, related to hyperexpansion in the lungs (Ball et al., 2017; Pickles & DiVincenzo, 2015).

Clinical Aspects

ASSESSMENT

The most important areas to assess in young children presenting with RSV bronchiolitis are the child's airway and respiratory function. This can be done using good observation skills noting how quickly the infant is breathing and whether retractions are noted, and by using pulse oximetry to determine oxygenation (Ball et al., 2017). Infants with RSV bronchiolitis can progress into severe disease quite easily, but identifying which patients will exhibit a progressively worse disease is difficult (Mejias & Ramillo, 2015), making the need for close observation of subtle changes in patient's status important. Parent and caregiver education also becomes very important, as many children with an RSV infection can be managed at home. The families need to help their child by encouraging rest, proper fluid intake and comfort, while being able to recognize when the patient's status may be declining (Potts & Mandleco, 2012). Children who are showing signs of respiratory distress and/or dehydration may require hospitalization. A hospitalized infant with RSV bronchiolitis may require humidified oxygen, nasal suctioning, intravenous (IV) fluids, intake and output (I&O) monitoring, and daily weights (Ball et al., 2017).

As mentioned, treatments for RSV are mostly supportive therapies. At this time, there is no specific treatment for RSV, and medications are generally not prescribed for RSV infections (Ball et al., 2017). Palivizumab (Synagis) is a medication given to protect infants from RSV, but it is reserved for only high-risk infants who meet criteria outlined by the American Academy of Pediatrics (Walsh, 2016). This medication is given monthly, up to five times, during an infant's first winter, and it provides a passive immunity protection (Ball et al., 2017; Walsh, 2015).

NURSING INTERVENTIONS, MANAGEMENT, AND IMPLICATIONS

One of the most important nursing-related problems surrounding RSV of the hospitalized infant is being careful not to spread this contagious disease from one patient to another. Proper handwashing and isolation precautions for the RSV patient are crucial. These patients require contact precautions, which include gloves and gowns (Walsh, 2016). It is also important to continually promote adequate respiratory status, fluid balance, nutrition, rest, and comfort (Ball, Bindler, Cowen, & Shaw, 2017). Finally, nursing professionals must educate the parents and caregivers about the disease and it's normal progression. Parents will need guidance in understanding bronchiolitis and respiratory distress, and recognizing signs and symptoms that their infant's disease is getting more severe or improving. In addition, parents and family may need emotional support due to the stress of the child's hospitalization, and caring for a sick infant (Ball & Bindler, 2017).

OUTCOMES

The expected outcome of nursing care for an infant infected with RSV is complete recovery without further complications. Within 24 to 72 hours, the production of mucus will begin to decrease, aiding in improved respiratory function (Ball & Bindler, 2017). Once the virus runs its course, most infants and young children return to their pre-RSV health. Their breathing and feeding patterns should return to normal, and any weight lost due to poor feeding should be regained quickly. The incidence of reinfection can occur, but as the child grows, the severity of the disease will lessen. As noted, there is a higher incidence of children acquiring asthma later in life who were severely infected with RSV and required hospitalization (Meijias & Ramilo, 2015), making an RSV infection an important component of the patient's medical history.

Summary

A RSV infection in infants and young children can differ in its severity, making it vital for health care professionals to recognize subtle changes in the patient's status, especially related to respiratory function. Early recognition, supportive nursing interventions, and thorough parent/caregiver teaching are crucial in managing a patient infected with RSV.

Ball, J., Bindler, R., Cowen, K., & Shaw, M. (2017). *Principles of pediatric nursing: Caring for children*. Hoboken, NJ: Pearson.

Bont, L., Checchia, P., Fauroux, B., Figueras-Aloy, J., Monzoni, P., Paes, B., … Carbonell-Estrany, X. (2016). Defining the epidemiology and burden of severe respiratory syncytial virus infection among infants and children in western countries. *Infectious Disease Therapy, 5*(3), 271–298.

Centers for Disease Control and Prevention. (2016). Respiratory syncytial virus. Retrieved from https://www.cdc.gov/rsv/research/us-surveillance.html

Figueras-Aloy, J., Monzoni, P., Paes, B., Simoes, E., Bont, L., Checchia, P., . . . Carbonell-Estrany, X. (2016). Defining the risk and associated morbidity and mortality of severe respiratory syncytial virus infection among preterm infants without chronic lung disease or congenital heart disease. *Infectious Disease Therapy, 5*(4), 417–452.

Mejias, A., & Ramilo, O. (2015). New options in the treatment of respiratory syncytial virus disease. *Journal of Infection, 71*, S80–S87.

Pickles, R., & DeVincenzo, J. (2015). Respiratory syncytial virus (RSV) and its propensity for causing bronchiolitis. *Journal of Pathology, 235*(2), 266–276.

Potts, N., & Mandleco, B. (2012). *Pediatric nursing: Caring for children and their families.* Clifton Park, NY: Delmar.

Walsh, E. (2016). Respiratory syncytial virus infection. *Clinics in Chest Medicine, 38*(1), 29–36. doi:10.1016/j.ccm.2016.11.010

Zhou, L., Xiao, Q., Zhao, Y., Huang, A., Ren, L., & Liu, E. (2015). The impact of viral dynamics on the clinical severity of infants with respiratory syncytial virus bronchiolitis. *Journal of Medical Virology, 87*(1), 1276–1284.

■ CANCERS OF CHILDHOOD

Breanne M. Roche

Overview

Cancer develops when a single cell proliferates uncontrollably and the cell is independent of the laws governing the remainder of the body. The balance between cellular division and cellular loss is disrupted, leading to uncontrolled cellular growth. In 2016, according to the National Cancer Institute, there were an estimated 10,380 new cases of cancer in children ages 0 to 14 years in the United States. Childhood cancer is a devastating diagnosis that can affect family dynamics. Nurses are at the forefront of care when it comes to caring for the child with an oncological disease.

Background

Fewer than 1% of all cancers are in children (American Cancer Society, 2016). Out of the over 10,000 new cases annually, about 10% of these children will die from their disease (National Cancer Institute, 2016).

Although survival rates continue to improve, and more than 80% of children with cancer will survive 5 years or more, cancer remains the leading cause of death from disease among children (American Cancer Society, 2016). The types of cancer that develop in children are different than those in adults. The most common types of childhood cancers in ages 0 to 14 years include acute lymphocytic leukemia (ALL), brain tumors, and neuroblastoma. The adolescent and young-adult (AYA) population aged 15 to 29 years is a unique group of patients. The incidence of cancer in this age group represents 2% of all cancers. The most common types of cancers in the United States for patients aged 15 to 19 years include lymphoma, germ cell tumors, brain tumors, malignant melanoma, and ALL (Kline, 2014).

The etiology of childhood cancer is unknown although it is likely that the interaction among many different factors both environmental and host contribute to its development (Kline, 2014). Only 5% of all childhood cancers are caused by an inherited mutation (National Cancer Institute, 2016). With an inherited mutation, there are DNA changes within every cell in the body that may be linked to an increased risk to develop cancer, or these inherited mutations lead to syndromes that can predispose a child to cancer (American Cancer Society, 2016). For example, children with Down syndrome are at increased risk for the development of ALL and acute myelogenous leukemia (Frangkandrea, Nixon, & Panagopoulou, 2013). Most pediatric cancers are not caused by inherited DNA changes, but rather they develop as a result of an acquired mutation that is a mutation that occurs within one cell in the body during cellular division and it has the potential to escape apoptosis and proliferate uncontrollably (American Cancer Society, 2016). Unlike adult cancers, lifestyle factors are not associated with the development of childhood cancer. There are a few environmental factors, such as radiation exposure, that may increase a child's risk for the development of cancer.

Cancer diagnosis in children is often delayed because the presenting symptoms are nonspecific and resemble benign conditions like a common viral illness (Frangkandrea et al., 2013). The diagnosis of pediatric cancer includes a thorough history and exam, labs, imaging, or tissue biopsy. There is oftentimes a lag time between presenting symptoms and diagnosis, which creates a great deal of uncertainty for the family. Treatment varies according to the type of malignancy and may include chemotherapy, radiation therapy, surgery, or bone marrow transplant.

Clinical Aspects

ASSESSMENT

Nursing assessment is a vital component in caring for the oncological child and may vary depending on the type of malignant process. Most signs and symptoms of childhood cancer are due to the following: changes in blood cell production due to bone marrow infiltration by tumor or an acute or chronic disease, a mass resulting in compression of vital structures or organs, and tumor by-products causing electrolyte disturbances or altered immunologic responses (Kline, 2014). Effective nursing care for pediatric oncology patients includes accurate records of history, physical exam, and lab values. The nurse must be able to recognize abnormal laboratory findings in association with physical exam findings in order to create and execute an effective nursing care plan.

Physical examination findings will be correlated to common chief complains. Exam findings related to alterations in blood cell production include pallor (conjunctivae, oral mucosa, nail beds, skin), petechiae or purpura, fever, infection, or fatigue (Kline, 2014). Dermatological findings are oftentimes associated with bone marrow function (Frangkandrea et al., 2013). A mediastinal mass may be present in a newly diagnosed patient with leukemia, lymphoma, neuroblastoma or other abdominal/pelvic tumors, which can cause respiratory compromise. Examination may indicate signs of respiratory distress, including retractions, nasal flaring, grunting, and wheezing. An abdominal mass could be indicative of a tumor, hepatosplenomegaly, distended bladder, or retained stool (Kline, 2014). Symptoms associated with an abdominal mass may include gastrointestinal (nausea, vomiting, constipation or diarrhea), urinary (hematuria, retention), or respiratory (dyspnea related to increased abdominal pressure). Signs and symptoms of central nervous system (CNS) tumors vary according to the location of the tumor but may include loss of developmental milestones, irritability, early-morning or postnap headaches, cranial nerve palsies, diplopia, nystagmus, or ataxia (Kline, 2014).

Accurate record of vital signs is imperative in the oncological child. A fever is a medical emergency and is not a symptom in these patients, but rather an indication of an underlying problem, which has the potential to rapidly progress to life-threatening sepsis in an immunocompromised patient (Kline, 2014). Rectal temperatures are avoided in these patients due to potential injury of the rectal mucosa and a patient's risk of thrombocytopenia and neutropenia leading to unintentional bleeding or infection. Chills are a serious implication that a fever is brewing and could be one of the first signs of the showering of bacteria in the bloodstream. Tachycardia is a common sign that may be from anemia, anxiety, hypovolemia, shock, fever, or pain. Tachypnea may be a sign caused by anxiety, hypoxia, fever, pain, or respiratory compromise. Hypotension is a medical emergency and rapid fluid resuscitation is critical to prevent septic shock, hemorrhage, or dehydration.

Nursing assessment also includes monitoring for signs of toxicity related to therapy and oncological emergencies. Chemotherapeutic agents, radiation therapy, or biological response modifiers can all cause toxicity to the child with cancer (Kline, 2014). Understanding therapy-related side effects helps the nurse develop a safe nursing care plan. Oncological emergencies are life-threatening events that can occur during the treatment course of the child with cancer (Kline, 2014). Oncological emergencies include hyperleukocytosis, tumor lysis syndrome, septic shock, typhlitis, spinal cord compression, and inappropriate antidiuretic hormone secretion syndrome (Kline, 2014). Thorough nursing assessment can lead to early recognition of oncologic emergencies and rapid intervention preventing complications.

Proper assessment of the child with cancer is ongoing from diagnosis through survivorship. Children who have survived cancer are at risk for late effects of cancer treatment, and therefore meticulous assessment of late effects is imperative. Late effects of cancer treatment depend upon the type of therapy used, which may affect every organ of the body.

NURSING INTERVENTIONS, MANAGEMENT, AND IMPLICATIONS

Every organ system in the body can be compromised with an oncological process. Nursing care of the child with cancer should focus on the prevention of infection, education, and anticipatory guidance to the patient and caregivers regarding diagnosis, treatment, and medications. Some of the more common nursing-related problems include bone marrow suppression, impairment of the immune system leading to increased risk of infection, altered electrolytes as a result of malignancy or therapy, nausea and vomiting associated with chemotherapeutic agents, and altered family dynamics related to a cancer diagnosis.

Nursing management for the child with cancer is comprehensive and family centered. Nursing management is focused on managing the treatment side effects while providing ongoing education to the patient and family. With chemotherapy, bone marrow suppression is an expected side effect, and therefore nurses must be comfortable educating families regarding blood counts and routine administration of blood products. Nursing interventions also include assessing for evidence of infection, and understanding that fever is a medical emergency. With a fever, nurses should anticipate clinician orders such as obtaining blood cultures from each lumen of a central line and antibiotic administration. Nursing care also includes providing emotional support to the patient and family during this vulnerable time period. Supportive care measures must be part of the nursing care plan. These measures, including managing pain (postoperative pain from surgical resection, a new central-line placement, advanced disease leading to pain), nausea, vomiting, constipation, fatigue, and mucositis.

OUTCOMES

Outcomes when caring for the child with cancer include safe chemotherapy administration, improved treatment delivery, and proper education for the patient and family regarding the diagnosis and treatment, minimizing side effects from therapy, improving the quality of life for the child, and monitoring for late effects of cancer treatment in the pediatric cancer survivor. Palliative care plays a crucial role for these children and their families. If a child reaches the end-of-life spectrum, outcomes include a safe transition to the end-of-life continuum, respecting and honoring the patient and family, and effective symptom management control.

Summary

Childhood cancer is rare, but the nurse caring for these children and families has a pivotal role from diagnosis through treatment and survivorship. Accurate physical exams, assessment of vital signs and potential complications, and recognizing anticipated side effects of therapy are crucial components for the oncology nurse.

American Cancer Society. (2016). What is cancer in children? Retrieved from http://www.cancer.org/cancer/cancerin children/detailedguide/cancer-in-children-key-statistics

Frangkandrea, J., Nixon, J. A., & Panagopoulou, P. (2013). Signs and symptoms of childhood cancer: A guide for early recognition. *American Family Physician, 88*(3), 195–192.

Kline, N. (Ed.). (2014). *Essentials of pediatric hematology/ oncology nursing.* Chicago, IL: Association of Pediatric Hematology/Oncology Nurses.

National Cancer Institute. (2016). Childhood cancers. Retrieved from https://www.cancer.gov/types/ childhood-cancers

■ CEREBRAL PALSY

Rachael Weigand

Overview

Cerebral palsy (CP) is defined as "a group of disorders of the development of movement and posture, causing activity limitation that are attributed to non-progressive disturbances that occurred in the developing foetal or infant brain. The motor disorders of CP are often accompanied by disturbances of sensation, cognition, communication, perception, or behavior, and may be accompanied by a seizure disorder" (Jackson Allen, Vessey, & Schapiro, 2010, p. 326). The damage to the brain is nonprogressive, however; the effects of CP can worsen with time, growth, and maturity.

Cerebral palsy occurs in approximately two out of every 1,000 births, and is the most common physical disability in childhood (Kirby et al., 2011). The incidence, prevalence, and most common causes of cerebral palsy vary over time because of continuing changes in prenatal and pediatric care. Cerebral palsy is a chronic disorder affecting multiple different body systems. Many different elements must be dealt with in order to manage the children diagnosed with this disorder, including motor disability.

Background

The classification of CP is based upon the type and distribution of the motor disruption. The damage occurs in the motor cortex and pyramidal tracts in the brain. The severity and distribution of the neurological impairments vary significantly among children. There are four types of movement disorders seen in children with CP. These types are spastic, dystonia, athetosis, and ataxia. Children can fall under a "mixed" category, but only if there is a clear description of each type of movement disorder present (Jackson Allen et al., 2010).

Spasticity is characterized by increased muscle tone and is the most common motor difficulty (Hasnat & Rice, 2015). Signs of spastic CP include persistent primitive reflexes, such as an ongoing Moro reflex, rooting reflex, palmar reflex, exaggerated stretch reflexes, positive Babinski reflex, ankle clonus, and development of contractures as the child grows (Jackson Allen et al., 2010). Spastic CP affects 70% to 80% of children with CP (Delgado et al., 2010). Spasticity can be further broken down based on limb distribution: diplegia, hemiplegia, or quadriplegia.

Diplegia refers to the dysfunction of all extremities with the lower extremities more affected than the upper extremities. Children with spastic diplegia may have relatively intact hand function (Patterson, 2016). *Hemiplegia* is dysfunction of one side of the body, with the upper extremity more affected that the lower extremity. *Quadriplegia* refers to all extremities affected by increased muscle tone. These quadriplegic children are often severely handicapped with deficits of intellectual disability, communication, vision, epilepsy, feeding difficulties, and possible pulmonary disease (Patterson, 2016).

Dystonia is defined as slow and twisting, abnormal movements of the trunk or extremities that may involve abnormal posturing and can remain in that position. Dystonia can occur in dyskinetic CP but also is commonly present in spastic CP. Dyskinesia is described as abnormal involuntary movements after initiation of voluntary movements. Children experience manifestations of rigid muscle tone when awake, although they experience decreased tone when asleep or idle. In athetosis, the basal ganglia are damaged, which is illustrated by slow, writhing movements. Choreoathetoisis is a form of athetosis that includes erratic, rapid, and random movements (Jackson Allen et al., 2010).

There are many risk factors that are associated with the development of CP. Risks can occur during prenatal period, birth, perinatal, childhood, or an unknown period. Prematurity and low birth weight represent the largest risk factors. In addition, risk factors that could be prevented include teratogens and infections during pregnancy. CP is multifactorial and many risk factors can contribute to its development (Jackson Allen et al., 2010). For babies who are born at full term, risks for CP development include placental abnormalities, birth defects, low birth weight, meconium aspiration, instrumental/emergency cesarean delivery, birth asphyxia, neonatal seizures, respiratory distress syndrome, hypoglycemia, and neonatal infection (McIntyre et al., 2012).

There are many associated problems related to CP, which include disabilities with motor function, cognitive function, feeding and nutrition, bowel and gastrostomy-tube dependence, bladder, dental, osteoporosis, pulmonary, skin, pain, behavior, and emotional and intellectual disability (Jackson Allen et al., 2010). Epilepsy occurs in about 25% to 45% of patients with CP, and seizures are most commonly seen in spastic quadriplegia and hemiplegia (Patterson, 2016). Children with CP can get tired or frustrated faster than other children without the disorder. Due to the prolonged reflexes, children can overreact to stimulation much more frequently. They also can become more demanding or uncooperative (Jackson Allen et al., 2010).

Clinical Aspects

ASSESSMENT

The evaluation of children who are suspected of CP begins with a thorough history and physical exam. CP is diagnosed based on physical, functional, and developmental abilities. There is no specific test confirming the diagnosis. Clinical manifestations noted are delayed gross motor development, abnormal cognitive performance, alterations of muscle tone, abnormal postures, reflex abnormalities, and other associated disabilities such as learning disability, seizures, and sensory impairment (Jackson Allen et al., 2010).

Specific clinical signs that warrant suspicion of CP include poor head control and clinched hands at 3 months, no side protective reflexes at 5 months, extended Moro and atonic neck reflexes past 6 months, no parachute reflex after 10 months, crossing of the midline to reach objects before 12 months, and hand preference before 18 months (Jackson Allen et al., 2010). Behavioral manifestations during infancy, such as irritability, weak cry, poor extraction, excessive sleep patterns, and little interest in surroundings, may indicate CP. A diagnosis is not given until the child is 18 to 24 months old due to development and the rapid changes that can occur. Research shows that it is difficult to diagnose a specific CP syndrome until around age 5 years, because many of the developmental milestones have not been reached so as to see the true delays caused by CP (Patterson, 2016).

NURSING INTERVENTIONS, MANAGEMENT, AND IMPLICATIONS

Children diagnosed with CP may experience impaired physical mobility related to decreased muscle strength and control, sensory/perceptual alteration related to cerebral damage, altered nutrition, and less-than-bodily requirements related to difficulty in chewing, swallowing, high metabolic needs, and seizure activity. Children may experience ineffective management of therapeutic regimens related to excessive demands made on the family. The children have complex care needs. They may experience diversional activity deficit related to poor social skills, altered learning, language development, and reasoning (Sparks & Taylor, 2011).

The first objective is the early identification of CP, and then to accelerate the process of referrals to the proper community resources (Liptak & Murphy 2011). Positive signs of CP that nurses may observe are ongoing primitive reflexes, and absent or delayed developmental milestones. Nurses need to be aware of the basic red flags that indicate CP.

Basic management of children with CP requires a patient- and family-centered medical home, physiotherapy, physical therapy, speech therapy, occupational therapy, and orthotics. Treatment goals are aimed at promoting social and emotional development, communication, education, nutrition, mobility, and maximal independence in activities of daily living (Patterson, 2016). After proper assessment of the child and the child's needs, interventions should be implemented beginning with the least invasive method. Studies show that effective treatments include medications; functional therapies, including physiotherapy, occupational therapy, speech therapy, and constraint-induced movement therapy; orthoses; casting and splinting; weight-bearing exercises; and multilevel orthopedic surgery (Jackson Allen et al., 2010).

The primary goal of management is to increase the child's function. Nurses should promote optimal growth and development, maximize joint range of motion, optimize muscle control and balance, provide means of communication and locomotion, and promote childhood independence (Jackson Allen et al., 2010). Research has also shown that the combination of interventions from all areas of management can improve a child's function, self-care, and activities of daily living.

Children with CP often struggle with dysphagia, and therefore may not meet nutritional requirements (Liptak & Murphy 2011). A child's ability to feed him- or herself can range based on the severity of the child's condition. The degree of oral motor function, however, may require tube feeding. Gastroesophageal reflux disease (GERD) is also common in children with this condition, and nurses should assess risk for aspiration. Educating families on this issue as well as

appropriate posture when eating is a key intervention. Drooling can be excessive and persistent in children with CP. Psychosocially, this excessive drooling can be embarrassing. Working with the children to help them swallow, remind them how to swallow, and assessment of posture (i.e., head control, positioning and mouth closure) can help to maintain secretions.

OUTCOMES

Evidence shows that high-quality health care for children with CP depends on collaborations among parents and health care providers, including dentists and community agencies (i.e., educational services, recreation programs, parent groups) with ongoing monitoring of the child's health and function (Liptak & Murphy, 2011, p. e1324). Optimizing health and well-being for children with CP and their families involves family-centered care provided in the medical home (Liptak & Murphy 2011). If an infant or child is hospitalized, the nurse should maintain the at-home regimen as much as possible.

There are a variety of notable responsibilities that a parent must take on when raising and caring for a child with CP. The first aspect addressed is the psychological effect on siblings and parents. There is a direct impact on the quality of life that affects the family members of the child who is suffering from CP. The family members often requires their own psychological help and support. The nurse should help guide children and their families in the right direction to help find a strong support system, including parent support and advocacy groups, respite programs, and community programs for recreational and adaptive sports (Liptak & Murphy 2011).

Summary

Cerebral palsy is the most common motor disability condition in children and adolescents. CP represents a distressing and difficult condition that is experienced by a multitude of families throughout the world. However, with proper treatment and care, this disease can be combated to preserve a high level of function and a suitable quality of life. Providers and families affected by this disease must work together in order to treat diagnosed children with the utmost personal, financial, and medical responsibility.

Delgado, M. R., Hirtz, D., Aisen, M., Ashwal, S., Fehlings, D. L., McLaughlin, J., . . . Vargus-Adams, J. (2010). Practice parameter: Pharmacologic treatment of spasticity in children and adolescents with cerebral palsy (an evidence-based review): Report of the Quality Standards Subcommittee of the American Academy of Neurology and the Practice Committee of the Child Neurology Society. *Neurology, 74,* 336–343. doi:10.1212/WNL.0b013e3181cbcd2f

Hasnat, M. J., & Rice, J. E. (2015). Intrathecal baclofen for treating spasticity in children with cerebral palsy. *Cochrane Database of Systematic Reviews, 2015*(11), CD004552. doi:10.1002/14651858.CD004552.pub2

Jackson Allen, P., Vessey J. A., & Schapiro, N. (2010). *Primary care of the child with a chronic condition* (5th ed., pp. 326–341). St. Louis, MO: Mosby.

Kirby, R., Wingate, M., VanNaarden Braun, K., Doernberg, M., Arneson, C., Benedict, R., ... Yeargin-Allsopp, M. (2011). Prevalence and functioning of children with cerebral palsy in four areas of the United States in 2006: A report from the Autism and Developmental Disabilities Monitoring Network. *Research in Developmental Disabilities, 32,* 462–469. doi:10.1016/j.ridd.2010.12.042

Liptak, G. S., & Murphy, N. A.; The Council on Children with Disabilities. (2011). Providing a primary care medical home for children and youth with cerebral palsy. *American Academy of Pediatrics, 128,* 1321–1329. doi:10.1542/peds.2011-1468

McIntyre, S., Taitz, D., Keogh, J., Goldsmith, S., Badawi, N., & Blair, E. (2012). A systematic review of risk factors for cerebral palsy in children born at term in developed countries. *Developmental Medicine & Child Neurology, 55,* 499–508. doi:10.1111/dmcn.12017

Patterson, M. C. (2016). Clinical features and classification of cerebral palsy. *UpToDate.* Retrieved from http://www.uptodate.com/content/clinical-features-and-classification-of-cerebral-palsy

Sparks, S., & Taylor, C. M. (2011). *Nursing diagnosis pocket guide.* Philadelphia, PA: Lippincott Williams & Wilkins.

■ CYSTIC FIBROSIS

Karen Vosper

Overview

Cystic fibrosis (CF) is a complex and multisystem disease, characterized by thickened tenacious secretions in the respiratory tract, sweat glands, gastrointestinal tract, pancreas, and other exocrine tissue. It is the most common life-shortening autosomal recessive disorder of the exocrine glands. Typical respiratory manifestations of CF include persistent, productive cough, difficulty in clearing secretions and frequent respiratory infections. Typical gastrointestinal manifestations include large bulky malodorous stools; impaired absorption of fat, protein and carbohydrates resulting in poor weight gain and growth and malnutrition; and excess losses of sodium and chloride in sweat (National Heart, Lung, and Blood Institute, 2016).

Background

In the United States, CF occurs in approximately one in 3,000 Caucasians, predominately of European decent; one in 9,200 Hispanics; one in 10,900 Native Americans; one in 15,000 African Americans; and one in 100,000 Asian Americans (Lahiri et al., 2016). Gender is not a factor in the disease incidence. Median predicted survival for CF patients in the United States in 2015 was 41.6 years (95% confidence interval: 38.5–44.0 years) and the median age at death was 29.1. Overall, 5% of deaths occur in individuals younger than age 13 (Cystic Fibrosis Foundation, 2015). Although CF is a multisystem disease, lung involvement is the major cause of morbidity and more than 90% of mortality.

The gene that causes CF was discovered in 1989 and is located on the long arm of chromosome 7, known as the *CF transmembrane regulator* (*CFTR*) gene (Stern, 2006). People with CF either have too few CFTR proteins at the cell surface, CFTR proteins that don't work properly, or both. The defective CFTR proteins result in poor flow of salt and water into and out of the cells. As a result, abnormally thick and sticky mucus forms and obstructs the epithelial tissues throughout the body, such as the lungs, sinuses, pancreas, intestine, reproductive system, and sweat glands—thick and sticky airway secretions, a combination of mucus and pus, build up in the lungs causing chronic lung infections and progressive lung damage. In the gastrointestinal tract, there is a reduced ability to absorb nutrients and digestive enzymes from the pancreas that are critical to the breakdown and absorption of fats and calories, and nutrients do not reach the small intestine, resulting in malabsorption, steatorrhea, and malnutrition (Davis, 2006).

The sweat test is considered the gold standard for diagnosing CF. The sweat test can be done on an individual of any age. The sweat test generally has three technical parts: localized sweat stimulation induced by iontophoresis of pilocarpine, collection, and analysis. The preferred site for sweat collection is the flexor surface of the forearm. The chance of uticaria or burn to the skin after iontophoresis is possible. For all patients, sweat chloride values greater than or equal to 60 mmol/L are considered positive for CF. A positive result on the sweat chloride test indicates that CF is nearly certain (Collie, Massie, Jones, LeGrys, & Greaves, 2014).

Currently, all 50 states and the District of Columbia screen newborns for CF, but the method for screening may differ from state to state. All screening algorithms in current use in the United States rely on testing for immunoreactive trypsinogen (IRT) as the primary screen for CF. The presence of high levels of IRT, typically elevated in CF-affected infants, indicates the need for a second tier of testing, which determines the positive or negative outcome of the screen. The second-tier testing relies on IRT again or DNA testing. All babies with a positive newborn screen will be required to have a confirmatory sweat test. As a characteristic of all newborn screening (NBS), most infants with a positive CF NBS result will not have CF (Farrell, et al., 2008).

Clinical Aspects

ASSESSMENT

Assessment of the child with CF focuses on respiratory and gastrointestinal function. Typical respiratory manifestations of CF include a persistent cough, cough with sputum production, and pulmonary function tests consistent with obstructive airway disease. Onset of clinical symptoms varies widely due to differences in *CFTR* genotype and other individual factors, but pulmonary function abnormalities often are detectable even in the absence of symptoms. As the disease progresses, chronic bronchitis and progressive bronchiectasis develop and are accompanied by acute exacerbations, characterized by increased cough, tachypnea, increased sputum production, malaise, anorexia, and weight loss. Digital clubbing is often seen in patients with moderate to advanced lung disease. Clinicians need to inquire about the frequency and character of the patient's cough as well as the quality and quantity of sputum production. Auscultation of the chest for breath sounds, crackles, and wheezes accompanies assessment of respiratory rate, work of breathing, use of accessory muscles position of comfort, any cyanosis or clubbing of the extremities.

NURSING INTERVENTIONS, MANAGEMENT, AND IMPLICATIONS

Nurses in the outpatient, inpatient, home care, and school settings need to help others understand the increased calorie and salt requirements of those with

CF and support the plan of care. Maintaining infection control practices in the primary care provider's office, schools, and hospital setting is the key to minimizing the risk for acquisition and spread of pathogens. The nurse is in a position to help people with CF and their families fit the complex medical care into their daily routines. Promoting health, quality of life, and education about the signs and symptoms of potential problems is a primary focus of a nurse.

Management of CF focuses on minimizing pulmonary complications, promoting growth and development, and facilitating coping and adjustment of the child and family. Early intervention and monitoring for respiratory and gastrointestinal disease in children with CF is vital to improve outcomes. Evidence-based nutrition goals and pulmonary and nutritional care guidelines for children with CF have been published by the CF Foundation. More than 85% of patients are pancreatic insufficient at birth and others often gradually loose function over time. If the patient is taking pancreatic enzymes, evaluating response to enzymes should be a routine part of the nutritional assessment. Inquire about pancreatic enzyme dose and amount, appetite, weight loss, stool history, steatorrhea, flatus, abdominal bloating, constipation, and abdominal pain.

For infants and children with CF, airway clearance at least twice daily is a critical intervention that is increased during illness. Airway clearance for infants involves manual percussion, vibration, and postural drainage. For older infants and children, a high-frequency chest compression vest may be used. Inhaled hypertonic saline may be used to assist with mobilization of secretions. Inhaled recombinant human DNase (Pulmozyme) is given daily to decrease sputum viscosity and help clear secretions. Inhaled bronchodilators and anti-inflammatory agents are prescribed for some children. Aerosolized antibiotics are often prescribed and may be given in the home as well as in the hospital. *Pseudomonas aeruginosa* has been long recognized as a significant pathogen in the disease progression. Other pathogens can lead to worsening symptoms and can speed the decline in lung function (Lahiri et al., 2016).

Pancreatic enzymes must be administered with all meals and snacks to promote adequate digestion and absorption of nutrients. In the infant and young child, the enzymes capsule can be opened and mixed with a small amount of applesauce. Supplemental fat-soluble vitamins are prescribed to promote adequate digestion and absorption of nutrients, and optimize nutritional status. Increased-calorie, high-protein diets are recommended, and sometimes supplemental high-calorie formula, either oral or via tube feeding, is needed. It can be difficult to maintain a schedule that requires hours of treatments daily as well as close attention to a high-calorie diet, enzyme supplementation, vitamins, and oral and aerosolized antibiotics (Schindler et al., 2005).

OUTCOMES

The expected outcomes for CF respiratory management are aimed at slowing the progression of the lung disease, minimizing pulmonary complications, maximizing lung function, and preventing infection. The expected outcomes of evidence-based nutritional goals are centered on maintaining 50th percentile weight/length from birth to 24 months and body mass index (BMI) at the 50th percentile for 2 to 20 years of age (Schindler, Mitchell, & Wilson, 2005).

Summary

Advances in science have led to increased survival among patients with CF such that currently, nearly half of the CF population in the United States is older than age 18 years, which far exceeds survival rates of previous decades. The disease demands significant adaptations by children and their families, many of which can be challenging and stressful. Families commonly face a set of significant obstacles accessing CF care. Obtaining and maintaining adequate health insurance, paying for prescription medications, disease-related out of pocket expenses, lost work days as well as travel to specialists and CF care centers can tax family resources. Delays in or denial of coverage for medications and treatment can be extremely difficult.

Children face their own challenges associated with medication and nutrition regimens, pulmonary therapy, missed school days due to illness, and difficulty engaging in extracurricular activities with peers, often resulting in a sense of social isolation. Affective partnerships among children, families, clinicians, and community agencies are critical to quality of life and sustained health. The nurse plays an essential and long-lasting role throughout the life of a person with CF contributing direct care, advocacy, and education to help each individual achieve his or her best health and quality of life.

Collie, J. T. B., Massie, J. R., Jones, O. A. H., LeGrys, V. A., & Greaves, R. F. (2014). Sixty-five years since the New York heat wave: Advances in sweat testing for cystic fibrosis. *Pediatric Pulmonology, 2014*(49), 106–117.

Cystic Fibrosis Foundation. (2015). Patient registry annual data report. Retrieved from https://www.cff.org/Our -Research/CF-Patient-Registry/2015-Patient-Registry -Annual-Data-Report.pdf

Davis, P. B. (2006). Cystic fibrosis since 1938. *American Journal of Respiratory and Critical Care Medicine, 173*(5), 475–482.

Farrell, P. M., Rosenstein, B. J., White, T. B., Accurso, F. J., Castellani, C., Cutting, G. R., . . . Campbell, P. W. (2008). Guidelines for diagnosis of cystic fibrosis in newborns through older adults: Cystic Fibrosis Foundation Consensus Report. *Journal of Pediatrics, 153*, S4–S14.

Lahiri, T., Hempstead, S. E., Brady, C., Cannon, C. L., Clark, K., Condren, M. E., . . . Davis, S. D. (2016). Clinical practice guidelines from the cystic fibrosis foundation for preschoolers with cystic fibrosis. *Pediatrics, 3*(22), Retrieved from https://pediatrics.aappublications.org/ content/early/2016/03/22/peds.2015-1784

National Heart, Lung, and Blood Institute. (2016). What are the signs and symptoms of cystic fibrosis? Retrieved from https://www.nhlbi.nih.gov/health/health-topics/ topics/cf/signs

Schindler, T., Mitchell, S., & Wilson, A. (2005). Nutrition management of cystic fibrosis in the 21st century. *Nutrition in Clinical Practice, 30*(4), 488–500.

Stern, R. (2006). The diagnosis of cystic fibrosis. *New England Journal of Medicine, 336*(7), 487.

■ DEVELOPMENTALLY APPROPRIATE COMMUNICATION

Nanci M. Berman

Overview

Developmentally appropriate communication applies skills of communication that are aligned with the developmental stage of the patient as defined by the theoretical frameworks of Piaget, Erikson, and Freud (Ball, Bindler, & Cowen, 2013, 2014). Effective, developmentally appropriate communication can affect the emotional well-being, medical compliance, and preparation of the patient to care for themselves into adulthood (Bell & Condren, 2016; Brand, Fasciano, & Mack, 2016). Developmentally appropriate communication in nursing keeps the patient at the center of triadic communication between nurse, parent, and child, which is a unique factor within the pediatric population (Brand et al., 2016).

Background

Communication is a process whereby the sender encodes a message, which is sent to the receiver, who decodes the message and responds, providing feedback to the original sender for decoding (D'Amico & Barbarito, 2015). Communication can have positive and negative effects on behavior. In pediatric nursing, the way the message is encoded and sent can make a significant difference in the behavior and emotion, which result during decoding. The patient's developmental age and previous experience contribute to his or her ability to decode information (Bell & Condren, 2016). Nurses who identify the patient's developmental age and exhibit appropriate approaches to interactions and communication gain a greater trust from the parent/caregiver and have a greater effect on the future nurse-to-patient encounters (Salmani, Abbaszadeh, & Rassouli, 2014). These encounters provide an opportunity to build and sustain a relationship that provides mutual respect between patient, parent, and nurse, each in his or her significant role promoting well-being and providing care (Salmani et al., 2014).

Communication can be verbal, nonverbal, or abstract. Verbal communication includes pace, intonation, simplicity, clarity, timing, and adaptability that accompanies the spoken words (Ball et al., 2013; Pearson Education, 2015). Nonverbal communication, posture, gait, facial expression, and gestures can be interpreted during the process of communication to be supportive or contradictory to verbal communication (Ball et al., 2013; Pearson Education, 2015). Verbal and nonverbal messages should be consistent and congruent in order for the nurse to gain trust and credibility. Children who play with dolls or cars as they see others do, or teenagers who dress to make a statement, are exhibiting abstract communication (Ball et al., 2013).

Therapeutic communication is the process of interacting and sharing information within a professional–patient relationship; for the purpose of this discussion, the focus is on the relationship between nurse and child or nurse and family. This relationship is founded on mutual respect and trust between the patient/parent and nurse (Pearson Education, 2015). Therapeutic communication includes verbal and nonverbal communication, which is meaningful and adjusted to the situation. Techniques include use of broad open-ended statements, active listening, physical presence, and clarification (Pearson Education, 2015).

Clinical Aspects

ASSESSMENT

Developmentally appropriate communication is specific to the patient's developmental and cognitive age, which may differ from one's chronological age. Humans communicate from birth, initially with cries, followed by pointing and grunting, and proceeding eventually to putting words together to create meaningful sentences. Communication aids in alleviating fears, building trusting relationships, and developing confidence to sustain treatment plans. Erik Erikson's theory of psychosocial development and Jean Piaget's theory of cognitive development are most often utilized as frameworks for nursing care of the pediatric patient. Erikson (1979) categorizes the stages of psychosocial development as birth to 1 year of age: trust versus mistrust; ages 1 to 3 years: autonomy versus shame and doubt; ages 3 to 6 years: initiative versus guilt; ages 6 to 12 years: industry versus inferiority; and ages 12 to 18 years: identity versus role confusion. Piaget (1976) provides four stages of cognitive development: birth to 2 years: sensory motor; ages 2 to 7 years: preoperational; ages 7 to 11 years: concrete operational; and 12 years of age and older: formal operational.

In order to organize the following presentation of a developmentally appropriate approach to communication, Erikson and Piaget's stages are combined. Examples are presented for the newborn, infant, toddler and preschooler, school-age child, and adolescent. Newborns communicate with cries to get their basic needs, such as feeding, clean clothes, and comfort, met (Ball et al., 2013). Human voice and touch and kangaroo care gain a greater importance for this stage, especially for those born prematurely (Ball et al., 2013). Infants continue to need comforting touch and predominately communicate nonverbally, making it important for nurses caring for this patient to use voice inflection and facial expression to engage (Ball et al., 2013). Toddlers and preschoolers need time to process their thoughts without interruptions and are gaining their independence, requiring time commitments from the nurse (Ball et al., 2013). Nurses who provide simple responses, simple directions, and choices that result in the acceptable decision of the child, while carving out time for responses, will allow for the greatest exchange with this age group. School-age children are exploring the world around them, initiating activities, and engaging in groups (Ball et al., 2013). Patients at this stage like to take part in decisions that affect them. Nurses should clarify the extent of patient involvement in decision making prior to initiating conversations (Brand et al., 2016). Communicating at the same physical level of the patient and including the patient in a conversation allows the patient the ability to answer the question, allowing the parent/caregiver to answer after the patient offering any required clarification (Ball et al., 2013). Adolescents are seeking their position into adulthood (Ball et al., 2013). Nurses should build a rapport with this age group by active listening and presenting a nonjudgmental attitude.

NURSING INTERVENTIONS, MANAGEMENT, AND IMPLICATIONS

Adjustments of the approach and techniques for communication may vary based on the physiological, psychological, and emotional state of the patient. For example, patients diagnosed with autism spectrum disorder, attention deficit disorder, mental retardation, or developmental delay requiring an adjustment to the approach may combine skills from more than one stage to produce meaningful communication, trust, and respect. As another example, children with chronic conditions may regress to an earlier stage or mature to a higher cognitive or developmental stage that requires tailoring to individual needs.

OUTCOMES

Outcomes of developmentally appropriate communication are increasingly reported. Relationship-based care provides an example of an approach to improving patient safety, satisfaction, and motivation, which are grounded in trusting relationships with a foundation in developmentally appropriate, highly individualized communication (Bell & Condren, 2016). Research has established that patients are more likely to take appropriate doses of medication at the correct intervals for the prescribed amount of time when their education is presented in ways that are appropriate for their stage of cognition and development (Bell & Condren, 2016).

Summary

Nurses play an integral role in the relationship, satisfaction, and adherence to medical treatment, and are more effective when they apply developmentally appropriate communication and approaches with patients. As children mature and seek input into their medical care,

shared decision-making frameworks should be considered as a means to maintain the therapeutic relationship, promote satisfaction, and achieve adherence to treatment plans.

Ball, J. W., Bindler, R. C., & Cowen, K. J. (2013). *Child health nursing: Partnering with children and families* (3rd ed.). Upper Saddle River, NJ: Pearson.

Ball, J. W., Bindler, R. C., & Cowen, K. J. (2014). *Principles of pediatric nursing: Caring for children* (6th ed.). Upper Saddle River, NJ: Pearson.

Bell, J., & Condren, M. (2016). Communication strategies for empowering and protecting children. *Journal of Pediatric Pharmacology and Therapeutics*, 21(2), 176–184. doi:10.5863/1551-6776-21.2.176

Brand, S. R., Fasciano, K., & Mack, J. W. (2016). Communication preferences of pediatric cancer patients: Talking about prognosis and their future life. *Support Care Cancer*, 10, 769–774. doi:10.1007/s00520-016-3458-x

D'Amico, D. T., & Barbarito, C. (2015). *Health and physical assessment in nursing* (3rd ed.). Upper Saddle River, NJ: Pearson.

Erikson, E. (1979). *Childhood and society* (2nd ed.). New York, NY: W. W. Norton.

Pearson Education. (2015). *Nursing a concept-based approach to learning* (2nd ed.). Upper Saddle River, NJ: Pearson.

Piaget, J. (1976). *The child and reality: Problems of genetic psychology* (A. Rosin, Trans.). New York, NY: Grossman.

Salmani, N., Abbaszadeh, A., & Rassouli, M. (2014). Factors creating trust in hospitalized children's mothers towards nurses. *Iranian Journal of Pediatrics*, 24(6), 729–738. Retrieved from https://www.ncbi.nlm.nih.gov/pmc/articles/PMC4442835/pdf/IJP-24-729.pdf

■ DIABETES

Julia E. Blanchette

Overview

Diabetes mellitus (DM) is a chronic metabolic disorder in which the body does not metabolize carbohydrates, fats, and proteins because of progressive loss or function of pancreatic beta cells resulting in hyperglycemia (American Diabetes Association [ADA], 2017). The majority of pediatric patients with diabetes have type 1 diabetes (T1D), though some have type 2 diabetes (T2D) or other forms (ADA, 2017). Despite medical advances, a majority of children with T1D do not obtain optimal glycemic control resulting in higher mortality rates, shortened average life spans, and risk of long-term complications (ADA, 2017; Juvenile Diabetes Research Foundation [JDRF], 2016). Nurses focus on the prevention of decline in health status and future complications. Care delivery is focused on family-centered self-management care to maintain optimal and safe glycemic control for children with DM (ADA, 2017).

Background

There are more than 200,000 Americans younger than the age of 20 years living with T1D (JDRF, 2016). Over the past decade, there has been a 21% increase in the prevalence of childhood T1D (CDC, 2014; JDRF, 2016). The annual increase in the prevalence of childhood T2D is expected to quadruple in the next 40 years (CDC, 2014). Both types of DM are polygenic and have many disease progression factors (ADA, 2017). Common environmental factors associated with the development of T1D and T2D include dietary factors, endocrine disruption, environmental toxins, gut microbiome composition, and infection (ADA, 2017). Children who are at risk for T1D are those who have a family member with T1D or autoimmune diseases such as celiac disease or Hashimoto's thyroiditis (ADA, 2017). A majority are Caucasian and have inherited complex risk factors from both the parents though there may be no prior family history of DM (ADA, 2017). Children at risk for T2D include the following: those who have a body mass index (BMI) greater than the 85th percentile for gender and age; weight greater than the 120% for ideal height; a family history of T2D in first- and second-degree relatives; and are Native American, African American, Hispanic, or Asian/South Pacific Islander ethnicity (ADA, 2017).

The onset of T1D occurs suddenly and most frequently in children younger than 4 years and during adolescence (ADA, 2017). It is a multifactorial disease caused by autoimmune destruction of insulin-producing pancreatic beta cells in those who are predisposed to it (ADA, 2017). Hyperglycemia, or increased blood glucose, occurs due to decreased secretion of insulin (ADA, 2017). Fat is then used as an energy source when glucose is unavailable to the cells for metabolism, causing diabetes ketoacidosis (DKA), an acute life-threatening form of metabolic acidosis, which presents in at least one third of T1D onset (ADA, 2017). The onset of T2D is less common than T1D in childhood and occurs due to insulin resistance and the relative decrease in insulin secretion resulting in elevated glucose levels (ADA, 2017). Insulin resistance occurs when the body is less able to utilize insulin resulting in reduced absorption of glucose into the cells for fuel (ADA, 2017). Insulin resistance causes excess production of glucose from the liver and dysfunction or total loss of function of the pancreatic beta cells (ADA, 2017).

Diabetes management for optimal glycemic control includes insulin administration, blood glucose monitoring, carbohydrate counting, treatment of hyperglycemia, treatment of hypoglycemia, exercise, nutrition therapy, family counseling, stress management, and self-monitoring of trends in insulin requirement and glucose levels (ADA, 2017). In the hospital, diabetes management includes a monitored initiation of insulin therapy via hospital protocol, fluid replacement, and family-centered diabetes education (ADA, 2017). Basal and bolus insulin administration occur through intravenous lines (IVs), insulin pumps, insulin syringe, or insulin pen. Basal insulin delivers a continuous insulin in small doses over a 24-hour period (ADA, 2017). Basal administration occurs via infusion of rapid-acting or one daily dose of long-acting insulin analogs (ADA, 2017). Bolus insulin is for hyperglycemia and carbohydrate corrections, and is determined based on the patient's weight and blood sugar targets; a sliding scale regimen is strongly discouraged for inpatient settings (ADA, 2017). However, those with T2D may not be insulin dependent and may have tailored pharmacological treatment such as administration of metformin and increased physical activity (ADA, 2017).

Despite knowledge of risk factors, medical advances and technology advances in diabetes care, children with DM still have higher mortality rates due to complications than the rest of the population especially during pubertal years due to increased insulin sensitivity (ADA, 2017). Of the children living with DM, fewer than one third obtain the recommended glycemic control targets, placing them at high risk for DKA and complications (JDRF, 2015).

Clinical Aspects

ASSESSMENT

The child's history, key physical assessment findings, and laboratory data are vital components of nursing care for children with DM. Children with both types of DM often present with polydipsia, polyphagia, blurred vision, and polyuria (ADA, 2017). Many children present with weight loss and flu-like symptoms, which have been present for several weeks (ADA, 2017). Diagnosis of DM in children occurs when symptoms manifest, and A1C is greater than or equal to 6.5%, a casual plasma glucose level is greater than or equal to 200 mg/dL, or a fasting plasma glucose level is greater than or equal to 126 mg/dL (ADA, 2017). Though DM diagnosis occurs under the same glycemic criteria, classification of the type of diabetes is important in determining therapy. Children with T2D may have conditions or signs associated with insulin resistance such as acanthosis nigricans (dark velvety patches) on the skin folds, hypertension, dyslipidemia, polycystic ovarian syndrome, history of small for gestational age at birth, or maternal history of gestational DM (ADA, 2017). Children at risk should be screened every 3 years after the age of 10 or at the onset of puberty if DM occurs earlier (ADA, 2017). Those with T2D do not typically present with DKA (ADA, 2017).

Physical assessment for a hospitalized child with DM should focus on detecting and preventing DKA. Children with T1D often present with DKA at diagnosis though infection, insulin pump failure, expired insulin, omission of insulin and inadequate insulin, mental health issues, and lack of family or social support after trauma or after surgery (ADA, 2017). Assessment should focus on the following: changes in the cardiovascular system (hypotension, arrhythmias, widening pulse rate), respiratory system (Kussmaul respirations, respiratory rate, acid–base disturbance), neurologic system (pupillary changes, altered level of consciousness), and integumentary system (dry mucous membranes, sunken eyes, decreased skin turgor; ADA, 2017). A child in DKA may also complain of abdominal pain, nausea, vomiting, and have fruity breath (ADA, 2017). Diagnosis of DKA occurs when plasma glucose is greater than 250 mg/dL, arterial pH is greater than 7.3, serum bicarbonate is greater than 15 mEq/L, and moderate or greater ketonuria is present (ADA, 2017). Management of DKA includes isotonic IV fluids, electrolyte replacement, regular IV insulin (0.1 unit/kg/hr), potassium supplementation, and phosphate supplementation (ADA, 2017). If cerebral edema occurs, it must be treated with mannitol (ADA, 2017).

Blood glucose is monitored at least every hour and is managed based on hospital protocols to prevent hyperglycemia and hypoglycemia (ADA, 2017). Young children may not be able to communicate hypoglycemia symptoms efficiently. In addition, children with complications may have hypoglycemia unawareness (ADA, 2017). Children who are not new to diabetes may have continuous blood glucose monitors to prevent hypoglycemia unawareness. The child is not required to take off a continuous monitor though one should still monitor the child's blood glucose via the hospital's policy.

A plan for preventing and treating hypoglycemia (blood glucose below 70 mg/dL) is established for each patient, and episodes are documented (ADA, 2017). Signs of hypoglycemia include sudden heart palpitations, fatigue, pallor, shakiness, anxiety, diaphoresis, hunger, and irritability (ADA, 2017). Hypoglycemia occurs from a sudden reduction of corticosteroids, reduced oral intake, extra insulin, and increased physical activity (ADA, 2017). It typically requires treatment of 15 g of fast-acting carbohydrates and when the blood sugar rises, a complex carbohydrate (ADA, 2017). If a patient is unresponsive with severe hypoglycemia (under 40 mg/dL), glucagon or IV dextrose may be administered.

NURSING INTERVENTIONS, MANAGEMENT, AND IMPLICATIONS

Nursing care of the hospitalized child with DM should focus on prevention of DKA and severe hypoglycemia. Priority nursing-related problems include imbalanced nutrition less than body's requirements, fluid volume deficit, the risk of injury (for hypoglycemia), the risk of infection, fatigue, and knowledge deficit related to new diabetes diagnosis or self-management skills.

Evidence-based practice supports interventions to improve glycemic control. According to evidence-based practice, diabetes self-management education includes medical nutrition therapy and psychosocial support at diagnosis and regularly thereafter in a developmentally appropriate manner. These interventions result in a less-frequent decline in health status and improved glycemic control (ADA, 2017). The use of a team-based approach and shared decision making between the youth and family members results in improved diabetes self-efficacy, protocol adherence, and positive metabolic outcomes (ADA, 2017). In addition, evidence-based practice suggests that the child should have periodic assessments to determine the need for self-care skills education. Premature transfer of diabetes care from the parent to the child can result in nonadherence and deterioration in glycemic control (ADA, 2017). Psychosocial and family issues should also be assessed to ensure that adherence to diabetes self-management is not impacted; early detection of depression, anxiety, and eating disorders can minimize adverse effects on diabetes management and improve glycemic control (ADA, 2017).

OUTCOMES

The results of evidence-based nursing care are to incorporate family-centered self-management to reach optimal glycemic control to prevent DKA and severe hypoglycemia. Monitoring for changes in physical assessment and blood glucose changes can provide evidence for intervening with blood glucose levels. It is vital to monitor children's blood glucose levels frequently, and to pay attention to signs and symptoms of decline in health status.

Summary

Treatment plans for optimal glycemic outcomes incorporate family dynamics, mental health, developmental readiness, and physiological changes. Hospitalized children with DM can rapidly progress into DKA or severe hypoglycemia if not monitored and managed appropriately. Changes in glucose and insulin patterns can be related to physical growth, puberty, insulin pump failure, a decline in mental health, and children beginning to provide their own self-care. Educating families to recognize these developmental changes and the signs and symptoms of DKA, hyperglycemia, and hypoglycemia are vital in the prevention of poor health outcomes.

American Diabetes Association. (2017). Standards of medical care in diabetes—2017. *Diabetes Care, 40*(1), S4–S5. doi:10.2337/dc14-S014

Centers for Disease Control and Prevention. (2014). National diabetes statistics report, 2014. Retrieved from https://www.cdc.gov/diabetes/pdfs/library/diabetes reportcard2014.pdf

Juvenile Diabetes Research Foundation. (2015). JDRF 2015 annual report. Retrieved from http://www.jdrf.org/annualreport/2015

Juvenile Diabetes Research Foundation. (2016). JDRF 2016 annual report. Retrieved from http://www.jdrf.org/annualreport/2016/html5/index.html?page=1&noflash

■ FAILURE TO THRIVE

Mary Alice Dombrowski

Overview

Failure to thrive (FTT) describes the occurrence of insufficient weight gain over a period of time. Although there are varying definitions, commonly used criteria for FTT includes a consistent weight less than the 3% to 5% on the standardized growth curve, and/or crossing over two major percentiles with consecutive measurement over a period of time (Jaffe, 2011; Keane, 2015). Although FTT can occur in any age group, FTT in pediatrics is typically reserved to describe poor weight gain during the first 2 to 3 years of life. Untreated FTT is associated with poor linear growth (height), disease, behavioral challenges, and cognitive delay. All children, regardless of socioeconomic status or race, should be monitored for FTT. Careful nursing assessment, application of appropriate nursing intervention, and comprehensive parental education are essential components of nursing care. Successful and early interventions have life-long implications for improved mental and physical health (Cole & Lanham, 2011; Kirkland, Motil, & Duryea, 2015).

Background

In the United States, FTT occurs in approximately 5% to 10% of children in primary care settings, and 3% to 5% of those in the hospital setting (Cole & Lanham, 2011; Kirkland et al., 2015). Eighty percent of children present with FTT in the first 18 months of life (Cole & Lanham, 2011). Poor linear growth, a natural consequence of early FTT, is estimated to be much higher throughout the world, especially in developing countries given poor access to adequate nutrition and medical care (Karra, Subramanian, & Fink, 2016). Gender is affected equally (Habibzadeh, Jafarizadeh, & Didarloo, 2015). During this period of critical brain growth, untreated FTT can lead to significant developmental delay (Jaffe, 2011; McLean & Price, 2015). FTT may occur secondary to underlying biological, psychosocial, and environmental circumstances, or a combination of these circumstances (Jaffe, 2011; Kirkland et al., 2015). Regardless of its contributing factors, FTT occurs when there are too little calories ingested to meet energy demands of the body (Jaffe, 2011).

Biological risk factors may begin prenatally. Intrauterine growth retardation and exposure to a harmful substance in utero puts an infant at risk for developing FTT. Children born with chromosomal disorders or birth defects, such as cleft lip, can have early challenges with feeding mechanics. Others may have medical conditions with high-energy demands (i.e., heart disease, chronic infection, or endocrine disorders) or poor intestinal absorption (i.e., cystic fibrosis, short bowel syndrome) necessitating high-calorie diets (Jaffe, 2011; McLean & Price, 2015).

Many psychosocial conditions contribute to the development of FTT. Children raised in poverty with little food or poor living conditions may find it difficult to obtain food (Habibzadeh et al., 2015). Parents with mental illness, addiction, poor education (Habibzadeh et al., 2015), or little social support are at increased risk of having children with FTT. Lack of parental guidance and role modeling may encourage children to develop disordered eating patterns (Jaffe, 2011; McLean & Price, 2015) or choose foods with little nutritional value. Often, parents have unrealistic expectations regarding food. Some very young children develop phobias associated with eating (Kirkland et al., 2015).

Many children with FTT are not identified or go untreated. Poor access to medical care, no or limited insurance, inaccurate measurements, or dismissal of growth concerns by primary care providers prevent children from receiving nutritional intervention. Untreated FTT may cause growth stunting, immune disorders, medical complications, developmental delay, and lower cognitive function throughout the life span (Jaffe, 2011; Kaneshiro, 2016). There is even some evidence that early FTT increases the likelihood of hostility as an adult (Jaffe, 2011). Interventions include aggressive nutritional supplementation, family education (Jaffe, 2011; McLean & Price, 2015), and sometimes, medications like cyproheptadine are used to stimulate appetite (Sant'Ana et al., 2014).

Clinical Aspects

ASSESSMENT

Assessment of FTT is multifaceted and includes careful consideration of the child, family, and environment. Medical history, including complications of pregnancy and labor, gestational age, birth weight, birth length, and birth head circumference should be obtained as well as newborn screening results. Feeding method, food intolerances, feeding difficulties, vomiting, diarrhea, sleep difficulties, history of illness, and achievement of developmental milestones should be recorded. Caregiver cultural beliefs and feeding practices should be discussed. Parental ability to make formula or food, feeding routine, and family living conditions as well as other child care providers are important factors to consider in FTT (Wilson, 2015; McLean & Price, 2015).

The most important aspect of the physical exam includes appropriate measurement of weight, length, and head circumference. Infants and toddlers should be undressed and in dry diapers before measurement. Measurements need to be plotted on the appropriate pediatric growth chart, the World Health Organization (WHO) growth chart is used for children 2 years and under, whereas the Centers for Disease Control and Prevention (CDC) growth chart is used for children older than age 2 years (Keane, 2015). Medical conditions associated with unique growth patterns, including prematurity, Down syndrome, or Turner syndrome, have their own charts, which should be used (Jaffe, 2011). Physical exam findings common in FTT include small head size and prominent forehead (Keane, 2017), thin appearance, decreased activity, thin hair, and rash. Bruising, burns, or scaring may be signs of physical abuse. The child may appear to have a syndrome face suggesting an underlying genetic condition. Mouth mucous membranes may appear dry, teeth discolored, and atypical smelling breath. Abdomens may look distended and bowel sounds may be more or less active. Genitals should be examined for trauma. Infant muscle tone, ability to suck and swallow, and quality of movement must be documented. Behaviors of concern include inability to meet eyes and poor responsiveness to visual, verbal, or tactile stimuli (Wilson, 2015). There is very little evidence to support the use of laboratory testing in FTT; however, it may be used to screen for other associated conditions of poor nutrition, including anemia and celiac disease (McLean & Price, 2015). The practitioner may want to consider reviewing a complete blood count, comprehensive metabolic panel, and stool studies for fats and reducing substances (Jaffe, 2011; McLean & Price, 2017).

NURSING INTERVENTIONS, MANAGEMENT, AND IMPLICATIONS

The primary nursing problem is ensuring the child's nutritional needs are being met. Nursing interventions should focus on identifying contributing factors to pediatric FTT, correcting the child's nutrition deficit, and addressing parental educational and social needs. Nursing interventions include parental education regarding growth and development, assisting health care providers in developing plan of care, implementing the plan of care, and encouraging parental participation in feeding goals. In many cases, this involves parent education and setting realistic short- and long-term goals for weight gain. Implementing a plan of care may include demonstrating proper mixing and administration of infant or toddler formula, placement and assessment of nasogastric tube placement, assessment of gastrostomy tube sites, management of enteral feeding, and administration of medications used to stimulate appetite (Wilson, 2015; Sparks Ralph & Taylor, 2014). Depending on contributing factors and circumstances of FTT, nursing diagnoses may include insufficient breast milk, ineffective breastfeeding, ineffective infant feeding pattern, imbalanced nutrition, less than body requirements, impaired swallowing, risk for electrolyte imbalance, feeding self-care deficit, impaired parenting, risk for disproportionate growth, and risk for delayed development (Sparks Ralph & Taylor, 2014).

OUTCOMES

Weight gain is the primary expected outcome for pediatric FTT. Also, parents should be able to describe weight goals and interventions to achieve those goals. Nursing interventions include ensuring that the child receives adequate nutrition and/or working with a team of providers to correct underlying obstacles to obtaining adequate nutrition. This may include intensive parental nutrition and feeding skills education, working with the medical team to treat underlying medical conditions, addressing social factors, providing home nursing visits, and, in some cases, assisting with the removal of the child from its home (McLean & Price, 2015).

Summary

Pediatric FTT occurs when there is insufficient caloric intake, and its effects may lead to poor cognitive and physical health outcomes for the child. Its etiology is often multifaceted and stems from underlying biological and psychosocial circumstances. Primary nursing goals include correction of nutritional deficiency and family education. Successful interventions and corrected nutritional deficiencies have lifelong implications for improved mental and physical health.

Cole, S. Z., & Lanham, J. S. (2011). Failure to thrive: An update. *American Family Physician, 83*(7), 829–834.

Habibzadeh, H., Jafarizadeh, H., & Didarloo, A. (2015). Determinants of failure to thrive (FTT) among infants aged 6–24 months: A case-control study. *Journal of Preventative Medicine and Hygiene, 56*, E180–E186.

Jaffe, A. (2011). Failure to thrive: Current clinical concepts. *Pediatrics in Review, 32*, 100–107. doi:10.1542/pir.32-3-100

Karra, M., Subramanian, S. V., & Fink, G. (2016). Height in healthy children in low- and middle-income countries: An assessment. *American Journal of Clinical Nursing, 105*, 121–126.

Keane, V. (2015). Assessment of growth. In R. M. Kliegman, B. F. Stanton, J. W. St. Germe III, & N. F. Schor (Eds.), *Nelson textbook of pediatrics* (20th ed.). Philadelphia, PA: Elsevier.

Kirkland, R. T., Motil, K. J., & Duryea, T. K. (2015). Failure to thrive, under nutrition, in children younger than two years: Etiology and evaluation. In J. E. Drutz, C. Jensen, & C. Bridgemohan (Eds.), *UpToDate*. Retrieved from http://www.uptodate/home

Sant'Ana, A. M. G. A., Hammes, P., Porporino, M., Martel, C., Zygmuntowicz, C., & Ramsay, M. (2014). Use of cyproheptadine in young children with feeding difficulties and poor growth in a pediatric feeding program. *Journal of Pediatric Gastroenterology and Nutrition, 59*(5), 674–678.

Sparks Ralph, S., & Taylor, C. M. (2014). *Nursing diagnosis reference manual*. Philadelphia, PA: Wolters Kluwer Health/Lippincott Williams & Wilkins.

Wilson, D. (2015). Health problems of the infant. In M. J. Hockenberry & D. Wilson (Eds.), *Wong's nursing care of infants and children* (10th ed., pp. 452–487). St. Louis, MO: Mosby/Elsevier.

■ INFLAMMATORY BOWEL DISEASE

Sharon Perry

Overview

Inflammatory bowel disease (IBD) is a chronic inflammatory disorder of the gastrointestinal tract that includes Crohn's disease, ulcerative colitis (UC), and inflammatory bowel disease unclassified (IBD-U). The location and degree of inflammation as well as histological findings determine the diagnosis. The incidence of IBD is increasing in children, and an up-to-date investigation, diagnosis, and management are essential (Kammermeier et al., 2015). The role of the nurse in IBD is to educate patients and their families so that they are successful in the management of their disease.

Background

Around 25% of patients are diagnosed with IBD within the first two decades of life, with the most common occurrence between 13 to 18 years, with the incidence increasing in the early second decade of life (Ye, Chen, Ju, & Zhou, 2015). The incidence of pediatric IBD is increasing worldwide; the highest rise occurring in developing countries is thought to be due to the influence of Western culture (Ye et al., 2015). In the United States, IBD in children and adolescents accounts for 30% of all patients diagnosed; in Canada, the incidence of pediatric IBD increased from 9.5/100,000 in 1994 to 11.4/100,000 in 2005 (Ye et al., 2015).

The exact etiology of IBD is unknown. The current concept is that IBD has a multifactorial etiology, consistency of an overlap among genetics, environment, dysregulation of the immune system, and the microbiome. It has been linked to several genes, including *NOD2/CARD15* gene. Although the link between genetics and environment is unknown, previous research suggests that nonpathogenic intestinal bacterial trigger and perpetuate an uncontrolled inflammatory response. Microorganisms, including Mycobacterium avium subspecies *paratuberculosis* (MAP) and *Escherichia coli* adherent-invasive organisms have also been linked to IBD.

Crohn's disease and UC share many features, but do have some distinct differences. Clinical presentation, radiologic findings, and histological patterns can allow for differentiation of the two, but there can still exist clinical ambiguity between them in a single patient. In pediatric patients, IBD demonstrates unique characteristics in phenotype and severity. In Crohn's disease, the terminal ileum is most often involved and disease progression within the first decade of diagnosis is well documented, along with more extensive disease than found in adults with Crohn's disease. In UC, pancolitis is the most common finding at diagnosis and is more likely to progress in the first decade.

Diagnosis is made by history, physical exam, laboratory results, and endoscopic findings. Once the diagnosis is made, there are several treatment options for patients, including steroids, exclusive enteral nutrition, immunomodulator medications, and biologic agents to induce and maintain remission. The role of the nurse is to provide support throughout the journey.

Clinical Aspects

ASSESSMENT

Diarrhea, rectal bleeding, abdominal pain, weight loss, and growth failure are common presenting symptoms of IBD. Patients may also present with extraintestinal manifestations, including aphthous ulcers, fever, anemia, joint pain, or skin rashes. Lab work is done to identify anemia, hypoalbuminemia, and elevated inflammatory markers. Stool studies to rule out an infectious process, including *Clostridium difficile* and bacterial infections, are part of the routine work up. Esophagogastroduodenoscopy (EGD) and colonoscopy remain the gold standard of IBD, and can determine disease location and extent. Small-bowel imaging, such as magnetic resonance enterography, is obtained to rule out abscess, strictures, or fistulas in the portion of the small bowel out of reach from standard endoscopes. Video-capsule endoscopy can also be obtained to survey the mucosal lining of the small bowel. In most cases, this workup is done in the outpatient setting.

For IBD in the outpatient setting, the nurse is seen as a "first point of contact" for patients and their families. The nurse is responsible for recognizing a change in symptoms and early intervention during acute exacerbations, which may reduce admissions and emergency room visits (Leach et al., 2014). The nurse also coordinates medical management, future endoscopic procedures, and development of self-management strategies.

In the inpatient setting, effective nursing care is based on physical exam, interpretation of labs, recognition of medication reactions, and education. A change in abdominal exam (increased pain, abdominal tenderness, or abdominal distention), increase in stool pattern, and/or onset of hematochezia are concerns related to an exacerbation or worsening disease. In addition, changes in albumin, hemoglobin, and inflammatory markers may indicate changes in disease status.

NURSING INTERVENTIONS, MANAGEMENT, AND IMPLICATIONS

Nursing care of the pediatric patient with IBD in the inpatient setting is focused on education, allowing the patient to be discharged home with basic knowledge of the disease. The focus of the outpatient nurse is disease management, medication adherence, and promotion of self-care, with the ultimate goal of successful transition to adult care at the appropriate time.

OUTCOMES

Research has shown that IBD nurse specialists have a positive impact on outcomes of patients with IBD. As valuable and cost-effective members of the health care team, nurses excel in providing educational materials on lifestyle, health maintenance, medications, and diagnostic testing, which help to improve patient education, satisfaction, and disease management. Hospital stays were also shown to decrease by 38% and length of admissions decreased by 19% when an IBD specialist was involved in the patient's care (Stretton, Currie, & Chauhan, 2014).

Summary

Adolescents and children with IBD can thrive when detected early in the disease process and managed with the most effective medications. Diagnosis is multifactorial and treatment options are continually expanding. The nurse plays a crucial role in providing the education necessary for IBD patients to achieve and sustain remission.

Kammermeier, J., Morris, M., Garrick, V., Furman, M., Rodrigues, A., & Russell, R. (2015). Management of Crohn's disease. *British Journal of Medicine, 101*(5), 1–6.

Leach, P., De Silva, M., Mountifield, R., Edwards, S., Chitti, L., Fraser, R., & Bampton, P. (2014). The effect of an inflammatory bowel disease nurse position on service delivery. *Journal of Crohn's and Colitis, 8*, 370–374.

Stretton, J., Currie, B., & Chauhan, U. (2014). Inflammatory bowel disease nurses in Canada: An examination of Canadian gastroenterology nurses and their role in inflammatory bowel disease care. *Canadian Journal of Gastroenterology and Hepatology, 28*(2), 89–93.

Ye, Y., Chen, W., Ju, S., & Zhou, C. (2015). The epidemiology and risk factors of inflammatory bowel disease. *International Journal of Clinical and Experimental Medicine, 8*(12), 22529–22542.

■ OBESITY

Rosanna P. Watowicz

Overview

Pediatric obesity is a major concern in the United States, affecting approximately 17% of children between 2 and 19 years of age. Defined as a body mass index (BMI) at the 95th percentile or higher, obesity has been linked to several serious comorbidities, both physiological and psychological. Nurses play an important role in educating families about specific guidelines that have been developed for children with obesity.

Background

In children, obesity is defined as having a BMI at or greater than the gender-specific 95th percentile according to the Centers for Disease Control and Prevention (CDC; 2016) BMI-for-age growth charts. Most recent estimates indicate that 17% of the U.S. population between the ages of 2 and 19 years are obese. The prevalence of obesity is higher for non-Hispanic Black children (19.5%) and Hispanic children (21.9%), compared to non-Hispanic White children (14.7%). The overall prevalence is also higher for 6- to 11-year-old children (17.5%) and 12- to 19-year-old children (20.5%).

Obesity comorbidities may include hypertension, sleep apnea, type 2 diabetes, hyperinsulinemia, non-alcoholic fatty liver disease, dyslipidemia, polycystic ovarian syndrome and other menstrual irregularities, and orthopedic conditions such as Blount's disease and slipped capital femoral epiphysis. Psychosocial comorbidities, including bullying or isolation from peers, decreased quality of life, and anxiety or depression, are also common (Barlow & Expert Committee, 2007).

In 2013, the American Heart Association brought attention to the additional health risks for children and adolescents with severe obesity. Consequently, a standardized definition of severe obesity was recommended (Kelly et al., 2013). Based on this recommendation, the most widely accepted definition of severe obesity is now 120% of the 95th percentiles of gender-specific BMI-for-age (i.e., 1.2 times the absolute BMI at the 95th percentile for the child's gender and age). Estimates indicate that 5.8% of the U.S. population ages 2 to 19 years have severe obesity (Ogden et al., 2016). Mirroring the trends for obesity overall, prevalence is higher for non-Hispanic Black and Hispanic children compared to non-Hispanic White children, and also for older children compared to younger children.

The etiology of obesity is extremely complex and most likely involves both environmental and genetic factors (Kumar & Kelly, 2017). Collectively referred to as lifestyle behaviors, diet and physical activity play a large role in the development of obesity. High caloric consumption from sugar-sweetened beverages, fast foods or restaurant foods, and large portion sizes can contribute to energy imbalance. In addition, reduced physical activity and increased screen time contribute to decreased energy expenditure. Several additional environmental factors that are further outside of individual control, such as parental feeding styles, perinatal factors (i.e., maternal weight gain during pregnancy), breastfeeding status, antibiotic use, gut microbiota, and adverse life experiences have also been implicated as causes of obesity. However, multiple gene sites related to appetite, satiety, and fat distribution have been identified as being associated with obesity, clearly indicating heritability (Barlow & Expert Committee, 2007). Certain medications, particularly antipsychotics, are known to contribute to weight gain, and for a small percentage of children, obesity may be related to a genetic syndrome such as Prader–Willi syndrome (Kumar & Kelly, 2017).

Clinical Aspects

ASSESSMENT

Nurses and other health care professionals should use BMI percentile to identify obesity in children 2 years and older. Weight and height should be measured at least annually, and BMI percentile should be calculated at each measurement. Many electronic health record systems can be configured to automatically calculate and display the BMI percentile for children, which removes the burden of calculating BMI percentile from the medical staff. If BMI percentile is not available in the electronic health record, gender-specific BMI for age, CDC growth charts, or the CDC's (2016) online BMI percentile calculator should be used. The American Academy of Pediatrics does not recommend screening children for obesity before the age of 2 years.

Severe obesity is more difficult to assess as growth charts defining 120% of the 95th percentile are not readily available, nor are they easily configured into electronic health records. Clinicians may use an absolute BMI of 35 kg/m² or greater as a proxy for severe obesity in children. However, young children with severe obesity may not approach this BMI cutoff. For clinicians to whom it is important to know whether a child has obesity versus severe obesity, a manual calculation of 120% of the BMI at the 95th percentile for that child may be necessary (Kelly et al., 2013).

If a child is found to have obesity, the nurse may look for physical signs of the comorbidities related to obesity, such as elevated blood pressure, acanthosis nigricans (a darkening of the skin around the neck, which can be indicative of hyperinsulinemia), or problems with gait. The nurse may also ask about snoring, which may be a sin of obstructive sleep apnea. Common laboratory assessments for children with obesity include fasting blood glucose and/or hemoglobin A1c (HbA1c), fasting lipid panel, alanine transaminase (ALT), and aspartate aminotransferase (AST). Elevated values for any of these studies may indicate an obesity-related comorbidity (Kumar & Kelly, 2017).

Health care professionals should also assess diet and physical activity behaviors for children with obesity. Nutrition-related assessment may include sugar-sweetened beverage consumption, frequency of dining out, fruit and vegetable consumption, and typical composition and portion size of meals and snacks. Physical activity behaviors may include the amount of daily or weekly active play or vigorous activity as well as the amount of daily screen time. Due to the psychosocial comorbidities that are common among children with obesity, quality of life is often assessed as well. Several validated tools exist to assess the quality of life in children, including the Pediatric Quality of Life Inventory (Peds-QL) and the Impact of Weight on Quality of Life–Kids (IWQOL–Kids; Bryant et al., 2014). The nurse may also ask the child about teasing or bullying experiences.

NURSING INTERVENTIONS, MANAGEMENT, AND IMPLICATIONS

Nursing-related problems for the child with obesity may include a knowledge deficit and/or imbalanced nutrition. To address these problems, nurses and other health care professionals should provide education around eight specific guidelines for families and children with obesity: (a) consume five or more servings of fruits and vegetables per day, (b) minimize sugar-sweetened beverages, (c) limit screen time to 2 hours per day or fewer, (d) participate in 1 hour or more of physical activity per day, (e) eat breakfast daily, (f) limit meals outside the home, (g) eat family meals at least five or six times per week, and (h) allow the child to self-regulate his or her meals and avoid overly restrictive behaviors (Spear et al., 2007). In addition, children with obesity should be referred to a primary care provider or registered dietitian with additional training in pediatric weight management and behavioral counseling. Older children, or those with more severe obesity, may benefit from a referral directly to a multidisciplinary pediatric weight management clinic or tertiary care center where more aggressive options, such as pharmacological treatment or weight loss surgery, can be discussed.

OUTCOMES

In the early stages of obesity treatment, the goal is for the child to maintain his or her weight while age and height increase, thereby decreasing their BMI and BMI percentile. If a child loses weight, weight loss should be limited to an average of 2 pounds per week, with lesser weight loss suggested for younger children (Spear et al., 2007).

Summary

Pediatric obesity is a common yet complex disease with a variety of potential causes. Nurses play an important role in ensuring that BMI percentile is assessed and that the recommended education is provided. Children with obesity should also be referred to health care professionals with training in pediatric obesity management. The high prevalence of obesity has led to the existence of multidisciplinary weight management centers where nurses who specialize in obesity are part of the treatment team. The goal for children with obesity should be weight maintenance or weight loss of no more than 2 pounds per week.

Barlow, S. E., & Expert Committee. (2007). Expert committee recommendations regarding the prevention, assessment, and treatment of child and adolescent overweight and obesity: Summary report. *Pediatrics, 120*(Suppl. 4), S164–192. doi:10.1542/peds.2007-2329C

Bryant, M., Ashton, L., Brown, J., Jebb, S., Wright, J., Roberts, K., & Nixon, J. (2014). Systematic review to identify and appraise outcome measures used to evaluate childhood obesity treatment interventions (CoOR): Evidence of purpose, application, validity, reliability and sensitivity. *Health Technology Assessment, 18*(51), 1–380. doi:10.3310/hta18510

Centers for Disease Control and Prevention. (2016). BMI percentile calculator for child and teen. Retrieved from https://nccd.cdc.gov/dnpabmi/calculator.aspx

Kelly, A. S., Barlow, S. E., Rao, G., Inge, T. H., Hayman, L. L., Steinberger, J., . . . Daniels, S. R. (2013). Severe obesity in children and adolescents: Identification, associated health risks, and treatment approaches: A scientific statement from the American Heart Association. *Circulation, 128*(15), 1689–1712. doi:10.1161/CIR.0b013e3182a5cfb3

Kumar, S., & Kelly, A. S. (2017). Review of childhood obesity: From epidemiology, etiology, and comorbidities to clinical assessment and treatment. *Mayo Clinic Proceedings, 92*(2), 251–265. doi:10.1016/j.mayocp.2016.09.017

Ogden, C. L., Carroll, M. D., Lawman, H. G., Fryar, C. D., Kruszon-Moran, D., Kit, B. K., & Flegal, K. M. (2016). Trends in obesity prevalence among children and adolescents in the United States, 1988–1994 through 2013–2014. *Journal of the American Medical Association, 315*(21), 2292–2299. doi:10.1001/jama.2016.6361

Spear, B. A., Barlow, S. E., Ervin, C., Ludwig, D. S., Saelens, B. E., Schetzina, K. E., & Taveras, E. M. (2007). Recommendations for treatment of child and adolescent overweight and obesity. *Pediatrics, 120*(Suppl. 4), S254–S288. doi:10.1542/peds.2007-2329F

■ ORAL HEALTH

Marguerite DiMarco

Overview

Tooth decay, or dental caries, are one of the most prevalent chronic diseases in children, five times more common than asthma. Dental caries are an infectious disease that can be transmitted from mother or primary care-taker to infant. Many health care professionals do not know about the pathology behind dental caries, or how serious oral disease can affect systemic health. In fact, the surgeon general called dental caries the "silent epidemic" especially affecting poor children. Many Americans lack a dental home and children are 2.5 times more likely than adults not to have dental coverage. The number of dentists is declining and many do not accept Medicaid, making it difficult for poor families to access dental care. Therefore, health professionals, including dentists/hygienists, physicians, physician assistants, nurse practitioners, nurses, and dieticians, need to work together to meet the oral health needs of infants, children, and adolescents (Office of Disease Prevention and Health Promotion, 2014).

Background

The primary cause of tooth decay is the bacterium *Streptococcus mutans*, which is the main contributor to tooth decay. Adults may have higher amounts of *S. mutans* in their mouths and can transmit it to an infant or child through the exchange of saliva. Frequent sugary snacking and drinking interact with *S. mutans*, producing acids that can cause mineral loss from teeth, increasing the risk for tooth decay. Dental caries affect more children in the United States than any other chronic infectious disease. Tooth decay and other oral diseases that can affect children are preventable. Fluoride varnish can reduce cavities in preschool children by 30% to 40%. The American Dental Association (ADA) currently recommends rinsing with 2.26% fluoride varnish for prevention of dental caries in children aged 6 years and younger. School-age children in second and sixth grades can have dental sealants placed on healthy molars, which has reduced the amount of caries in school-age and adolescent children. Unfortunately, rates of caries continue to rise in the preschool age group. Tooth decay in baby teeth contributes to an increased amount of decay in the permanent teeth (DiMarco, et al., 2016).

Tooth decay of the top front teeth is referred to as *early childhood caries (ECC)* formerly called *baby bottle tooth decay*. Causes of ECC include poor oral hygiene; not enough fluoride; sleeping with a bottle or sippy cup; frequent snacking; bottle/sippy cup feedings containing beverages high in sugar, milk, or formula during the day or night; coating pacifiers with sweeteners like sugar or honey; and having a mother/caregiver or sibling who has had active tooth decay in the past 12 months. ECC and tooth decay in general is a multifactorial disease, and a child could have a few of these factors and not have decay, whereas other children may have only one factor and have decay. Also, some foods called *cariogenic foods*, such as cookies, juice or sweet drinks, chips, fruit rollups, and chewy candy, cause tooth decay more than others. ECC develop in young children who use sippy cups or baby bottles constantly, and have poor nutrition with a history of eating frequently or eating the wrong foods (DiMarco, et al., 2016).

The process of decay is mostly influenced by sugars that can be fermented by the bacteria in the mouth, causing a lower pH, or an acidic environment. This environment works on deteriorating the enamel of the tooth. This demineralization will incite a cavity. Caries, in the primary dentition, lead to the same in permanent teeth. Another source of caries, aside from poor nutrition choices, is infection. Mothers who pick up a child's pacifier and put the pacifier in their mouth to clean it off may inadvertently pass on the bacteria *Mutans streptococci*, which causes dental caries. Along with passing the infection by saliva and mouth when kissing the baby, the frequency of eating significantly increases the presence of *Mutans streptococci*. The constant change of the acidity of the mouth's saliva will wear down of the protective enamel setting up the possibility of decay. A human's saliva has the ability to cause remineralization of the tooth's enamel. Eating foods that keep the acidity of saliva high continues to cause demineralization and the potential for dental caries. The more the teeth are bathed in anything other than water or healthy saliva, the greater the chance of demineralization. Despite our understanding of the risk factors associated with caries in early childhood, caries remains one of the largest untreated conditions in preschool children (Griffin, Barker, Liang, Li, Albuquerque, & Gooch, 2014).

Oral health has been linked to physical health, social acceptance, and well-being. During the early years of physical growth, appropriate nutrition is essential. If chewing is painful, children will refuse to eat crunchy fresh fruit or vegetables because they cause too much discomfort. Socially, children are sensitive to being different from others. If teeth are decayed or eroded, it sets them up for social bullying, even at a young age. Normal eruption of teeth permits successful language development in children. Proper speech, sturdy teeth, and attractive smiles permit children greater access to their social worlds, and help them achieve not only physical health but social acceptance as well. Lack of access to care and untreated dental conditions in children contribute to emergency room visits, expensive treatments, dysfunctional speech, compromised nutrition and growth, and an estimated 52 million missed hours of school per year, 189 million hours of lost work, not to mention the pain and suffering. Untreated caries can lead to infection, and infections in the mouth can spread to the blood causing infections in the brain, mouth abscesses, sinus infections, cellulitis, endocarditis, and sepsis, to mention a few. Unborn babies are affected if their mother has dental disease and periodontal disease; the infant could be born having a low birth weight, be premature, or even stillborn (Norris, DiMarco, & Thacker, 2013).

Clinical Aspects

The American Academy of Pediatric Dentistry (AAPD) and the American Academy of Pediatricians (AAP) recommend that primary care providers and other health professionals include the following oral health prevention strategies: (a) perform periodic risk assessments to determine the child's relative risk of developing dental caries; (b) provide anticipatory guidance to parents about oral hygiene, diet, and fluoride exposure; (c) apply appropriate preventive therapies, such as fluoride varnish; and (d) help parents establish a dental home for their children by 12 months of age (Griffin et al., 2014).

ASSESSMENT

Nurses can perform a screening oral assessment of the lips, tongue, teeth, gums, inside the cheeks, and the roof of the mouth to assess for dental caries or other oral conditions such as abscesses or trauma. An oral health screening takes about 2 minutes; no diagnosis is made that takes a dentist and the nurse can provide guidance for management. The nurse can do a knee-to-knee exam with the parent facing them and the child lying down on the nurses and parent's knees facing the parent. With a gloved hand, the nurse lifts the lip, views the soft tissue, the teeth, and the entire mouth. Any light, such as a flashlight, can be used for a screening. A tongue blade or toothbrush can be used to move the tongue and view the teeth (Norris, et al., 2013).

NURSING INTERVENTIONS, MANAGEMENT, AND IMPLICATIONS

Anticipatory guidance to parents and the child should be given not only during well-child exams but also in the hospital when doing an oral exam and/or brushing the child's teeth. Children who are at high risk are special-needs children, children with cancer, and/or children on ventilators. Nurses should follow special hospital procedures to prevent ventilator-associated pneumonia (VAP) with children on ventilators. Oral care with chlorhexidine has been studied and meta-analyses suggest that oral care with chlorhexidine can reduce VAP rates in this population by 10% to 30%. The American Dental Association recommends beginning oral hygiene a few days after birth. Wipe the gums with a gauze pad after each feeding to remove plaque and residual formula that could harm erupting teeth. When teeth erupt, brush them gently twice a day with a child-size toothbrush and water. Fluoride toothpaste is recommended for children older than 2. After oral hygiene, rinse and suction the mouth. Keep the oral mucosa and lips clean, moist, and intact using sponge-tipped applicators dipped in nonalcohol nonperoxide mouth rinse (Klompa, et al., 2014). Here are some tips for well or stable children:

1. Have your very own toothbrush that no one else uses.

2. Brush at least 2 minutes twice a day (after breakfast and before bed) with an adult brushing the child's teeth before bedtime until age 7 years.

3. Use a smear of fluoride toothpaste on a soft toothbrush until child spits well.

4. Once able to spit well and not swallow, increase fluoride paste to a small pea size or the size of the child's smallest fingernail.

5. Drink water after eating sweets to rinse off the teeth.

6. If a toddler carries a sippy cup around while playing, fill it with water only.

7. If going to bed, fill bottles or sippy cups with water only.

8. Be cautious, when nursing your baby, that you take the baby off the breast once asleep.

9. Limit fruit juice to 4 ounces daily, 3 cups of milk, and otherwise, DRINK WATER.

10. Encourage fresh vegetables and protein-rich foods as snacks, and limit candy (Norris, DiMarco, & Thacker, 2013).

OUTCOMES

Dental problems can have deadly outcomes if not treated. Help parents establish a dental home. If a dental problem is assessed that needs the immediate attention of a dentist, be aware of the resources available in your hospital or community. Some hospitals have a dentist on call or a dental clinic affiliated with the hospital. Dental schools, safety net clinics, and health departments are other sources. If these are not available in your community, make a list of private dentists and what types of insurance they accept.

Summary

Dental caries and oral health problems are common with children. It is often difficult for poor families to access a dentist. Interprofessional collaboration is needed to help address the oral health problem. Nurses working in every area can help with the oral health problem. Nurses have initiated Smiles for Life: A National Oral Health Curriculum. This program presents oral health education to nurses and other health professionals in web-based modules. This entry touched on some of the problems of oral health with children. A free curriculum, Smiles for Life, is available online with more detail than is discussed here (http://smilesforlifeoralhealth.org/buildcontent.aspx?tut=555&pagekey=62948&cbreceipt=0).

DiMarco, M. A., Fitzgerald, K., Taylor, E., Marino, D., Huff, M., Mundy, E., & Biordi, D. (2016). Improving oral health of young children: An interprofessional demonstration project. *Pediatric Dental Care, 1,* 113.

Griffin, S., Barker, L., Liang, W., Li, C., Albuquerque, M., & Gooch, B. (2014). Use of dental care and effective preventive services in preventing tooth decay among U.S. children and adolescents—Medical expenditure panel survey, United States, 2003–2009 and National Health and Nutrition Examination Survey, United States, 2005–2010. *Morbidity and Mortality Weekly Report, 63*(Suppl. 2), 54–60.

Klompas, M., Branson, R., Eichenwald, E. C., Greene, L. R., Howell, M. D., Lee, G.,...Berenholtz, S. M. (2014). Strategies to prevent ventilator-associated pneumonia in acute care hospitals. *Infection Control and Hospital Epidemiology, 35*(8), 915–936.

Norris, M., DiMarco, M. A., & Thacker, S. A. (2013). Open wide: Tips for performing oral health screening on young children during fluoride varnish application. *Nurse Practitioner, 38*(9), 14–21.

Office of Disease Prevention and Health Promotion. (2014). *Healthy people 2010: Progress reviews area 21 oral health presentations.* Washington, DC: U.S. Department of Health and Humans Services. Retrieved from https://www.cdc.gov/nchs/healthy_people/hp2010/focus_areas/fa21_oral2.htm

■ ORTHOPEDICS

Michelle Calabretta
Emily Canitia
Michelle A. Janas

Overview

Pediatric orthopedic nursing encompasses care of both the trauma and the surgical patient. Patients of all ages are affected by orthopedic issues, from the infant with congenital club foot to the teenager with a femur fracture from a motor vehicle accident. Surgeries can range from correction of a spinal deformity to acute treatment of a fracture. Predominant focus of the pediatric orthopedic specialty focuses on fracture care. An increase in physical activity, such as sports and recreational activities, places the pediatric population at high risk for orthopedic injury, specifically upper extremity fractures (Shah, Buzas, & Zinberg, 2014). Many of these patients will require surgical nursing care in an inpatient hospital setting. Specialized pediatric orthopedic nursing care and knowledge are to the successful treatment and recovery of these patients.

Background

Fractures in children are an important public health issue and a frequent cause of emergency room visits and inpatient hospital stays. According to the National Electronic Injury Surveillance System (NEISS), nearly one in every five children will experience a fracture sometime during childhood or adolescence (Naranje, Erali, Warner, Sawyer, & Kelly, 2016). The annual incidence of fractures increases with age, with children between 10 and 14 years of age having the highest incidence of fractures. There is no gender difference in younger age groups; however, for older age groups, fractures are more prevalent in males. Children in urban areas or lower socioeconomic status are also at an increased risk (Shah et al., 2014).

Fractures of the upper extremity in children are much more common than those of the lower extremity. The most common anatomic area for fracture is the distal radius, followed by the elbow and fingers. For lower extremities, the tibia is more commonly fractured than the femur. Supracondylar humerus fractures are the most common in children 7 years and younger. Fractures of the femur are most prevalent for ages 0 to 3 years. Falls from playground equipment, trampolines, bicycles, and sports account for a majority of fractures, and there is a higher incidence of these injuries during summer and school holidays (Shah et al., 2014).

Fracture diagnosis is usually made with a plain radiograph. Although a majority of pediatric fractures can be treated nonoperatively, some fractures that are open, displaced, or unstable may require surgical treatment. Surgical treatment depends on the severity of the fracture and ranges from closed reduction to open reduction and internal fixation with hardware. Most orthopedic injuries require a period of immobilization by casting.

Although most pediatric patients recover completely and return to full function after treatment for a fracture, all fractures are associated with a significant potential for complications. Some serious complications can include vascular injury, peripheral nerve injury, pain, and compartment syndrome. Fortunately, most neuropraxias resolve spontaneously over time with adequate fracture reduction. Compartment syndrome can occur with the initial injury if the swelling is greater than the compartment of the muscle and tissues, or postoperatively, if the cast material becomes too tight (Nguyen, McDowell, & Schlechter, 2016). Any of these complications can lead to premature disability and decreased quality of life. Nursing assessment and clinical knowledge in the care of pediatric fractures can contribute to timely and safe treatment for the patient.

Clinical Aspects

ASSESSMENT

Key elements of the nursing assessment of the pediatric orthopedic patient include a thorough pain assessment and neurovascular checks. Pain management can pose a particular challenge during the acute stage of care. Children and parents are often fearful following an injury, which can make pain assessment challenging. Ineffective pain management can play a major role in patient recovery time, cost of stay, and overall patient satisfaction. Consistent communication and collaboration with the patient and caregiver(s) are crucial in maintaining pain control (Schroeder et al., 2016).

The use of pain scales such as the face, legs, activity, cry, consolability (FLACC), Wong's faces, or a 1–10 numerical scale are key elements in assessing patient pain. The use of these pain scales requires a detailed assessment of physiological, behavioral, and patient/caregiver verbal reports. Behavioral assessment is often helpful in measuring pain in the young child, especially after a surgical procedure when measuring sharp procedural pain (Wilson, Curry, & Hockenberry, 2009). Older children are usually able to describe the presence and nature of their pain.

Neurovascular monitoring is a fundamental part of the postoperative assessment and recognition of neurovascular deterioration is crucial. Early recognition of neurovascular compromise prevents detrimental damage such as functional loss, contractures, amputation, infection, and renal failure (Large, Agel, Holtzman, Benirschke, & Krieg, 2015). It is important to know that neurovascular deterioration can occur late after trauma, surgery, or cast application. Neurovascular checks include frequent assessment of the six Ps of acute compartment syndrome: pain, pressure, pallor, paresthesia, pulselessness, and poikilothermia (Howard-Hill, 2014). Postoperative pain is to be expected, however, pain that is not consistent with the surgery or is not relieved by pain medication should raise concern. The feeling of pins and needles is concerning and should not be dismissed. Pulses should be monitored closely so should color and temperature; a pale, cool limb should be examined thoroughly.

Neurovascular checks in the pediatric patient can prove to be most difficult due to lack of language skills and the patient's inability to articulate signs and symptoms of discomfort. Therefore, a meticulous assessment of the limb is vital. Visually assess the limb, checking for color and swelling. Check for temperature with superficial touch. The limb should be warm to the touch and pink in color. Capillary refill should be less than 3 seconds. Pulses should be palpated thoroughly, and strength of pulses should be documented.

NURSING INTERVENTIONS, MANAGEMENT, AND IMPLICATIONS

Immobilization of a fracture is achieved with a type of cast applied to the extremity or area of the fracture. Most often a two-sided plaster splint with a mold on the posterior and anterior aspects of the extremity is used. Having only two solid sides of a cast allows for swelling of the extremity. The fracture causes a significant amount of swelling in the first 24 to 48 hours. If the cast were solid circumferentially during this time, in the event of excessive swelling a tourniquet effect of the limb can be created. A hard cast is applied later for better protection. Although casting provides the stability required to facilitate musculoskeletal healing, there are certain risks associated with immobilization by casting. Excessive internal swelling remains a potential

risk once a hard cast is applied. The fascia compartments of the limb or the hard cast may not be able to accommodate a large amount of swelling. Frequent assessment is needed by the nurse to provide early diagnosis and intervention is required with casting complications. It is imperative that the nurse be able to accurately identify and intervene if complications arise. It is important to first calm the family and the child to improve the accuracy of the initial evaluation. This includes identifying and assessing the pain of the child (Wilson, Curry, & Hockenberry, 2009).

If there is a change in the neurovascular assessment of the patient and acute compartment syndrome is suspected, call the patient's medical team for an urgent review. If the limb has a bandage or plaster cast, completely split the cast and cut the dressing to skin level. Elevate the limb to the height of the heart, and continue to assess neurovascular status as your facility deems necessary but usually every 15 to 30 minutes. If there is a circumferential cast in place, the cast can be valved. Valving a cast is a noninvasive procedure, which can be done quickly at the bedside. The cast is cut on one or two sides as well as on the bottom layer, and slightly opened to allow increased room for swelling and circulation. High-energy fractures carry a higher risk for significant swelling to the extremity than an injury caused by a low energy force (Nguyen et al., 2016). It is important to understand the etiology of the injury in order to anticipate the potential complications and interventions.

OUTCOMES

Orthopedic injuries are often painful and traumatic for both the patient and the family. The nurse plays a vital role in the care of these patients. If the complications of an orthopedic injury are caught early, the proper interventions can be initiated and the damage to the patient can be limited. Without early identification of a complication, the patient may require further surgical intervention and can have lasting physical consequences.

Summary

Nursing care of the pediatric orthopedic patient requires a specialized knowledge of not only the population, but also the orthopedic condition itself. The developmental level of the patient must be taken into consideration when caring for these patients. Orthopedic injuries and conditions are often painful. The nurse must know how to most appropriately assess and treat the pain associated with either an orthopedic surgical intervention or injury. This includes the use of the correct pain scale corresponding to the developmental level of the patient, attention to the external environment contributing to the pain or stress of the patient, and appropriate use and dosage of medications. Nursing care of the pediatric orthopedic patient requires patience and vigilance by the nurse. With appropriate observation, assessment, and intervention, these patients can recover well following an orthopedic surgery or injury.

Howard-Hill, A. (2014). Acute compartment syndrome. *Dissector, 42*(3), 20–22.

Large, T. M., Agel, J., Holtzman, D. J., Benirschke, S. K., & Krieg, J. S. (2015). Interobserver variability in the measurement of lower leg compartment pressures. *Journal of Orthopaedic Trauma, 29*(7), 316–320.

Naranje, S. M., Erali, R. A., Warner, W. C., Sawyer, J. R., & Kelly, D. M. (2016). Epidemiology of pediatric fractures presenting to emergency departments in the United States. *Journal of Pediatric Orthopaedics, 36*(4), 45–48.

Nguyen, S., McDowell, M., & Schlechter, J. (2016). Casting: Pearls and pitfalls learned while caring for children's fractures. *World Journal of Orthopedics, 7*(9), 539. doi:10.5312/wjo.v7.i9.539

Schroeder, D. L., Hoffman, L. A., Fioravanti, M., Medley, D. P., Zullo, T. G., & Tuite, P. K. (2016). Enhancing nurses' pain assessment to improve patient satisfaction. *Orthopaedic Nursing, 35*(2), 108–117.

Shah, N. S., Buzas, D., & Zinberg, E. M. (2014). Epidemiologic dynamics contributing to pediatric wrist fractures in the United States. *Hand, 10*(2), 266–271. doi:10.1007/s11552-014-9710-2

Wilson, D., Curry, M., & Hockenberry, M. (2009). The child with musculoskeletal or articular dysfunction. In M. Hockenberry D. Wilson, & C. Rodgers (Eds.), *Wong's essentials of pediatric nursing* (8th ed.). St. Louis, MO: Mosby/Elsevier.

■ SEIZURE DISORDER

Kathleen Maxwell

Overview

The majority of seizures are idiopathic. Seizures can present at any age and clinically, seizures can be described as convulsions, staring spells, muscle spasms, and odd sensations. Seizure types include febrile seizures, benign familial neonatal seizures, focal seizures, and generalized seizures, including absence epilepsy and juvenile myoclonic epilepsy (JME). *Epilepsy* has been defined by the International League Against Epilepsy (ILAE) as at least two unprovoked seizures occurring greater than 24 hours apart, one unprovoked seizure, and the probability of further seizures similar to the general recurrence risk (at least 60%) after two unprovoked seizures occurring over the next 10 years and a diagnosis of an epilepsy syndrome (Fisher et al., 2014). Seizures that are provoked by changes in electrolytes, high fevers, or alcohol or drug withdrawal are generally not classified as epilepsy. Individuals can have a combination of provoked and unprovoked seizures. In children, brain malformations, intracranial lesions, or trauma can provoke seizures.

Background

Seizure disorders can be a chronic condition for many individuals and chronic seizures can cause problems that impact social development and feelings that they are not like everyone else. This perceived feeling of social difference could also impact their psychological development. Further, cognitive development can be impacted as a consequence of seizure frequency and medication side effects.

Clinical Aspects

ASSESSMENT

The evaluation of a patient with a seizure disorder consists of getting a detailed history of the event. This description includes what the child looked like before the event (if it was witnessed from the start), details of the event itself, whether or not the child lost consciousness and continence, how long the event lasted, and how long it took the individual to return to baseline. A thorough medical and developmental history will be obtained. Labs, including a complete blood count (CBC), toxicology screen, and comprehensive metabolic panel (CMP), may be ordered depending upon the circumstances surrounding the seizure. Neuroimaging studies, a head MRI, and an EEG are indicated.

Seizure disorders can be broken down into two main groups: focal and generalized. Generalized seizures involve both sides of the brain. They are associated with a loss of consciousness, but not necessarily with shaking or convulsions. Generalized seizures are further delineated as absence (brief staring that may have associated automatisms) or tonic (stiffening), atonic (loss of tone), myoclonic (sudden, quick jerks), or clonic (jerking). The definition of *status epilepticus* includes the length of the seizure, the continuity of the seizure, and the time after which there is risk of long-term consequences (Trinka et al., 2015).

There are certain childhood epilepsies that are considered benign. These entities generally remit and require shortened or no medical intervention. Benign familial neonatal seizures affect otherwise healthy neonates. In general, seizures are brief and are associated with a period of apnea, causing cyanosis, and generalized tonic–clonic or focal–clonic movements (Park, Shahid, & Jammoul, 2015). The majority of infants with this seizure type have their seizures abate spontaneously. The infants can be started on phenobarbital with about 75% of infants responding to this treatment and continued for several weeks before weaning. Parents need to be aware of the increased risk of seizure recurrence later in life (Kaddurah, Kao, Moorjani, Talavera, & Riviello, 2017).

Febrile seizures are a common occurrence in childhood affecting 2% to 5% of the pediatric population between 6 and 60 months of age. Febrile seizures occur in the presence of a fever not concomitant with an intracranial infection, a metabolic disorder, or in children who have a history of afebrile seizures (Shinnar & Shinnar, n.d.). Daily anticonvulsant therapy is not recommended for children with simple febrile seizures. Treatment options include the use of a benzodiazepine such as clonazepam orally disintegrating tablets, rectal diazepam gel, or buccal midazolam. These treatments can shorten the duration of the febrile seizure and are generally tolerated with less potential side effects than a daily anticonvulsant.

Sudden unexplained death in epilepsy (SUDEP), is defined as an unexpected, witnessed or unwitnessed, death in patients with epilepsy, with or without evidence of a seizure, an excluding documentation of status epilepticus, drowning, or trauma, with no toxicological or anatomic cause for death found on postmortem (Keddie et al., 2016). Individuals with epilepsy have a 24- to 28-fold increase of dying unexpectedly compared to the general population. Risk factors to SUDEP include poor seizure control, especially generalized tonic–clonic seizures, nighttime seizures, decreased supervision, polytherapy with antiepileptic medications, comorbid psychiatric conditions, and increased incidence of medication noncompliance (Tomson, Surges, Delamont, Haywood, & Hesdorffer, 2016).

Focal seizures generally arise from the temporal lobe and can be termed *temporal lobe epilepsy*. Children can demonstrate automatisms and motor manifestations as part of their seizure patterns. These motor behaviors can change depending on the age of the child. In the 0- to 3-year-old age group, the child's motor manifestations may be difficult to differentiate from generalized seizures as the behaviors seen may be bilateral and symmetric, appearing more consistent with seizures arising from the frontal lobe. Children in the 3- to 6-year age range may have automatisms that are easier to disseminate, such as dystonic posturing, eye/mouth or head deviation, as well as having an awareness of an aura. Children over the age of 6 years and into adolescence may report similar automatisms and auras as adults. Auras may include a confusion state prior to seizure onset, a feeling of déjà vu, an olfactory aura, lip-smacking, dystonic posturing of an extremity, or aimless movements (Nickels, Wong-Kisiel, Moseley, & Wirrell, 2012).

Treatment options for focal seizures include, but are not limited to, the following medications: carbamazepine, oxcarbazepine, phenytoin, levetiractetam, zonisamide, and perampanel. Multiple factors influence medication choice. Children often require a medication that either comes in a liquid preparation or one that can easily be chewed or crushed. In general, medications that are administered daily or twice a day have a greater likelihood of compliance compared to three times a day or four times a day regimens. Any seizure medication has the potential to cause lethargy, so it is often advantageous to start with a bedtime dose and titrate up slowly to improve tolerability.

Childhood absence epilepsy is the most common of all childhood epilepsies with females having a higher rate of occurrence than males. Absence seizures are brief staring spells that may or may not have associated automatisms. The associated automatisms may include a repetitive eye blink, lip movement, finger picking/rubbing, trunk arching, or eyelid twitching (Park et al., 2015). This type of seizure will generally manifest between 4 and 10 years of age with the highest prevalence between 5 and 6 years of age (Park et al., 2015). The prognosis for this type of seizure is generally good as the majority of children with just absence seizures have their seizures abate after 6 to 7 years (Vrielynck, 2013). Studies have shown about 40% of individuals with absence seizures will develop a generalized tonic–clonic seizure. It may initially be thought to be inattentiveness or attention deficit hypertensive disorder (ADHD). Parents need to monitor the child for accidental injury, such as falling, when the child experiences a seizure, as well as comorbid conditions, including ADHD, anxiety, self-esteem issues, and depression (Tenney & Glauser, 2013). Treatment options include ethosuximide, valproate, and lamotrigine. Ethosuximide is often the first choice as it has a high rate of treatment success with minimal side effects. When ethosuximide has tolerability issues, it is usually with the gastrointestinal (GI) system. Most often, dosing twice a day or three times a day and taking with food can minimize GI upset. Valproate is an option especially if the individual has also had a generalized convulsion.

JME consists of bilateral myoclonic jerks, usually most prevalent in the early morning after waking, generalized convulsions, and absence seizures. JME syndrome occurs most frequently in individuals aged 13 to 15 years (Park, Shahid, & Jammoul, 2015). Long-term seizure control on medication has been seen in as many as 75% to 90% of patients with a diagnosis of JME (Rossi, 2013). Individuals with JME should adopt lifestyle changes to maximize seizure control. This includes maintaining a regular eating and sleeping schedule, minimizing alcohol consumption, and maintaining a high percentage of medication compliance (Mantoan & Walker, 2011).

NURSING INTERVENTIONS, MANAGEMENT, AND IMPLICATIONS

Nursing intervention starts with the identification of the seizure. It is important to document how the patient looked at the start of the seizure, duration of the seizure, and duration until the child was back to baseline. Parental education is a crucial nursing function. There are several elements to seizure first aid and safety to be discussed with families. In addition to timing and noting the description of the event, parents should be instructed to lay the child down on a flat surface once the seizure starts. The child should be turned on his or her side to maintain a patent airway and to prevent aspiration as the child may vomit during or immediately after the seizure. Keep the airway open and clear, and instruct the parents never to place anything, including their own fingers, in the child's mouth. The child's glasses and nearby safety hazards should be removed. Safety issues for the child in the wheelchair are a bit different. These children are safer if they remain in the wheelchair. Make sure that the brakes of the wheelchair are engaged and that the seat belt is secured. Hold the wheelchair in place and upright while the child is seizing.

Nursing education of anticonvulsants includes more than discussing potential side effects. Compliance issues can be addressed by determining the route and frequency of medication administration that will work best for each patient. When checking anticonvulsant levels, instruct families to obtain levels first thing in the morning or late in the day as a trough level. A trough level may be more beneficial than obtaining a peak level. It is important for the nurse to know the reference range and parameters so that the lab value is interpreted correctly. A thorough medication history, including over-the-counter medications and herbal supplements, is taken to determine any potential drug interactions.

Individuals with seizure disorders should be encouraged to take showers rather than baths so the drain is always open, and standing water cannot accumulate. Nonskid strips on the tub or shower floor are often helpful in preventing falls, and bathroom doors should never be locked in the event an emergency occurs. Swimming needs to be supervised with an adult present who can remove the child from the water if a seizure occurs. Schools will often require a seizure action plan for students with epilepsy. In addition to the student and parent's name, this should include several contact numbers for the family as well as for the treating provider. Medications, including routine and as needed (pro re nata [PRN] rescue medications, as well as instruction for use, are imperative. The plan needs to dictate when 9-1-1 is to be called as well as how to manage the child in the postictal period until able to return to the classroom.

The last restriction that should be discussed with the family is the driving privilege. Each state has its own protocol with regard to getting and maintaining a license when there is a history of seizure disorders. Generally, the individual needs to demonstrate that he or she has been seizure free for at least 6 months. The individual needs to have a measurable blood level of anticonvulsant(s). It is recommended that this level be checked randomly as a trough rather than at a scheduled or predetermined visit. The random check will give the provider a better sense of patient compliance rather than giving the patient the opportunity to take an oral load to catch up for missed doses. The state bureau of motor vehicle forms are completed every 6 to 12 months.

OUTCOMES

There are several medication choices for the treatment of seizure disorders. Medication choice depends on seizure type, patient age, functional level, and comorbid conditions. The outcome of medication treatment is to balance the therapeutic levels with toxic side effects. The patients' and families' quality of life will depend upon their perceived feeling of social difference and the cognitive, physical, and social development of the child.

Summary

Seizure disorders can affect individuals throughout the life span and the diagnosis can be challenging for both the patient and family. It is imperative to provide support for the patient and all concerned. There are several community-based resources that can and should be made available to the family. The local Epilepsy Foundation (www.epilepsy.com) will provide additional educational materials as well as in-services for schools, day cares, and employers. The American Epilepsy Society (www.aesnet.org) can also provide helpful information. Prescription medication can be costly to families, and programs, such as www.Rxassist.org, should be discussed with the family. Finally, additional resources for insurance coverage, such as state health departments, should be made available to families.

Fisher, R. S., Acevedo, C., Arzimanoglou, A., Bogacz, A., Cross, J. H., Elger, C. E.,...Wiebe, S. (2014). ILAE Official Report: A practical clinical definition of epilepsy. *Epilepsia, 55*(4), 475–482. doi:10.1111/epi.12550

Kaddurah, A., Kao, A., Moorjani, B., Talavera, F., & Riviello, J. (2017). Benign childhood epilepsy: Overview, benign familial neonatal convulsions, benign idiopathic neonatal convulsions. Retrieved from http://emedicine.medscape.com/article/1181649-overview#a1

Keddie, S., Angus-Leppan, H., Parker, T., Toescu, S., Nash, A., Adewunmi, O., & Liu, R. (2016). Discussing sudden unexpected death in epilepsy: Are we empowering our patients? A questionnaire survey. *Journal of the Royal Society of Medicine Open, 7*(9). doi:10.1177/2054270416654358

Mantoan, L., & Walker, M. (2011). Treatment options in juvenile myoclonic epilepsy. *Current Treatment Options in Neurology, 13*(4), 355–370. doi:10.1007/s11940-011-0131-z

Nickels, K. C., Wong-Kisiel, L. C., Moseley, B. D., & Wirrell, E. C. (2012). Temporal lobe epilepsy in children. *Epilepsy Research and Treatment, 2012*, 1–16. doi:10.1155/2012/849540

Park, J. T., Shahid, A. M., & Jammoul, A. (2015). Common pediatric epilepsy syndromes. *Pediatric Annals, 44*(2), e30–e35. doi:10.3928/00904481-20150203-09

Rossi, M. A. (2013). Juvenile myoclonic epilepsy: When will it end. *Epilepsy Currents, 13*(3), 148–149. doi:10.5698/1535-7511-13.3.148

Shinnar, S., & Shinnar, R. (n.d.). Febrile seizures. Retrieved from http://www.childneurologyfoundation.org/disorders/febrile-seizures

Tenney, J. R., & Glauser, T. A. (2013). The current state of absence epilepsy: Can we have your attention? *Epilepsy Currents, 13*(3), 135–140. doi:10.5698/1535-7511-13.3.135

Tomson, T., Surges, R., Delamont, R., Haywood, S., & Hesdorffer, D. C. (2016). Who to target in sudden unexpected death in epilepsy prevention and how? Risk factors, biomarkers, and intervention study designs. *Epilepsia, 57*, 4–16. doi:10.1111/epi.13234

Trinka, E., Cock, H., Hesdorffer, D., Rossetti, A. O., Scheffer, I. E., Shinnar, S.,...Lowenstein, D. H. (2015). A definition and classification of status epilepticus—Report of the ILAE task force on classification of status epilepticus. *Epilepsia, 56*(10), 1515–1523. doi:10.1111/epi.13121

Vrielynck, P. (2013). Current and emerging treatments for absence seizures in young patients. *Neuropsychiatric Disease and Treatment, 13*(9), 963–975. doi:10.2147/NDT.S30991

■ SICKLE CELL DISEASE

Valerie Cachat

Overview

Sickle cell disease (SCD) is a group of chronic genetic disorders that affect an estimated 70,000 to 100,000 Americans (National Heart, Lung, and Blood Institute, 2014). SCD is characterized by an abnormal hemoglobin, called *hemoglobin S (HbS)* or *sickle hemoglobin*, in the red blood cells (RBCs). The most common form of SCD is homozygous (SS) allele. Other variants are the result of compound heterozygotes for HbS and other β-globin variants, including sickel cell (SC), Sβ⁺ thalassemia, and Sβ⁰ thalassemia. Patients with SCD are at high risk for acute and chronic complications that may result in disability or death.

Background

SCD is a group of inherited hemoglobinopathies associated with hemolytic anemia and vasoocclusive complications. All forms of SCD are inherited in an autosomal recessive pattern. Normally, two β-globin chains combine with two α-globin chains to form the predominant normal Hb in adults (HbA). SCD involves a mutation in the β-globin genes. An amino acid substitution of valine from glutamic acid occurs (Piccone, 2011). In deoxygenated conditions, the polymerization of HbS results in the characteristic sickle shape of the RBCs. These sickled cells are stiff, and adhere to one another and to the vasculature, leading to occlusion of the microvasculature and causing decreased oxygen delivery to tissues. This impaired oxygen delivery effects multiple organ systems. Organ damage occurs because of the sickling of the RBCs and chronic hemolysis throughout the life span (Ware, 2010). Affected children in the United States now increasingly survive into adulthood because of increased knowledge and advances in disease therapy; however, the average life span remains 20 to 30 years less than those without SCD (National Heart Lung and Blood Institute, 2017). Although the life span has increased, SCD continues to cause significant morbidity and mortality. Acute complications, such as sudden anemia, vaso-occlusive pain crisis (VOC), splenic sequestration, acute chest syndrome (ACS), and stroke, occur. In addition, chronic hemolysis effects all organ systems and can lead to kidney, liver, and cardiac decompensation among other complications.

Clinical Aspects

SCD is now diagnosed based on newborn screen in the United States. Early diagnosis has led to a decrease in complications, in particular the risk of sepsis. Patients with SCD have functional asplenia. Shortly after birth, they are diagnosed with SCD and antibiotic prophylaxis is started to decrease the risk of sepsis due to encapsulated organisms (*Streptococcus pneumoniae* in particular). Febrile illness in a patient with SCD is considered an emergency due to risk of bacterial sepsis. Fever may be the result of acute and sometimes life-threatening conditions such as ACS and osteomyelitis. Often, the cause of a fever is not clear. Patients with fever require evaluation, including history and physical, complete blood count (CBC) with differential, reticulocyte count, blood culture, and urine culture when urinary tract infection is suspected. Patients presenting with respiratory symptoms or chest pain should have a chest radiograph done to rule out developing ACS. Prompt administration of empiric parenteral antibiotics with coverage for *S. pneumoniae* is necessary. Patients who appear ill should be hospitalized for observation and continued antibiotic administration, and intravenous fluids. Close attention should be paid to additional symptoms concerning the development of ACS, including hypoxia, tachypnea, fever, increased work of breathing and osteomyelitis, including localized pain, fever, swelling, and erythema (Piccone, 2011).

ASSESSMENT

Pain is perhaps the hallmark of sickle cell disease, with both acute and chronic pain being a significant cause of morbidity. Occlusion of the microvasculature leads to poor perfusion causing hypoxia, ischemia, and ultimately, tissue damage (Ballas et al., 2012). Inflammation occurs as inflammatory mediators are released from damaged cells. In addition to the physical effects of dealing with pain, psychological well-being is often affected, particularly due to the unpredictable nature of the disease.

Some common triggers of VOC are illness, temperature changes, stress, dehydration, and high altitude. Often, there is no identifiable cause. One of the first presentations of pain in infants with SCD is called *dactylitis*, which is swelling of the hands and/or feet due to occlusion of the microvasculature. Pain can occur anywhere in the body and in more than one spot at a time. Although VOC is often the reason for pain, other differential diagnoses should be considered depending on the location of the pain. Most children are pain free between painful crises, but adolescents and adults may also suffer from ongoing chronic pain.

NURSING INTERVENTIONS, MANAGEMENT, AND IMPLICATIONS

Pain is best treated by a combination of nonsteroidal anti-inflammatory drugs (NSAIDs) and opiates. Patients should have a home-pain regimen established and attempt to manage pain at home with the use of NSAIDs, opiates, if needed, and rest, hydration, and warmth. If they are unable to manage at home, they present to the hospital for further care, including evaluation, administration of pain medications, hydration, and monitoring. Treatment with parenteral opioids can often lead to sedation, increasing the risk of developing ACS. A balance between adequate pain control and lack of sedation is needed. The nurse must closely monitor for oversedation when administering opiates for pain control. The nurse should also encourage ambulation, and bronchial hygiene should be used routinely to prevent atelectasis and decrease the risk of developing ACS (Ballas, Gupta, & Adams-Graves, 2012).

Patients with sickle cell disease live with chronic mild to moderate anemia. At times, they may present with severe anemia, which may be life threatening. Some episodes of anemia are caused by rapid hemolysis during a VOC. However, in children, the cause of severe anemia is often splenic sequestration or aplastic crisis.

Splenic sequestration is a serious and potentially life-threatening complication of SCD. Splenic sequestration is defined as a decrease in Hb with a rapidly enlarging spleen. Parents need to be educated during infancy on palpation of the spleen and symptoms of splenic sequestration to decrease morbidity and mortality (Piccone, 2011). Rapid enlargement of the spleen can lead to hypovolemic shock. Patients who present for anemia should be evaluated for splenic sequestration. A patient admitted with splenic sequestration should have frequent, regular assessment of the spleen size by palpation as well as laboratory monitoring of CBC. The nurse must remain vigilant to signs of worsening sequestration, including tachycardia, pallor, hypotension, and altered mental status. Treatment may include fluid resuscitation and blood transfusion. Children with recurrent splenic sequestration may require chronic transfusions or splenectomy.

Aplastic crisis is another cause of acute anemia. This is usually caused by parvovirus B19 infection (also called *fifth's disease*), a very common childhood illness. Patients with SCD are dependent on rapid replacement of red blood cells due to hemolysis. A virus, such as parvovirus B19, which causes reticulocytopenia, can lead to significant anemia in a patient with SCD. Patients present with pallor, headache, and fatigue and a marked decrease in their Hb with associated low reticulocyte count. Frequent laboratory assessment to evaluate for return of reticulocytosis is necessary to determine course of treatment. Patients may require red cell transfusion until bone marrow activity increases.

ACS is a potentially life-threatening complication of SCD. ACS is defined by respiratory symptoms (i.e., cough, chest pain), fever, and evidence of pulmonary infiltrate on chest radiography (Piccone, 2011). Patients admitted for pain management are at high risk of developing ACS due to decreased respiratory effort secondary to pain as well as sedation from parenteral opioids. Aggressive bronchial hygiene is needed for prevention of ACS. Treatment includes antibiotics, which would include the coverage of *S. pneumoniae* and atypical organisms. Patients with ACS require frequent and close monitoring of respiratory symptoms to identify when more aggressive treatment is required.

Stroke is a major complication of SCD, and approximately 11% of pediatric patients are at risk for this occurrence. The most common cause of pediatric stroke related to SCD is vasoocclusion of the cerebral vasculature. Signs and symptoms may vary from very mild weakness to obvious hemiparesis, visual and speech disturbances, seizures, and altered mental status (Piccone, 2011). Patients presenting with symptoms of stroke require emergent evaluation. Treatment for patients with stroke is red blood cell transfusion to decrease the present HbS to less than 30%. Exchange transfusion is often used to avoid the risk of hyperviscosity that can lead to further cerebral injury.

Priapism, sometimes seen in patients with SCD, is defined as a sustained, painful penile erection. Priapism is caused by an obstruction of venous drainage from the penis. Prolonged priapism (longer than 3 hours) is considered an emergency requiring urological consultation. Treatment should include hydration and pain control, and medications, such as α-agonists and β-agonists, have been used and prolonged episodes may require penile aspiration (Piccone, 2011).

Care for the child with sickle cell is ongoing. Children with SCD must stay up to date with childhood immunizations. Patients receive the 23-valent pneumococcal vaccine at age 2 years with a booster at age 5 years. They should also receive the flu shot annually. Penicillin prophylaxis is started shortly after birth and continued until the age of 5 at minimum. Daily folic acid supplementation of 1 mg/day is recommended to increase RBC production. Stroke screening begins at age 2 years with the use of transcranial Doppler ultrasonagraphy (TCD). Those with abnormal velocities indicating risk for stroke will be initiated on a chronic transfusion protocol to decrease HbS and reduce the risk of stroke. Routine ophthalmologic exams should be done to evaluate for sickle retinopathy (National Heart, Lung, and Blood Institute, 2014).

There are few treatments to decrease the severity of sickle cell disease. Hydroxyurea is a medication used to increase fetal Hb levels, therefore increasing oxygen-carrying capacity, decreasing sickled Hb levels, and reducing morbidity related to chronic hemolysis and hypoxia (Ware, 2010). Bone marrow transplant (BMT) is curative but has not become standard practice because of treatment-related complications and morbidities.

OUTCOMES

Neonatal screening and early diagnosis, family education, and routine comprehensive care are necessary to reduce the morbidity and mortality associated with this chronic disease. Sickle cell disease affects every organ system. Due to anemia and hemolysis, growth and puberty are often delayed. Avascular necrosis can occur, most often in the femoral and humeral head.

Routine monitoring of kidney function, liver function, pulmonary function, and cardiac function is important.

Summary

SCD has a variable presentation in pediatrics. Despite significant anemia, many patients are clinically well between acute complication episodes. Infection is the most common cause of mortality in the pediatric sickle cell population. Research is ongoing to identify ways to lessen the complications and cure this unpredictable disease.

Ballas, S. K., Gupta, K., & Adams-Graves, P. (2012). Sickle cell pain: A critical reappraisal. *Blood, 120,* 3647–3656.

National Heart, Lung, and Blood Institute. (2014). Evidence-based management of sickle cell disease: Expert panel report, 2014. Retrieved from https://www.nhlbi.nih.gov/health-pro/guidelines/sickle-cell-disease-guidelines

National Heart, Lung, and Blood Institute. (2017). What is sickle cell disease? Retrieved from https://www.nhlbi.nih.gov/health/health-topics/topics/sca

Piccone, C. M. (2011). Sickle cell disease. In T. A. Florin, S. Ludwig, P. Aronson, & H. Werner (Eds.), *Netter's pediatrics* (pp. 326–330). Philadelphia, PA: Elsevier.

Ware, R. E. (2010). How I use hydroxyurea to treat young patients with sickle cell anemia. *Blood, 115*(26), 5300–5311.

Perioperative Nursing

Perioperative nursing has a long credible history in providing crucial nursing care to the surgical patient throughout the continuum of care. Formerly referred to as operating room nursing, this nursing specialty assumes significant responsibilities for the patient and surgical team each time a surgical or invasive procedure is performed. This specialty nursing care includes care provided in the preoperative, intraoperative, and postoperative periods.

Perioperative nurses specialize often in just one area of perioperative practice: preoperative, intraoperative, or postoperative. Considered one of the most complex, technical specialty areas, perioperative nurses provide patient care within the same nursing process framework as nurses in other specialty areas. Patient assessment, care planning, intervention, and evaluation occur with each patient. Perioperative nurses demonstrate specialized skills, knowledge, competence, and advocacy.

Essential successful surgical intervention requires a team effort. Working closely and collaborating on the care plan, surgeons, the anesthesiologist, certified registered nurse anesthetist, surgical technologists and others recognize the importance of this interprofessional team. Each team member has specific activities that she or he performs as a member of the surgical team. For example, the surgeon's immediate consideration is providing and obtaining informed consent from the patient. The scheduling secretary's role is to correctly schedule the procedure indicating site-specific information if appropriate, for example, left total hip arthroplasty. The perioperative nursing staff ensures that all supplies, including implants, are available on the day of the surgery. The goal is to ensure that safe, quality care is delivered each day and for each patient.

Perioperative nurses perform various roles (scrubbing or circulating). The nurse's priority starts with the needs of the patients. It is routine to witness a perioperative nurse supporting and advocating for the patients and families when the patients and families are often incapable of advocating for themselves, especially while undergoing a surgical or invasive procedure.

The entries included in the perioperative nursing section provide a small overview of surgical procedures and nursing care considerations for patients. From traditional surgical procedures to the most complex and advanced, the entries highlight the transformation occurring as a result of technology, medical advancement, and perioperative nursing involvement.

■ Ethics and Advocacy for Surgical Patients *Michelle McHugh Slater*

■ Infection Control *Joan Rotnem and Rebecca M. Patton*

■ Perioperative Patient Safety *Janet S. Duran*

■ Surgical Interventions in Cancer Care *Carol Pehotsky, Mary Szostakowski, and Jacob Runion*

■ Surgical Interventions in Parkinson's Disease *Karyn L. Boyar*

■ Surgical Interventions Using Emerging Technologies *Carol Pehotsky, Mary Szostakowski, Jacob Runion, Florin Sgondea, and Dena L. Salamon*

■ Traditional Surgical Interventions *Michelle McHugh Slater*

■ ETHICS AND ADVOCACY FOR SURGICAL PATIENTS

Michelle McHugh Slater

Overview

"The very first requirement in a hospital is that it should do the sick no harm" (Nightingale, 1863, p. iii). This direct quote from the founder of modern nursing, Florence Nightingale, illustrates one of the basic tenets in ethics for nursing practice. Ethics is a broad concept associated with sociological morality that focuses on beliefs and behaviors that guide decision making (Blais & Hayes, 2016; Catalino, 2015; Cherry & Jacob, 2008). Ethics offers a formal, structured, effective process to apply moral perspectives to determine right and wrong conduct (Blais & Hayes, 2016; Catalino, 2015; Cherry & Jacob, 2008). There are no absolute rules governing ethics and moral philosophy, only context-based norms and practices within a society.

Advocacy is an ethical concept that is the cornerstone of the nursing profession. By definition, advocacy is a provision of nursing support for a patient's rights and best interests to facilitate patient autonomy in all health care decisions (Blais & Hayes, 2016). Nurses advocate for the patient when the patient cannot advocate for himself or herself as an expectation of nursing practice. The perioperative setting stands out as an environment in which patient advocacy is essential because often patients are under anesthesia and unable to advocate for themselves. Advocacy occurs in many forms: legal advocacy, self-advocacy, collective advocacy, and client advocacy. Advocacy may require immediate intervention, crucial conversations, and/or political action, all based on the context of the situation. The nursing profession requires advocacy on the client's behalf as an obligation for competent nursing practice. Failure to carry out a duty owed to a client is a cause for legal consequences for negligence and/or malpractice based on the specific situational context.

Background

The nurse must understand and evaluate her or his own personal value and belief systems to determine professional versus personal ethics before decision making. When making this determination, a professional code of ethics is invaluable to delineate boundaries for nursing practice. Ethical professional practice focuses on the moral principles of autonomy, beneficence, nonmaleficence, justice, fidelity, and veracity. Standards and provisions of practice encompass these moral principles within interpretive statements.

Ethics transcend the law as value behaviors and beliefs that govern professional conduct. Ethics outline the standards by which a profession operates. These ethical standards form the basis of a profession's contract with society that defines boundaries and scope of the profession. Codes of ethics are professional value statements of conduct that guide decision making for its members. These codes are dynamic as the needs and demands within a society may change over time.

The practice of nursing occurs within a complex system of multicultural and multiethnic populations that are highly contextual to the individual client. The American Nurses Association (ANA) *Code of Ethics for Nurses with Interpretive Statements* functions as a nonnegotiable ethical standard of nursing care with statements reflecting its commitment to society, ethical standards, professional obligation, and duties (2015). This code clearly defines the role of the professional nurse with nine provisions for care. The International Council of Nurses (ICN) *Code of Ethics for Nurses* also provides a framework for professional standards of ethical conduct in nursing based on four essential, universal obligations: "to promote health, to prevent illness, to restore health and to alleviate suffering" (2012, p. 1). The Canadian Nurses Association (CNA) *Code of Ethics for Registered Nurses* provides an outline for ethical relationships, ethical behavior, and ethical decision making when used in combination with professional laws and regulations in nursing practice (2008). Each code of ethics is based on the premise of nursing advocacy for the health and well-being of society with specific standards to describe the duty of the nurse in the nurse–patient relationship.

In all situations, the nurse is required to respect patient autonomy through advocacy. Advocacy is the nurse's specific actions and strategies implemented to protect client rights, interests, and beliefs (Galuska, 2016). The nurse demonstrates advocacy in every interaction with the client, the family, the health care team, and society. Advocacy for the client is shown when the nurse supports client rights in care planning, nursing interventions, therapeutic treatments, and advance directives. Advocacy for the family is demonstrated when the nurse incorporates cultural and ethnic traditions in the treatment plan of the client. Advocacy within the health care team is demonstrated when the nurse requests adequate resources and staffing from administration or when the nurse participates in interdisciplinary patient rounds. Advocacy in society is demonstrated when the nurse actively participates in education, research, and public policy on behalf of the community stakeholders.

Clinical Aspects

The perioperative nurse is the epitome of a patient advocate in the practice environment. Perioperative nurses are moral agents accountable to provide for patient safety throughout the surgical services experience. The Association of periOperative Registered Nurses' (AORN) position statement on patient safety describes perioperative nursing's promise to reduce patient harm and surgical error through collaboration on safe practice (AORN, 2016). This statement further delineates the perioperative nurse's belief in every client receiving excellence in surgical care as well as every client receiving professional nursing care from an RN throughout the experience (2016).

With the ANA *Code of Ethics for Nurses* as the guiding framework, the AORN Ethics Taskforce provides perioperative explications to clarify the nonnegotiable ethical standards for perioperative decisions (AORN, 2015). Perioperative nurses must first recognize ethical issues to be able to intervene accordingly. The following explications will further explain the nine provisions within the context of perioperative nursing.

The perioperative nurse respects human dignity without prejudice in all professional interactions. This ethical belief includes recognition of a patient's right to self-determination. Perioperative examples include respect for patient decisions (informed consent, advance directives, end-of-life organ procurement); universal application of nursing standards regardless of patient disability, disease process, surgical procedure, race, religion, age, sexual preference, or socioeconomic status; integration of cultural and ethnic patient values with the care plan (AORN, 2015). The perioperative nurse has a primary commitment to protect patient autonomy, dignity, and human rights. Perioperative examples include patient collaboration; identification of an individualized plan of care with patient specific outcomes; inclusion of the family within the process; patient advocacy when respecting patient decisions for interventions; abstention from influence of outside sources (vendors, gifts, gratuities, favors); collaboration with the perioperative team, interdisciplinary teams, and professional colleagues (anesthesia, critical care, home health, RN first assistants); avoidance of unprofessional behaviors and respect for professional boundaries in relation to both the patient and other health care professionals (AORN, 2015). The perioperative nurse has a duty to protect patient privacy, confidentiality, and health and safety of every surgical patient. Perioperative examples include safeguarding physical, personal, and identifiable information (body exposure, restriction of access to unauthorized persons, appropriate documentation, limitation to access of surgical information via the main schedule or personal chart); confirmation of consent and adherence to protocols for research; compliance with professional standards of practice as well as regulatory practices; protection from incompetent or unethical practices; intervention to protect patient safety (removal of unsafe providers, refusal to perform intervention, consultation with team to resolve concerns; AORN, 2015).

The perioperative nurse is accountable for nursing practice in all forms: delegation, nursing judgment and actions, competency, professional growth, and quality improvement in health care. The perioperative nurse assumes primary accountability for nursing care given to the patient. Perioperative examples include maintenance of licensure and certification; continuing education, on-call and workforce staffing, and competent patient care; warning team of risks with appropriate intervention (environmental hazards, positioning injury, blood loss, patient safety); delegation to assistive persons based on established competency and scope of practice; and supervision of unlicensed assistive personnel (AORN, 2015).

The perioperative nurse has a duty to advance the profession, collaborate for public health needs and human rights, and articulate nursing values to maintain the integrity of the nursing profession (ANA, 2015). Perioperative examples include: "doing what is right and doing it well"; speaking up against unsafe practice; standing up against harassment and abuse; advocating and participating in the community, local, and national levels of health care; donating to health care-related organizations; collaborating with elected officials; participating in the legislative process; collaborating with professional health care organizations (nursing, medical, administrative); exhibiting positive portrayal of nursing in the community; and valuing volunteer time and talent (AORN, 2015).

Summary

The perioperative nurse is ethically bound in all situations to advocate on behalf of the patient and family, to speak up to colleagues to ensure patient safety, and to represent the nursing profession in a positive manner. Codes of conduct, ethical standards, practice guidelines, and explication statements are meant to provide a consistent framework for decision making; however, the professional nurse has the duty to ensure ethical practice. "Rather, ten times, die in the surf, heralding the way to a new world, than stand idly on the shore" (Nightingale, personal communicartion).

American Nurses Association. (2015). Code of ethics for nurses with interpretive statements. Retrieved from http://www.nursingworld.org/code-of-ethics

Association of periOperative Registered Nurses. (2015). *Perioperative standards and recommended practices.* Denver, CO: Author.

Association of periOperative Registered Nurses. (2016). AORN position statement: Patient safety. Retrieved from: https://www.aorn.org/-/media/aorn/.../position-statements/posstat-safety-patient.pdf

Blais, K., & Hayes, J. (2016). *Professional nursing practice: Concepts and perspectives* (7th ed.). Boston, MA: Pearson.

Canadian Nurses Association. (2008). Code of ethics for registered nurses. Retrieved from https://www.cna-aiic.ca/en/on-the-issues/best-nursing/nursing-ethics

Catalino, J. (2015). *Nursing now!: Today's issues, tomorrow's trends* (7th ed.). Philadelphia, PA: F. A. Davis.

Cherry, B., & Jacob, S. (2017). *Contemporary nursing: Issues, trends, & management* (7th ed.). St. Louis, MO: Mosby Elsevier.

Galuska, L. (2016). Advocating for patients: Honoring professional trust. *AORN Journal, 104*(5), 410–416.

International Council of Nurses. (2012). The ICN code of ethics for nurses. Retrieved from http://www.icn.ch/who-we-are/code-of-ethics-for-nurses

■ INFECTION CONTROL

Joan Rotnem
Rebecca M. Patton

Overview

The operating room (OR) environment is a high-paced environment that requires strong teamwork to provide the quality of care that each patient deserves. According to the Office of Disease Prevention and Health Promotion (ODPHP), one out of every 25 hospitalized patients will contact a health care-associated infection (HAI) related to hospital care. HAI resulted in hundreds of thousands of preventable deaths annually (ODPHP, 2017; James, 2013). Despite improvement with infection-control strategies, including OR ventilation, sterilization methods, surgical technique, and antimicrobial prophylaxis, HAIs remain a substantial cause of morbidity, lengthened hospitalization, and death (CDC, 2016). To achieve desired outcomes and prevent infection, strict infection-control practices are vital in the OR environment. Not only does this benefit the patient, but it also benefits each of the team members caring for the patient.

Background

Florence Nightingale, as early as the 1870s, urged nurses to wash their hands and discussed the use of antiseptic precautions (Small, 2017). Robert Koch, physician and pioneering microbiologist, reported in 1878 that microbes carrying infection were not airborne but were transferred by contact. This and the following discoveries resulted in much of today's principles to reduce and eliminate pathogenic microorganisms in the OR environment. Even though surgeons washed their hands with soap or alcohol, the use of surgical gloves did not come into use until the 1890s. This began at Johns Hopkins University in Baltimore, where a surgeon ordered two pairs of gloves, one for himself and one for his scrub nurse, who had an allergy to the soap products being used. By 1897, all the surgeons at Johns Hopkins were wearing gloves and the rest of the nation soon followed the trend (Johns Hopkins Medicine, 2017).

Other forms of protection (personal protection equipment [PPE]) have been introduced over the years to provide protection in a germ environment. As the exposure to both blood-borne pathogens and disease can occur, it is crucial that the entire team wear PPE and practice stringent aseptic technique. There is no gray area in the OR when it comes to sterility. An item is either sterile or it is not. This principle is consistently practiced in all situations where surgical or invasive procedures are performed.

Clinical Aspects

ASSESSMENT

All surgical team members must monitor and reduce risks that can result in HAI. The circulating nurse plays a significant role in managing most activities in the room while monitoring infection control processes and sterile supplies. This nurse must have the ability to address strong personalities in the surgical team while functioning in a fast-paced environment. This expected job performance can be challenging, difficult to achieve, and essential to minimize risks for HAI.

NURSING INTERVENTIONS, MANAGEMENT, AND IMPLICATIONS

The Association of periOperative Registered Nurses (AORN) has established recommended guidelines and practices to reduce risks associated with infections (AORN, 2017a). Using evidence-based practices and associated research, these recommendations are reviewed and revised routinely. In addition to the recommended guidelines and practices, surgical nurses are competent in infection-reduction strategies including but not limited to patients' antiseptic showers; perioperative hair removal; antimicrobial stewardship/antibiotic selection, dosing, timing; antimicrobial irrigation; antimicrobial sutures and dressings; and surgical attire/surgical scrubs. Specific AORN- and Centers for Disease Control and Prevention (CDC)-recommended guidelines address sterile practices, hand hygiene, PPE, and sharps safety and prevention strategies for transmittable diseases.

Hand hygiene has been recognized as the primary strategy to prevent the spread of infection and is the basic standard to reduce infections within and outside surgical environments (Institute for Healthcare Improvement, 2014). It is recommended that caregivers wash their hands before and after every patient contact. Hand hygiene involves the use of soap and water when the hands are visibly soiled, and when there is no visible soil, an alcohol-based product can be used to clean hands (AORN, 2017b).

The surgical gloves, gowns, and surgical drapes function as barriers to prevent the spread of infection to the patient and surgical team. These barriers meet strict standards for protection against blood-borne pathogens. Manufacturers must provide a consistent standard with each type of barrier, that is high quality, meets intended purposes, and has a low chance of failure.

Surgical gloves should be changed periodically during a procedure (every 90–150 minutes; AORN, 2017c). AORN has established the following guidelines for when surgical gloves should be changed.

- After each patient procedure
- After potential or actual contamination occurs with gastric content
- After touching a nonsterile item such as surgical helmet system hoods and visors
- Immediately after direct contact with certain substances, like methyl methacrylate
- When gloves begin to swell, expand, and become loose on the hands as a result of the material's absorption of fluids and fats
- When a visible defect or perforation is noted or a suspected perforation from a needle, suture, bone, or other object occurs

Surgical gowns are worn by the surgical team during the procedure and changed in between each patient. These gowns are made from either disposable or fabric material. Disposable material gowns are discarded after each patient or more often during the procedure. Fabric gowns are seldom used and require established protocols for washing, sterilizing, and maintaining the quality of these gowns. All gowns must be resistant to tear and provide a barrier for protection.

Recommended practices (AORN, 2017d) provide guidance on whether the gowns and drape barriers are considered sterile or not. Similar to gloves, if suspected or actual contamination occurs with a nonsterile item or if a visible defect or perforation is noted, the gown and drape barrier are changed as soon as possible to reduce surgical infection risk. The recommended practice provides guidance on a multitude of infection risk-reduction strategies that include what portion of gown and drape are considered sterile when in use. In addition to gowns and gloves, all OR personnel must wear hats and hospital-provided surgical attire. The purpose of hats and attire is to cover staff hair and any skin shedding.

Jewelry can conceal microorganisms and can be a source of surgical site infection. Therefore, for both staff and patients, jewelry should be at a minimum, and rings, watches, bracelets should be completely removed from staff before scrubbing, gowning, and gloving (Arrowsmith & Taylor, 2014).

During surgical procedures, surgical smoke or plume is created as a byproduct from thermal destruction of tissues when using an electrosurgical unit or laser. The smoke that is generated during a surgical procedure is similar to other smoke plumes containing toxic gases (Occupational Safety and Health Administration, 2017). This smoke can cause allergic reactions, respiratory problems, and spread viruses. Infection-risk strategies include specialized vacuums and protective masks that meet the recommendation for the type of procedure being performed (Dobrogowski et al., 2015).

Needlesticks and other sharps-related exposures to blood-borne pathogens (including HIV, hepatitis B virus [HBV], and hepatitis C virus) pose a significant risk for health care workers. Largely preventable, these incidents create significant concern even when there is no resulting infection. Sharps-related injuries are one of the greatest concerns for OR nurses today. The CDC estimates that about 385,000 sharps-related injuries occur annually, with the OR environment having the greatest incidence (CDC, 2015). AORN-recommended guidelines provide strategies for sharps safety (AORN, 2017e). One strategy is the creation of a "no pass" of sharps on the sterile field. This means that the scalpels, needles, and so on will not be passed from individual to individual by hand. Instead, these instruments will be placed on a tray where they can then be picked up and utilized. A neutral zone should be established where these items are going to be placed to avoid injury and potential infections.

Studies have shown that limiting traffic in the surgical environment and specifically in the OR will reduce risks for surgical site infections (SSIs). Personnel traffic in and around the surgical environment leads to airflow disruptions and airborne contamination that may increase the risk of SSIs. OR ventilation systems are designed to reduce airborne contaminants. But these mechanical systems cannot work effectively if the doors are opened frequently with excessive personnel traffic. Reducing the number of times the doors are opened is essential (AORN, 2017f).

All instrument processing needs to be monitored to ensure sterility. Biologic testing is done on the sterilizers used as well as on each individual instrument tray. Decontamination is a two-step process involving thorough cleaning followed by a process, such as disinfection or sterilization, that will kill microorganisms to render items safe to handle. All instruments should be examined for sterility before use (Association of periOperative Registered Nurses, 2017a).

OUTCOMES

Practices and techniques in the OR can help to prevent SSIs for the patient as well as undesired outcomes for the staff involved. HAIs acquired during a health care experience may not be apparent until after the patient has been released from care or discharged. The source of these infections may be endogenous (from one's own tissues: self-infection) or exogenous (from objects or other persons: cross-contamination). HAI can proliferate in health care environments due to the population of susceptible hosts, presence of infective agents, and the existence of various modes of transmission. Health care professionals must understand the chain of infection so that practices can be implemented to reduce the transmission of pathogens (Steris, 2017).

Summary

SSIs are one of the most prevalent hospital-acquired infections and can result not only in an increase in health care-associated costs—even more significant—death. Intentional practices and learned techniques in the OR can reduce risks and prevent SSIs as well as undesired outcomes for the staff. All SSIs are now reportable and made available to the public, which can influence hospital reputation and revenue. It is the responsibility of all perioperative personnel to prevent infection and injury to the patient as well as to each other. Recommended practices provide guidance on a multitude of infection risk-reduction strategies that include traffic, food prohibition, and personal belongings.

Arrowsmith, V. A., & Taylor R. (2014). Removal of nail polish and finger rings to prevent surgical infection. *Cochrane Database of Systematic Reviews*, 2014(8), CD003325. doi:10.1002/14651858.CD003325.pub3

Association of periOperative Registered Nurses. (2017a). Recommended practices for prevention of transmissible infections. In *Perioperative standards and recommended practices for inpatient and ambulatory settings* (2017 ed.). Denver, CO: Author. doi:10.6015/psrp.15.01.419

Association of periOperative Registered Nurses. (2017b). Guideline for hand hygiene in the perioperative setting. Guidelines for perioperative practice. In *Perioperative standards and recommended practices for inpatient and ambulatory settings* (2017 ed.). Denver, CO: Author. doi:10.6015/psrp.16.01.e27

Association of periOperative Registered Nurses. (2017c). Recommended practices for sterile technique. In *Perioperative standards and recommended practices for inpatient and ambulatory settings* (2017 ed.). Denver, CO: Author. doi:10.6015/psrp.15.01.067

Association of periOperative Registered Nurses. (2017d). Guideline for surgical attire. Guidelines for perioperative practice. In *Perioperative standards and recommended practices for inpatient and ambulatory settings* (2017 ed.). Denver, CO: Author. doi:10.6015/psrp.15.01.097

Association of Perioperative Registered Nurses. (2017e). Recommended practices for sharps safety. In *Perioperative standards and recommended practices for inpatient and ambulatory settings* (2017 ed.). Denver, CO: Author. doi:10.6015/psrp.15.01.365

Association of periOperative Registered Nurses. (2017f). Recommended practices for traffic patterns in the perioperative practice setting. In *Perioperative standards and recommended practices for inpatient and ambulatory settings* (2017 ed.). Denver, CO: Author. doi:10.6015/psrp.17.01.269

Centers for Disease Control and Prevention. (2015). Sharps safety for healthcare settings. Retrieved from https://www.cdc.gov/sharpssafety

Centers for Disease Control and Prevention. (2016). National health statistics report: Surgical site infection (SSI) event. Retrieved from http://www.cdc.gov/nhsn/PDFs/pscManual/9pscSSIcurrent.pdf

Dobrogowski, M., Wesolowski, W., Kucharska, M., Paduszyńska, K., Dworzyńska, A., Szymczak, W., ... Pomorski, L. (2015). Health risk to medical personnel of surgical smoke produced during laparoscopic surgery. *International Journal of Occupational Medicine and Environmental Health*, 28(5), 831–840. doi:10.13075/ijomeh.1896.00374

Institute for Healthcare Improvement. (2014). How-to guide: Improving hand hygiene. Retrieved from http://www.ihi.org/resources/Pages/Tools/HowtoGuideImprovingHandHygiene.aspx

James J. T. (2013). A new, evidence-based estimate of patient harms associated with hospital care. *Journal of Patient Safety*, 9(3), 122–128. doi:10.1097/PTS.0b013e3182948a69

Johns Hopkins Medicine. (2017). The four founding physicians. The Johns Hopkins University. Retrieved from http://www.hopkinsmedicine.org/about/history/history5.html

Occupational Safety and Health Administration. (2017). Laser/electrosurgery plume. Retrieved from https://www.osha.gov/SLTC/laserelectrosurgeryplume/index.html

Office of Disease Prevention and Health Promotion. (2017). Overview of health care-associated infections. Retrieved from https://health.gov/hcq/prevent-hai.asp

Small, H. (2017). *A brief history of Florence Nightingale: And her real legacy, a revolution in public health (Brief Histories)*. London, UK: Robinson.

■ PERIOPERATIVE PATIENT SAFETY

Janet S. Duran

Overview

Patient safety fundamentally refers to the patient's freedom from accidental or preventable injuries produced by medical care (Agency for Healthcare Research and Quality [AHRQ], 2017). The Institute of Medicine (IOM) reports that the number of deaths due to medical errors may be as high as 98,000 patients per year in the United States (James, 2013). The Joint Commission (TJC) reports that there are more than 40 incidents of preventable medical errors known as *never events* reported each week by medical institutions. The perioperative environment and patient care processes are unique and present safety challenges. By providing a culture of safety, effective communication, and standardizing workflow, nursing can improve patient safety while serving the foundation for effective interdisciplinary teamwork. Perioperative nurses are focused on error and injury reduction.

Background

Health care errors, known as never events, are more common than health care providers and patients understand. Prevention of errors requires an environment of safety and interdisciplinary communication regarding the patients' care, especially in the perioperative setting. Challenging variables create this environment with extensive complexity and high opportunity for safety-related adverse events. The American College of Surgeons (ACS) along with the World Health Organization (WHO), TJC, and the Association of peri-Operative Registered Nurses (AORN) in 2003 developed the surgical/procedural safety checklist known as a *universal protocol*. In 2004, the universal protocol for preventing never events became operational for accredited hospitals, in the United States as a National Patient Safety Goal (NPSG). The universal protocol applies to all invasive procedures performed in the operating room, procedure room, and at the patient's bedside. Universal protocol has three components that the health care team follows with every patient in these areas: (a) conducting a preprocedure verification process, (b) marking or identifying the procedure site if applicable, and (c) performing a time-out or final verification before starting the procedure (Mallett, Conroy, Zaidain, & Bruce, 2012). The goal behind the universal protocol is to reduce errors that occur and include patient and surgical site misidentification.

System factors, such as standardized implementation, incomplete or inaccurate time-out, and a culture of safety, continue to impact the outcomes of never events in the surgical and procedural setting (TJC, 2010). Universal protocol in the health care setting starts at the micro level implementing the protocol at the bedside, operating room, or procedural areas for all invasive procedures. Macro- and meso-level support regarding strict adherence to universal protocol is needed by supporting the staff and patient safety advocacy with the use of the universal protocol. Never events adversely affect the surgical patient population, the surgical/procedural and bedside team members involved, hospital reputation, and finances as hospitals have not received reimbursement for these events since 2009 by Medicaid and Medicare as well as private insurers (AHRQ, 2013). Errors during medical care can be catastrophic even though theoretically they are 100% preventable and should never occur with the implementation of the universal protocol. Universal protocol, checklist standardization, and universal protocol policy are evidenced-based practice solutions to guide procedural and surgical staff members to zero tolerance for never events in the surgical and procedural setting.

The objective of zero tolerance not being met is in direct correlation to the lack of standardization of education and workflow while implementing and using universal protocol in the procedural endoscopy setting. Areas of improvement to decrease medical errors are (a)

communication, (b) not taking the time to complete each element in the universal protocol, and (c) required paperwork not being signed by physician or patient before the time-out. Although none of the preceding issues may become never events, they are identified as near misses and room for improvement regarding universal protocol and promotion of a culture of safety is needed.

Wrong-site surgery and human factors regarding universal protocol suggest that one in 5,000 surgical cases are reported in the United States as being a never event (Feldman, 2008). There is a significant research by the IOM, AORN, and the American Medical Association (AMA) that universal protocol does decrease harm to patients in procedural areas; however, medical errors involving the wrong site/procedure or patient is on the rise.

Clinical Aspects

The ACS recognizes patient safety as being an item of the highest priority and strongly urges hospitals to develop guidelines to ensure patient safety (ACS, 2002). Universal protocol guidelines and checklists are aimed at achieving zero tolerance for severe reportable never events in procedural/surgical areas or bedside procedures to safeguard patient safety. The universal protocol is a well-established evidenced-based standard of practice proven to decrease patient harm and increase patient safety. Providing a culture of quality and commitment to diminish errors in the surgical suite requires an environment of safety and interdisciplinary communication with the surgical team regarding the patient. The use of the universal protocol as a standard of practice by the interdisciplinary team can prevent adverse events such as (a) wrong patient, (b) wrong surgery, and (c) wrong site (TJC, 2010).

OUTCOMES

Universal protocol is an evidenced-based practice used to guide nursing to be the patient's advocate, increase safety, and reduce medical error and possible injury in patients. Systems factors increasing medical error and decreasing patient safety include lack of nursing practice standardization, education, and evaluation when universal protocol is being used hospital-wide. Universal protocol, when initiated, should be standardized and not fluctuate in timing, combine universal protocol elements, and should be documented in the electronic medical record as being completed. Standardization is essential to decrease human error and harm patients. Hospitals should create a strengths, weaknesses, opportunities, and threats (SWOT), analysis, which can identify gaps in compliance, education, and understanding as well as incomplete or inaccurate communication regarding universal protocol and patient safety initiatives. Monitoring compliance regarding universal protocol elements should be conducted using the electronic medical record for the evaluation of universal protocol. Findings collected by electronic chart review can be shared with staff regarding compliance with individual documentation compliance. The overall goal of universal protocol as an evidenced-based nursing practice is to enhance safety, patients' advocacy, and quality standards to achieve a culture of safety for all patients.

Summary

Patient safety initiatives during surgical interventions are being implemented in an effort to ensure a culture of safety and reduce patient harm. Perioperative nurses play a role in improving patient safety and preventing surgical errors. Regardless of mandated initiatives from TJC to prevent harm in health care settings, there are more than 40 never events, preventable medical errors reported every week (TJC, 2010). Medical errors and deaths are avoidable with the implementation and use of the universal protocol in medical centers and hospitals. Barriers surrounding health care procedural and surgical settings achieving a zero tolerance to never events regarding errors in care continue to be caused by lack of communication, lack of standardization workflows, and lack of compliance with universal protocol.

Evidenced-based practice shows that the use of the universal protocol in the surgical/procedural and bedside setting does work to decrease errors and increase patient safety. Implementation of a standardized workflow, including a universal protocol and checklist increases advocacy for patient safety. Standardized evidenced-based practices in the clinical setting using strategic planning, implementation of an electronic health care record, universal protocol tools, and mandatory staff education may facilitate a zero tolerance policy regarding never events in the perioperative setting.

American College of Surgeons. (2002). Statement in ensuring correct patient, correct site, and correct procedure surgery. Retrieved from http://www.facs.org

Agency for Healthcare Research and Quality. (2013). Eliminating CLABSI, a national patient safety imperative. Retrieved from http://www.ahrq.gov

Agency for Healthcare Research and Quality. (2017). Patient safety network, AHRQ. Retrieved from http://www.psnet.ahrq.gov

Feldman, D. (2008). PSNET, patient safety network. Retrieved from https://www.psnet.ahrq.gov/webmm/case/177

James, J. (2013). A new evidence-based estimate of patients with hospital care. *Journal of Patient Safety*, 9(3), 122–128. doi:10.1097/PTS.0b013e3182948a69

The Joint Commission. (2010). The wrong site surgery project. Retrieved from http://www.centerfortransforminghealthcare.org/UserFiles/file/CTH_Wrong_Site_Surgery_Project_6_24_11.pdf

Mallett, R., Conroy, M., Zaidain, L., & Bruce, S. (2012). Preventing wrong site, procedure, and patient events using a common cause analysis. *American Journal of Medical Quality*, 27(1), 21–29. doi:10.1177/1062860611412066

■ SURGICAL INTERVENTIONS IN CANCER CARE

Carol Pehotsky
Mary Szostakowski
Jacob Runion

Overview

The Commission on Global Cancer Surgery estimates that there were 15.2 million new cancer diagnoses in 2015 (Sullivan et al., 2015). Of those diagnosed, 80% required surgical treatment. Cancer surgery may be curative or palliative in nature and is conducted in a variety of ways to best target the cancer while maximizing overall functioning of the patient. Nursing care for a patient during cancer surgery includes preventing injury related to positioning during surgery, interacting with technologies for delivering surgical cancer care, and ensuring safe transitions throughout the perioperative setting.

Background

It is projected that surgery can be curative in approximately 50% of all cancer diagnoses, thus making surgery an important part of any cancer treatment plan (Sullivan et al., 2015). Surgical care for those with cancer diagnoses can take on many forms. There are currently almost 300 distinct surgical procedures across complexity levels for surgical cancer care, with half of those procedures requiring surgical cancer expertise (Sullivan et al., 2015).

Surgical cancer care may focus on removing a tumor, reducing the size of the tumor, or decreasing cancer symptoms (National Cancer Institute [NCI], 2015). For certain cancers, surgery may be the only form of treatment; for others, it is part of a comprehensive treatment approach that also includes chemotherapy, hormone therapy, immunotherapy, or radiation (DeSantis et al., 2014). The surgery used for cancer care also varies based on the type of cancer, the extent of the surgery, and the extent to which the cancer has spread. The goal of cancer surgery is not only to remove or treat the cancer, but also to minimize the destruction of healthy cells and organs surrounding the tumor.

Solid tumors that are clearly demarcated, with easily identified borders, that have not metastasized are most responsive to surgical removal. Surgeons may remove a wider area of tissue beyond the cancer, known as a *margin*, to ensure the removal of as many cancer cells as possible (DeSantis et al., 2014). Even one remaining cancer cell can continue to grow and place the patient at risk for tumor growth after surgery. The surgical team may use imaging equipment, such as fluoroscopy (a continuous x-ray) or computer-assisted navigation devices, to pinpoint the exact location of the tumor during the surgery.

When removing a cancerous tumor, the surgical team also considers the best course of action for maintaining function and healthy tissues following surgery. For example, removing a tumor from a bone or tissues surrounding a bone can leave the remaining bone susceptible to fractures; the remaining bone may be filled with medical cement to ensure that it can properly heal. Cancer surgery may also necessitate removing the tumor and portions of affected organs as well to maximize function. In these types of procedures, surgical bypasses may need to be created. A *pancreaticoduodenectomy*, or *whipple* procedure, for example, includes the removal of the gall bladder along with portions of the pancreas, duodenum, and stomach. The remaining portions of the stomach and pancreas are then attached to the jejunum to maintain gastrointestinal function.

Tumor debulking, or reducing the size of a cancer tumor, is done when it is not possible to remove the entire tumor. This may be because the surgeon cannot safely remove the tumor due to its proximity to other organs or blood vessels. Debulking can still aid the patient in allowing other types of cancer treatment to work.

Advances in recent years have allowed surgical teams to treat cancer in surgery using minimally invasive techniques. These techniques may result in small or no incisions, reducing the impact to surrounding tissues, decreasing risk of complications, and speeding recovery times. Examples of these types of procedures are the use of lasers in surgery and intraoperative chemotherapy.

Lasers can be used surgically to either destroy or shrink tumors. Surgical approaches often use endoscopes and either the body's natural openings (such as the nose, mouth, vagina) or small incisions that allow for the laser to be directed at the tumor. The laser is used to heat the tumor until it is liquefied. In addition to using lasers to destroy cancer tumors, laser surgery can be used to shrink cancer tumors. Shrinking a tumor, while not removing it, may allow other treatment modalities to work more effectively, or may be used to ease symptoms such as pain or obstructions caused by tumors in patients seeking palliative care.

Chemotherapy may be part of the surgical procedure as well and can be used to treat bladder, gynecological, and abdominal cancers. Intraoperative chemotherapy is often preceded by surgical removal of tumors before instillation. *Heated intraperitoneal chemotherapy*, or *HiPEC*, is high-temperature, highly concentrated chemotherapy instilled into the abdominal cavity during surgery to kill cancer cells too small to be seen or removed surgically.

Clinical Aspects

Nursing care of the patient undergoing surgical cancer care is focused on both safety of the patient and safety of the surgical team. Patients with cancer may experience immunosuppression both before and after surgery as a part of their treatment plan. Perioperative nurses have the responsibility to ensure that the utmost sterile techniques are used for every surgery; that charge becomes even more important for those who are immunocompromised. Safeguarding aseptic technique in surgery includes providing the surgical team with sterilized instruments, supplies, and equipment in a way that does not compromise sterility; monitoring all members of the team for proper technique; and ensuring proper hand hygiene, movement within the operating room (OR), and surgical attire (Burlingame et al., 2016).

Cancer surgery may place patients at increased risk for skin injuries due to the length of the surgical procedure, the position required for the surgery, or both (Burlingame et al., 2016). Perioperative nurses must also assess patients having cancer surgery for other factors that could increase the risk of pressure injury, such as bony prominences from cachexia or existing skin injuries from radiation treatment. Positioning devices or pressure-reducing dressing should be used to reduce the risk of skin injury for these patients (Spruce & VanWicklin, 2014).

The use of lasers and chemotherapy within a surgical procedure requires the perioperative nurse to provide for the safety of both the patients and caregivers within the OR. The perioperative nurse must know the wavelength of the laser being used to determine the type and extent of safety equipment needed (Burlingame et al., 2016). Patients and caregivers will need eye protection specific to the laser wavelength, and nonreflective instruments and endotracheal tubes are used to reduce the risk of fire with the laser. Intraoperative chemotherapy requires the same careful handling as that administered outside of the OR, and the surgical team dons chemotherapy personal protective equipment when handling this medicine or bodily fluids. The perioperative nurse must be sure to communicate the need for chemotherapy precautions in handoff communication to subsequent nursing care areas (NIOSH, 2014).

Specimen handling is an important component of the care a perioperative nurse provides the patient having cancer surgery. Surgical specimens received during a cancer surgery may range from a biopsy to a lymph node to larger sections of the tumor. Accurate analysis of these specimens is crucial to ensure that patients receive the appropriate oncological care. The specimen must be received from the surgical field and handled in such a way as not to disrupt or contaminate it (Burlingame et al., 2016). Nurses must know how the specimen must be preserved or prepared, and ensure that it is labeled correctly and sent to the correct location for timely analysis (Burlingame et al., 2016).

OUTCOMES

Surgical intervention is an important part of a patient's cancer treatment. Positive patient outcomes resulting from perioperative nursing care include an absence of injury, related to positioning or use of devices such as lasers. Prevention of surgical site infections is also an important outcome for the surgical team (Burlingame et al., 2016).

Surgery can be curative in 50% of cancer care, and also remains part of the treatment approach for patients with metastatic cancer. Surgical interventions for those with metastatic cancer have declined slightly over the last 10 years, with accompanying decreases in morbidity and mortality following these surgeries (Bateni et al., 2015). Researchers attribute this to improvements in the way patients are screened for and educated about surgical options, especially in instances of incurable cancers (Bateni et al., 2015).

Summary

Surgery is an important component of the treatment plan for patients with cancer. Several options and modalities are available to patients, dependent on whether the goal is to remove the cancer or to make it more amenable to other treatments. Perioperative nursing care for these patients focuses primarily on injury prevention, whether related to infection, positioning, or the surgical intervention.

Bateni, S. B., Meyers, F. J., Bold, R. J., & Canter, R. J. (2015). Current perioperative outcomes for patients with disseminated cancers. *Journal of Surgical Research, 197*(1), 118–125. doi:10.1016/j.jss.2015.03.063

Burlingame, B., Denholm, B., Link, T., Ogg, M. J., Spruce, L., Spry, C., . . . Wood, A. (2016). *AORN Guidelines for Perioperative Practice*. Denver, CO: Association of periOperative Registered Nurses.

DeSantis, C. E., Lin, C. C., Mariotto, A. B., Siegel, R. L., Stein, K. D., Kramer, J. L., . . . Jemal, A. (2014). Cancer treatment and survivorship statistics, 2014. *A Cancer Journal for Clinicians, 64*, 252–271. doi:10.3322/caac.21235

National Cancer Institute. (2015). Cancer treatment: Surgery. Retrieved from https://www.cancer.gov/about-cancer/treatment/types/surgery

National Institute for Occupational Safety and Health. (2014). *NIOSH list of antineoplastic and other hazardous drugs in healthcare settings, 2014* (NIOSH Publication No. 2014–138). Atlanta, GA: Author. Retrieved from http://www.cdc.gov.ccmain.ohionet.org/niosh/docs/2014-138/pdfs/2014-138.pdf

Spruce, L., & Van Wicklin, S. A. (2014). Back to basics: Positioning the patient. *AORN Journal, 100*(3), 298–305.

Sullivan, R., Alatise, O. I., Anderson, B. O., Audisio, R., Autier, P., Aggarwal, A., . . . Purushotham, A. (2015). Global cancer surgery: Delivering safe, affordable, and timely cancer surgery. *Lancet Oncology, 16*(11), 1193–1224. doi:10.1016/S1470-2045(15)00223-5

■ SURGICAL INTERVENTIONS IN PARKINSON'S DISEASE

Karyn L. Boyar

Overview

Parkinson's disease (PD) is a chronic, progressive, neurological disorder triggered by a degeneration of the dopamine-producing cells in the brain. There is no known cure. A diagnosis is established based on the presence of at least two out of four motor symptoms: tremor at rest, muscle rigidity, bradykinesia, and balance/gait problems. A robust response to the dopamine replacement drug carbidopa/levodopa aids in confirming the diagnosis. Other nonmotor symptoms may include mood disorders, cognitive loss, autonomic disorders, gastrointestinal complaints, and sleep disturbance. Although the mainstay of disease management remains the use of dopaminergic therapies after 5 to 7 years, these drugs often lose efficacy. In advanced PD even as medications are increased, drugs often fail to control symptoms, last for increasingly shorter periods of time, and are frequently associated with debilitating side effects such as daily motor fluctuations and dyskinesia (unwanted, involuntary movements). For certain patients with advanced PD, a surgical intervention may be indicated with deep brain stimulation (DBS), and to a lesser extent, pallidotomy and thalamotomy ablative procedures. Ablative surgery has been performed since the 19th century but provided limited success and carried a high risk of complications. With the discovery of the synthetic dopamine agent levopdopa in the 1960s, these interventions were mostly abandoned (Rossi, Cerquetti, Mandolesi, & Merello, 2015). However, the surgical pendulum has swung back into favor due to a number of factors, including the knowledge that medications often lose potency over time, MRI-assisted brain mapping became available, and a more defined selection process of suitable surgical candidates was constructed. Furthermore, current research studies demonstrate that surgery improves motor function and quality of life, allowing patients to decrease medications that cause the adverse side effects often associated with dopaminergic replacement therapy (Godden, 2014; Hu, Moses, Hutter, & Williams 2016; Rossi et al., 2016). Nurses who manage the care of Parkinson's patients and those involved in the perioperative care of these patients are required to have an in-depth knowledge of PD medication management and the unique concerns involved in taking care of this population. Trained movement-disorder nurses and nurse practitioners may also be responsible for the postoperative programming, adjustment, and maintenance of optimal DBS settings, and medications in the outpatient setting.

Background

Parkinson's disease affects as many as 1 million people in the United States, with more than 60,000 new cases reported each year. Worldwide estimates show PD affecting more than 10 million people (Parkinson Disease Foundation, 2015), whereas the number of undiagnosed cases may run into the thousands. A small percentage of people (4%) is diagnosed with young-onset PD, in which symptoms appear before age 50 years. Men are more than one and half times more likely to receive a diagnosis of PD than women (Parkinson Disease Foundation, 2015). Although the incidence of PD increases with age, a later onset generally presages a milder course of progression. A recent systematic review and meta-analysis examined age-specific PD incidence rates showing a peak incidence in those between 70 and 79 years (Hirsch, Jette, Frolkis, Steeves, & Pringsheim, 2016). In addition to age and gender, risks for PD include a familial component, genetic factors, occupational exposures, traumatic brain injury, and drug use. In the United States, the cost of PD in terms of both direct and indirect costs of disability is estimated at nearly $25 billion per year. The estimated costs for medications run upwards of $2,500 per patient a year, whereas surgical costs may spiral toward $100,000 per patient with insurance covering most procedures (Parkinson Disease Foundation, 2015).

Parkinson's disease may be considered one of the most challenging neurological disorders. For people with advanced PD experiencing motor fluctuations and dyskinesia, symptoms can grievously affect the quality of life. Moreover, research studies have established that caregiver burden rises when the patient in the dyad experiences both motor and nonmotor symptoms with increased strain correlating with social and economic loss, as well as increased rates of depression among caregivers (Grün, Pieri, Vaillant, & Diederich, 2016; Rozina, 2014).

The importance of surgery in the management of people with advanced PD cannot be underestimated. Thousands of patients have achieved substantial control over symptoms with two Food and Drug Administration (FDA)-approved surgeries: DBS and stereotactic ablation (Martinez-Ramirez et al., 2015). DBS was pioneered in France in 1987 for essential tremor and approved for use in PD in the United States in 2002 (Kalia, Sankar, Lozano, 2013). Both procedures aim to modulate abnormal activity within targeted brain circuits and thus provide relief from symptoms. (Martinez-Ramirez et al., 2015). Ablative surgeries include thalamotomy, subthalamotomy, or pallidotomy and are used far less frequently than DBS, and then only when DBS is not a viable option. Ablative surgery is permanent and more invasive; therefore, DBS has evolved as the preferred treatment as patients may be continuously reprogrammed to achieve better results and turning off the stimulators allows for reversibility.

Most recent, other minimally invasive therapies have come into use and include continuous subcutaneous apomorphine infusion (CSAI) and levodopa–carbidopa intestinal gel (LCIG). Both of these procedures use implantable devices placed in the abdomen that provide a constant stimulation of dopamine receptors allowing for a decrease in the number of motor fluctuations. Common side effects include nausea, vomiting, and possible bradycardia and postural hypotension (De Rosa, Tessitore, Bilo, Peluso, De Michele, 2016). Because these procedures are performed far less frequently than DBS, the remaining discussion is chiefly focused on the use of DBS.

Clinical Aspects

As discussed, DBS remains the predominant surgical option for people with advanced PD. The exact mechanism of action remains unclear. Patients with medication-induced complications refractory to care are most likely to benefit from DBS. The neurosurgeon performs a stereotactic mapping of the brain, targeting preselected areas that correspond to the individual's main complaints. The four most common areas employed include the subthalamic nucleus (STN), globus pallidus interna (GPI), the pedunculopontine nucleus (PPN), and a subdivision of the thalamus or VIM (ventral intermediate nucleus). Stimulation of the globus pallidus or subthalamic nucleus may achieve a reduction in tremor, rigidity bradykinesia, gait disorder, and dyskinesia. The PPN is a new, investigational target that may be appropriate for patients with gait freezing, and is currently under investigation in several clinical trials (Rizzone et.al. 2014). For most patients, DBS of the globus pallidus or subthalamic nucleus is the most appropriate choice as stimulation of these targets affects a broader range of symptoms. Until recently, the long-term efficacy and safety of STN–DBS were unclear but an 11-year follow-up study assessed the long-term outcomes in 26 PD patients, indicating that motor complications were still well controlled as compared to their baseline data. Dyskinesia showed an 84% improvement, and motor fluctuations were also well controlled (Rizzone et al., 2014).

Appropriate selection of surgical candidates is critical to achieving successful outcomes in DBS, but many patients may not fit the exacting criteria. Current consensus on the ideal candidate for DBS requires that patients should have had PD for at least 5 years; have experienced a robust response to levodopa, but suffer from daily "off" periods when medications fail to control symptoms; have experienced dyskinesia from dopaminergic therapy; be younger than 75 years; have no comorbidities; have normal brain scans; be free from cognitive or depressive disorders; and have a supportive family network. Patients undergo a battery of tests called the Core Assessment Program for Surgical Interventional Therapies in PD (CAPSIT-PD). These tests assess both the motor and neuropsychological function of surgical candidates using specific scales to measure function: the Unified Parkinson's Disease Rating Scale (UPDRS) "on/off" home diaries, quality-of-life scales, and neuropsychological evaluations (Rossi et al., 2016). Nurses should also be aware of possible disparity in patient selection. There is growing concern that African Americans do not receive medical and surgical care as often as their White counterparts. In terms of DBS, disproportionately fewer surgeries were performed for African Americans, with less access to care, cultural biases, or socioeconomic status identified as causative factors (Chan et al., 2014).

NURSING INTERVENTIONS, MANAGEMENT, AND IMPLICATIONS

In order to educate and provide support to patients undergoing DBS and their families, nurses should be familiar with the prescreening process and well versed in the procedural details of DBS surgery. Patients should be counseled that surgery may provide relief from symptoms commensurate with the best response they achieve when their medications work. As with any surgery, patients should be informed of the risks and benefits. Patients may be reassured that DBS is generally well tolerated with few complications. Less than 2% of DBS patients experience complications, but these may include hemorrhage, infection, cerebrospinal fluid (CSF) leakage, lead breakage, and failure of the battery. DBS may be performed either awake or asleep (Godden, 2014) with the majority of surgeries performed awake under local anesthesia. The advantage to awake surgery is that a patient's response may be assessed during surgery. Electrodes are implanted using MRI mapping techniques and then connected to an internal pulse generator similar to a pacemaker. Often this small battery-powered generator is implanted in the chest or less frequently, the abdomen. By delivering small high-frequency electrical stimulation, the patient may achieve moderate to significant control over symptoms (Godden, 2014). An external handheld device controls the on/off function of the stimulator.

Nursing care for patients undergoing surgery includes interventions that reduce preventable errors and injuries such as those related to positioning. Before electrode implantation, a "beach chair" position is utilized with care to pad any bony prominences or pressure areas. A local anesthetic numbs the scalp surface. A custom-made platform is affixed to the skull using screws and small holes are drilled allowing placement of the electrodes. Once electrodes are implanted, the neurosurgeon may ask that the patient perform simple maneuvers in order to assess efficacy or side effects. After the surgeon determines correct electrode placement, the patient will be sedated, allowing for permanent lead placement and implantation of the battery. The procedure usually takes less than 6 hours, and patients can be expected to spend 1 or 2 nights in the hospital (Godding, 2016). During this time, perioperative nurse will focus on monitoring patients for sensations of cold or pain induced by long periods of sitting in one place, any side effects from the stimulation or procedure that may include dyskinesia, paresthesia, double vision or sustained muscle contractions. As with all surgical intervention, perioperative nurses have the responsibility to reduce risks for surgical site infections that includes aseptic technique with all supplies, instruments, and equipment. Postoperative care will focus on assessing the patient for pain, sleep, infection, constipation, urinary disorders, as well as monitoring the patient for any motor fluctuations and "off" periods (De Rosa et al., 2016). The surgical team has responsibilities for safe transitions throughout the perioperative setting.

OUTCOMES

Positive patient outcomes include an absence of injury, and surgical site infections are important for the surgical patient (Burlingame et al., 2016). Within 1 to 2 weeks following surgery, patients are assessed in the ambulatory setting. They participate in an elaborate number of visits to discover optimal stimulation programming and parameters. Patients and families may need reassurance that programming sessions will ultimately result in maximum benefit and relief from symptoms. Nursing provides essential help during this time by maintaining frequent communication with patients and families in order to assess the effectiveness of DBS and monitor for skin infections or erosions. The nurse may also be involved in parameter programming and assess the efficacy of stimulator settings (De Rosa et al., 2016).

Summary

Surgery can be an important option in the treatment plan for patients with PD. It is essential that the perioperative nurse focuses on error and injury prevention through good communication. Nurses caring for people undergoing surgical procedures for advanced PD assume vital roles in the ongoing, interdisciplinary management of care while managing the needs of both patient and caregiver. Valuable resources, such as support groups, exercise programs, and cognitive, voice and balance training, impart great benefit and should be strongly encouraged. Finally, to improve surgical selection and management in this population, nurse researchers can further explore and disseminate the factors limiting people from receiving equal and optimal care.

Burlingame, B., Denholm, B., Link, T., Ogg, M. J., Spruce, L., Spry, C., . . . Wood, A. (2016). *AORN guidelines for perioperative practice.* Denver, CO: Association of peri-Operative Registered Nurses.

Chan, A. K., McGovern R. A., Brown, L. T, Sheehy J. P., Zacharia B. E., Mikell C. B., . . . McKhann G. M. (2014). Disparities in access to deep brain stimulation surgery for Parkinson disease: Interaction between African American race and medicaid use. *JAMA Neurology, 71*(3), 291–299 doi:10.1001/jamaneurol.2013.5798

De Rosa, A., Tessitore, A., Bilo, L., Peluso, S., & De Michele, G. (2016). Infusion treatments and deep brain stimulation in Parkinson's disease: The role of nursing. *Geriatric Nursing, 37*(6), 434–439. doi:10.1016/j.gerinurse.2016.06.012

Godden, B. (2014). Deep brain stimulation for Parkinson's disease. *Journal of Perianesthesia Nursing, 29*(3), 230–233. doi:10.1016/j.jopan.2014.03.006

Grün, D., Pieri, V., Vaillant, M., & Diederich, N. J. (2016). Original Study: Contributory factors to caregiver burden in Parkinson Disease. *Journal of the American Medical Directors Association, 17,* 626–632. doi:10.1016/j.jamda.2016.03.004

Hirsch, L., Jette, N., Frolis, A., Steeves, T., & Pringsheim, T. (2016). The incidence of Parkinson's disease: A systematic review and meta-analysis. *Neuroepidemiology, 46,* 292–300 doi:10.1159/000445751

Hu, K., Moses, Z., Hutter, M., & Williams, Z. (2017). Short-term adverse outcomes after deep brain stimulation treatment in patients with Parkinson Disease. *World Neurosurgery, 98,* 365–374. doi:10.1016/j.wneu.2016.10.138

Kalia S., Sankar, T., & Lozano, A. (2013). Deep brain stimulation for Parkinson's disease and other movement disorders. *Current Opinion in Neurology, 26,* 374–380

Martinez-Ramirez, D., Wei, H., Bona, A. R., Okun, M. S., & Shukla, A. W. (2015). Update on deep brain stimulation in Parkinson's disease. *Translational Neurodegeneration,* 4(1), 1. doi:10.1186/s40035-015-0034-0

Parkinson Disease Foundation. (2015). Understanding Parkinson's. Retrieved from http://www.pdf.org/en/understanding_pd

Rizzone, M. G., Fasano, A., Daniele, A., Zibetti, M., Merola, A., Rizzi, L., & Albanese, A. (2014). Long-term outcome of subthalamic nucleus DBS in Parkinson's disease: From the advanced phase towards the late stage of the disease? *Parkinsonism & Related Disorders,* 20(4), 376–381. doi:10.1016/j.parkreldis.2014.01.012

Rossi, M., Cerquetti, D., Mandolesi J., & Merello, M. (2016). Parkinson's disease: Current and future therapeutics and clinical trials. Cambridge, UK: Cambridge University Press. Retrieved from https://www.cambridge.org/core/books/parkinsonsdisease/29D3044B24C127BC5AF148E74B0AC83A

Rozina, B. (2014). Understanding the burden on caregivers of people with Parkinson's: A scoping review of the literature. *Rehabilitation Research and Practice, 2014,* Article ID 718527. doi:10.1155/2014/718527

■ SURGICAL INTERVENTIONS USING EMERGING TECHNOLOGIES

Carol Pehotsky
Mary Szostakowski
Jacob Runion
Florin Sgondea
Dena L. Salamon

Overview

Innovations in surgical procedures have impacted virtually every surgical specialty. Emerging technologies allow surgical teams to better meet the needs of patients with minimal complications, smaller incisions, and decreased hospital stays. Surgical nurses are challenged to stay informed of these technological advances to ensure that they are adequately trained and prepared to care for patients undergoing innovative procedures.

Background

A review of patents and publications related to surgical technology over the course of 30 years yielded more than 50,000 patents and 1.8 million publications (Hughes-Hallett et al., 2014), confirming the omnipresence of innovation and technology in surgery. Minimally invasive surgical techniques have been a long-standing area of exploration; robotic-assisted surgery and imaging-guided surgical techniques are on the rise (Hughes-Hallett et al., 2014).

Minimally invasive surgical techniques involve the use of one or several small incisions in which specially designed cameras and surgical instruments are inserted (Burlingame et al., 2016). The placement and number of incisions are dictated based on the type of surgery to be performed. Once focused on abdominal procedures, minimally invasive surgery innovation now includes surgery using existing openings into the body, such as the mouth, nose, or anus. Recent innovations in minimally invasive surgery include single incision site procedures, including those for gall bladder surgery, kidney surgery, and colon resections. There are several patient benefits with the use of any minimally invasive surgery technique, whether using one or several incisions. This includes decreased pain due to fewer and smaller incisions, decreased blood loss, shorter length of stay, and decreased scarring (Rockall & DeMartines, 2014).

The addition of robotic-assisted technologies has further enhanced minimally invasive surgical approaches. This technology increases the depth perception for surgeons and allows greater flexibility and control. Robotic-assisted surgery makes use of separate components: the console where the surgeon sits separately from the surgical team and manipulates the robotic instrumentation, the tower where the camera and display are housed, and the cart containing the robotic camera "arm" as well as "arms" with surgical instruments attached (Burlingame et al., 2016). Each component is connected via network cables to allow communication between devices as well as with the vendor if troubleshooting needs arise.

Robotic surgery can result in superior outcomes, such as lower blood loss, shorter length of hospital stay, and lower complication rates when compared to traditional incision surgeries, but fare only slightly better than minimally invasive surgical techniques in some studies (Tan et al., 2016). Robotic-assisted surgery may result in increased cost, both in terms of equipment and supplies, as well as in training of surgeons and the surgical team.

Surgical teams are increasingly using image-guided surgery techniques to aid in visualization and localization of the operative site (Brown, 2016). An example of this emerging technology is interventional magnetic resonance imaging (IMRI). Before IMRI, surgeons would utilize preoperative radiological imaging to determine the location of tumors and lesions. The surgical resection would be completed, and postoperative imaging would reveal how much resection was completed. The use of IMRI within the operating room (OR) allows for real-time feedback of tumor resection or lesion ablation, enabling the surgeon to continue the resecting when appropriate. This approach has been used successfully with brain tumor resections, deep-brain stimulator placement, and ablation of epilepsy focal tissues.

Clinical Aspects

Nurses must be aware of the implications technology has on their practice and the unique challenges technology presents. During minimally invasive or robotic-assisted surgeries, the surgical team may use gas, such as carbon dioxide or helium to distend the abdomen to improve visualization and, space in which to operate. Perioperative nurses can help prevent patient injuries by ensuring proper use of the gas insufflator and assessing for signs and symptoms of gas emboli. If gas emboli are suspected, the treatment includes large volume intravenous fluid infusion and position change (Burlingame et al., 2016).

Fluids may also be used either for surgical site irrigation or to create additional space within the cavity or joint during a minimally invasive or robotic-assisted surgery (Burlingame et al., 2016). Perioperative nurses verify that the correct irrigation fluid is used, assess the patient's overall risk of fluid management issues, and monitor fluid dispensed and irrigated (Burlingame et al., 2016). An imbalance in fluid output merits notification of the surgical team to address the issue.

Each of these emerging technologies may require unique patient positioning during the surgical procedure. With these unique positions come challenges in protecting patient skin integrity. The perioperative nurse assesses patient's skin position as the patient arrives at the OR, and provides positioning devices and skin protective devices while placing the patient in the correct surgical position (Burlingame et al., 2016). In addition, the operating room table may be moved or tilted during the procedure; it is the responsibility of the perioperative nurse to ensure that the patient is secured safely as part of the positioning process (Burlingame et al., 2016).

Minimally invasive and robotic-assisted procedures may require the steep Trendelenburg position. The perioperative nurse assesses for risk of sheering forces and shifting of patient position. Extreme positions should be tested before draping to ensure that the patient does not slide (Burlingame et al., 2016). During this extreme positioning, the patient may also experience decreased chest expansion, decreased air exchange, and decreased blood return if the insufflation pressure is too high. The perioperative nurse assesses the patient for these risks and works collaboratively with the rest of the surgical team to prevent or treat them.

OUTCOMES

It is important for perioperative nurses to understand the technology with which they are working, and to ensure that they have been trained properly before its use. This is true for any surgical innovation, and the emerging technologies discussed in this entry are no exception. For robotic-assisted surgery, the surgical team needs to have a safety plan in place if the robot shuts down while in use. Both minimally invasive and robotic-assisted surgery require specialized surgical instrumentation; the perioperative nurse needs to be familiar with these instruments and their safe use.

The use of IMRI must be accompanied by a collaboration between radiology and surgical specialties. Each specialty must fully understand how the other operates to have a successful program. From a radiology perspective, this personnel must adapt and understand the process of an operation and the importance of sterile technique. The surgical team must go through in-depth training on the inherent risks in working around a high-powered magnet. Perioperative nurses undergo additional training before work in an IMRI environment to ensure that they know how to provide care that ensures both patient and caregiver safety. This includes the use of nonferrous metallic instruments and oxygen tanks (because they are not magnetic), and how to ensure patient safety when the MRI is active.

Summary

Innovation is a hallmark of the surgical specialty, as surgeons seek to minimize disruption of healthy tissue and speed recovery for their patients. Techniques, such as minimally invasive and robotic-assisted surgery, allow the surgical team to operate with great precision in most of the surgical specialties. Image-guided surgery allows the surgical team to use real-time information to ensure correct and adequate localization of the area on which to be operated. Perioperative nurses play an important role in the safe care of patients undergoing innovative procedures. It is important for nurses working in the perioperative setting to ensure that they have received adequate training before use of emerging technologies to best advocate for their patients.

Brown, S. (2014). Image-guided surgery. *Medscape.* Retrieved from http://emedicine.medscape.com/article/875524-overview

Burlingame, B., Denholm, B., Link, T., Ogg, M. J., Spruce, L., Spry, C., . . . Wood, A. (2016). *AORN guidelines for perioperative practice.* Denver, CO: Association of periOperative Registered Nurses.

Hughes-Hallett, A., Mayer, E. K., Marcus, H. J., Cundy, T. P., Pratt, P. J., Parston, G., . . . Darzi, A. W. (2014). Quantifying innovation in surgery. *Annals of Surgery, 260*(2), 205–211. doi:10.1097/SLA.0000000000000662

Rockall, T. A., & Demartines, N. (2014). Laparoscopy in the era of enhanced recovery. *Best Practice & Research Clinical Gastroenterology, 28*(1), 133–142.

Tan, A., Ashrafian, H., Scott, A. J., Mason, S. E., Harling, L., Athanasiou, T., & Darzi, A. (2016). Robotic surgery: Disruptive innovation or unfulfilled promise? A systematic review and meta-analysis of the first 30 years. *Surgical Endoscopy, 30*(10), 4330–4352. doi:10.1007/s00464-016-4752-x

■ TRADITIONAL SURGICAL INTERVENTIONS

Michelle McHugh Slater

Overview

The perioperative phase of patient care for traditional surgical interventions consists of three distinct phases: preoperative care, intraoperative care, and postoperative care. The surgical setting may be either inpatient or outpatient based on the type of procedure, anesthesia requirements, level of urgency, and patient's health status. Traditional surgical procedures are classified according to the reason for the intervention, urgency of the intervention, degree of risk to the patient, and extent of procedural area involvement. Each category for classification may be further described. Reasons for surgical procedures fall into five distinct types: diagnostic, curative, restorative, palliative, and cosmetic. The urgency for an intervention is determined as elective (not acute), urgent (requires intervention within 24–48 hours), or emergent (requires immediate intervention due to its life-threatening nature). Degree describes the amount of risk associated with a procedure in which a minor degree is without significant risk and a major degree is with greater risk. *Extent* describes for the surgical team the amount of tissue resection anticipated as simple (involves obvious area), radical (extends beyond the obvious area to the tissue root), or minimally invasive surgery (procedure within a body cavity with minimal wounds and use of endoscopes).

Background

Surgical care is provided across the life span; the World Health Organization (WHO; Weiser et al., 2016) estimates one procedure for every 25 persons globally. In 2004, the worldwide estimate of surgical operations was 234.2 million procedures (McDowell & McComb, 2014; Weiser et al., 2016). A majority of these surgeries (58.9% = 138 million) occurred in countries with high health care costs and a lower portion of the entire global population (Weiser et al., 2016). In 2012, global surgical volumes increased to an estimated 312.9 million procedures, which resulted in a 38.2% increase over 8 years (2016). The high-health-care-cost countries accounted for 59.8% of the 2012 surgical volume and only 17.7% of the world population (2016). In contrast, the very-low-health-care-cost countries accounted for 6.3% of the 2012 surgical volume and 36.8% of the world population (2016). The rates of surgical volume growth within the very-low and low-health-care-cost groups were highest. The very-low-health-care-cost countries group saw a 69% increase from 394 to 666 procedures per 100,000 people per year, whereas the low-health-care-cost countries group increased by 114.6% from 1,851 to 3,973 procedures per 100,000 people per year (2016). No significant changes in surgical volume are noted for the middle or high-health-care-cost countries.

Perioperative mortality rates (POMR) within 30 days of surgery demonstrate variation based on the classification and type of procedure performed. In developed countries, the POMR ranges from 0.2 (lowest) to 9.8 (highest) per 100 procedures (McDowell & McComb, 2014; Watters, 2014). POMR demonstrate the level of urgency as a determinant of mortality with the lowest POMR for elective procedures and the highest POMR for emergent/emergency cases (Watters, 2014). Mortality risk increases by 11% for patients, with a postoperative surgical site infection (SSI), with an estimated treatment cost of $62,000 per event in the United States (WHO, 2016). Research shows SSIs as the most common type of hospital-acquired infection (HAI) with a global rate of 11.8 per 100 surgical patients (WHO, 2016).

Surgical patients are a vulnerable population by definition: Groups with an increased risk of developing adverse health outcomes based on contributing factors such as human capital, social determinants, health status, and poverty (Stanhope & Lancaster, 2014). The interaction and number of these contributing factors relate to the degree of risk for a surgical patient. Industrialized countries have an estimated surgical complication rate from 3% to 16% (McDowell & McComb, 2014). In the United States, 35% of 8,275 reported patient safety events over a 10-year period from 2004 to 2014 occurred in the perioperative setting (Office of Quality Monitoring, 2014). Based on the complexity of perioperative services, patient safety is the primary goal for all surgical patients.

Perioperative nursing interventions focus on individualized nursing diagnoses to promote optimal patient outcomes regarding the patient's safety, physiological responses, and behavioral responses to surgical care. This conceptual framework for perioperative nursing practice is illustrated in the Association of periOperative Registered Nurses (AORN) Perioperative Patient Focused Model (AORN, 2008). This model guides patient care and is the basis for the clinical information infrastructure, the Perioperative Nursing Data Set (PNDS; AORN, 2007). AORN's PNDS is the working vocabulary for perioperative nursing care used in the implementation of the nursing process and workflows for outcome-based patient care (2007).

Clinical Aspects

Perioperative patient assessment is based on the phase of perioperative care. During each transition of care, a thorough caregiver handoff report is provided to ensure continuity of care. Standardized tools optimize this communication process. Two examples of standardized processes include SBAR (situation, background, assessment, recommendation) and I PASS the BATON (introduction, patient, assessment, situation, safety, background, actions, time, ownership, next). Along with written checklists, standardized tools for communication are an effective strategy to prevent surgical never events and adverse surgical outcomes (Criscitelli, 2013).

The preoperative phase is a critical time for both the patient and perioperative team. The preoperative nursing assessment includes the traditional head-to-toe assessment along with review of the history and physical, laboratory values, diagnostic studies, medication history, physician orders, surgical consent, patient and surgical site verification, and advance directive documentation. Additional assessment data are required specific to the surgical procedure to prevent patient injury. This data includes signs and symptoms of infection, contraindications for anesthesia, nothing-by-mouth status, patient allergies, skin preparation, bowel

and bladder preparations, implanted surgical devices, and removal of all personal items (piercings, dentures, jewelry). Preoperative teaching is a primary focus for patient preparation. Common topics for patient education include anesthesia, surgical procedure, preoperative routine, pain management, anxiety, coughing and deep breathing, blood transfusions, postoperative exercises, and prevention of postoperative complications. Nursing interventions during the preoperative phase focus on both physical and psychosocial preparation of the patient and family for the surgical procedure.

The intraoperative phase begins when the patient is transported from the preoperative area to the surgical suite. Standardized patient care plans do not address the needs of every surgical patient. The intraoperative nurse must consider the preoperative assessment findings in conjunction with age-specific outcomes to individualize the patient plan of care. The following nursing diagnoses are universal for most surgical procedures and are the basis of the care plan: acute pain; anxiety; risk for infection; risk for injury and delayed surgical recovery related to an unintended retained foreign object; risk for injury related to wrong patient, side, site and level; risk for perioperative positioning injury. From the nursing diagnosis, the nurse implements nursing interventions to best meet the desired outcome. The intraoperative nurse advocates for the patient and provides leadership for the surgical team. The intraoperative nurse must collaborate within an interdisciplinary team (physician, anesthesia, technicians, radiologists, advanced practice providers) to plan, deliver, and evaluate the perioperative care plan.

OUTCOMES

The postoperative phase begins when the patient is transported from the surgical suite to the postanesthesia care unit (PACU). The PACU nurse requires advanced medical surgical skills and situational awareness to recognize postoperative complications and intervene promptly. Patients are vulnerable in this phase as the anesthetic medications abate while respiratory control and neurological functions return. The critical PACU assessment is of the respiratory function of the patient. Before any interventions, the PACU nurse must then focus on the surgical site, pain level, cardiovascular and peripheral vascular function, neurological status (motor and sensory function), hydration status, and gastrointestinal function assessments. The PACU phase is typically 1 hour followed by transport to an inpatient unit or to a phase-two recovery area for discharge. Discharge criteria from the PACU require a patent airway, stable vital signs, tolerable pain, arousable, conscious, oriented, and free from active bleeding. The highest incidence of postoperative complications occurs between 1 and 3 days after a surgical procedure (Ignatavicius & Workman, 2016).

Summary

The perioperative nurse is the cornerstone of patient care who is responsible for reducing surgical risks and delivering safe outcomes for every patient. Traditional surgical procedures begin in the preoperative phase, transition to the intraoperative phase, and conclude in the postoperative phase. Each phase of care requires distinct skill sets and integration of technology, along with a comprehensive knowledge base of pharmacology, anatomy, and physiology. In perioperative services, constant change requires flexibility, ingenuity, and adaptation skills for the surgical team. Technology often outpaces evidence-based practice implementation methods but is necessary as a tool to enhance traditional surgical procedures. Cutting-edge procedures, advanced technologies, and contemporary research require the perioperative nurse to ardently pursue knowledge and currency in practice. The perioperative nurse is adept at patient advocacy, leadership, care coordination, communication, and medical surgical nursing. Moreover, in perioperative services, every nurse is a leader.

Association of periOperative Registered Nurses. (2007). *Perioperative nursing data set: The perioperative nursing vocabulary.* Denver, CO: Author.

Association of periOperative Registered Nurses. (2008). *Perioperative standards and recommended practices.* Denver, CO: Author.

Criscitelli, T. (2013). Patient safety first: Safe patient hand-off strategies. *AORN Journal* 97(5), 582–585.

Ignatavicius, D., & Workman, M. L. (2016). *Medical surgical nursing: Patient centered collaborative care* (8th ed.). St. Louis, MO: Saunders.

McDowell, D., & McComb, S. (2014). Safety checklist briefings: A systematic literature review. *AORN Journal* 99(1), 125–137. doi:10.1016/j.aorn.2013.11.015

Office of Quality Monitoring. (2014). The Joint Commission: Sentinel event data. Retrieved from https://www.joint commission.org/sentinel_event.aspx

Stanhope, M., & Lancaster, J. (2014) *Foundations of nursing in the community: Community oriented practice* (4th ed.) St. Louis, MO: Elsevier.

Watters, D., Hollands, M., Gruen, R., Maoate, K., Perndt, H., McDougall, R., . . . McQueen, K. (2015). Perioperative mortality rate (POMR): A global indicator of access to safe surgery and anesthesia. *World Journal of Surgery,* 39(4), 856–864. doi:10.1007/s00268-014-2638-4

Weiser, T., Haynes, A., Molina, G., Lipsitz, S., Esquivel, M., Uribe-Leitz, T., . . . Gawande, A. (2016). Bulletin of the World Health Organization: Size and distribution of the global volume of surgery in 2012. Retrieved from http://www.who.int/bulletin/volumes/94/3/15-159293/en

World Health Organization. (2016). *Global guidelines for the prevention of surgical site infection.* Geneva, Switzerland: Author. Retrieved from http://www.who.int/gpsc/ssi-guidelines/en

Psychiatric-Mental Health Nursing

This section's content is focused on clinical aspects of care that involve mental health. The topics cover the common areas of concern seen in psychiatric care settings. Psychiatric-mental health care can be delivered to clients in inpatient units, outpatient clinics, home-health programs, correctional facilities, group homes, and on medical units via a mental health consultation/liaison nurse. This most recent model of mental health treatment, integrated medical/mental health care, has become a mandate for most major health care organizations, including the Department of Veteran Affairs. This initiative is the result of data showing that client outcomes are significantly improved when mental health care needs are addressed along with medical issues, often at the same time (National Alliance on Mental Illness, 2015).

The delivery of care in the psychiatric mental health nursing field is highly specialized and requires specific education, skill sets, and temperament. By and large, it is relationship-based care in its purest form. That is, the nurse delivers the care through the establishment and maintenance of a therapeutic relationship. In this psychiatric mental health nursing section, you will find entries on common illnesses, such as bipolar disorders, depression, anxiety, and so forth, as well as important areas of practice such as maintaining therapeutic boundaries. If you are interested in more in-depth study in this area of nursing practice, please refer to Jones, Fitzpatrick, and Rogers (2017).

Jones, J. S., Fitzpatrick, J. J., & Rogers, V. L. (2017). *Psychiatric-mental health nursing: An interpersonal approach* (2nd ed.). New York, NY: Springer Publishing.

National Alliance on Mental Illness. (2015). The benefits of integrating behavioral health into primary care. Retrieved from https://www.nami.org

- Anxiety Disorders *Susan Phillips*
- Bipolar Disorder *Julie A. Berg*
- Boundary Management *Jeffrey S. Jones*
- Dementia *Stephanie R. Martin*
- Depression *Jeffrey S. Jones*
- Eating Disorders *Kathryn E. Phillips*
- Impulse Control Disorders *Lisa L. Salser*
- Obsessive Compulsive Disorder *Susan Phillips*
- Posttraumatic Stress Disorder *Danette L. Core and Denise Chivington*
- Schizophrenia *Sharon L. Phillips*
- Substance Use Disorders *Chikodiri Gibson and Se Min Um*
- Suicide *Jeffrey S. Jones*
- Vulnerable Populations *Melanie S. Lint*

■ ANXIETY DISORDERS

Susan Phillips

Overview

Anxiety is a normal emotional reaction to worry or fear and is beneficial in that it protects us from danger. However, excessive anxiety can interfere with a person's ability to live life fully and can have a significant impact on one's physical health. When anxiety becomes excessive and affects a person's daily functioning, it is a disorder. There are many types of anxiety disorders and, according to the National Institute of Mental Health (NIMH), 18.1% of adults in the United States suffer from some type of anxiety disorder. Nurses play an important role in recognizing anxiety and in reducing the disabling effects of an anxiety disorder (NIMH, 2016).

Background

Occasional anxiety is a normal part of life. You might feel anxious when faced with a problem at work, before taking a test, or making an important decision. However, anxiety disorders involve more than temporary worry or fear. An "anxiety disorder" is defined as excessive worry or fear about one or more events or activities, with intensity, frequency, and duration that is out of proportion to the actual likelihood or impact of the anticipated event (American Psychiatric Association [APA], 2013). With an anxiety disorder, the emotion of anxiety can get worse over time and can interfere with vocational, social, and family activities. Anxiety disorder often begins in childhood and is associated with deficits in the quality of life related to personal growth, social functioning, and achievement (Cohen, Jensen, Dryman, & Heimberg, 2015).

Children and adolescents most often worry about competence in academic and athletic performance, and adults worry about job duties, their health, or the health and well-being of their family members. There are several different types of anxiety disorders. Examples include social anxiety disorder (excessive anxiety limited to social settings), phobias (acute anxiety in response to specific situations or objects), posttraumatic stress disorder (excessive anxiety in response to reminders of a traumatic event), separation anxiety (persistent anxiety in response to separation from a loved one), generalized anxiety disorder (excessive worry for months to years in most situations), and anxiety associated with the use of or withdrawal from certain medications or substances. Panic disorder is a type of anxiety associated with intense fear and is characterized by recurrent and unexpected acute anxiety attacks with palpitations, sweating, trembling, and a feeling of suffocation and impending doom (APA, 2013).

Of the several types of anxiety disorders, generalized anxiety disorder is the most common with a prevalence of 0.9% among adolescents and 2.9% of adults in the United States. Generalized anxiety disorder is two times more prevalent among women than men. Adults of European descent are more likely than adults of non-European descent to experience anxiety and people from developed countries are more likely than those from nondeveloped countries to report symptoms of anxiety during their lifetime (APA, 2013).

Worry, the first core feature of anxiety, is characterized by catastrophic thinking, obsessive thoughts, and apprehension. Several neurotransmitters modulate these cognitive features, including serotonin, gamma-aminobutyric acid (GABA), norepinephrine, dopamine, and glutamate. The availability of these neurotransmitters in the brain is associated with genotype and a person's vulnerability to developing an anxiety disorder (Stahl, 2013).

The physical response to worrisome thoughts, anxiety is thought to be a part of the evolutionary "fight or flight" response for survival. The amygdala plays an important role in the cognitive understanding of sensory input to determine whether a fear response is necessary. The persons' previous life experiences play an important role in the perception of danger. For example, a child who experienced a vicious dog bite is more likely to experience anxiety in the presence of a dog as an adult. The perception of fear is associated with the autonomic nervous system and motor responses affecting muscle contractibility and breathing. Therefore, the perception of fear is associated with increased respirations, muscle tension, increase in cortisol levels, and an increase in heart rate and blood pressure. For the person experiencing chronic anxiety, there is an increased risk of medical comorbidity such as cardiovascular disease, stroke, or diabetes. Anxiety can exacerbate respiratory conditions such as asthma and chronic obstructive pulmonary disease (Stahl, 2013).

Substance abuse and depression often complicate an anxiety disorder. Loss of functioning, social isolation, increased risk of chronic disease, and increased risk of suicide make anxiety a potentially serious disabling disease. The global burden of mental illness was estimated in 2013 as the fifth leading cause of disability-adjusted life years (DALYs) and the leading cause of years lived with disability globally. The most prevalent of these disorders were anxiety and depression (Whiteford, Ferrari, & Degenhardt, 2016).

Clinical Aspects

ASSESSMENT

Providing care for the person with anxiety disorder begins with an assessment of health data. The symptoms associated with anxiety disorder include restlessness, feeling wound up or irritable, muscle tension, feeling fatigued, difficulty falling or staying asleep, poor concentration, inability to control worry or fear, and depressed mood with or without suicidal ideation.

In addition, review of the person's physical health status, past psychiatric history, and understanding of how anxiety affects the patient's self-esteem, role in the family, vocational functioning, and spiritual/cultural beliefs is important. Anxiety can be a symptom of physical diseases such as arrhythmia, hyperthyroidism, or abuse of substances. Medical causes and drug-induced anxiety must be ruled out.

The nurse should be competent in meeting quality and safety standards related to the assessment. This includes assessing for suicidal thoughts, self-mutilation, depression, and substance use, and documenting findings in the medical record using recognized terminology so that communication occurs among all members of the treatment team, including the patient's family. Lastly, the nurse needs to be aware of and monitor her or his own anxiety, as not doing so can exacerbate the client's anxiety (Jones, Fitzpatrick, & Rogers, 2017).

NURSING INTERVENTIONS, MANAGEMENT, AND IMPLICATIONS

Nursing problems should reflect the person's response to anxiety disorder in the context of his or her role in the family, at work, and in the community. This includes information derived from an assessment of the patient's needs, preferences, values, and knowledge about situations that exacerbate anxiety and techniques to reduce anxiety. Examples of nursing problems related to anxiety are:

- Ineffective coping related to disruption in social or vocational abilities
- Knowledge deficit related to anxiety-reduction techniques
- Disturbance in sleep patterns because of chronic worry

Treatment of anxiety disorder involves psychiatric medications that reduce the symptoms associated with anxiety and psychotherapy that addresses cognitions contributing to the physiological response. Nursing interventions in the treatment of anxiety disorder are assessing for environmental and cognitive triggers; educating about relaxation skills and thought-stopping techniques; educating about psychotropic medication and side effects; providing empathetic responses that support dignity and self-control, and an ongoing assessment for the presence of suicidal thoughts and substance abuse.

OUTCOMES

The desired outcomes of the treatment of anxiety are the reduction of the frequency and intensity of symptoms, and patient safety with regard to use of substances and risk of suicide. This is accomplished through an understanding of environmental factors and associated cognitions that exacerbate anxiety along with the use of effective coping strategies to mitigate its intensity.

Summary

Anxiety is a normal and useful emotion until it interferes with daily functioning and physical health. The core features of anxiety are worrisome cognitions and associated fear that triggers the "fight or flight" response. Anxiety is often comorbid with depression, substance abuse, and cardiovascular disease, making anxiety disorder a leading cause of disability. We need a better understanding of what environmental factors impact the development of anxiety. Nurses play an important role in identifying anxiety and in providing education around the treatment of anxiety disorder.

American Psychiatric Association. (2013). *Diagnostic and statistical manual of mental disorders* (5th ed.). Arlington, VA: American Psychiatric Publishing.

Cohen, J. N., Jensen, D., Dryman, M. T., & Heimberg, R. G. (2015). Enmeshment schema and quality of life deficits: The mediating role of social anxiety. *Journal of Cognitive Psychotherapy, 29*(1), 20–31.

Jones, J. S., Fitzpatrick, J. J., & Rogers, V. L. (2017). *Psychiatric-mental health nursing: An interpersonal approach* (2nd ed.). New York, NY: Springer Publishing.

National Institute of Mental Health. (2016). Anxiety disorders among adults. Retrieved from https://www.nimh.nih.gov/health/statistics/prevalence/any-anxiety-disorder-among-adults.shtml

Stahl, S. M. (2013). *Stahl's essential psychopharmacology: Neuroscientific basis and practical applications* (4th ed.). New York, NY: Cambridge University Press.

Whiteford, H., Ferrari, A., & Degenhardt, L. (2016, June). Global burden of disease studies: Implications For mental and substance use disorders. *Health Affairs, 35*(6), 1114–1120.

■ BIPOLAR DISORDER

Julie A. Berg

Overview

Bipolar disorder is a complex psychiatric illness that is distinguished by episodes of mania alternating with episodes of depression. Patients with bipolar disorder can present with a wide array of symptoms, such as mood swings, anxiety, insomnia, racing thoughts, and depression, making it challenging for those caring for the individual (Culpepper, 2014). The symptoms of bipolar disorder can be debilitating for the person experiencing this roller coaster of emotions, and these patients require collaborative medical care. The nurse caring for the patient with bipolar disorder plays an important role in the assessment and monitoring of symptoms and in implementing interventions to minimize the burden of this chronic illness (Culpepper, 2014).

Background

According to the National Institute of Mental Health (2016), bipolar disorder affects approximately 5.7 million adult Americans annually, or about 2.6% of the U.S. population aged 18 years and older. The median age of onset of the disease is 25 years, but the illness can start in early childhood or as late as age 50 years (National Institute of Mental Health, 2016). The illness is equally distributed among men and women and is found in all social classes, races, and ethnicities (National Institute of Mental Health, 2016).

The *Diagnostic and Statistical Manual of Mental Disorders, Fifth Edition* (*DSM-5*; American Psychiatric Association [APA], 2013) presents criteria for the diagnosis of bipolar disorder. The patients who suffer from bipolar disorder have recurrent episodes of mood states, which are defined as manic, hypomanic, or depressed (APA, 2013). There is a distinction between bipolar I disorder and bipolar II disorder. According to the *DSM-5* (APA, 2013), patients diagnosed with bipolar I disorder have experienced at least one episode of mania, and those diagnosed with bipolar II disorder have experienced at least one episode each of hypomania and depression.

A patient in a manic state often has increased energy, irritability, insomnia, racing thoughts, pressured speech, and risky behavior (APA, 2013). These symptoms are often severe enough to cause impairment in the patient's daily life. Patients experiencing hypomania can present with the same symptoms, but the symptoms are not severe enough to significantly impact daily living. Patients in the depressed episode of this cycle may complain of low mood, loss of interest in activities, poor motivation, fatigue, poor concentration, and suicidal ideations (APA, 2013).

Patients who suffer from this disorder are prone to increased rates of co-occurring psychiatric disorders such as personality disorders, anxiety disorders, attention deficit hyperactivity disorder (ADHD), and substance abuse (Culpepper, 2014). In addition to being predisposed to psychiatric disorders, patients with bipolar disorder also have an elevated rate of certain physical conditions that complicate treatment such as cardiovascular and metabolic disorders (Culpepper, 2014). It is possible that these conditions are co-occurring because of the lifestyle and symptoms associated with bipolar disorder, leading to increased morbidity.

Treatment for the patient with a diagnosis of bipolar disorder is multifactorial and requires various treatment modalities. Pharmacological interventions are the cornerstone of treatment for these patients, and multiple classifications of medications can be used with good response. Medications are not only crucial in the acute phases of the mania or depression but are used for maintenance therapy to prevent recurrences of mood episodes. Mood stabilizers, such as lithium and Depakote, are approved for the treatment of bipolar disorder, and require laboratory testing to monitor blood levels and other pertinent values. Atypical antipsychotics, such as olanzapine, quetiapine, and aripiprazole, are Food and Drug Administration (FDA) approved and can be used alone or in conjunction with a mood stabilizer for treatment. Conventional antidepressants can be used but must be used vigilantly, as they can precipitate mania in some patients (McCormick, Murray, & McNew, 2015).

Pharmacological intervention alone is not enough to treat these complicated patients. According to Hirschfeld, Bowden, and Gitlin (2002):

At this time there is no cure for bipolar disorder; however, treatment can decrease the associated morbidity and mortality. Initially, the psychiatrist should perform a Diagnostic evaluation and assess the patient's safety and level of functioning to Arrive at a decision about the optimum treatment setting. Subsequently, specific Goals of psychiatric management include establishing and maintaining a therapeutic Alliance, monitoring the patient's psychiatric status, providing education regarding Bipolar disorder, enhancing treatment compliance, promoting regular patterns of Activity and of sleep, anticipating stressors, identifying new episodes early, and minimizing functional impairments. (p. 9)

Clinical Aspects

ASSESSMENT

The nurse plays an important role in the assessment of the patient with suspected bipolar disorder. He or she needs to perform a comprehensive interview to obtain pertinent information. The interview should consist of the patient's chief complaint, history of present illness, alcohol and substance abuse history, medical history family history, developmental history, and social history (O'Brien, Kennedy, & Ballard, 2008). This information is vital in determining whether the patient meets the criteria for the diagnoses.

The nurse then needs to assess various aspects of the patient such as affect and physical behavior. For example, patients in a depressive episode may have facial expressions of sadness, poor eye contact, and speak low and slow. Patients in a manic episode may speak quickly and loudly, appear agitated, have a labile mood, and may appear restless. The nurse must also assess the patient's thought process for suicidal and homicidal thoughts, poor judgment, poor concentration, pressured speech, or flight of ideas. Finally, the nurse should inquire about how the patient is sleeping, appetite, risky behaviors, insight, judgment, and overall ability to remain safe.

NURSING INTERVENTIONS, MANAGEMENT, AND IMPLICATIONS

After completing a thorough interview and assessment, the nurse must develop nursing interventions to help aid the patient. According to Nettina (2013), nursing interventions for the patient in a depressive episode include strengthening coping skills, fostering a sense of hope, maintaining safety, and encouraging participation in activities of daily living (ADL), facilitating sleep, providing individual and family education, and encouraging health maintenance. Nursing interventions for the patient in a manic or hypomanic episode consist of improving impulse control, decreasing disturbed thoughts, improving sleep patterns, improving the effect of bipolar illness on the family, and ensuring adequate nutrition (Nettina, 2013).

OUTCOMES

There are several expected outcomes for the patient with bipolar disorder. According to Nettina (2013), "for the patient in a depressed episode, expected outcomes are that the patient will report an improvement in mood and an increase in daily activities, the patient remains free from self-harm, the patient can accomplish ADLs in an independent manner, and obtains a minimum of 5 hours of uninterrupted sleep" (p. 1823). Expected outcomes for the patient in a manic or hypomanic episode are, "improved thought processes demonstrated by clear sentences with no evidence of flight of ideas, completion of simple tasks, 5 hours of sleep and no weight loss noted" (Nettina, 2013, p. 1825).

Summary

Bipolar disorder is an ongoing battle for patients who deal with the roller coaster of emotions it causes. The nurse plays a vital and important role in caring for these individuals. Proper assessment and initiation of nursing interventions are central to maintaining the highest level of functioning for these patients.

American Psychiatric Association. (2013). *Diagnostic and statistical manual of mental disorders* (5th ed.). Arlington, VA: American Psychiatric Publishing.

Culpepper, L. (2014). The diagnosis and treatment of bipolar disorder: Decision making in primary care. *Primary Care Companion for CNS Disorder, 16*(3), PCC.13r01609. doi:10.4088/PCC.13r01609

Hirschfeld, R. M., Bowden, C. L., & Gitlin, M. J. (2002). *Practice guideline for the treatment of patients with bipolar disorder* (2nd ed.). Washington, DC: American Psychological Association.

McCormick, U., Murray, B., & McNew, B. (2015). Diagnosis and treatment of patients with bipolar disorder: A review for advanced practice nurses. *Journal of the American Association of Nurse Practitioners, 27,* 530–542.

National Institute of Mental Health. (2016). Bipolar disorder among adults. Retrieved from http://www.nimh .nih.gov/health/statistics/prevalence/bipolar-disorder -Among-adults.shtml

Nettina, S. M. (2013). *Lippincott manual of nursing practice* (10th ed.). Philadelphia, PA: Wolters Kluwer Health, Lippincott Williams & Wilkins.

O'Brien, P. G., Kennedy, W. Z., & Ballard, K. A. (2008). *Psychiatric mental health nursing: An introduction to theory and practice* (2nd ed.). Burlington, MA: Jones & Bartlett.

Schultz, J. M., & Videbeck, S. L. (2013). *Lippincott's manual of psychiatric nursing care plans* (9th ed.). Philadelphia, PA: Wolters Kluwer Health, Lippincott Williams & Wilkins.

■ BOUNDARY MANAGEMENT

Jeffrey S. Jones

Overview

Boundary management is one of the essential components in the interpersonal nurse/patient relationship. The ability to therapeutically interact in a way that is interpersonally healthy for the patient as well as for the nurse is integral to the concept of relationship-based care. The term "boundary" typically refers to the physical and psychological space that a person has that separates him or her from others. Each patient's boundaries are unique to that person and reflect his or her self. The nurse must gain the trust and respect of the patient by presenting himself or herself as genuine and empathic yet maintaining therapeutic boundaries, which is the space between the nurse's power and the patient's vulnerability (National Council of State Boards of Nursing [NCSBN], 2014).

Background

As mentioned earlier, the reason that boundary management is such an important factor in the practice of nursing is that there is an imbalance of power in the nurse–patient relationship. Patients, by nature of their illness, are dependent on nurses for some aspects of their care. In psychiatric-mental health nursing, the patient is also vulnerable because of the mental illness. This vulnerability is even more evident for patients who are psychotic, have problems with communication, or have been involuntarily committed. Juxtaposed to this are nurses, who, because of their knowledge, experience, and status, are in the positions of power.

The nurse–patient relationship must remain professional because of this imbalance of power. The patient assumes that he or she is safe with the nurse and that a nurse will protect the patient while in his or her care. Owing to this implied dynamic in the nurse–patient interpersonal relationship, the nurse must abstain from obtaining personal gain at the patient's expense, as well as refraining from inappropriate involvement in the patient's relationships.

The American Nurses Association's (ANA) *Code of Ethics for Nurses* (Section 2.4) describes the nurse–patient relationship, addressing boundaries in this relationship: The work of nursing is inherently personal. Within their professional role, nurses recognize and maintain appropriate personal relationship boundaries (ANA, 2015, p. 6).

Owing to the potential damage to the patient, emotionally, or otherwise, failure to maintain professional boundaries can result in a disciplinable offense by a state board of nursing (BON). Most states' BONs have language regarding the need to maintain professional boundaries in the nurse–patient relationship. In the United States, the NCSBN has taken a strong position about failing to maintain professional boundaries and issued the following to facilitate disciplinary action at the local level:

Professional boundaries are the spaces between the nurse's power and the patient's vulnerability. The power of the nurse comes from the professional position and the access to sensitive personal information. The difference in personal information the nurse knows about the patient versus personal information the patient knows about the nurse creates an imbalance in the nurse–patient relationship. Nurses should make every effort to respect the power imbalance and ensure a patient-centered relationship. (NCSBN, 2014, p. 4)

Clinical Aspects

ASSESSMENT

Nursing is fortunate in that it has many conceptual models that can guide our practice. Concerning boundary management and nurse–patient relationships, the archetype model is that of Hildegard Peplau. She was a nurse theorist who designed a conceptual model for nursing practice describing four phases of the nurse–patient relationship: orientation, identification, exploitation, and resolution (Peplau, 1991). For more in-depth information regarding practice from this model, please refer to Jones, Fitzpatrick, and Rogers (2017).

NURSING INTERVENTIONS, MANAGEMENT, AND IMPLICATIONS

Adding to the challenge of maintaining healthy boundaries is the fact that nurses often find themselves working in a fast-paced environment, such as the emergency department or intensive care unit, with little time for reflective analysis of relationship dynamics. This can lead to impulsive and spontaneous responses to patients rather than thoughtful and planned interactions. There is no shortcut to healthy boundary management. The thoughtful practice of boundary management to understand nuances of a boundary crossing versus a boundary violation is purposeful (Glass, 2003). Nurses need to be alert for some early-warning signs that may indicate the need to step away and take some additional time to process what is going on. These can include (a) over or inappropriate use of self-disclosure, (b) feeling as though the relationship with a patient is "special," (c) getting personal needs met (e.g., admiration, physical compliments) through a relationship with the patients, and (d) becoming distant and secretive from the peers.

Meeting with a mentor or clinical supervisor on a regular basis to discuss cases is a healthy way to manage boundaries. Problems arising from poor boundaries or testing of boundaries in therapeutic relationships may occur at any time in the course of treatment, but they are best dealt with as they occur. It is helpful to think of boundaries as rules or expected behaviors that guide healthy conduct between nurses and patients. Establishing healthy boundaries at the onset of the nurse–patient relationship is particularly important in psychiatric nursing because some symptoms of various illness may result in the testing of boundaries. Thus, it is the responsibility of the nurse to set clear boundaries for the therapeutic relationship. For example, sexually explicit or vulgar language violates boundaries and should never be used. In addition, the nurse and patient need to mutually negotiate and agree on whether to use first or full names. This decision typically reflects the customs where the treatment takes place. How do you greet each other, a handshake? When is it okay to offer a hug or physical comfort? When is it okay to reveal something about yourself? Physical contact and self-disclosure by the nurse, very powerful tools, must be done appropriately and only when its purpose is to model, educate, foster a therapeutic alliance, or validate a patient's reality. Physical contact and self-disclosure are never to be used to meet the nurse's own needs. Misuse or overuse of touching and self-disclosure could lead to overinvolvement and a weakening of the professional relationship (Jones et al., 2017).

Sometimes boundaries in the relationship will be tested by a patient. Some examples of boundary-testing behaviors include (a) attempting to initiate a social relationship, (b) attempting role reversal in which the patient offers care to the nurse, (c) soliciting personal information about the nurse, and (d) violating the personal space of the nurse. The nurse is responsible for maintaining the structure of the therapeutic relationship by reinforcing the boundaries.

Not all therapeutic relationships run smoothly. Patients are dynamic human beings who experience a wide range of emotions and feelings such as fear, sadness, or frustration. Being the recipient of health care can leave one feeling helpless and vulnerable. In addition, the stressors of dealing with an illness, physical or emotional, can lead to challenges in the therapeutic relationship. One of the biggest challenges to boundaries occurs when patients attempt to convert therapeutic relationships into social ones, thereby testing the boundaries of therapeutic encounters. At times in the therapeutic relationship, brief social exchanges are appropriate, for example, greetings or in social situations, for example, the medication line, waiting room, or dining room.

Testing behavior challenges the nurse to remain focused and goal oriented. Careful, self-assessment in such situations enables the nurse to use what the patient is saying and doing to intervene therapeutically. Adhering to the guidelines for professional boundaries aid in maintaining and stabilizing the boundaries of the therapeutic interpersonal relationship.

OUTCOMES

In addition to the earlier strategies, it is important to remember that you may also be held to the following patient-centered care practice knowledge and skills, in accordance with QSEN initiatives: (a) explore ethical and legal implications of patient-centered care, (b) recognize the boundaries of therapeutic relationships, (c) describe the limits and boundaries of therapeutic patient-centered care, and (d) facilitate informed patient consent for care (Cronenwett et al., 2007).

Summary

Establishing and maintaining healthy and therapeutic boundaries in the nurse–patient relationship is not only ethically expected but also legally required as part of a nurse's practice. Failure to do so can result in harm to the patient (exploitation, abuse, and so forth) and possible disciplinary action for the nurse. Approaching care from a relationship-based perspective grounded in an interpersonal nursing theory helps the nurse to competently maintain this important aspect of practice.

American Nurses Association. (2015). Code of ethics for nurses. Retrieved from http://www.ana.org

Cronenwett, L., Sherwood, G., Barnsteiner J., Disch, J., Johnson, J., Mitchell, P., . . . Warren, J. (2007). Quality and safety education for nurses. *Nursing Outlook, 55*(3), 122–131.

Glass, L. L. (2003). The gray areas of boundary crossings and violations. *American Journal of Psychotherapy, 57*(4), 429–444.

Jones, J. S., Fitzpatrick, J. J., & Rogers, V. L. (Eds.). (2017). *Psychiatric-mental health nursing: An interpersonal approach* (2nd ed.). New York, NY: Springer Publishing.

National Council of State Boards of Nursing. (2014). *A nurse's guide to professional boundaries.* Chicago, IL: Author. Retrieved from https://www.ncsbn.org/Professional Boundaries_Complete.pdf

Peplau, H. E. (1991). *Interpersonal relations in nursing: A conceptual frame of reference for psychodynamic nursing* (Rev. ed.). New York, NY: Springer Publishing.

■ DEMENTIA

Stephanie R. Martin

Overview

Dementia is a general term that refers to a range of neurocognitive impairments that affect a person's ability to perform activities of daily living independently. There are more than 10 types of specific dementias, each with various constellations of symptoms, cause, course, and prognosis. The symptoms can range from mild to severe, can start insidiously or abruptly, and can be progressive and irreversible or reversible depending on the cause. Aspects of a person's functioning that may be affected include memory, nutrition, the sleep cycle, the ability to work, driving skills, ambulation, socialization, communication, comprehension of written/ spoken word, financial decision making, and personal hygiene. Nurses may encounter patients with dementia in all types of health care settings. Patient-centered care necessitates the involvement of significant others in all aspects of the nursing process when the patient is a poor historian or unable to communicate. The assessment of symptoms, response to interventions, and management of comorbid diseases can provide challenges to the health care team.

Background

The diagnosis of dementia is based on criteria identified by the *Diagnostic and Statistical Manual of Mental Disorders,* Fifth Edition (*DSM-5*; American Psychiatric Association, 2013). Symptoms vary depending on the specific area of the brain affected. Overall, the symptoms indicate a decline in functioning from the person's previous baseline in one or more of the following cognitive domains: learning and memory, language, executive functioning (planning, organizing, working memory, impulse control), complex attention (difficulty retaining new information), perceptual–motor, and/or social cognition. In addition, the person demonstrates symptoms related to aphasia (impairment in the ability to communicate orally or written), apraxia (motor speech disorder), or agnosia (impairment in recognition/meaning of sensory stimuli). Discerning symptoms related to dementia versus delirium or depression is important as symptoms may be overlapping but with different timelines and treatments.

Alzheimer's is the most commonly occurring type of progressive, irreversible dementia comprising 50% to 75% of dementia cases. The Centers for Disease Control and Prevention (CDC) reported that 5 million people were diagnosed with Alzheimer's in 2013 and expect the number to increase to 14 million by the year 2050. Alzheimer's is the sixth leading cause of death (CDC, 2013). Other progressive, permanent types of dementia include vascular (20%–30%), Lewy body (10%–25%), frontotemporal (10%–15%), mixed type, Parkinson's dementia, HIV induced, substance induced, Creutzfeldt-Jakob disease, Huntington's disease, and Wernicke–Korsakoff's syndrome. There are a few types of reversible dementias in which cognitive function can be restored if treated in a timely manner, that is, metabolic imbalances, endocrine imbalances, infections, toxic effects of medications, drug interactions, vitamin deficiencies, traumatic brain injury, neurological disorders, or normal pressure hydrocephalus (National Institute on Aging, 2014).

There are several factors that are thought to cause or contribute to the development of dementia. Possible factors include brain atrophy, accumulation of abnormal amyloid protein plaques, changes in the brain's white matter, chronic or acute decreased vascular perfusion, abnormal protein deposits (Lewy bodies), and disruption of the dopamine/acetylcholine neurotransmitter balance, viral-induced toxins, opportunistic infections, cancerous tumors, autosomal dominant genes, or trauma to brain structures during a sudden injury.

Age is the biggest risk factor for dementia. The other risk factors include family history of Alzheimer's, cardiovascular disease, smoking, stroke, Parkinson's disease, brain injury, diabetes, hypertension, obesity, chronic stress, females who are postmenopausal, hypercholesterolemia, and high homocysteine levels (Alzheimer's Association, 2014). Social factors contributing to the problem of dementia include stigma, which may decrease the willingness of the patients to report early symptoms; geographical spread of families who may then be unaware of symptoms; society's emphasis on privacy, which may contribute to the patients' refusing to allow significant others to be involved in their care. Biologically, patients may have multiple comorbid conditions such as chronic pain, cancer, chronic obstructive pulmonary disease (COPD), diabetes, or arthritis. The presence of other disorders can make the diagnosis of dementia difficult, whereas the presence of dementia can make the treatment of other conditions challenging. Patients may be poor historians, confabulate to cover memory loss, forget to take medication as directed, may be unable to follow directions, forget appointments, or cannot maneuver through the health care system as they once did.

Quality-of-life issues include loss of independence triggering grief reactions, loss of dreams about expectations of "the golden years," having to accept help/assistance with personal care, loss of driving, increased isolation, feelings of shame related to loss of bladder or bowel control, stigma, loss of ability to participate in lifelong hobbies. Patients may experience increased levels of anxiety knowing that something is not quite right and may fear nursing home placement, boredom, loss of home and belongings if a move to assisted living is needed, downsizing from a whole house to one room. Loss of privacy and loss of dignity ("time to change your diaper") are common experiences.

Clinical Aspects

ASSESSMENT

Care of patients with cognitive impairment requires ongoing assessment. It is important not to make assumptions and to clarify information as patients confabulate and may use humor to cover lapses in memory. Assessment needs to include a thorough history to ascertain baseline behavior and cognitive abilities, collaborative information from those familiar with the patient, physical assessment findings, and laboratory data. Screening tools can be used to indicate possible cognitive impairment, such as the Montreal Cognitive Assessment (MoCA), the Mini-Mental State Exam (MMSE), and the Saint Louis University Mental Status Examination (SLUMS). The Functional Assessment of Staging Test (FAST) can be used to quickly stage the extent of cognitive impairment on daily living. Questionnaires are also available to quickly assess caregiver burnout, which can prompt discussions about respite services and resources to help with placement options. These are screening tools with which nurses need to be familiar and comfortable in administering.

Pain may need to be assessed using alternative methods other than asking the patient to rate it using the traditional pain scale. Observe patients for grimacing or other facial changes, stiff posture, squirming or fidgeting more than usual, frequently placing a hand on a specific body part, changes in eating or sleeping, increased irritability or crying spells, moaning, sighing frequently, grunting, or changes in breathing that may indicate the patient is experiencing pain. Family members can usually identify when the patient with dementia is acting differently or seems to be uncomfortable so be sure to ask for their input.

NURSING INTERVENTIONS, MANAGEMENT, AND IMPLICATIONS

Patient-centered care must also include assessing safety issues such as driving, cooking, medication routines, wandering from home, getting lost, and incidence of agitation at home or in the community. Providing education to the family about recommended levels of supervision may be necessary. Nurses can also empower families to use creative alternative approaches such as music, art, brain games, exercise, sensory stimulation, validation, cognitive stimulation therapy, aromatherapy, massage, and reminiscence activities to enhance the patient's quality of life (Alzheimer's Association, 2015).

OUTCOMES

Knowledge of resources is important in empowering the patient and family to learn how to manage the diagnosis of dementia and improve their quality of life. Resources can include the local Area Office on Aging, the National Institute on Aging, Adult Protective Services, the Alzheimer's Association, health care providers specializing in geriatrics, Meals on Wheels, adult day care services, the National Alliance on Mental Illness, driving evaluation services, hospice, palliative care, transportation services for the elderly, and home health services. Caregiver stress is common and often involves depression and anxiety for the patient's family member assuming primary care of the patient. Caregivers also grieve the loss of their lifestyle and routines because of the patient's diagnosis (McDermott, 2015).

Summary

The current life expectancy is 78.8 years (CDC, 2015) and is expected to continue to increase. As people live

longer, the incidence of dementia increases and nurses come into contact with this population in every facet of health care. Each step of the nursing process must take the patient's cognitive impairment into account to provide quality patient-centered care. A thorough assessment of daily functioning needs to be obtained at each visit to identify changes in cognition or needs and collaborative data from significant others is invaluable. Patients may exhibit symptoms of grief, anxiety, fear, agitation, and/or loss of filter, resulting in inappropriate comments or sexual behaviors, changes in sleep or eating patterns, decrease in personal hygiene, all of which may require nursing interventions. Education is important to both the patient and family to empower them to understand and manage dementia, as well as to implement creative ways to improve quality of life. Caregiver stress and burnout are also a nursing concern that impacts the patient's overall treatment plan. The presence of comorbid illnesses creates additional challenges in providing health care to patients with dementia and often requires more time and resources.

Alzheimer's Association. (2014). Alzheimer's disease facts and figures. Retrieved from https://www.alz.org/downloads/facts_figures_2014.pdf

American Psychiatric Association. (2013). *Diagnostic and statistical manual of mental disorders* (5th ed.). Arlington, VA: American Psychiatric Publishing.

National Institute on Aging. (2013–2014). Alzheimer's disease progress report. Retrieved from https://www.nia.nih.gov/alzheimers/publication/2013-2014

Centers for Disease Control and Prevention. (2016). *Healthy brain initiative*. Atlanta, GA: Division of Population Health. National Center for Chronic Disease Prevention and Health Promotion.

McDermott, O. (2015). A psychological intervention for family carers of people with dementia is clinically and cost effective at reducing carer depression and anxiety levels over 2 years follow-up. *Evidence Based Nursing, 18*(4), 128.

■ DEPRESSION

Jeffrey S. Jones

Overview

Depression can be described as a change in mood or emotion and is closely related to feelings of sadness or discouragement. Most people experience occasional episodes of depressed moods throughout their lives. Fluctuations in the mood, especially during times of loss, change, and other social stressors, are normal. However, changes occurring and lasting for an extended period, 2 to 3 weeks, could indicate a more serious problem. Nurses, in the course of their daily practice, undoubtedly interact with clients undergoing some form of depression. In mental health care, the prevalence is higher. One of the major practice concepts for nursing is the utility and awareness of our empathy and sympathy toward our patients (Travelbee, 1971). If one of the tasks of nursing is to alleviate physical pain and suffering (postoperative, cancer, injuries, and so forth), then surely addressing a patient's emotional pain and suffering from depression falls squarely in the nursing domain.

Background

Depression has been reported in medical history as early as the 4th century BCE, when Hippocrates referred to it as *melancholia* and described sad/dark moods in some of his patients. Recent statistics regarding depression reveal the following: Approximately 20.9 million American adults, or about 9.5% of the population of the United States aged 18 years and older, are diagnosed with depression. The average age of diagnosis is 30 years. Depression is often seen with anxiety disorders and substance misuse disorders, and is the leading cause of disability in the United States for people between ages 15 and 44 years. Depression seems to be more common in females than males (National Institute of Mental Health, 2010).

One of the ongoing debates in health care concerns the actual cause of depression. Is it the age-old question of nature versus nurture? Is it psychologically driven or biological in origin? Before the 1950s most of the theories about depression came from the psychology field. Sigmund Freud and other therapists, for example, felt that anger turned inward or that prolonged exposure to stress could lead to depression. Childhood experiences and attachment to parents was also thought to possibly predispose an individual to more episodes of depression (Freud, 1920).

In the mid-1950s the first antidepressant was trialed (tricyclic) with some modest success, which led to the further development of biological theories. Interest in serotonin, dopamine, and norepinephrine began. It has been suggested that patients who are suffering from depression may have altered levels of these neurotransmitters. However, the exact role of the neurotransmitters is still not known. In fact, many of these neurobiological theories are now under scrutiny. There is very little actual scientific data to support that depression has anything to do with altered levels of serotonin, norepinephrine, or dopamine. To date, there is no double-blind, placebo-controlled studies to support these theories (Whitaker, 2011).

Clinical Aspects

ASSESSMENT

Although each person suffering from depression experiences the symptoms in his or her unique way based on culture, age, current life situation, and support system, and so forth, there are some clusters of symptoms that can be viewed as common enough to serve as warning signs to indicate a need for treatment or intervention. They are:

- Feelings of prolonged sadness
- Feelings of hopelessness and helplessness
- Change in appetite (either decreased or increased)
- Change in sleep (either decreased or increased)
- Decreased motivation or energy
- Lack of pleasure in previously pleasurable activities
- Difficulty with focus and concentration
- Thoughts of self-harm or ending your life (NIMH, 2010)

These symptoms (can be just a few, does not have to be all) lasting longer than 2 to 3 weeks should be viewed as serious and in need of professional intervention. This can be in the form of counseling, medication, or in cases in which safety is at risk, hospitalization.

Current recommended treatment for depression usually involves a combination of psychotherapy and medication management. The therapeutic aspect can be individual or in a group setting. The types of individual therapy can vary from therapist to therapist, but some examples are:

- Interpersonal
- Psychodynamic
- Cognitive behavioral therapy (CBT)
- Insight oriented

The types of group therapy that can be offered may be:

- Support
- Psychoeducational
- Traditional process group

Medication options also vary from prescriber to prescriber but can include:

- Selective serotonin-reuptake inhibitors (SSRIs) such as fluoxetine, paroxetine, sertraline, and escitalopram

- Serotonin/norepinephrine-reuptake inhibitors (SNRIs) such as duloxetine and venlafaxine

- Selective reuptake inhibitors (also known as serotonin 2 antagonist reuptake inhibitors [SARIs]) such as trazodone

- Selective atypical antidepressants such as bupropion and mirtazapine

- Tricyclic antidepressants such as amitriptyline, imipramine, amoxapine, and doxepin

- Monoamine oxidase inhibitors (MAOIs) such as tranylcypromine, phenelzine, and isocarboxazid (rarely used)

- Mood stabilizers such as lithium and anticonvulsants (carbamazepine, divalproex sodium, and lamotrigine) are sometimes added to augment the antidepressant regimen (Jones, Fitzpatrick, & Rogers, 2017).

NURSING INTERVENTIONS, MANAGEMENT, AND IMPLICATIONS

Most of the nursing concerns involving the care of clients suffering from depression have to do with medication monitoring for effectiveness or side effects and worsening of the condition and potential risk for self-harm (suicidality). The aspect of suicide is discussed at more length in a separate entry. Some of the common side effects that nurses need to monitor in antidepressant medication are:

- Weight gain

- Sexual dysfunction

- Sedation

- Cognitive fogging (memory impairment and difficulty focusing and concentrating)

- Activation/anxiety

- Cardiac changes (prolongation of QT interval)

- Lack of motivation/apathy (Jones et al., 2017)

Along with the responsibilities mentioned earlier is the role of the nurse in establishing and maintaining a therapeutic relationship. The nurse–patient relationship can be a source of comfort and healing for clients suffering from emotional pain. The nurse, through forging relatedness with the patient, can bring clarity, education, and validation to the client's experience (Travellbee, 1971).

OUTCOMES

Caring for clients who are depressed and potentially suicidal carries with it multiple responsibilities for nurses. The outcomes for clients who are depressed obviously are a reduction in depression, maintenance of safety, and an improvement of function. Some mutual goals may be the return to their desired previous state of functioning without the use of medication. Others may need guidance in finding a use of medication for a longer term that reduces the risk of side effects (weight gain, sexual dysfunction, drowsiness/sedation, cognitive fogging, or feeling numb). Outcomes are unique to each client and need to be established and carefully arrived at in concordance with the client and the nurse.

Summary

Depression can be present in almost any clinical situation or area of nursing practice. It is the responsibility of our profession to recognize and treat this suffering as we would any other physical condition that causes pain. Through early and proper intervention most clients notice an improvement. The nurse's empathic ability to monitor progress, medication issues, and any safety concerns as the client recovers can be a powerful and rewarding experience for both the client and nurse.

Freud, S. (1920). *An introduction to psychotherapy*. New York, NY: Horace Liveright.

Jones, J. S., Fitzpatrick, J. J., & Rogers, V. L. (Eds.). (2017). *Psychiatric-mental health nursing: An interpersonal approach* (2nd ed.). New York, NY: Springer Publishing.

National Institute of Mental Health. (2010). The numbers count: Mental disorders in American. Retrieved from http://www.nimh.nih.gov/health/publications/the-numbers-count-mental-disorders-in-america/index.shtml#Mood

Travelbee, J. (1971). *Interpersonal aspects of nursing* (2nd ed.). Philadelphia, PA: F. A. Davis.

Whitaker, R. (2011). *Anatomy of an epidemic: Magic bullets, psychiatric drugs, and the astonishing rise of mental illness in America*. New York, NY: Broadway Books.

■ EATING DISORDERS

Kathryn E. Phillips

Overview

Eating disorders are serious psychiatric conditions with mental and physical manifestations that require nursing care. Psychiatric complications of eating disorders include an altered body image, low self-esteem, dread of weight gain, and emotional distress. Physiologically, those with restricting disorders may display symptoms of hypotension, bradycardia, and amenorrhea, whereas those with purging behaviors may experience a loss of dental integrity, acid reflux, and electrolyte imbalances that can lead to cardiac dysfunction (Mehler, Krantz, & Sachs, 2015). Nursing care for individuals with eating disorders is focused on ensuring patient safety, medical stabilization, restoration of healthy-eating behaviors, and addressing the complex psychopathology underlying these conditions.

Background

The lifetime prevalence of anorexia nervosa (AN) is 0.9%, bulimia nervosa (BN) is 1.5%, and binge eating disorder (BED) is 3.5% for females, whereas the estimates for males are lower at 0.3%, 0.5%, and 2%, respectively (Hudson, Hiripi, Pope, & Kessler, 2007). Despite the low prevalence rates, these disorders are associated with significant economic implications. There are the obvious treatment costs of eating disorders, with studies showing individuals with eating disorders as having $1,869 higher annual health costs than those without eating disorders (Samnaliev, Noh, Sonneville, & Austin, 2015). Furthermore, new research indicates that there are even effects on earnings and employment rates (Samnaliev et al., 2015).

Eating disorders are most prevalent in females with the onset occurring in late adolescence to early adulthood (Hudson et al., 2007). Numerous risk factors have been implicated in the etiology of these disorders with the likely source stemming from an interaction of multiple factors. One often-cited risk factor is the sociocultural environment that promotes a thin body ideal in the media, creating pressure to be slim (Bakalar, Shank, Vannucci, Radin, & Tanofsky-Kraff, 2015). Genetic and biological factors, such as alterations in serotonin function, and psychological factors, such as personality traits like perfectionism and negative urgency, may also play a role (Bakalar et al., 2015). Other risk factors include depressive symptoms, a history of trauma, and excess body weight or changes in weight (Bakalar et al., 2015).

Eating disorders are identified according to criteria outlined in the *Diagnostic and Statistical Manual of Mental Disorders*, Fifth Edition (*DSM-5*; American Psychiatric Association [APA], 2013). AN is characterized by a restriction of caloric intake resulting in a body weight below the ideal for the individual's age and height. Heightened anxiety about weight gain causes individuals with AN to use extreme methods to alter their body weight and shape, including excessive exercise regimens and abuse of laxatives or diet pills. A distorted body image makes them believe that they are overweight or obese despite evidence to the contrary. These behaviors can result in anemia, osteopenia, and delayed gastric emptying (Mehler et al., 2015).

Another eating disorder described in the *DSM-5* is BN, which is characterized by cycles of binge eating large amounts of food in a short period while feeling out of control (APA, 2013). As a result of binge eating, individuals with BN often feel guilt, shame, and fear of weight gain. These feelings cause them to compensate for the high caloric intake by engaging in behaviors such as purging, misusing laxative or diuretics, and fasting. Along with these physical manifestations, individuals with BN are preoccupied with their weight and shape, which affects their self-esteem. Some medical complications of this disorder include hypokalemia, metabolic alkalosis, and hypovolemia (Mehler et al., 2015).

Individuals with BED exhibit similar eating pathology to those with BN whereby they have cycles of binge eating with an associated lack of control (APA, 2013). Those with BED experience significant emotional distress about binge eating but do not engage in compensation behaviors as those with BN do. Several medical comorbidities of BED have been identified, including obesity, metabolic syndrome, hypertension, dyslipidemia, and type 2 diabetes (Kornstein, Kunovac, Herman, & Culpepper, 2016).

Clinical Aspects

ASSESSMENT

When patients with eating disorders present for treatment, a thorough biopsychosocial evaluation should be conducted. The assessment should include the patient's chief complaint; mental status; developmental milestones; family history and function; medical and psychiatric history, including medication trials; treatment history; as well as current and past eating and compensation behavior(s) (Wolfe, Dunne, & Kells, 2016). Another important consideration during the assessment process is to evaluate the patient for symptoms of commonly co-occurring disorders like mood, anxiety, substance use, and impulse control disorders (Hudson et al., 2007). Throughout the assessment, the nurse is seeking to identify the most significant problems, strengths of the patient, as well as social supports.

The other component of a comprehensive assessment is a physical examination, with a focus on evaluating the patient for physical manifestations of the eating disorder. Orthostatic vital signs should be taken because dehydration is common. Other important examination components include auscultation of heart rate and rhythm, as well as bowel sounds. During the skin assessment, the nurse wants to look for edema, lanugo, and any evidence of self-harm. The oral examination should assess for dental integrity and parotid gland swelling. By conducting a thorough assessment, a holistic care plan can be developed based on the individual's presenting problems.

NURSING INTERVENTIONS, MANAGEMENT, AND IMPLICATIONS

Nursing care for those with eating disorders begins with ensuring the safety of the patient. This includes removing any objects from their environment that could be used for self-harm and monitoring the patient periodically to ensure their safety. Other immediate concerns include addressing medical complications resulting from restriction of caloric intake and/or dysfunctional elimination behaviors (e.g., purging, laxative use). Nurses may need to administer tube feedings and fluid boluses. Central to the care of every patient with an eating disorder is assisting the patient in restoring a normal body weight, halting disordered eating and compensation behaviors, improving self-esteem and body image, and addressing the patient's emotional concerns.

The specific nursing interventions implemented to care for the patient with an eating disorder depend on the presenting symptoms and concerns of the patient. However, nursing care typically includes monitoring weight gain, administering psychopharmacological interventions, and assessing vital signs. The majority of patients also require supervision around meal times and trips to the bathroom. Nursing oversight at these times is meant to ensure patients are not engaging in pathological behaviors around food/fluid intake and elimination.

Another key component of nursing care is the nurse–patient relationship. Nurses are responsible for establishing a trusting relationship with the patient that becomes the foundation of their therapeutic work together. In a study of female adolescents receiving treatment for eating disorders, the two most cited aspects in the development of trust were a genuine concern for the patient and allowing the patient to convey her or his feelings rather than making assumptions (Zaitsoff, Yiu, Pullmer, Geller, & Menna, 2015). A good rapport with the patient allows the nurse to engage the patient in the treatment process actively. A strong nurse–patient relationship also makes it possible to address the altered thought processes and emotional concerns driving the disordered-eating behaviors.

OUTCOMES

Although the specific outcomes of nursing care for the patient with an eating disorder are related to the symptoms assessed at the beginning of treatment, all patients should be making progress toward the establishment and maintenance of an ideal body weight for age and height. By the end of treatment, patients should be experiencing elevated levels of self-esteem and improvements in their body image. Any concerns of self-harm should have subsided and patients are better able to express their emotions and regulate their mood. Other outcomes include the development of healthy coping mechanisms to handle stressors and the establishment of physiologic homeostasis, including vital signs and lab values that are in normal limits.

Summary

Individuals with eating disorders present with a host of mental and physical concerns that require nursing attention. Nurses are responsible for ensuring patient safety, stabilizing any medical complications, engaging the patient in the treatment process, and addressing the underlying emotional aspects and disturbed thought processes associated with these disorders.

American Psychiatric Association. (2013). *Diagnostic and statistical manual of mental disorders* (5th ed.). Arlington, VA: American Psychiatric Publishing.

Bakalar, J. L., Shank, L. M., Vannucci, A., Radin, R. M., & Tanofsky-Kraff, M. (2015). Recent advances in developmental and risk factor research on eating disorders. *Current Psychiatry Reports, 17*(42). doi:10.1007/s11920-015-0585-x

Hudson, J., Hiripi, E., Pope, H., & Kessler, R. (2007). The prevalence and correlates of eating disorders in the national comorbidity survey replication. *Biological Psychiatry, 61*, 348–358.

Kornstein, S. G., Kunovac, J. L., Herman, B. K., & Culpepper, L. (2016). Recognizing binge-eating disorder in the clinical setting: A review of the literature. *The Primary Care Companion for CNS Disorders, 18*(3). doi:10.4088/PCC.15r01905

Mehler, P. S., Krantz, M. J., & Sachs, K. V. (2015). Treatments of medical complications of anorexia nervosa and bulimia nervosa. *Journal of Eating Disorders, 3*(15). doi:10.1186/s40337-015-0041-7

Samnaliev, M., Noh, H. L., Sonneville, K. R., & Austin, S. B. (2015). The economic burden of eating disorders and related mental health comorbidities: An exploratory analysis using the U.S. Medical Expenditures Panel Survey. *Preventative Medicine Reports, 2,* 32–34. doi:10.1016/j.pmedr.2014.12.002

Wolfe, B. E., Dunne, J. P., & Kells, M. R. (2016). Nursing care considerations for the hospitalized patient with an eating disorder. *Nursing Clinics of North America, 51,* 213–235. doi:10.1016/j.cnur.2016.01.006

Zaitsoff, S., Yiu, A., Pullmer, R., Geller, J., & Menna, R. (2015). Therapeutic engagement: Perspectives from adolescents with eating disorders. *Psychiatry Research, 230,* 597–603. doi:10.1016/j.psychres.2015.10.010

■ IMPULSE CONTROL DISORDERS

Lisa L. Salser

Overview

An impulse is a wish or urge, particularly a sudden one, and can be considered a normal part of the human thinking process. The ability to control the desire to act on impulsive thoughts is an important factor in personality, socialization, human behavior, and decision making. Deferred gratification, also known as impulse control, is often lacking in mental health disorders such as substance misuse, aggression, paraphilias, attention deficit disorder, mania, and some personality disorders. When lack of impulse control results in behaviors that violate the rights of others and/or creates conflict with societal norms or authority figures, the individual is considered to have an impulse control disorder (American Psychiatric Association [APA], 2013).

We discuss the diagnosis of pyromania, kleptomania, and intermittent explosive disorder. Although impulse control disorders have not been well studied, there are no Food and Drug Administration (FDA)-approved medications at this time for these disorders (Grant & Leppkin, 2015).

The disruptive impulse control disorders are more commonly seen in the male population. The disorders tend to have a childhood or adolescent age of onset. They present to the nursing population across multiple age spectrums and are found in multiple areas such as the school system, jails, hospitals, and doctor's offices. Nurses must be educated on the possibility of these diagnoses so that they can be recognized and offer the proper recommended treatment.

Background

The process of impulse control has been explained through multiple perspectives—psychoanalytic; neurobiologic, including genetic influences; cognitive; behavioral; and developmental. As with many behavioral constructs, impulsivity is multifaceted. There may be a failure of motor inhibition (impulsive action), acceptance of immediate small rewards versus delayed large ones (impulsive choice) and risky behavior regarding impulsive decision making. In many situations, alternative actions and impulsive thoughts require inhibition to allow the emergence of goal-directed behaviors (Bari & Robbins, 2013).

Intermittent explosive disorder (IED) and pyromania are rare, but when they occur, it is believed to be more prominent in males. Kleptomania is also rare, constituting fewer than 5% of impulse control disorders; however, most shoplifters are female. The behavior can be sporadic with brief episodes or prolonged periods that are more chronic. The items stolen are usually of little value.

Many times, contributing factors to all the earlier conditions are related to a traumatic childhood. There can also be a history of obsessive compulsive mental illness in the family. These are the populations of individuals that are identified as most at risk. If left untreated, morbidity and mortality could be heightened because of excessive unhappiness and dissatisfaction with themselves, leading to suicidal behavior. It can also result in a life in jail or prison. All diagnoses affect personal relationships, which could lead to a lifetime of havoc and loneliness. Many of these diagnoses accompany other mental illnesses (Tusaie & Fitzpatrick, 2016).

Clinical Aspects

Pyromania

Pyromania is defined as behavior that is purposeful with fire-setting behaviors on more than one occasion. The fire setter feels a tension and an effective arousal before the act and has a feeling of relief and pleasure after the act. There is a fascination with a sustained interest and curiosity about the fire. Pyromaniacs are attracted to the out-of-control damage, chaos, and intensity that occurs with the fire. The individual reports and receives pleasure and gratification when constructing a fire or witnessing the harmful effects of his or her actions. This reward leads to the cycle repeating itself. Fire setting in the juvenile population is frequently associated with a conduct disorder, attention deficit hyperactivity disorder (ADHD), or an adjustment disorder, or other comorbid psychiatric problems that include mental retardation, conduct disorder, alcohol and substance use disorder, personality disorders and schizophrenia, depression, or other impose control disorders (Grant, Odlaug, & Kim, 2007).

Kleptomania

Kleptomania is demonstrated as repetitive, uncontrollable acts of stealing items for the result of personal gratification and not of need. It often begins in adolescence to early adulthood. The course of the illness is chronic with waxing and waning of symptoms. Most people with kleptomania try unsuccessfully to stop stealing, which often leads to feelings of shame and guilt. They may have another mental illness such as anxiety disorder (Grant & Leppkin, 2015).

Many people with kleptomania return stolen items. Many of the behaviors lead to arrest with criminal records that can be debilitating for future social and economic stability.

Many with kleptomania (64%–87%) have been arrested because of their stealing behavior. A smaller percentage (15%–23%) has been incarcerated. Suicide attempts are common among such patients (Grant & Leppkin, 2015). Kleptomania is best understood in light of conditioning theory. The problem behavior arises in the arousal and tension stage and then is reinforced by the relaxed feeling that follows, therefore promoting occurrence of the behavior again and again (Rinsho, 2015).

The Kleptomania Symptom Assessment Scale (K-SAS) is a 12-question assessment of the past week's events. It is available online. The questions cover the areas of urges, frequency, stealing, and the extent of time that was involved with thoughts in these areas. The K-SAS asks questions such as: What kind of items do you steal? Are there any triggers that increase your urge to steal? How is stealing affecting your life, work, and personal relationships? Do you have any close relatives with a similar problem or mental disorder? Do you have any substance abuse problems? Have you received treatment for any other mental disorders or substance abuse that may also be occurring? Addictions, depression, anxiety, and stress can contribute to these cycles.

There are no controlled studies of psychological treatments for kleptomania. Case reports suggest

that cognitive behavioral therapy may be effective. It increases subjective adaptation that can be helpful to control the behavior (Rinsho, 2015). Covert sensitization combined with exposure and response prevention have shown some reduction in stealing frequency. Imaginal desensitization may result in a remission of symptoms over a prolonged period (Grant & Leppkin, 2015).

Intermittent Explosive Disorder

IED is defined by outbursts of anger that are more aggressive than expected in response to a stressor, which may lead to a physical assault against a person or property.

The symptoms tend to begin in adolescence and appear to be chronic. The outbursts usually last less than 30 minutes but may occur several times in a month's span. These behaviors frequently lead to legal and/or relationship problems. The disorder rarely begins for the first time in adulthood, usually presenting in childhood or adolescence. The diagnosis is usually a diagnosis of exclusion. Other aggressive behavior diagnoses have to be ruled out. Patients with a history of substance use disorders (especially alcohol) and neurological disorders (especially severe head trauma) are prone to IED. It appears to follow a chronic and persistent course over many years.

Individuals with IED recognize their behavior as problematic and distressing. Gender studies reveal males are more likely to be diagnosed with the disorder. A substantial genetic influence for impulsive aggression has been demonstrated with relatives. Environmental and genetic factors that could cause outbursts should be considered.

Individuals with IED likely grew up in a family in which explosive behavior and verbal and physical abuse were used. Patients with IED may also have other comorbid disorders such as ADHD, so nurses should ask patients about having other disorders. Ask about problems with impaired relationships, physical abuse, or arguments. Ask about trouble at work, home, or school. There could be a job loss, school suspension, financial problems, or trouble with the law (Tusaie & Fitzpatrick, 2016). Patients may experience problems with alcohol or other substance use.

Other questions to include would be (Tusaie & Fitzpatrick, 2016):

1. How often do you have explosive episodes?

2. What triggers your outbursts?

3. Have you ever injured or verbally abused anyone?

4. How have your outbursts affected your family or work life?

5. Is there anything that helps to calm you when an outburst occurs?

6. Has anyone in your family ever been diagnosed with a mental illness?

7. Have you ever had a severe head injury?

Fluoxetine may be considered an effective treatment for IED. Oxcarbazepine has shown some promise for symptom improvement. Results have shown that cognitive behavioral therapy is the best therapy option to reduce symptom severity for this disorder (Grant & Leppkin, 2015).

ASSESSMENT

A general psychosocial examination should be completed for any diagnosis (pyromania, kleptomania, and IED). During the assessment interview, the patient may try to alter their story in efforts to avoid legal consequences.

The clinician must look for a possible repetitive pattern in the history of the patient. There is often a history of maltreatment during childhood (Tusaie & Fitzpatrick, 2016).

Specific for pyromania: Assess for anger—Juveniles are frequently upset with someone such as their parents. A diagnosis of pyromania would not be given in the presence of a major neurocognitive disorder, intellectual disability, or substance intoxication (Burton, McNiel, & Bender, 2012).

NURSING INTERVENTIONS, MANAGEMENT, AND IMPLICATIONS

1. Develop a treatment plan that is acceptable to the clinician and the patient. The patient should be able to achieve some success early on in efforts to maintain treatment. The patient must see the benefits or the rewards.

2. Educate the client about the illness as a psychiatric disorder that is treatable.

3. Assist the patient in identifying situations, thoughts, and feelings that may trigger urges so that the patient can manage those situations better.

4. Address any other mental illness or substance abuse.

5. Discover healthy outlets to replace the unhealthy behaviors.

6. Teach relaxation and stress management.

7. Help the patient to stay focused on his or her goal. Recovery can take time. Keeping a diary can help to remind that he or she is getting better.

OUTCOMES

1. The patient will experience a decrease in impulsive feelings.

2. The patient will replace unhealthy behaviors with healthy outlets.

3. The patient will experience control over the irresistible urges.

4. The patient will report a decrease in the unwanted behavior.

5. The patient will understand that the chance of being arrested has lessened and see improvements in personal relationships (Tusaie & Fitzpatrick, 2016).

Summary

Impulse control and conduct disorders share many symptoms with other psychiatric diagnoses. Many of these diagnoses share a commonality in that the patient has experienced a harmful and disorganized childhood and is at risk because of some genetic factors. Controlling these childhood traumatic events is probably the main key to disrupting the development of the disorders.

Impulsive control disorder patients usually fail to resist an impulse that increases tension leading to completing the act followed by the pleasure/gratification response and release of tension, which then encourages the impulsive acts to go on and on and on.

Selective serotonin-reuptake inhibitor (SSRI) medication and behavioral therapies such as cognitive behavioral therapy and educational training have proven helpful at times. Nonpharmacological interventions are emerging as acceptable forms of treatment. The clinician should demonstrate knowledge in benefits, appropriate usage, side effects, and risks of the treatments they propose. Cultural beliefs and behaviors must always be employed when treating a patient. Presenting oneself in a positive manner is the greatest healing tool that one can use to help provide hope and healing (Tusaie & Fitzpatrick, 2016).

American Psychiatric Association. (2013). *Diagnostic and statistical manual of mental disorders* (5th ed.). Arlington, VA: American Psychiatric Publishing.

Bari, A., & Robbins, T. (2013). Initiation and impulsivity: Behavioral and neural basis of response control. *Neurobiology, 108,* 44–79.

Burton, P. R., McNiel, D. E., & Bender, R. L.(2012). Fire setting, arson, pyromania, and the forensic mental health expert. *Journal of the American Academy of Psychiatric Law, 40*(3), 355–356.

Grant, J. E., & Leppkin, E. W. (2015). Choosing a treatment for disruptive, impulse control, and conduct disorders. *Current Psychiatry, 14*(1), 29–36.

Grant, J. E., Odlaug, B. L., & Kim, S. W. (2007). Impulsive control disorders, clinical characteristics, and pharmacological management. *Psychiatric Times, 24*(10), 64–69.

Rinsho, N. (2015). Kleptomania and compulsive buying. *Oishi M, 73*(9), 1580–1584.

Tusaie, K., & Fitzpatrick, J. J. (2016). *Advanced practice psychiatric nursing:* psychotherapy, psychopharmacology, and complementary and alternative approaches across the life span (2nd ed.). New York, NY: Springer Publishing.

■ OBSESSIVE COMPULSIVE DISORDER

Susan Phillips

Overview

Obsessive compulsive disorder (OCD) is characterized by obsessive thoughts (or preoccupations) and compulsive behaviors (or rituals) in response to the preoccupying thoughts. The prevalence of OCD in the United States is 1.2% with females slightly more affected than males, and males more likely to develop symptoms in childhood (American Psychiatric Association [APA], 2013). The persistent preoccupations and associated rituals can occupy so much of a person's time that he or she cannot work, maintain relationships, or engage in everyday tasks (National Institute of Mental Health [NIMH], 2016). Nurses play an important role in recognizing OCD and in reducing the disabling effects of the disorder (Jones, Fitzpatrick, & Rogers, 2017).

Background

OCD is defined by the APA as a severe anxiety disorder in which people have recurring, unwanted thoughts, ideas, or sensations that make them feel driven to do something repetitively (APA, 2013). There are two opposing hypotheses regarding the formation of OCD. One widely held hypothesis is that compulsive behaviors are performed to reduce anxiety that is associated with obsessive thoughts to regain control. These behaviors are performed although the person is aware that the behavior is not particularly helpful in reducing anxiety. A second, newer hypothesis is that obsessive thoughts are used to rationalize compulsive behaviors. In this hypothesis, compulsive behaviors are learned responses and therefore can be unlearned through therapy designed to stop the behavior and thereby reduce the anxious thoughts (Stahl, 2013). In the United States, approximately 25% of people with OCD develop the disorder by the age of 14 years, with 25% of males with OCD experiencing onset by the age of 10 years. It is unusual for persons with OCD to experience onset after the age of 35 years. The onset of OCD is gradual, and without treatment, remission of the OCD in adults is less than 20% 40 years after onset. For persons with OCD who experience onset in childhood or adolescence, remission rates are near 40% (APA, 2013).

The lives of people who suffer from OCD can revolve around the compulsive behaviors. For example, obsessions involving a need for order can make it difficult to complete projects because the results never seem good enough or objects never seem properly placed. The person will likely engage in compulsive behaviors designed to bring order to the environment. Obsessions about contamination lead to compulsive hand washing, showering, or avoidance of places where contamination is perceived (such as health care facilities). The person suffering from OCD experiences intense urges to perform ritualistic acts although he or she has full insight into the senselessness and excessiveness of the behavior (Stahl, 2013). OCD is associated with comorbidities such as depression, panic disorder, body dysmorphic disorder (preoccupation with perceived flaws in one's physical appearance), hoarding (inability to discard items of little value leading to significant distress and overaccumulation of possessions), and shame. As a result, suicidal thoughts are often present because the person cannot live life fully (Weingarden, Renshaw, Wilhelm, Tangney, & DiMauro, 2016). In addition, some compulsive acts can be detrimental to the person's health because of poor nutrition or ingestion of foreign objects.

Clinical Aspects

ASSESSMENT

Early identification of OCD provides the best opportunity for remission. This requires assessment of associated symptoms, including recurrent and unwanted thoughts that cause significant distress, the performing of repetitive behaviors in an attempt to suppress the thoughts or fears, thoughts or behaviors that are time-consuming and impair social or occupational functioning, and the presence of depression with or without suicidal thoughts. In addition, a careful review of the person's physical health and past psychiatric history should be completed; health may be affected by compulsive behaviors. An assessment of how OCD affects the person's daily functioning in vocational, social, and family roles should also be made.

The nurse should be competent in meeting quality and safety standards related to the assessment. This includes assessing for suicidal thoughts, self-mutilation, depression, and substance use, and documenting findings in the medical record using recognized terminology so that communication occurs among all members of the treatment team, including the patient's family.

NURSING INTERVENTIONS, MANAGEMENT, AND IMPLICATIONS

Nursing problems should reflect the person's response to OCD in the context of his or her role in family and community. This includes information derived from an assessment of the patient's needs, preferences, and values. Examples of nursing problems related to OCD anxiety are:

- Information misinterpretation as evidenced by exaggerated behaviors
- Decreased role functioning related to nonproductive behaviors
- Feelings of hopelessness related to nonproductive behaviors

Treatment of OCD disorder involves psychiatric medications that reduce the symptoms associated with anxiety and cognitive behavioral therapy directed at breaking the pattern of compulsive behavior and reducing the anxiety. Nursing interventions in the treatment of OCD guide the person toward an understanding of the association between anxiety-producing triggers and associated compulsive behaviors, the use of empathetic responses that support dignity and self-control, educate the patient about psychotropic medications and side effect management, educate about relaxation skills and thought-stopping techniques, encourage involvement of family or other sources of support, and provide an ongoing assessment for suicidal ideation and substance abuse.

OUTCOMES

The desired outcomes for the treatment of OCD are a reduction of the intensity and frequency of symptoms, and patient safety with regard to use of substances and risk of suicide. This is accomplished through an understanding of environmental factors that are associated with obsessive thoughts and replacement of compulsive behaviors with healthier coping behaviors.

Summary

OCD is characterized by obsessive thoughts and compulsive behaviors. The lives of people who suffer from OCD can revolve around the compulsive behaviors although they have an awareness that the behaviors are not effective in reducing anxiety. OCD is often comorbid with body dysmorphic disorder and hoarding. As a result, shame, depression, and suicidal thoughts are often present because the person cannot live life fully. Substance use is common in an attempt to cope with unwanted thoughts. As OCD often develops in childhood, early intervention is essential to attain remission of this disorder. Nurses play an important role in identifying OCD and in providing alternatives to ritualistic behaviors.

American Psychiatric Association. (2013). *Diagnostic and statistical manual of mental disorders* (5th ed.). Arlington, VA: American Psychiatric Publishing.

Jones, J. S., Fitzpatrick, J. J., & Rogers, V. L. (2017). *Psychiatric-mental health nursing: An interpersonal approach* (2nd ed.). New York, NY: Springer Publishing.

National Institute of Mental Health. (2016). *Obsessive-compulsive disorder: When unwanted thoughts or irresistible actions take over* (NIH Publication No. TR 16-4676). Bethesda, MD: Author. Retrieved from https://www.nimh.nih.gov/health/publications/obsessive-compulsive-disorder-when-unwanted-thoughts-take-over/index.shtml

Stahl, S. M. (2013). *Stahl's essential psychopharmacology: Neuroscientific basis and practical applications* (4th ed.). New York, NY: Cambridge University Press.

Weingarden, H., Renshaw, K. D., Wilhelm, S., Tangney, J. P., & DiMauro, J. (2016). Anxiety and shame as risk factors for depression, suicidality, and functional impairment in body dysmorphic disorder and obsessive compulsive disorder. *Journal of Nervous and Mental Disease, 204*(11), 832–839.

■ POSTTRAUMATIC STRESS DISORDER

Danette L. Core
Denise Chivington

Overview

Posttraumatic stress disorder (PTSD) is a mental health condition that some people develop after experiencing or witnessing a life-threatening event such as combat, natural disaster, motor vehicle crash, or sexual assault (U.S. Department of Veterans Affairs, National Center for PTSD, 2016a). The symptoms of PTSD encompass a number of psychological distress symptoms that can either be vague or very distinct. These symptoms show a prevalence that has been reported in the *Diagnostic and Statistical Manual of Mental Disorders, fifth edition* (*DSM-5*) as demonstrating a lifetime risk of 8.7% for PTSD (American Psychiatric Association [APA], 2013). It has been estimated that approximately 20% of all military personnel are troubled with PTSD (Hanrahan et al., 2017). Although it is normal to experience an intense reaction to any traumatic event, the intensity usually fades over time. With PTSD, the symptoms can be acute or chronic but are typically long-lasting. The reaction to an offending experience that involves a life-threatening event becomes coupled with an intense fear response. These symptoms can involve both psychological and physical sequelae. People can develop PTSD at any age; however, symptom expression differs based on genetic background and life experience. Determining whether a person develops PTSD after a traumatic event depends on certain risk factors and the person's resilience. The effects of PTSD can invade most (if not all) aspects of a sufferer's life. The reactions range from mild to severe and can have long-lasting deleterious influences on personal and professional relationships.

Background

Although strong physical and emotional reaction are normal after experiencing a life-altering event, for most people, the reaction lessens over time (APA, 2013). With PTSD, it does not. Symptoms can occur a few months to a few years after the portentous event. The signs and symptoms of PTSD are highly individualized but do have common features and may include recurring dreams or nightmares of either actual or comparable events. Experiencers may eventually try to avoid similar situations that remind them of their bad experience. The expression of their emotional journey may also take on different forms. They may have unusual anger and irritability over things that would not normally bother them. They can lose patience with loved ones for no reason. Various manifestations of anxiety and depression abound in PTSD casualties.

Avoidance takes on many forms from totally changing one's life situation to simply not going to celebratory public events where loud noises or other triggering events may occur. The things in life that remind the sufferer of the offending event are either simply avoided or eliminated from his or her life. PTSD symptoms involve a reexperiencing of the terrible event. This can include nightmares or night terrors, almost out-of-body flashbacks, or feelings of impending doom (APA, 2013). The triggers may occur in everyday life, or the person's thoughts may initiate the same intense emotion experienced at the time of the original event (APA, 2013).

Reactivity and hyperarousal are also symptoms of PTSD (APA, 2013). Loud noises and crowds can be very disturbing to these individuals. These people may be easily startled and feel tensed or on edge. They can have difficulty sleeping and have angry outbursts about normally unimportant issues. Many times this intense attention can cause issues with activities of daily living. Mood and cognition may be affected as well. People living with PTSD can experience anhedonia, the lack of feelings of pleasantness while engaging in activities that used to bring enjoyment (APA, 2013). They can have trouble relaxing and feel uneasy. Many times it is difficult for them to verbalize how they feel. Lack of focus and difficulty concentrating are also common symptoms of PTSD (APA, 2013). Disturbing thoughts race through their minds producing negative emotional and physical reactions. Resilience and present risk factors both play a factor in who may acquire PTSD (APA, 2013). It is believed that an individual's genetic structure can predispose him or her to suffer from PTSD. Increased prevalence has been found among Latinos, African Americans, and American Indians, whereas Asian Americans have reported fewer instances (APA, 2013). A person's gender can be a predisposition to developing PTSD; females tend to develop PTSD more frequently than males (U.S. Department of Health and Human Services, National Institutes of Health, National Institute of Mental Health, 2016). Cultural, temperamental, and environmental factors also play a role in who will develop PTSD (APA, 2013).

Other factors are protective against developing PTSD (APA, 2013). These include a strong social support and/or network, having positive feelings about one's actions during the event, and having the ability to react appropriately although one may be experiencing fear (APA, 2013). Cultural dynamics come into play as well, such as perceptual interpretations and the meaning one gives to an event (APA, 2013). As with any mental health issue, the subject of suicidality must always be evaluated and effectively addressed.

Nursing concerns involving the care of clients who have PTSD may involve multiple physical and psychosocial symptoms. The patients often present with depression, anxiety, and sleep disorders (APA, 2013). This multisymptomatic presentation often leads to the patient's feelings of hopelessness and helplessness, which elicit suicidal ideation, which places these individuals at risk for potential self-harm. Nursing care requires careful monitoring for subtle changes in the mood and behavior to ensure client safety. Comprehensive treatment includes medications and therapy (APA, 2013).

Special consideration must be given to children as they express a slightly different set of signs and symptoms (APA, 2013). Expression of symptoms can often be conveyed by acting out during the medico-legal discovery process, demonstrations with childhood play, or when exhibiting other negative effects, such as bed wetting, having issues with separating from a parent, or regressing back into a previous developmental stage (APA, 2013). The diagnostic criteria are slightly different for children younger than 6 years old, but remain similar (APA, 2013).

Clinical Aspects

NURSING INTERVENTIONS, MANAGEMENT, AND IMPLICATIONS

The treatment of PTSD involves psychotherapy (individual and/or group) and/or pharmacotherapy. One of the most effective evidence-based treatments is cognitive behavioral therapy (CBT). Two main types of CBT are used to process the symptoms of PTSD: *prolonged exposure* (PE) and *cognitive processing therapy* (CPT; U.S. Department of Veterans Affairs, National Center for PTSD, 2016b). CPT uses techniques to explore the actual thoughts and feelings of a person living with PTSD to positively change the perception of the traumatic event (U.S. Department of Veterans Affairs, National Center for PTSD, 2016b). This approach works by uncovering the person's beliefs about *self-esteem*, *trust*, *control*, *power*, and *safety*. The goal of PE therapy is to decrease the effect that triggers have on the person living with PTSD by exposing them to a similar situation, but one that is safe in which the patient can be successful in overcoming the previous traumatic event's hold on his or her emotions and reactions (U.S. Department of Veterans Affairs, National Center for PTSD, 2016b).

Another modality, *symptom management*, is very individualized and customized to match the most effective therapy with the most distressing symptom (U.S. Department of Veterans Affairs, National Center for PTSD, 2016b). Providers collaborate in team meetings to discuss the treatment plans and outcomes. Two other therapies used for PTSD include stress inoculation therapy (SIT) and eye movement desensitization and reprocessing (EMDR; U.S. Department of Veterans Affairs, National Center for PTSD, 2016c). SIT teaches skills to help manage stress and anxiety symptoms, and EMDR involves performing rapid eye movements with guided imagery.

In addition, multiple self-help options are available for people living with PTSD to help manage their symptoms. Physical exercise is a very therapeutic and effective treatment not only for PTSD but also for the comorbid conditions that many times accompany it (U.S. Department of Veterans Affairs, National Center for PTSD, 2016b). PTSD has very high rates of comorbidity usually involving depression, anxiety, substance abuse, and dissociation. Taking a positive view on treatment goals and outcomes and having realistic expectations of oneself goes far toward improving the negative aspects of the experienced traumatic event (U.S. Department of Veterans Affairs, National Center for PTSD, 2016b). For many, simply sharing the experience with family and friends seems to lessen the deleterious effects of the experience (U.S. Department of Veterans Affairs, National Center for PTSD, 2016b).

Pharmacological interventions comprise discovering the right dose and the right formulation to decrease the intensity of the emotional reactions and negative thoughts surrounding PTSD. Selective serotonin-reuptake inhibitors (SSRIs), serotonin/norepinephrine-reuptake inhibitors (SNRIs), and tricyclic antidepressants (TCAs) are first-line treatments for PTSD as these groups of medications are more tolerable and have fewer side effects than other classes (U.S. Department of Veterans Affairs, U.S. Department of Defense, 2010). Mood stabilizers and antiadrenergic medications may be helpful as well. Sleep hygiene is also an important part of an effective treatment plan for PTSD. Prazosin is used for nightmare relief and hypnotics for short-term insomnia relief (U.S. Department of Veterans Affairs, U.S. Department of Defense, 2010).

Summary

PTSD can develop at any age or in any person after either witnessing or experiencing a traumatic event such as a sexual assault, combat, a natural disaster, or a major health-threatening situation. People living with PTSD have a wide range of emotional reactions that are either short-term or long-lasting after the event. The key points addressed in this entry include the history and background of PTSD; the idea that PTSD affects people of all ages across the life span and that many people experiencing significant life traumas may be vulnerable to developing PTSD; its presentation follows established patterns with some variability based on age, genetic composition, cultural background, and life experience; treatments are multimodal and include various forms of psychotherapy, self-help methods, social support, physical activity, and medications. Early intervention and client/family psychoeducation are essential factors in achieving effective client outcomes.

American Psychiatric Association. (2013). *Diagnostic and statistical manual of mental disorders* (5th ed.). Arlington, VA: American Psychiatric Publishing.

Hanrahan, N., Judge, K., Olamijulo, G., Seng, L., Lee, M., Herbig, P.,…Longmire, W. (2017). The PTSD toolkit for nurses: Assessment, intervention, and referral of veterans. *Nurse Practitioner, 42*(3), 46–55. doi:10.1097/01.NPR.0000488717.90314.62

U.S. Department of Health and Human Services, National Institutes of Health, National Institute of Mental Health. (2016). *Post-traumatic stress disorder*. Bethesda, MD: Author. Retrieved from https://www.nimh.nih.gov/health/topics/post-traumatic-stress-disorder-ptsd/index.shtml

U.S. Department of Veterans Affairs, National Center for PTSD. (2016a). PTSD overview [Web page]. Retrieved from http://www.ptsd.va.gov/public/PTSD-overview/basics/what-is-ptsd.asp

U.S. Department of Veterans Affairs, National Center for PTSD. (2016b). *PTSD: Treatment basics.* [Web page]. Washington, DC: Author. Retrieved from http://www.ptsd.va.gov/public/treatment/therapy-med/index.asp

U.S. Department of Veterans Affairs, National Center for PTSD. (2016c). *What is PTSD?* [Web page]. Washington, DC: Author. Retrieved from http://www.ptsd.va.gov/public/index.asp

U.S. Department of Veterans Affairs, U.S. Department of Defense. (2010). *Clinical practice guideline for management of PTSD* (Version 2.0). Washington, DC: Author.

■ SCHIZOPHRENIA

Sharon L. Phillips

Overview

Schizophrenia is a serious mental illness affecting approximately 1% of the world's population with a lifetime incidence of about one per 100. The etiology of the disorder is a genetic predisposition that is released by the impact of environmental factors. The health needs of people with schizophrenia are often complex as it impacts both mental and physical health, as well as the functioning and interpersonal relationships. Therefore, nursing care is best provided from a holistic perspective.

Background

Schizophrenia, a serious mental illness, affects one's cognition, emotions, and behavior. Onset usually occurs in late adolescence to young adulthood between the age of 16 and 30 years. It tends to occur earlier in males than females and is rarely found in children before the age 13 years. It can emerge later in adulthood after 45 years of age; however, it is uncommon (National Institute of Mental Health, 2016). Presentation of symptoms is usually insidious but can occur abruptly. Early onset of symptoms suggests a more chronic course and a poor outcome.

The predominant symptoms of schizophrenia are categorized into three dimensions: positive, negative, and disorganized (Black & Andreasen, 2014). The positive symptoms are the classic psychotic symptoms of hallucinations and delusions. These symptoms are considered as something that is there but should normally be absent. In contrast, negative symptoms are an absence of something such as motivation, which is normally present. The disorganization, or cognitive dimension, includes inappropriate affect, disorganized behavior, and speech (Black & Andreasen, 2014). Schizophrenia is defined by the presence of positive, negative, and disorganized symptoms along with disturbance of functioning in areas of work, interpersonal relationships, or self-care that persist for at least 6 months (American Psychiatric Association, 2013).

The clinical course of schizophrenia often proceeds to a chronic outcome. Typically, it progresses in three stages: the prodromal, active, and residual phases (Black & Andreasen, 2014). It is during the prodromal phase that initial symptoms begin. Early signs of the disorder include depression, social withdrawal and isolation, poor hygiene, and disturbance in performance at work or school. Interpersonal relationships are also affected by these behavioral changes. As the disorder progresses to the active phase, a more acute presentation is evident with hallucinations, delusions, and disorganized thinking. Other symptoms, such as reduced expression of emotion, ambivalence, difficulty in focusing and staying on task, bizarre speech, and loose associations, tend to become more prominent as the disorder progresses. Early treatment of the first psychotic episode can dramatically alter the trajectory of the illness, which makes an early diagnosis important. It is during this time that most individuals or their families seek help.

Before the diagnosis of schizophrenia is made, other disorders that cause hallucinations, delusions, and bizarre behavior must be ruled out, such as depression with psychotic features, substance use disorder, tumors, infections, personality disorders, temporal lobe epilepsy, and metabolic and endocrine disorders (Black & Andreasen, 2014). For an accurate diagnosis, MRI and lab tests (complete blood count, liver enzymes, serum creatinine, blood urea nitrogen [BUN], thyroid function tests, serologic tests to rule out HIV or syphilis, urinalysis, and urine or serum toxicology screen to rule out substance intoxication) should be done (Black & Andreasen, 2014).

The etiology of schizophrenia is considered to have genetic predisposition that can be altered or influenced by environmental factors. Research findings have long proposed genetics as a causative factor. Studies of monozygotic twins indicate that when one twin has schizophrenia, the incidence of schizophrenia in the other twin is between 40% to 50% (Cunningham & Peters, 2014). Research findings also indicate that children of two biological parents with schizophrenia have an incidence rate of 46% (Black & Andreasen, 2014). In addition, brain injury related to prenatal malnutrition and perinatal complications is a risk factor for the development of this disorder (Black & Andreasen, 2014). Low socioeconomic status, homelessness, and exposure to environmental agents, such as viruses, have also been proposed as environmental contributing factors in neurodevelopmentally predisposed individuals (Nielsen, Laursen, & Agerbo, 2016). Alterations in neurotransmitters, particularly dopamine, glutamate, and serotonin, also play a part in the development of schizophrenia (Black & Andreasen, 2014).

Clinical Aspects

ASSESSMENT

Complex medical and mental health needs of people with schizophrenia exemplify the need for a holistic approach to nursing care. Medical conditions may go unnoticed and untreated because of inadequate assessment. Complaints of medical symptoms are often vague and overshadowed by psychotic symptoms. Medical conditions, such as hypertension, cardiovascular disease, and diabetes, are more prevalent with a higher mortality rate among people with schizophrenia than the general population (Strassnig & Harvey, 2014). The delay in seeking early medical care is an important factor related to the increased mortality rates among individuals with schizophrenia. Often, disorganized thinking and hallucinations interfere with the individual's ability to make his or her needs known; therefore, it imperative for the nurse to consider both mental and medical conditions when gathering the assessment data.

NURSING INTERVENTIONS, MANAGEMENT, AND IMPLICATIONS

Using a client-centered approach to data collection, such as motivational interviewing, can be a useful tool. This approach to assessment focuses on the client's perception of the problem, thereby helping to increase his or her likelihood of adherence to a proposed care plan. Cultural influences on presentation cannot be underestimated, as it is in an individual's culture that illness and behavior are defined. Schizophrenia and its accompanying symptoms may go unrecognized or viewed as less of a problem in some cultures. Symptoms such as hallucinations or what may appear as bizarre behavior or speech are interpreted in the norms of one's culture. Thus, nurses must consider the client's cultural background when providing nursing care.

Suicide risk is a nursing priority in all populations of mentally ill clients and is particularly important when working with people with schizophrenia. The suicide rate in younger adult males with schizophrenia, particularly during the early phase of the illness, is higher than the general population. The lifetime incidence of suicide attempts is also higher (Gabbard, 2014). It is estimated that the suicide risk is 50 times higher in people with schizophrenia compared with the general population. Approximately one third of the people with schizophrenia attempt suicide with the rate of completed suicide being one in 10 (Black & Andreasen, 2014). Risk factors include male gender, age less than 30 years, unemployed, history of previous depression, history of substance abuse, chronicity, and recent hospital discharge (Black & Andreasen, 2014). Assessing the content of auditory hallucinations is important as the individual may be experiencing command hallucinations telling him or her to harm self or others. The nurse needs to ask the client to divulge the content of the auditory hallucination in a respectful, yet direct manner. For example, the nurse could ask: "What are the voices saying to you? Are they telling you to harm yourself or someone else?" Protecting a client from harming self or others is an essential part of nursing care. The goal of treatment should be the least restrictive environment, which, dependent on the severity of the illness and risk of harm, may require involuntary admission and the administration of antipsychotic medications.

OUTCOMES

Conventional antipsychotics, such as haloperidol, and atypical antipsychotics—risperidone, olanzapine, and quetiapine—are commonly used to treat acute psychosis. They are also beneficial in treating disruptive behaviors and distorted thinking that influence self-care and social functioning. It is important for the nurse to know each medication's use, actions, side/adverse effects, and expected outcomes. Fostering the client's cooperation in adhering to a medication regimen is a vital component in providing evidence-based care. The use of antipsychotics agents is considered the standard of care in the treatment of schizophrenia. Psychoeducation; skills training; and psychotherapy, such as cognitive behavioral therapy and supportive therapy, are found to be helpful in treating the negative symptoms of the disorder (Carbon & Correll, 2014). Therefore, evidence-based nursing care incorporates psychoeducation for the client and family regarding the importance of medication compliance, early signs of decompensating, treatment, symptom management, and supportive community resources.

Summary

Schizophrenia is a serious chronic mental illness that affects every aspect of the person's life. It is theorized to be an interaction between biology and environment. There is no cure; however, management of symptoms with antipsychotic medications, psychotherapy, and psychoeducation can improve and often restore function to help people with the disorder to live a fulfilling life. Early diagnosis and intervention are imperative in the management of this mental illness.

American Psychiatric Association. (2013). *Diagnostic and statistical manual of mental disorders* (5th ed.). Arlington, VA: American Psychiatric Publishing.

Black, D. W., & Andreasen, N. C. (2014). *Introductory textbook of psychiatry* (6th ed.). Arlington, VA: American Psychiatric Publishing.

Carbon, M., & Correll, C. U. (2014). Cognitive and negative symptoms in schizophrenia. *CNS Spectrums, 19*, 38–53.

Cunningham, C., & Peters, K. (2014). Etiology of schizophrenia and implications for nursing practice: A literature review. *Issues in Mental Health Nursing, 35*, 732–738.

Gabbard, G. O. (2014). *Gabbard's treatments of psychiatric disorders* (5th ed.). Arlington, VA: American Psychiatric Publishing.

National Institute of Mental Health. (2016). *Schizophrenia* (NIH Publication No. 15-3517). Bethesda, MD: Author. Retrieved from http://www.nimh.nih.gov/health/publications/schizophrenia-booklet/index.shtml

Nielsen, P. R., Laursen, T. M., & Agerbo, E. (2016). Comorbidity of schizophrenia and infection: A population-based cohort study. *Social Psychiatry and Psychiatric Epidemiology, 51*(12), 1581–1589.

Strassnig, M. T., & Harvey, P. D. (2014). Treatment resistance in schizophrenia. *CNS Spectrums, 19*, 16–24.

■ SUBSTANCE USE DISORDERS

Chikodiri Gibson
Se Min Um

Overview

Addiction is a compulsive need for and use of a habit-forming substance. It is accepted as a mental illness that results in substantial health and socioeconomic problems. Addiction is characterized by the inability to consistently abstain, impairment in behavioral control and craving, diminished recognition of significant problems with one's behaviors and interpersonal relationships, and a dysfunctional emotional response. Like other chronic diseases, addiction often involves cycles of relapse and remission. It is diagnosed when the use of substances (or reward-seeking behaviors) continues despite adverse consequences.

Background

Throughout history, humans have discovered paths to pleasure, euphoria, and alternate realities through substances. Psychoactive substances that were ingested, chewed, inhaled, or smoked have played an important part in cultural rituals across the millennia. Early humans also discovered that substances derived from plants (e.g., opium from the poppy plant) could relieve pain. All of these substances that benefit humanity can also be abused either intentionally or inadvertently (Cleary & Thomas, 2017).

Substance use disorders (SUDs) are psychiatric disorders defined to be chronic health disorders with similar rates of relapse or exacerbation as other chronic conditions, such as congestive heart failure, chronic obstructive pulmonary disease, asthma, and diabetes mellitus (National Institute on Drug Abuse, 2015). Approximately 10% of people who use illicit substances develop an SUD (Worley, 2017).

In 2016, the World Health Organization described the global burden of disease resulting from substance use as amounting to 5.4% of the total burden of disease worldwide. In the United States, the total economic cost of substance use is estimated at $700 billion (National Institute on Drug Abuse, 2015). Since the 1990s, the high prevalence of SUDs comorbid with mental health disorders (MHDs) has emerged as a major concern for drug and alcohol and mental health services (Lai, Cleary, Sitharthan, & Hunt, 2015). Increased awareness of the importance of recognizing SUDs and MHDs in different populations can facilitate more effective comprehensive assessment to support treatment and recovery from SUDs and/or MHDs.

There are many more forms of addiction, but we will mention many of the widely known and abused substances that can lead to addiction as follows:

- Ethyl alcohol, or ethanol, is an intoxicating ingredient found in beer, wine, and liquor. Alcohol is produced by the fermentation of yeast, sugars, and starches (Centers for Disease Control and Prevention, 2016b). Alcohol arguably is the most common "gateway drug" for other substances.

- Nicotine, an ingredient in tobacco, causes physiological addiction to tobacco products like cigarettes, cigars, and chewing tobacco, and continues to be a public health concern across the globe, as it results in nearly 6 million deaths per year worldwide.

- Marijuana or cannabis is the plant that tetrahydrocannabinol (THC) is derived from, which is a mind-altering psychoactive drug. Whether organic or synthetic versions of the drug, users can become addicted despite the legalization of use for certain medical conditions.

- Crystal methamphetamine (informally known as *ice, glass, meth,* and *crystal*) is a colorless form of d-methamphetamine, a powerful highly addictive synthetic psychostimulant.

- Methylenedioxymethamphetamine (MDMA), also known as *ecstasy* and *molly*, is an illegal psychoactive drug that has both stimulant and hallucinogenic effects.

- Cocaine is a powerfully addictive stimulant drug made from the leaves of the coca plant native to South America (National Institute on Drug Abuse, 2016a). Its intense effect, as well as the need for more of the drug to achieve the effect, makes cocaine a dangerously addictive substance.

- Heroin is an illegal, highly addictive opioid. Heroin use has more than doubled among young adults (ages 18–25 years) in the past 10 years, and heroin-related overdose deaths have more than tripled since 2010 (Centers for Disease Control and Prevention, 2016a).

- Internet addiction can include addictions *on* the Internet (excessive use of Internet because it affords access to social media, gambling, shopping, or gaming) and addictions *to* the Internet itself.

Addiction to any substance can impact the following negatively: health (causes a decline of health and other medical conditions to develop), psychological (changes in behavior and mental status), financial (inability to sustain or maintain employment coupled with the need for money to buy the substance), social/family (strained relationship with friends, family, and change in social status), and community (financial and social burden to the community).

Clinical Aspects

Addiction is an issue across the entire life span, beginning with babies who are born addicted, either exhibiting neonatal abstinence syndrome (NAS) produced by prenatal exposure to opioids in utero or fetal alcohol syndrome (FAS) produced by prenatal exposure to alcohol.

ASSESSMENT

Assessment of an individual with addiction and SUDs begins with a physical and psychosocial examination. A variety of tools is used in determining the level of withdrawal and related treatment, such as CIWA (Clinical Institute Withdrawal Assessment for Alcohol) and COW (Clinical Opiate Withdrawal Scale). Medication therapy often involves tapering doses to alleviate withdrawal symptoms during the detoxification process as well as maintenance dosing so that patients may be able to retain a higher quality of life in long-term treatment.

The choice between maintaining abstinence and sobriety versus induction and stabilization depends on the patient. Each case should be evaluated on a case-by-case basis with support toward treating both SUD and/or MHD factors.

NURSING INTERVENTIONS, MANAGEMENT, AND IMPLICATIONS

As nurses, we need to understand the meaning of the terminologies that are used when referring to SUDs, and we need to take care to use the most accurate and scientific terminology that also reduces stigma. Some of the nursing concerns for patients suffering from addiction include understanding the behaviors and personality associated with SUDs; knowledge of treatment of comorbid medical and mental conditions; societal stigma; constantly evolving medical terminology in SUDs treatment; understanding street jargon; knowing how to assess patients' quality of life, self-efficacy, and spirituality; and understanding the factors associated with treatment success and recovery.

Continuous professional development across all disciplines is important to interdisciplinary teamwork as well as the provision of best practice, including person-centered care to support patient and family recovery in the treatment of addiction. Addiction treatments include the use of medication-assisted treatment (MAT) such as methadone and suboxone; motivational interviewing; and group, family, and individual therapy. Long-term treatment of addiction includes long-term inpatient programs, Alcoholics Anonymous, Narcotics Anonymous, Cocaine Anonymous, outpatient treatment programs, spiritual support, and medication therapy.

OUTCOMES

In dealing with patients with SUDs, it is very important for nurses to understand some of the behaviors and characteristics that are common with addiction, such as manipulative behaviors, deception, and countertransference, as a care provider. Overall, nurses should maintain hopeful and positive patient-centered approaches when working with patients with SUDs, and guide them in their recovery (Worley, 2017). The expected outcomes of patients with SUDs is abstinence with the goal to achieve sobriety and sustained remission. The long-term desired goals would be for the patient to return to optimal physical and psychosocial health and obtain and maintain financial independence.

Summary

Addiction as a global health issue is unprecedented as discussed in this entry. Before treatment can be provided, adequate substance use and mental status assessments should be completed. Given the immense scope and complexity across the life span, it is clear that much work remains to develop more enlightened public policies, greater access to evidence-based treatments, clinical guidelines and recovery programs, and increased societal compassion toward individuals with SUDs and/or comorbid MHDs.

Centers for Disease Control and Prevention. (2016a). Heroin overdose data. Retrieved from http://www.cdc.gov/drugoverdose/data/heroin.html

Centers for Disease Control and Prevention. (2016b). Increases in drug and opioid overdose Deaths—United States, 2000–2014. *Morbidity and Mortality Weekly Report, 64*(50), 1378–1382. Retrieved from http://www.cdc.gov/mmwr/preview/mmwrhtml/mm6450a3.htm

Cleary, M., & Thomas, S. P. (2017). Addiction and mental health across the lifespan: An overview of some contemporary issues. *Issues in Mental Health Nursing, 38*(1), 2–8.

Lai, H. M. X., Cleary, M., Sitharthan, T., & Hunt, G. E. (2015). Prevalence of comorbid substance use, anxiety and mood disorders in epidemiological surveys, 1990–2014: A systematic review and meta-analysis. *Drug and Alcohol Dependence, 154*, 1–13.

National Institute on Drug Abuse. (2015). Trends and statistics: Cost of substance abuse. Retrieved from https://www.drugabuse.gov/relatedtopics/trends-statistics

National Institute on Drug Abuse. (2016a). Synthetic cannabinoids (K2/spice). Retrieved from https://www.drugabuse.gov/drugs-abuse/synthetic-cannabinoids-k2spice

National Institute on Drug Abuse. (2016b). Synthetic cathinones ("bath salts"). Retrieved from https://www.drugabuse.gov/publications/drugfacts/synthetic-cathinones-bath-salts

Worley, J. (2017). Recovery in substance use disorder: What to know to inform practice. *Issues in Mental Health Nursing, 38*(1), 80–91.

■ SUICIDE

Jeffrey S. Jones

Overview

Nowhere else in the area of nursing or mental health care will you be challenged on a personal level than when dealing with the issue of suicide. The subject matter often triggers strong emotions and opinions based on one's own beliefs. This phenomenon has touched most nurses, either they knew someone who took his or her own life (family member or friend) or may have encountered it in any number of client populations and settings (emergency department, psych, intensive care, and so forth). Regardless of one's own current belief, the fact is that the act of ending one's own life has been around since the beginning of time. Belief and opinions around this differ from culture to culture and generation to generation. Some feel, based on their own religious beliefs, that killing yourself is a sin. Others may allow that in cases of terminal illnesses an individual has a right to choose when to end the suffering. Several states now allow physician-assisted euthanasia in such cases (Jones, Fitzpatrick, & Rogers, 2017). This entry gives an overview of this aspect of care primarily in patients who are depressed.

Background

There is no one single cause for suicide. However, most often, the act of ending one's own life seems to occur when stressors exceed the current coping abilities of someone who is also suffering from depression. Current statistics regarding suicide indicate that it is the tenth leading cause of death in the United States; approximately 44,193 Americans die by suicide each year, and for every 25 attempts, there is one that is successful (National Institute of Mental Health, 2016).

Further statistics reveal:

■ The annual age-adjusted suicide rate is **13.26 per 100,000** individuals.

■ Men die by suicide **3.5** times more often than women.

■ On average, there are **121** suicides each day.

■ White males accounted for **seven** out of 10 suicides in 2015.

■ Firearms are used **in almost 50%** of all suicides.

■ The rate of suicide is **highest in middle age**—White men in particular (www.nimh.nih.gov).

Clinical Aspects

ASSESSMENT

People who complete suicide usually exhibit one or more of the following warning signs, either through what they say or what they do. The more warning signs present, the greater the risk.

These warning signs include talking about suicide:

■ Killing himself or herself

■ Having no reason to live

■ Being a burden to others

■ Feeling trapped

■ Feeling unbearable pain

A person's suicide risk is greater if a certain behavior is new or has increased, especially if it is related to a painful event, loss, or change. A person is suicidal if he or she engages in these behaviors:

■ Increased use of alcohol or drugs

■ Looking for a way to kill themselves, such as searching online for materials or means

■ Acting recklessly

■ Withdrawing from activities

■ Isolating from family and friends

■ Sleeping too much or too little

■ Visiting or calling people to say goodbye

■ Giving away prized possessions

■ Acting aggressively

People who are considering suicide often display one or more of the following moods. Be on the lookout for:

■ Depression

■ Loss of interest

■ Rage

■ Irritability

■ Humiliation

■ Anxiety

■ Sudden brightening of mood, as if they are at peace (American Foundation for Suicide Prevention, 2015)

NURSING INTERVENTIONS, MANAGEMENT, AND IMPLICATIONS

Here is what you can do as a nurse. Many suicidal individuals report feeling alone and disconnected from others. Travelbee, a nurse theorist, suggested that patients may only be able to tolerate pain and suffering so long before falling into despair and apathy (Travelbee, 1971). Remembering that most patients who contemplate suicide are suffering from emotional pain and have reached a stage of hopelessness, as a nurse, you could do the following:

1. Establish and maintain a therapeutic relationship with the client. It is imperative that you come across as honest and real.

2. Manage your feelings about the subject matter and be nonjudgmental.

3. Convey a calm, caring attitude and try to understand from an empathic standpoint where the client's emotional pain is coming from.

4. Understand that this takes time, you have to be willing to sit and talk. Sometimes just allowing the client to talk, cry, and get rid of some of the pain is enough to avert a crisis.

5. Explore issues of safety. (Does the person have a plan and the means to carry it out?) You only learn this once you have gained his or her trust.

6. Determine whether you need to take immediate steps to avert an attempt (put on suicide watch, remove potentially harmful objects, and so forth). If so, this must be done as an act of caring, not as a punishment (Jones et al., 2015).

OUTCOMES

Caring for someone who is depressed and potentially suicidal carries with it multiple responsibilities. If you think of a client who is depressed as someone who is in pain and may be potentially suicidal as a means to end the pain, then the following Quality and Safety Education for Nurses (QSEN) nursing behaviors apply:

- Assess presence and extent of pain and suffering

- Assess levels of physical and emotional comfort

- Elicit expectations of patient and family for relief of pain, discomfort, or suffering

- Initiate effective treatments to relieve pain and suffering in light of patient values, preferences, and expressed needs (Cronenwett et al., 2007)

Summary

This section has provided a very brief overview on the complex topic of suicide. Although the numbers can be overwhelming, it is important to remember that early detection and treatment can translate to successful intervention. The first step in being able to address this issue in clients is to come to terms with it yourself first. Remember that as a nurse you are more effective at suicidal interventions if

you can present yourself as open, unbiased, and caring. As mentioned in the text on depression, it may be helpful to think of suicide as a symptom of suffering. If the nurse's primary function is to alleviate suffering, physical or emotional, then being educated and prepared to identify and intervene in suicidal matters is a nursing function.

American Foundation for Suicide Prevention. (2015). Suicide statistics and prevention. Retrieved from https://afsp.org

Cronenwett, L., Sherwood, G., Barnsteiner J., Disch, J., Johnson, J., Mitchell, P., . . . Warren, J. (2007). Quality and safety education for nurses. *Nursing Outlook*, 55(3), 122–131.

National Institute for Mental Health. (2016). NIMH answers questions about suicide. Retrieved from https://www.nimh.nih.gov/health/publications/nimh-answers-questions-about-suicide/index.shtml

Travelbee, J. (1971). *Interpersonal aspects of nursing* (2nd ed.). Philadelphia, PA: F. A. Davis.

■ VULNERABLE POPULATIONS

Melanie S. Lint

Overview

Vulnerable populations in nursing are those that are typically defined by gender, age, geography (urban or rural), race or ethnicity, or socioeconomic status. These populations include, but are not limited to, children, elderly, homeless individuals, incarcerated individuals, and those with intellectual disabilities according to the *Healthy People 2020* report (Office of Disease Prevention and Health Promotion, 2010). Disparity or lack of equality in health care often occurs in these populations. Some of the reasons for disparity in health care may be because of lack of access to health care services, lack of public transportation, lack of education regarding mental health problems and the availability of treatment, stigma regarding receiving mental health treatment, language barriers, cultural barriers, age, gender and sexual identity, inadequate housing, economic circumstances, exposure to violence, and general mistrust of medical and mental health professionals.

Background

The first report by the surgeon general on mental health was published by the U.S. Department of Health and Human Services in 1999. Its purpose was to promote an understanding of mental health as an important component of general health, and to enhance its status in the United States by putting forth an anti stigma campaign. In focusing on a "vision of mental health for the future" (p. 6) one assertion was that for diagnosis and treatment of mental illness to be effective, it must take into account age, gender, race, culture, and individual circumstances. It also emphasized the importance of understanding information about ethnic and racial groups, their traditions, beliefs, histories, and value systems, to provide culturally competent care (U.S. Department of Health and Human Services, 1999). In 2003, the President's New Freedom Commission on Mental Health looked at areas where improvement had occurred, and issues that still needed to be adequately addressed. A major goal for the future was to eliminate disparities in mental health care.

Clinical Aspects

ASSESSMENT

Nurses in all practice areas are ethically bound to provide care to patients regardless of their level of functioning, age, race, gender, economic status, medical, or mental health diagnoses (Jones, Fitzpatrick, & Rogers, 2017). The nurse acts as an advocate for all patients, but particularly for those in vulnerable groups who may not be able to advocate for themselves. The youngest and oldest people in society are often the most vulnerable and at a potential risk for neglect and abuse. Mental health settings are often the first point of contact for these individuals.

NURSING INTERVENTIONS, MANAGEMENT, AND IMPLICATIONS

Children

Children may grow up in homes where there is not adequate food or heat; where there is a lack of adult supervision; or they may have parents who have mental health, physical health, and/or substance abuse issues of their own. Children and adolescents may have mental health problems such as depression, anxiety, eating disorders, autism spectrum disorders, anger, attention deficit hyperactivity disorder (ADHD), substance abuse, or suicidal thoughts, and may have difficulty expressing their concerns and feelings to parents, teachers, or school counselors. Families may not have health insurance or the financial resources for counseling and medication. Sometimes other children in school may bully a child. The nurse may see the child in the school health clinic and obtain information from the child, family, and teachers, to understand more about the child's growth and development, current progress, and any problems in school, home life, and any changes in usual behavior. Planning for the care of children is often done in collaboration with family members, social workers, teachers, and primary care providers. The nurse needs to be alert for any signs and symptoms of physical, emotional, or sexual abuse of the child and is legally required to report any suspected abuse to the local authorities.

The Elderly

Elderly people often experience chronic physical illness, insomnia, pain, functional decline, stress, and loneliness related to the loss of loved ones and friends. They may experience depression and anxiety as well (Jones et al., 2016). The nurse might work with an elderly individual who has dementia along with the individual's family to make sure that the living environment is as safe as possible for the patient. The nurse would plan interventions that help maintain the patient's independence as much as possible, but also take into account those things that the patient may need assistance with. For example, the nurse could arrange for a home health aide to help with personal care, or make arrangements for a program that delivers meals to the homebound elderly. A nurse might work at a senior center or assisted living facility to provide teaching about medications or health topics such as coping with depression and anxiety, exercise, and nutrition. Nurses providing home health care services for the elderly would teach patient and family about medications and how to cope with illness, and screen for suicidal thoughts and other symptoms of depression or anxiety, and to monitor any physical health problems. It is also the responsibility of the nurse to be alert for signs and symptoms of potential elder abuse, whether in a home setting or when the patient comes in for a clinic appointment, or to the hospital or a mental health unit.

Intellectual Disabilities

The nurse may encounter individuals with intellectual disabilities in any health care setting. An individual with an intellectual disability might also have a co-occurring physical health, mental health and/or substance abuse diagnosis. Some individuals may be higher functioning and able to live independently and hold jobs. Others may live in a supervised, safe living environment, and require assistance with activities of daily living. They may be at risk of being victimized by others.

The Homeless

It is very difficult to obtain accurate statistics regarding the number of homeless people in the United States at any one particular moment in time. Different local and federal agencies that attempt to help the homeless keep their statistics. This population is often transient, which can affect keeping an accurate count. Nurses care for clients who are living in homeless shelters, in tent communities often seen in urban areas, or those who may be living in other temporary housing. There is a significant correlation between homelessness and mental health problems. The nurse might be part of a hospital- or clinic-based homeless outreach team that goes to locations where patients are living temporarily to provide medical and mental health services. Various agencies in major cities in the United States work to help place homeless individuals in permanent supportive housing and to provide food, clothing, substance abuse, and mental health treatment, and assist in job training and placement.

Incarcerated Patients

In a jail or prison setting, the nurse might provide medical information to patients and administer psychotropic and other medication. Another responsibility might include providing educational information for incarcerated patients about topics such as managing stress and anxiety, sleep hygiene, exercise, anger management, and 12-step groups. It is important for the nurse to assess incarcerated individuals for thoughts of suicide, thoughts of harming others, and the presence of psychotic symptoms on an ongoing basis. Setting clear boundaries is of vital importance in the nurse–patient relationship, particularly when working with the incarcerated patient population.

OUTCOMES

Regardless of age group, living situation, socioeconomic status, race, or ethnicity, the nurse advocates for and provides nursing care to all individuals who need

services. Vulnerable populations, such as the elderly or the homeless, are frequently seen in mental health as the first point of contact. Providing a safe living environment, adequate hydration and nutrition, access to mental health care and physical health care, with the goal of improving health and level of functioning of each patient is the ultimate goal.

Summary

Eliminating disparities in health care in the United States is an ongoing goal. Some current initiatives include the National Prevention Strategy for Elimination of Health Disparities by the Office of the Surgeon General, *Healthy People 2020*, the National Academies of Science Communities in Action: Pathways to Health Equity projects, and those by the National Alliance for the Mentally Ill (NAMI) and Mental Health America consumer groups. Nurses can help by becoming culturally competent and work in their local communities and states to help eliminate barriers to mental health care for all. Nurses continue to provide excellent health care services to individuals in vulnerable populations and to others.

Jones, J. S., Fitzpatrick, J. J., & Rogers, V. L. (Eds.). (2017). *Psychiatric-mental health nursing: An interpersonal approach* (2nd ed.). New York, NY: Springer Publishing.

Office of Disease Prevention and Health Promotion. (2010). *Healthy People 2020* objectives. Retrieved from http://www/healthpeople.gov2020/about/foundation-health-measures/Disparities

The President's New Freedom Commission on Mental Health. (2003). *Achieving the promise: Transforming mental health care in America*. Rockville, MD: Substance Abuse and Mental Health Services Administration. Retrieved from http://govinfo.library.unt.edu/mentalhealth commission/reports/FinalReport/downloads/downloads .html

U.S. Department of Health and Human Services. (1999). *Mental health: A report of the surgeon general.* Rockville, MD: U.S. Department of Health and Human Services, Substance Abuse and Mental Health Services Administration, Center for Mental Health Services, National Institutes of Health, National Institute of Mental Health. Retrieved from https://profiles.nlm.nih .gov/ps/retrieve/ResourceMetadata/NNBBHS

AACN Synergy Model for Patient
Care, 51–52
abdominal aortic aneurysm (AAA),
5–7, 148
abdominal pain, 8–10, 13, 15
abnormal uterine bleeding, 112
ABO incompatibility, 416–418
bilirubin levels, 417
in infants, 417–418
mechanism leading to, 417
acetyl-cholinesterase inhibitors, 185
acid–base imbalances, 10–12
active management of third-stage labor
(AMTSL), 574
activities of daily living (ADL),
689, 692
acupuncture, 555
acute abdomen, 13–15
signs and symptoms of, 284
acute chest syndrome (ACS),
522, 523
acute coronary syndrome (ACS), 16–18,
39–40, 42
acute exacerbation of a chronic
condition, 19–20
acute hepatic failure (AHF), 89, 90, 91
acute kidney injury (AKI), 48, 161–162
acute low-back pain (ALBP), 30, 32, 33
acute lung injury (ALI), 273, 502, 512
acute lymphoblastic leukemia
(ALL), 349
acute mountain sickness (AMS), 76, 77
acute myeloid leukemia (AML), 349
acute pancreatitis (AP), in adults,
21–23
Acute Physiological and Chronic Health
Evaluation (APACHE II), 57
acute renal failure (ARF), 419–421,
622–624
causes of, 419
in infants, 419
nephrotoxin-induced, 419
prevention of, 420

postrenal, 420
prerenal, 419
acute respiratory distress syndrome
(ARDS), 23–25, 273
acute respiratory failure (ARF), 25–27,
124, 126
acute severe asthma, 628
acute urinary retention (AUR), 161
Addison's disease, 266–267
common cause of, 266
darkening of skin in, 266
destruction of the adrenal
glands, 266
glucocorticoid replacement
therapy, 267
hydrocortisone therapy, 267
mineralocorticoid replacement with
fludrocortisone therapy, 267
patient education about, 267
adenocarcinomas, 280, 315
adrenal crisis, 74
adrenal insufficiency (AI), 28–29
adrenocorticotropic hormone (ACTH),
28, 266–267
adrenocorticotropic hormone
(ACTH)-secreting pituitary tumors,
298–299
adult difficult airway management,
482–484
advance care planning (ACP),
586–587, 588
advance directives, 586–588
adverse childhood experiences
(ACEs), 43, 67
adverse drug events (ADEs), 195
advocacy, 216–219, 666–667
collaboration and, 218
communication for, 218
influence, significance of, 218
by nurses, 216
problem solving and, 218
professional, 217
resource identification in, 218

skills required for, 218
for surgical patients, 666–668
age-related changes, 174–176
atypical presentation of signs and
symptoms, 174
aging in place, 176–178
effectiveness of, 178
goal of supporting, 177
meaning, 177
airway, breathing, and circulation
(ABC), 9
AKI Network (AKIN), 622
alkaline phosphatase (ALP), 373
alveolar resorption atelectasis, 273
Alzheimer's dementia, 589, 618
Alzheimer's disease (AD), 184
Alzheimer-type dementia, 184
amyotrophic lateral sclerosis (ALS),
268–270
association with lead and
formaldehyde exposure, 268
bowel and bladder function in, 268
end-of-life care, 269–270
symptoms, 269
anaphylactic shock, 141
anemia in adults, 270–272, 330–332,
392, 503, 522, 523
medical management and nursing
care, 272
pernicious, 271
predisposing factors, 271
treatment of, 272
anemia of prematurity, 421–423
hemoglobin (Hb) or hematocrit (Hct)
concentration in, 421
iron supplementation for, 422
angiotensin receptor blockers (ARB), 18
angiotensin-converting enzyme (ACE)
inhibitors, 420
anorexia and weight loss, 589–591
anorexia nervosa (AN), 697
anti-A and anti-B antibodies, 417
anticholinergics, 147, 595, 599, 619

anticoagulation, and anesthesia, 490–492
antidiuretic hormone (ADH), 81
antidiuretic hormone secretion syndrome, 635
anxiety disorders, 686–688, 689
anxiety in advanced illness, 592–594
apnea of prematurity (AOP), 423–425
    and anemia, 425
    factors contributing to, 424
    and gastroesophageal reflux, 424
    hypercapnic ventilatory response, 424
appendicitis, 624–626
aquagenic pruritus, 387
arrythmogenic right ventricular cardiomyopathy (ARVC), 288
arrhythmogenic right ventricular dysplasia (ARVD), 287
ask-tell-ask strategy, 597
asleep–awake–asleep (AAA) techniques, 493
Asperger syndrome, 630
aspiration pneumonia, 605
assistive reproductive therapy (ART), 546, 547
asthma, 627–629
atelectasis, 272–274
    airway obstruction in, 273
    surfactant impairment, 273
atherosclerosis, 275–277, 296
    atherosclerotic plaque, 275
    pathogenesis of, 276
    poststroke disability, 275
    risk factors, 276
    risk of developing cardiovascular disease, 275
    treatment guidelines, 277
atrial septal defect (ASD), 452–453
atrioventricular canal (AVC) defect, 452–453
attention deficit hypertensive disorder (ADHD), 658, 689
autism spectrum disorder (ASD), 630–631
autoimmune hemolytic anemia (AIHA), 331
autonomic dysreflexia (AD), 144
awake craniotomy, 493–494

bacillus Calmette–Guérin (BCG) vaccine, 411
back pain, 30–33
bacterial pneumonia, 193
Bakas Caregiving Outcomes Scale, 180

Bakri balloon, 575
benign prostatic enlargement (BPE), 278
benign prostatic hyperplasia (BPH), 161, 277–280
    adverse effect of chronic urinary retention, 278
    cause of, 278
    lower urinary tract symptoms (LUTS), 277, 278, 279
    risk for developing, 278
    symptoms, 278
bereavement, grief and, 611–613
biliary tract disease, 314–316
bilirubin-induced encephalopathy (BIND), 443
binge eating disorder (BED), 697
bipolar disorder, 688–690
birth, home, 538–540
bladder cancer, 280–282
    clinical and pathological stage, 281
    risk factors, 280–281
Blalock–Taussig shunt, 429
blood pressure (BP), 96–97
blunt traumatic eye injuries, 114
bone health, 559–560
bone marrow transplant (BMT), 662
boundary management, 690–692
    nurse–patient relationship, 690
    professional boundaries, 691
boundary-testing behaviors, 691
bowel obstruction, 282–284, 594–596
    common cause of, 283
    large (LBO), 283
    signs and symptoms of acute abdomen, 284
Braden Scale, 210
brain tumors, 285–287
    common nonmalignant, 285
    primary malignant, 285
BRCA1 gene, 526–528, 562
BRCA2 gene, 526–528, 562
breast cancer and BRCA, 526–528
breastfeeding, 550–553
bronchiolitis respiratory syncytial virus, 632–633
bronchopulmonary dysplasia (BPD), 425–428
    antenatal steroid therapy, 426
    presentation of, 426
    pulmonary changes, 426
    risk factors of, 426
brown adipose fat (BAT), metabolism of, 478
bulimia nervosa (BN), 697

bupropion, 696
Burch-Wartofsky Point Scale (BWPS), 153
burns, 33–36
    classification and severity, 36–39
    depth, 36–37
    first-degree burns, 37
    second-degree burns, 37

calcium and neuromuscular function, 82
calcium intake, 560
Canadian Study of Health and Study (CSHA) Frailty Index, 191
cancer care, surgical interventions in, 673–675
cancers of childhood, 634–636
carbon dioxide, 11, 25, 26–27
carbon monoxide (CO) poisoning, 34
cardiac anesthesia, 495–496
cardiac shunting, 452
cardiomyopathies, 287–289
    classification of, 287
    diagnostic tests for, 288
    prescribed medication regimen, 289
cardiopulmonary resuscitation (CPR), 121, 167, 587–588
cardiovascular (CV) disease, 544, 555, 571
caregivers
    agency-based, 179
    educational interventions and resources, 180
    family, 179, 180
catheter-associated urinary tract infections (CAUTI), 227–228
cauda equina syndrome (CES), 31
central line associated blood stream infection (CLABSI), 227
central nervous system (CNS) tumors, 635
cerebral palsy (CP), 636–638
cerebral perfusion pressures (CPP), 156–157
cervical cancer, 528–531
chemical burns, 37
chemoreceptor trigger zone (CRTZ), 517
chemotherapy, 674–675
    and menopause, 554
chest pain, 17, 39–42
child abuse and neglect, 42–45
childbearing
    delayed, 576
    optimal age, 576

childhood absence epilepsy, 658

Childhood Asthma Control Test (C-ACT), 628

childhood cancers, 634–636

chlamydia, 578, 579

cholangiocarcinoma, 315, 351

chronic back pain (CBP), 30

Chronic Care Model, 258

chronic hepatic failure (CHF), 90

chronic kidney disease (CKD), 289–292
  causes of, 290
    financial burden with, 290
    PD complications in, 291

chronic low-back pain (CLBP), 30, 32

chronic lymphocytic leukemia (CLL), 349–350

chronic myelogenous leukemia (CML), 349–350

chronic obstructive pulmonary disease (COPD), 19–20, 124–125, 292–294, 301, 592, 607–608
  inflammation of lung and airways, 293
  risk factors for development, 292–293

chronic pelvic pain (CPP), 535, 563–564

circadian sleep–wake rhythm disorders, 211

CIWA (Clinical Institute Withdrawal Assessment for Alcohol), 709

Clostridium difficile infection, 46–48, 193, 227, 337, 604

cognitive behavioral therapy (CBT), 555, 593, 701, 705

cognitive processing therapy (CPT), 705

COLDSPA (character, onset, location, duration, severity, pattern and associated factors), 125

colorectal cancer, 294–296
  early stage, 294
  epidemiologic pattern of, 294
  evaluation of, 295
  genetic conditions and, 294
  risk of, 294

combined hormonal contraceptives (CHCs), 533

combined oral contraceptives (COCs), 533

communication, 517, 528, 588, 596–598, 602
  developmentally appropriate, 641–643

community acquired ARF, 623

community-acquired pneumonia (CAP), 192

compartment syndrome, 38, 117, 313, 655–656

compensatory volume expansion (CVE), 502

complete blood count (CBC), 625, 647, 657, 661

compound muscle action potential (CMAP), 499

Confusion Assessment Method (CAM), 601

congenital hyperinsulinism, 447

conjunctivitis, 115

constipation, 598–600, 618, 619

Consumer Assessment of Healthcare Providers and Systems (CAHPS), 236

continuous RRT (CRRT), 49, 50

continuous veno-venous hemodialysis (CVVHD), 48–49

continuous veno-venous hemofiltration (CVVH), 48–50

contraception, 532–534

Coombs-direct antibody test (DAT), 417

coronary artery disease (CAD), 40, 296–298
  cardioprotective medications, 297
  imaging studies of, 297
  laboratory tests, 297
  modifiable and nonmodifiable risk factors, 296
  obstruction in blood flow associated with, 295

COWS (Clinical Opiate Withdrawal Scale), 147, 709

C-reactive protein (CRP), 625

Crohn's disease, 648, 649

crystal methamphetamine, 709

crystalloids, 84
  fluid management of, 502

CT angiography (CTA), 21

Cushing syndrome, 298–300
  adrenal enzyme inhibitors for, 299
  alterations in coagulation factors and, 300
  laboratory test for, 299
  surgical intervention, 299

cystic fibrosis (CF), 639–641

cystic fibrosis transmembrane regulator (CFTR) gene, 639

decompression sickness (DCS), 76

decreased pulmonary blood flow, 428–431
  congenital heart defects (CHD), 428, 429

deep vein thrombosis (DVT), 38, 145, 300–302
  complications, 301
  endothelial damage/dysfunction, 301
  goals of therapy, 302
  hypercoagulable causes of, 301
  risk factors, 301
  signs and symptoms for, 301

deferred gratification, 699

define, measure, analyze, improve, and control (DMAIC) model, 242

definitions of emergency and critical care nursing, 50–52

degenerative disc disease (DDD), 400

delirium, 71, 122, 595, 600–602
  as a neurocognitive disorder (NCD), 181

delta hepatitis, 93

dementia, 67, 122, 184, 692–694
  Alzheimer-type, 184
  cardiovascular risk factors, 184
  care planning and outcomes, 185
  characteristics specific to, 185
  cognitive deficits, 184
  costs of, 184–185
  quality of life issues, 693
  risk factors, 184, 693
  vascular, 184

dental caries, 652–654

dental emergencies, 52–54

depression, 687, 694–696
  antidepressant medication, 696
  group therapy, 695
  individual therapy, 695
  medication options, 695–696

developmentally appropriate communication, 641–643

diabetes insipidus (DI), 303–304
  complications of, 304
  risk for developing, 305
  types of, 303

diabetes ketoacidosis (DKA), 644

diabetes mellitus (DM), 73, 95, 110–111, 454, 509, 643–646
  laboratory studies, 305
  type 1 DM (T1DM), 304
  type 2 DM (T2DM), 304

diabetic embryopathy, 455

diabetic ketoacidosis (DKA), 73–74, 84, 85, 95, 305

diarrhea, 599, 603–604

dilated cardiomyopathy (DCM), 287–288

diplegia, 637

disability adjusted life years
(DALYs), 687
disaster response, 55–57
disc herniation, 400–402
cervical, 400–401
lumbar, 401
disseminated intravascular coagulation
(DIC), 57–59, 574
distal limb ischemia, 105
diverticular disease, 307–309
clinical course of, 307
etiology of, 307–308
domestic violence (DV), 59–62
do-not-resuscitate (DNR) form, 587
Down syndrome, 634, 647
drug hypersensitivity syndrome
(DHS), 101
drug-induced hepatitis, 89
drug rash with eosinophilia and
systemic symptoms (DRESSs)
syndrome, 101–102
dyskinesia, 637
dysphagia, 590, 605–607
dyspnea, 607–609
dystonia, 637

ear, nose, and throat (ENT)
emergencies, 63–65
early-onset sepsis (EOS), 472
neonatal EOS calculator, 474
eating disorders, 696–698
nurse–patient relationship, 698
psychiatric complications,
696–697
risk factors, 697
E. coli sepsis, 472
ectopic pregnancy, 8, 9, 112
elder abuse and neglect,
66–69, 186
early signs and symptoms of, 187
economic impact of, 186
estimated number of victims, 186
types, 186–187
electrolyte imbalances, 81–84, 96
encephalopathy, 71–72
endocardial cushion defect, 452
endocarditis (IE), 310–311
endocrine emergencies, 72–75
endometriosis, 535–536
enhanced recovery after anesthesia
(ERAA), 496–498
enhanced recovery after surgery
(ERAS), 496–497
envenomation injuries, 76
environmental emergencies, 75–78

enzyme-linked immunoabsorbent assay
(ELISA), 632
epilepsy, 637, 657–659
episiotomy, 536–538
epithelial ovarian tumors, 561
estrogen, 533, 535, 554, 555, 559–560,
562, 570
ethics, 609–611
for surgical patients, 666–668
ethyl alcohol, 709
evoked potentials (EPs), 498–501
exertional heat illness (EHI), 77
exertional heat stroke (EHS), 77
extracorporeal life support
(ECLS), 78–81
extracorporeal membrane oxygenation
(ECMO), 25, 78–79
extremely low-birth-weight (ELBW)
infants, 431–433
care of, 431
goal of delivery resuscitation, 432
long-term morbidity in, 431–432
neurodevelopmental impairment
in, 432
proper management and care of, 432
risk for death, 431–432
at risk for experiencing skin shearing
and denuding, 432–433
subgroups of, 431
thermoregulation, 432
eye movement desensitization and
reprocessing (EMDR), 705

failure to thrive (FTT), 646–648
Fall Risk Assessment Tool (FRAT), 205
falls, 188
etiology of, 188
gender differences and, 188
pain and, 188
prevention of, 189
risk factors, 188–189
Falls Risk Assessment and Falls Plan of
Care, 189
familial adenomatous polyposis
(FAP), 294
family caregivers
assessing effects of caregiving, 180
complexity and intensity of care, 179
educational interventions and
resources, 180
health risks associated with family-
provided care, 179
Family Violence Prevention and Services
Act, 60
febrile seizures, 657–658

Federation of International
Gynecologists and Obstetricians
(FIGO) system, 562
Felty syndrome, 392
fetal alcohol syndrome, 475
fetal hyperinsulinemia, 456
fluid and electrolyte imbalance, 81–84
fluid and transfusion management, in
anesthesia care, 501–503
fluid resuscitation, 84–86
fondaparinux, 491, 492
fractures, 312–314
categorizations and classifications
of, 312
healing process, 313
pathophysiology of, 313
risk factors for, 315
traumatic and nontraumatic,
312–313
frailty, 190–191
frontotemporal dementia (FTD), 268
Functional Assessment Staging
of Alzheimer's disease scale
(FAST), 693
functional bowel obstruction, 283
functional residual capacity (FRC), 509
fundoplication, 435

gallbladder disease, 314–316
malignant and benign tumors in, 315
risk factors associated with, 315
surgical intervention, 315
types of gallstones, 314–315
gastric cancer, 316–318
clinical manifestations, 317
common sites of, 317
dietary and lifestyle factors impact
on, 317
types of, 317
gastritis, 319–320
signs and symptoms of, 319
types, 319–320
gastroesophageal reflux (GER),
433–435
clinical guidelines for
management, 434
symptoms, 434
gastroesophageal reflux disease
(GERD), 321–323, 493, 509, 638
costs associated with, 321
signs and symptoms, 321
gastrointestinal stromal tumors, 317
gastroschisis and omphalocele,
436–437
genetics of, 436

risk of, 437
general adaptation syndrome (GAS), 43
general anesthesia, 486, 487, 493, 497, 499, 502, 507–510, 518
generalized anxiety disorder, 686, 687
geriatric syndromes, 175
germ cell tumors, 561
gestational diabetes, 455
Glasgow Coma Scale (GCS) score, 494
glioblastoma (GBM), 285
glucocorticoids, 74, 143
gout, 323–325
    genetic and environmental risk factors, 323
    nonpharmacological pain management, 325
    urate-lowering therapy, 324
    urates and, 323–324
Graves' disease, 342
grief and bereavement, 611–613
group B Streptococcus (GBS) infection, 472
    intrapartum antibiotic (IPA) treatment for, 472
    maternal chorioramnionitis and, 473
Guillain–Barré syndrome (GBS), 325–327

health behavior, 250–252
    promotion of, 250
    smoking cessation, 251
Health Belief Model, 250
health care–associated infection (HAI), 226–227, 668
    burden of, 227
    from hospitals, 227
    patient risk of, 227
    risk assessment categorization of patients, 227
health economics, 219–221
    cost-benefit analysis, 220
    cost-consequence analysis, 220
    cost-effectiveness analysis, 220
    cost-effectiveness ratio, 220
    economic evaluations of interventions, 219–220
    evaluations of health policies, 219
    return on investment (ROI), 220
health education, 253–254
    evaluation process, 254
    in prevention of chronic illnesses, 253
    teaching–learning plan, 253–254
health literacy, 254, 255–257

low health literacy and/or limited basic literacy, 255, 256
    tools for measuring, 256
health policy, 222–224
    big "P" policies, 222, 223
    evidence-based practice (EBP) approach, 223
Health Promotion Model (HPM), 250
health-related quality of life, 199, 318, 348
heart failure (HF), 16, 86, 327–329
    laboratory tests, 328
    pathophysiologic process of, 328
    systolic or diastolic, 327
heart transplantation, 86–88, 166
heated intraperitoneal chemotherapy (HiPEC), 674
Helicobacter pylori infection, 317, 319, 375, 379
HELLP syndrome, 485, 486
hemiplegia, 637
hemoglobin S, 521–522, 660
hemolytic anemia (HA), 330–332
    causes of, 231–232
    hemolysis of red blood cell, 330–331
    laboratory features of, 331
hemorrhage, 540, 549, 573–575
Hendrich II Fall Risk Model, 189
heparin-induced thrombocytopenia (HIT), 332–334
    central features of, 332
    clinical signs of, 333
    guidelines and evidence-based interventions, 334
    risk for developing, 333
    standard for anticoagulation and heparin therapy, 334
hepatic failure (HF), 89–91
hepatitis, 92–94
hereditary nonpolyposis colorectal cancer syndrome (HNPCC), 294
heroin, 709
herpes simplex virus (HSV), 115
herpes zoster, 115, 193
hiatal hernia, 335–337
    classification, 335
    risk factors for developing, 336
    symptoms, 335
Hirschsprung's disease (HD), 283, 438–440
    clinical presentation of, 438–439
    rectal dilation treatment in, 439
    rectal examination, 439
    symptoms, 439

home birth, 538–540
homicide, 121–124, 544
hormonal contraceptive methods, 533
hormone-replacement therapy (HRT), 555
hospital accreditation, 224–226
    Agency for Healthcare Research and Quality (AHRQ), 225
    award recognition for nursing standards, 225
    The Joint Commission (TJC) standards, 224–225
    Magnet Standards, 225
    National Patient Safety Goals (NPSGs), 225
    Quality and Safety Education for Nurses (QSEN) competencies, 225
    review on behalf of CMS, 224
hospital birth, 539
Hospital Elder Life Program (HELP), 317
human immunodeficiency virus (HIV), 337–339
    psychosocial implications, 337
    staging of, 338
    types of, 337
human leukocyte antigen (HLA) tissue typing, 103
human papilloma virus (HPV), 528
hydronephrosis, 440–442
    antibiotic therapy, 441
    bilateral, 440–441
    etiology of, 440
    grading of unilateral or bilateral, 440
    prenatal, 440
    ultrasonography findings, 441
hyperbilirubinemia, 417–418, 442–444
    Bhutani nomogram for, 443
    bilirubin levels in, 442
    clinical signs of, 442
    educating families about, 444
    guidelines for management of, 443
    in IDM, 456
    phototherapy for, 443
    rate of RBC destruction in, 442
hyperglycemia, 94–96, 643, 644, 645
hyperglycemic hyperosmolar state (HHS) trauma, 84, 85, 95
hyperglycemic hyperosmolar syndrome (HHS), 304
hypernatremia, 82
hyperosmolar hyperglycemia syndrome (HHS), 73, 74

hypertension (HTN), 96–98, 339–341, 444–447, 485
   BP measurements, 445
   lifestyle changes for preventing, 446
   long-term complications, 446
   neonatal, 445
   signs and symptoms, 340
   types of, 340
hypertensive crisis, 96–98, 340
hyperthyroidism (HT), 342–344
   in children, 342
   common cause of, 342
   subclinical, 342
   thyroid hormone (TH) level, 342
hypertrophic cardiomyopathy (HCM), 287
hypoglycemia, 74, 94–96, 447–449, 461, 645
   common cause of, 447
   neonatal, 447–449
   postprandial, 447
   risk of, 448
hyponatremia, 82
hypotension, 635, 645, 662
hypothalamic–pituitary–adrenal axis, 28
hypothermia, 38, 99–100, 498, 501, 505, 507, 522, 523
hypothyroidism, 344–346
hypovolemia, 82, 83, 85
hypovolemic shock, 139, 140
hypoxic ischemic encephalopathy (HIE), 448, 449–451
   categorization of, 450
   hypothermia therapy, 450
   perinatal, 450
   therapeutic hypothermia/cooling therapy, 450
hypoxic pulmonary vasoconstriction (HPV), 513

idiopathic thrombocytopenic purpura (ITP), 150
immunosuppressant therapy, 88, 141
impulse control disorders, 699–701
in vitro fertilization (IVF), 542, 546–548
increased pulmonary blood flow, 452–454
   common congenital cardiac lesions related to, 452
   defects related to, 452
   symptoms and signs, 453
Infant Breast Feeding Assessment Tool (IBFAT), 552

infant of a diabetic mother (IDM), 454–457
   with cardiomyopathy, 456
   complications associated with, 455
   hyperbilirubinemia in, 456
   risk for complications, 456
infection, 192–194
   immunity and, 192
   prevention and control, 226–229, 668–671
   social and environmental factors and, 192
infective endocarditis (IE), 310–311
   approaches to treating, 311
   epidemiology of, 310
   major risk factor for, 310
   nosocomial infections, 310
   at risk factors, 310
   signs and symptoms, 310
infertility, 541–543, 546–547
inflammatory bowel disease (IBD), 315, 347–348, 648–650
   etiology of, 347
inflammatory bowel disease unclassified (IBD-U), 648
influenza, 193
insomnia, 211
Instrumental Activities of Daily Living (IADL) scale, 177
integumentary emergencies, 101–103
intermittent explosive disorder (IED), 699, 700–701
interventional magnetic resonance imaging (IMRI), 679–680
intimate partner violence (IPV), 544–545
intra-aortic balloon pump (IABP), 104–106
intracranial hemorrhage (IVH), 457–459
   cerebral blood flow and pressure in, 458
   grading of, 458
   progression of, 459
   screening for, 458
intracranial pressure (ICP), 155, 493, 494, 501
intraductal papillary mucinous neoplasms (IMPN), 374
intravenous patient-controlled analgesia (IVPCA), 519
intraventricular hemorrhage, 457–459

jaundice, 442–443
Jean Piaget's Theory of Cognitive Development, 642
juvenile myoclonic epilepsy (JME), 657

Katz Index of Activities of Daily Living, 177
Kegal exercises, 555
Kleihauer–Betke test, 113
kleptomania, 699, 700

labor and delivery, 548–550
lactation, 550–553, 570
laryngeal chemoreflex, 423–424
LATCH tool, 552
late preterm infant (LPI), 460–462
   brain growth, 461
   care of, 462
   risks, 460
latent tuberculosis infection (LTBI), 193
late-onset sepsis (LOS), 472–473
leukemia, 349–350
   examinations and testing, 350
   prognosis and treatment plan, 349
   symptoms, 349
liver cancer, 351–353
   risk factors for developing, 351, 352
   signs and symptoms, 352
   stage and type, 351
liver transplant and anesthesia, 504–506
low-back pain (LBP), 30–31
lung cancer, 353–355
   causes of, 353
   forms, 354
   screening criteria, 354
   symptomatic treatment and palliative care, 355
luxation injuries, 53
lymphoma, 317, 355–357
   alterations in lymphocytes, 356
   common sign of, 356
   genetic and environmental factors, 356
   nurse/patient navigator, role in patient education, 357
   patient's prognosis of, 356
   prevention of infection, 357

major depressive disorders (MDD), 592, 616
malignant hyperthermia, 506–508
Malnutrition Universal Screening Tool (MUST), 197
mammalian target of rapamycin (mTOR), 143
MaZaFi 3-project, 528
Meckel's diverticulum, 307
meconium aspiration syndrome (MAS), 462–464

clinical signs and symptoms, 463–464
signs of recovery, 464
symptoms, 463
Medication Appropriateness Index (MAI), 207
medication reconciliation, 194–196
Medications at Transitions and Clinical Handoffs (MATCH) Toolkit for Medication Reconciliation, 196
Memorial Delirium Assessment Scale (MDAS), 601
menopause, 554–556
mental and behavioral health emergencies, 106–109
metabolic acidosis, 11–12
metabolic alkalosis, 12
methicillin-resistant *Staphylococcus aureus* (MRSA) infections, 227
methylenedioxymethamphetamine (MDMA), 82, 709
migraine, 109
mild cognitive impairment (MCI), 184
Mini Nutrition Assessment (MNA), 197–198
Mini-Mental State Exam (MMSE), 693
Model for End-stage Liver Disease (MELD), 504–505
Model for Improvement, 242
monitored anesthesia care (MAC), 493, 497
monoamine oxidase inhibitors (MAOIs), 97, 696
Montreal Cognitive Assessment (MoCA), 693
mood stabilizers, 689, 696, 705
morbid obesity and anesthesia, 508–510
Morse Fall Scale, 205
Mother Baby Assessment Tool (MBA), 552–553
motherhood, 556–558, 571
motor evoked potentials (MEPs), 499
motor vehicle injuries, 158
mucinous neoplasms (MCNs), 374
mucositis, 614–615
multidisciplinary evidence-based bone health education program, 560
multiple organ dysfunction syndrome (MODS), 139–141
multiple sclerosis (MS), 357–359
adverse effects of, 358
etiology of, 358
physical deterioration of patients in, 358
social, environmental, and biological factors, 358
muscle-invasive bladder cancer (MIBC), 281
muscle-specific tyrosine kinase (MUSK), 360
musculoskeletal injuries, 117
Mutans streptococci, 653
myasthenia gravis (MG), 360–362
classification, 360
clinical forms, 360–361
medication adjustment and immunotherapy treatments, 360
nursing problems related to care, 361
symptoms, 361
myeloproliferative neoplasms (MPN), 387
myocardial infarction (MI), 16, 110, 276
myoclonic seizures, 129
myofascial pelvic pain, 564, 565

National Kidney Disease Education Program (NKDEP), 290
natural killer (NK) cell activity, 192
necrotizing enterocolitis (NEC), 465–467
morbidity and mortality rates associated with, 465
pathogenesis of, 465
prenatal strategies for prevention, 466
risk factors of, 465
surveillance for, 466
necrotizing fasciitis, 101
Neisseria gonorrhea, 579
Neisseria meningitis, 101
neonatal abstinence syndrome (NAS), 475–477, 709
clinical signs, 475
effects of infant exposure to chemical substances, 475
future risk of addictive behaviors, 476
methadone exposure symptoms, 476
nonpharmacologic nursing therapies, 476
screening of, 476
neonatal intensive care unit (NICU), 423, 431, 436, 445, 448, 449, 460, 465, 467, 470, 479
nephrotoxic-induced ARF, 623
neurogenic shock, 141
neuromuscular blocking agents (NMBAs), 500–501, 510
neuromuscular blocking drugs (NMBDs), 511–512
neurotrauma, 109–111
nicotine, 709
NOD2/CARD15 gene, 648
nonalcoholic, fatty liver disease (NAFDL), 504
noninvasive positive pressure ventilation (NPPV) devices, 126
nonmuscle invasive bladder cancer (NMIBC), 281
nonnociceptive pain, 564
nonoperating room anesthesia (NORA), 487
non-small cell lung cancer (NSCLC), 354
non-ST elevation MI (NSTEMI), 16
nonsteroidal anti-inflammatory drugs (NSAIDs), 32, 102, 420, 617
nucleic acid amplification tests (NAAT), 580
nucleus tractus solitarius (NTS), 517
Numerical Pain Scale, 199
nursing leadership, 229–231
design of structure, 229
The Joint Commission (TJC) leadership standards, 229
nursing management, 231–233
classical style, 232
leadership and, 232
neoclassical style, 232
patient care, 232
resource management, 233
responsibility for addressing personnel issues, 232
systems management model, 232
nursing process, 234–236
evaluation phase of, 235
knowledge, skills, and attitude (KSAs) dimensions, 234
plan, do, study, and act (PDSA) cycle, 235
planning phase of, 235
QSEN competency of safety, 234–235
specific, measurable, achievable, realistic, and timely (SMART) statement, 235
treatment phase of, 235
nutrition, 197–198
adults at risk of malnutrition, 197
importance of nutrition, 196
nonpharmacologic methods to improve, 198

obesity, 362–364, 508–510, 650–652
    body mass index (BMI) in, 362–363
obesity hypoventilation syndrome
    (OHS), 509
obsessive compulsive disorder (OCD),
    702–703
obstetrical anal sphincter injuries
    (OASIS), 537
obstetrical and gynecological (OB/
    GYN) emergency care, 112–114
obstructive apnea, 423
obstructive shock, 139, 140
obstructive sleep apnea (OSA),
    493, 509
older adults, 186, 206
    common infections in, 193
    genetic and lifestyle choices, impact
        of, 204
    risk of chronic conditions and
        falls, 204
one-lung ventilation (OLV), 512–514
open-book pelvic fractures, 117
ophthalmic emergencies, 114–116
opioids, 30, 32, 595, 599–600, 608,
    617, 709
    withdrawal, 475–477
OPQRST (onset, provocation, quality,
    severity, timing) mnemonic, 8, 125
oral glucose tolerance test (OGTT), 305
oral health, 652–654
oral rehydration therapy (ORT), 604
orthopedic emergencies in adults,
    117–119
orthopedics, 655–657
osteoarthritis (OA), 365–366
    genetic, environmental, metabolic,
        and biochemical factors, 365
    nonpharmacological intervention,
        365, 366
    risk factors, 365
    symptoms, 365
osteomyelitis (OM), 367–369
    antibiotic therapy with antibiotic-
        impregnated beads, 368
    bacterial organisms causing, 367
    classification, 368
    etiology of, 368
    pathophysiology and clinical
        presentation, 367
    risk factors, 367
    surgical management, 368
    vertebral, 368
osteoporosis, 369–371, 555, 558–561
    common sites for fractures, 369
    fall prevention strategies, 371

modifiable risk factors, 369–370
nonmodifiable risk factors, 369
nutritional and lifestyle
    counseling, 371
process of bone remodeling, 370
types, 369
otalgia, 63
otitis externa, 64
otitis media, 63, 64, 65
ovarian cancer, 527–528, 561–563
ovarian hyperstimulation syndrome
    (OHSS), 547

Paget's disease, 372–374
    cause of, 372
    common sites affected, 372
    serum levels of alkaline phosphatase
        (ALP) in, 373
    signs and symptoms, 372
pain, 536, 537, 558
    control, 9, 116
    defined, 564
    nociceptive, 564
    nonnociceptive, 564
    pelvic, 563–565
pancreatic cancer, 374–376
    biological features, 374
    chemotherapy and radiation
        therapy, 376
    risk factors, 375
    surgical resection, 375
    symptoms, 375
pancreatic ductal adenocarcinoma, 375
pancreatic endocrine tumors, 374
panic disorder, 686
paraesophageal hernias (PEH), 335
Parkinson's disease (PD), 283,
    376–378
    definitive characteristic of, 376
    genetic predisposition and
        environmental influences, 377
    signs associated, 377
    surgical interventions in, 675–678
patent ductus arteriosus (PDA),
    429, 452
pathologic jaundice, 442–443
patient controlled analgesia (PCA),
    519–521
patient controlled epidural analgesia
    (PCEA), 521
patient experience, 236–238
    CMS patient satisfaction
        survey, 236
pediatric emergencies, 119–121
pelvic fractures, 117, 118

pelvic inflammatory disease (PID), 112,
    541, 546, 579
pelvic pain, 112, 529, 563–565
penicillin prophylaxis, 662
peptic ulcer disease (PUD), 378–380
    complications of, 378
    risk factors, 379
pericarditis, 381–383
    acute, 381
    classification of, 381
    symptoms, 381
perinatal mood disorders (PMDs),
    565–567
perinatal nurse, 548–550
perioperative mortality rates
    (POMR), 681
perioperative patient safety, 671–673
peripartum cardiomyopathy
    (PPCM), 288
peripheral artery disease (PAD), 275,
    383–385
    cause of, 383
    clinical symptoms and signs, 383
    risk factors, 383
peripheral nerve blocks, 497, 510,
    515–516
peripheral vascular disease, 275
periventricular leukomalacia
    (PVL), 458
pernicious anemia (PA), 385–386
    causes, 386
    evidence-based nursing care, 386
    symptoms associated, 386
persistent hyperinsulinemic
    hypoglycemia of infancy
    (PHHI), 447
persistent oncogenic HPV
    infection, 529
persistent pain, 199–200, 616–617
    and depression, 199
    guided imagery for reducing, 200
    intensity scale measurements, 199
    mindfulness-based meditation
        program, 200
    noncancer pain, 199
    relaxation for reducing, 200
persistent pulmonary hypertension of
    the newborn (PPHN), 463
personality disorders, 689
pervasive developmental disorders
    not otherwise specified
    (PDD-NOS), 630
pharmacokinetic changes in geriatrics,
    201–204
    drug clearance, 201

drug distribution, 201–202
gastrointestinal (GI) absorption, 201
health and population changes, 201
metabolism of drugs, 202
risk for toxicity, 202
risk of adverse drug events, 202
physical activity, 204–206
impact of, 205
physical exercise, 705
physiologic jaundice, 442
placenta previa, 113
placental abruption, 113
Pneumocystis pneumonia, 337
pneumonia, 227
poisoning injuries, 76
polycystic kidney disease, 290
polycystic ovary syndrome (PCOS),
541, 568–569
polycythemia vera (PV), 386–388
at risk for thrombosis, 387
symptoms, 387
polypharmacy, 176, 188, 203, 204,
206–208
Beers Criteria, 207
biophysiological/functional
factors, 207
demographic and social
factors, 207
medication review and reconciliation,
207–208
multidisciplinary care, 208
screening protocol to address, 207
socioeconomic/environmental
factors, 207
population health, 238–240, 246
approach to optimizing health system
performance, 239
as a type of health, 238–239
portal hypertension (PH), 90
postoperative nausea and vomiting
(PONV), 494, 498, 517–519
postpartum, 570–573
postpartum hemorrhage (PPH), 549,
573–575
posttraumatic stress disorder (PTSD),
616, 686, 703–706
preeclampsia, anesthesia for, 484–486
pregnancy, 530, 576–578
"no risk" pregnancy philosophy, 539
normal pregnancy, 540
prevention of, 533
-related death, 571
pregnancy-induced hypertension
(PIH), 112
pressure injury, 208–210

hospital costs, 209
risk factors for development of, 209
stages of, 209
priapism, 662
primary sclerolsing cholangitis
(PSC), 315
progesterone, 551, 554, 555, 570
progestin-only pills (POPs), 533
prolonged exposure (PE), 695
prostate cancer, 389–391
early stages of, 389
geographic factor as risk of
developing, 389
manifestations, progressive course,
and prognosis, 389
primary risk factors, 389
proton pump inhibitors
(PPIs), 380
pseudobulbar palsy, 268
pseudomonas aeruginosa, 640
psychiatric disorders, 121–124
psychosis, 121–124
pulmonary over-inflation syndrome
(POIS), 76–77
pyelonephritis, 160–161
pyromania, 699–700, 701

quadriplegia, 637
Quality and Safety Education for
Nurses (QSEN), 234–235, 712
activities, 245
competencies and their
definitions, 244
and improvement in quality and
safety of patient care, 244
quality improvement (QI) movement,
240, 244–245
QI competency, 241
QI models and methods, 242

radiation emergencies, 56
rape, 133–136
rectal cancer, 295
regional anesthesia, 486, 492, 493,
497, 510, 515, 523
remote locations, anesthesia in,
487–488
renal calculi, 161
renal failure, 48, 90
renal replacement therapies
(RRTs), 48–50
respiratory acidosis, 11
respiratory alkalosis, 11
respiratory depression and patient-
controlled analgesia, 519–521

respiratory distress syndrome (RDS),
460, 467–469
antenatal corticosteroid therapy, 468
pathogenesis of, 468
signs and symptoms, 468
stages of fetal lung development, 468
respiratory emergencies, 124–126
respiratory failure, 20, 124–125
acute respiratory failure, 25–27
respiratory syncytial virus (RSV),
632–633
restrictive cardiomyopathy
(RCM), 288
retinopathy of prematurity (ROP),
469–471
hyperoxia as contributing factor
of, 470
reasons for development of, 470
screening and management
guidelines, 471
therapeutic management of
severe, 471
Rett syndrome, 630
reversible dementias, 693
rheumatoid arthritis (RA), 391–393
complications of, 391–392
early signs and symptoms, 392
pain management, 392
Rh isoimmunization, 417
right middle lobe (RML)
syndrome, 273
robotic surgery, and anesthesia,
489–490
Rocky Mountain spotted fever
(RMSF), 101

Saint Louis University Mental Status
Examination (SLUMS), 693
Schistosoma haematobium
infection, 281
schizophrenia, 706–708
Screening Tool of Older Person's
Prescriptions (STOPP), 203, 207
Screening Tools to Alert Right
Treatment (START), 207
seatbelt syndrome, 5
seizure disorder, 657–660
seizures, 129–131
prevention and control of, 486
selective atypical antidepressants, 696
selective reuptake inhibitors, 696
selective serotonin reuptake inhibitors
(SSRIs), 555, 560, 695, 701
self-management, 257–259
of chronic illness, 257–258

sepsis, 23, 57, 393–395, 472–474
  in adult, 131–133
  of hospitalized adults, 131–132, 395
  increased susceptibility to, 393
  intrapartum antibiotic (IPA)
    treatment for, 472
  manifestations of infection
    in, 394
  maternal risk factors, 473
  skin care in neonates, 473
septic shock, 132, 133, 141
Sequential Organ Failure Assessment
  (SOFA), 57
seronegative myasthenia gravis
  (SNMG), 360
serotonin reuptake inhibitors (SSRIs),
  695, 696, 701
serotonin 2 antagonist reuptake
  inhibitors (SARIs), 696
serotonin-norepinephrine reuptake
  inhibitor (SNRI), 32, 695, 696
sexual assault, 133–136
sexually transmitted infections (STIs),
  528, 578–581
shock and multiple organ dysfunction
  syndrome, 139–141
short-acting beta2-agonists
  (SABAs), 628
sickle cell disease (SCD), 396–398,
  521–523, 660–663
  complications from, 396
  long-term effects of, 396–397
  screening for, 396
Simple Descriptive Pain
  Scale, 199
Simplified Nutritional Appetite
  Questionnaire (SNAQ), 198
Sjögren's syndrome, 392
skin aesthetics, 581–584
skin rashes, 101
sleep apnea (SA), 398–399
  cause of, 399
  clinical characteristics of OSA and
    CSA, 399
  common form of, 398
  conditions for, 398
  risk for occupational injury, 398
sleep disorders, 211–212
  behavioral and pharmacologic
    therapies, 212
  categories of, 211
  cost of, 211
  predisposing factors to, 211
  rapid eye movement (REM) cycle
    in, 211

small bowel obstruction (SBO),
  282, 594
small cell lung cancer (SCLC), 354
social anxiety disorder, 686
social determinants of health (SDH),
  246–247
  factors determining, 246
  impact of, 246
sodium and water balance, 82
solid organ transplantation, 141–143
somatosensory evoked potentials
  (SSEPs), 499
speech therapists, 590, 591, 605, 606
spermicides, 532
SPICES, 176
spinal cord injuries (SCIs), 143–146
spinal stenosis, 400–402
  cervical, 401
  lumbar, 400–401
splenic sequestration, 661–662
spontaneous bacterial peritonitis
  (SBP), 90
squamous cell carcinoma, 280, 281
staphylococcal scalded skin syndrome
  (SSSS), 101
staphylococcal/streptococcal toxic
  shock syndrome (TSS), 101
status asthmaticus, 628
status epilepticus, 129, 658
Stevens–Johnson Syndrome (SJS), 101
Streptococcus mutans, 652–653
stroke, 109–110, 492, 502, 509, 662
stromal tumors, 562
substance abuse, 147, 169, 170,
  475–477, 687, 713
substance use disorders (SUDs),
  146–148, 703, 707, 708–710
suicide, 121–124, 707, 710–712
supracondylar humerus fractures, 655
surgical interventions
  in cancer care, 673–675
  in Parkinson's disease, 675–678
  using emerging technologies,
    679–680
surgical patients, ethics and advocacy
  for, 666–668
surgical site infections (SSIs), 670, 672,
  675, 678
symptomatic uncomplicated
  diverticular disease (SUDD), 307
syndrome of inappropriate antidiuretic
  hormone (SIADH) secretion, 82,
  83, 402–404
  malignancy-associated, 403
  pathophysiology, 403

syphilis, 578–579
systemic inflammatory response
  syndrome (SIRS), 57
systemic lupus erythematosus (SLE),
  290, 405–407
  cause of, 405
  nursing care goals, 406
  symptoms, 405
  types of lupus, 405

tachycardia, 635, 662
tachypnea, 635, 661
tacrolimus, 143
Takotsubo cardiomyopathy, 288
temperature-targeted therapy,
  127, 157
testicular torsion (TT), 162
tetralogy of Fallot (TOF)
  classic description of, 429
therapeutic hypothermia, 127–128
thermoregulation, 432, 477–480
  central thermoregulatory mechanisms
    at birth, 478
thermoregulation injuries, 76
thoracic aortic aneurysms (TAAs),
  148–150
thrombocytopenia, 407–409
  in adults, 150–152
  heparin-induced, 332–334
thromboembolism, 492
thymoglobulin, 143
thyroid crisis, 152–154
thyrotoxicosis, 74, 152, 153–154
tonic–clonic seizure, 129
total intravenous anesthetic (TIVA)
  techniques, 500, 518
toxic epidermal necrolysis (TEN), 101
tracheal intubation, 484, 486, 492, 493
traditional surgical interventions,
  681–683
transcranial Doppler ultrasonagraphy
  (TCD), 662
transitional care coordination,
  248–249
transitional cell carcinoma, 280
transtheoretical model (TTM), 251
traumatic brain injury (TBI), 155–157
traumatic injury, 158–159
tricuspid atresia, 429, 430
tuberculosis (TB), 193, 409–411
tumor debulking, 674
tumor lysis syndrome (TLS), 357

ulcerative colitis (UC), 648, 649
urinary incontinence (UI), 617–619

bladder sphincter injury or neurological dysfunction in, 212–213
lifestyle changes to prevent, 213
psychosocial factors of, 213
types of, 213
urinary tract infections (UTIs), 193, 227, 555, 578
urologic emergencies, 160
acute kidney injury (AKI), 161–162
acute urinary retention (AUR), 161
pyelonephritis, 160–161
renal calculi, 161
testicular torsion (TT), 162
urinary tract infection (UTI), 160

valvular heart disease (VHD), 411–413
comorbidities with, 412

risk of thromboembolic events, 412
symptoms, 412
types, 412
venous thromboembolic event (VTE), 300–301, 490–491
ventilator-associated pneumonia (VAP), 163–165, 654
ventilator-induced lung injury (VILI), 24
ventricular arrhythmias, 287
ventricular assist device (VAD), 165–168
ventricular septal defect (VSD), 452–453
violent patient, 168–171
Virchow's triad, 301
visual acuity, 116
Visual Analog Scale, 199

visual evoked potentials (VEPs), 499–500
vulnerable populations, 712–714
children, 713
elderly people, 713
homeless, 714
incarcerated patients, 714
intellectual disabilities, 713–714

wellness, 259–261
efforts in nursing, 259–260
lifestyle behavior changes and, 260
programs and outcomes, 260–261
wheezing, 627–628
Whipple procedure, 376, 674
workplace violence, 169